# DENTAL LABORATORY PROCEDURES
## REMOVABLE PARTIAL DENTURES

To
those who inspired us along the way

VOLUME THREE

# DENTAL LABORATORY PROCEDURES
## REMOVABLE PARTIAL DENTURES

**KENNETH D. RUDD,** D.D.S., F.A.C.D., F.I.C.D.

Associate Dean for Continuing Dental Education,
Professor of Prosthodontics, Department of Prosthodontics,
The University of Texas Health Science Center
at San Antonio, Dental School,
San Antonio, Texas

**ROBERT M. MORROW,** D.D.S., F.A.C.D., F.I.C.D.

Associate Dean for Advanced Education,
Professor and Head, Postdoctoral Division, Department of Prosthodontics,
The University of Texas Health Science Center
at San Antonio, Dental School,
San Antonio, Texas

**HAROLD F. EISSMANN,** D.D.S., F.A.C.D.

Clinical Professor, Department of Fixed Prosthodontics,
University of California at San Francisco,
School of Dentistry,
San Francisco, California

with **2258** illustrations

## The C. V. Mosby Company

ST. LOUIS • TORONTO • LONDON    1981

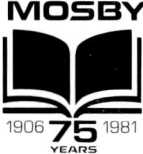

**MOSBY**
1906 **75** 1981
YEARS

A TRADITION OF PUBLISHING EXCELLENCE

Editor: Darlene A. Warfel
Manuscript editor: Sandra L. Gilfillan
Design: Susan Trail
Production: Margaret B. Bridenbaugh

Copyright © 1981 by The C. V. Mosby Company

All rights reserved. No part of this book may be reproduced in any manner without written permission of the publisher.

Printed in the United States of America

The C. V. Mosby Company
11830 Westline Industrial Drive, St. Louis, Missouri 63141

**Library of Congress Cataloging in Publication Data**
Main entry under title:

Dental laboratory procedures.

   Includes bibliographies and index.
   Contents: v. 1. Complete dentures.
v. 3. Removable partial dentures.
   1. Dental technology. I. Morrow, Robert M.,
1931-    . II. Rudd, Kenneth D. III. Eissmann,
Harold F. [DNLM: 1. Denture, Complete—Laboratory
manuals. 2. Technology, Dental—Laboratory
manuals. WU530 R914d]
RK652.D47      617.6'92      79-16785
ISBN 0-8016-3513-6 (v. 1)      AACR2
ISBN 0-8016-3516-0 (v. 3)

C/CB/B  9 8 7 6 5 4 3 2 1   03/C/302

# CONTRIBUTORS

**Sam R. Adkisson, B.S., D.D.S., F.A.C.D.**
Associate Professor, Department of Prosthodontics, The University of Texas Health Science Center at Houston, Dental Branch, Houston, Texas

**William B. Akerly, B.S., D.D.S., M.S.**
Associate Professor, Department of Restorative Dentistry, The University of Mississippi Medical Center, School of Dentistry, Jackson, Mississippi

**William C. Berlocher, D.D.S.**
Assistant Professor, Department of Pediatric Dentistry, The University of Texas Health Science Center at San Antonio, Dental School, San Antonio, Texas

**James D. Browning, D.M.D.**
Associate Professor, Department of Reconstructive Dentistry, Oral Roberts University, School of Dentistry, Tulsa, Oklahoma

**James S. Brudvik, D.D.S.**
Associate Professor, Department of Prosthodontics, University of Washington School of Dentistry, Seattle, Washington

**Ambrocio V. Espinoza, C.D.T.**
Department of Prosthodontics, The University of Texas Health Science Center at San Antonio, Dental School, San Antonio, Texas

**James A. Fowler, Jr., B.S., D.D.S., M.S.**
Assistant Program Director, Postdoctoral Division, Department of Prosthodontics, The University of Texas Health Science Center at San Antonio, Dental School, San Antonio, Texas

**Ennis Howard, C.D.T.**
Department of Prosthodontics, The University of Texas Health Science Center at San Antonio, Dental School, San Antonio, Texas

**David L. King, B.S., D.D.S., Ph.D.**
Associate Professor and Acting Chairman, Department of Pediatric Dentistry, The University of Texas Health Science Center at San Antonio, Dental School, San Antonio, Texas

**George Knight, C.D.T.**
Instructor, Dental Laboratory Technology Education, The University of Texas Health Science Center at San Antonio, Dental School, San Antonio, Texas

**William A. Kuebker, D.D.S., M.S., F.A.C.P.**
Associate Professor, Department of Prosthodontics, The University of Texas Health Science Center at San Antonio, San Antonio, Texas

**Merrill C. Mensor, Jr., B.A., D.D.S., F.I.C.D.**
Formerly, Assistant Clinical Professor, Department of Fixed Prosthodontics, University of the Pacific School of Dentistry, San Francisco, California; Consultant in Removable Prosthodontics, Veterans Administration, Wadsworth and Palo Alto, California; International Circuit Courses Faculty, American Prosthodontic Society; Private Practice, San Mateo, California

**Ralph (Monty) Montalvo**[*]
Senior Master Sergeant (retired), United States Air Force, San Antonio, Texas

---
*Created original artwork.

**Robert M. Morrow, D.D.S., F.A.C.D., F.I.C.D.**

Associate Dean for Advanced Education, Professor and Head, Postdoctoral Division, Department of Prosthodontics, The University of Texas Health Science Center at San Antonio, Dental School, San Antonio, Texas

**Brett H. Mueller, D.D.S.**

Clinical Associate Professor, Department of Pediatric Dentistry, The University of Texas Health Science Center at San Antonio, Dental School, San Antonio, Texas

**Lowell Y. C. Park, C.D.T.**

Instructor, Dental Laboratory Technology Education, The University of Texas Health Science Center at San Antonio, Dental School, San Antonio, Texas

**Connie A. Reisbick, C.D.A.**

Clinic Coordinator, Departments of Pedodontics and Orthodontics, University of Southern California School of Dentistry, Los Angeles, California

**Kenneth D. Rudd, D.D.S., F.A.C.D., F.I.C.D.**

Associate Dean for Continuing Dental Education, Professor of Prosthodontics, Department of Prosthodontics, The University of Texas Health Science Center at San Antonio, Dental School, San Antonio, Texas

**Joe J. Simmons, D.D.S., F.A.C.D., F.I.C.D.**

Private Practice, Dallas, Texas

**Wade D. Smith, B.S., D.D.S., M.S.**

Clinical Assistant Professor, Department of Prosthodontics, The University of Texas Health Science Center at San Antonio, Dental School; Private Practice, San Antonio, Texas

**Kenneth L. Stewart, D.D.S., F.A.C.D.**

Professor and Head, Removable Partial Denture Division, Department of Prosthodontics, The University of Texas Health Science Center at San Antonio, Dental School, San Antonio, Texas

**Jack H. Swepston, D.D.S., F.A.C.D., F.I.C.D.**

Professor, Department of Fixed Prosthodontics, Baylor College of Dentistry, Dallas, Texas; Regional Consultant, Fixed Prosthodontics, Wilford Hall United States Air Force Hospital, Lackland Air Force Base, San Antonio, Texas

# PREFACE

As in most prosthodontic procedures, the fabrication of high-quality, professionally acceptable restorations depends on the knowledge and skill of a dental team. The dentist, dental assistant, and laboratory technician working in harmony with precision and concern are each responsible for the patient's dental happiness. To fully understand the restorative process, each member of the team must be aware of the procedures involved. Many overlap, and in this volume we have tried to describe the complete laboratory procedure for fabricating removable partial dentures. It was our concern to provide dental professionals with precise technical guidelines, using ample illustrations to explain procedures.

This book represents the accumulation of knowledge over many years from many different people and sources. From the beginning, our goal has been to make this book simple, yet detailed, and to write it in a step-by-step format that was easy to follow. We have wanted it to be a text that would benefit those who have knowledge by stimulating a few new ideas. We have hoped that those who lack experience could refer to it when in question about a procedure and arrive at a solution.

Francis Bacon, in *Essays*, wrote, "Some books are to be tasted, others to be swallowed, and some few to be chewed and digested." If our ideas are digested and help make your job easier, then our goal has been reached.

We are indebted to our contributors who have been outstanding in assembling knowledge in their fields. We acknowledge with thanks the support we received from Mrs. Wanita Morrow who was responsible for typing our scribbled notes. To thank everyone connected with making this book a reality would take more space than is available. You know who you are, but more important, we know who you are; for your effort, contribution, and dedication, we thank you.

**Kenneth D. Rudd**
**Robert M. Morrow**
**Harold F. Eissmann**

# CONTENTS

**1 Care of impressions and making casts,** 1
KENNETH D. RUDD and ROBERT M. MORROW

Requisites for casts, 1
Alginate irreversible hydrocolloid impressions, 2
   Care of the impression, 4
   Pouring the stone, 12
   Trimming the cast, 19
Agar reversible hydrocolloid impressions, 23
   Care of the impression, 23
   Pouring the stone, 24
Elastomeric impressions, 26
   Care of the impression, 26
Summary, 29

**2 Pouring corrected cast impressions,** 30
WILLIAM A. KUEBKER, JAMES A. FOWLER, Jr., and LOWELL Y. C. PARK

Boxing corrected cast impression with plaster/pumice mix and wax, 30
Beading and boxing corrected cast impression with wax, 36
Beading corrected cast impression with wax and two-stage pour, 42
North Carolina technique, 49
Summary, 57

**3 Stock and custom impression trays,** 58
KENNETH D. RUDD, ROBERT M. MORROW, and GEORGE KNIGHT

Requirements for impression trays, 58
Stock trays, 58
Custom trays, 60
   Acrylic resin trays, 62
   Thermoset vinyl trays, 68
Summary, 71

**4 Record bases and mounting casts,** 72
JAMES A. FOWLER, Jr., and WILLIAM A. KUEBKER

Record base requirements, 72
   Clinical application, 72
Record base materials, 73
Autopolymerizing resin record bases, 73
   Sprinkle-on method, 74
   Sprinkle-on method with framework, 80
   Finger-adapted dough method, 86
   Wax-confined dough method, 91
Shellac record bases, 96
   Stabilized shellac record bases, 100
   Record bases stabilized with zinc oxide–eugenol impression paste, 100
   Record bases stabilized with elastomeric impression material, 106
   Record bases stabilized with autopolymerizing resin, 109
Vacuum-adapted thermoplastic resin record bases, 113
Wax record bases, 119
Wax occlusion rims, 124
Modeling plastic occlusion rims, 128
Summary, 128

**5 Survey and design,** 130
KENNETH D. RUDD, GEORGE KNIGHT, and KENNETH L. STEWART

Classification of removable partial dentures, 130
   Class I (bilateral distal extension), 130
   Class II (unilateral distal extension), 131
   Class III, 132
   Class IV (anterior edentulous area), 132
Materials for cast frameworks, 134
Removable partial denture components, 134
   Clasps, 135
   Connectors, 144
   Minor connectors, 148

Denture bases, 150
Anterior tooth replacement, 152
Posterior replacement, 155
Principles of surveying, 158
Surveyor, 158
Surveying instruments, 159
Orientation of the cast, 160
Cast tilting, 160
Procedure for design of diagnostic casts for removable partial dentures, 170
Armamentarium, 170
Color code, 170
Summary, 180

## 6 Design transfer, blockout, relief, and beading, 181

KENNETH D. RUDD, ROBERT M. MORROW, and GEORGE KNIGHT

Design transfer, 181
Blockout and duplication, 188
Preparing the casts for duplication, 188
Summary, 202

## 7 Duplication and refractory casts, 203

KENNETH D. RUDD, ROBERT M. MORROW, and GEORGE KNIGHT

Reversible hydrocolloid (agar) molds, 203
Investment cast, 214
Treating the refractory cast, 222
Summary, 227

## 8 Waxing and spruing, 228

KENNETH D. RUDD, ROBERT M. MORROW, and GEORGE KNIGHT

Design transfer, 228
Waxing the framework, 230
Waxing the maxillary cast, 233
Waxing the mandibular cast, 249
Spruing, 254
Summary, 266

## 9 Wrought wire clasps, 267

JAMES S. BRUDVIK

Definition, 267
Description, 267
Materials, 268
Precious metal alloys, 268
Nonprecious metal alloys, 268
Armamentarium, 268
Wire selection, 269
Construction techniques, 269
Clasp contouring, 270
Clasp attachment, 282

## 10 Investing, burnout, and casting, 293

KENNETH D. RUDD, ROBERT M. MORROW, GEORGE KNIGHT, and ENNIS HOWARD

Investing the sprued pattern, 293
Burnout, 308
Casting, 313
Recovering the casting, 315
Cleaning the casting, 316
Pickling the casting, 318
Summary, 320

## 11 Finishing and polishing the framework, 321

KENNETH D. RUDD, ROBERT M. MORROW, GEORGE KNIGHT, and ENNIS HOWARD

Finishing the framework, 321
Summary, 338

## 12 Selecting and arranging teeth, 339

WADE D. SMITH, WILLIAM A. KUEBKER, and JAMES A. FOWLER, Jr.

Selecting the artificial teeth, 339
Arranging the artificial teeth, 344
Anterior teeth, 344
Posterior teeth, 346
Setting artificial posterior teeth to a functionally generated path template, 354
Mounting the template, 357
Arranging the artificial teeth and adjusting the occlusion to a functionally generated path occlusion, 358

## 13 Flasking, processing, deflasking, and finishing, 363

KENNETH D. RUDD, ROBERT M. MORROW, and GEORGE KNIGHT

Flasking, 368
Wax elimination, 372
Packing, 376
Processing, 380
Deflasking, 383
Remounting and correcting processing errors, 387
Finishing and polishing, 390
Duplicate master casts, 398
Summary, 399

## 14 Relining and rebasing, 400

WILLIAM A. KUEBKER, JAMES A. FOWLER, Jr., and AMBROCIO V. ESPINOZA

Relining, 400
Reline master cast, 400
Reline using a reline jig, 403
Rebasing, 413
Reconstruction of removable partial dentures, 425
Making a reconstruction cast, 425
Summary, 426

## 15 Repairs, 427
JAMES S. BRUDVIK

Metal repairs, 427
   Precious metal solders, 427
   Nonprecious metal solders, 428
   Soldering techniques, 428
   Major connector repair, 430
   Rest and minor connector repair, 431
   Clasp repair, 433
   Repair with wrought alloys, 433
   Repair with cast clasps, 434
   Resin retention repairs, 437
Resin repair, 441
   Autopolymerizing repair resins, 441
   Denture base fractures, 441
Fractured and missing teeth, 444
Tooth and denture base additions, 445

## 16 Frictional wall precision attachment partial prosthesis, 448
JACK H. SWEPSTON

Goals, 448
Indications, 449
Contraindications, 449
Advantages, 449
Technical procedures, 449
Treatment planning, 450
Preoperative procedures, 454
Transfer procedure, 458
Alternate procedure, 462
Verifying parallelism, 469
Care of refractory cast, 472
Framework wax-up, 472
Investing, burnout, and casting, 472
Fitting the framework, 473
Framework and male attachment assembly, 474
   Tissue support, 476
Investing and soldering, 480
Replacement teeth, 483
Acrylic inserts, 486
Suggestions for the dentist, 488
Summary, 488

## 17 Swing-Lock, 491
JOE J. SIMMONS

Dentist and dental technician cooperation, 493
Diagnostic casts and preliminary design, 493
Impression technique procedure, 494
Requirements of master cast, 494
Pouring the master cast, 495
Examining the master cast, 495
Duplicate cast, 496
Casting the plastic patterns into metal, 496
Examining the attachment castings, 498
Placement of attachments, 500
Blockout of the master cast, 503
Waxing the framework, 503
Spruing and investing, 504

Metal requirements, 505
S/L single casting technique, 505
S/L double casting technique, 505
Burnout and casting, 505
Freeing attachments—opening the labial bar, 506
Finishing and polishing, 506
Completed framework (prefitted on the cast), 506
Adjustments, 508
Framework try-in, 508
Jaw relation registration, 509
Mounting the framework, 509
Setup and finishing, 509
Constructing and finishing labiogingival tissue acrylic
   veneer, 509
Other S/L procedures (simple to complex), 512
   Mandibular struts (interrupted), 512
   Maxillofacial prosthesis—unilateral abutments, 514
   S/L complete denture, 515
   Double bars, double hinges, single lock, pure
      periodontal splint, full arch labial gingival veneer, 516
   Maxillary coping overdenture, 516
   Sprue placement, 518
   Double labial bar, 518
Summary, 524

## 18 Reinforced facings and metal backings, 525
WILLIAM B. AKERLY

Indications for metal backings, 525
Techniques for metal backings, 525
   Technique for reverse-pin facings, 526
   Alternative approaches, 540
Summary, 549

## 19 Attachments for overdentures, 550
MERRILL C. MENSOR, Jr.

Telescope crowns and attachments, 550
Telescope crown (single crown), 550
Attachments, 554
   Stud attachment use, 555
   Activation, 570
   Bar attachments, 574

## 20 Orthodontic procedures, 587
WILLIAM C. BERLOCHER and BRETT H. MUELLER

**PART ONE**
**Interceptive orthodontic appliances, 587**

Section 1:  Components of the interceptive
   orthodontic appliance, 587

Orthodontic wire, 587
   Preactivated wire, 587
   Annealed wire, 587
Orthodontic pliers, 588
Wire bending, 588
Wire-bending procedures, 589
   Semicircular bend, 589
   Helical bend, 589

Closed end loop, 590
Right-angle bend, 591
Deflection bend, 592
Zigzag bend, 593
Smooth curve bend, 594
Orthodontic springs, 594
Simple finger spring, 594
Helical finger spring, 595
Labial bow spring, 596
Dumbbell spring, 598
Slingshot spring, 600
Orthodontic clasps, 601
Circumferential clasp, 601
Ball clasp, 602
Arrowhead clasp, 604
Adams clasp, 604
Stainless steel soldering, 607
Materials, 607
Soldering, 608
Acrylic resin preparation, 611
Materials, 611

Section 2: Fabrication of interceptive orthodontic appliances, 614

Accurate diagnosis, 614
Working cast, 614
Prescription, 614
Appliance construction, 614
Lingual arch appliance, 615
Transpalatal appliance, 617
Modified Nance appliance, 618
Rapid palatal expansion appliance, 620
W-arch appliance, 622
Hawley appliance, 624

**PART TWO**
**Preparation of diagnostic casts,** 626

DAVID L. KING

Requirements for study casts, 626
Summary, 632

## 21 Three-dimensional teaching aids, 634

CONNIE A. REISBICK

Silicone elastomer molds, 634
Constructing a silicone mold, 634
Constructing epoxy resin models, 644
Preparing silicone mold for epoxy pour, 645
Mixing ivory epoxy resin No. RF3503, 646
Pouring the ivory epoxy model, 648
Polyvinyl chloride elastomers, 650
Fabricating PVC duplicating molds, 650
Fabrication of copper epoxy models for PVC duplicating molds, 651
Fabricating PVC molds, 654
Summary, 658

## 22 Packing and shipping, 659

JAMES D. BROWNING and SAM R. ADKISSON

Packing materials, 659
Choosing a carrier, 668
Summary, 668

# CHAPTER 1

# CARE OF IMPRESSIONS AND MAKING CASTS

KENNETH D. RUDD and ROBERT M. MORROW

**agar** A gelatinous colloidal extract of a red alga used as a gelling agent and principal effective ingredient in reversible hydrocolloid impression materials.

**alginate** A salt of alginic acid, such as sodium alginate, which, when mixed with water in accurate proportions, forms an irreversible hydrocolloid gel used for making impressions.

**aqueous impression materials** Both agar and alginate material are included in this category because they contain, or are mixed with, large amounts of water. Agar is about 85% water, and alginate is about 70% water when it is mixed.

**elastomeric impression materials** A rubberlike impression material. The four types are polysulfide, silicone, polyether, and polysiloxane.

**hydrocolloid** A name applied to either alginate or agar impression materials because they yield a gel when mixed with water.

**irreversible hydrocolloid (alginate)** A hydrocolloid whose physical condition is changed by a chemical action that is not reversible.

**partial denture impression** An impression of part or all of a partially edentulous arch made for the purpose of designing or constructing a partial denture.

**preliminary impression** An impression made for the purpose of diagnosis or the construction of a tray for making a final impression.

**reversible hydrocolloid (agar-agar type)** A hydrocolloid whose physical condition is changed by temperature. The material is made fluid by heat and becomes an elastic solid on cooling.

The most frequently used material for making impressions for diagnostic casts and removable partial dentures is alginate irreversible hydrocolloid. Alginate is easy to use, requires no special equipment, and when proper procedures are followed can produce an acceptable cast (Rudd et al., 1970). Reversible hydrocolloid (agar) is also used to make impressions for removable partial dentures. Reversible hydrocolloid requires special equipment for liquefying, tempering, and storage and water-cooled trays and hoses; as a result, it is not used as frequently as alginate. Polysulfide, silicone, polyether, and polysiloxane impression materials may also be used for removable partial denture impressions, although their most common use is for fixed partial dentures and quadrant inlay and crown impressions. They are also used as secondary or wash materials for making complete denture impressions. In this chapter, methods for pouring casts in alginate irreversible hydrocolloid, agar reversible hydrocolloid, and elastomeric impressions will be described. See pp. 28 to 78 in *Dental Laboratory Procedures: Fixed Partial Dentures* for the methods used in making impressions and casts from hydrocolloid and elastomeric materials for fixed restorations.

## REQUISITES FOR CASTS

All casts for removable partial dentures should exhibit the following qualities:

1. All surfaces to be contacted by the prosthesis should be accurate and free of voids or nodules. Removal of nodules resulting from voids or bubbles in the impression is essential, but hand carving in critical areas is, of course, not acceptable.

2. The surface of the cast should be hard, dense,

and free of any grinding sludge left by the cast trimmer.

3. The cast extensions should include all of the area available for denture support, for example, 3 to 4 mm beyond the hamular notches on the maxillary cast and 3 to 4 mm beyond the retromolar pad on the mandibular cast.

4. The peripheral roll should be complete and approximately 3 to 4 mm deep.

5. Side walls of the cast should be vertical and may be tapered slightly outward but should not be undercut.

6. The base of the cast should be not less than 15 mm thick at the thinnest place, and the lingual region of mandibular casts should be trimmed flat and smooth. The lingual peripheral roll, however, should not be removed. The cast should show no indications of having been wet, washed, or brushed in tap water.

## ALGINATE IRREVERSIBLE HYDROCOLLOID IMPRESSIONS

The impression should be examined critically before pouring to determine that the alginate has not pulled loose from the tray (Fig. 1-1). The impression should also be checked for voids in critical areas, metal tray show through, and any indication that the impression has been allowed to set too long before sending it to the laboratory (Fig. 1-2). It is more economical for everyone concerned to obtain another impression at this point rather than accept a questionable impression and perhaps remake a framework later.

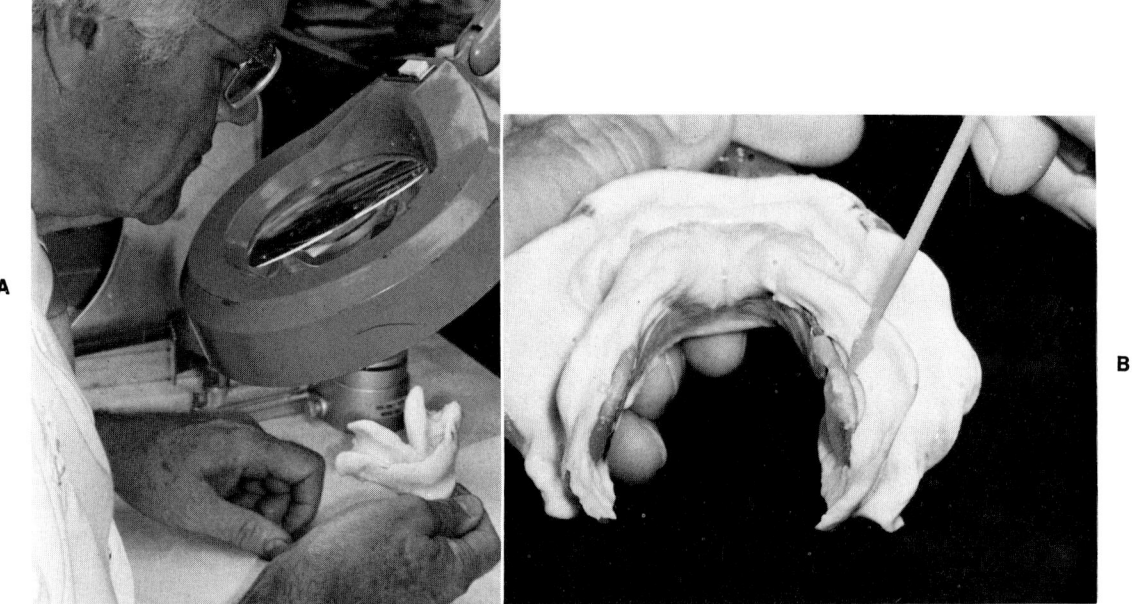

**Fig. 1-1. A,** Examining impression critically. **B,** Alginate impression material has pulled away from tray. It cannot be repositioned accurately, and new impression should be obtained.

*Care of impressions and making casts* 3

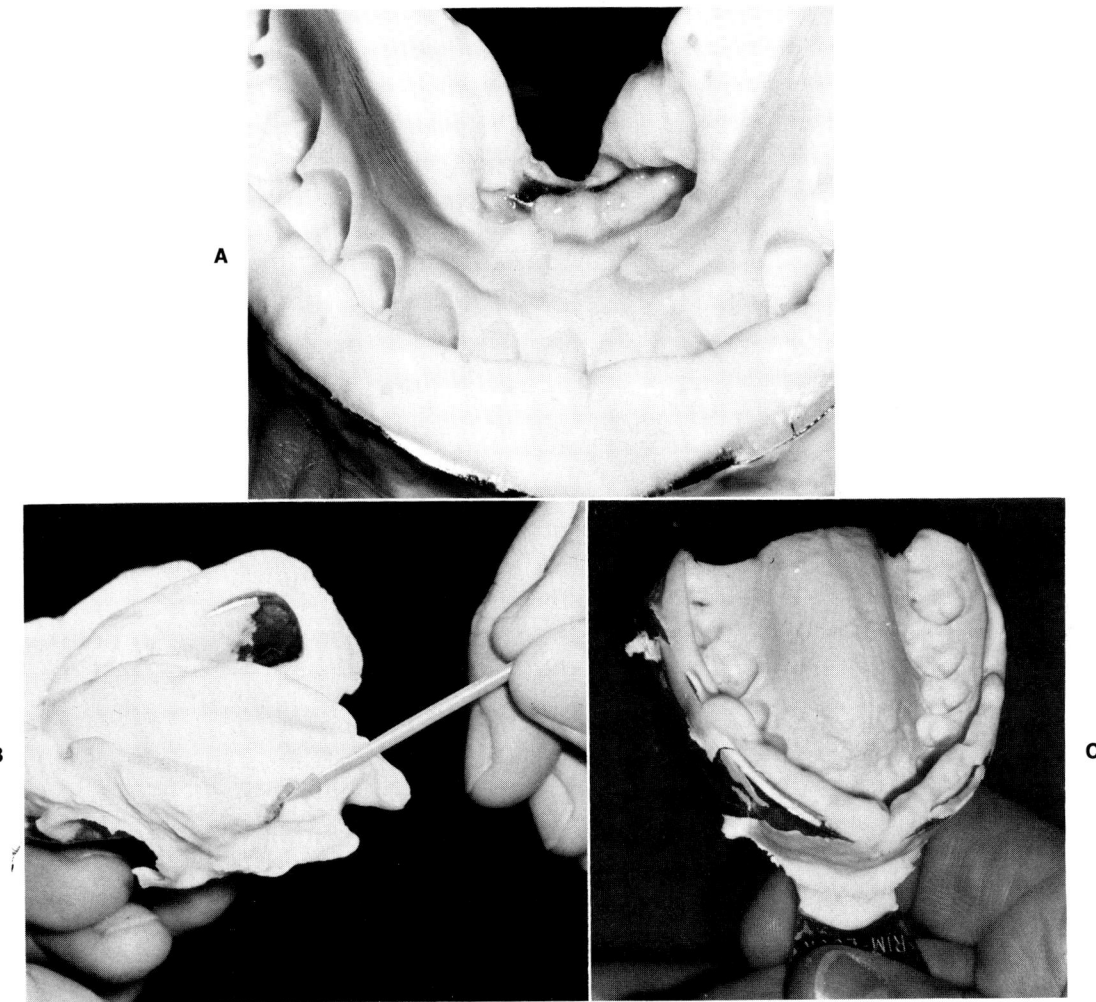

**Fig. 1-2. A,** Impression has void in critical area and should be remade. **B,** Metal tray shows through due to faulty positioning of tray when making impression. Resultant cast will be inaccurate. **C,** Too much time has elapsed between making and pouring impression. Note shrinkage as result of drying. Pour alginate impression within 15 minutes.

# Care of the impression
**PROCEDURE**

1. Examine the impression to determine its acceptability.
2. With a sharp knife, trim excess alginate extending beyond the back of the tray. Cut toward the tray to negate the possibility of pulling the alginate loose from the tray. Alginate extensions should not touch the bench top when resting on it, or the impression may be distorted (Fig. 1-3).

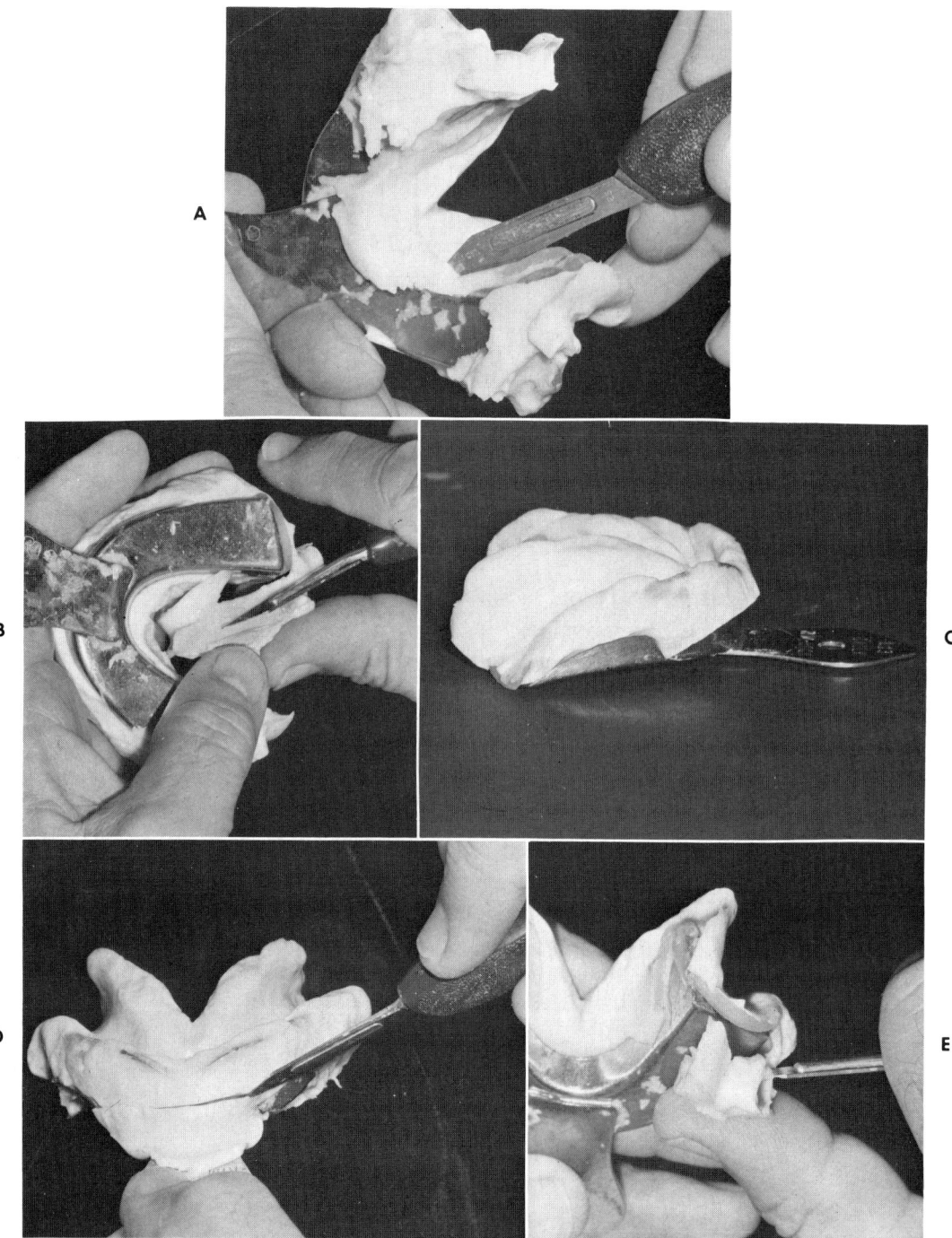

**Fig. 1-3. A,** Alginate extends beyond tray and will be distorted if placed on bench top. **B,** Alginate is trimmed with sharp No. 25 blade. Take care to not remove needed portions of impression. **C,** Trimmed impression will not be distorted if placed on bench top. **D,** Remove alginate extending onto sides. **E,** Alginate on top of tray is cut away.

3. Suspend the tray by its handle if excess alginate cannot be trimmed (Fig. 1-4). While mixing and setting the stone, place the handle of the tray in a holder to eliminate the need to rest the tray on the bench.

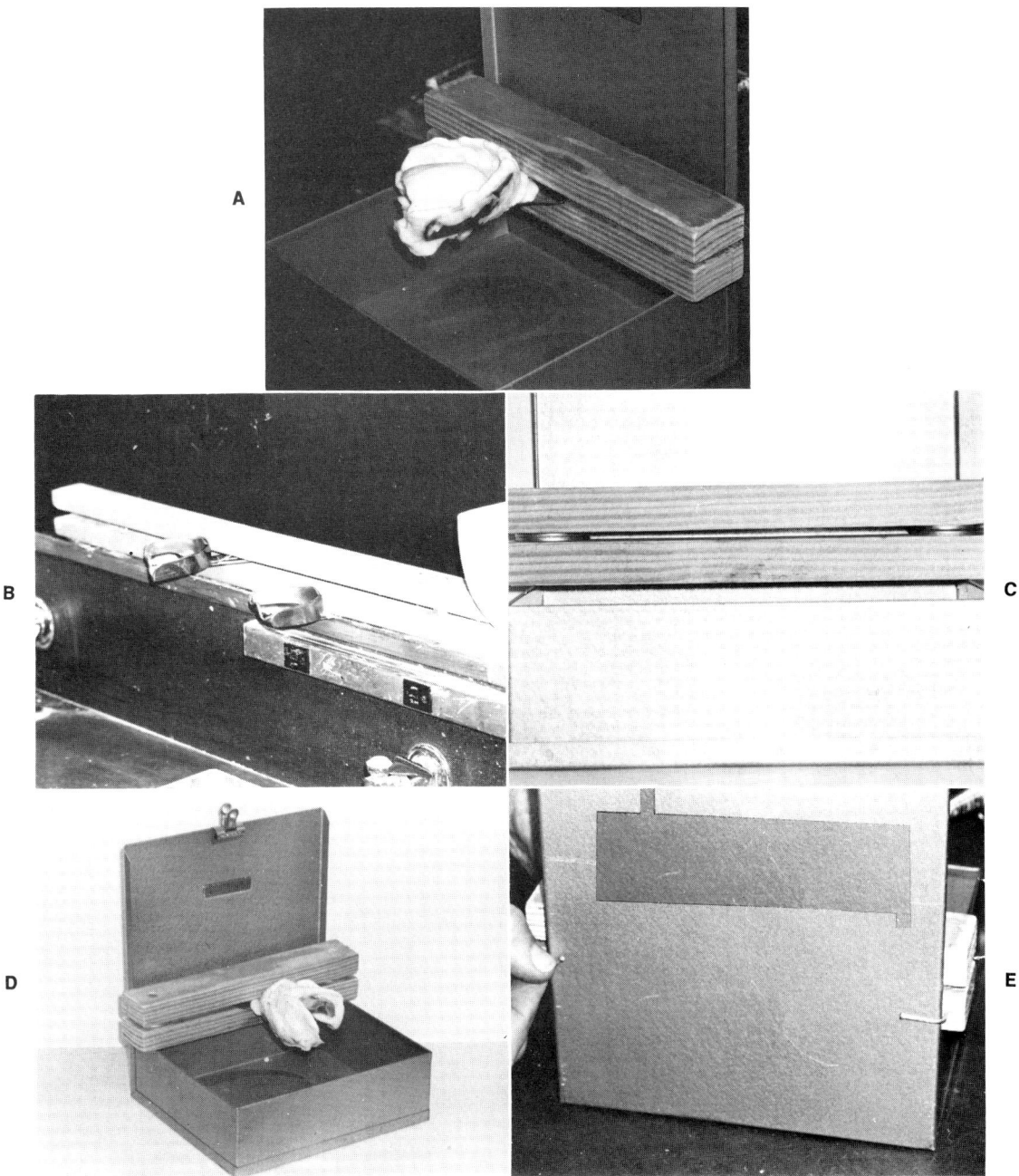

**Fig. 1-4. A,** Tray is suspended in tray holder to prevent distortion of alginate. **B,** Bench holder is made by placing suitable spacers between two 1 × 2-inch (2.5 × 5-cm) boards and attaching it to back of bench. In this case, thicker spacer was placed in top slot for water-cooled trays. Slot between bottom board and bench is narrower and will accommodate standard trays. **C,** Smaller tray holder for case pan is made by attaching two 1 × 2-inch (2.5 × 5-cm) boards together. **D,** Tray in position in small tray holder. **E,** Bent nails secure holder to case pan and permit easy removal.

**6** *Dental laboratory procedures: removable partial dentures*

4. Do *not* wrap the impression in a wet cloth or paper towel, since uneven weight or pressure on the alginate and uneven distribution of moisture may produce distortion (Fig. 1-5).

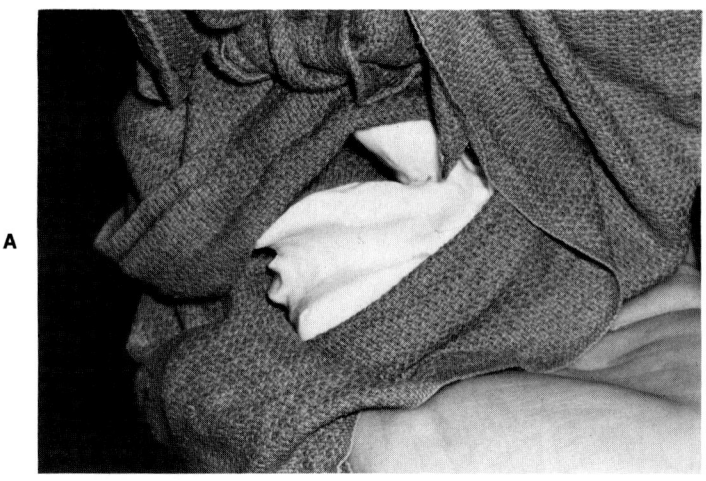

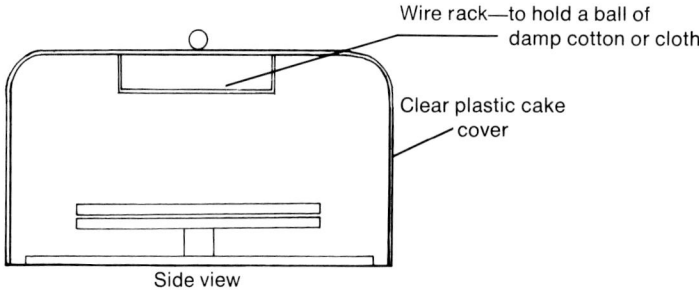

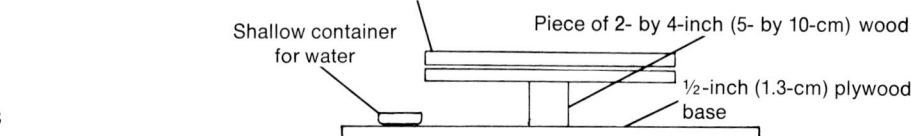

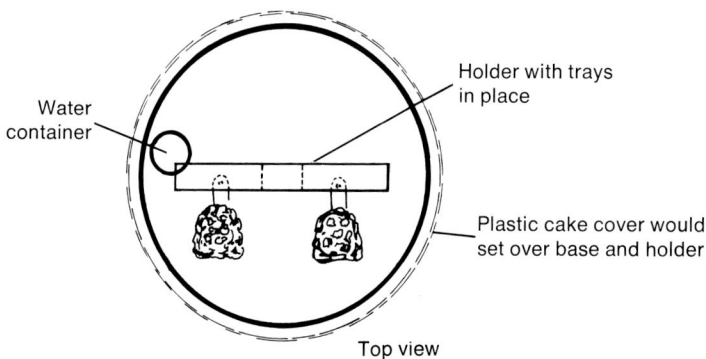

**Fig. 1-5. A,** Wrapping impression in wet cloth or paper towel is no substitute for immediate pouring. Uneven application of weight and moisture may ruin otherwise acceptable impression. **B,** Humidor is made by modifying plastic cake keeper. Wet cotton develops high humidity storage environment suitable for short time. Impression should be poured within 15 minutes.

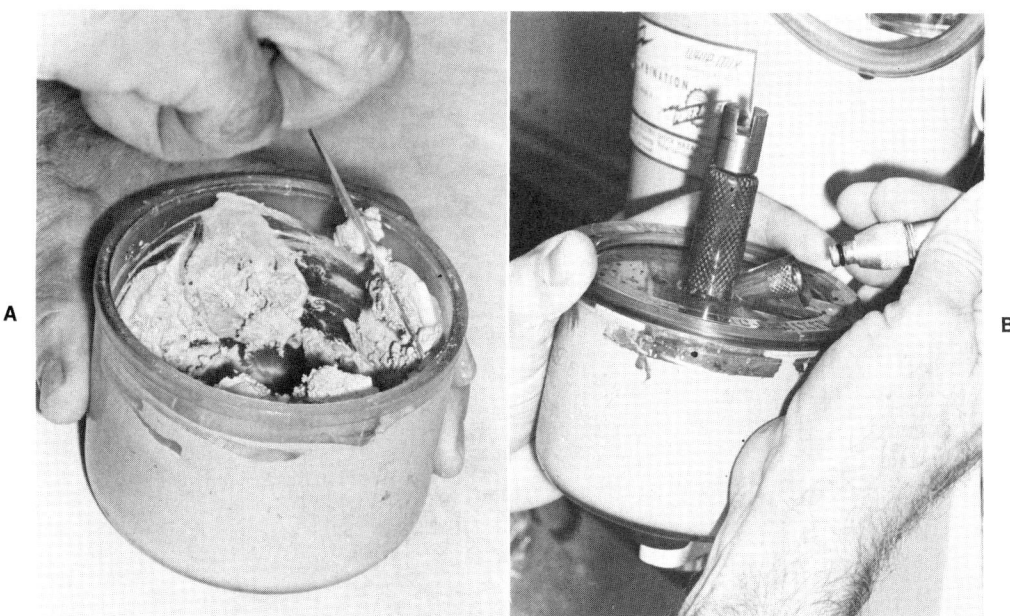

**Fig. 1-18. A,** Stone is added to water and hand spatulated to incorporate powder and liquid. **B,** Lid is placed on bowl, and hose is attached.

## Pouring the stone

Pouring the cast in two stages can result in improved cast surfaces over the one-stage method (Young, 1975). The entire anatomical portion of the impression is covered in the first pour. Then the first stage is permitted to set, after which the second stage, or base, is added.

### PROCEDURE

1. Add the preweighed stone to the proper volume of distilled water in a mixing bowl. A mechanical spatulator,* which mixes the stone under reduced atmospheric pressure, is recommended because it results in a smooth mix with minimal air inclusions (Fig. 1-18).
2. Mix the stone in the power mixer for 15 to 20 seconds (Fig. 1-19).
3. Use gentle vibration, and carefully flow stone into the impression (Fig. 1-20). Do not permit the alginate to touch the vibrator.
4. Add stone in small amounts to one distal corner of the impression, and tilt the impression to allow the stone to flow into each tooth indentation (Fig. 1-21). Watch the leading edge of the stone as it flows into the indentations to prevent bridging and resultant voids (Fig. 1-22).

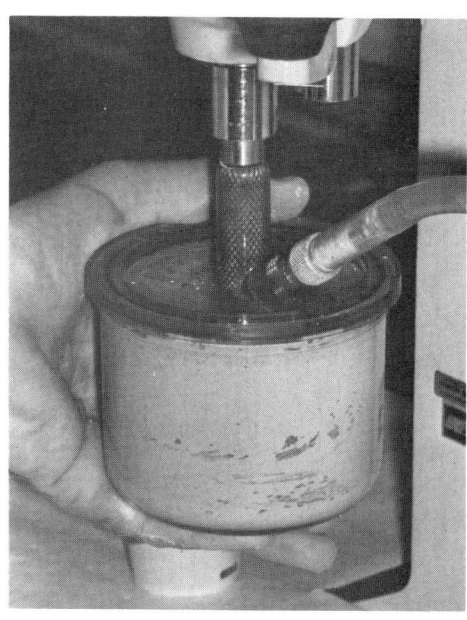

**Fig. 1-19.** Mix is spatulated for 15 to 20 seconds.

---

*Combination Vac-U-Vestor/Power Mixer, Whip-Mix Corp., Louisville, Ky.

Care of impressions and making casts  11

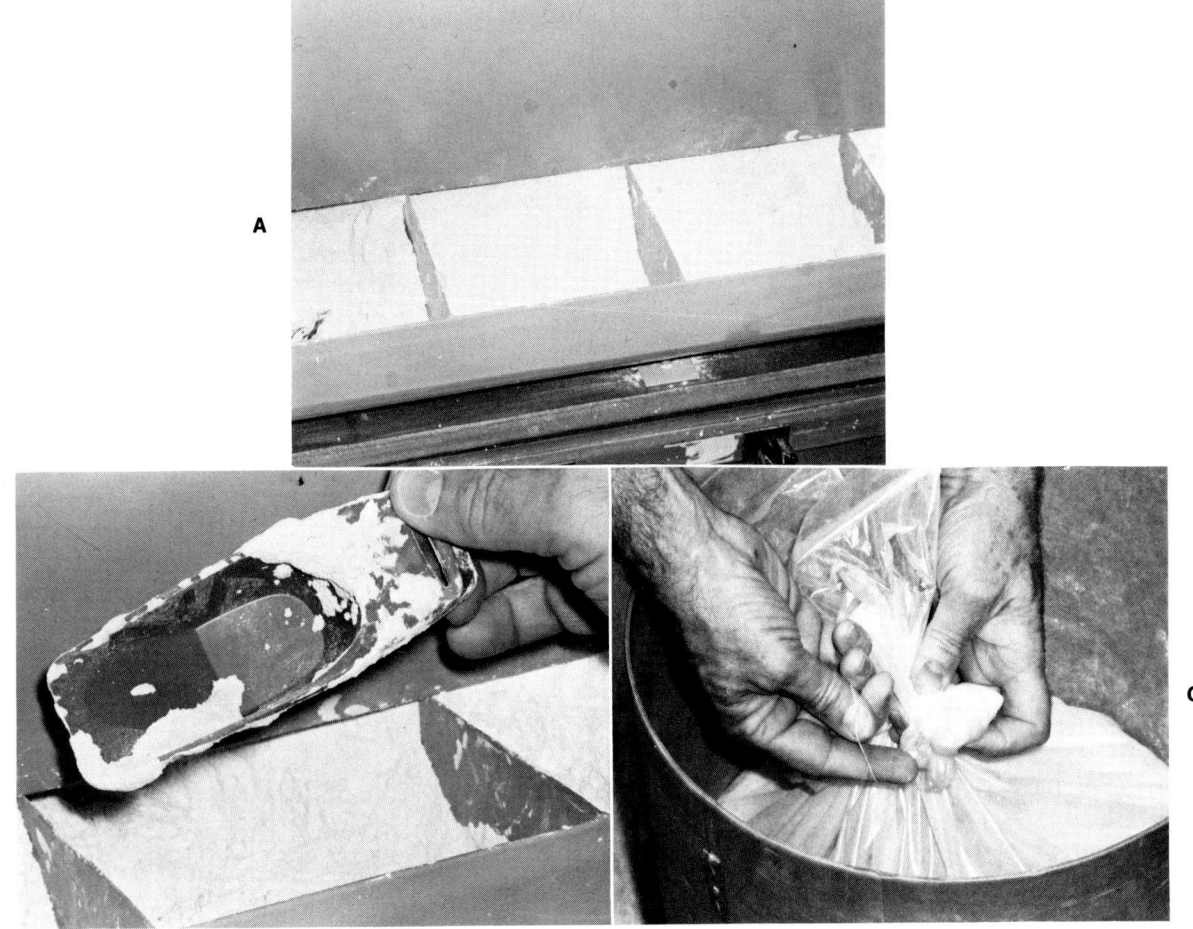

**Fig. 1-17. A,** Stone stored in bins can be contaminated with water droplets if near faucet or when humidity is high. **B,** Stone may be contaminated by other types of stones or plaster if scoop is interchanged. **C,** Seal bulk stone in plastic bag until it is used.

the label the amount of water required for the mix (Fig. 1-15). Stone used for making casts should be stored in tightly sealed foil or plastic bags or sealed in jars (Fig. 1-16). Do not use stone from open bins or open cardboard containers for pouring casts, since stone stored in this manner is subject to contamination by water droplets and other types of stones if the scoop is interchanged (Fig. 1-17). Stone stored in bins can be used to mount casts and pour indexes and flask dentures, but should not be used for casts. Preweighed stone stored in sealed containers eliminates the problem of contamination and, when mixed with the proper volume of water, permits uniform stone mixes. In addition, properly proportioned stone mixes permit development of the maximum physical properties of the particular stone. Thus preweighing the stone and storing it in sealed containers are highly recommended.

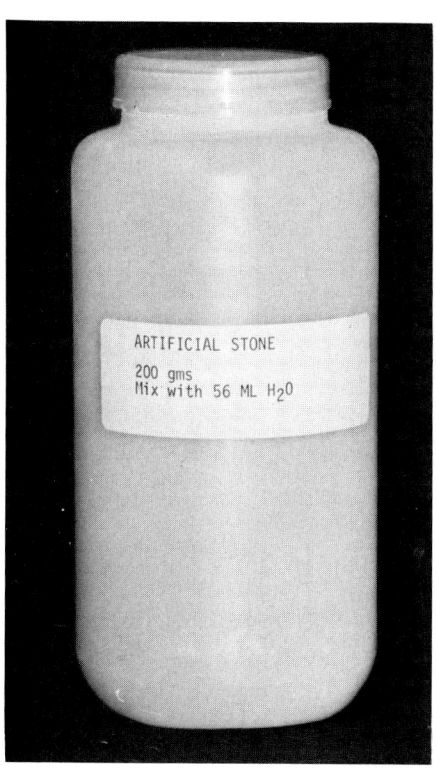

Fig. 1-15. Label should indicate volume of water required to make mix, thus assuring uniformity.

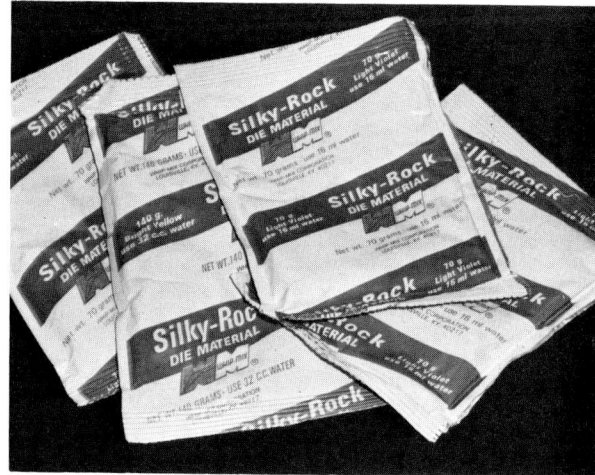

Fig. 1-16. Stone may be purchased in preweighed packets although usually at higher cost than bulk stone.

9. Do *not* box an alginate impression with wax or plaster/pumice. Wax will not adhere to the alginate, and plaster/pumice mixes may dehydrate the impression, resulting in distortion.

10. Pour the impression immediately with preweighed artificial stone mixed with the recommended volume of distilled water (Fig. 1-13). Weight out 100- and 200-gm portions of artificial stone, and store them in a 112-gm (4-ounce) ointment jar or a plastic bottle (Fig. 1-14). Indicate on

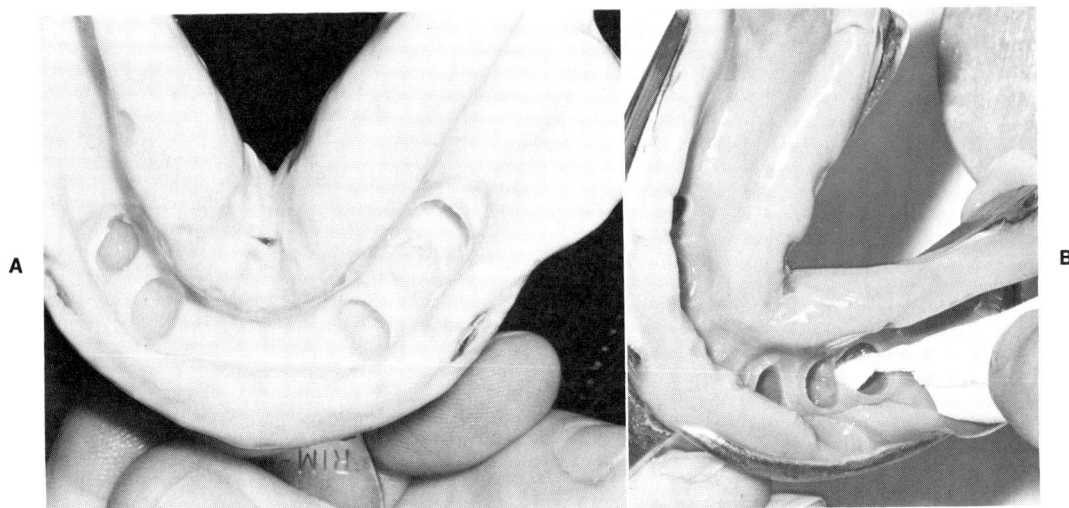

**Fig. 1-12. A,** Excess moisture accumulations in cusp indentations may produce soft chalky surfaces on cast. **B,** Strip of absorbent tissue is used to remove moisture from cusp indentations.

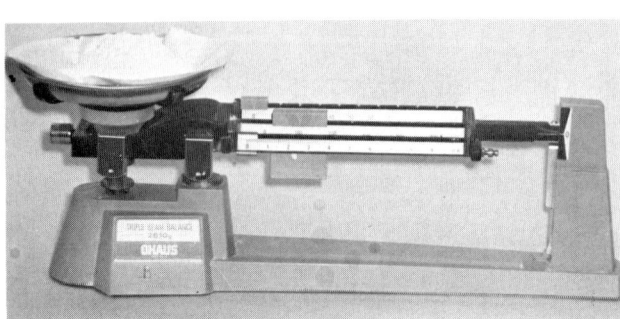

**Fig. 1-13.** Stone is weighed to permit accurate proportioning and resultant improved physical properties.

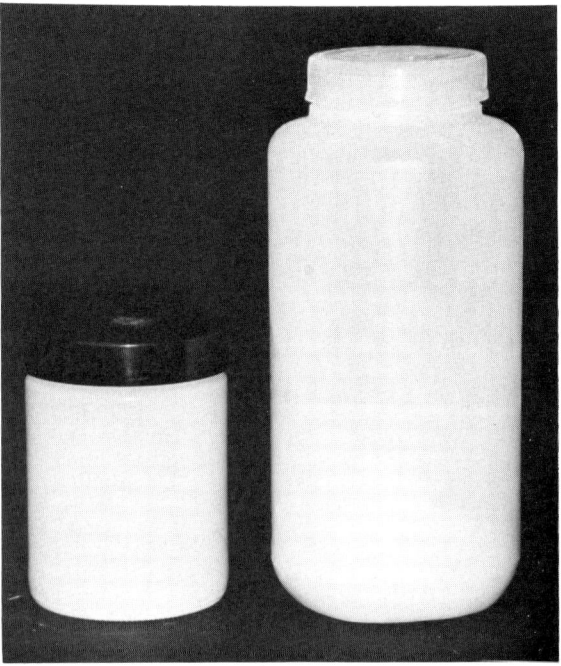

**Fig. 1-14.** Portions of 100 gm of stone (left) are used for small impressions. Portions of 200 gm are stored in plastic bottle (right) and are used for most impressions.

7. Remove all stone by flowing cold tap water over the impression, and scrub it with a soft camel's hair brush (Fig. 1-9). Although most manufacturers do not recommend placing alginate impressions in a 2% potassium sulfate solution, most cast surfaces are improved when this procedure is followed.

8. Remove excess moisture from the impression with a gentle stream of air (Fig. 1-10). Use caution, since a strong blast of air can separate the alginate from the tray (Fig. 1-11). Take care to not overdry the impression. The impression surface should glisten. There should, however, be no visible accumulation of liquid on the impression and particularly in the tooth indentations (Fig. 1-12). A small strip of absorbent tissue paper can be used to blot excess moisture from tooth indentations.

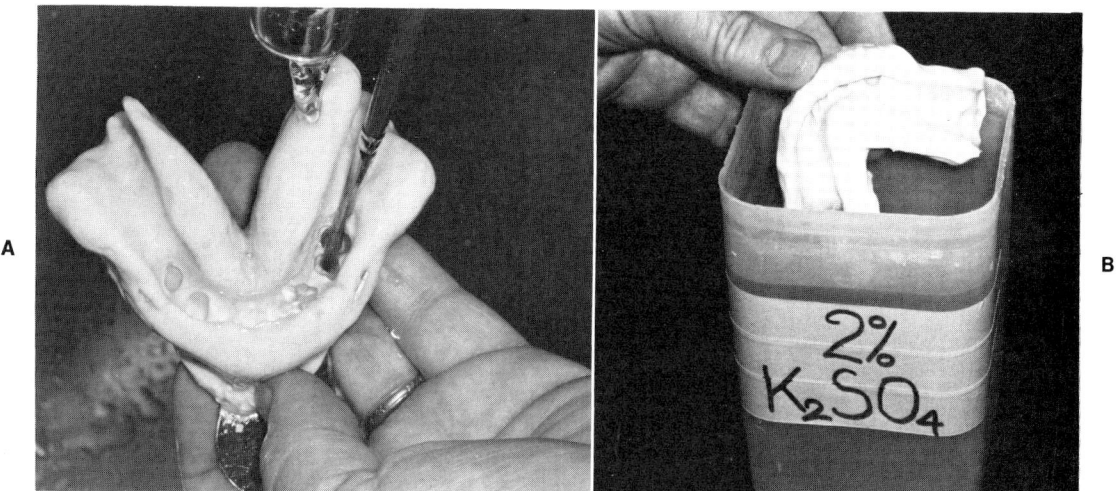

Fig. 1-9. **A,** All stone must be removed from impression surface. Use soft camel's hair brush if necessary. **B,** Rinse impression thoroughly in 2% potassium sulfate solution.

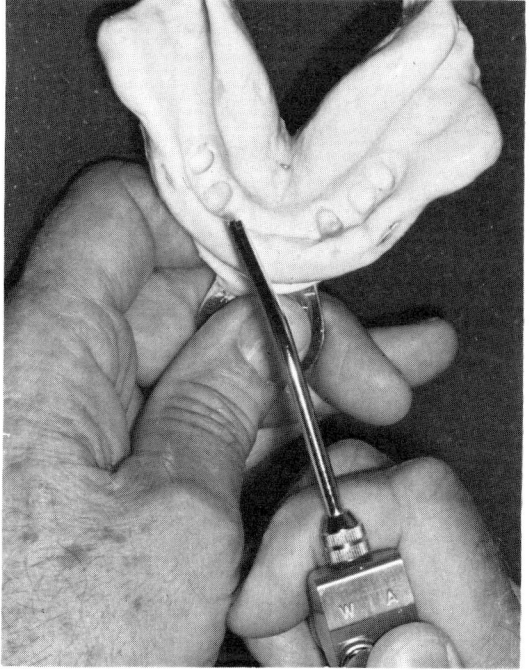

Fig. 1-10. Gentle stream of air is used to remove excess moisture.

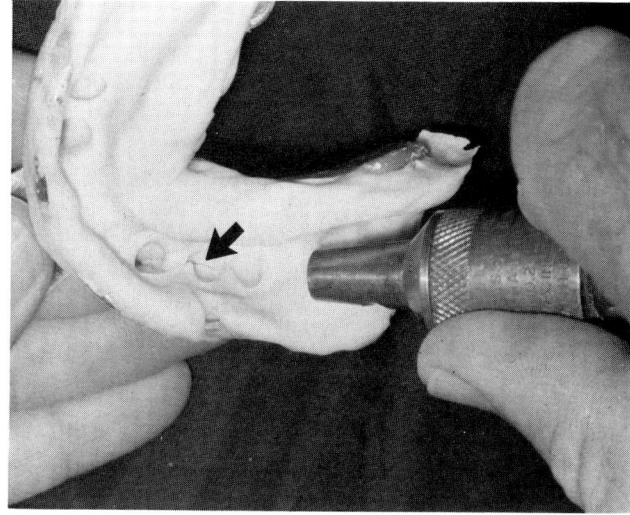

Fig. 1-11. Impression can be ruined by strong blast of air. Note separation of alginate from tray (arrow).

5. Run cold tap water gently over the impression to rinse saliva from it (Fig. 1-6).

6. Sprinkle artificial stone into the impression, and scrub it lightly with a soft camel's hair brush to disclose saliva and react with the surface of the alginate, which will make a smoother surface on the cast (Fig. 1-7). A plastic mustard or catsup container is a handy dispenser for the stone (Fig. 1-8).

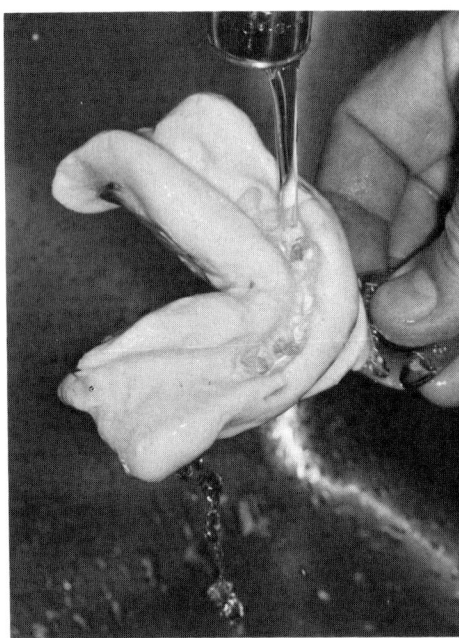

**Fig. 1-6.** Saliva remaining in impression is rinsed with cold tap water. Do not use forceful stream of water.

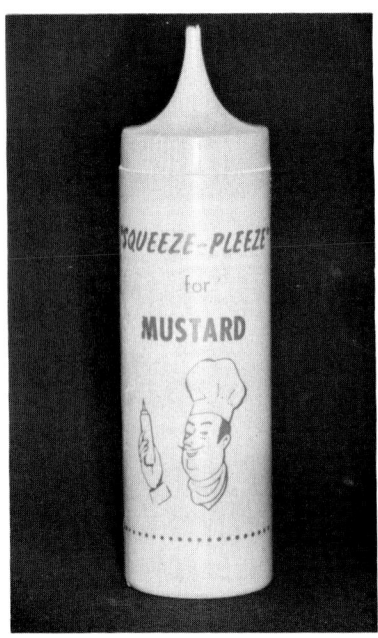

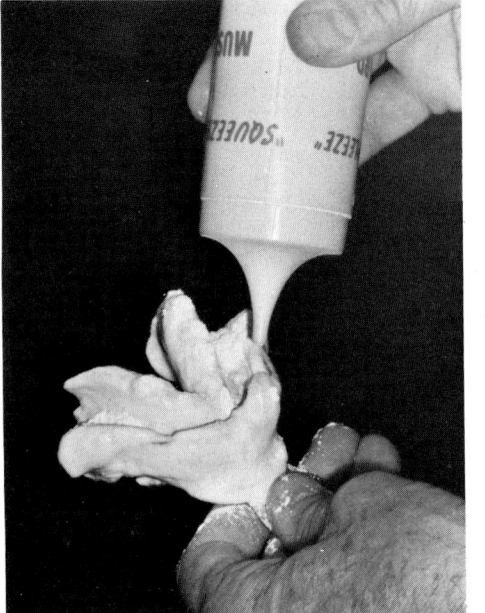

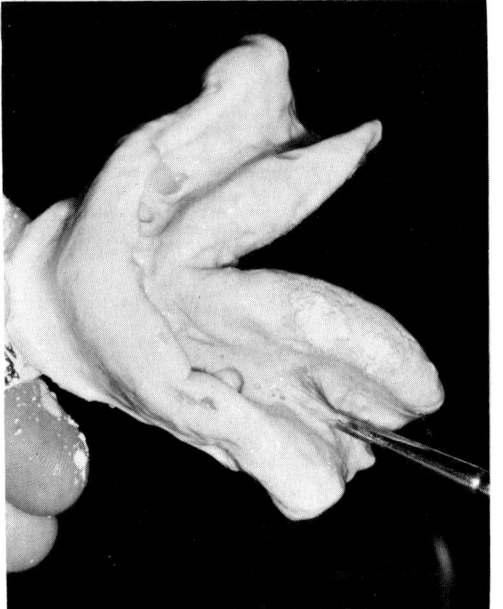

**Fig. 1-7. A,** Artificial stone sprinkled on impression surface discloses saliva films otherwise difficult to see. **B,** Soft camel's hair brush and water are used to gently scrub impression surface with stone.

**Fig. 1-8.** Plastic catsup or mustard containers can be used when sprinkling stone.

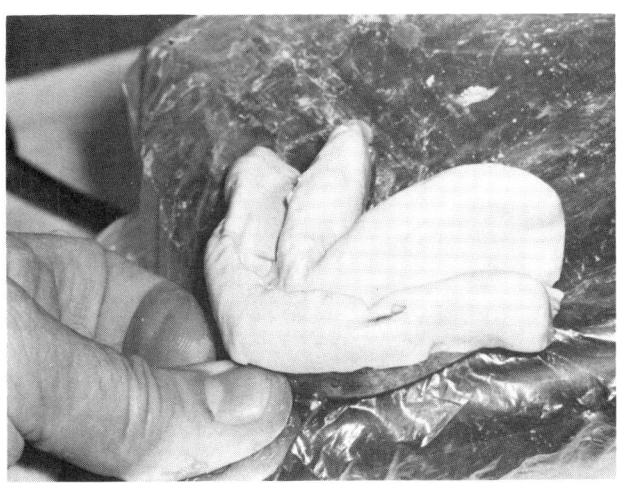

**Fig. 1-20.** If mechanical vibrator has adjustable settings, it is set for gentle vibration, and stone is flowed into impression.

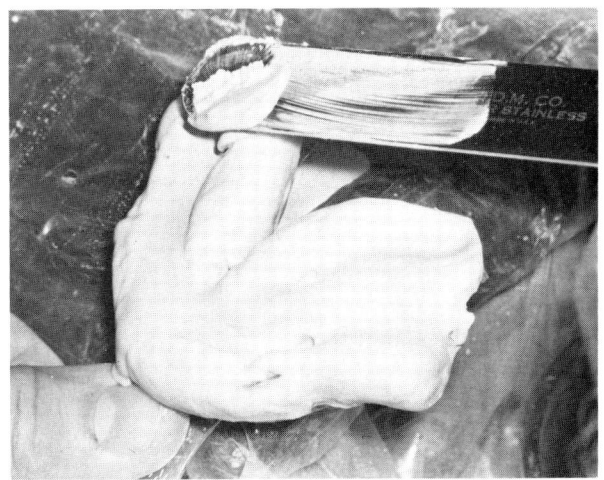

**Fig. 1-21.** Stone is added to one distal region of impression, and impression is tilted as needed to control flow.

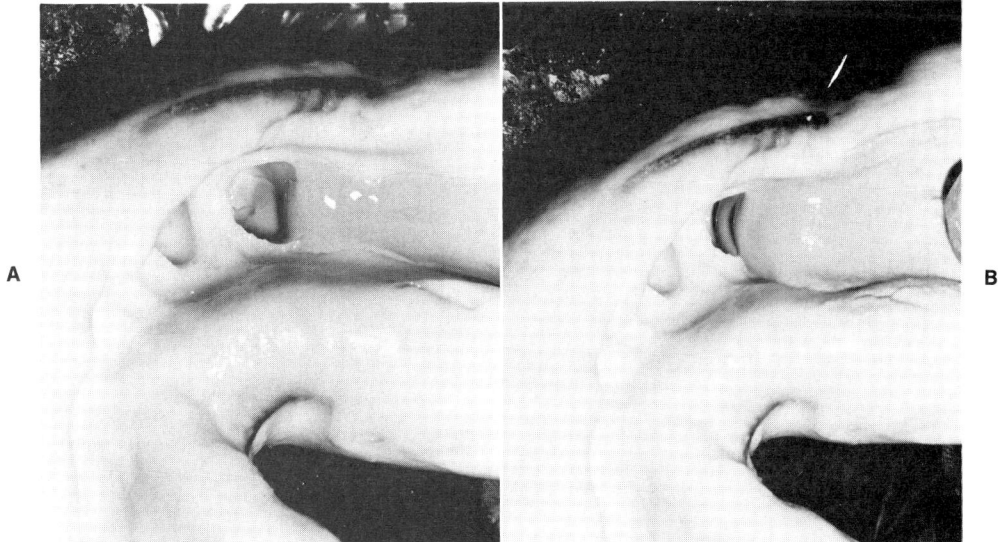

**Fig. 1-22. A,** As stone flows into impression, carefully watch leading edge of stone to determine that stone flows into each indentation, filling it completely. **B,** If tooth indentation is bridged and air entrapped, air must be expelled by tilting tray or by using small brush to release trapped air.

5. After all indentations are filled, the stone can be added more rapidly until the impression is full.

6. Place droplets of stone onto the upper stone surface to create irregularities with undercuts (Fig. 1-23). The upper surface of the stone should be rough to facilitate a firm bond between the two stages of the pour.

7. Suspend the poured impression by the handle in the tray holder (Fig. 1-24). Allow the stone to set.

8. While the stone is still warm from the heat of crystallization, place the poured impression in clear slurry water* for 3 to 5 minutes (Fig. 1-25). Slurry water will not dissolve the stone surface. Tap water can ruin an otherwise accurate cast by dissolving

---

*Tap water in which stone casts or debris have been allowed to soak for 48 hours. The resultant supernatant solution is slurry water.

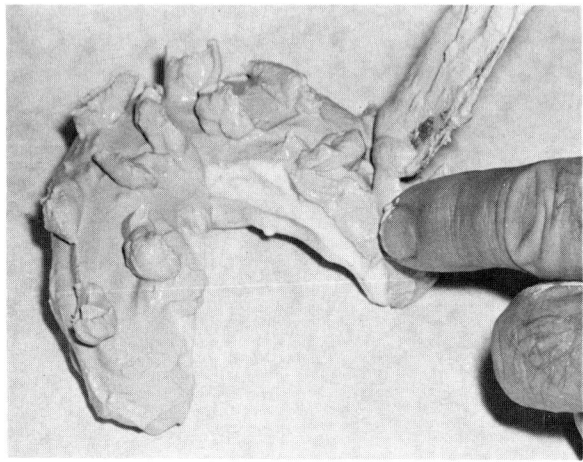

**Fig. 1-23.** After impression is completely filled, small droplets of stone are placed on upper surface to make undercuts.

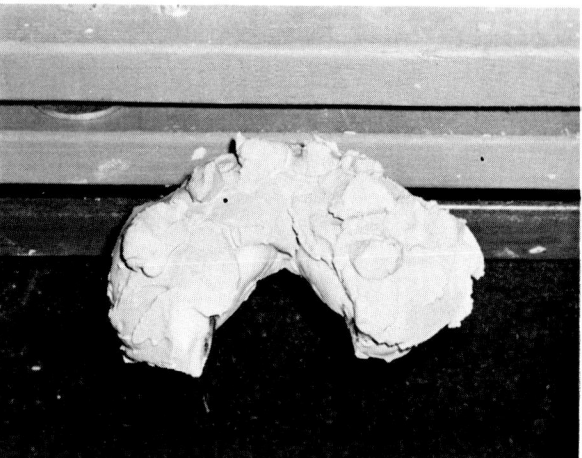

**Fig. 1-24.** Poured impression is suspended in tray holder.

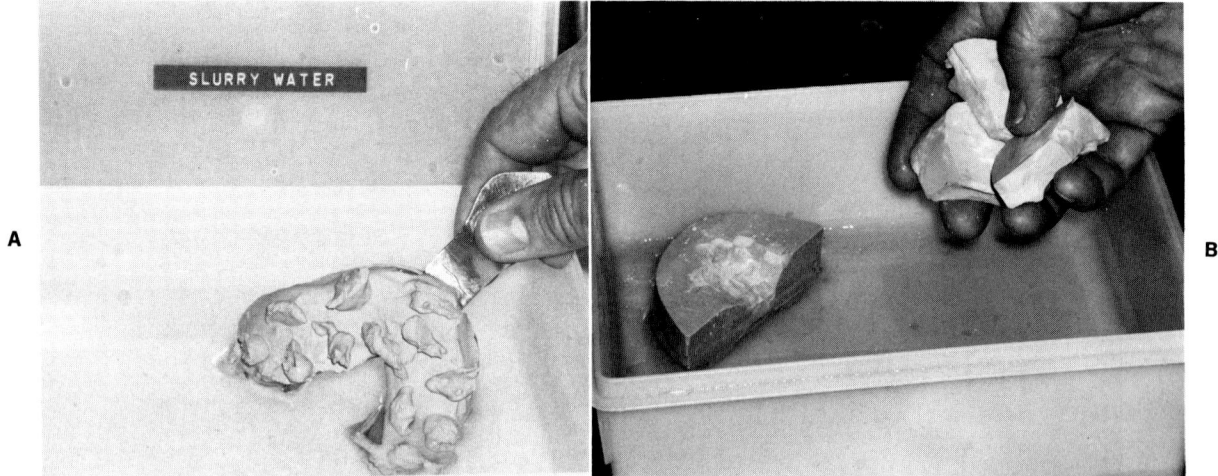

**Fig. 1-25. A,** Impression with first stone pour is placed in clear slurry water for 3 to 5 minutes to wet stone. **B,** Clear slurry water is made by soaking stone in tap water for 48 hours. Resultant solution is used to wet casts and will not dissolve cast surface.

some of the surface stone, thus casts should not be needlessly exposed to tap water (Rudd et al., 1970).

9. Remove the impression and stone from the slurry water, and blow off excess liquid with a stream of air (Fig. 1-26).

10. Make another mix of stone using the same kind of stone and the same water-powder ratio. Place the second mix of stone on a plastic or glass plate, and shape the stone to the appropriate shape and thickness to serve as a base (Fig. 1-27).

11. Add a small amount of stone to the base of the cast in the impression, taking care to *wipe* the stone into the undercuts (Fig. 1-28).

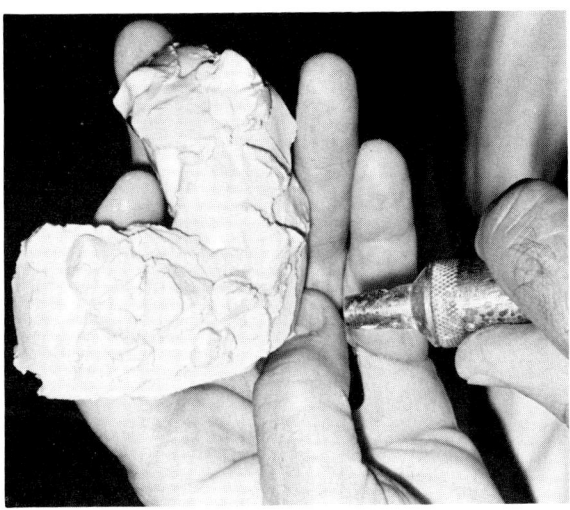

Fig. 1-26. Excess moisture is removed with stream of air.

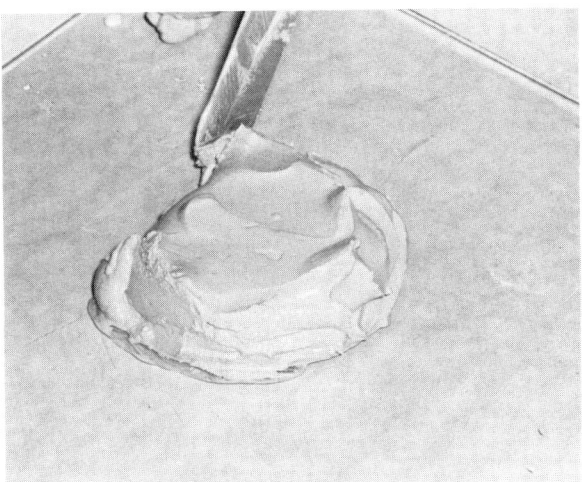

Fig. 1-27. Stone is shaped to approximate form of cast base.

Fig. 1-28. Stone is wiped into undercuts with spatula.

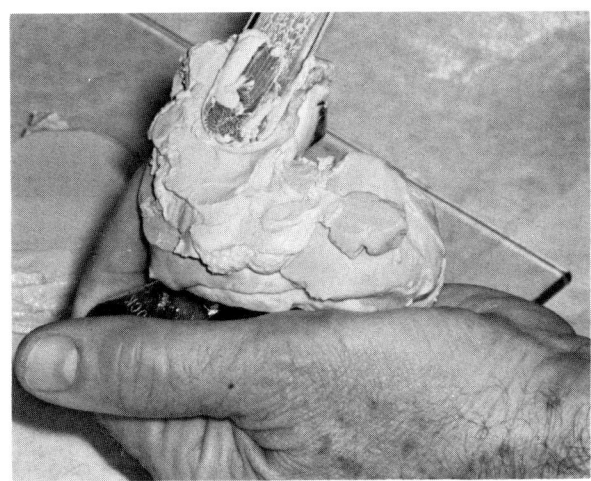

12. Invert the cast and impression, and settle them into the new mix of stone on the glass plate (Fig. 1-29). Do not attempt to remove the first stone pour from the impression before adding the base, otherwise it may be broken.

13. With the spatula, pull the stone up around the sides of the impression (Fig. 1-30). Smooth the area lingual to the mandibular ridge so that it is flat and smooth (Fig. 1-31).

14. After 45 minutes to 1 hour from the first pour, separate the impression from the cast (Fig. 1-32).

15. After the cast has been separated from the impression, carefully remove any remaining alginate (Fig. 1-33). Do not, however, wash or trim the cast for at least 12 hours, and preferably 24 hours or more, after separation. The cast should never be wet, rinsed, or soaked in distilled or tap water because artificial stone is soluble in water, and invariably the surface of the cast will be etched. Only clear slurry water should be used to wet casts, since

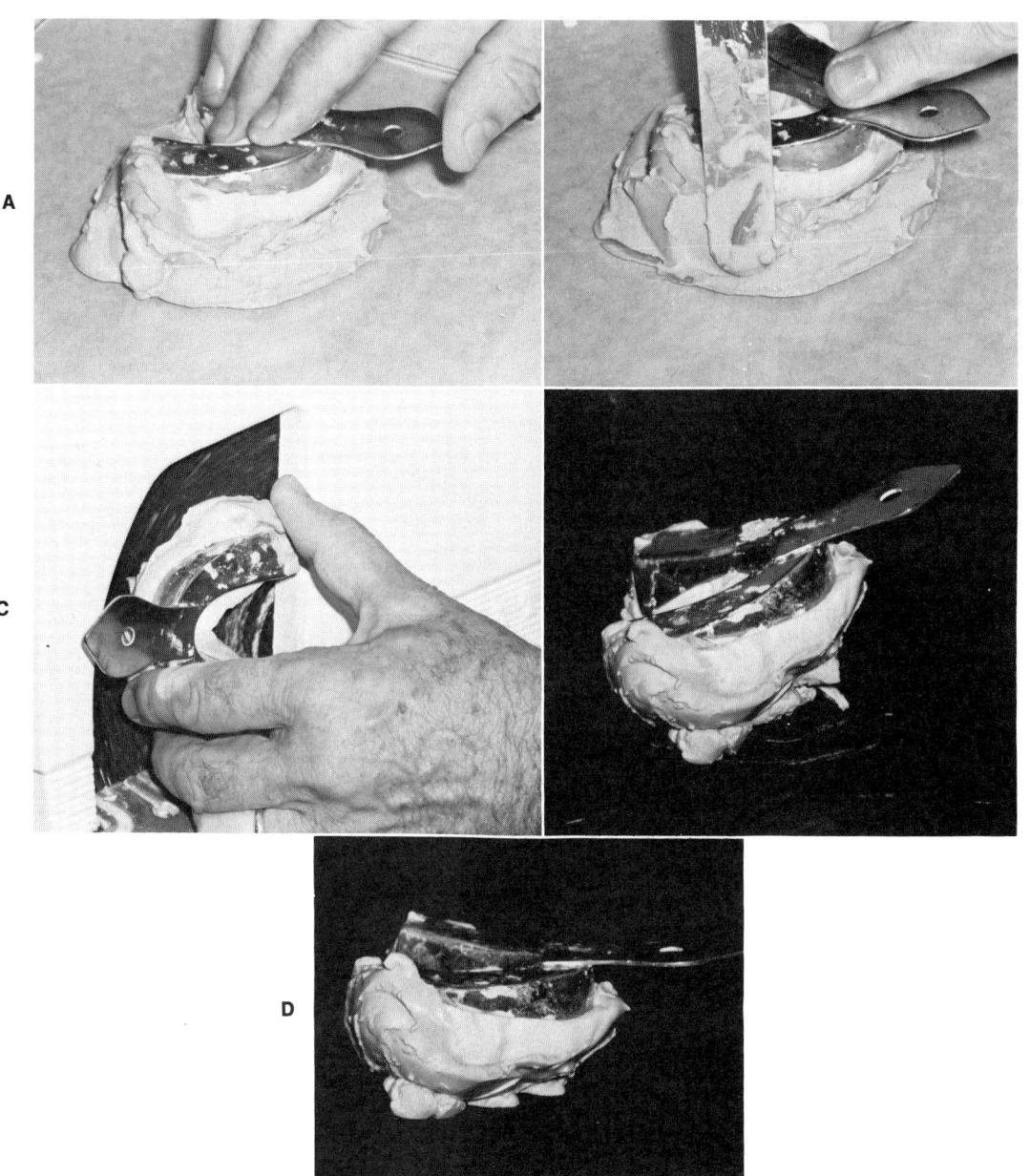

Fig. 1-29. **A,** Impression and cast are settled into base mix, keeping tray handle parallel to bench top. **B,** Cast thickness is controlled by distance impression is settled into second pour. **C,** If undercut droplets on first pour were too high, it may be necessary to trim them on cast trimmer before adding base (left). If this is not done, cast may be too thick (right). **D,** Trimmed stone droplets are now proper height.

## Care of impressions and making casts 17

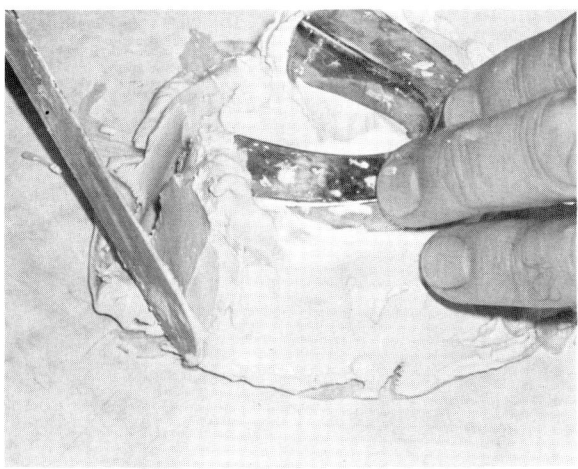

**Fig. 1-30.** Spatula is used to pull stone around sides of impression. Do not, however, lock tray in stone by making sides too high.

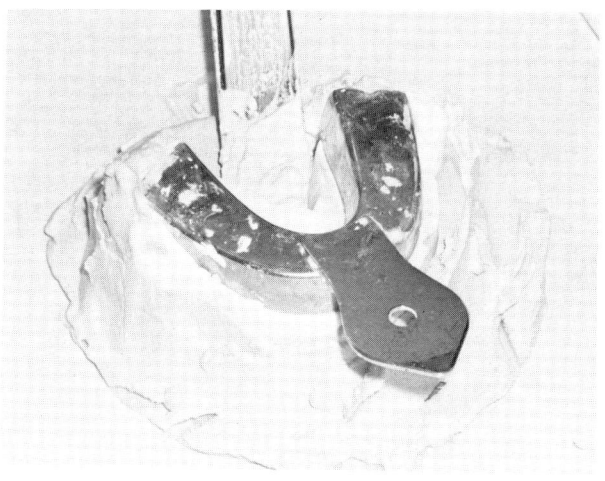

**Fig. 1-31.** Mandibular cast in lingual region should be smooth and not too high, otherwise difficult trimming will be required later.

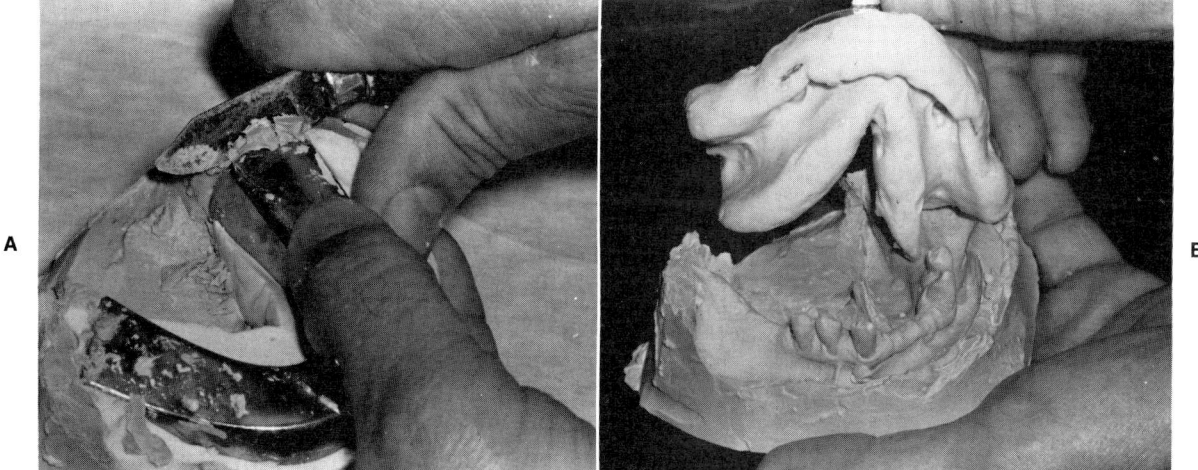

**Fig. 1-32. A,** Tray is freed by trimming stone with knife. **B,** Cast is separated from impression 45 minutes to 1 hour after first pour.

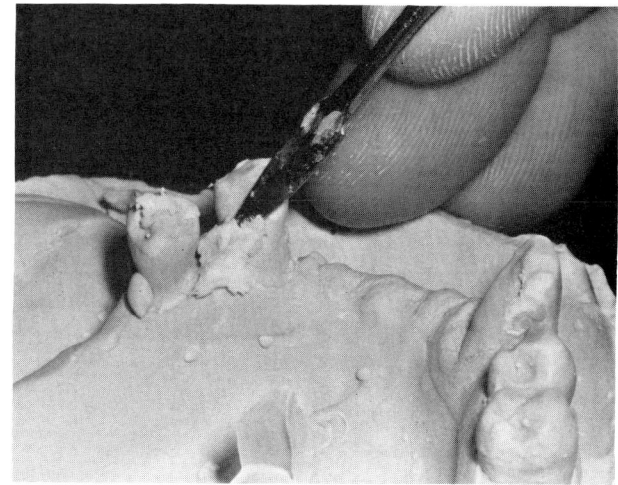

**Fig. 1-33.** Alginate remaining between teeth on cast is removed.

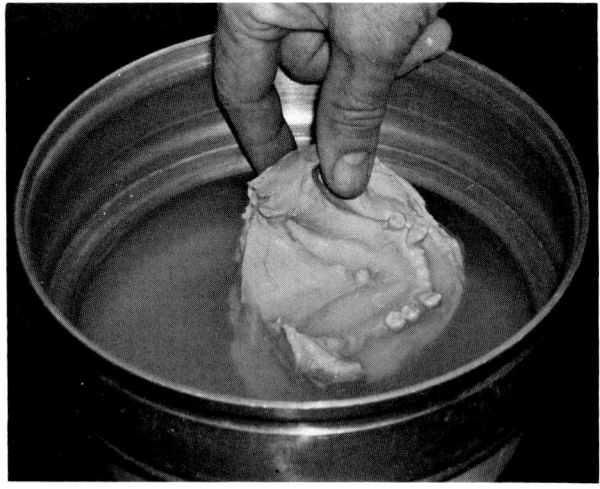

Fig. 1-34. Cast is soaked 3 to 5 minutes in container of clear slurry water prior to trimming on cast trimmer.

this solution, being saturated with stone, will not dissolve the cast.

16. Before trimming, soak the cast in clear slurry water for 3 to 5 minutes (Fig. 1-34). Soaking prior to trimming the cast on a cast trimmer will permit the sludge created during trimming to be rinsed off by swishing the cast in a pan of slurry water (Fig. 1-35). The cast should be rinsed again in slurry water on completion of the trimming. Remove any sludge remaining on the cast with a soft camel's hair brush (Fig. 1-36). Do not use a denture brush, toothbrush, or hand brush, since the stiff bristles may remove part of the surface of the cast, making it inaccurate (Fig. 1-37). Failure to soak the cast in slurry water prior to trimming it on the cast trimmer or letting the cast dry with sludge on it will make removal of the sludge produced during trimming extremely difficult with damage to the cast (Fig. 1-38).

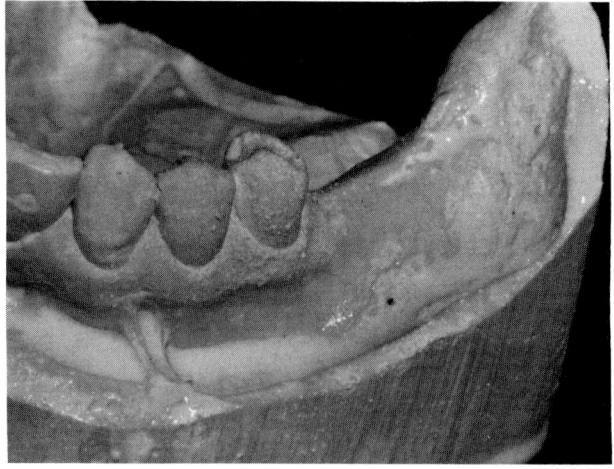

Fig. 1-35. Sludge from cast trimmer will not stick to wet cast if rinsed off immediately.

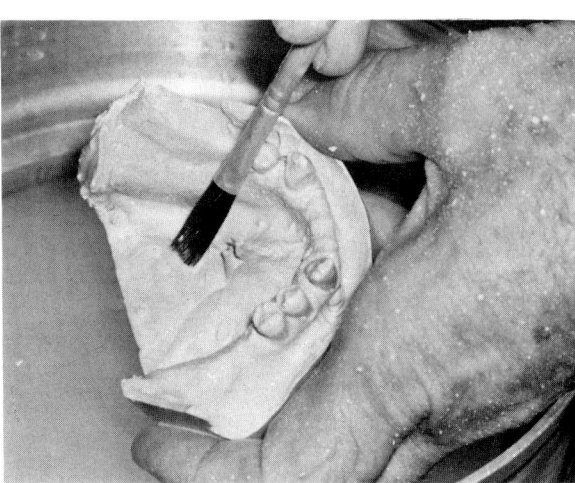

Fig. 1-36. Soft brush can be used to remove stone sludge.

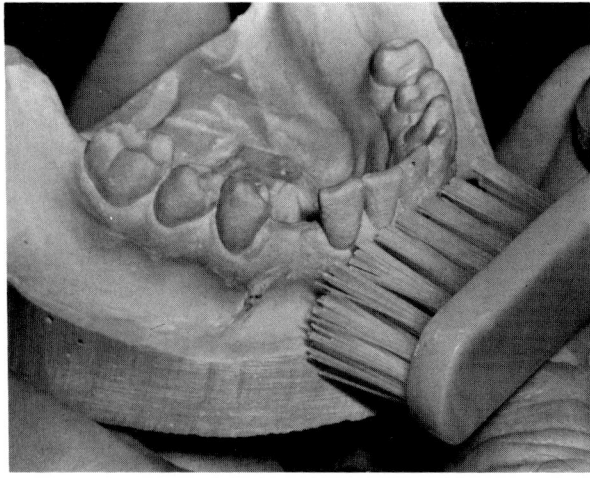

Fig. 1-37. Stiff brush can ruin cast.

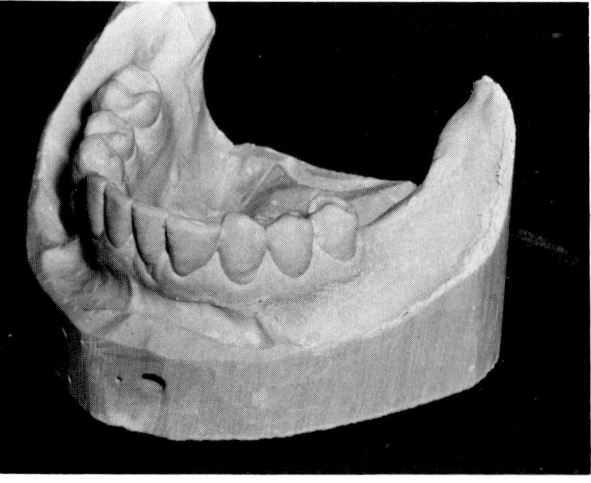

Fig. 1-38. Cast with dried sludge is ruined.

## Trimming the cast
**PROCEDURE**

1. Trim the cast so that its base is 15 to 16 mm thick at the thinnest part (Fig. 1-39).
2. Trim the sides of the base of the cast vertically; they should not be tilted inward or outward (Fig. 1-40).

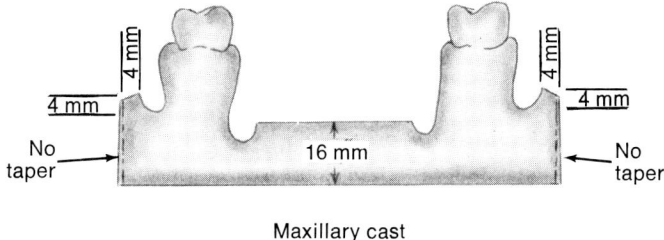

Maxillary cast

**Fig. 1-39.** Cast base is trimmed so that cast is 15 to 16 mm thick at thinnest point. Base is trimmed parallel to occlusal plane or residual ridges.

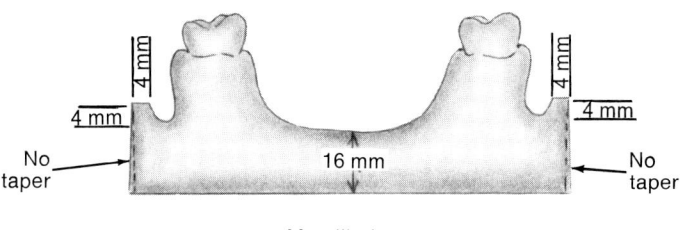

Mandibular cast

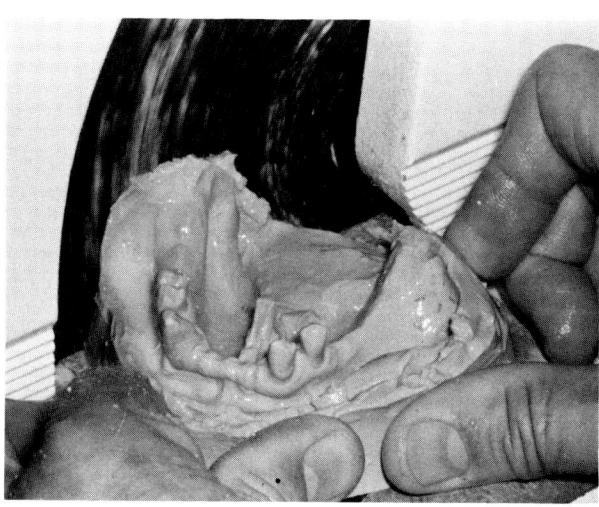

**Fig. 1-40.** Sides of cast are trimmed vertically, perpendicular to base. Do not overtrim removing essential portions of cast.

3. Trim the cast to form a border area of 3 to 4 mm high around the anatomical portion of the cast, and smooth the tongue area of the mandibular cast (Fig. 1-41).

4. Trim the borders of the cast vertically to preserve the border extension and thickness of the original impression (Fig. 1-42).

5. After the cast is dry, inspect it carefully, and remove any nodules of stone present using a sharp instrument or a dental explorer (Fig. 1-43).

6. Identify the cast by marking it with an indelible pencil (Fig. 1-44).

7. Methods for packing and mailing casts to prevent damage in transit are given in Chapter 22.

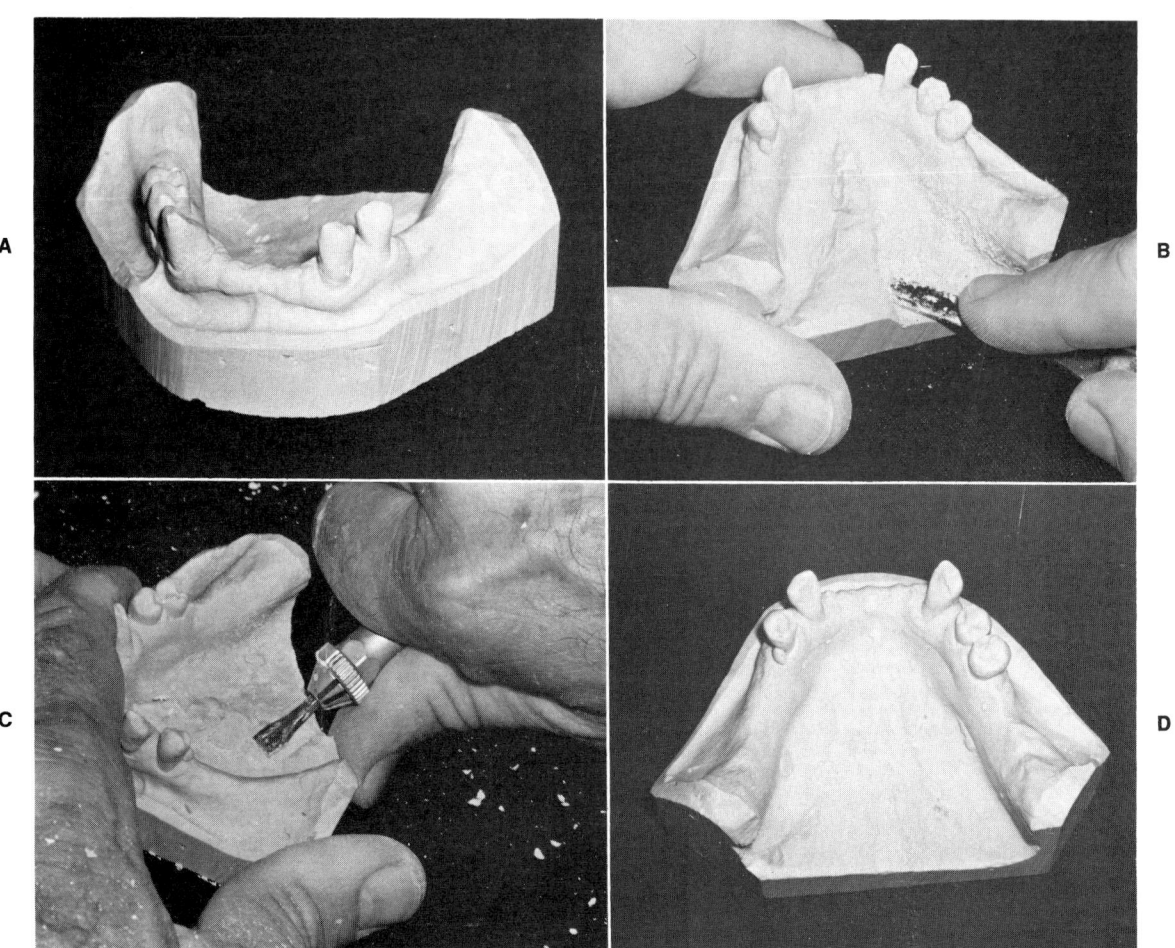

**Fig. 1-41. A,** Where possible, cast border should preserve impression border thickness. **B,** Use of knife to trim tongue area. **C,** Use of pneumatic chisel to trim tongue area. **D,** Smooth tongue area.

*Care of impressions and making casts* 21

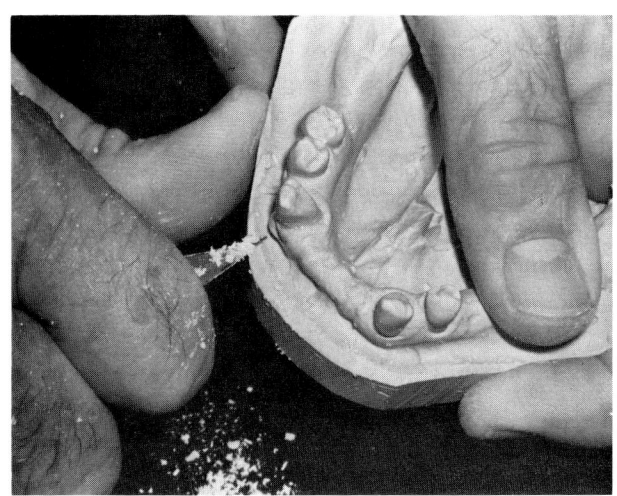

**Fig. 1-42.** Borders are trimmed to form vestibular sulcus 3 to 4 mm deep.

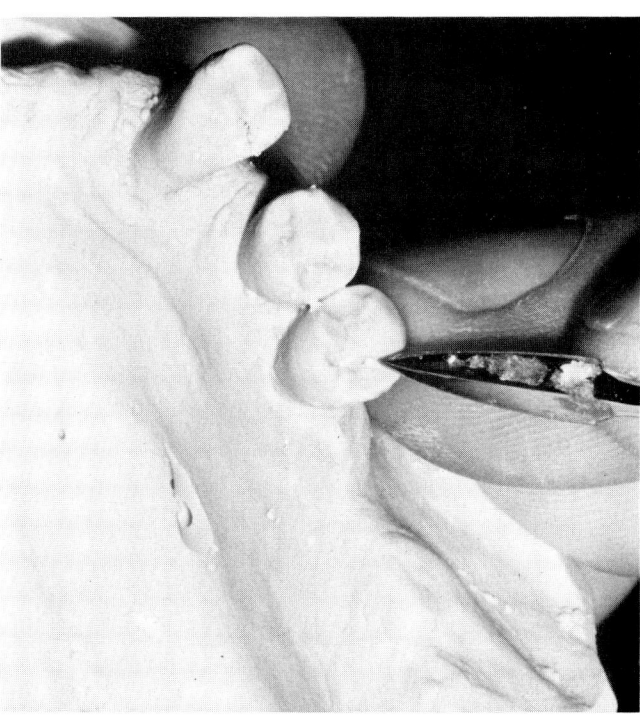

**Fig. 1-43.** Nodules of stone are removed with Roach carver or explorer. Do not carve cast surfaces however.

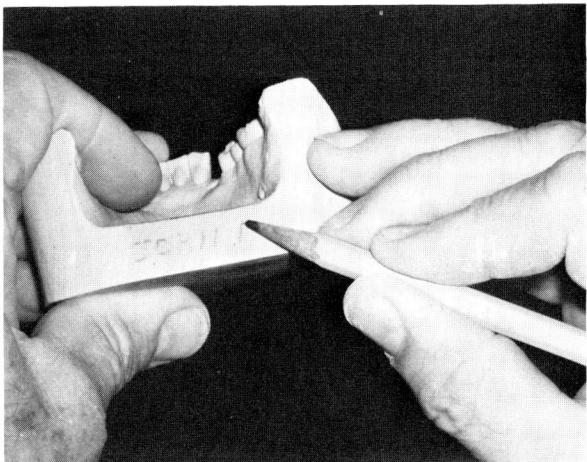

**Fig. 1-44.** Cast is identified with indelible pencil.

## PROBLEM AREAS

The principal problems with pouring impressions and making casts are related to the individual procedures involved in the care and handling of the alginate impression and pouring and trimming of the resultant cast (Table 1-1). Each step in the chain can be accomplished incorrectly with subsequent compromised cast quality. Although all procedures have been carefully executed, the stone and alginate used may not be compatible. Some brands of artificial stone give better cast surfaces when poured into impressions made with certain alginate impression materials than with others. It is then axiomatic that if the best stone cast surfaces are desired, compatible stone-alginate combination should be used. If, after careful examination of the

**Table 1-1.** Pouring impressions and making casts

| Problem | Probable cause | Solution |
|---|---|---|
| Surface of cast is soft or chalky | Saliva in impression when stone was poured | Identify saliva with sprinkled stone and remove before pouring cast |
| | Water from rinsing remained in impression when cast was poured | Remove excess water with stream of air; use tissue paper to absorb water in tooth indentations before pouring cast |
| | Incompatible stone-alginate combination used | Use compatible stone-alginate combination for best results |
| | Cast not separated from impression within 1 hour | Remove impression from cast within 1 hour of initial pour |
| | Improper water-powder ratio used for stone | Use manufacturer's recommended water-powder ratio for stone |
| Cast appears to be distorted, or isolated teeth on cast appear distorted | Impression material separated from tray | Do not accept impressions that have separated from tray |
| | Air inclusion in impression with thin wall that bulges when stone is poured into it | Impression material should be loaded carefully in tray to minimize air entrapment |
| Cast base is too thin | Cast base not poured thick enough | Pour base to assure 15 to 16 mm thickness |
| | Cast base overtrimmed on cast trimmer | Use care when trimming cast to avoid overtrimming |
| Cast surface is rough | Slurry splatter from cast trimmer stuck to cast | Rinse cast in clear slurry during trimming to prevent slurry splatter from adhering to cast surface |
| Numerous voids in poured cast | Stone hand spatulated with air inclusion | Mix stone with mechanical spatulator under reduced atmospheric pressure |
| | Air trapped during pouring of cast | Use vibrator; exercise care when pouring cast to avoid air entrapment |
| Cast is weak and easily broken | Incorrect water-powder ratio used for stone | Follow manufacturer's recommendations for water-powder ratio; weigh stone on scale and mix with recommended volume of water |
| Numerous positive stone nodules on cast | Failure to place alginate in vestibules and on teeth with finger before seating tray | Wipe alginate into vestibules and palate before seating tray to reduce air entrapment and resultant stone nodules on cast |

cast, the cast does not meet all specifications, it should be discarded, and another impression should be obtained. It is much less time consuming and costly to start over at this time than to take a chance on making an ill-fitting removable partial denture that will necessitate repeating the entire procedure. Accepting a cast of doubtful quality is poor economy for all concerned.

## AGAR REVERSIBLE HYDROCOLLOID IMPRESSIONS

Agar reversible hydrocolloid is widely used in dentistry, particularly for making casts and dies for fixed partial dentures and for duplicating casts in dental laboratories. It is not used as frequently to make impressions for removable partial dentures; however, it is used, and the resultant casts can be of excellent quality. The principal disadvantage to using agar reversible hydrocolloid is the requirement for specialized equipment to liquefy, temper, and store it.

Since impression procedures and pouring techniques vary with the individual manufacturers, the manufacturer's recommendations should be closely followed.

### Care of the impression
PROCEDURE

1. The agar reversible hydrocolloid impression should be poured immediately. As with alginate impressions, lengthy exposure of the reversible hydrocolloid impression to air can result in dehydration and corresponding distortion.

2. Examine the agar reversible hydrocolloid impression critically for deficiencies that would result in a poor cast.

3. In accordance with the manufacturer's suggestions, soak the impression in the recommended solution, such as 2% potassium sulfate, for the recommended period of time (Fig. 1-45).

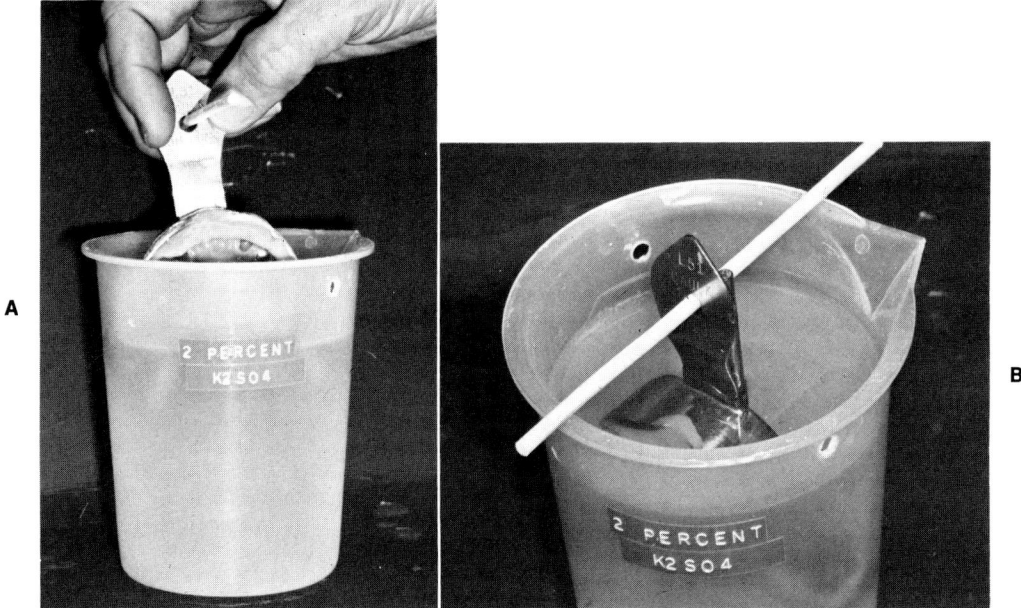

Fig. 1-45. A, Reversible hydrocolloid impression is soaked in 2% potassium sulfate solution prior to pouring. B, Stick or instrument can be placed through hole in tray to suspend it in solution.

**24**  *Dental laboratory procedures: removable partial dentures*

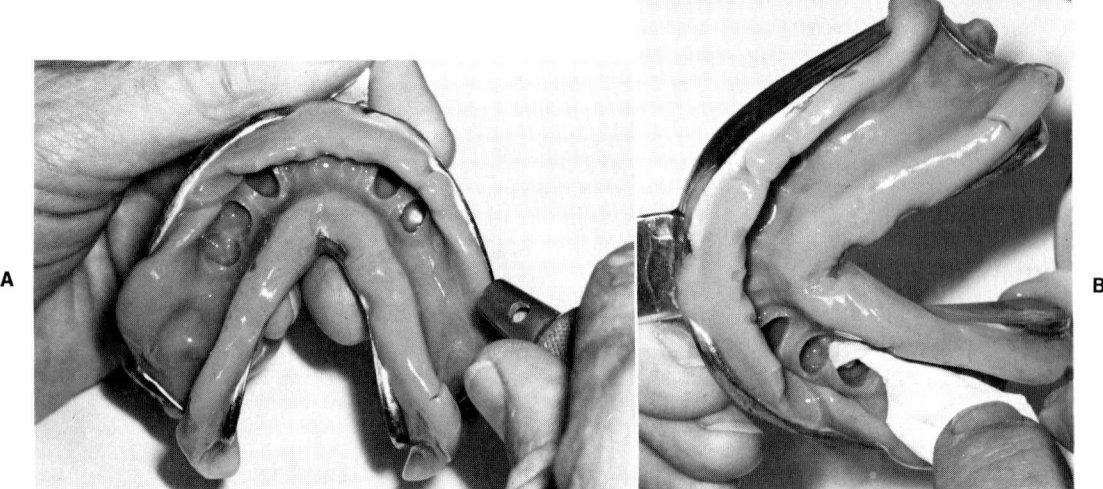

**Fig. 1-46. A,** Excess solution is removed from impression with stream of air. **B,** Strip of absorbent tissue can aid in removing moisture.

4. Remove excess moisture from the impression with a gentle stream of air (Fig. 1-46). Do not use a strong blast of air, since the impression may be separated from the tray. Moisture accumulation in tooth indentations may be removed with absorbent tissue or an air syringe.

## Pouring the stone

As with alginate impressions, there is much more to pouring a cast than just vibrating an arbitrary mix of stone into it. Following exact procedures can greatly improve the accuracy and surface characteristics of the cast.

### PROCEDURE

1. Proportion the stone as previously discussed, and mix the stone in a mechanical spatulator under reduced atmospheric pressure (Fig. 1-47).

2. Use the two-stage pouring technique, and pour the anatomical portion of the impression as previously described for alginate impressions.

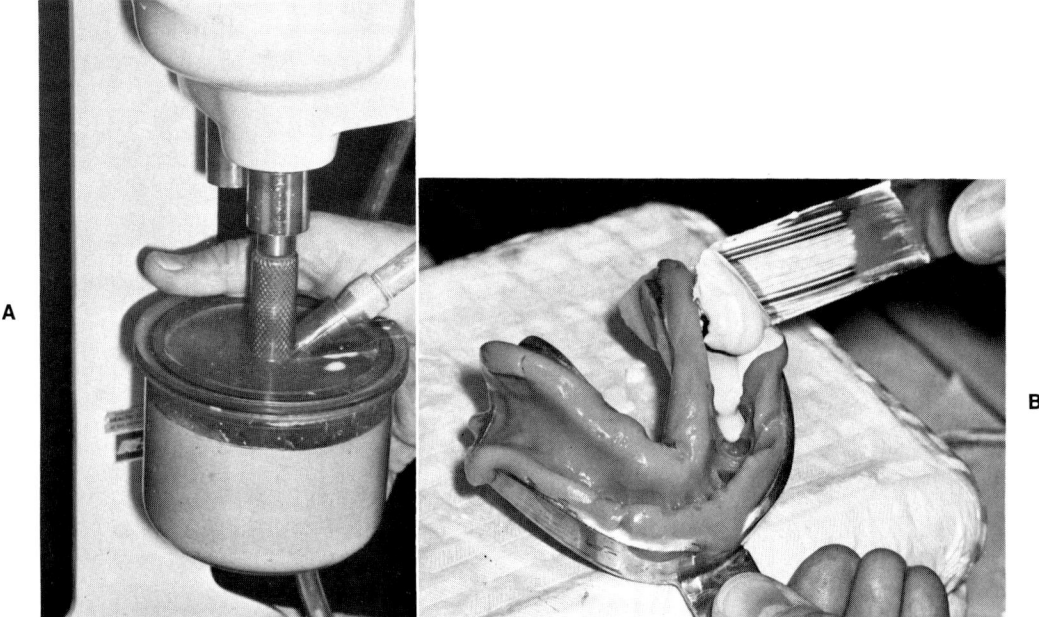

**Fig. 1-47.** Stone is mixed in mechanical spatulator **(A)** and vibrated into impression **(B)**.

# Care of impressions and making casts

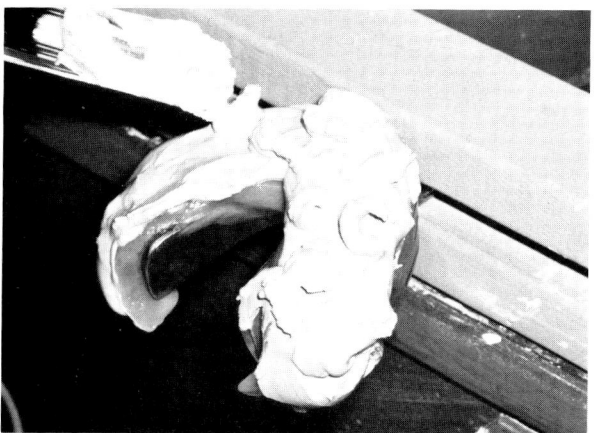

Fig. 1-48. Undercuts are created on stone surface.

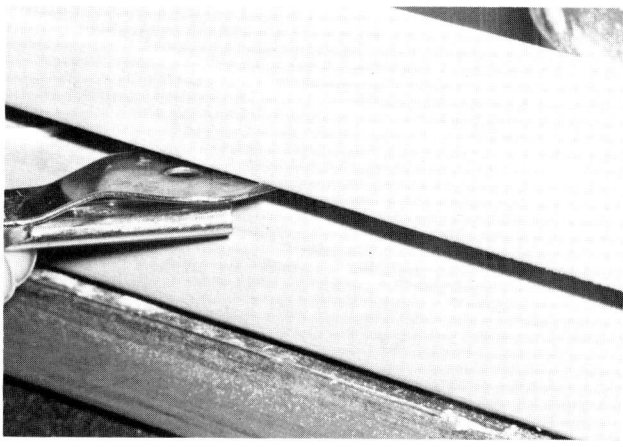

Fig. 1-49. Tray holder for water-cooled trays must be wider to accommodate tube attachment.

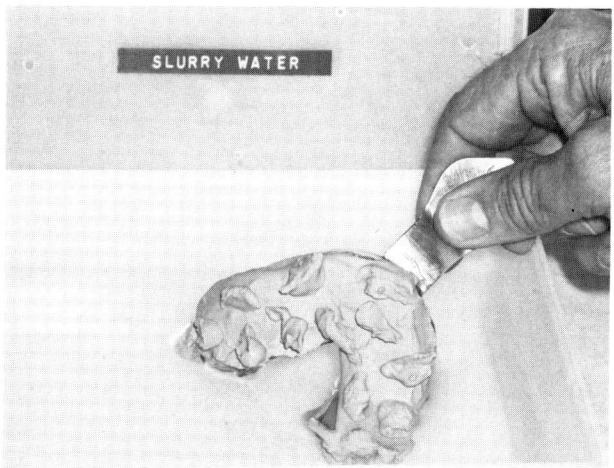

Fig. 1-50. Impression and first pour are soaked in clear slurry water for 3 to 5 minutes.

3. Build rough areas with undercuts on the upper surface of the stone of the first stage (Fig. 1-48).

4. Suspend the poured impression in a tray holder to prevent contact of any hydrocolloid with the bench top (Fig. 1-49).

5. After the first pour has set and the heat of crystallization is beginning to cool, place the impression with the stone in clear slurry water for 3 to 5 minutes (Fig. 1-50).

6. Make a mix of stone using the same water-powder ratio as before, add the stone to the first stage, and pour the base as previously described for alginate impressions (Fig. 1-51).

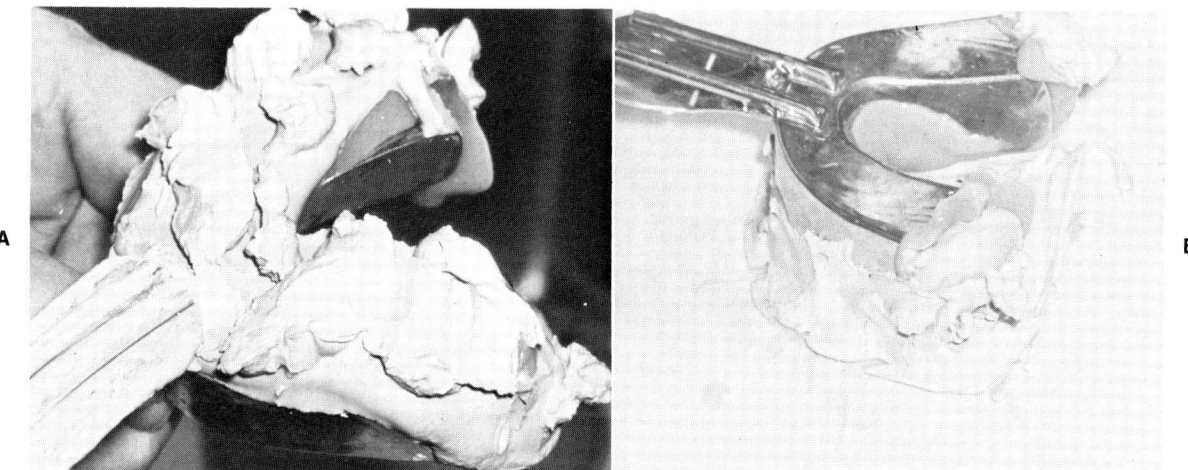

Fig. 1-51. Base of cast is poured. **A,** Add stone mix to bottom of first pour with spatula. **B,** Invert it on patty of stone and pull stone around edges with spatula.

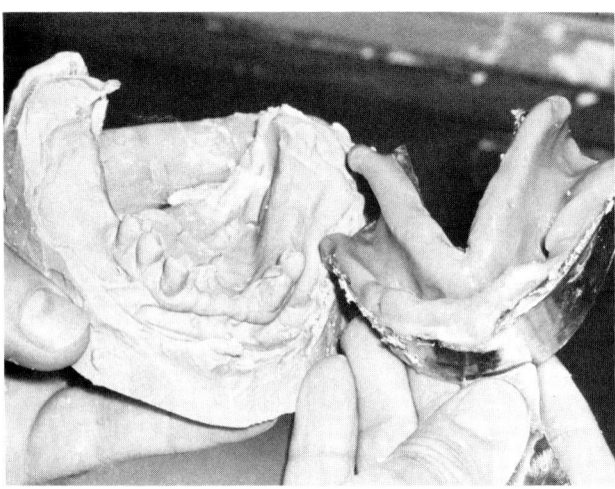

Fig. 1-52. Cast and impression are separated 45 minutes to 1 hour after first pour.

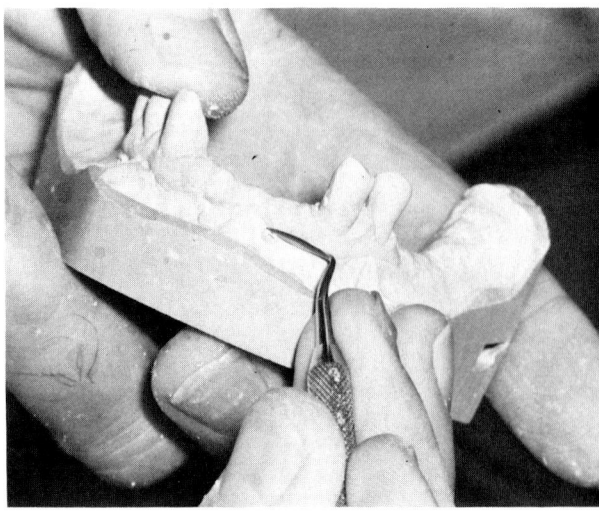

Fig. 1-53. Nodules on cast are removed with sharp instrument.

7. Separate the impression from the cast 45 minutes to 1 hour after pouring the first stage (Fig. 1-52).

8. After separating the cast from the impression, do not touch the cast for at least 12 hours, then trim as previously described for alginate impressions.

9. Examine the cast critically to determine its acceptability, and remove any nodules with a sharp instrument such as a dental explorer (Fig. 1-53).

10. Permit the cast to dry, and identify it with an indelible pencil.

### PROBLEM AREAS

Principal problem areas associated with pouring irreversible hydrocolloid impressions are the same as those for alginate impressions. Careful adherence to the suggested procedures will result in minimal problems and quality casts.

## ELASTOMERIC IMPRESSIONS

Since elastomeric impression materials are rubberlike when they set, they should be boxed before they are poured. However, the casts will be more accurate if they are poured as soon as they are removed from the mouth. Impressions made from these materials are subject to pressure distortion as well as distortion from the release of strains and the continuation of the vulcanizing process. Some of these materials are easily displaced by saliva as the impression is being made, so they have a tendency to contain more voids than hydrocolloid impressions.

### Care of the impression
#### PROCEDURE

1. Examine the impression critically to determine its acceptability.

2. Trim the excess material with scissors or a very sharp knife.

3. Suspend the handle of the tray in a holder as described for alginate impressions. The rubberlike consistency of the impression material may lull the operator into thinking that the material is impervious to distortion. However, these materials are subject to pressure distortion, as are the hydrocolloid materials, and should not be permitted to touch the bench or the vibrator.

4. Dry the impression so the wax used in boxing will stick to it better (Fig. 1-54).

5. Fill in the tongue space of the lower impression with baseplate wax (Fig. 1-55).

6. Adapt beading wax or othodontic wax around the periphery of the impression, and seal it in place (Fig. 1-56). The wax should be approximately 4 mm wide and 3 to 4 mm below the peripheral roll of the impression (Fig. 1-57).

7. Level the impression on the workbench by using balls of wax or Plasticine (Fig. 1-58).

8. Notching the boxing wax makes it easier to adapt to the beading (Fig. 1-59).

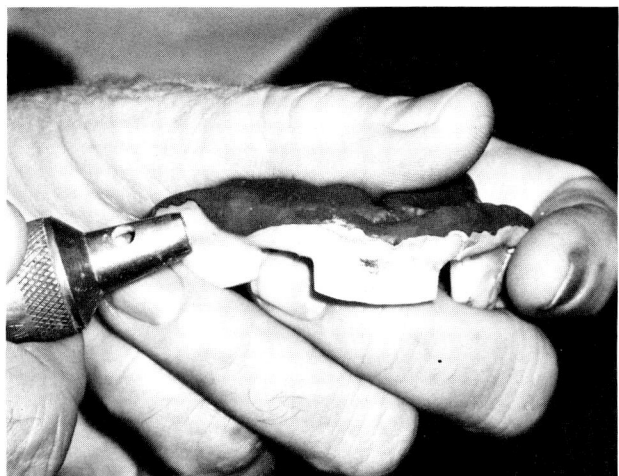

**Fig. 1-54.** Elastomeric impression should be thoroughly dry so wax will stick to it.

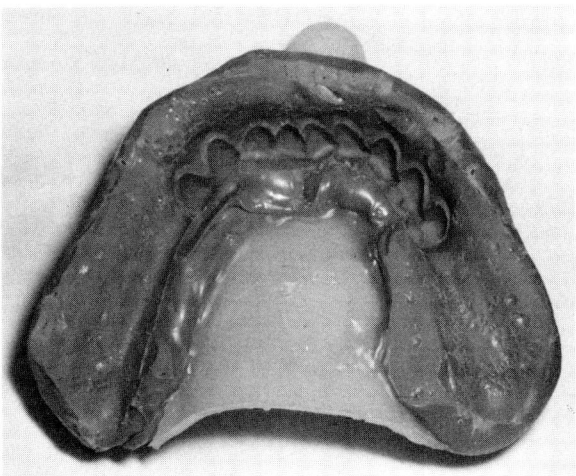

**Fig. 1-55.** Pink baseplate wax is sealed into tongue space of lower impression.

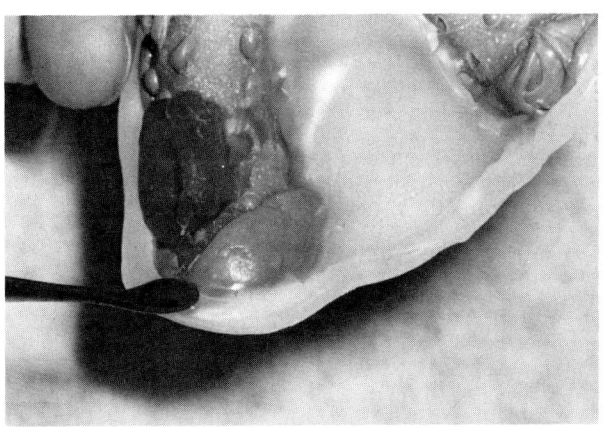

**Fig. 1-56.** Round or square beading wax is sealed to periphery of impression.

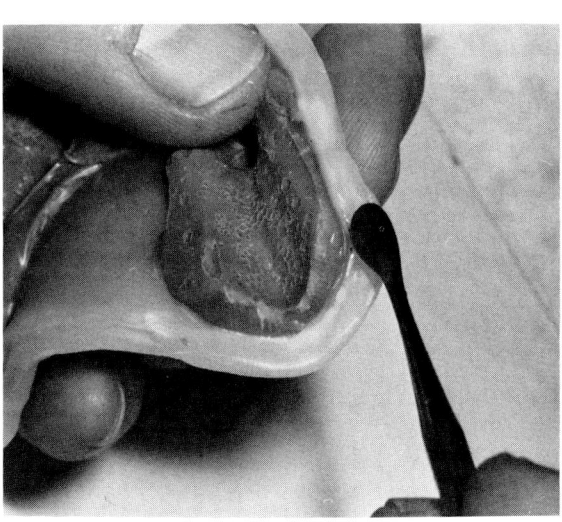

**Fig. 1-57.** Beading wax should be 4 mm wide and 3 to 4 mm below peripheral border.

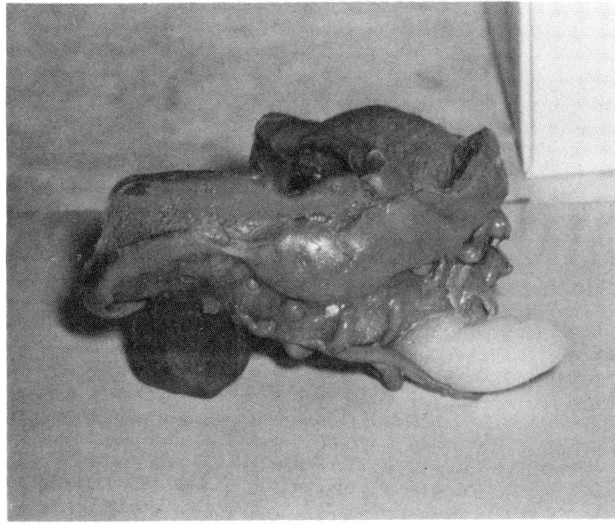

**Fig. 1-58.** Occlusal plane of teeth and ridges in impression are made parallel with bench top by supporting impression with wax or Plasticine.

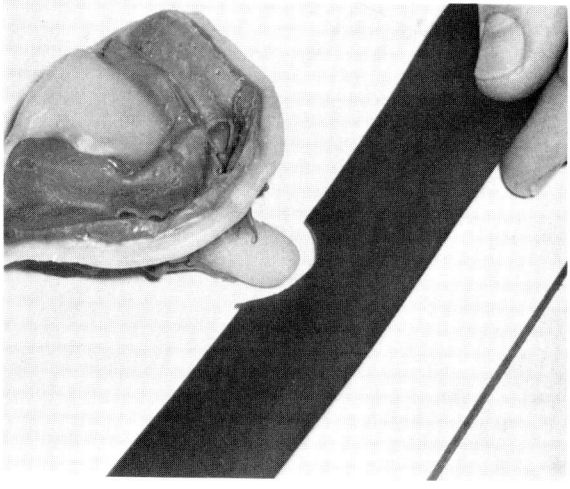

**Fig. 1-59.** Notch in boxing wax facilitates placing it over handle of tray.

9. Carefully wrap the boxing wax around the impression and wax beading, using the bench top as a guide (Fig. 1-60). Handle the impression carefully, so it is not distorted due to excessive pressure.

10. Seal the boxing wax to the beading wax with a hot spatula (Fig. 1-61).

11. Make sure that the boxing is watertight, and vibrate a stone mix into the dry impression to form the cast (Fig. 1-62). It may be advisable to use a small amount of surface tension–reducing agent before pouring the cast.

12. Separate the cast from the impression in 1 hour.

13. Lay the cast aside; do not trim it for at least 12 hours.

14. Remove nodules on the cast with a sharp instrument, and the cast is ready for surveying (Fig. 1-63).

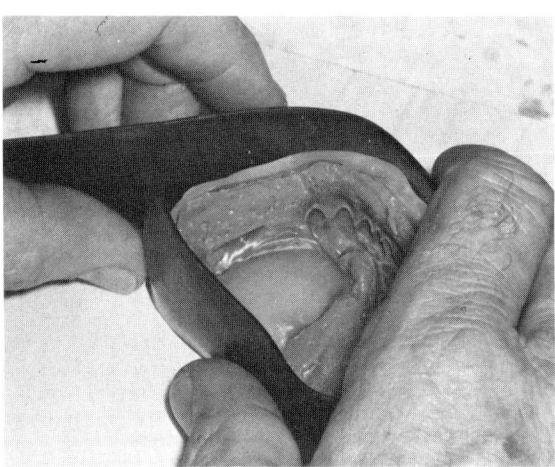

**Fig. 1-60.** Impression is wrapped with boxing wax and sealed in place. Do not distort impression by using too much pressure.

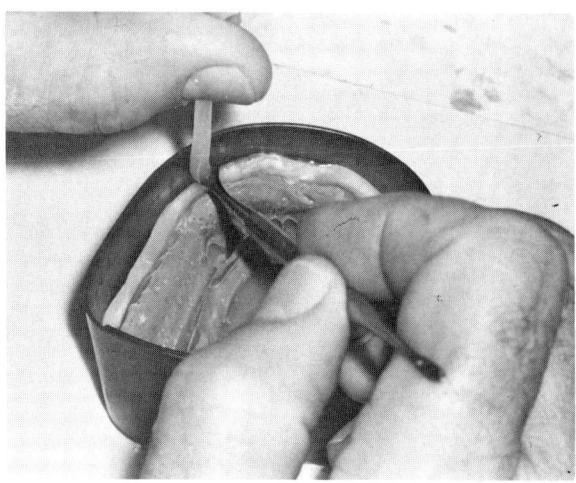

**Fig. 1-61.** Boxing wax is sealed watertight.

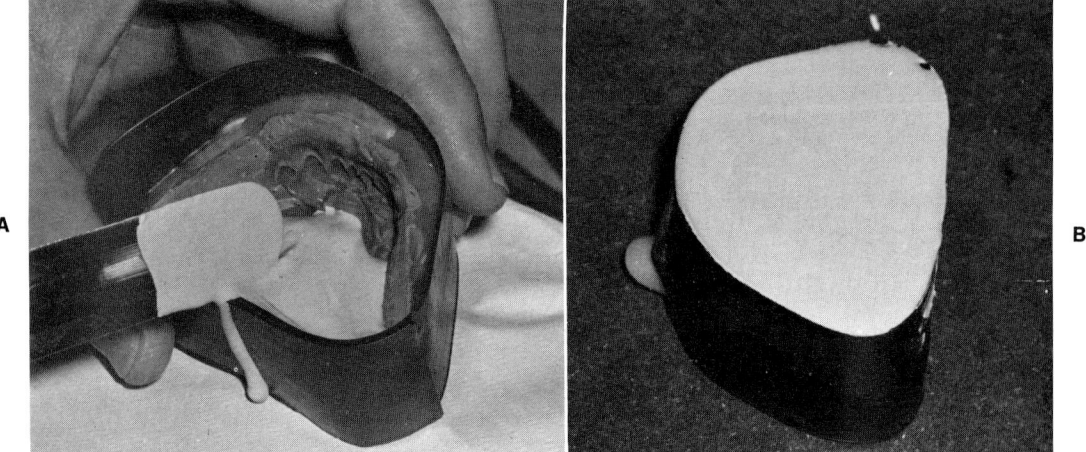

**Fig. 1-62. A,** Mix of stone is vibrated into boxed impression using care to avoid entrapment of air. **B,** Mold filled. Use of surface wetting agent (debubblizer) may help to eliminate voids.

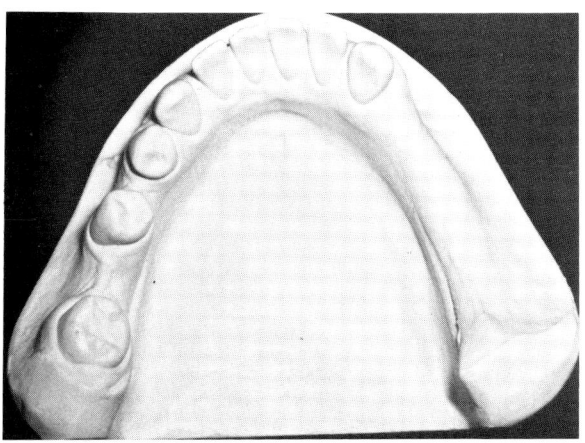

**Fig. 1-63.** Trimmed nodule-free cast ready for surveying.

## SUMMARY

Methods for pouring alginate irreversible hydrocolloid, agar reversible hydrocolloid, and elastomeric impressions, and construction of the casts were described in this chapter. Excellent casts can be obtained with these impression materials. Alginate, despite its relatively easy technique, can be easily abused. To assure the best results, it is important to follow the procedure outlined, which is known to be effective for producing superior casts. This detailed procedure is extremely important, since the cast is the first step in obtaining a successful prosthesis.

## REFERENCES

Rudd, K. D., Morrow, R. M., Brown, C. E., et al.: Comparison of effects of tap water and slurry water on gypsum casts, J. Prosthet. Dent. **24**:563-570, Nov., 1970.

Young, J. M.: Surface characteristics of dental stone: impression orientation, J. Prosthet. Dent. **33**(3):336-341, 1975.

# CHAPTER 2

# POURING CORRECTED CAST IMPRESSIONS

WILLIAM A. KUEBKER, JAMES A. FOWLER, Jr., and LOWELL Y. C. PARK

**corrected (altered) cast** A cast made from a master cast on which the residual ridges have been recorded by means of a functional impression technique.

**functional (corrected) impression** A secondary impression that is made for the purposes of recording the residual ridges in their functional form and recording the optimum length and width of the flanges of the denture bases.

A functional impression is generally made by adding an impression base to the removable partial denture framework. Usually, the functional impression is made for a distal extension base, whereas the master cast is adequate for most tooth-supported edentulous areas. A variety of impression materials is used for making functional impressions.

The laboratory procedure involves making a corrected, or altered, cast. Ridge areas that have been recorded in the functional impression are removed from the cast. The framework is seated on the cast, and new ridge areas are poured in dental stone. There are four techniques for pouring corrected cast impressions: boxing with a plaster/pumice mix and wax, beading and boxing with wax, beading with wax and the two-stage pour, and the North Carolina technique.

## BOXING CORRECTED CAST IMPRESSION WITH PLASTER/PUMICE MIX AND WAX

Boxing with a plaster/pumice mix and wax works well with a corrected cast impression made with rubber base or elastomeric impression materials.

### PROCEDURE

1. A rubber base corrected cast impression is received in the laboratory. Use a sharp knife to trim away the excess impression material (Fig. 2-1).
2. Outline the master cast for removal of the ridge areas (Fig. 2-2).
3. Remove the residual ridge areas from the master cast, and cut retention areas into the cast (Fig. 2-3).
4. Place the framework with its impression on the master cast, and lute it (Fig. 2-4).

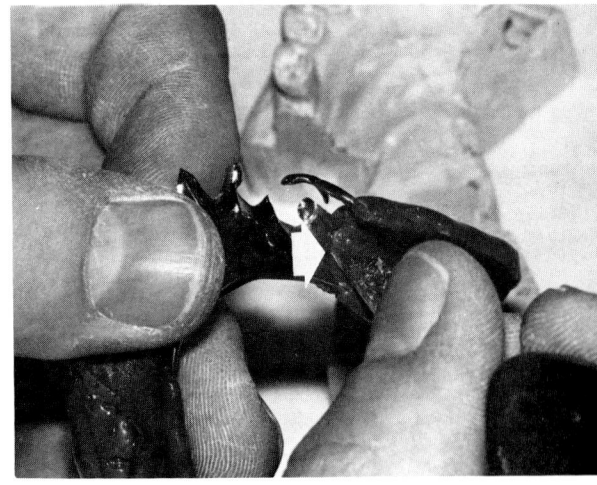

**Fig. 2-1.** Sharp knife is used to trim rubber base impression material that has flowed onto major and minor connector areas of framework.

**Fig. 2-2.** Pencil is used to outline residual ridge areas for removal by drawing line approximately 1 mm distal to abutment tooth and running from outer edge of cast (bottom arrow), crossing ridge to point approximately 5 mm lingual to ridge. Line is then extended distally paralleling residual ridge area (top arrow) and continuing to posterior border of cast.

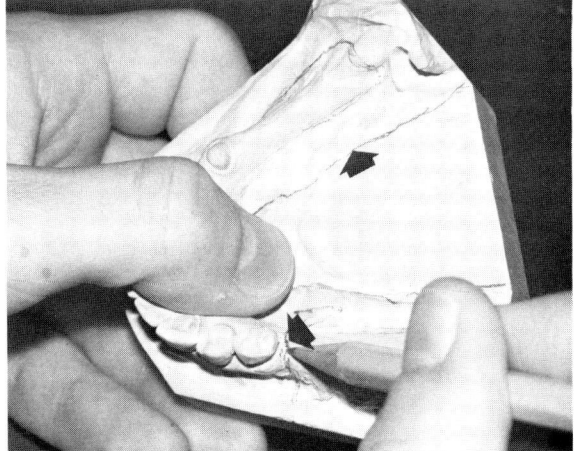

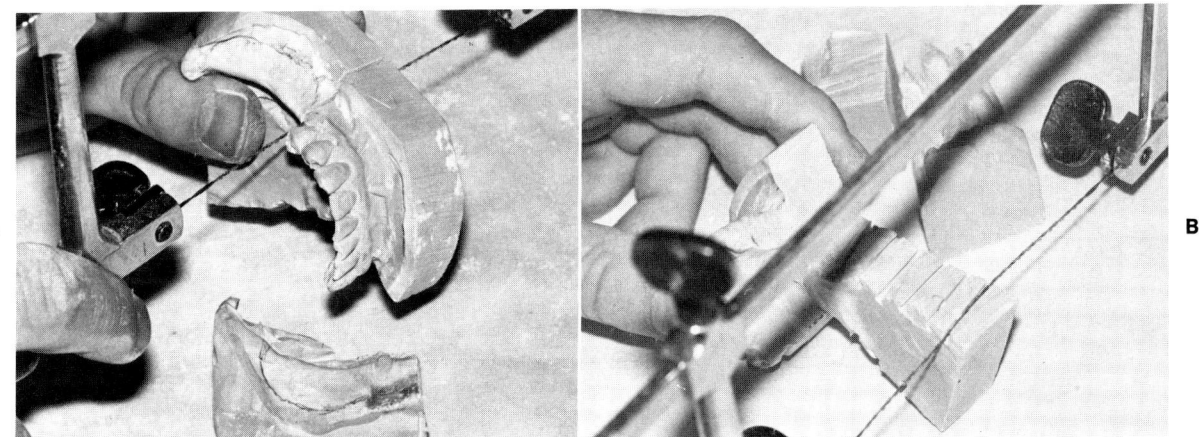

**Fig. 2-3. A,** Round spiral plaster saw blade is used to remove residual ridge areas by following lines that were placed on cast. **B,** Same saw is used to create retentive dovetails in cast.

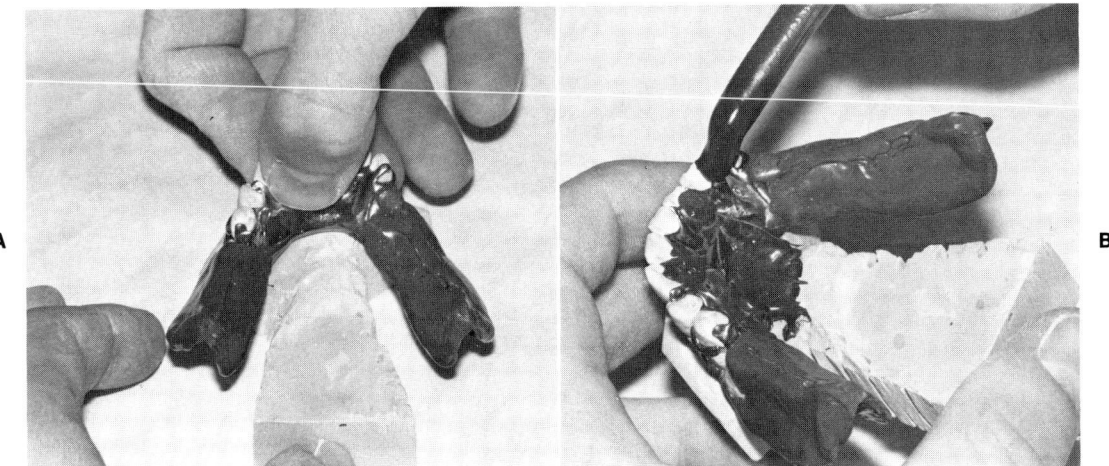

**Fig. 2-4. A,** Framework is seated on master cast and inspected to make certain that rests are completely seated. Functional impression must not contact cast. **B,** Framework is securely luted to cast using modeling plastic or sticky wax. This step is critical in preventing movement of framework during boxing and pouring procedures.

5. Soak the cast and framework in clear slurry water, and place it into a patty of a plaster/pumice mixture.* Form this mixture around the impression (Fig. 2-5).

6. After the plaster/pumice mixture has set, shape it to the outline of the cast. Paint the plaster/pumice area with a stone separating medium† (Fig. 2-6).

7. Use a strip of boxing wax to complete the boxing of the impression (Fig. 2-7).

8. Soak the boxed impression in clear slurry water for 5 minutes in preparation for pouring (Fig. 2-8).

9. Pour the boxed impression in improved stone* (Fig. 2-9).

---

*Laboratory Plaster, Whip-Mix Corp., Louisville, Ky., or equivalent.
†Super-Sep Separating Fluid, Kerr Manufacturing Co., Romulus, Mich.

*Vel Mix, Kerr Manufacturing Co., Romulus, Mich.

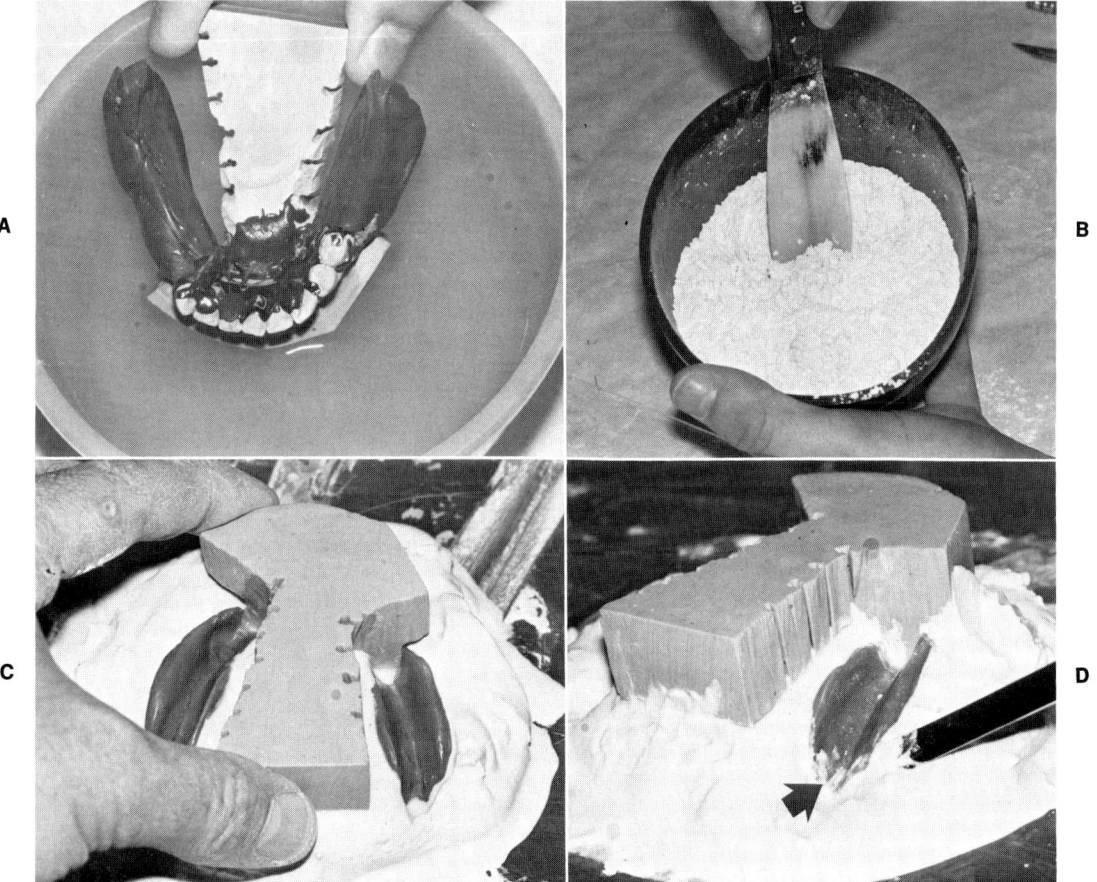

Fig. 2-5. **A,** Cast and impression are placed in clear slurry water to soak for 5 minutes. **B,** During soaking period, mixture of 50% laboratory plaster and 50% laboratory pumice is placed in rubber bowl. **C,** Powder is mixed with water to make rather heavy mixture, which is placed on glass slab. Impression and cast are placed into plaster/pumice mix. **D,** Cement spatula is used to shape plaster/pumice mix so as to close space between lingual roll of impression and tongue space area of cast. Same instrument is used to expose 2 to 3 mm of buccal roll of impression. Thin film of mixture that invariably gets on tissue surface of impression is easily removed with damp cotton or gauze after plaster has reached its final set. Special care is needed to prevent mixture from flowing onto tissue surface of impression in retromolar pad area.

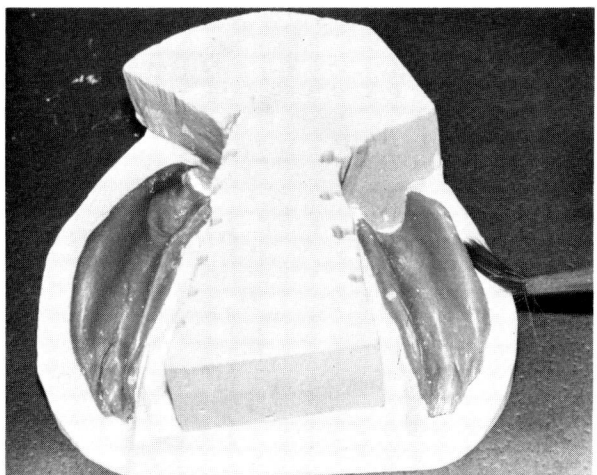

**Fig. 2-6.** Laboratory knife or cast trimmer is used to shape set plaster/pumice mixture to outline of cast. Stone separating medium is painted on all plaster/pumice surfaces that will be contacted by poured dental stone.

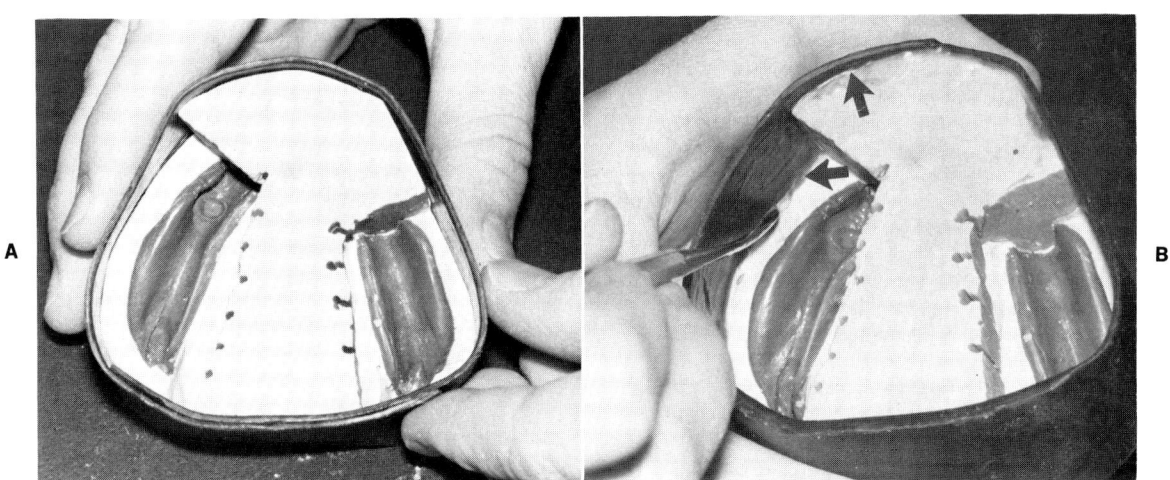

**Fig. 2-7. A,** Strip of boxing wax is adapted around cast and plaster/pumice mixture. **B,** Hot No. 7 spatula is used to seal wax to both cast and plaster/pumice mixture. This sealing should make boxed impression watertight.

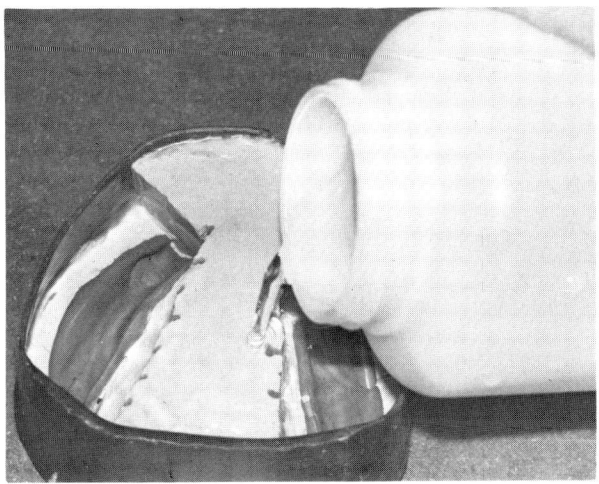

**Fig. 2-8.** Clear slurry water is poured into boxed impression and allowed to remain for 5 minutes to thoroughly wet cast. Water will also verify seal of boxed impression. Common problem associated with incomplete seal is flow of poured stone onto teeth of cast.

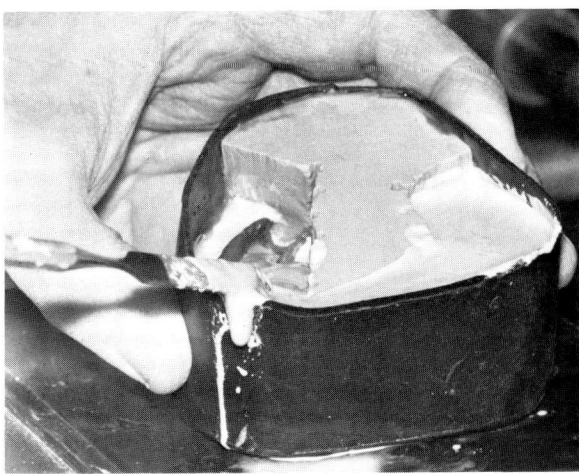

**Fig. 2-9.** Mix of properly proportioned improved stone is poured into boxed impression. Small amount of stone is added at a time to avoid entrapment of air and to allow stone to flow into retention areas of original cast.

**34** *Dental laboratory procedures: removable partial dentures*

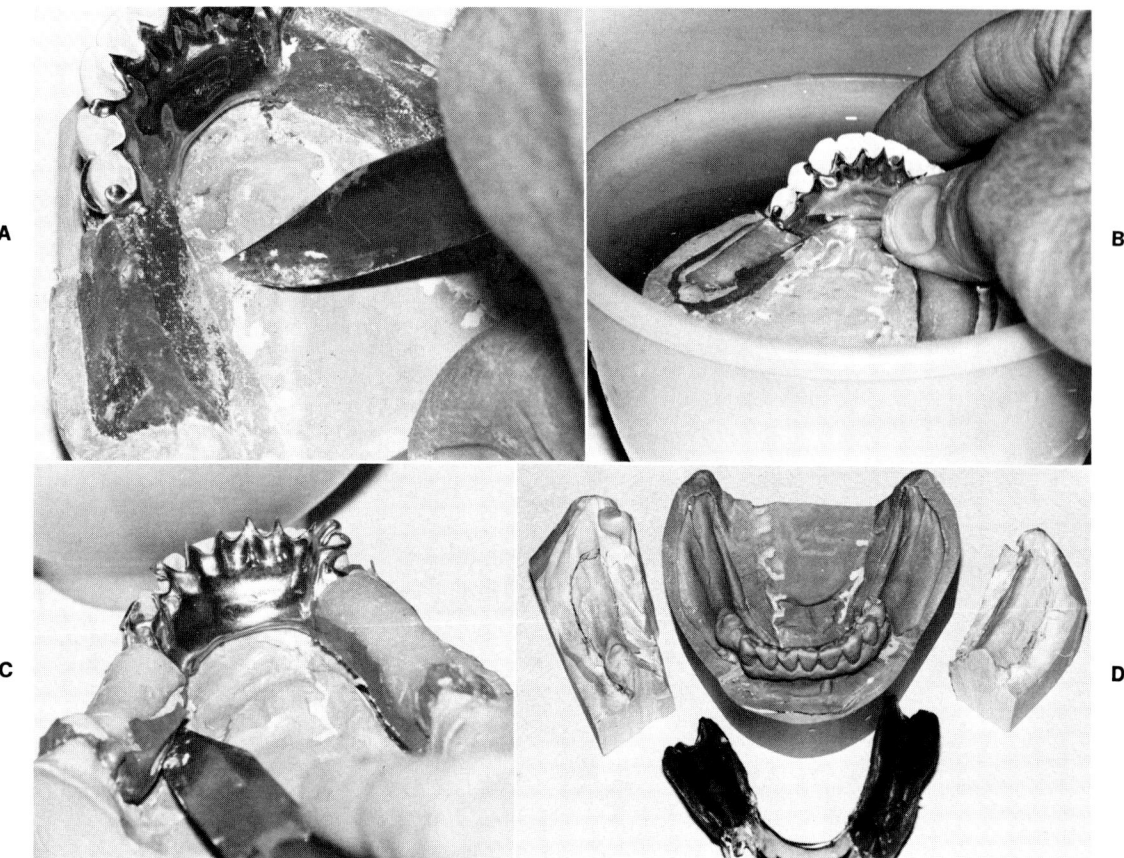

**Fig. 2-10. A,** Boxing wax is removed. Plaster/pumice mixture breaks away easily from corrected cast. Modeling plastic or sticky wax used in luting framework to cast is removed. Knife is used to remove plaster adhering to cast. **B,** Cast and framework are placed in hot water of approximately 130° to 140° F to soften modeling plastic used in border molding impression. **C,** Instrument is helpful in carefully lifting framework and impression off cast. **D,** Completed corrected cast. Next step is to remove impression material from resin bases and to burn resin off framework.

10. Remove the boxing wax and plaster/pumice mixture from the cast. Remove the framework and impression from the cast; the corrected cast is complete (Fig. 2-10).

### PROBLEM AREAS

The principal problems associated with this corrected cast procedure are related to incorrect or incomplete seating of the framework in the mouth or on the cast. These problems may occur when making the impression or when boxing the impression and pouring the cast. Other problems may occur if the proper procedures are not followed when using the plaster/pumice mix (Table 2-1).

**Table 2-1.** Boxing corrected cast impression with plaster/pumice mix

| Problem | Probable cause | Solution |
|---|---|---|
| Framework with impression does not seat completely on cast | Impression material under rest, or under minor connector, or ridge areas of cast not adequately trimmed | Remove all impression material from surfaces of framework that contact teeth; cut away entire residual ridge area of cast extending into tongue space to provide clearance for impression |
| Difficulty in removing plaster/pumice mix from cast and impression | Failure to soak cast before boxing with plaster/pumice mix | Soak cast and impression in clear slurry water for 5 minutes before boxing with plaster/pumice mix |
| | Dental stone used for pouring corrected cast sticks to plaster/pumice mix because of failure to use separating medium | Use separating medium to paint all surfaces of plaster/pumice mix that will be contacted by new dental stone |
| Difficulty in removing impression from corrected cast | Failure to heat modeling plastic used for border molding before separating | Place cast and impression in warm water (130° to 140° F; 54.5° to 60° C) for 3 to 4 minutes to soften modeling plastic |
| | Undercuts in impression tray | Remove undercuts from impression tray before border molding and making the corrected cast impression |
| | Impression tray locked into dental stone because too much of tray was exposed when boxing impression | Carry boxing material to within 2 to 3 mm of borders of impression |
| Voids in ridge areas of corrected cast | Air trapped when pouring corrected cast | Add small increments of properly proportioned and mixed dental stone; use light vibration when pouring corrected cast impression |
| New ridge areas separate from original cast | Failure to cut retention areas into cast | Prepare undercut retention areas into original cast using saw or bur |
| | Original cast dry when new stone was poured into ridge areas | Soak boxed cast and impression in clear slurry water for 5 minutes before pouring corrected cast impression |
| Completed partial denture rocks in mouth | Framework not completely seated when impression was made | Avoid overfilling tray or getting impression material under rests; seat framework with finger pressure over rests, making certain framework is completely seated |
| | Framework improperly oriented to teeth when making impression | Avoid holding impression with finger pressure over ridge areas; pressure should be over rest areas only |
| | Framework not completely seated on cast because of interference by impression material | Remove any impression material under rests or on minor connectors; cut away ridge areas of cast so that contact with impression is avoided |
| | Framework moved when pouring cast | Lute framework to cast with sticky wax or modeling plastic |

## BEADING AND BOXING CORRECTED CAST IMPRESSION WITH WAX

Beading and boxing the corrected cast impression with wax works well for zinc oxide–eugenol paste or plaster of Paris impressions.

### PROCEDURE

1. A zinc oxide–eugenol impression paste corrected cast impression is received in the laboratory. Remove all impression material that has flowed beyond the internal finish line of the framework (Fig. 2-11).

2. Cut the denture base areas off the cast, and prepare dovetailed retention grooves in the remainder of the cast (Fig. 2-12).

3. Seat the framework on the cast, and lute it (Fig. 2-13).

4. Place beading wax* 2 to 3 mm above the border of the entire periphery of the corrected cast impression. Seal the wax to the impression and to the tongue space of the cast on the lingual side (Fig. 2-14).

---

*Beading Grip Wax, The L. D. Caulk Co., Milford, Del., or equivalent.

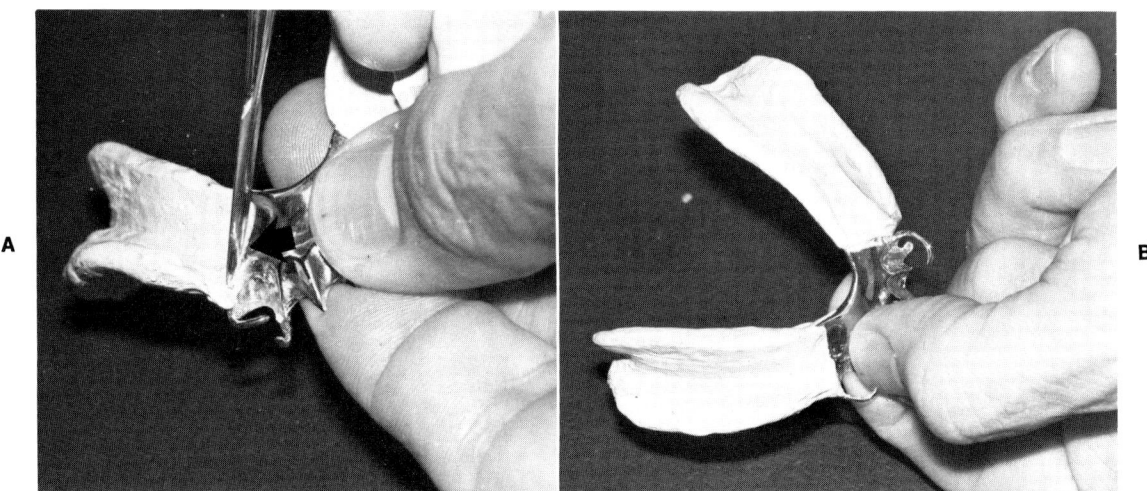

Fig. 2-11. **A,** Corrected cast impression is received in laboratory, and instrument is used to trim away impression paste that interferes with seating of framework. **B,** Impression is ready for beading and boxing.

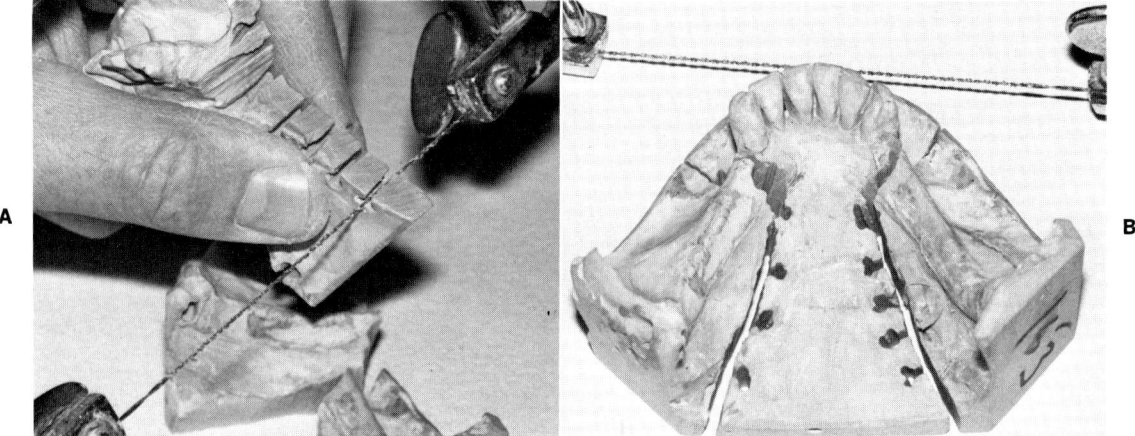

Fig. 2-12. **A,** Denture base areas of cast are cut off using plaster saw. Same instrument is used to prepare numerous dovetailed retention grooves in cast. **B,** Cast is sectioned and ready for seating of framework and impressions.

# Pouring corrected cast impressions 37

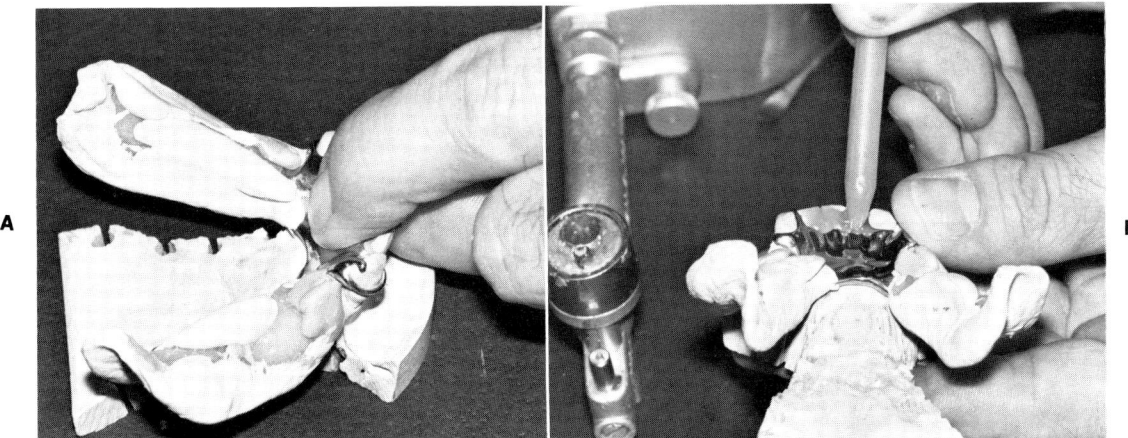

**Fig. 2-13. A,** Framework and impression are seated on cast. Areas of cast that contact impression are relieved to allow complete seating of framework. **B,** Modeling plastic or sticky wax is used to firmly lute framework to cast to prevent movement during boxing and pouring procedures.

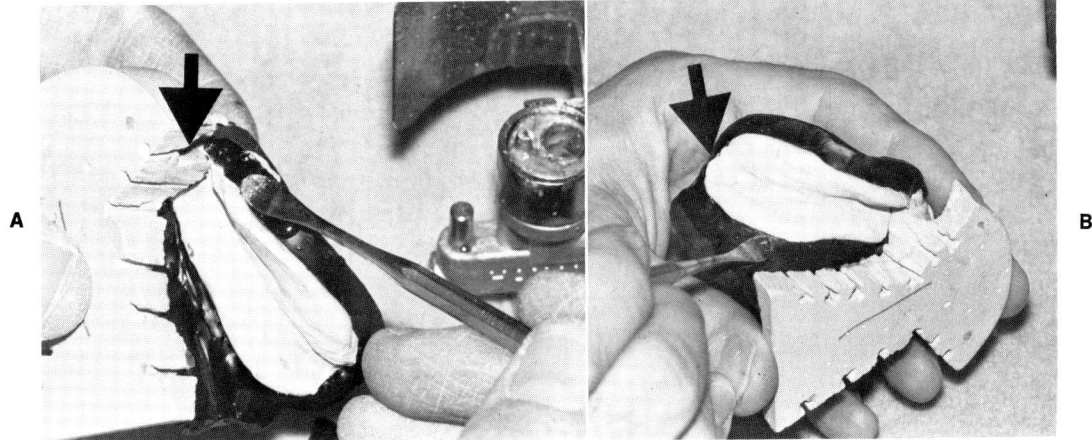

**Fig. 2-14. A,** Beading wax or white rope orthodontic wax is placed 2 to 3 mm above borders of impression. Wax is sealed to impression with hot No. 7 spatula. Care must be taken to completely seal anterior end (arrow) to prevent stone from flowing onto remaining teeth during pouring of cast. **B,** Usually more than one thickness of beading wax is needed to seal lingual aspect of beading to cast. Again, care must be taken in sealing anterior end of beading to prevent leakage. Common error is allowing beading wax to extend onto retromolar pad impression surface (arrow).

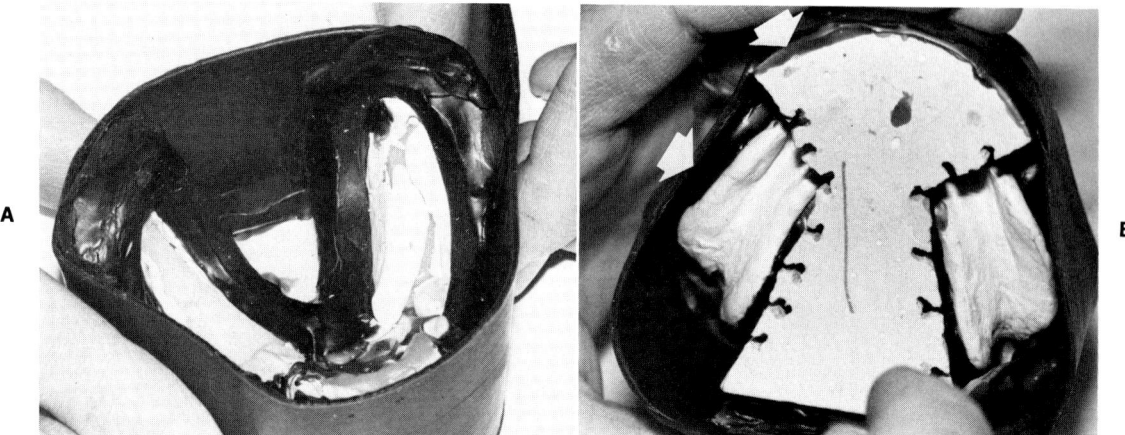

**Fig. 2-15. A,** Strip of boxing wax is adapted around cast and beaded impression bases. Care is taken to avoid excessive pressure that can displace beading wax. **B,** Hot No. 7 spatula is used to seal boxing wax to beading wax and cast (arrows). This is accomplished on both sides of beading wax. Holding boxed impression up to light or filling it with water will indicate watertightness of beading and boxing. If artificial stone used to pour impression leaks through beading and boxing, cast may be made unusable because of stone attached to remaining teeth.

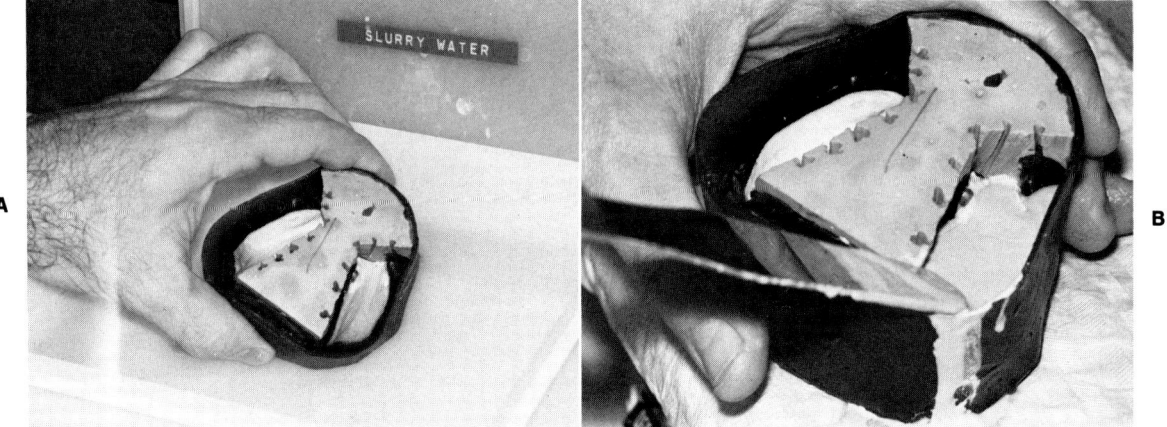

**Fig. 2-16. A,** Boxed impression is soaked in container of clear slurry water for 5 minutes. This step must be accomplished to ensure good union of new and old stone. **B,** Water is measured, and stone is weighed for mix of minimal expansion dental stone. Mixing is accomplished with mechanical vacuum mixer. Stone is added in small amounts and is lightly vibrated to allow stone to flow over impression surface and into retention grooves. Cast is allowed to set for minimum of 30 minutes.

5. Adapt a strip of boxing wax* around the beading wax and cast. Seal the wax with a hot instrument to make it watertight (Fig. 2-15).

6. Soak the boxed impression in clear slurry water for 5 minutes to saturate the original stone. Pour the corrected cast using a vacuum-mixed improved stone of a correct water-powder ratio (Fig. 2-16).

7. Remove the boxing and beading wax. Carefully remove the framework and impression from the cast to prevent breakage of the teeth or ridge areas (Fig. 2-17).

*Boxing Grip Wax, The L. D. Caulk Co., Milford, Del., or equivalent.

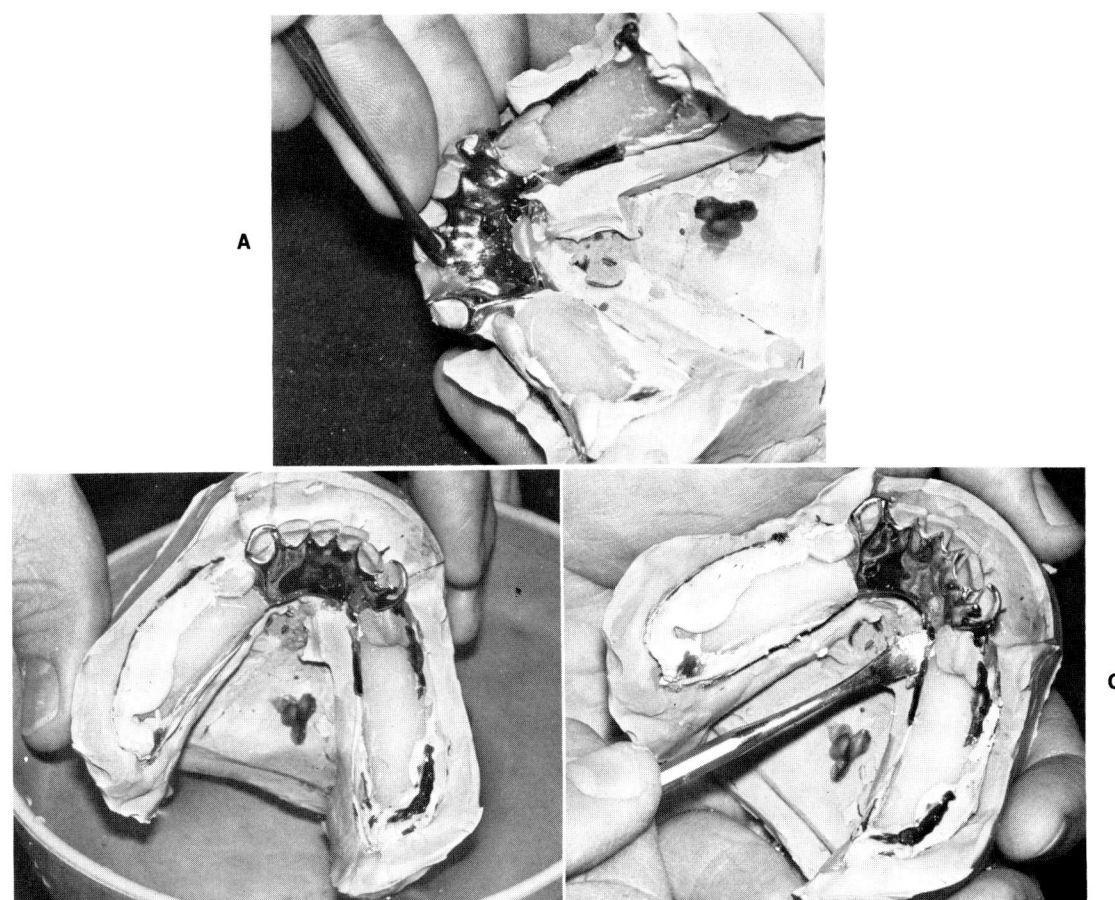

Fig. 2-17. **A**, After removal of beading and boxing wax, instrument is used to remove modeling plastic or sticky wax used for luting framework to cast. **B**, Cast is placed in hot water at 130° to 140° F for 3 to 4 minutes to soften impression material. **C**, Instrument is used to carefully lift framework and impression bases from cast. Care must be taken to avoid breakage of cast or distortion of framework.

**40** *Dental laboratory procedures: removable partial dentures*

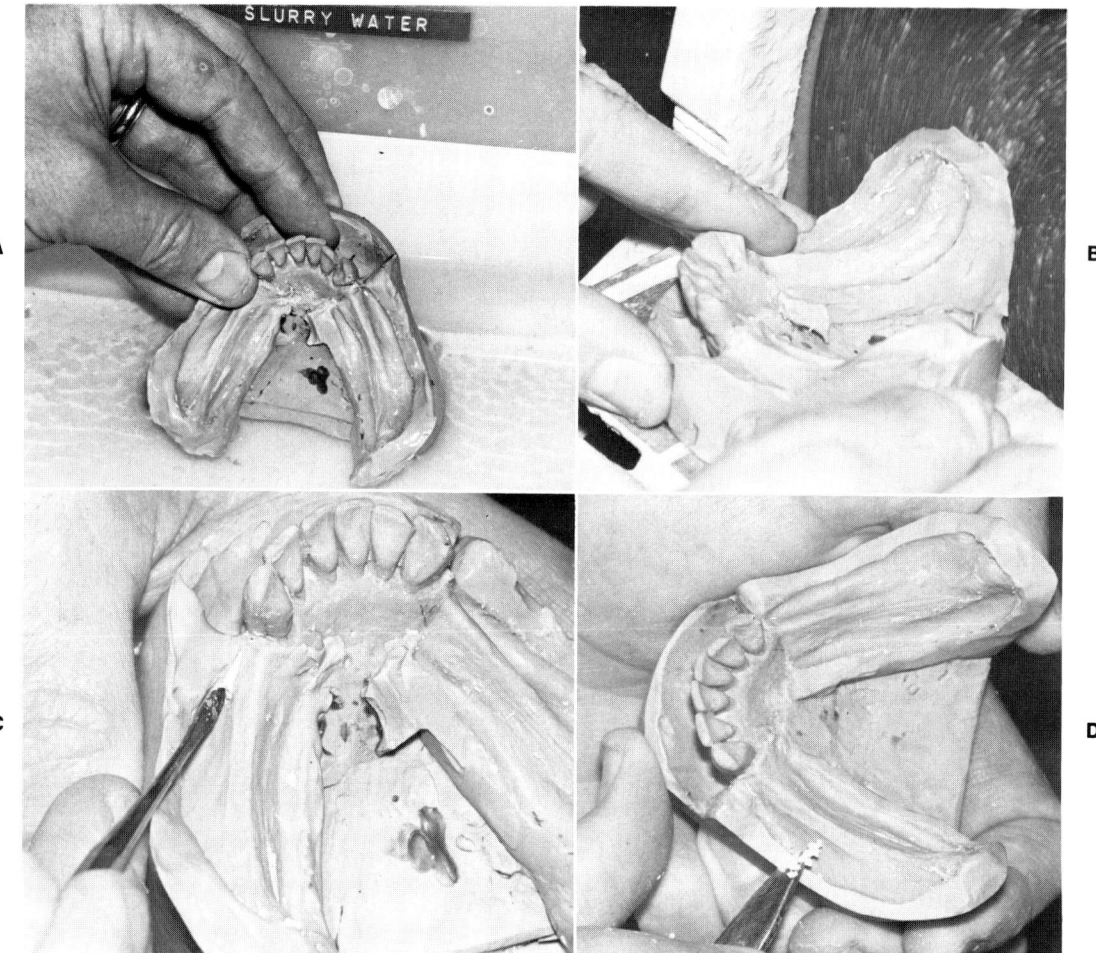

**Fig. 2-18. A,** Corrected cast is soaked in clear slurry water for 3 to 4 minutes to wet cast in preparation for trimming on model trimmer. **B,** Cast is shaped on model trimmer, taking care to preserve 3- to 4-mm land area and support for heels of cast. **C,** Instrument is used to remove impression material that remains on cast. **D,** Sharp laboratory knife is used to smooth land area.

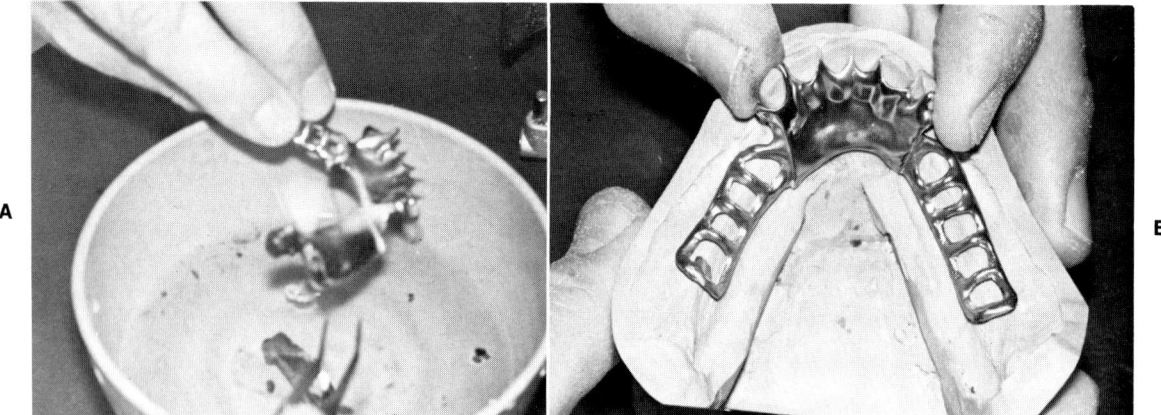

**Fig. 2-19. A,** Impression bases are cleaned of impression material and held in flame to burn off resin. When resin begins to flame, it should be placed over bowl of water. When resin has softened, it is removed from framework with instrument. **B,** Framework is polished if residue from burning resin remains on framework. Framework is seated on cast, and corrected cast procedure is complete.

8. Soak the corrected cast in clear slurry water, and shape it on a model trimmer. Use instruments to remove any impression material remaining on the cast and to smooth the land areas (Fig. 2-18).

9. Remove the resin impression bases from the framework. Seat the framework on the cast, and the corrected cast procedure is complete (Fig. 2-19).

## PROBLEM AREAS

The principal problem encountered when using this technique is failure to develop a good seal of the wax used in beading the impression, allowing dental stone to flow onto the teeth of the original cast (Table 2-2).

**Table 2-2.** Beading and boxing corrected cast impression with wax

| Problem | Probable cause | Solution |
|---|---|---|
| Dental stone on teeth of cast | Wax used for beading and boxing not completely sealed | Carefully seal beading wax around entire impression; seal boxing wax to cast and beading wax; pour clear slurry water into boxed impression to test integrity of seal |
| Framework with impression does not seat completely on cast | Impression material under rest, or under minor connector, or ridge areas of cast not adequately trimmed | Remove all impression material from surfaces of framework that contact teeth; cut away entire residual ridge area of cast extending into tongue space to provide clearance for impression |
| Difficulty in removing impression from corrected cast | Failure to heat modeling plastic used for border molding before separating | Place cast and impression in warm water (130° to 140° F; 54.5° to 60° C) for 3 to 4 minutes to soften modeling plastic |
| | Undercuts in impression tray | Remove undercuts from impression tray before border molding and making the corrected cast impression |
| | Impression tray locked into dental stone because too much of tray was exposed when boxing impression | Carry boxing material to within 2 to 3 mm of borders of impression |
| Voids in ridge areas of corrected cast | Air trapped when pouring corrected cast | Add small increments of properly proportioned and mixed dental stone; use light vibration when pouring corrected cast impression |
| New ridge areas separate from original cast | Failure to cut retention areas into cast | Prepare undercut retention areas into original cast using saw or bur |
| | Original cast dry when new stone was poured into ridge areas | Soak boxed cast and impression in clear slurry water for 5 minutes before pouring corrected cast impression |
| Completed partial denture rocks in mouth | Framework not completely seated when impression was made | Avoid overfilling tray or getting impression material under rests; seat framework with finger pressure over rests making certain framework is completely seated |
| | Framework improperly oriented to teeth when making impression | Avoid holding impression wih finger pressure over ridge areas; pressure should be over rest areas only |
| | Framework not completely seated on cast because of interference by impression material | Remove any impression material under rests or on minor connectors; cut away ridge areas of cast so that contact with impression is avoided |
| | Framework moved when pouring cast | Lute framework to cast with sticky wax or modeling plastic |

## BEADING CORRECTED CAST IMPRESSION WITH WAX AND TWO-STAGE POUR

Beading the corrected cast impression with wax and the two-stage pour procedure is similar to the wax beading and boxing procedure and can be used for metallic paste or plaster of Paris impressions.

### PROCEDURE

1. The impression is received in the laboratory and prepared for pouring (Fig. 2-20).
2. Draw lines as a guide for sectioning the cast, and cut off the ridge areas with a plaster saw (Fig. 2-21).
3. Carefully seat the framework on the sectioned cast, and securely lute it to the cast with sticky wax or modeling plastic (Fig. 2-22).
4. Use beading wax to seal the entire impression, exposing 2 to 3 mm of all the border areas (Fig. 2-23).

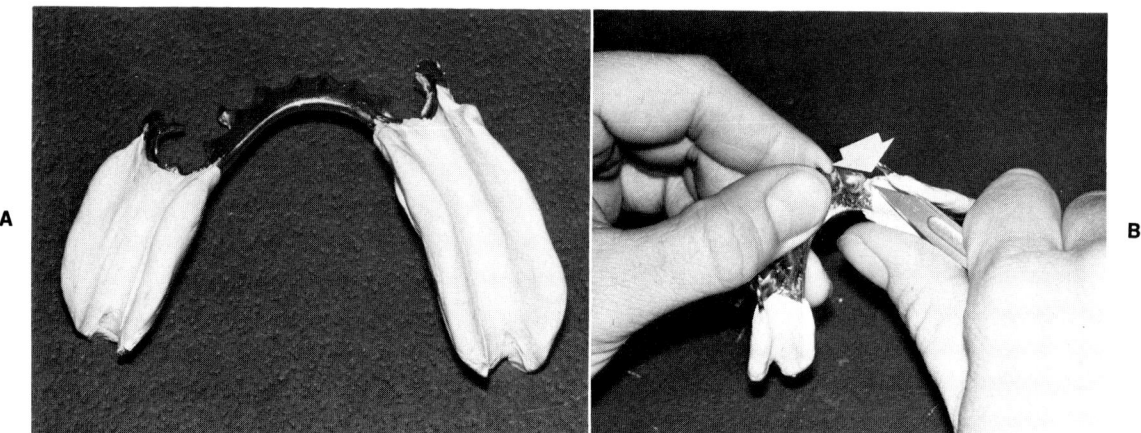

Fig. 2-20. **A,** Metallic paste–corrected cast impression is received in laboratory. **B,** Bard-Parker knife is used to trim impression material from areas of framework that contact teeth.

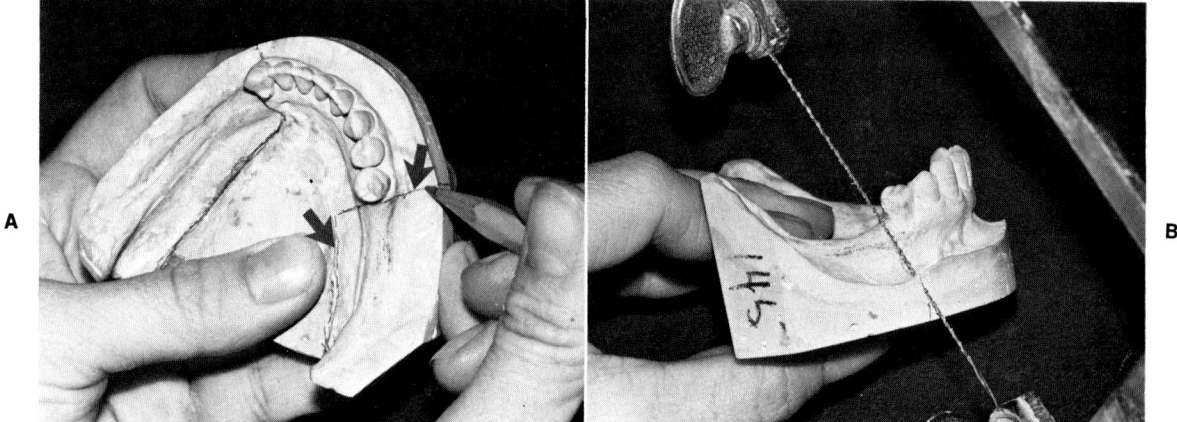

Fig. 2-21. **A,** Line is drawn approximately 1 mm distal to abutment tooth (top arrow) and is joined to line 3 to 4 mm lingual to and paralleling residual ridge (bottom arrow). **B,** Spiral plaster saw blade in saw frame is used to cut off residual ridge areas following outline penciled on cast. Retention grooves are prepared in cast.

Pouring corrected cast impressions **43**

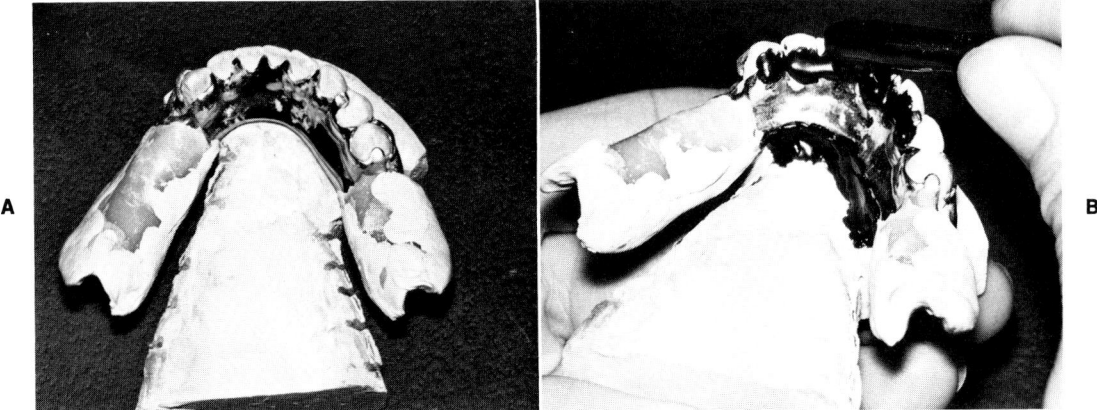

**Fig. 2-22. A,** Framework is seated on cast, making certain that it seats completely and that borders of corrected cast impression do not contact the cast. **B,** Framework is securely luted to cast with modeling plastic.

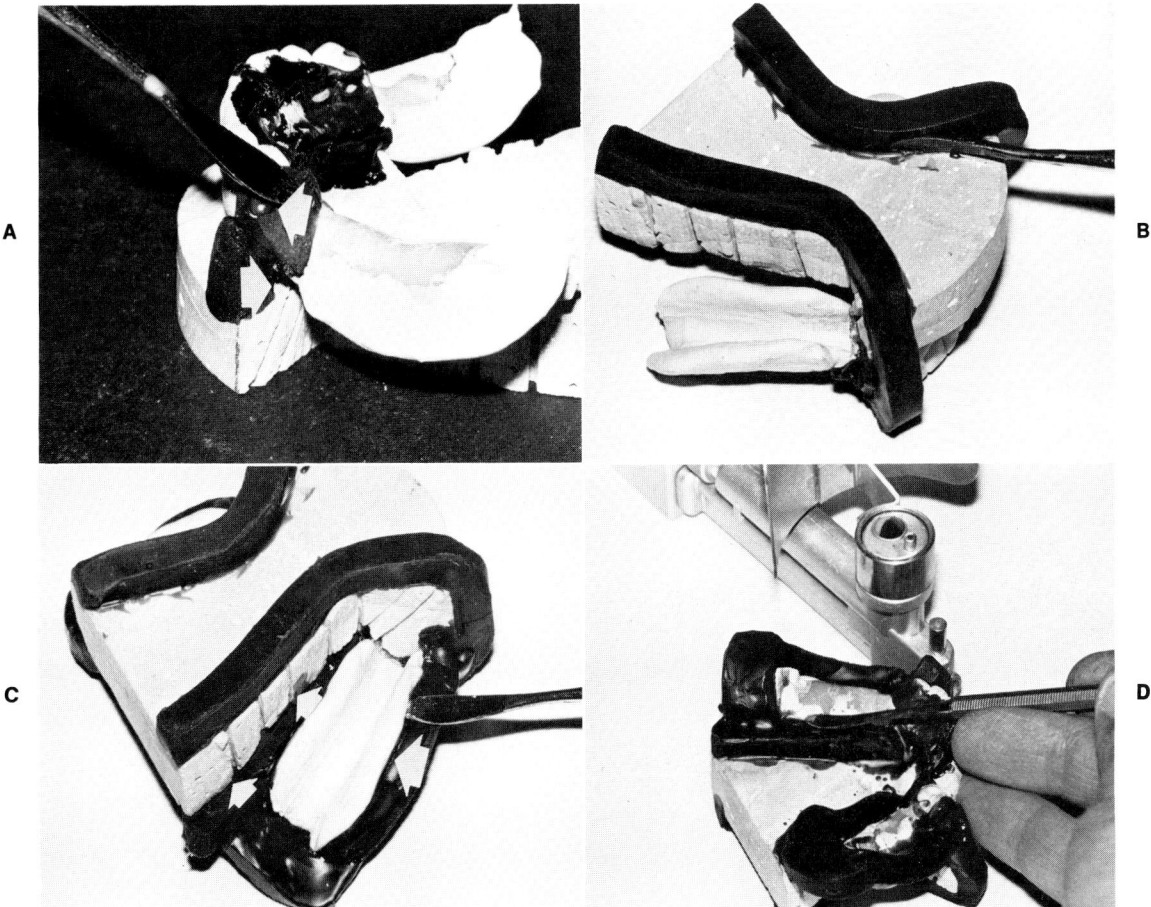

**Fig. 2-23. A,** Beading wax is used to seal anterior area of impression (arrow) and framework to cast to prevent dental stone from flowing onto teeth. **B,** Strips of beading wax are sealed to cast adjacent to cut margins. **C,** Beading wax is adapted around impression exposing 2 to 3 mm of all border areas. Wax is sealed to impression (arrow) and to tongue space (arrows) of cast. **D,** Sealing is accomplished on both sides of beading wax to prevent leakage of dental stone.

5. Soak the cast and impression in clear slurry water. Make the first pour, covering the entire impression area. Add retention for the second pour (Fig. 2-24).

6. Soak the first pour in clear slurry water. Complete the second stage of the pour by inverting the first pour into a patty of stone and shaping the cast (Fig. 2-25).

7. After the cast has reached its final set, soak it in clear slurry water, and trim it on a model trimmer (Fig. 2-26).

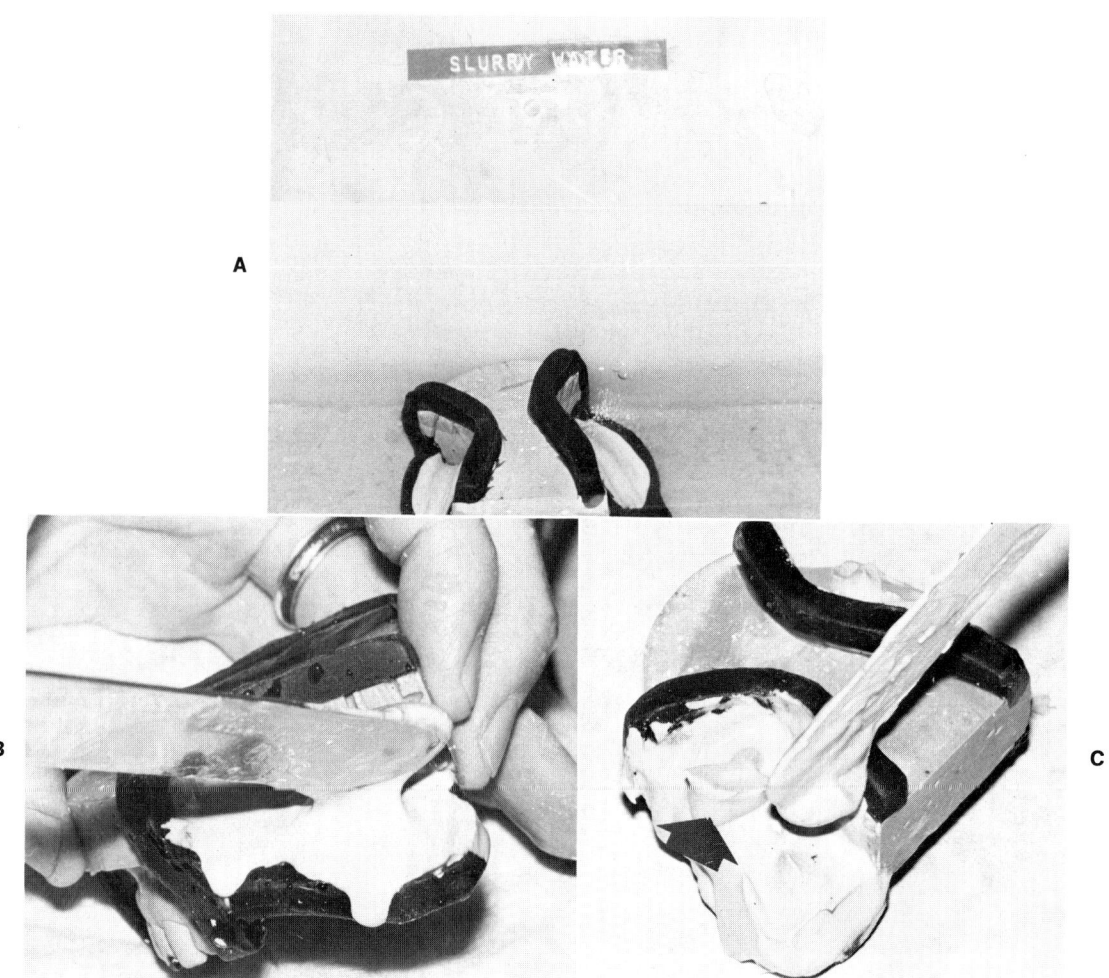

**Fig. 2-24. A,** Cast and impression are soaked in clear slurry water for 3 to 5 minutes to thoroughly wet cast. **B,** Small increments of properly proportioned and mixed improved dental stone are placed and vibrated onto surface of impression. Care is taken to cover all surfaces of impression with minimum of 3 to 4 mm of stone. **C,** Small irregular mounds of stone are added to provide retention for second pour.

## Pouring corrected cast impressions 45

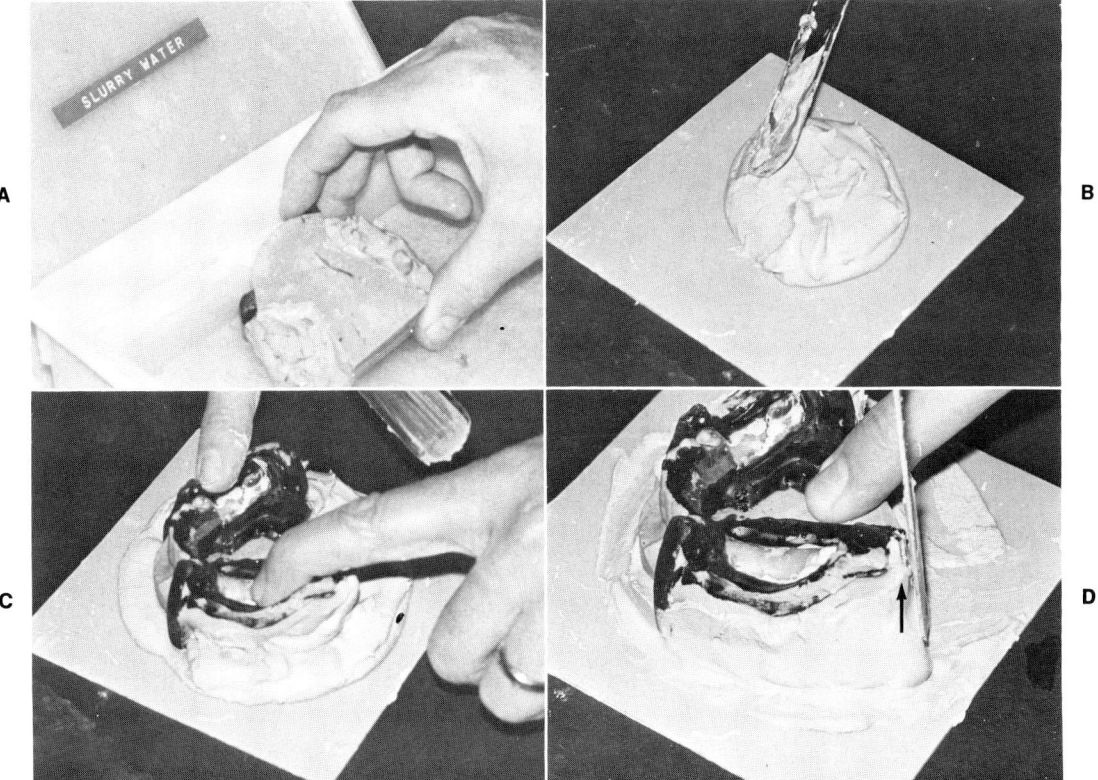

**Fig. 2-25. A,** Cast and first pour are placed in clear slurry water for 3 to 5 minutes to thoroughly wet first pour. **B,** Correctly proportioned mix of improved stone is placed on plastic or glass slab and shaped into patty approximately same size as cast. **C,** Cast and first pour are inverted and placed into patty of stone. **D,** Spatula is used to shape unset stone, making certain that adequate stone is present to support heels (arrow) of cast.

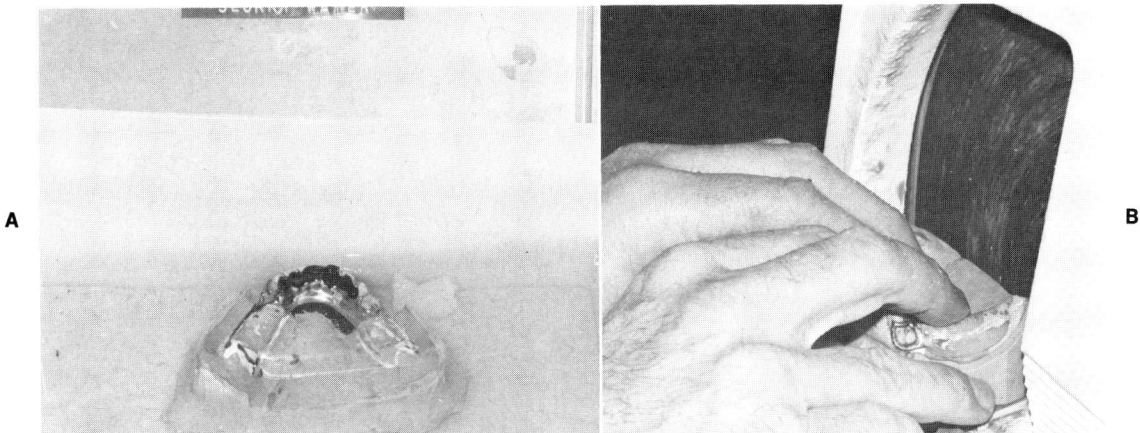

**Fig. 2-26. A,** Set cast is placed in clear slurry water for 3 to 4 minutes to thoroughly wet cast in preparation for trimming. **B,** Corrected cast is shaped on model trimmer.

8. Remove the material used for luting the framework to the cast. Remove the framework and impression from the cast after softening the impression material in warm water (Fig. 2-27).

9. Smooth the land areas and tongue space of the cast if necessary. Remove the impression material retained on the cast (Fig. 2-28).

10. Remove the impression bases from the framework (Fig. 2-29).

11. Inspect the corrected cast for obvious errors. Try the framework on the cast, and inspect it for possible distortion of the framework. The framework and corrected cast are ready for the next procedure in the construction of the prosthesis (Fig. 2-30).

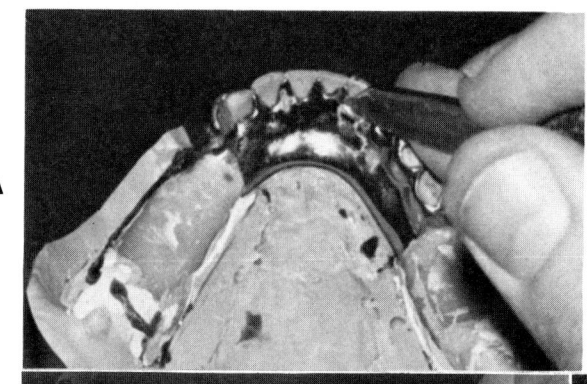
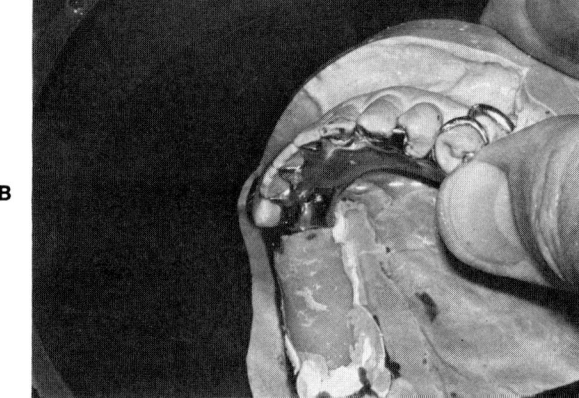
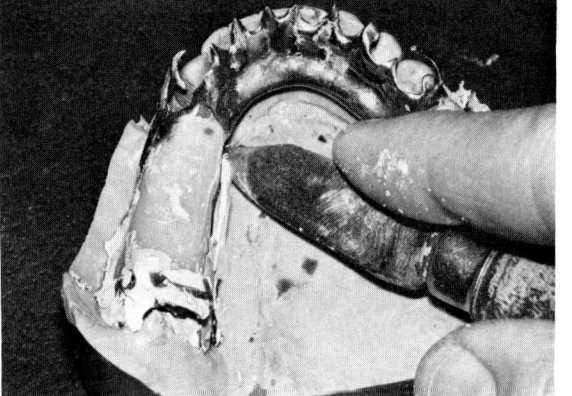

Fig. 2-27. **A,** Instrument is used to remove modeling plastic used to lute framework to cast. **B,** Cast and framework are placed in warm (130° to 140° F) water for 3 to 5 minutes to soften modeling plastic used for border molding impression. **C,** Knife is used to carefully tease framework and impression bases from cast. Care must be taken to avoid breaking teeth of cast or distorting framework.

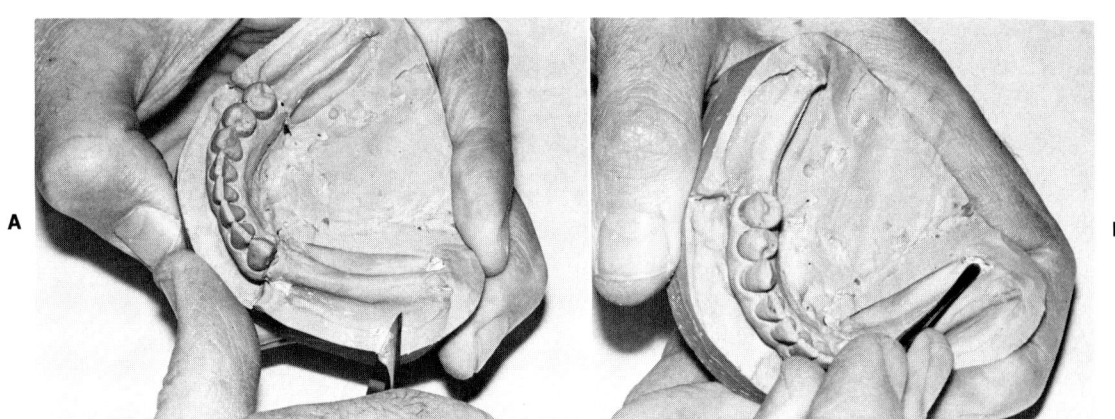

Fig. 2-28. **A,** Sharp laboratory knife is used to smooth irregularities of land areas or tongue space of cast. **B,** Blunt instrument is used to remove impression material retained on cast.

Pouring corrected cast impressions  **47**

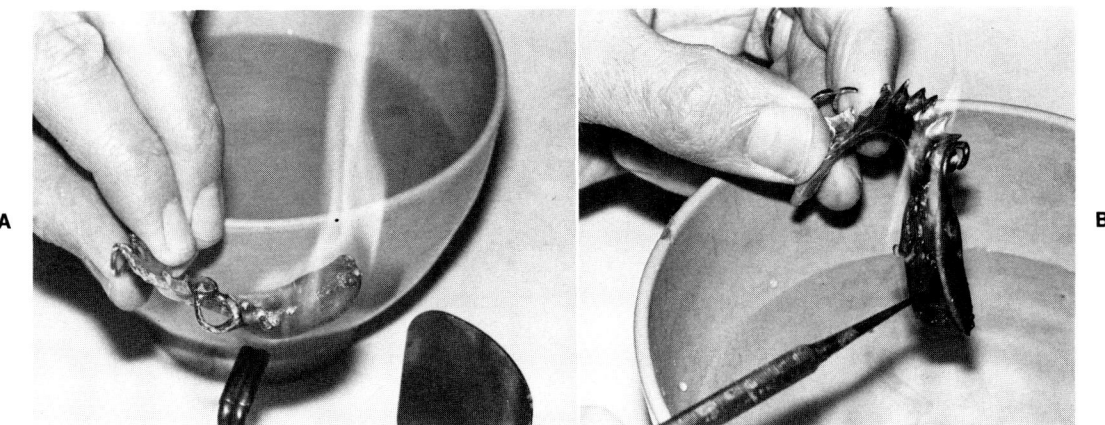

**Fig. 2-29. A,** After scraping impression material from acrylic resin impression base, the base is placed in flame to soften resin. **B,** Instrument is used to remove softened resin from framework. This should be accomplished over bowl of water as safety precaution as resin flames during softening procedure.

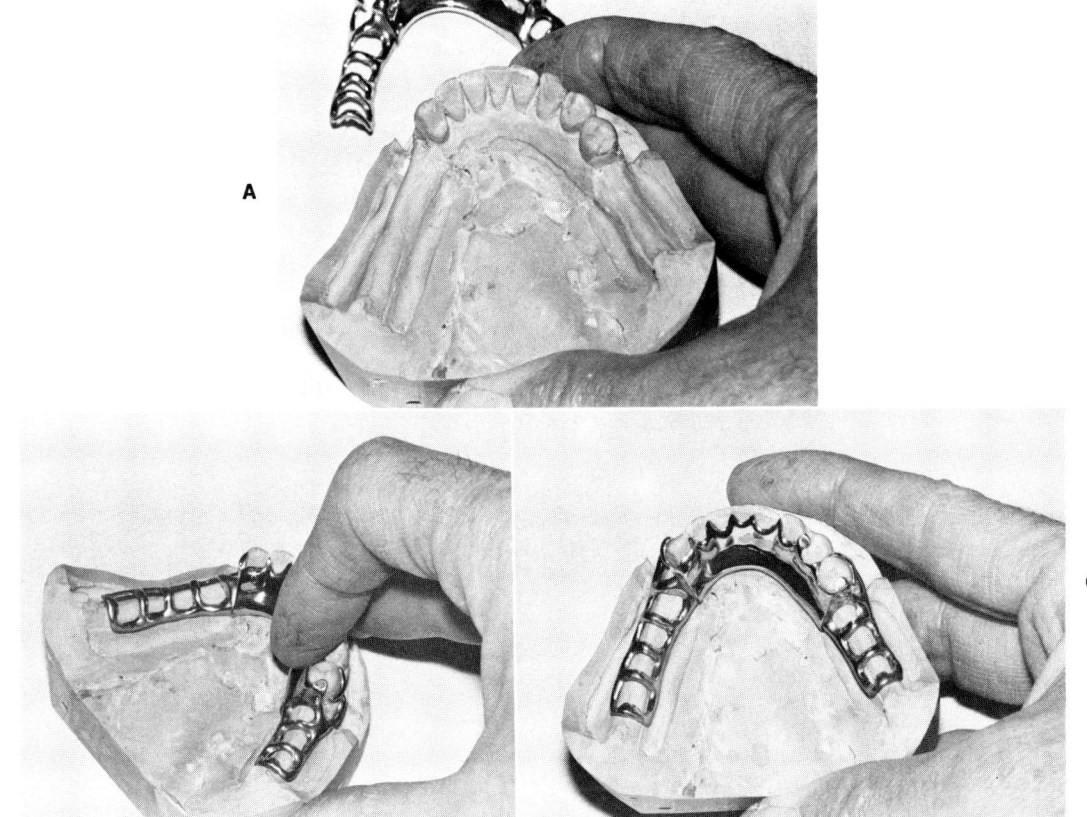

**Fig. 2-30. A,** Corrected cast is inspected for voids or other error. **B,** Framework is tried on cast to verify that distortion did not occur during laboratory procedures. **C,** Framework and cast are ready for next procedure.

**Table 2-3.** Wax beading and two-stage pour of corrected cast impression

| Problem | Probable cause | Solution |
| --- | --- | --- |
| Second pour separates from first pour and original cast | Retention not placed on surface of first pour | Place undercut mounds of dental stone on surface of first pour to retain second pour |
| | First pour and original cast were dry when making second pour | Soak original cast and first pour in clear slurry water for 3 to 5 minutes before making second pour |
| Small areas of surface of corrected cast break away during subsequent procedures | First pour of stone was too thin for necessary strength | Cover entire impression surface with minimum of 3 to 5 mm of stone when making first pour |
| Dental stone on teeth of cast | Poor seal of beading wax | Carefully seal beading wax around impression surface with special care at anterior junction with cast |
| Framework with impression does not seat completely on cast | Impression material under rest, or under minor connector, or ridge areas of cast not adequately trimmed | Remove all impression material from surfaces of framework that contact teeth; cut away entire residual ridge area of cast extending into tongue space to provide clearance for impression |
| Difficulty in removing impression from corrected cast | Failure to heat modeling plastic used for border molding before separating | Place cast and impression in warm water (130° to 140° F; 54.5° to 60° C) for 3 to 4 minutes to soften modeling plastic |
| | Undercuts in impression tray | Remove undercuts from impression tray before border molding and making corrected cast impression |
| | Impression tray locked into dental stone because too much of tray was exposed when boxing impression | Carry boxing material to within 2 to 3 mm of borders of impression |
| Voids in ridge areas of corrected cast | Air trapped when pouring corrected cast | Add small increments of properly proportioned and mixed dental stone; use light vibration when pouring corrected cast impression |
| New ridge areas separate from original cast | Failure to cut retention areas into cast | Prepare undercut retention areas into original cast using saw or bur |
| | Original cast dry when new stone was poured into ridge areas | Soak boxed cast and impression in clear slurry water for 5 minutes before pouring corrected cast impression. |
| Completed partial denture rocks in mouth | Framework not completely seated when impression was made | Avoid overfilling tray or getting impression material under rests; seat framework with finger pressure over rests, making certain framework is completely seated |
| | Framework improperly oriented to teeth when making impression | Avoid holding impression with finger pressure over ridge areas; pressure should be over rest areas only |
| | Framework not completely seated on cast because of interference by impression material | Remove any impression material under rests or on minor connectors; cut away ridge areas of cast so that contact with impression is avoided |
| | Framework moved when pouring cast | Lute framework to cast with sticky wax or modeling plastic |

## PROBLEM AREAS

The principal errors are the same as for the wax beading and boxing method with one additional problem area. The stone of the second pour may separate from the first pour and original cast if sufficient retention is not developed on the surface of the first pour, or, the same problem may occur if the original cast and first pour are not thoroughly soaked prior to making the second pour (Table 2-3).

## NORTH CAROLINA TECHNIQUE*
### PROCEDURE

1. A metallic paste impression is received in the laboratory. Remove impression material from the framework in areas that contact the teeth (Fig. 2-31).

2. Trim the master cast so that the functional impression can be poured in correct relationship to the remaining teeth (Fig. 2-32).

3. Seat the framework on the cast, and inspect it for contact between the functional impression and the cast. If contact is present, the cast must be trimmed until clearance is present (Fig. 2-33).

---

*This technique is similar to that described in Sowter, J. P.: Dental laboratory technology: prosthodontic techniques, Chapel Hill, 1968, The University of North Carolina Press.

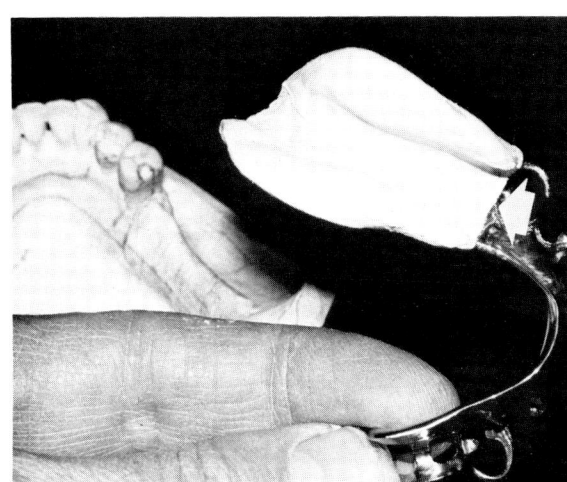

**Fig. 2-31.** Impression is received in laboratory. Sharp instrument is used to remove impression material from guide planes (arrow) or other framework areas that prevent framework from seating completely on abutment teeth.

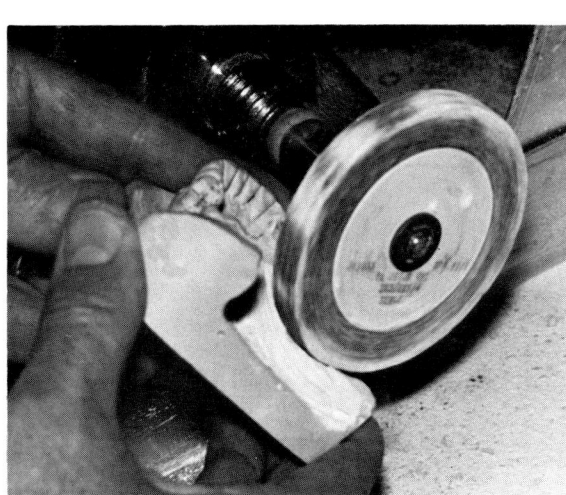

**Fig. 2-32.** Large Carborundum wheel is used to trim ridge area of master cast. Enough of cast must be removed so that no area of functional impression touches cast when framework is seated on cast.

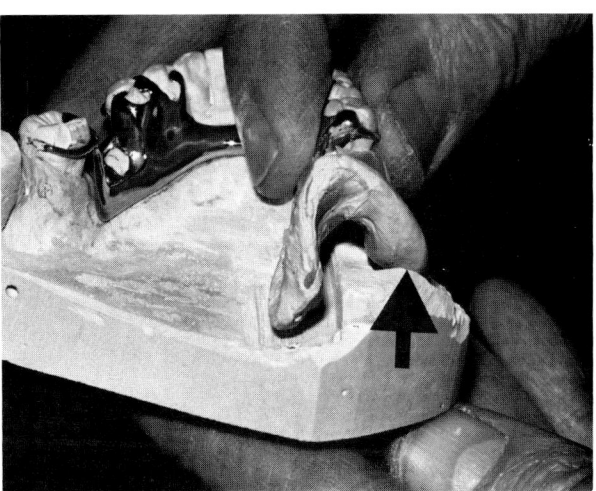

**Fig. 2-33.** Framework and functional impression are placed on master cast and inspected to determine if contact exists between cast and impression. If contact is present (arrow), cast must be trimmed until all contact is eliminated.

**50** *Dental laboratory procedures: removable partial dentures*

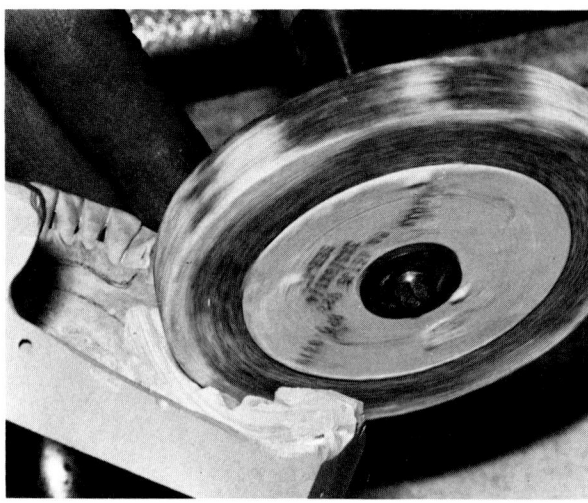

**Fig. 2-34.** Wheel stone is used to prepare retention grooves to enhance retention of new ridge area to cast.

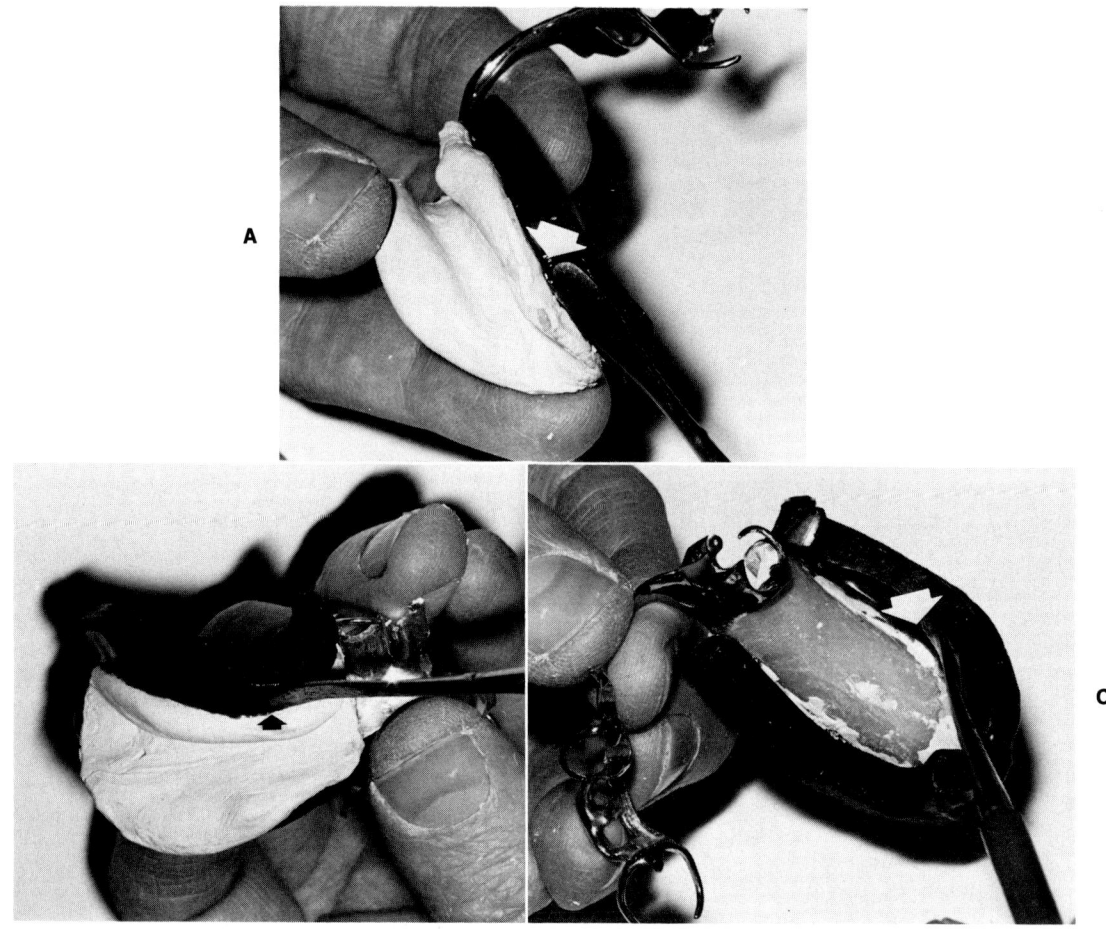

**Fig. 2-35.** Beading wax is adapted and sealed 2 to 3 mm above borders (arrow) of functional impression on lingual side **(A)** and on buccal side **(B)**. Wax beading is also sealed on its superior side (arrow) with wax spatula **(C)**.

4. Cut retention grooves into the areas of the cast that will be corrected when the functional impression is poured (Fig. 2-34).

5. Adapt and seal beading wax 2 to 3 mm above the borders of the functional impression (Fig. 2-35).

6. Seat the framework on the cast, and secure it in position with sticky wax (Fig. 2-36).

7. Seal the leading edge of the impression to the cast to prevent dental stone from flowing onto the teeth when the cast is poured (Fig. 2-37).

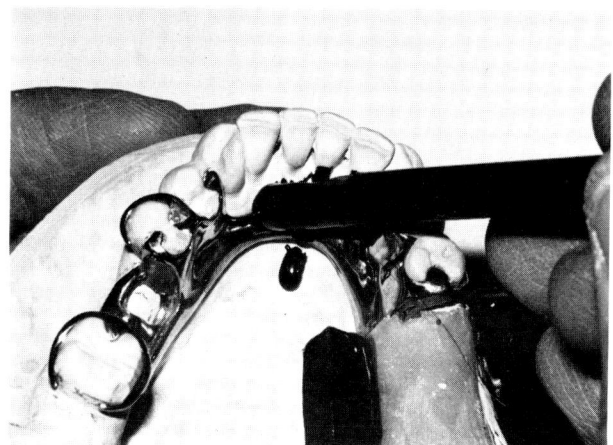

**Fig. 2-36.** Framework is seated on cast and luted to cast with sticky wax to prevent movement of framework during subsequent boxing and pouring procedures.

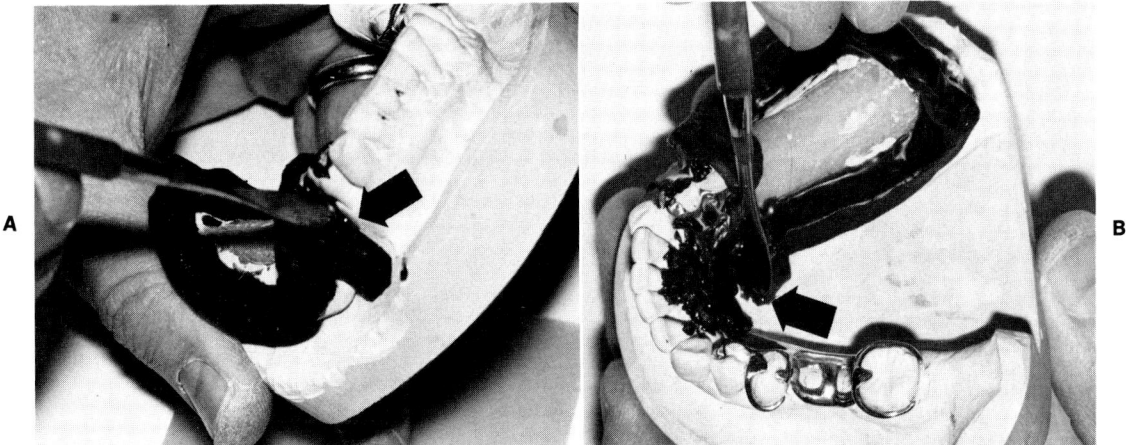

**Fig. 2-37. A,** Leading edge of impression is sealed to cast (arrow) to prevent stone from flowing onto teeth during pouring of new ridge area. **B,** Leading edge is also sealed on lingual side (arrow). Difficulty is encountered in developing complete seal because of relief area under major connector. Wax is flowed along superior and inferior borders of connector to help confine dental stone that may flow under connector.

8. Use strips of baseplate wax to complete the boxing of the impression on the buccal and lingual aspects (Fig. 2-38).

9. A tight seal of beading and boxing wax is critical in this pouring method and is difficult to attain. Test the completeness of the seal by pouring clear slurry water into the boxed impression. A difficult area to seal is the relief area under the major connector (Fig. 2-39).

10. Place the cast and impression in clear slurry water to soak for 4 to 5 minutes in preparation for pouring the corrected cast (Fig. 2-40).

11. Measure and mix the improved dental stone. Pour the boxed impression by adding small increments of stone and using light vibration. Sufficient stone must be used to support the heel of the cast (Fig. 2-41).

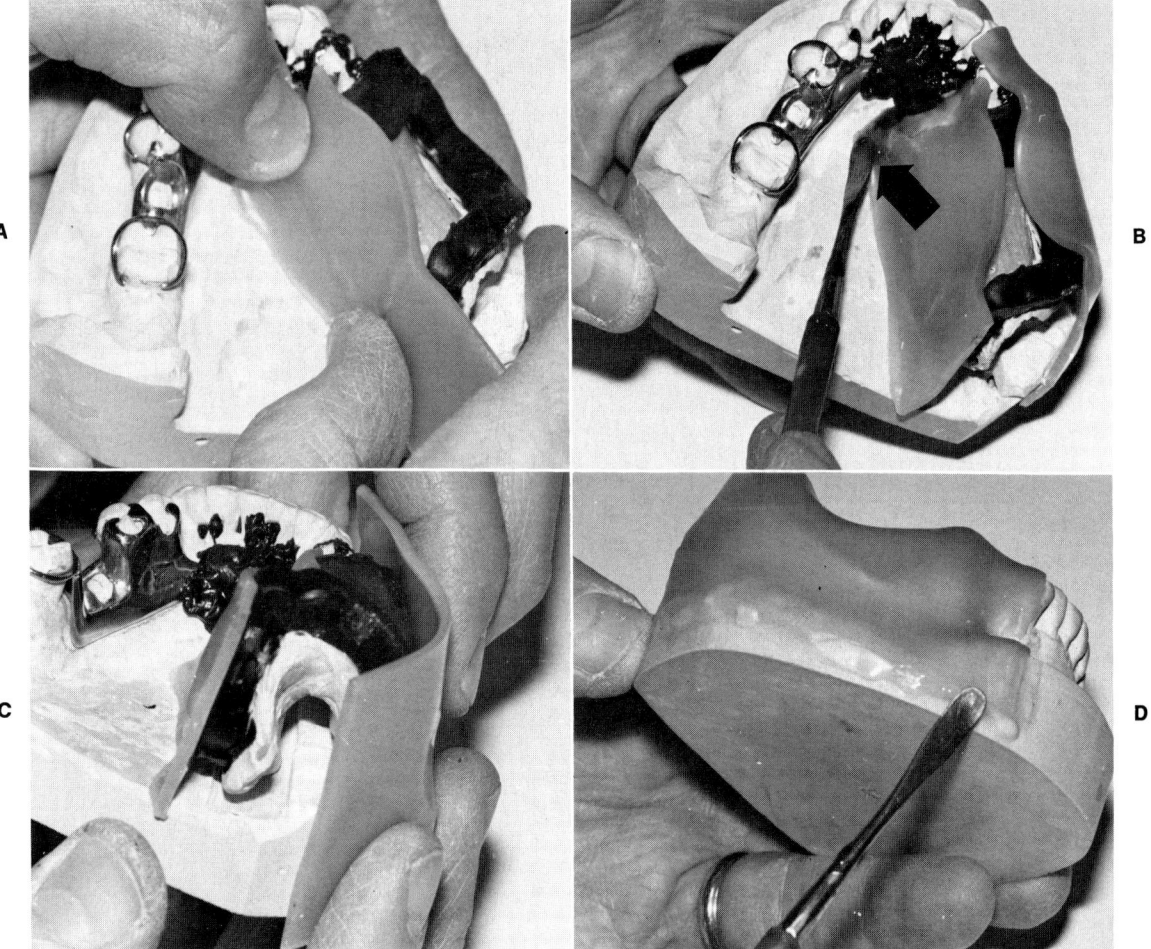

**Fig. 2-38. A,** Strip of baseplate wax is adapted to lingual side of impression. Wax is adapted so that it does not touch border of impression. It confines stone between lingual wax beading and tongue space area of cast. **B,** Wax spatula is used to seal wax to cast. **C,** Strip of wax is adapted to box buccal side of impression. Its purpose is to confine stone in area between buccal wax beading and base of cast. **D,** Wax is sealed to cast.

*Pouring corrected cast impressions* 53

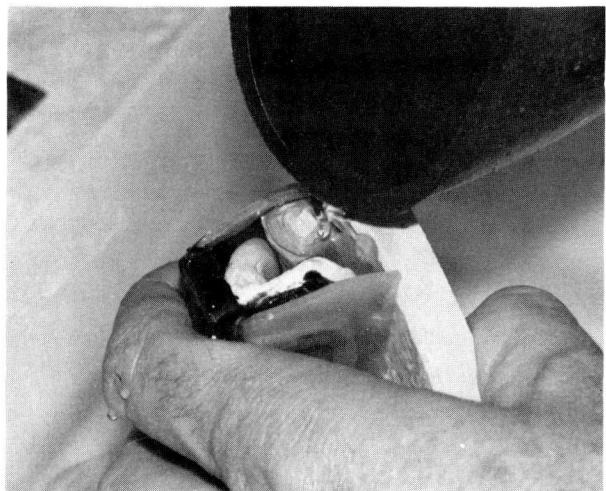

**Fig. 2-39.** Clear slurry water is poured into boxed impression to test integrity of seal. Most common problem area is on lingual side where it is difficult to seal because of relief under major connector.

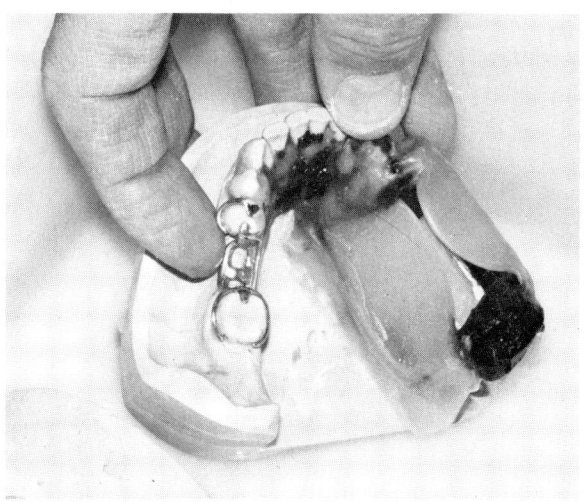

**Fig. 2-40.** Boxed impression and cast are placed in clear slurry water for 3 to 5 minutes to thoroughly soak cast. Failure to soak cast can result in inadequate union between new and old dental stone and can impede flow of new mix of dental stone to anterior portion of ridge area of cast.

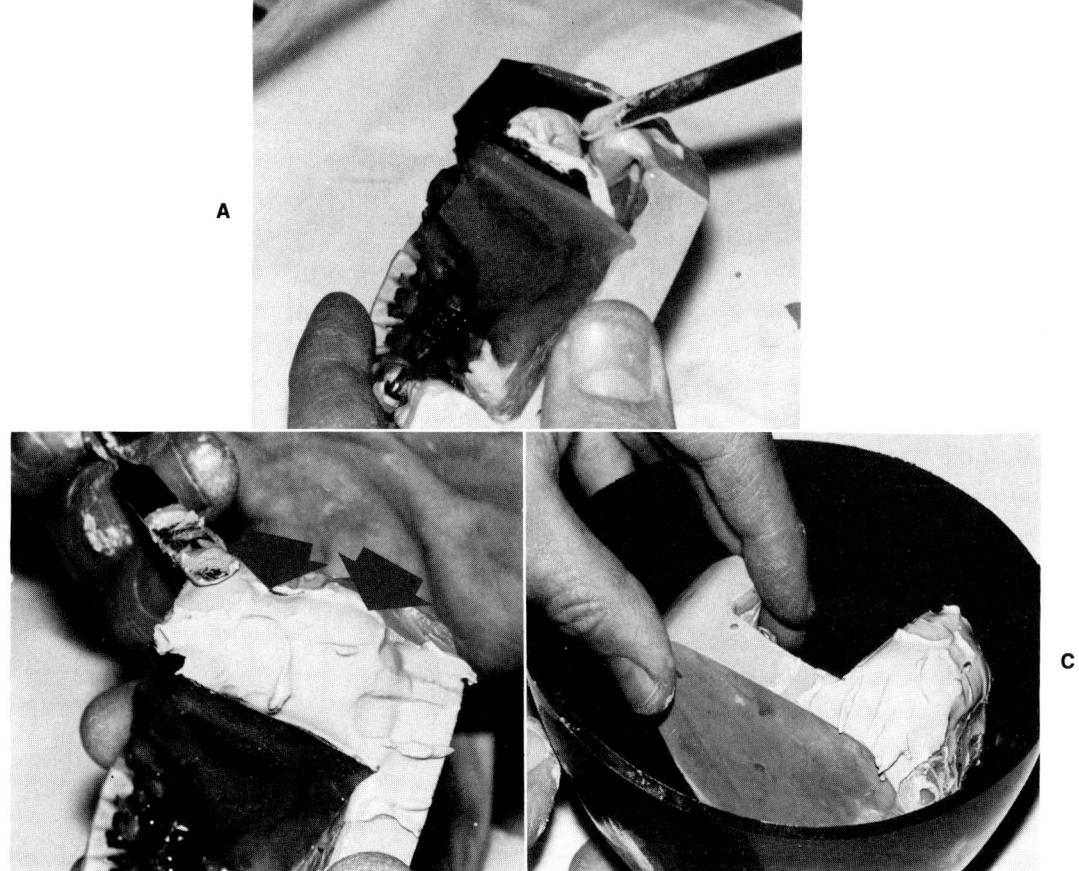

**Fig. 2-41. A,** Correctly proportioned and mixed improved dental stone is poured into boxed impression. Small increments of stone are added and lightly vibrated to avoid trapping air. **B,** Additional stone is added and shaped in heel area of cast (arrows) to ensure adequate support. **C,** Cast is supported during setting period to prevent dental stone from flowing out of boxed impression.

12. Remove the boxing and luting materials from the corrected cast. Shape the cast on a model trimmer (Fig. 2-42).

13. Soften the impression material in warm water, and remove the framework and impression tray from the corrected cast (Fig. 2-43).

14. Burn the impression tray off the framework, and place it on the cast. Smooth the land areas of the cast, and the corrected cast procedure is complete (Fig. 2-44).

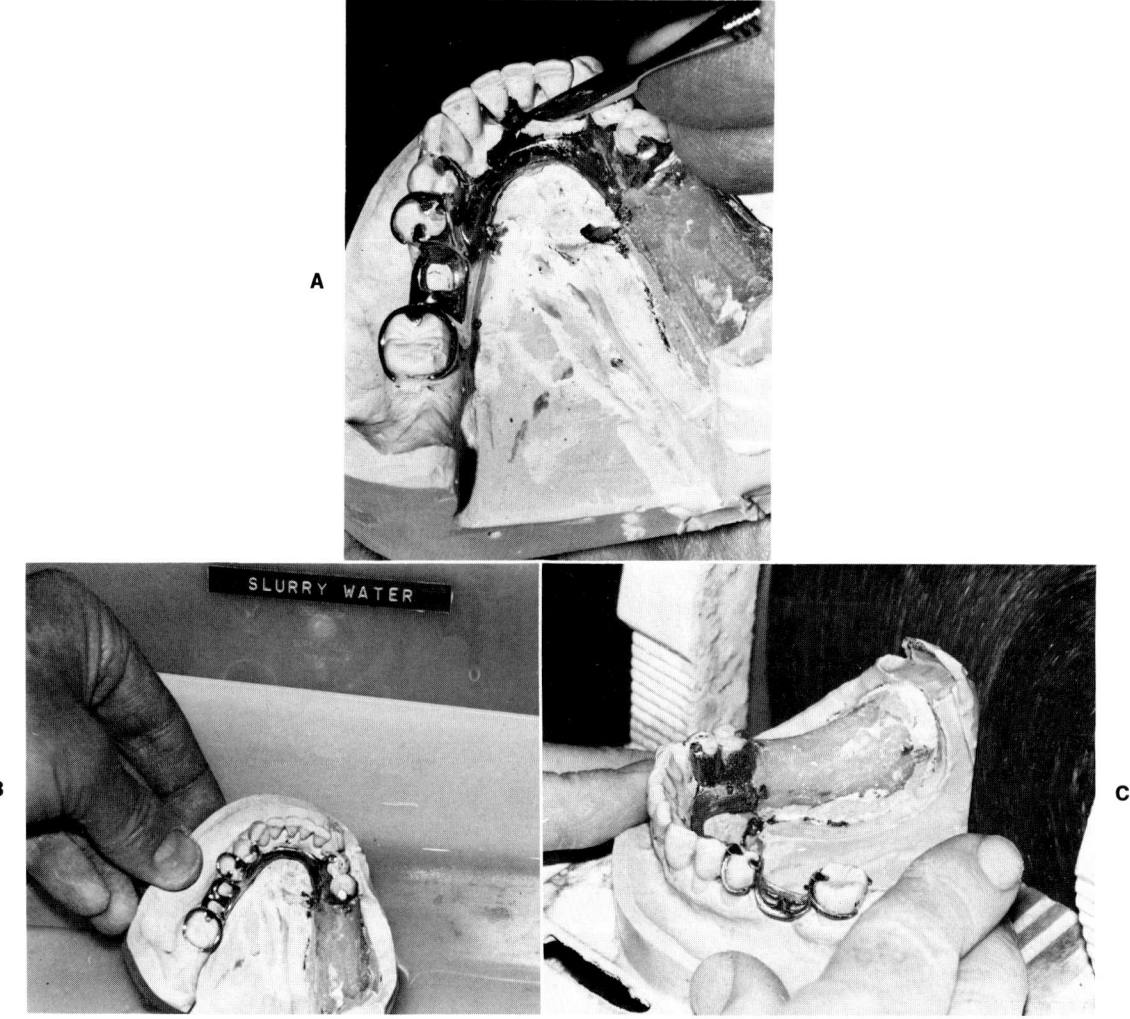

Fig. 2-42. **A,** Beading and boxing wax as well as sticky wax used for luting framework to cast are removed. **B,** Cast is soaked in clear slurry water for 3 to 5 minutes in preparation for trimming on model trimmer. **C,** Corrected area of cast is shaped on model trimmer.

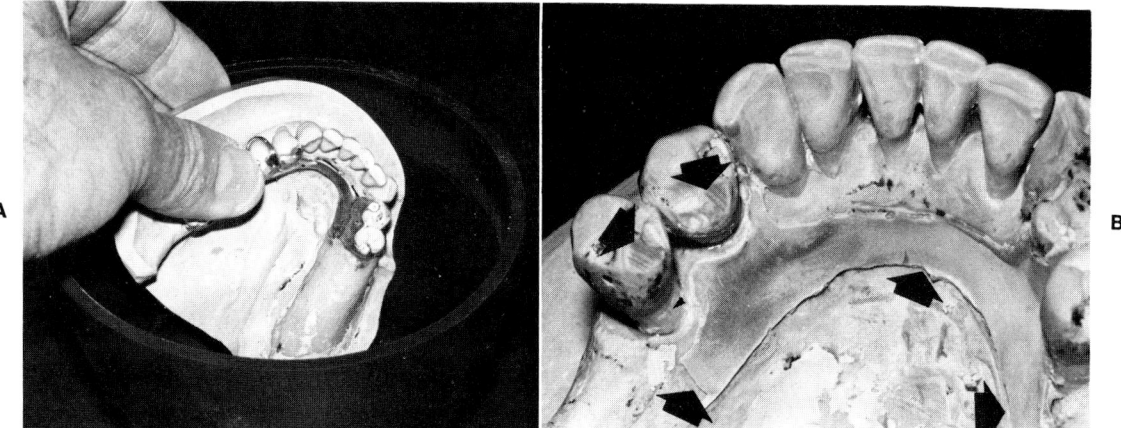

**Fig. 2-43. A,** Cast and impression are placed in 130° to 140° F water for 3 to 5 minutes to soften modeling plastic used for border molding impression. **B,** Framework and impression are removed from cast. Cast shows two errors that can occur using technique. Premolars were chipped (arrows) by large Carborundum wheel while trimming ridge area of cast. Dental stone flowed under major connector (arrows) during pouring of corrected cast because of lack of seal.

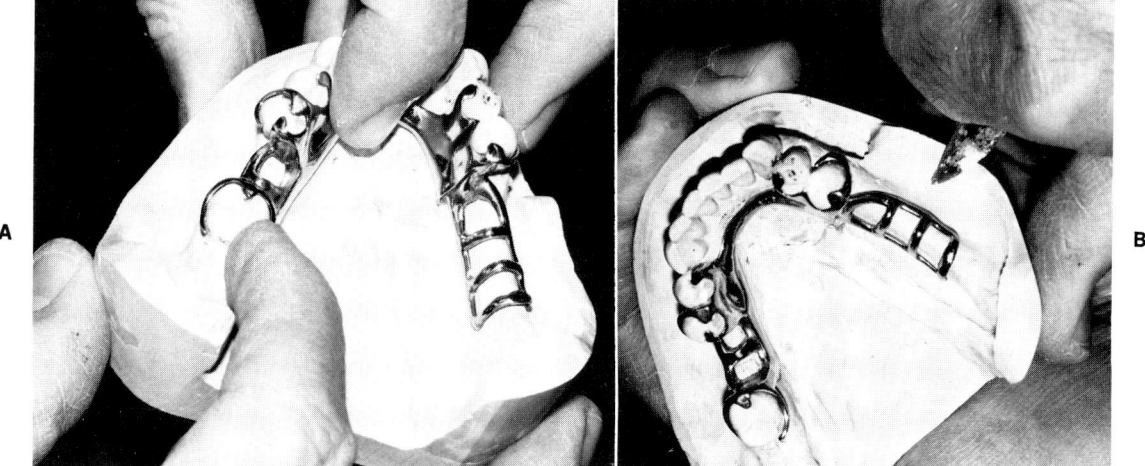

**Fig. 2-44. A,** Impression tray is burned off framework, and framework is seated on cast. **B,** Irregularities of land area of cast are smoothed. Corrected cast procedure is complete.

**Table 2-4.** North Carolina technique for pouring the corrected cast

| Problem | Probable cause | Solution |
| --- | --- | --- |
| Damaged teeth on cast | Large wheel stone used for trimming ridge areas touched teeth | Use great care when trimming cast, watching angle at which cast is held; use smaller wheel stone or plaster saw |
| New pour of stone on teeth of cast | Inadequate seal of beading and boxing wax | Seal anterior areas of impression to cast with wax; flow wax along margins of major connector to confine dental stone |
| Void in new ridge area of cast | Failure to soak cast before pouring | Soak cast in clear slurry water for 4 to 5 ninutes before pouring corrected cast |
| | Too much dental stone added at one time when pouring cast | Add small increments of dental stone and vibrate lightly |
| | Mix of dental stone too thick | Use correctly proportioned and mixed dental stone when pouring corrected cast |
| Framework with impression does not seat completely on cast | Impression material under rest, or under minor connector, or ridge areas of cast not adequately trimmed | Remove all impression material from surfaces of framework that contact teeth; cut away entire residual ridge area of cast extending into tongue space to provide clearance for impression |
| Difficulty in removing impression from corrected cast | Failure to heat modeling plastic used for border molding before separating | Place cast and impression in warm water (130° to 144° F; 54.5° to 60° C) for 3 to 4 minutes to soften modeling plastic |
| | Undercuts in impression tray | Remove undercuts from impression tray before border molding and making corrected cast impression |
| | Impression tray locked into dental stone because too much of tray was exposed when boxing impression | Carry boxing material to within 2 to 3 mm of borders of impression |
| Voids in ridge areas of corrected cast | Air trapped when pouring corrected cast | Add small increments of properly proportioned and mixed dental stone; use light vibration when pouring corrected cast impression |
| New ridge areas separate from original cast | Failure to cut retention areas into cast | Prepare undercut retention areas into original cast using saw or bur |
| | Original cast dry when new stone was poured into ridge areas | Soak boxed cast and impression in clear slurry water for 5 minutes before pouring corrected cast impression |
| Completed partial denture rocks in mouth | Framework not completely seated when impression was made | Avoid overfilling tray or getting impression material under rests; seat framework with finger pressure over rests, making certain framework is completely seated |
| | Framework improperly oriented to teeth when making impression | Avoid holding impression with finger pressure over ridge areas; pressure should be over rest areas only |
| | Framework not completely seated on cast because of interference by impression material | Remove any impression material under rests or on minor connectors; cut away ridge areas of cast so that contact with impression is avoided |
| | Framework moved when pouring cast | Lute framework to cast with sticky wax or modeling plasic |

## PROBLEM AREAS

The principal problems encountered in this technique are related to trimming the ridge areas of the cast and the development of a complete seal when beading and boxing the impression. The use of a large wheel stone to remove the ridge area can cause damage to the teeth of the cast if care is not taken. This is a greater problem when the dental arch is small.

A good anterior seal of the boxed impression is very imporant because of the direction of flow of the stone when pouring the corrected cast. The relief area under the major connector is the most difficult area to seal (Table 2-4).

## SUMMARY

Four methods of boxing and pouring corrected cast (functional) impressions were described in this chapter. All have several potential problems in common, and each has its own specific problems. Care must be taken in every laboratory step to avoid these problems. The fit of the removable partial denture depends on the procedures employed in pouring the functional impression. Complete success also depends on the quality of the prerequisite clinical procedures.

## BIBLIOGRAPHY

Air Force Manual 162-6. Dental laboratory technology, Washington, D.C., Jan. 22, 1975, U.S. Government Printing Office.

Bolouri, A., Hilger, T. C., and Gowrylok, M. D.: Boxing impressions, J. Prosthet. Dent. **33**:692-695, 1975.

Henderson, D., and Steffel, V. L.: McCracken's removable partial prosthodontics, ed. 6., St. Louis, 1981, The C. V. Mosby Co.

Holmes, J. B.: The altered cast impression procedure for distal extension removable partial dentures, Dent. Clin. North Am. **14**:(3):569-582, July, 1970.

Miller, E. L.: Removable partial prosthodontics, Baltimore, 1978, The Williams & Wilkins Co.

Morrow, R. M., Rudd, K. D., and Eissmann, H. F.; Dental laboratory procedures: complete dentures, vol. I, St. Louis, 1980, The C. V. Mosby Co.

Sowter, J. B.: Dental laboratory technology: prosthodontic techniques, Chapel Hill, N.C., 1968, The Universiy of North Carolina Press.

CHAPTER 3

# STOCK AND CUSTOM IMPRESSION TRAYS

KENNETH D. RUDD, ROBERT M. MORROW, and GEORGE KNIGHT

**impression** An impression of part or all of a partially endentulous arch made for the purpose of designing or constructing a partial denture.
**impression tray** A receptacle or device that is used to carry the impression material to the mouth, confine the material in apposition to the surfaces to be recorded, and control the impression material while it sets to form the impression.
**preliminary impression** An impression made for the purpose of diagnosis or the construction of a tray for making a final impression.

Properly selected impression trays contribute significantly to obtaining an acceptable impression and a resultant accurate cast.

## REQUIREMENTS FOR IMPRESSION TRAYS

Acceptable impression trays have the following qualities:
 1. They should confine the impression material to assure close adaptation to the teeth and soft tissues.
 2. They should permit the selection and control of impression material space between the tray and tissues to be recorded.
 3. They must be rigid to avoid distortion of the impression on removal.
 4. They should provide for mechanical locking of the impression material to the tray through rim-lock undercuts or perforations.
 5. They should be capable of being cleansed and sterilized if they are not disposable.
 6. They should be available in different sizes and shapes if they are stock trays.
 7. They must be inexpensive if they are disposable.

In this chapter the various trays, their advantages, and disadvantages will be described. Impression trays may be classified as follows:
 1. Stock trays
    a. Metal rim-lock trays: dentulous and edentulous
    b. Perforated trays: dentulous and edentulous
    c. Water-cooled trays: dentulous and edentulous
    d. Plastic stock trays: disposable
 2. Custom trays
    a. Tray resin trays
    b. Thermoplastic vacuum-adapted trays

## STOCK TRAYS

Many dentists prefer to modify stock trays with modeling plastic and use them for making impressions for removable partial dentures. They are available in several sizes for the maxillary and mandibular arches. Most commonly they are supplied in small, medium, large, and extra large sizes. If an odd shape or size is required, it is usually necessary to use a custom-made tray.

Stock trays are available in a variety of kinds (Fig. 3-1). The perforated metal rim-lock tray and the solid metal rim-lock tray are used with alginate ir-

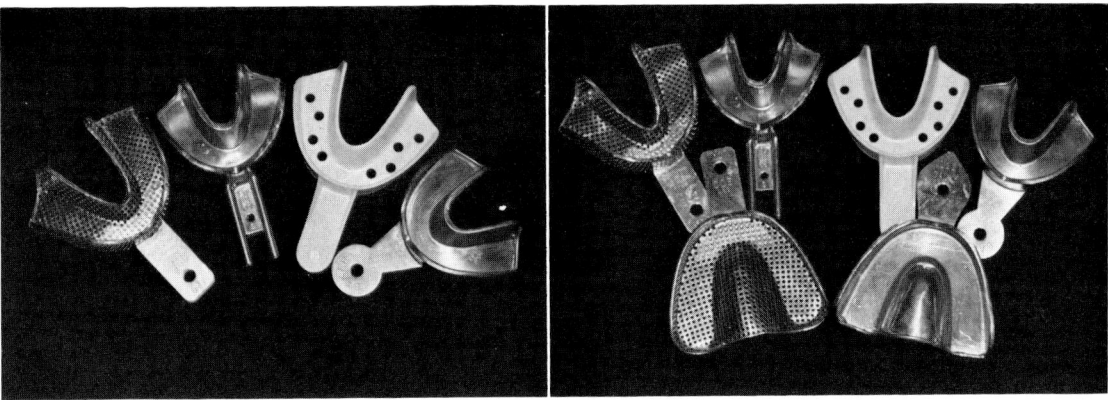

Fig. 3-1. Variety of mandibular and maxillary stock trays are available.

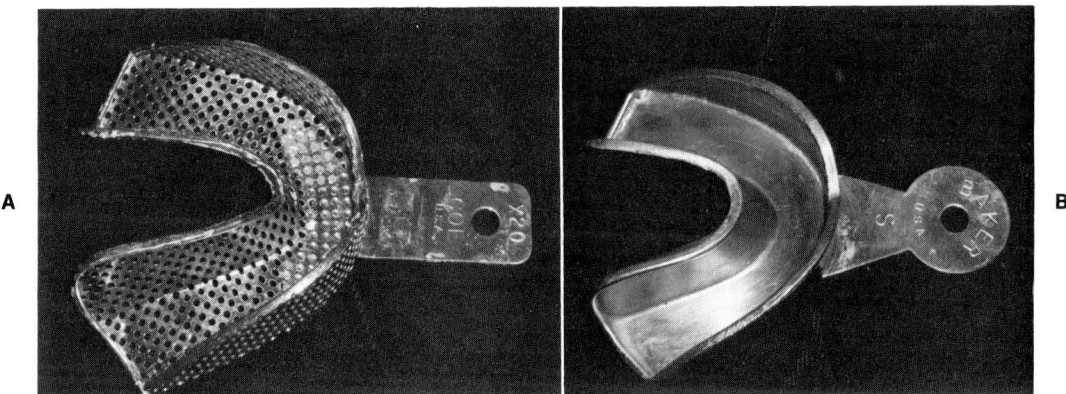

Fig. 3-2. **A,** Perforated metal rim-lock tray. **B,** Solid metal rim-lock tray.

reversible impression material (Fig. 3-2). These trays are usually modified or customized by the dentist by using modeling plastic to fill in the edentulous portions, palate, and postpalatal seal area. Metal trays are also made to use with agar reversible hydrocolloid impression material. This material is thermoset, so it must be cooled while it is in the mouth. These trays are made like the solid or perforated metal rim-lock trays just described except that they have metal tubing attached to the outside of the tray so cool water may be circulated around the impression material to cool it. Hoses are attached to the two water tubes protruding by the handle (Fig. 3-3).

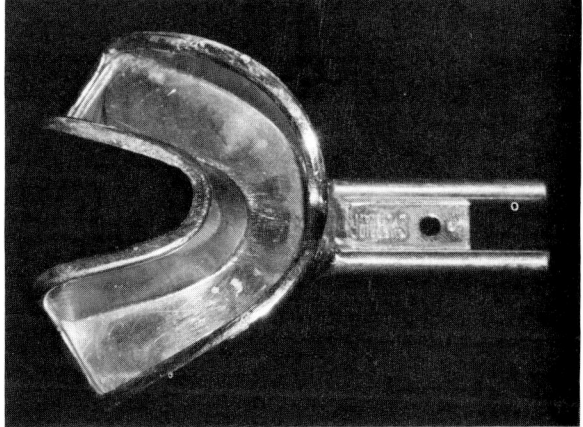

Fig. 3-3. Water-cooled tray used for reversible hydrocolloid impressions.

Many different types of plastic stock impression trays are available (Fig. 3-4). Some plastic trays are inexpensive enough that they can be used as disposable trays. One disadvantage of some of the plastic trays is that they are flexible. This may contribute to the inaccuracy of the impression. They have an advantage in that they may be ground with a stone or vulcanite bur to shorten the flange (Fig. 3-5).

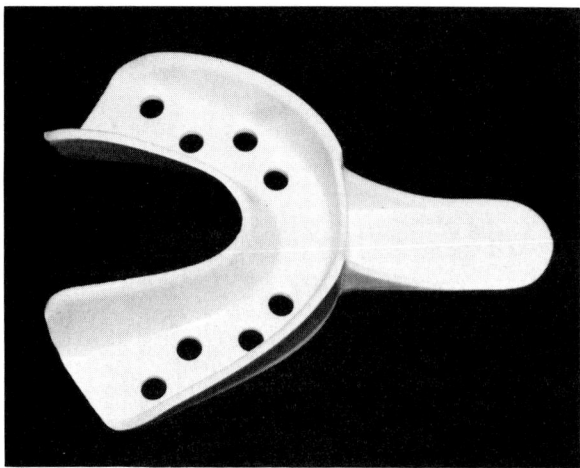

Fig. 3-4. Mandibular plastic stock impression tray.

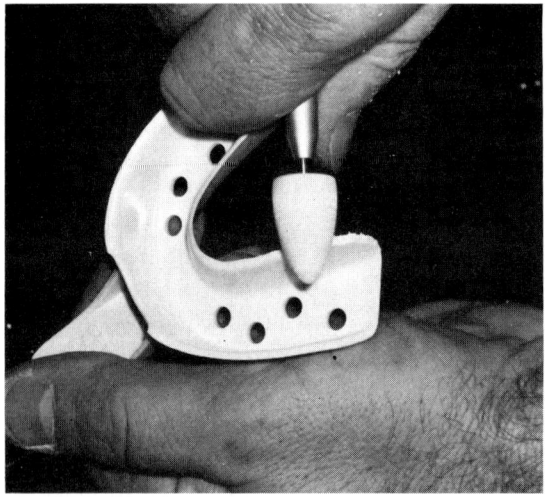

Fig. 3-5. Flanges of plastic trays may be altered by grinding.

## CUSTOM TRAYS

Custom trays are most commonly made from acrylic resin tray material or thermoset plastic vinyl sheets. These materials are usually not applied directly to the casts, since the elastic impression material, which will be used in the tray, requires room to expand when removed from an undercut. Therefore it is necessary to block out the cast with a spacing material such as wax or an asbestos substitute. Trays made for alginate require more relief than trays for elastomeric materials. When alginate is to be used in the tray, the relief should be about ¼ inch (0.6 cm) thick around the teeth and a lesser amount over the soft tissue. Some dentists prefer no relief at all over the soft tissue. If acrylic resin is to be adapted to the cast, a tinfoil substitute should be used (Fig. 3-6).

Elastomeric materials require a thickness of ⅛ inch (0.3 cm) when it is necessary for them to spring over undercuts. Wax should be adapted evenly over the teeth and soft tissue (Fig. 3-7).

An alternate method of applying wax relief is to dip the casts in molten wax. Do not use wax that is too hot. The ideal dipping temperature is about 130° F (54.5° C). Dip the cast repeatedly until the desired thickness is built up on the cast. Wax at 130° F will not burn the fingers, so the cast may be dipped by holding the base of the cast in the fingers (Fig. 3-8). The wax may be trimmed away from the base of the cast, and it may be cut out for stops (Fig. 3-9).

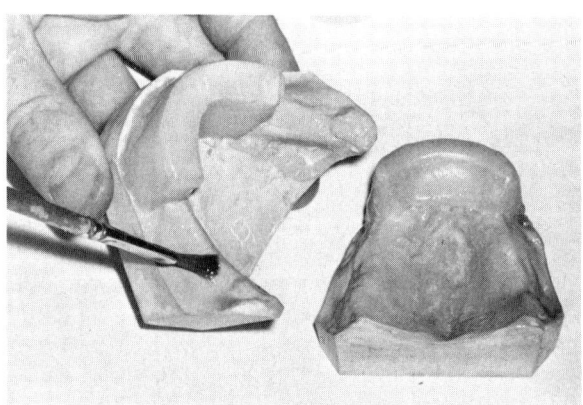

Fig. 3-6. Teeth are blocked out with wax about ¼ inch (0.63 cm) thick, and no relief is applied over the edentulous areas. Tinfoil substitute is applied to cast to prevent acrylic resin from sticking.

## Stock and custom impression trays 61

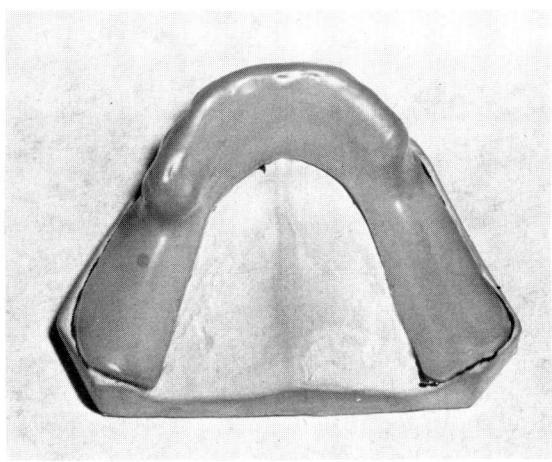

**Fig. 3-7.** Layer of wax ⅛ inch (0.3 cm) thick is adapted over teeth and cast when tray is to be used for elastomeric impression materials.

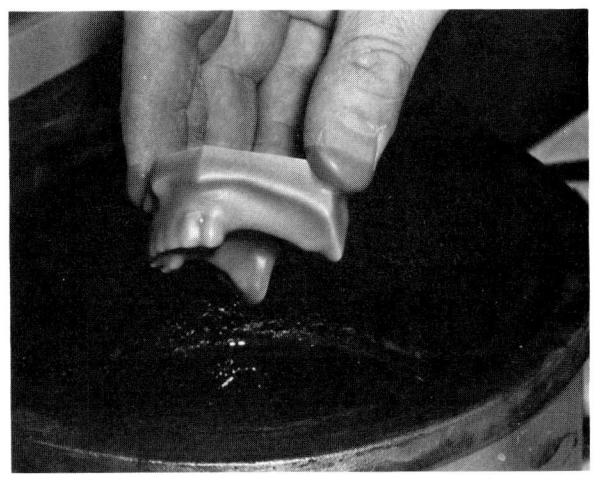

**Fig. 3-8.** Cast is dipped repeatedly in melted wax at 130° F (54.5° C). This temperature will not burn. Note wax on fingers.

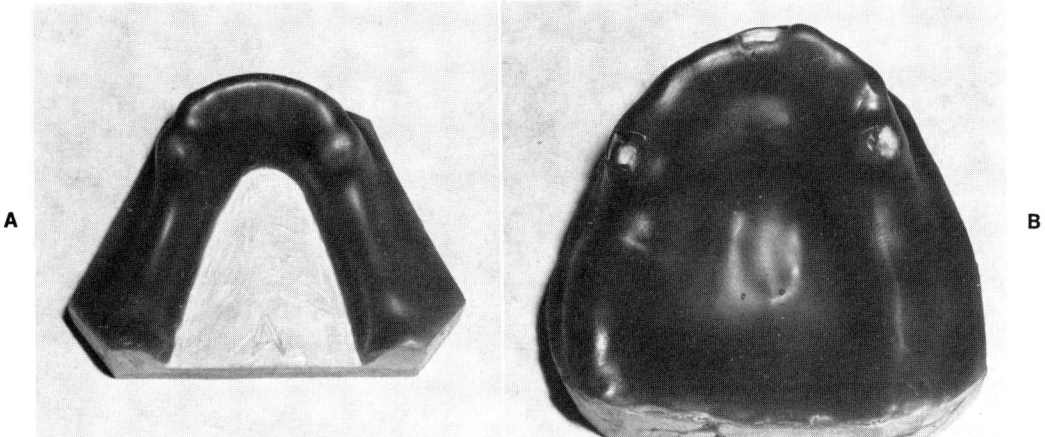

**Fig. 3-9. A,** Mandibular cast dipped in wax and trimmed around base area. **B,** Maxillary cast dipped, trimmed, and areas cut out of wax to form tissue stops in tray.

## Acrylic resin trays
### PROCEDURE

1. Outline the extent of the tray on the cast (Fig. 3-10).
2. Adapt the relief wax over the cast, and paint it and the cast with tinfoil substitute (Fig. 3-11).
3. Plastic tray material* is assembled along with a paper cup, spatula, tray formers, measuring devices, and a separating medium (Fig. 3-12).
4. Tray formers may be made by using baseplates and forming stone around them. Once made, they may be used many times if the mold is lubricated with petroleum jelly each time before the acrylic resin is used (Fig. 3-13).

---

*Coe Tray Plastic, Coe Laboratories, Inc., Chicago, Ill.

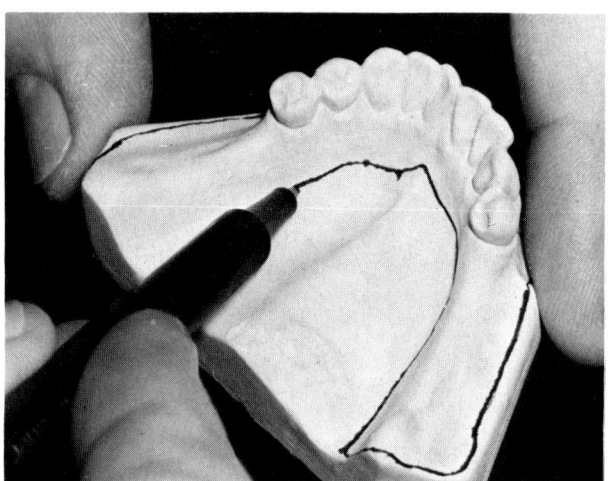

Fig. 3-10. Outline of relief is drawn on cast.

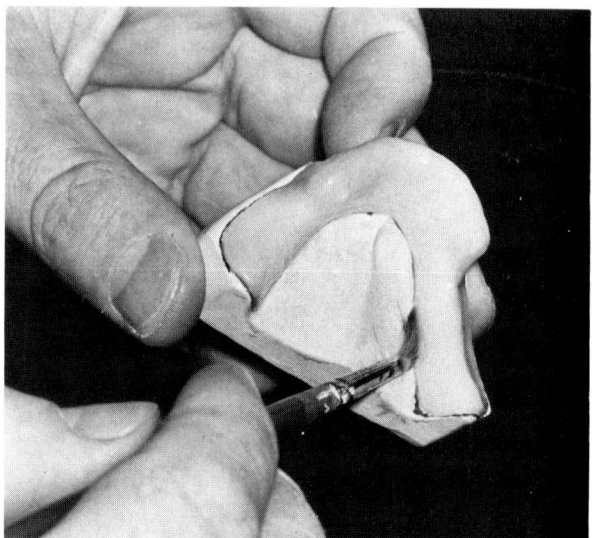

Fig. 3-11. Even layer of wax is adapted to cast and painted with tinfoil substitute.

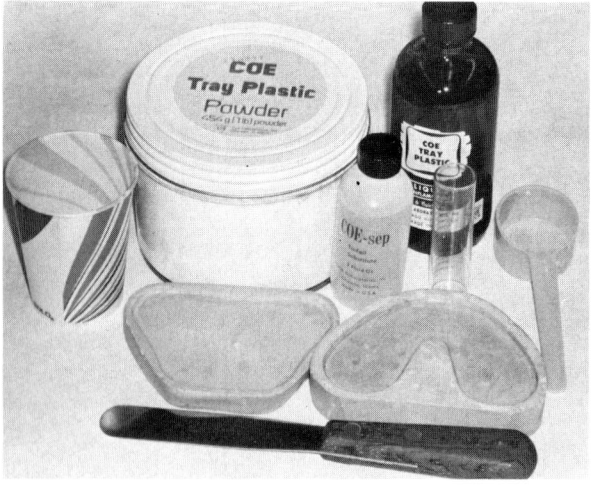

Fig. 3-12. Paper cup, tray powder and liquid, tinfoil substitute, measuring devices, tray formers, and spatula.

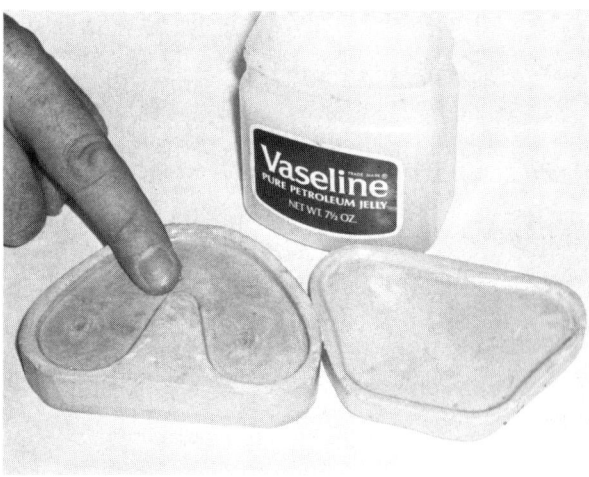

Fig. 3-13. Tray formers are lubricated with petroleum jelly.

5. Measure the powder and liquid according to the manufacturer's directions, and place them in the paper cup, liquid first. Stir with a spatula until they are thoroughly mixed (Fig. 3-14).

6. While the mix is still thin, pour it into the lubricated mold (Fig. 3-15).

7. Smooth the material with a spatula, and keep adding it until the mold is full (Fig. 3-16).

8. After the mold is filled with resin, allow it to set until it becomes plastic (Fig. 3-17).

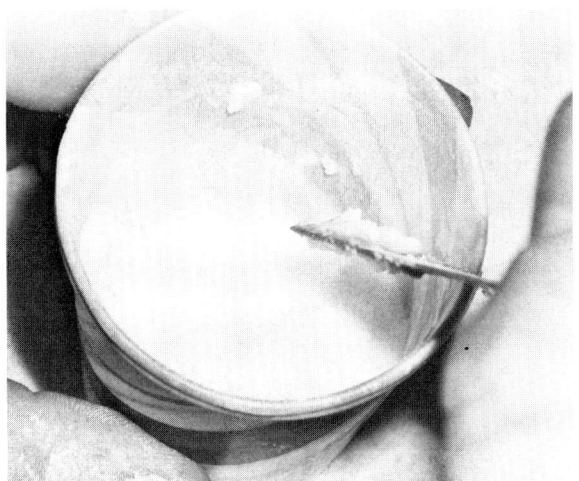

Fig. 3-14. Measured powder and liquid are mixed in paper cup.

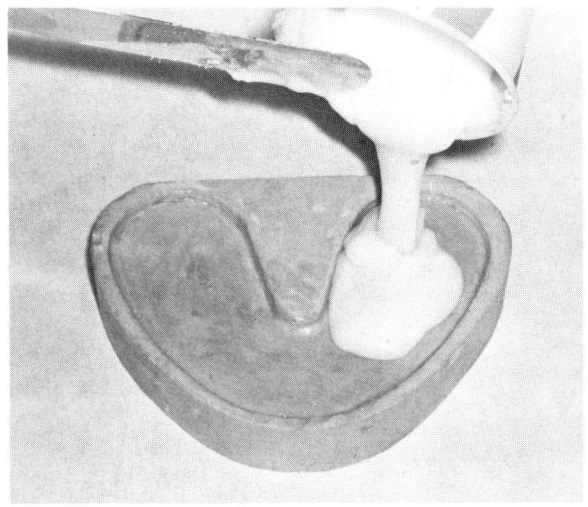

Fig. 3-15. Fluid resin mix is poured into lubricated mold.

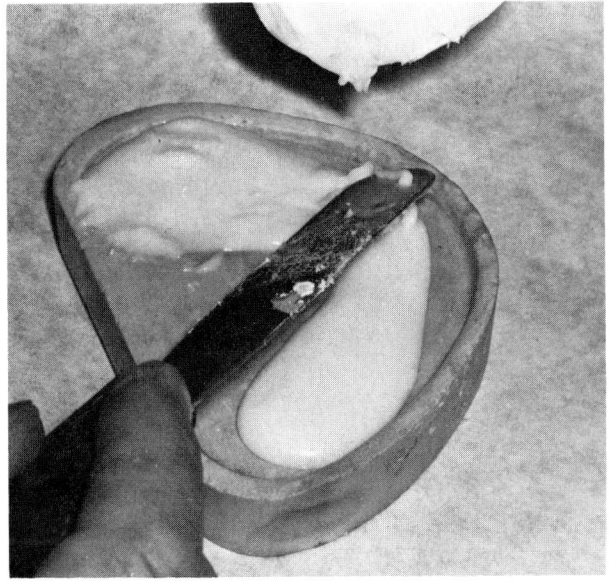

Fig. 3-16. Smooth resin with spatula as it is added to mold.

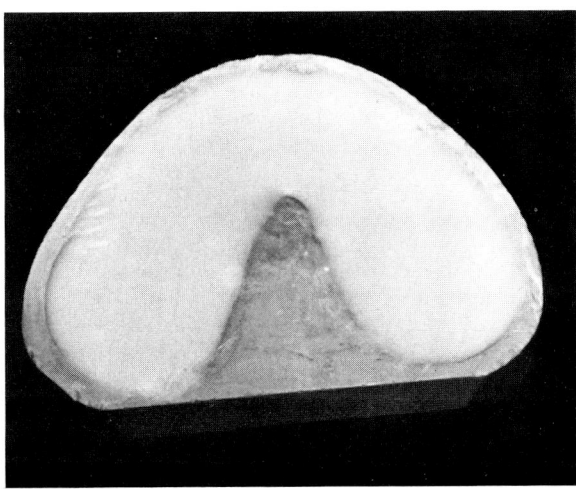

Fig. 3-17. Acrylic resin in mold must set until it becomes plastic and can be handled.

9. When the material holds together when it is lifted from the mold, it is ready to remove (Fig. 3-18).

10. Remove the formed acrylic resin sheet from the mold (Fig. 3-19).

11. Center the plastic sheet over the cast, making sure that it covers the entire area (Fig. 3-20).

12. Adapt the material to the cast, and hold it in position while it hardens enough to stay in place (Fig. 3-21).

13. Before the acrylic resin tray material sets completely, some of the material may be added to the front of the tray to form a handle. Excess monomer added to this area will help the material adapt and stick in place (Fig. 3-22).

14. After the tray material has been set, remove it from the cast. Note that when tinfoil substitute is used over the wax, the tray material will not stick to it and separates cleanly (Fig. 3-23).

15. To help in finishing the tray, use a pen or pencil to establish the length of the tray (Fig. 3-24).

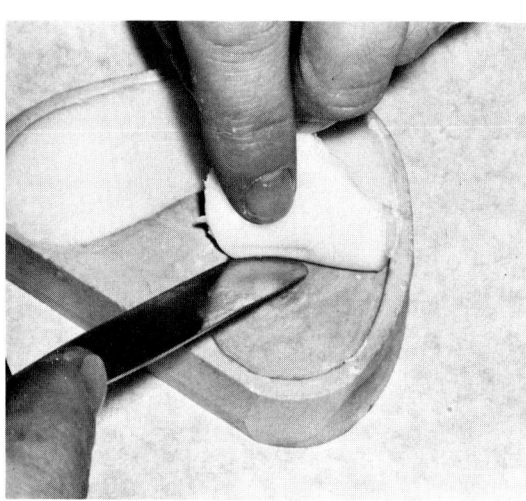

**Fig. 3-18.** Test material to see if it will hold together.

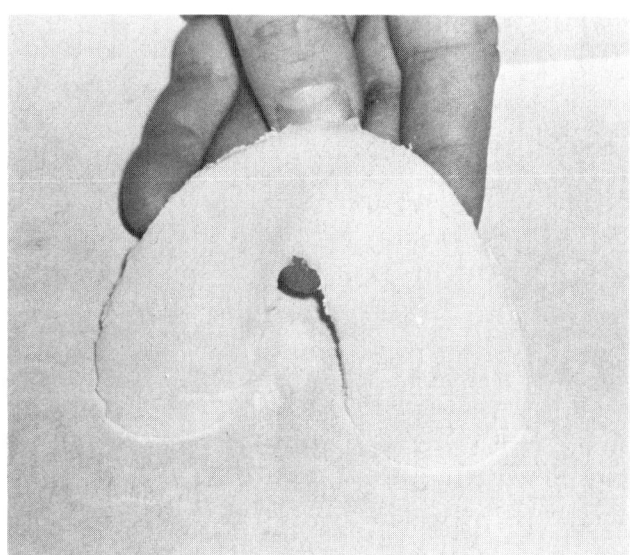

**Fig. 3-19.** Acrylic resin sheet removed from mold.

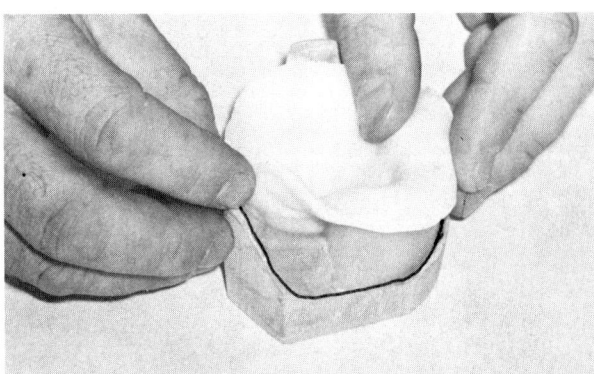

**Fig. 3-20.** Center plastic baseplate over cast, and cover entire outline that was placed on cast.

*Stock and custom impression trays* **65**

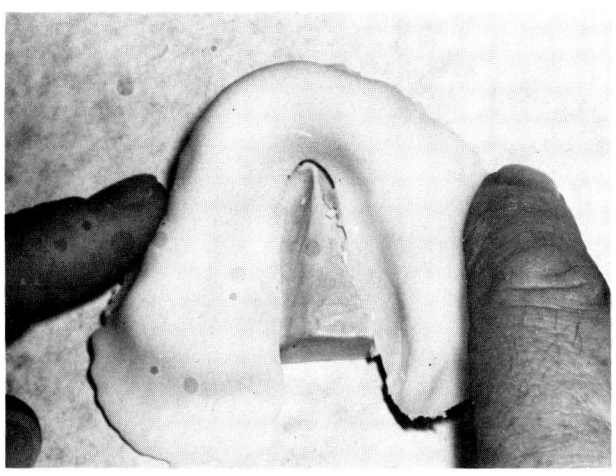

**Fig. 3-21.** Adapt plastic to cast with fingers, and hold it in place until it does not pull away from cast.

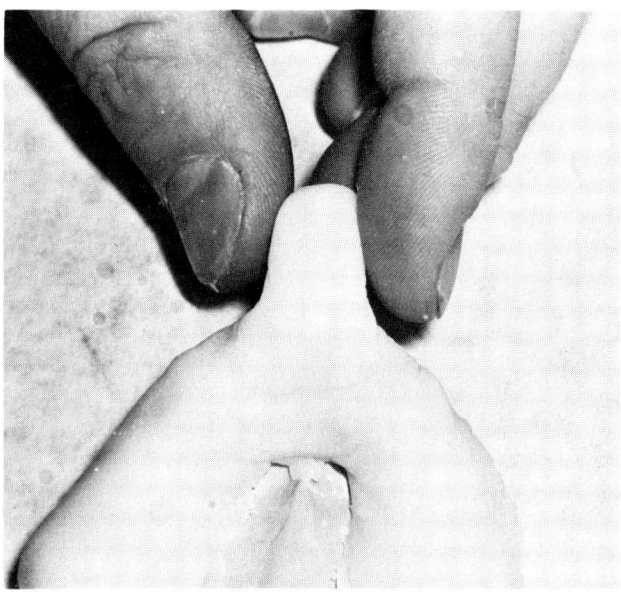

**Fig. 3-22.** Before material sets, some of excess may be added to form handle.

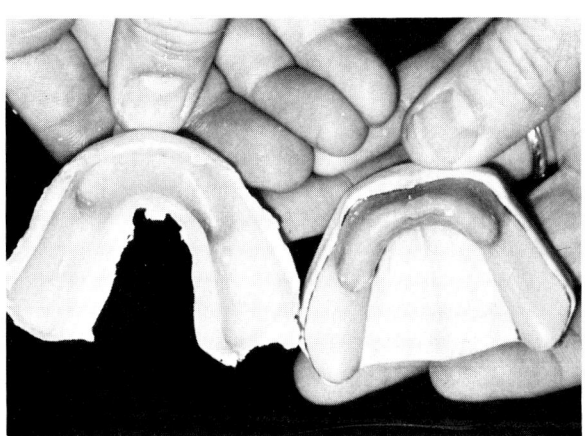

**Fig. 3-23.** Tray separated cleanly from cast and wax relief when tinfoil substitute is used.

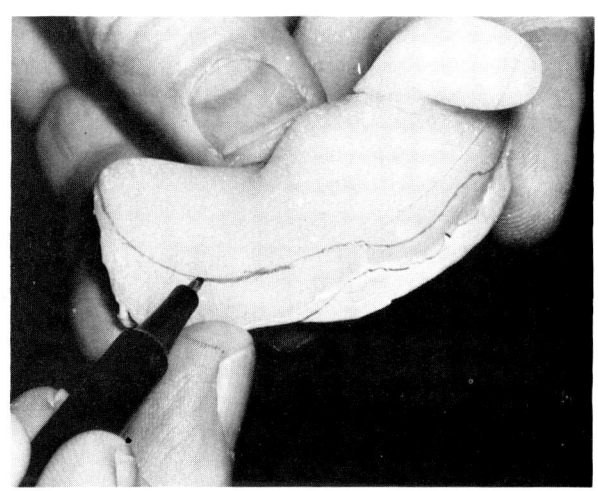

**Fig. 3-24.** Outline desired shape of tray on acrylic resin with pen or pencil.

**66** *Dental laboratory procedures: removable partial dentures*

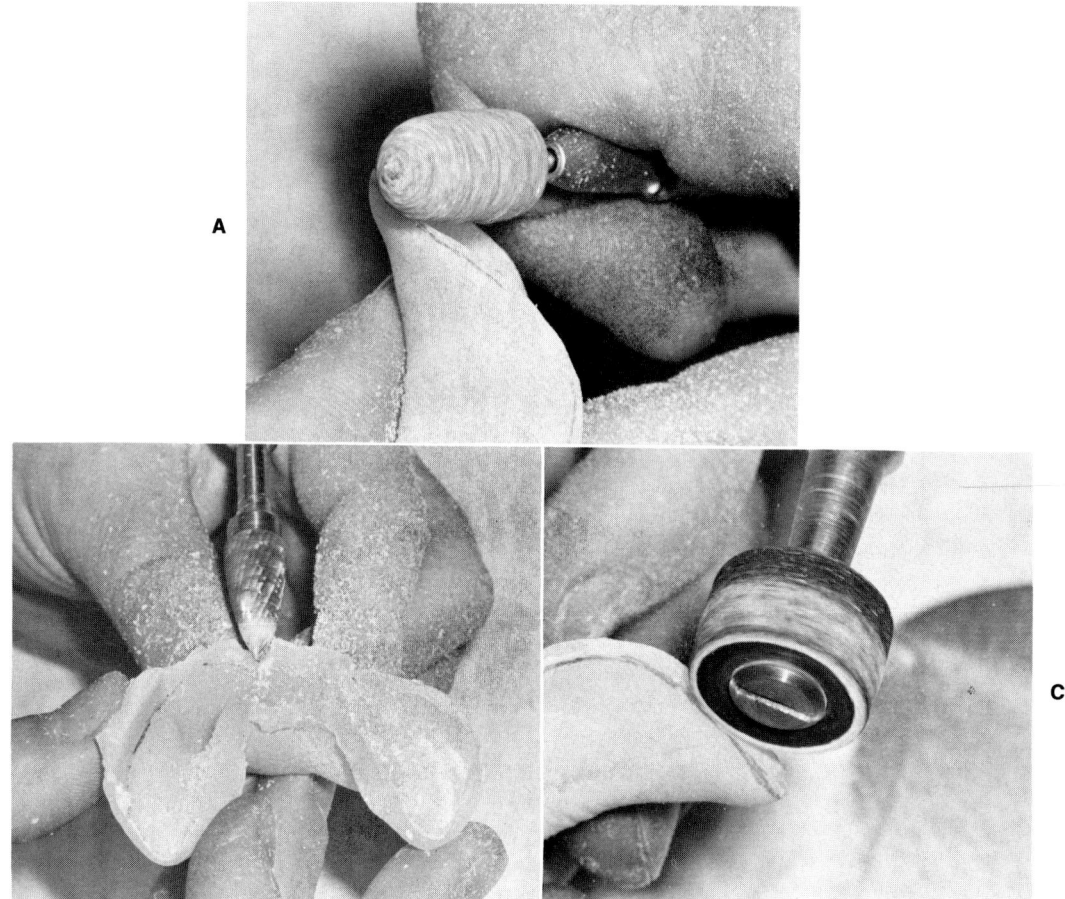

**Fig. 3-25.** Tray may be trimmed with stone or bur in handpiece **(A)**, it may be trimmed with lathe using carbide bur **(B)** or arbor band **(C)**.

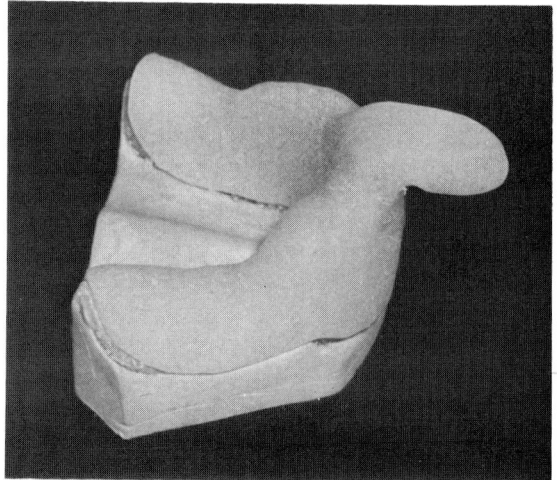

**Fig. 3-26.** Trimmed tray is placed back on cast to see if additional trimming is necessary.

16. Trim the tray material with a stone or vulcanite bur mounted in a handpiece or with a lathe-mounted carbide bur or an arbor band (Fig. 3-25).

17. After trimming, place the tray on the cast to see if all of the borders are in the proper position (Fig. 3-26).

18. When the desired length of the tray has been established, round the borders, and polish them with a rag wheel and pumice to remove any rough edges (Fig. 3-27).

19. The impression materials will not adhere to the smooth inside of the tray very well, so perforate the tray by using a bur. Make a large number of holes with a No. 6 or 8 round bur. They should be about ¼ inch (0.6 cm) apart (Fig. 3-28).

20. Neither alginate nor elastomeric impression materials will stick to wax. The last step in completing a custom impression tray is to flush it thoroughly with boiling water and detergent to remove all traces of wax (Fig. 3-29).

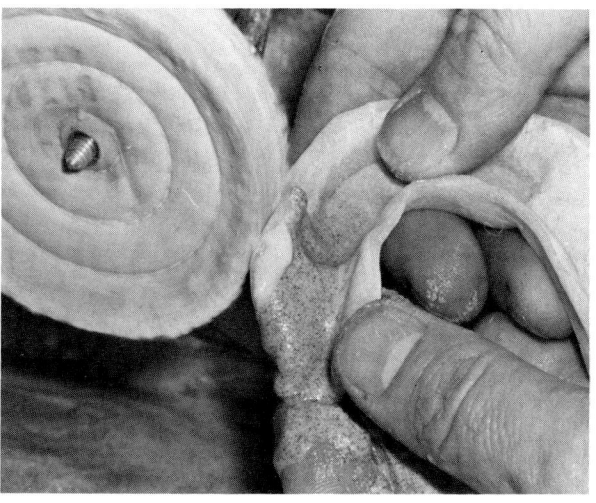

**Fig. 3-27.** Round borders of tray, and polish them with rag wheel and pumice to remove any sharpness.

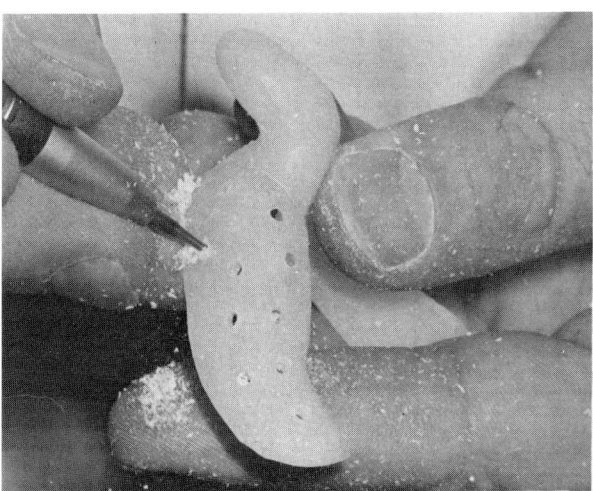

**Fig. 3-28.** Perforate tray with No. 6 or 8 round bur. This will enable impression material to adhere to tray more securely.

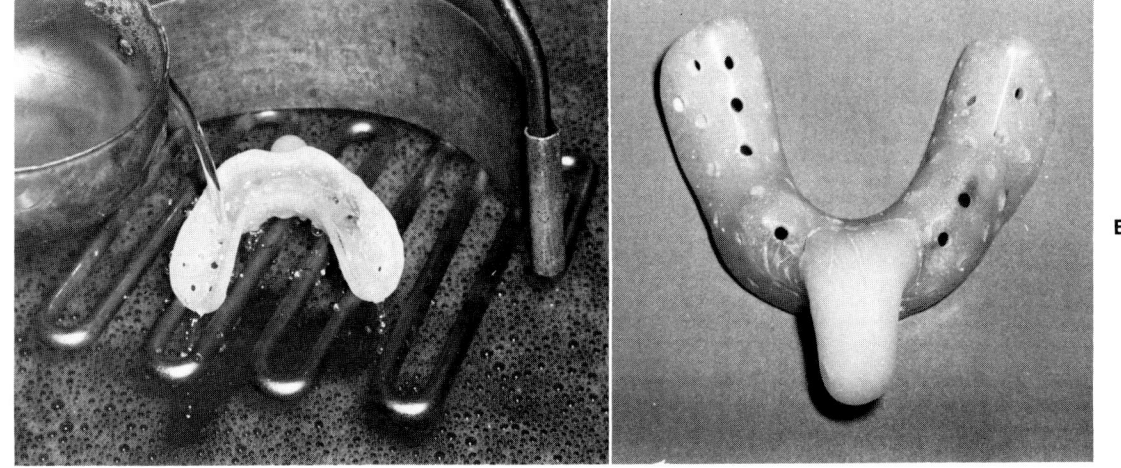

**Fig. 3-29. A,** Tray is flushed with boiling water and detergent to remove all traces of wax. **B,** Completed tray ready for impression material.

**Table 3-1.** Custom acrylic resin tray

| Problem | Probable cause | Solution |
|---|---|---|
| Teeth on cast broken when tray is removed | Insufficient blockout of teeth | Make certain that there is ¼ inch (0.6 cm) wax on cast for alginate tray and ⅛ inch (0.3 cm) for elastomeric impression material |
| Completed tray is too flexible | Tray is too thin | Make resin patty thicker; do not overthin when adapting to cast |
| Tray sticks to cast | Tinfoil substitute contaminated or not used | Paint cast with uncontaminated tinfoil substitute |
| Impression material pulls away from tray | Insufficient perforations or adhesive not used | Perforate tray with evenly spaced holes to periphery and use adhesive |

#### PROBLEM AREAS

Some of the more common problems encountered with this type of tray are mentioned in Table 3-1.

### Thermoset vinyl trays
#### PROCEDURE

1. Since material for adaptation must be very hot, wax cannot be used as a blockout material. Instead, use an asbestos substitute material* (Fig. 3-30).

2. Place the plastic sheet in a heater that is also a vacuum machine. Several are available and two are shown in Fig. 3-31: the Dentsply Vacu-Press* and Omnivac.†

3. When the plastic sheet sags about 1 inch (2.5 cm), lower it over the cast, and turn the vacuum on at the same instant (Figs. 3-32 and 3-33).

4. Use a vulcanite bur in a lathe to cut through the plastic sheet at the edge of the cast (Fig. 3-34).

---

*Kaoliner casting ring liner, Dentsply International, Inc., York Pa.

*Vacu-Press, Dentsply International, Inc., York, Pa.
†Omnivac, Buffalo Dental Manufacturing Co., Brooklyn, N.Y.

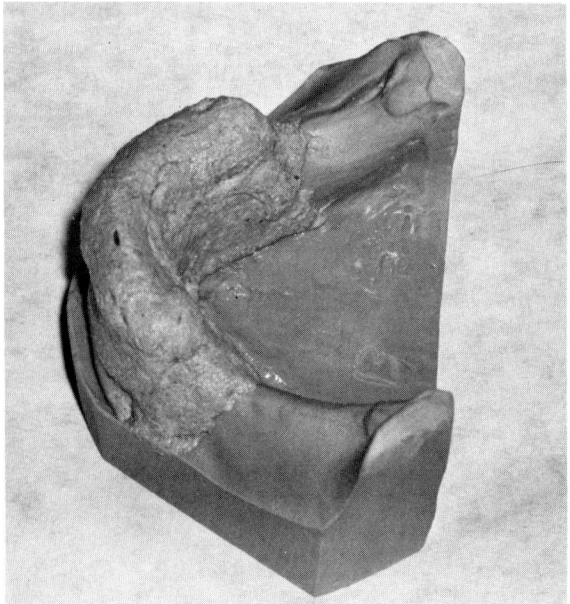

**Fig. 3-30.** Cast is blocked out with asbestos substitute material.

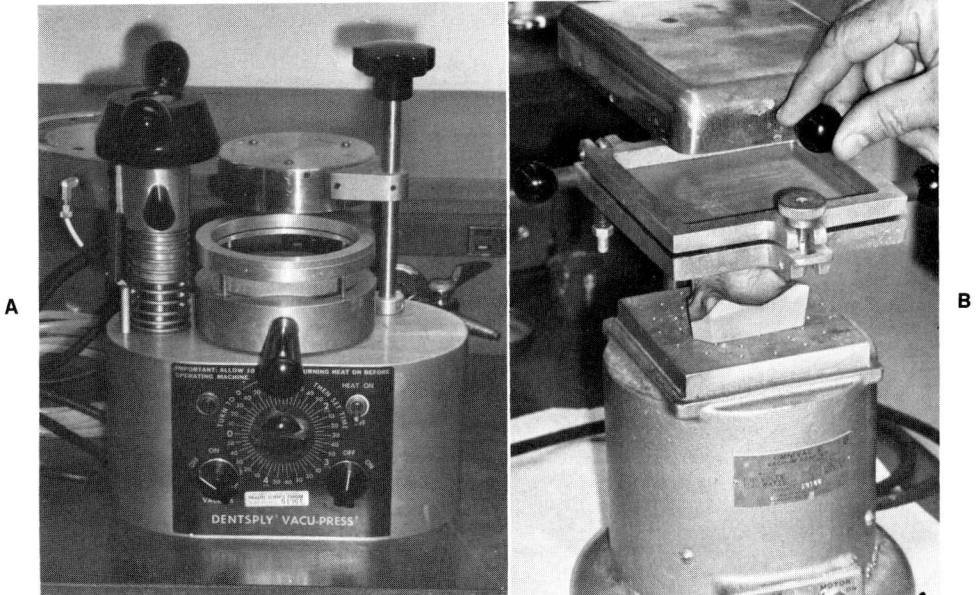

**Fig. 3-31.** Sheet of plastic is placed in heated vacuum machine. **A,** Dentsply Vacu-Press. **B,** Omnidental Omnivac.

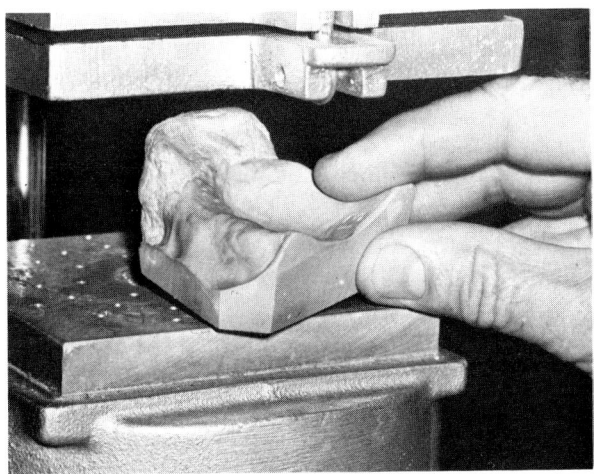

**Fig. 3-32.** Cast is placed on vacuum table, and machine is turned on.

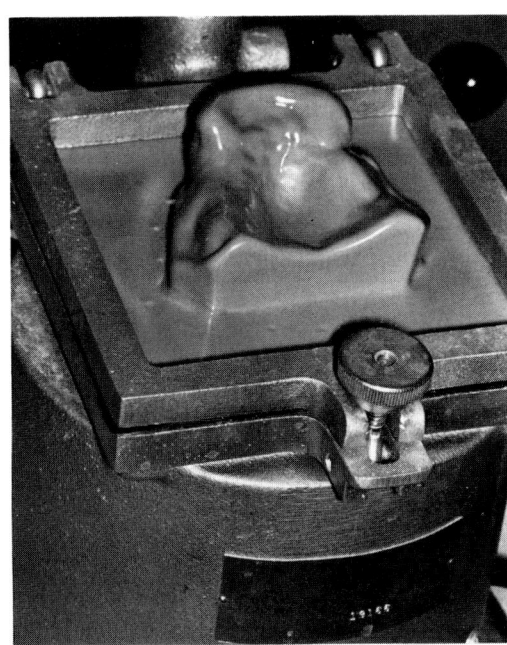

**Fig. 3-33.** Heated plastic sheet is adapted to cast by vacuum.

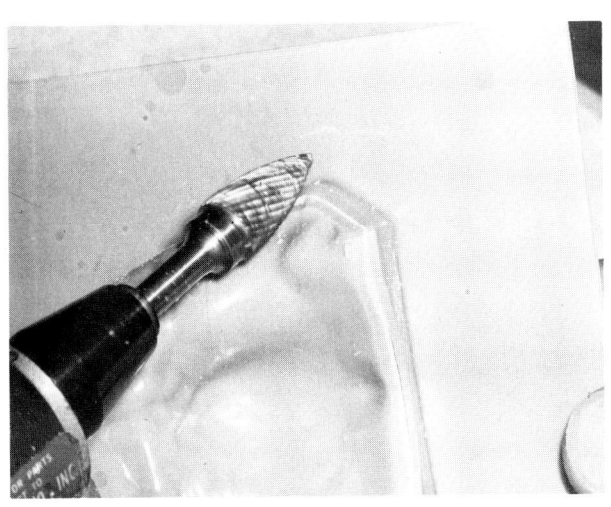

**Fig. 3-34.** Plastic is cut with vulcanite bur, and excess flash removed.

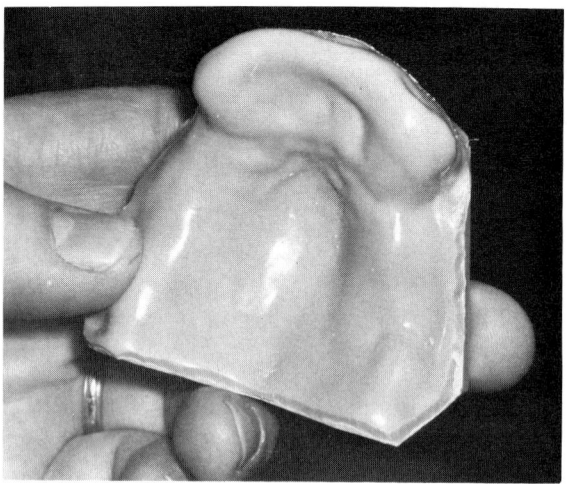

Fig. 3-35. Rough plastic tray is to be removed from cast.

5. After the excess plastic sheet is removed, remove the rough tray from the cast (Fig. 3-35).
6. Smooth the borders of the tray with a vulcanite bur or an arbor band in a bench lathe (Fig. 3-36).
7. Smooth and round the borders (Fig. 3-37). Usually the carbide bur or other arbor band will make them smooth enough. This kind of tray has a tendency to be flexible and may easily be distorted when the impression is made.
8. Try the tray on the cast, and adjust the borders if necessary (Fig. 3-38).
9. Drill numerous holes through the tray with a No. 6 or 8 round bur to lock the impression material in place when the impression is made (Fig. 3-39).

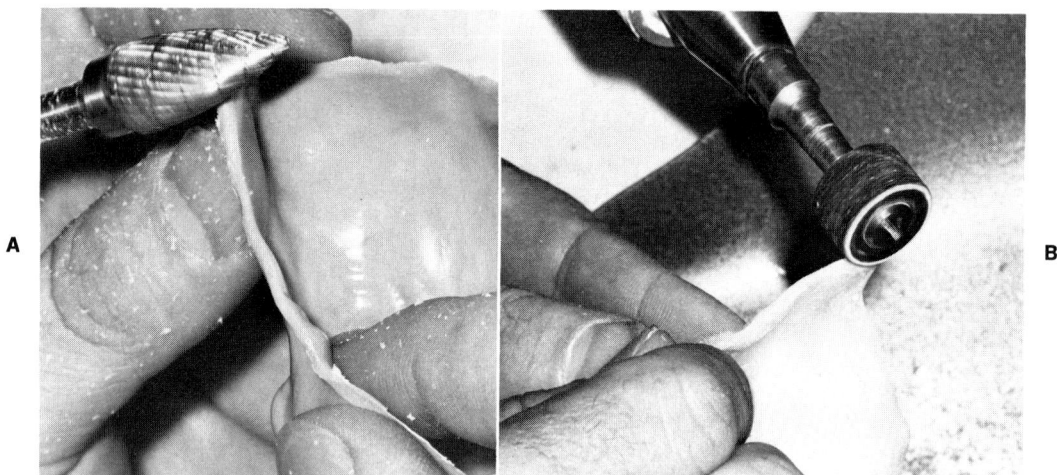

Fig. 3-36. Borders of tray are trimmed and smoothed in lathe with carbide bur **(A)**, or arbor band **(B)**.

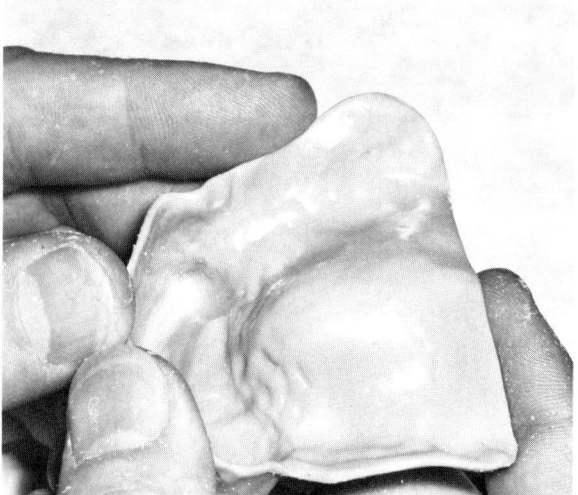

Fig. 3-37. Borders are rounded and smoothed.

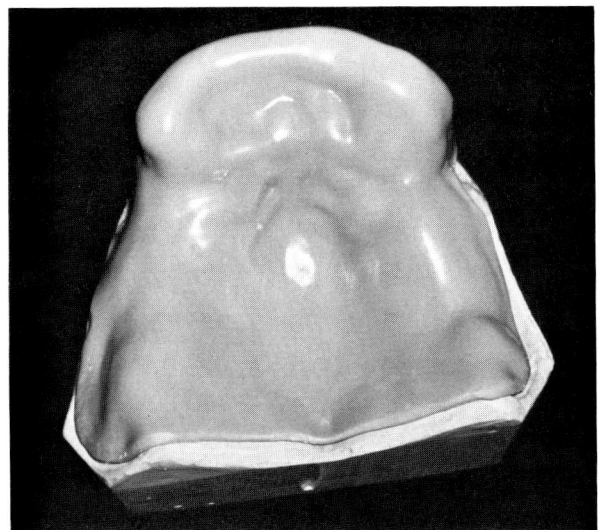

**Fig. 3-38.** Tray is replaced on cast, and borders are adjusted if necessary.

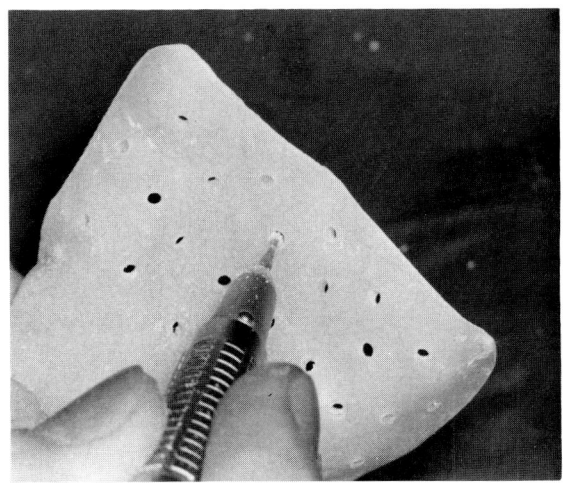

**Fig. 3-39.** Holes are drilled through tray with No. 6 or 8 round bur.

**Table 3-2.** Vacuum-adapted tray

| Problem | Probable cause | Solution |
| --- | --- | --- |
| Cast or tray broken on separation | Undercuts on teeth and cast not blocked out | Examine cast and block out teeth and undercuts with nonasbestos material |
| Tray not adapted to cast in some areas | Tray not heated sufficiently before vacuum adapting | Make certain recommended sag occurs in tray resin before activating vacuum |
| Tray too flexible | Stock material too thin | Use tray-weight resin sheet to ensure adequate rigidity |

### PROBLEM AREA

The major problem with this type of tray is its flexibility (Table 3-2).

### SUMMARY

In this chapter the requirements for impression trays for removable partial dentures, types of trays available, and methods for constructing trays from autopolymerizing resin and thermoplastic resin were described.

### BIBLIOGRAPHY

Air Force Manual 162-6: Dental laboratory technology, Washington, D.C., Jan. 22, 1975, U.S. Government Printing Office

Morrow, R. M., Rudd, K. D., and Eissmann, H. F.: Dental laboratory procedures: complete dentures, vol. 1, St. Louis, 1980, The C. V. Mosby Co.

Sowter, J. B.: Dental laboratory technology: Prosthodontic techniques, Chapel Hill, N.C., 1968, The University of North Carolina Press.

Stewart, K. L.: Removable partial denture manual, San Antonio, 1980, The University of Texas Health Science Center Dental School.

Zarb, G. A., Bergman, B., Clayton, J. A., and MacKay, H. F.: Prosthodontic treatment for partially edentulous patients, St. Louis, 1978, The C. V. Mosby Co.

# CHAPTER 4

# RECORD BASES AND MOUNTING CASTS

JAMES A. FOWLER, Jr., and WILLIAM A. KUEBKER

**diagnostic cast (study, preoperative cast)** A positive likeness of a part or parts of the oral cavity for the purpose of study and treatment planning.
**mounting** The laboratory procedure of attaching maxillary and/or mandibular casts to an articulator or similar instrument.
**occlusion rim (record rim)** Occluding surfaces built on temporary or permanent denture bases for the purpose of making maxillomandibular relation records and arranging teeth.
**record base (baseplate, temporary base, trial base)** A temporary substance, representing the base of a denture, that is used for making maxillomandibular (jaw) relation records and for the arrangement of teeth.
**stabilized record base** A baseplate lined with a plastic material to improve its fit and adaptation.

The dentist uses record bases with attached occlusion rims to record important information for the laboratory technician. The maxillomandibular jaw relationship and verification, occlusal plane, midline, and degree of vertical and horizontal overlap may be indicated on the occlusion rim that is attached to the record base. In certain instances, the record base, or baseplate, can support a platform for the development of a functionally generated path if that particular occlusal scheme is desired. Success of the partial denture treatment invariably depends on accurate transmission of the clinical findings and determinations to the laboratory for the appropriate technical phase. Certain requirements for record bases must be met to ensure that the information will be transmitted in an exacting manner.

## RECORD BASE REQUIREMENTS

Elder (1955) has suggested that record bases have the following requirements: (1) the same adaptation to the basal seat area as the finished denture base, (2) the same border form as the finished denture base, (3) sufficient rigidity to withstand occlusal forces, (4) dimensional stability, (5) construction that permits use as a base for tooth arrangement, (6) easy, quick, and inexpensive fabrication, and (7) a desirable color.

Additional requirements were specified by Tucker (1966). He stated that the record base should (1) not abrade the cast during removal or replacement, (2) take advantage of desirable undercuts present, and (3) be of a material that bonds with the material used to block out the undercuts so that it becomes an integral part of the record base.

### Clinical application

Record bases play a very important part in the diagnostic and therapeutic procedures involved in the clinical and laboratory phases of removable partial denture treatment. The dentist uses record bases in three separate phases of partial denture treatment (Fig. 4-1). In the planning phase of treatment record bases assist the dentist in obtaining an accurate mounting of the diagnostic casts. Some patients have sufficient remaining teeth to accurately hand relate the casts. In those patients with an inade-

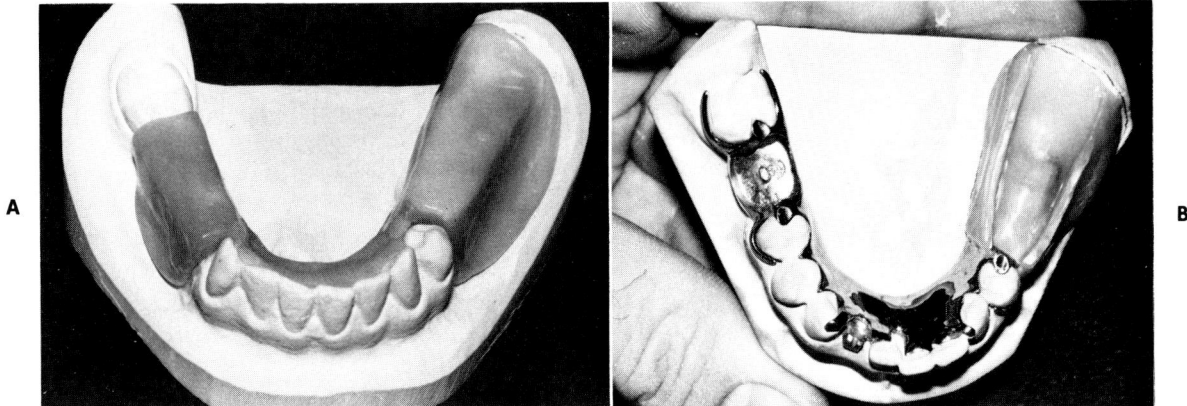

**Fig. 4-1. A,** Record bases with occlusion rims are used to accurately mount diagnostic casts for treatment planning and determine maxillomandibular relationship of master casts. **B,** Record bases stabilized with framework provide for accurate occlusal relations and tooth arrangements that satisfy functional and esthetic requirements.

quate number of teeth to confidently ascertain the maxillomandibular relationship, accurate fitting record bases may be indicated. During the second phase of treatment, record bases may be used to determine the maxillomandibular relationship of the master casts and aid the technician in fabricating the metal framework. In the third phase of treatment, the record base is attached to the cast metal framework, which will aid in the accurate occlusal relationship of the casts. Correct mounting of casts is essential for positioning the replacement teeth to satisfy functional and esthetic requirements.

In the first two treatment phases, record bases for the partially edentulous casts are essentially fabricated in the same fashion, except that in one instance the record base is made on the diagnostic cast, whereas in the second phase it is made on the master cast. During the third phase of treatment, the record base will be attached to the cast framework, and the overall stability should be improved. A stable well-fitting record base will enable the dentist to accurately record and verify the maxillomandibular relationship and later evaluate the esthetic composition of tooth arrangement.

## RECORD BASE MATERIALS

Various materials may be used to construct record bases for the removable partial denture patient: autopolymerizing resins, shellac baseplate material, heat-cured resins, baseplate wax, modeling compound, and metal. Record bases made for establishing the maxillomandibular relationship may require additional stabilization, especially if they are not attached to a partial denture framework. The stability of the record base may be enhanced by lining it with zinc oxide–eugenol impression paste,* elastomeric impression materials,† and autopolymerizing hard‡ or soft resin§ to improve the fit and provide rigidity. The rigidity can be enhanced by the addition of a stiff paper clip∥ wire in the anterior lingual area of the mandibular base and across the posterior border of the maxillary record base. The technician can also incorporate stainless steel wire clasps into the record base to provide additional stabilization.

## AUTOPOLYMERIZING RESIN RECORD BASES

Autopolymerizing resins have the same basic chemical composition as heat-cured acrylic resins, being composed of the powder polymer of methyl methacrylate and the liquid monomer of methyl methacrylate. A chemical activator such as $N,N$-dimethyl-$p$-toluidine is added to the liquid monomer to assure the liberation of a peroxide catalyst for the polymerization reaction without the addition of heat. These resins may be described as hard and rigid or soft and flexible according to the manufacturer's formulation. The flexibility of the soft resin is employed to good advantage in blocking out mild

---

*Opotow Standard ZOE impression paste, Teledyne Dental Products Co., Getz/Opotow Division, Elk Grove Village, Ill., or equivalent.
†Kerr Permlastic, Kerr Manufacturing Co., Romulus, Mich., or equivalent.
‡Fastcure, Kerr Manufacturing Co., Romulus, Mich., or equivalent.
§Coe-Soft, Coe Laboratories, Inc., Chicago, Ill., or equivalent.
∥Acco No. 1 clamps, Acco International, Inc., Chicago, Ill., or equivalent.

undercuts on the cast, whereas the hard resin makes up the bulk of the record base. Self-curing resins are frequently used to make record bases because of their reasonable cost, high degree of accuracy, and ease of manipulation. Three methods of fabricating record bases with autopolymerizing resin will be described: the sprinkle-on method, sprinkle-on method with framework, and finger-adapted dough method.

## Sprinkle-on method

In the sprinkle-on technique, the cast is thoroughly coated with a tinfoil substitute of a type that can be applied to a cold surface without leaving a thick or uneven film thickness. The polymer powder is sifted onto the cast surface and then saturated with the liquid monomer. This is done in an alternate fashion ensuring that the powder is well saturated by the liquid. After the desired thickness of resin has been attained, the cast is placed under an inverted rubber bowl, or it may be allowed to cure in a pressure pot.* Porosity of the record base may be reduced by removing it from the air and immersing it in warm water under pressure or allowing the resin to polymerize under a rubber bowl.

### PROCEDURE

1. Examine the cast carefully to identify any undercuts that may require relief (Fig. 4-2). The usual areas requiring blockout with baseplate wax or clay are the distolingual areas on the mandibular cast and the distobuccal and labial aspects of the maxillary cast. Additional wax is usually placed on the lingual interproximal tooth surfaces and around any small undercuts of the palatal rugae. The wax should be applied sparingly so as to not compromise the adaptation of the record base to the cast. Minimal undercuts can be handled through the use of a soft-curing autopolymerizing resin.* This soft resin will chemically bond with the hard resin to become an integral part of the record base, and it is possible to remove and replace the record base on the cast without abrading the surface.

2. Outline the peripheral extent of the record bases with a pencil. The outline should include the cingulum surfaces of the anterior teeth to facilitate accurate positioning of the record base in the mouth (Fig. 4-3).

3. Blockout any severe undercuts and the interproximal areas with baseplate wax to prevent the acrylic resin from extending into undercut areas (Fig. 4-4).

4. Adapt a heavy-duty wire paper clip to the lingual aspect of the mandibular cast from first molar to first molar area. The wire reinforcement will significantly improve the rigidity and strength of the record base (Fig. 4-5).

5. Place beading or utility wax along the pencil outline on the cast to confine the resin. Additional wax should be added to the proximal tooth surfaces to prevent their breakage (Fig. 4-6).

---

*Acri-Dense Pneumatic Curing Unit, Coe Laboratories, Inc., Chicago, Ill., or equivalent.

*Coe-Soft, Coe Laboratories, Inc., Chicago, Ill., or equivalent.

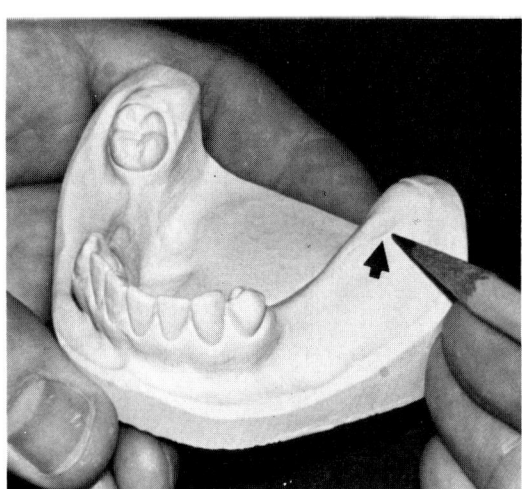

**Fig. 4-2.** Undercut requiring relief (arrow).

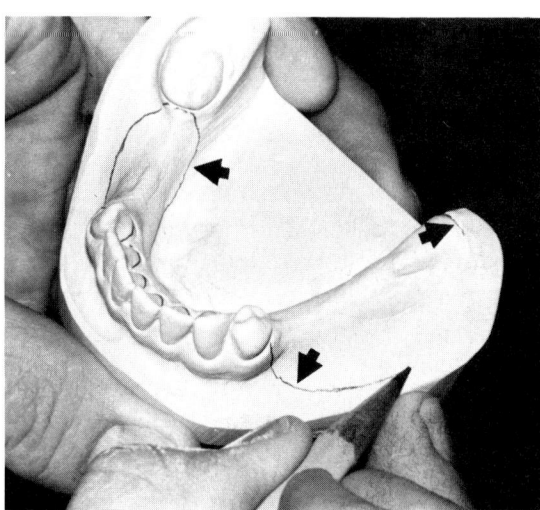

**Fig. 4-3.** Peripheral extent of acrylic resin record base is outlined with pencil (arrows).

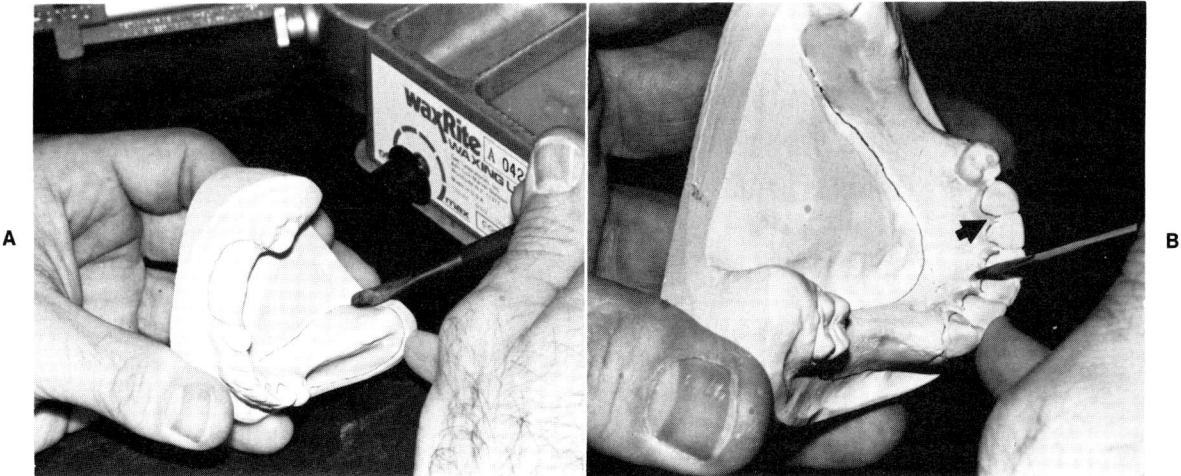

**Fig. 4-4. A,** Severe undercuts blocked out with baseplate wax. **B,** Additional wax is flowed into interproximal tooth areas (arrow).

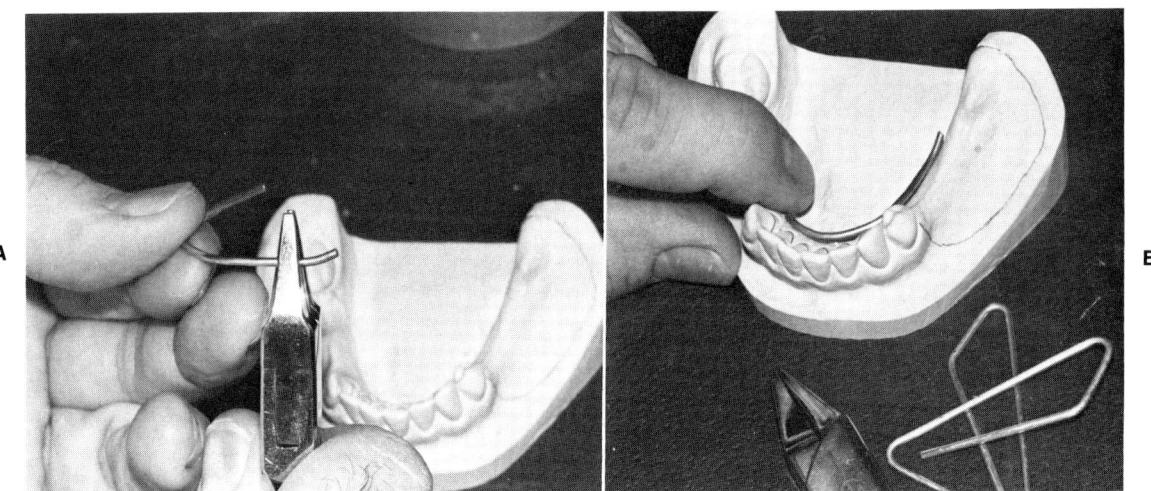

**Fig. 4-5. A,** Heavy-duty paper clip wire is adapted for reinforcement. **B,** Reinforcement wire is positioned on lingual aspect of mandibular cast from first molar to first molar.

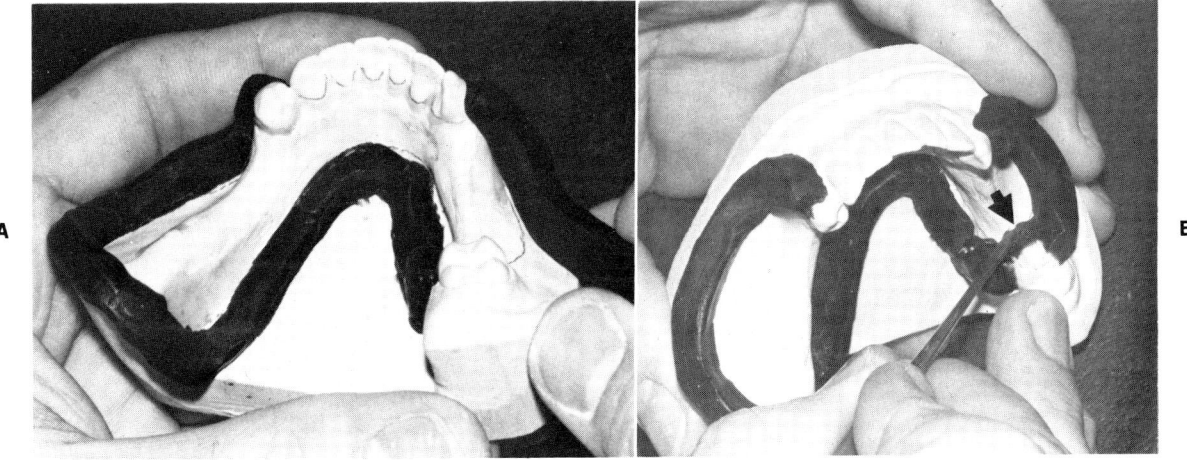

**Fig. 4-6. A,** Beading wax is placed along pencil outline to confine acrylic resin. **B,** Proximal tooth surfaces (arrow) are lightly covered with wax to protect tooth from fracture.

6. Place the cast in a slurry solution for 8 to 10 minutes (Fig. 4-7), shake off the excess moisture, and carefully paint a tinfoil substitute* on all areas that will be contacted by the acrylic resin (Fig. 4-8).

7. Fill minimal undercuts that exist with soft-curing autopolymerizing resin that will become a part of the finished record base. The soft-curing resin can be added to the cast by three means. Mix the resin powder and liquid together, and apply it to the undercuts with a spatula or other suitable instrument (Fig. 4-9). It can be brushed onto the surface by immersing the brush in the liquid monomer, picking up the polymer powder, and applying the soft resin to the undercut area (Fig. 4-10). The soft-curing resin can also be applied by alternately sprinkling on the monomer and polymer (Fig. 4-11).

8. Sometimes the soft-curing resin will tend to flow out of the undercut area, resulting in a thin covering that will not flex over the cast prominence. To offset this, apply heat carefully by either warming the resin surface with an alcohol torch or immersing the cast into hot water for a few seconds to accelerate surface polymerization and maintain the thickness (Fig. 4-12).

9. Sprinkle the autopolymerizing hard-resin powder onto the cast surface, and wet it with the liquid monomer. Select a resin with a nonfibered polymer to facilitate pouring the powder through the dispenser aperture. The powder can be readily applied from a plastic spray bottle or a large flexible plastic container such as a mustard dispenser (Fig. 4-13). An eyedropper or plastic bottle dispenser can

---

*Modern Foil, Modern Materials Manufacturing Co., St. Louis, Mo.; Alcote, The L. D. Caulk Co., Milford, Del., or equivalent.

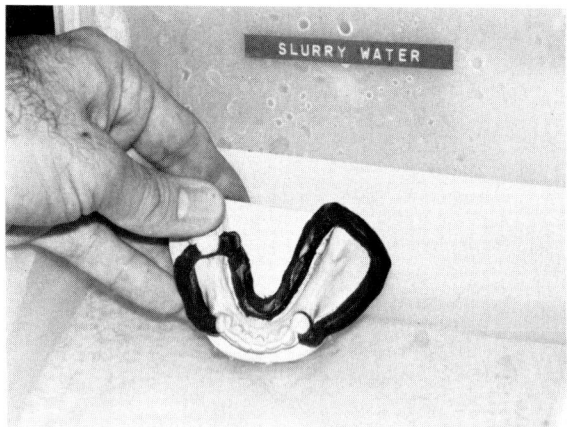

Fig. 4-7. Cast is soaked in slurry solution for 8 to 10 minutes.

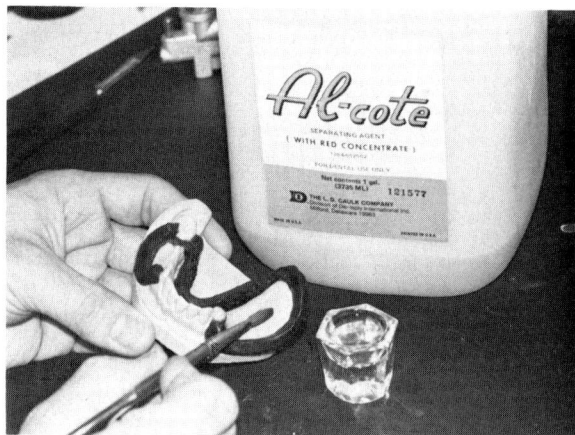

Fig. 4-8. Tinfoil substitute is painted on cast surface.

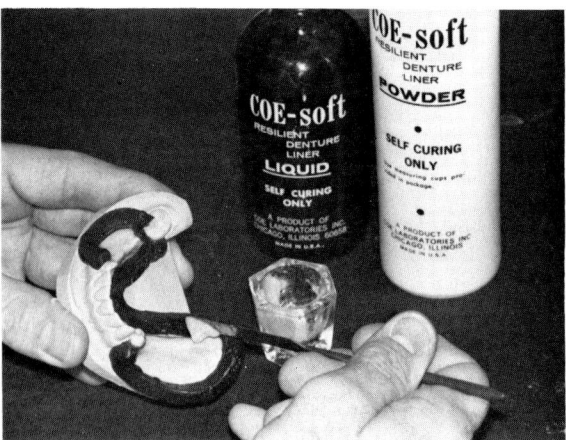

Fig. 4-9. Soft-curing autopolymerizing resin is placed into moderate undercuts with cement spatula.

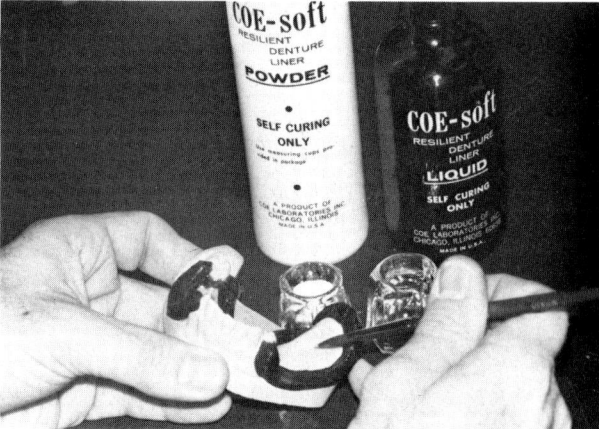

Fig. 4-10. Brush can be used to paint on soft-curing resin.

**Fig. 4-11.** Soft-curing autopolymerizing resin powder can be sifted onto cast surface and then moistened with monomer as alternate method.

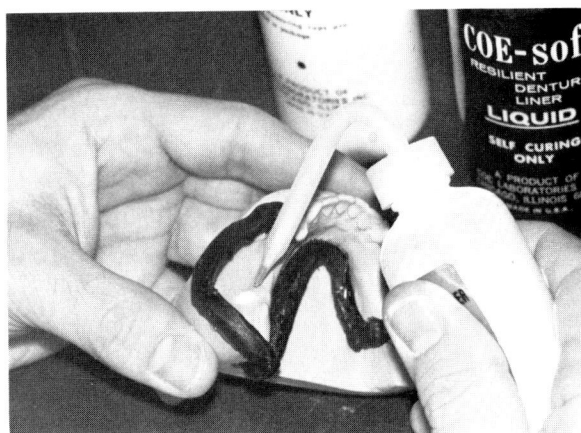

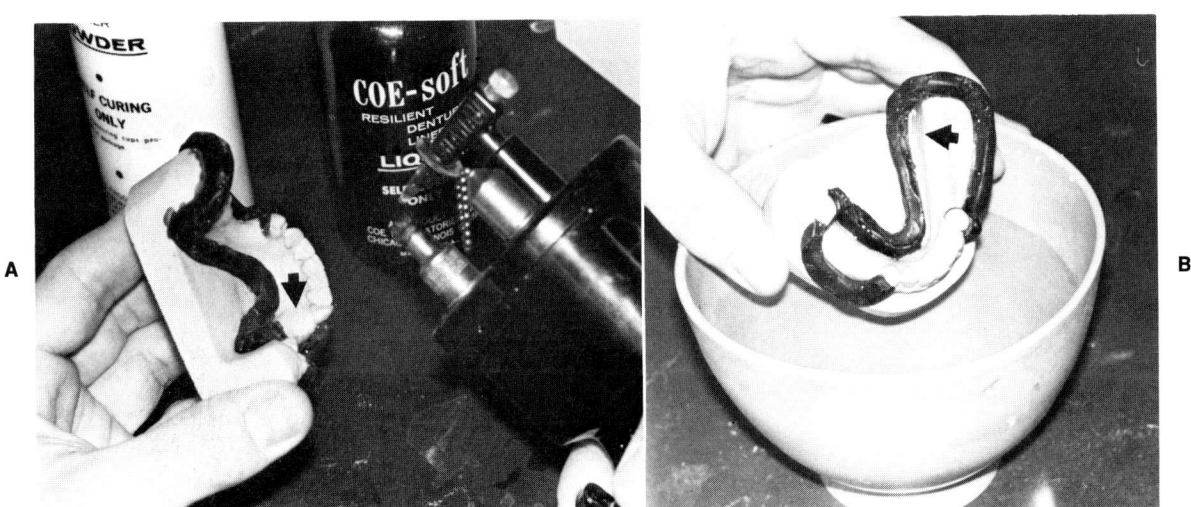

**Fig. 4-12. A,** Resin surface is warmed with torch to effect surface "set" (arrow). This will prevent resin from flowing out of undercut. **B,** Cast can be dipped into hot water to accelerate polymerization of resin and maintain its position (arrow).

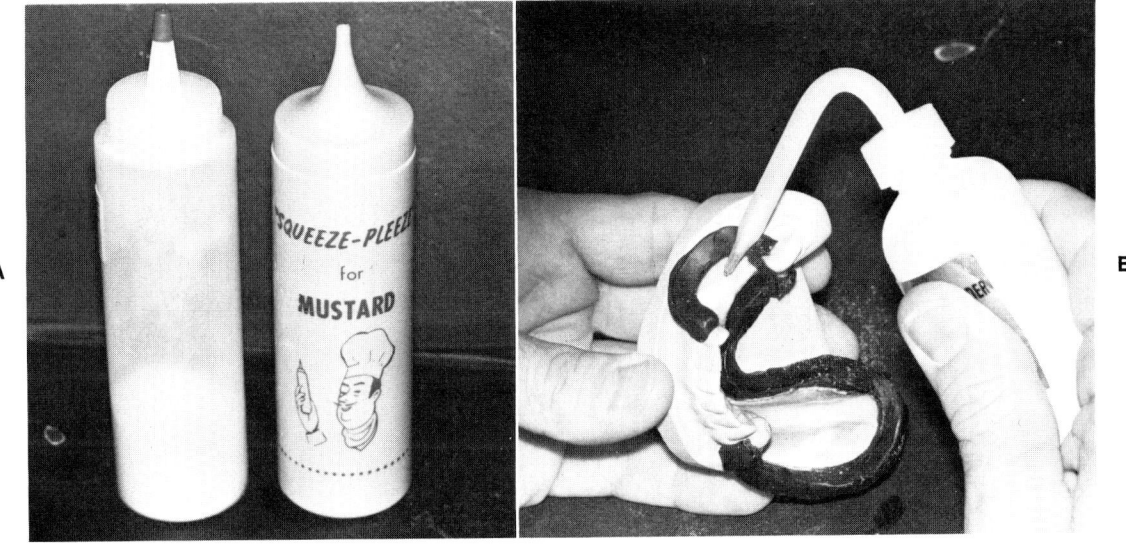

**Fig. 4-13. A,** Plastic mustard dispensers can be used to apply acrylic resin powder. **B,** Plastic dispenser bottle is also convenient means to sift polymer powder onto cast surface. Use of nonfibered acrylic resin powder will facilitate pouring.

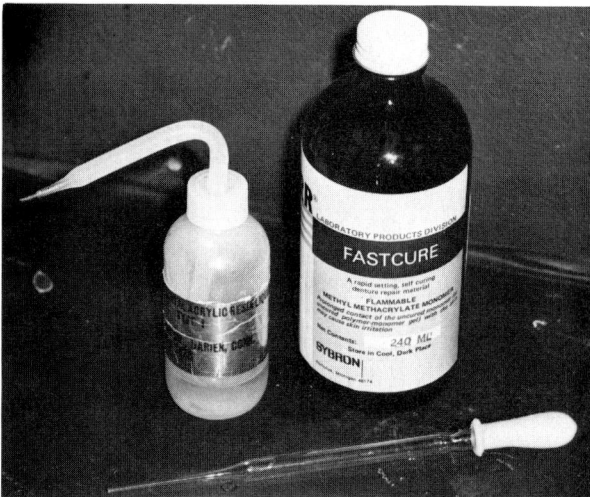

**Fig. 4-14.** Liquid monomer is applied from eyedropper or plastic dispenser bottle.

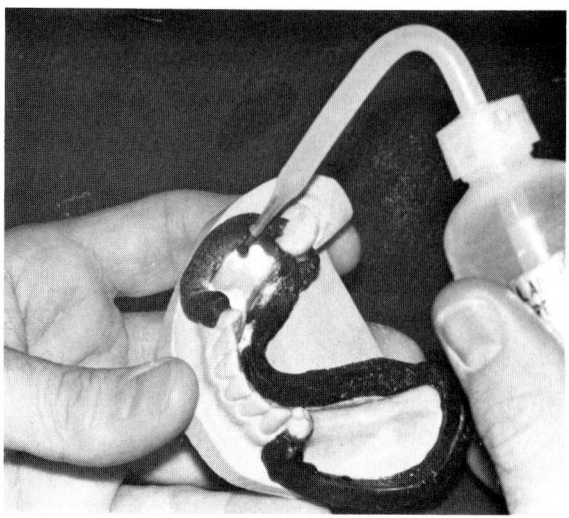

**Fig. 4-15.** Cast is tilted at 45-degree angle while applying resin, and then cast is tilted in opposite direction to control resin thickness.

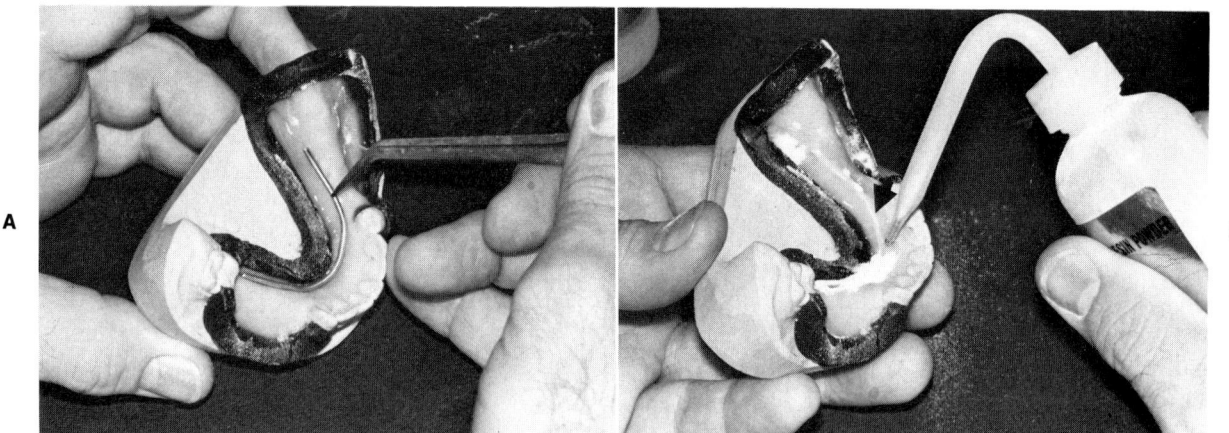

**Fig. 4-16. A,** Reinforcement wire is positioned on lingual aspect of cast. **B,** Additional acrylic resin is placed over wire (arrow) to ensure smooth contour.

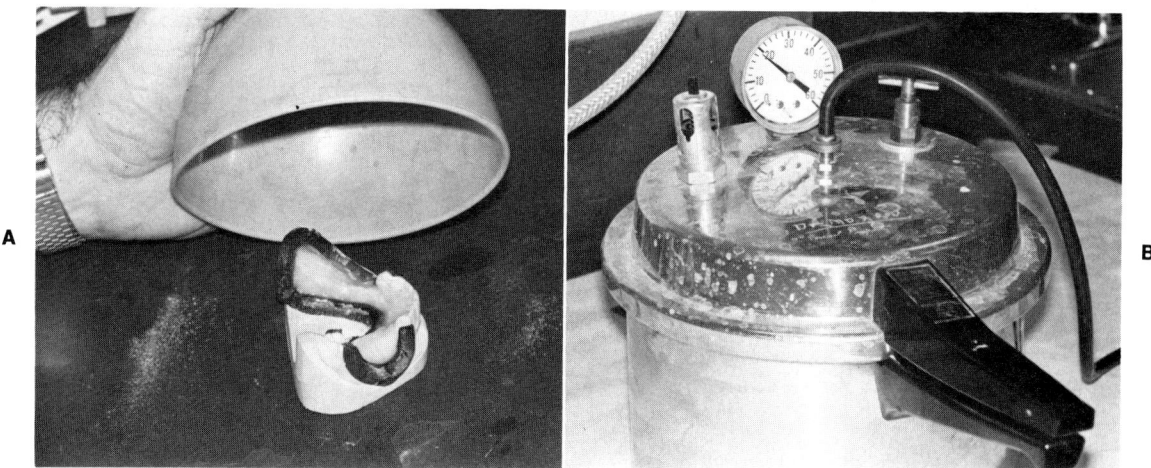

**Fig. 4-17. A,** Curing resin record base under inverted rubber bowl reduces porosity and improves fit. **B,** Curing record base at 20 psi significantly reduces porosity, but does not appear to fit cast as well as one cured at atmospheric pressure.

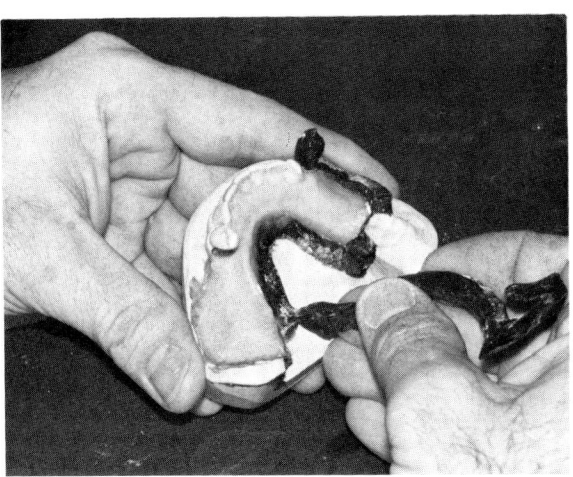

**Fig. 4-18.** After beading wax has been removed, adaption of record base is evaluated.

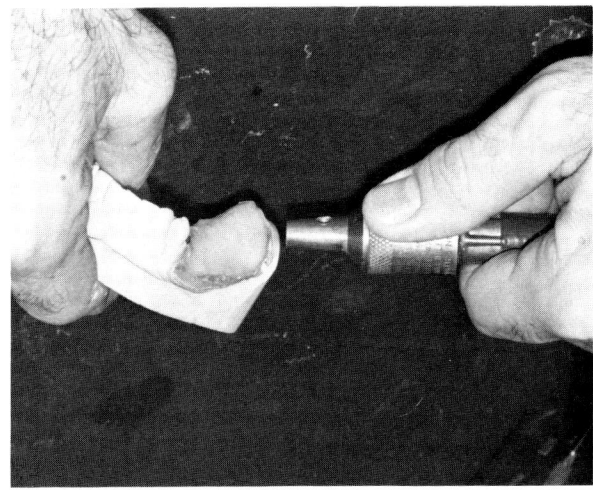

**Fig. 4-19.** In many instances, record base can be removed by directing blast of air under resin.

be used to apply the liquid monomer (Fig. 4-14). The powder and liquid are alternately applied until the desired uniform thickness of approximately 2 mm is achieved. To prevent an undesirable buildup of resin, tilt the cast at about a 45-degree angle (Fig. 4-15). Apply the resin to the upward surfaces, allow it to set for 1 or 2 minutes, and then tilt the cast in the opposite direction, and complete the remaining surfaces.

10. Embed the previously contoured wire to provide additional strength and stability. Cover the wire with additional acrylic resin to establish smooth contours (Fig. 4-16).

11. Cure the record base by covering it with an inverted rubber bowl, or place the cast in the pressure pot with warm water for 20 minutes at 20 psi (Fig. 4-17). Some surface porosity may be apparent when the record base is cured under normal atmospheric pressure, but the fit appears to be improved when compared to those cured in the pressure pot.

12. Remove the beading wax, and evaluate the adaptation of the cured record base on the cast (Fig. 4-18). The record base should be carefully removed from the cast. If no framework is attached, the record base can often be lifted from the cast by directing a blast of air under the periphery and then gently lifting (Fig. 4-19). When prying is required, it should be done on the side opposite the undercut (Fig. 4-20). To facilitate removal, the cast can be immersed in a solution of clear slurry water. The water flowing between the cast and the resin acts as a lubricant and aids in the separation.

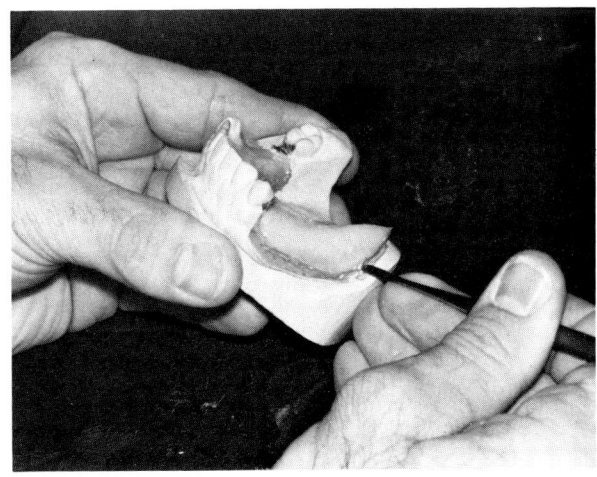

**Fig. 4-20.** When there is requirement to pry record base from cast, it should be done carefully on side opposite undercut to preclude breakage.

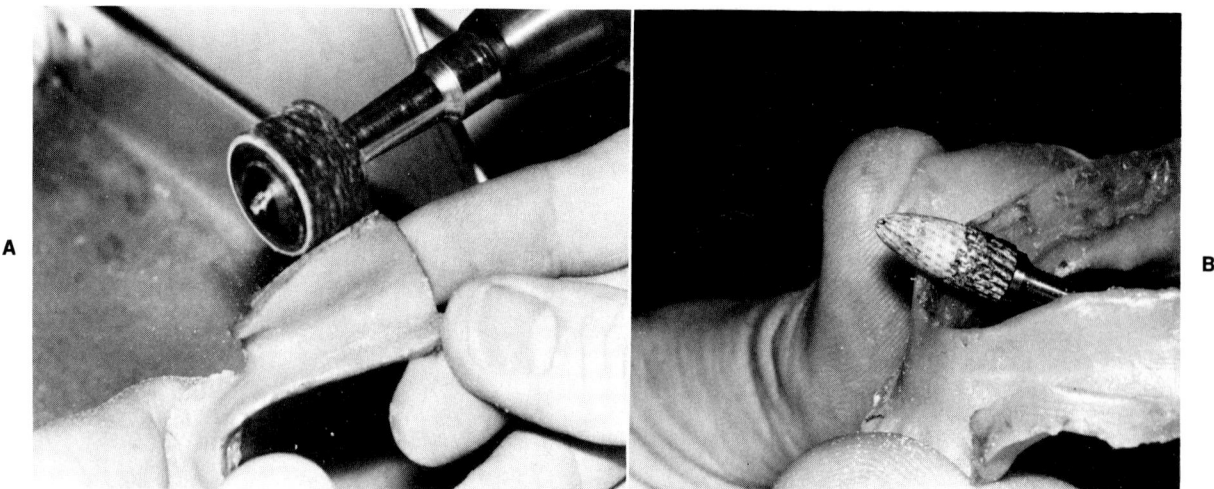

**Fig. 4-21. A,** Resin flash can be removed with lathe-mounted arbor band. **B,** Smaller, inaccessible border areas can be trimmed with carbide laboratory bur.

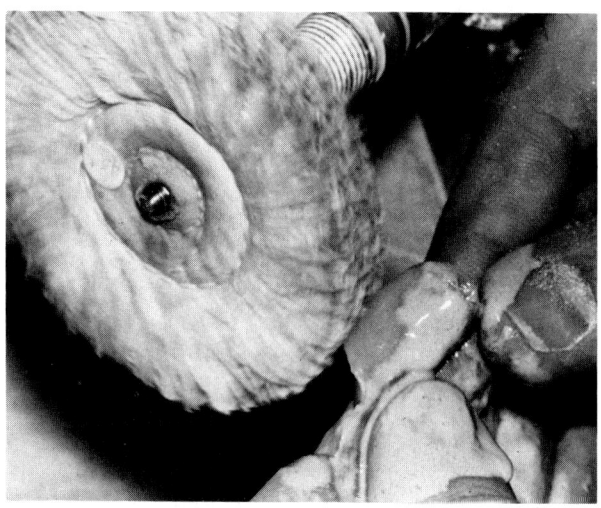

**Fig. 4-22.** Record base borders are polished with flour of pumice slurry and wet rag wheel at low (1740 rpm) speed to control heat buildup and diminish warpage.

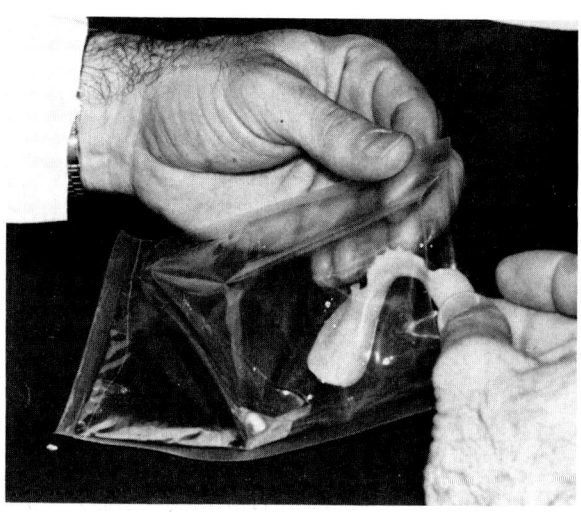

**Fig. 4-23.** Completed record base can be conveniently stored in sealed plastic bag with water until ready for use.

13. Remove the acrylic resin flash from the record base border by using a lathe-mounted arbor band, carbide laboratory bur, or resin-cutting stone (Fig. 4-21). The acrylic resin should be trimmed to create a border of approximately 2 mm thickness. Wear protective glasses during this procedure.

14. Smooth the record base borders using a slurry of water and flour of pumice applied with a wet rag wheel. A slow lathe speed (1740 rpm) will reduce heat buildup to the record base and facilitate its manipulation. Heat generated from polishing can affect the accuracy of fit by warping the record base; for this reason, the polishing should be intermittent and limited to the border extensions (Fig. 4-22).

15. Place the completed resin record base in a sealed plastic bag with water to prevent distortion due to dehydration (Fig. 4-23).

### Sprinkle-on method with framework

When the framework has been completed, it can be incorporated with the record base to provide a stable means for assisting the dentist in achieving the maxillomandibular relationship and determining tooth arrangement.

## Record bases and mounting casts 81

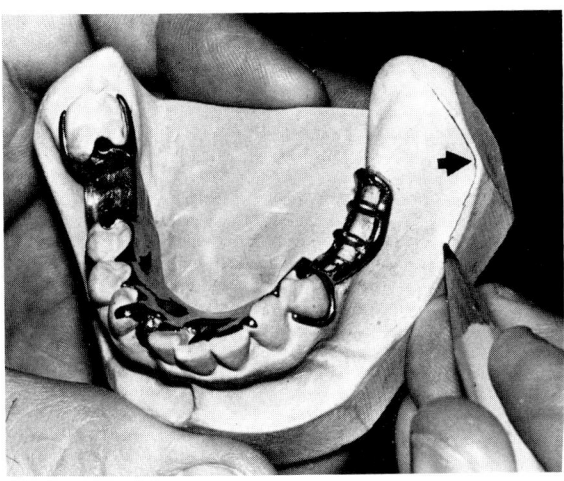

Fig. 4-24. With framework seated in its terminal position, peripheral extent of record base is outlined (arrow).

### PROCEDURE

The procedures for constructing an autopolymerizing resin record base attached to the framework are similar to making a record base for the diagnostic cast.

1. Seat the framework on the cast in its terminal position, and outline the peripheral extent (Fig. 4-24).

2. Remove the framework, identify any undercuts that require relief, and block out severe undercuts with baseplate wax (Fig. 4-25). Paint the edentulous area of the cast with tinfoil substitute (Fig. 4-26).

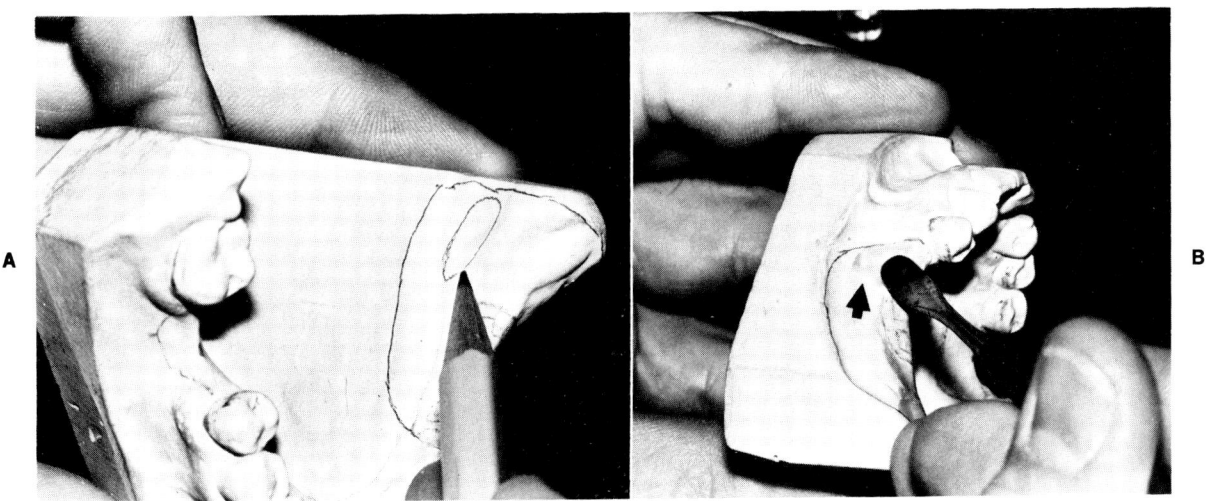

Fig. 4-25. **A,** Undercuts requiring relief are identified. **B,** Severe undercuts blocked out with baseplate wax (arrow).

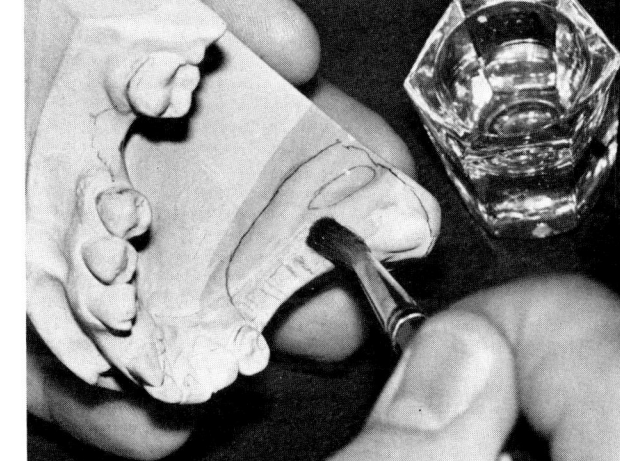

Fig. 4-26. Liberal coating of tinfoil substitute is painted onto cast surface.

3. Replace the framework, and place beading wax along the pencil outline to confine the acrylic resin when it is applied (Fig. 4-27).

4. Fill minimal undercuts with soft-curing autopolymerizing resin, and warm the resin surface slightly to accelerate the set (Fig. 4-28).

5. Sprinkle the hard-curing autopolymerizing resin powder onto the cast surface, and wet it with monomer (Fig. 4-29). Repeat this step until the desired thickness is attained.

6. Cure the record base under an inverted rubber bowl or in a pressure pot (Fig. 4-30).

7. Remove the beading wax, and inspect the adaptation of the resin to the cast (Fig. 4-31). Carefully remove the record base by teasing it and the clasps very gently to avoid damage (Fig. 4-32).

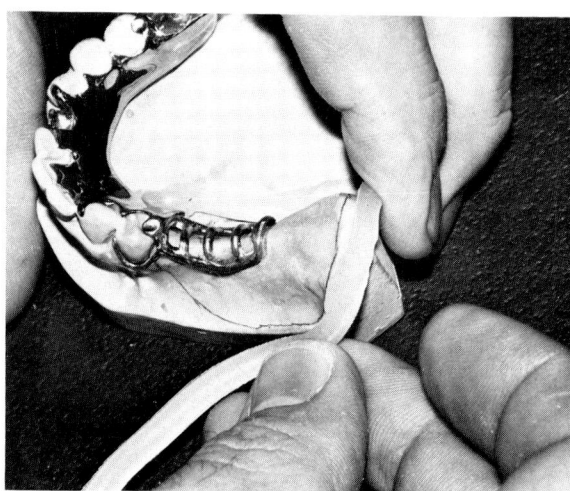

**Fig. 4-27.** Utility wax is placed along penciled outline to limit resin border.

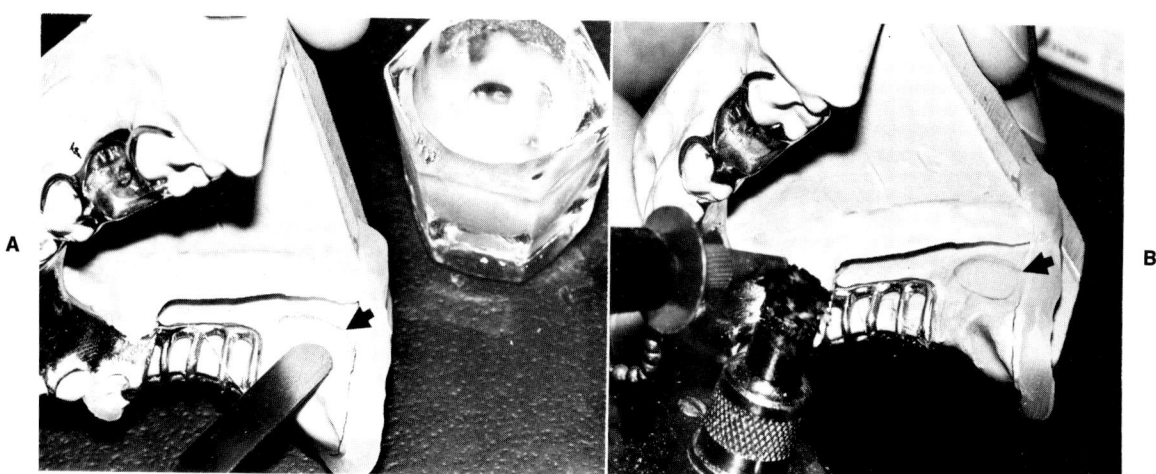

**Fig. 4-28. A,** Cement spatula is used to place soft-curing autopolymerizing resin into moderate undercuts (arrow). **B,** Soft-curing resin (arrow) is warmed slightly, producing surface "set" to control flow.

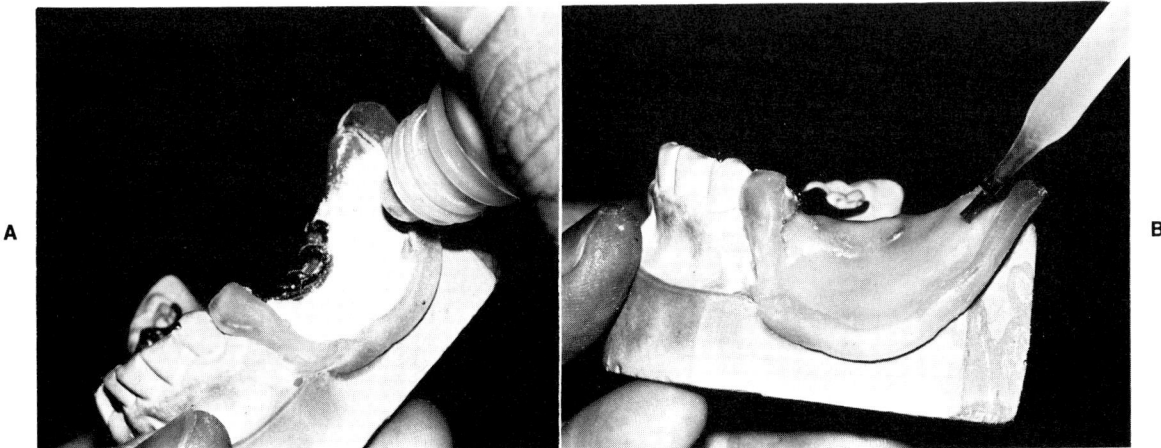

**Fig. 4-29. A,** Cast is tilted at 45-degree angle while powder is sifted onto cast. **B,** Plastic dispenser is used to control amount of monomer applied.

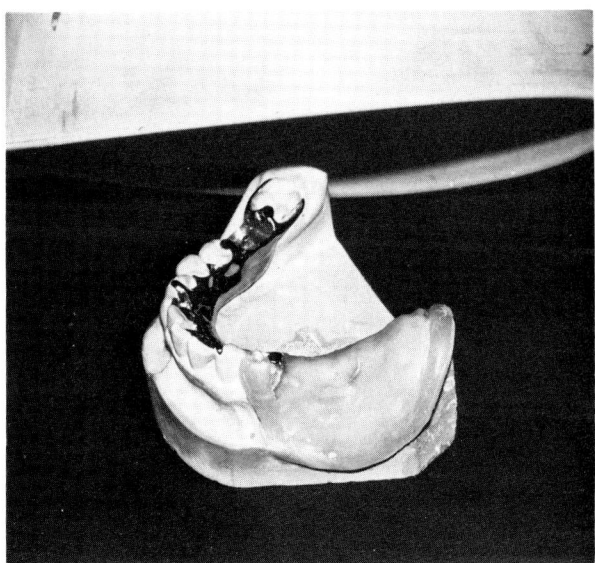

**Fig. 4-30.** Curing of resin record base is accomplished under inverted plaster bowl.

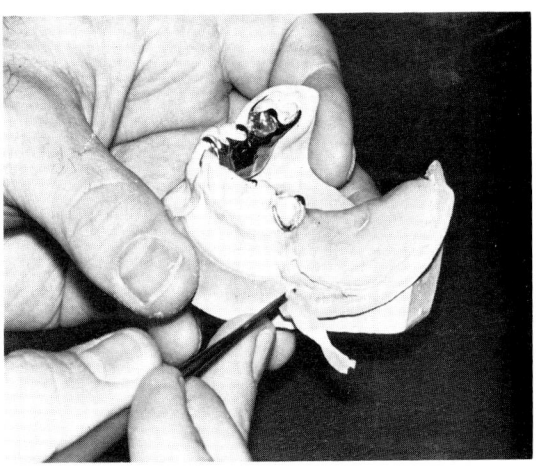

**Fig. 4-31.** Utility wax is removed and adaptation evaluated.

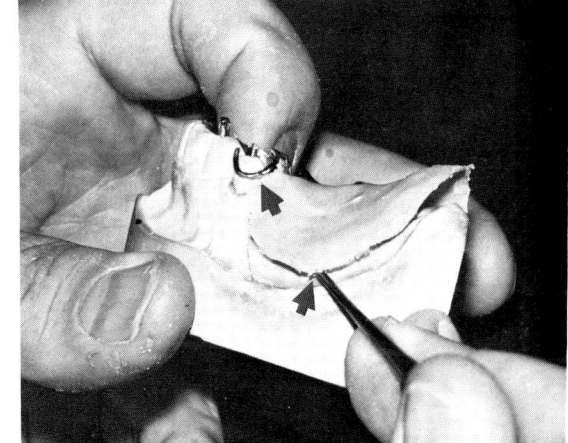

**Fig. 4-32.** Record base can be removed by gently prying on clasp shoulder and base (arrows) opposite any undercuts.

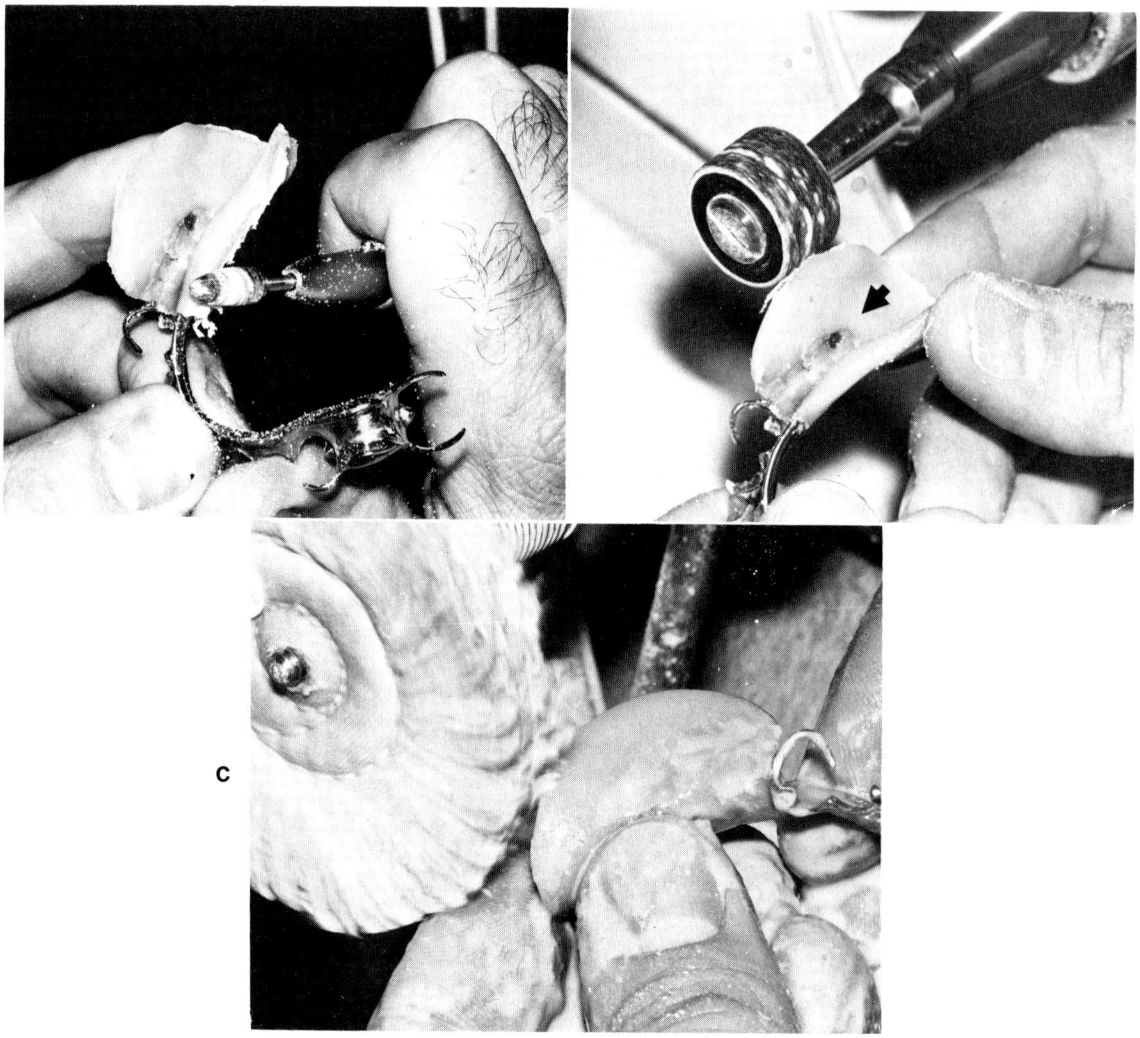

**Fig. 4-33.** **A,** Resin flash can be removed with carbide bur mounted in handpiece. **B,** Lathe-mounted arbor band can also be used to trim resin border. Note show through of tissue rest (arrow) that indicates complete seating of framework. **C,** Flour of pumice slurry and wet rag wheel are used to polish border of record base. Intermittent pressure and slow speed are used to minimize production of heat and subsequent warpage.

8. Trim the border areas with a carbide bur and/or arbor band, then smooth and lightly polish them with pumice (Fig. 4-33).

9. Place the record base back on the cast, and determine that the framework occlusal rests are fully seated (Fig. 4-34). Store the record base in a sealed bag with water to prevent distortion.

### PROBLEM AREAS

Occasionally, some difficulties can occur in constructing a record base using the sprinkle-on method. Table 4-1 lists the problem areas along with their probable causes and practical solutions.

1. *The record base cannot be separated from the cast without damage to one or both during removal.* The usual cause of this problem is failure to locate existing undercuts and block them out properly.

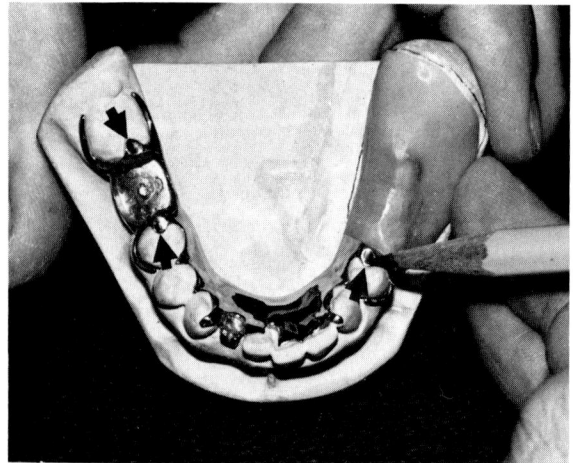

**Fig. 4-34.** Properly adapted record base should ensure complete seating of all framework occlusal rests (arrows).

**Table 4-1.** Sprinkle-on method

| Problem | Probable cause | Solution |
| --- | --- | --- |
| Teeth chipped or broken during removal | Interproximal and gingival tooth areas not blocked out with wax | Flow baseplate wax in gingival crest and interproximal areas to provide blockout |
| Record base removed from cast with difficulty | Insufficient blockout of undercuts | Block out moderate undercuts with soft-curing resin; extensive undercuts are blocked out with wax |
| Breakage of record base during removal | Cast coated with contaminated tinfoil substitute | Paint ample coating of uncontaminated tinfoil substitute before applying resin |
| Cast chipped or broken during separation | Cast coated with contaminated tinfoil substitute | Insure soft-curing resin is thick enough to spring over moderate undercuts |
| Record base lacks uniform thickness | Resin flows from prominent areas to lower peripheral areas of the cast | Control flow of resin by tilting cast while sprinkling on powder; use sufficient powder to prevent pooling |
| Completed record base too flexible | Improper ratio of soft-curing resin to hard-setting resin in undercut areas | Use only enough soft-curing resin to fill undercut; apply adequate overlay of hard-setting resin |
| | Use of wrong liquid or powder for hard-setting resin | Use correct liquid and powder for soft-curing and hard-curing resin systems |
| | Record base removed from cast before polymerization is complete | Allow adequate time interval for polymerization of resin |
| | Inadequate thickness of record base resin | Reinforce record bases by embedding heavy-duty paper clip wire |
| Porosity of record base | Drying out of resin during application | Keep all surfaces moist with monomer during resin buildup |
| | | Cure record base in atmosphere of monomer under inverted plastic bowl or covered with water in pressure pot |
| Failure of record base to fit cast | Removal of record base from the cast before adequate polymerization | Cure resin adequately before removing record base from cast |
| | Distortion of record base by excessive grinding and/or polishing | Do not overheat record base; use slow speed with slurry of water and flour of pumice |
| | Storage of record base in dry environment | Store finished record base in sealed plastic bag with water |
| | Warpage of record base from prying it off cast | Block out undercuts to facilitate removal of record base with minimal prying |

Use of a surveyor will help to identify the severe undercuts and confirm their proper blockout with wax. Interproximal and gingival tooth areas should be blocked out with wax to prevent breakage. Moderate tissue undercuts can be handled with a soft-curing resin, but there must be an adequate amount of the soft-curing resin present to spring over the undercut. The surface of the soft-curing resin can be warmed slightly with a torch to ensure that it is stationary until the hard-setting autopolymerizing resin is applied. Failure to paint the cast properly, or use of contaminated tinfoil substitute may allow the resin record base to adhere to the stone cast. When removal is attempted, the cast frequently fractures as it adheres to the acrylic resin surface. Contamination can be avoided by pouring a small amount of tinfoil substitute from the main container into a small cup and applying the solution to the cast from this source. After use, the remainder of this small contaminated portion is discarded, thus the effectiveness of the main supply is maintained.

2. *The record base lacks uniform thickness.* The fluid resin has a tendency to flow from prominent areas and pool in the lower peripheral areas and, in particular, the palatal area of the maxillary cast. By tilting the cast and controlling the viscosity with adequate polymer powder, the overall thickness of the record base can be controlled. Thinness over prominent cast areas can be avoided by exercising care when sifting the polymer powder in these regions.

3. *The record base lacks rigidity.* This situation may result from an inadequate thickness of the hard-setting acrylic resin. When too much soft-curing resin is used in proportion to the overlying application of hard-setting resin, the record base will lack strength. This is seen particularly in the lingual area of the mandibular record base. Use of the wrong liquid or powder when applying the overlying hard-setting resin will result in a record base that is too flexible. The respective hard and soft resin systems should be clearly identified and their use carefully monitored to prevent any mix-up during application. Mandibular bilateral distal extension record bases frequently are too flexible and require additional strength. A piece of heavy-duty paper clip wire can be suitably shaped and used for reinforcement. The wire should extend from first molar to first molar and be embedded within the lingual surface of the resin baseplate.

4. *The record base shows porosity.* Surface porosity is not critical unless it is so extensive that the strength is compromised and the record base is unhygienic. The polymer powder should be thoroughly wetted with the liquid monomer, and the construction procedure should not be interrupted until completion. The acrylic resin surface should be moistened continually and the last step in the sprinkle-on technique should be an overall saturation with monomer. The cast is covered with an inverted bowl to achieve final polymerization in a saturated monomer atmosphere that should reduce surface monomer evaporation. Surface porosity can also be reduced by curing the resin in a pressure pot at 20 psi for 20 to 30 minutes.

5. *The record base fails to accurately fit the cast.* This can occur when the record base is prematurely removed from the cast before sufficient polymerization has occurred. Warpage can also result from the production of heat through excessive trimming and polishing procedures and when the record base is stored in a dry environment. The cured record base can be distorted by excessive prying when removing it from the cast. Warpage can be diminished by allowing the acrylic resin to polymerize on the cast for $1/2$ hour. Avoid overheating the record base by using copious amounts of water and flour of pumice while polishing with the slow-speed (1740 rpm) lathe. Avoid prying the record base from the cast by properly blocking out the undercuts; if prying is required, use minimal pressure opposite the undercut on the cast.

### Finger-adapted dough method

Acrylic resin systems that are normally used in the fabrication of impression trays can also be used to make record bases. With this system, the polymer powder is mixed together with the liquid monomer until a dough consistency is reached. The resin dough can be rolled to a controlled thickness with a roller on a wooden block and then fitted to the cast using finger adaptation. This method for making record bases may take less time than the sprinkle-on method, but several disadvantages are apparent. Although this method begins with a resin of uniform thickness, the adaptation to the cast with the fingers often results in areas of varying resin thickness. Prominent areas over the ridge crest are frequently too thin, whereas the less accessible areas, such as the buccal and lingual vestibules and the palate, may be too thick. Unless the operator is protected with suitable gloves, the resin may be contaminated by contact with normal body oils from the skin surface. Another more serious complication is the development of contact dermatitis to the operator through exposure of the skin surface to the resin. It is has also been observed that as the polymerization reaction occurs, there is a tendency for the resin to rebound or pull away from the cast. To counter this the operator must continue adapting the resin until it has reached its final set. This procedure may result in some distortion of the resin record base to the cast.

#### PROCEDURE

1. Examine the cast, and evaluate the location and extent of undercuts present (Fig. 4-35). Control the extent of the record base periphery by adapting a caulking material* to the appropriate areas. This

---

*DAP Rope Caulk, DAP, Inc., Dayton, Ohio.

will prevent the resin from entering undercut areas that would lock the record base and prevent its removal from the cast. Block out other undercuts with baseplate wax (Fig. 4-36).

2. Soak the cast in a clear slurry solution for 10 minutes to aid in the separation of the record base from the cast. Shake off the excess moisture, and apply tinfoil substitute to the cast surface (Fig. 4-37).

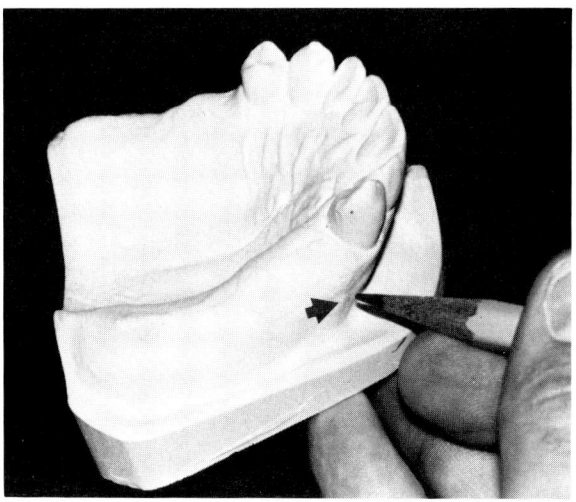

**Fig. 4-35.** Extent of any undercut (arrow) is determined on cast.

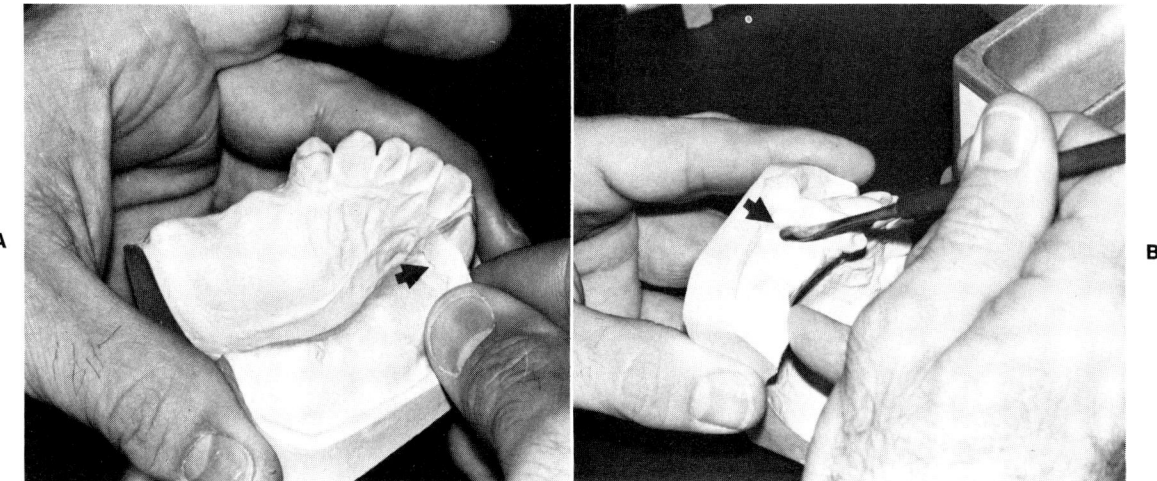

**Fig. 4-36. A,** Caulking material (arrow) is adapted to cast to confine resin. **B,** Baseplate wax is used to blockout severe undercuts (arrow).

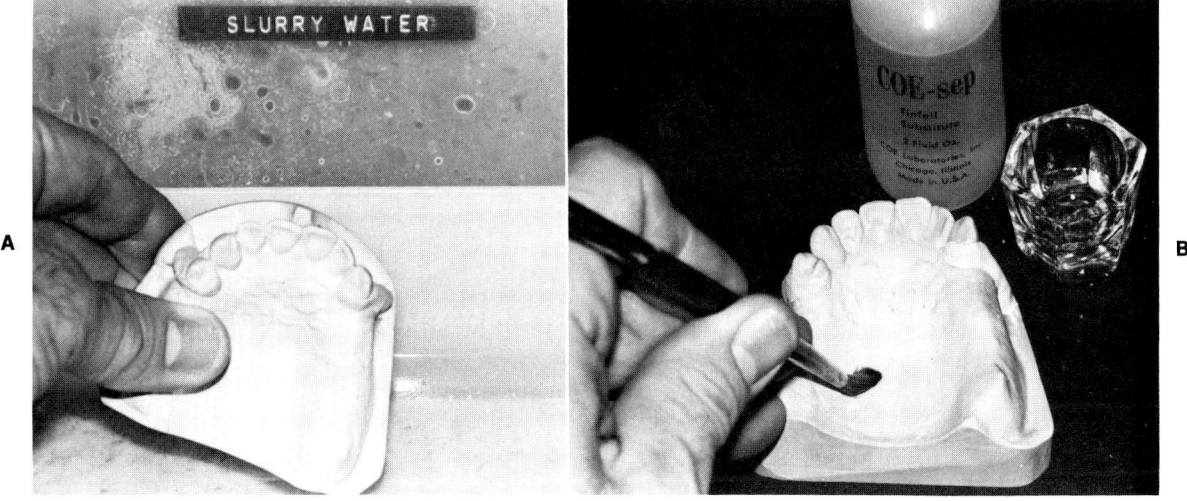

**Fig. 4-37. A,** Cast is soaked in clear slurry water for 10 minutes. **B,** Tinfoil substitute is painted on cast surface.

3. Coat the wooden tray and roller* with a silicone lubricant† to prevent the resin from sticking to the surface (Fig. 4-38).

4. Proportion the resin powder and liquid monomer,‡ and mix them together in a cup according to the manufacturer's directions (Fig. 4-39). When the resin reaches the dough stage, it should be placed on the wooden block (Fig. 4-40). Handling the resin can be facilitated by using a cellophane sheet. The thickness of the resin can be controlled initially by rolling it into a sheet on the wooden block (Fig. 4-41).

5. Trim the resin sheet into the appropriate shape, and adapt it to the prepared cast. Remove excess resin while in the dough stage by trimming with a cement spatula (Fig. 4-42).

6. Adapt the resin to the cast surface with the fingers (Fig. 4-43). Continue this finger adaptation until the resin does not rebound or pull away from the cast.

7. Cover the adapted record base on the cast with a rubber bowl while polymerization occurs. As an alternative, the record base and cast could also be placed in a pressure pot as previously described.

8. After polymerization has occurred, remove the record base from the cast, and determine the areas to be trimmed (Fig. 4-44). Trim the periphery of the record base with a lathe-mounted arbor band as described previously.

---

*Coe Tray Plastic, Coe Laboratories, Inc., Chicago, Ill.
†Masque, The Henry J. Bosworth Co., Chicago, Ill.
‡Rollette Unit, Kerr Manufacturing Co., Romulus, Mich.

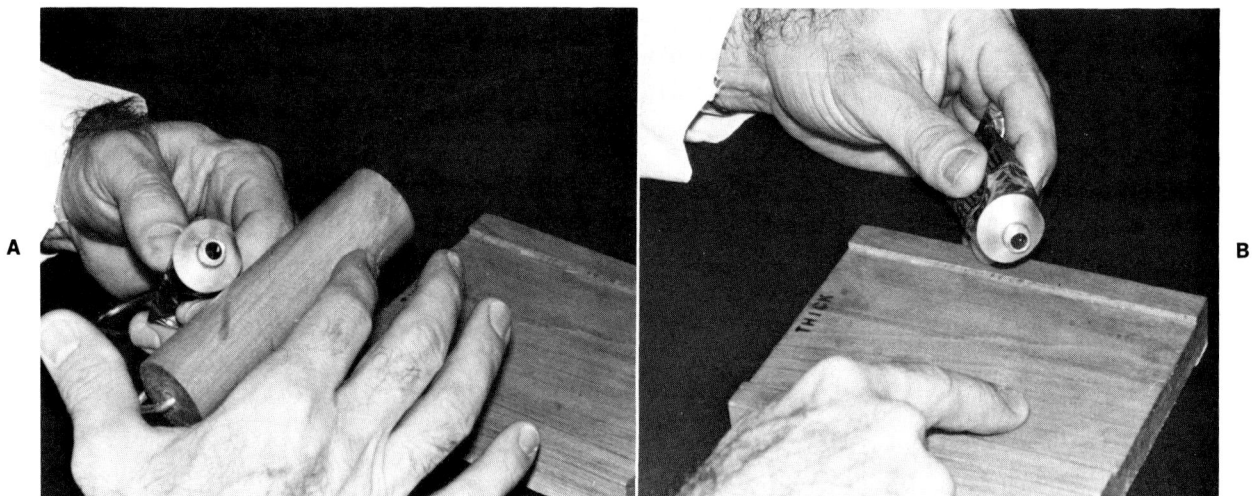

**Fig. 4-38. A,** Silicone lubricant is applied to roller to prevent sticking to resin. **B,** Wooden tray is coated with silicone lubricant.

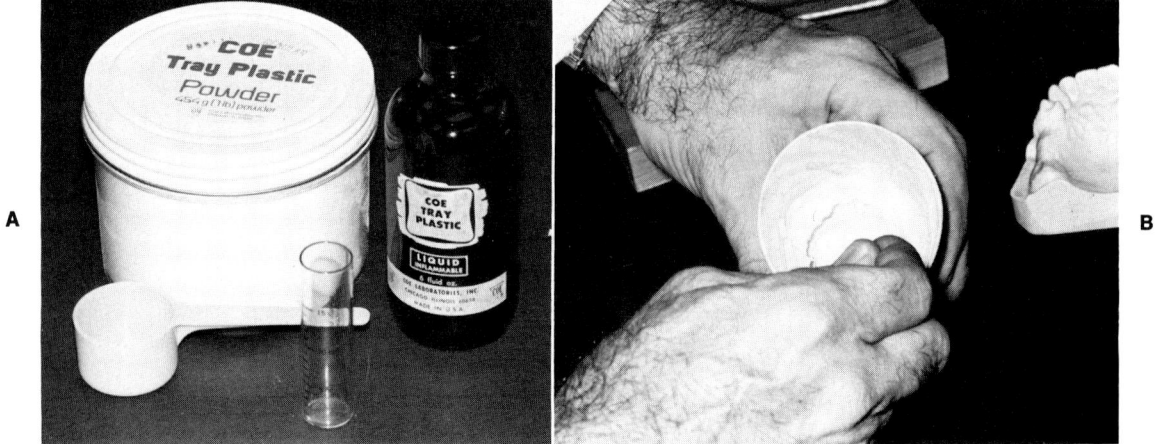

**Fig. 4-39. A,** Tray resin powder and liquid are proportioned according to manufacturer's directions. **B,** Mixing of materials is accomplished with spatula in paper cup.

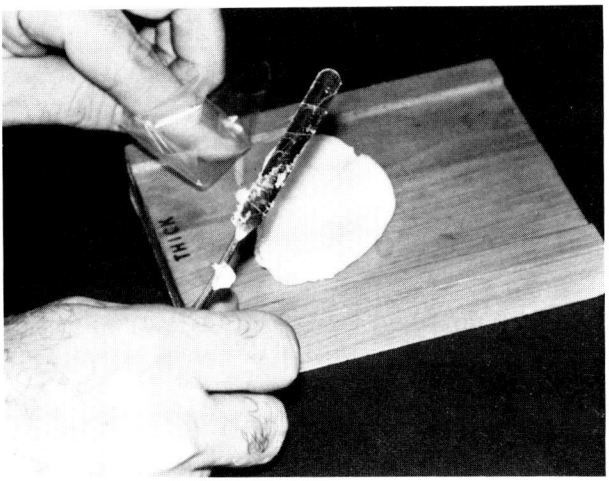

**Fig. 4-40.** In dough stage, resin is transferred to wooden block.

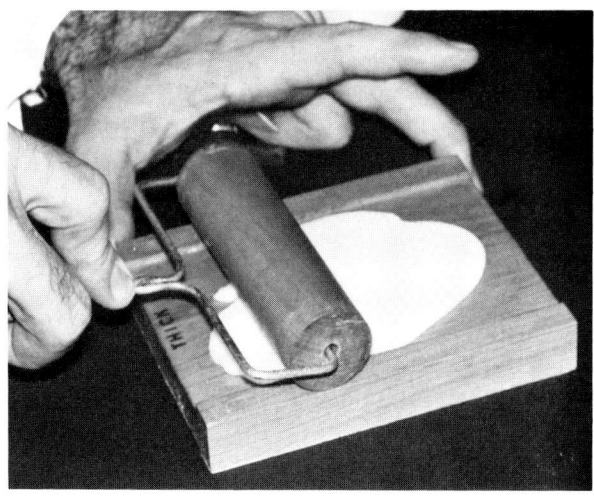

**Fig. 4-41.** Resin dough is rolled to desired thickness.

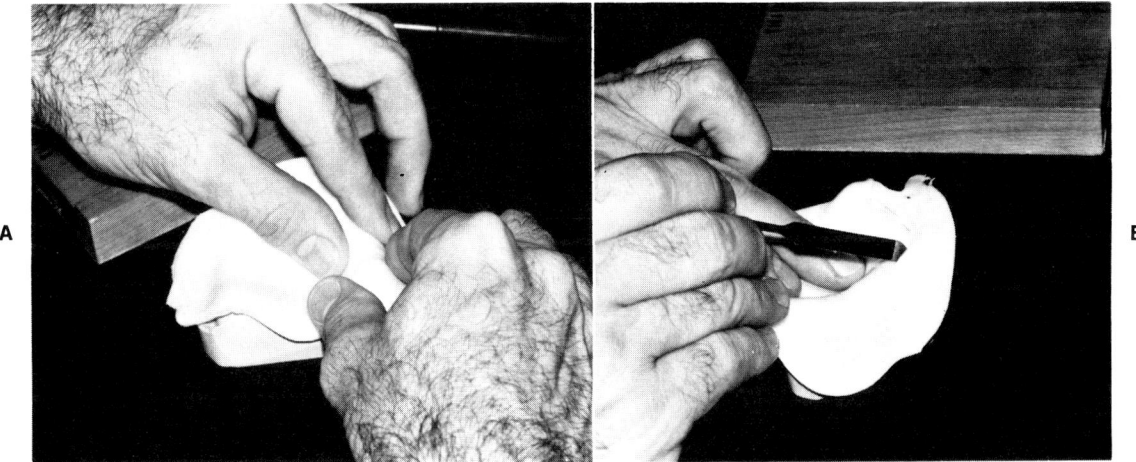

**Fig. 4-42. A,** Resin is removed from block and adapted onto cast. **B,** Cement spatula is used to trim away excess resin.

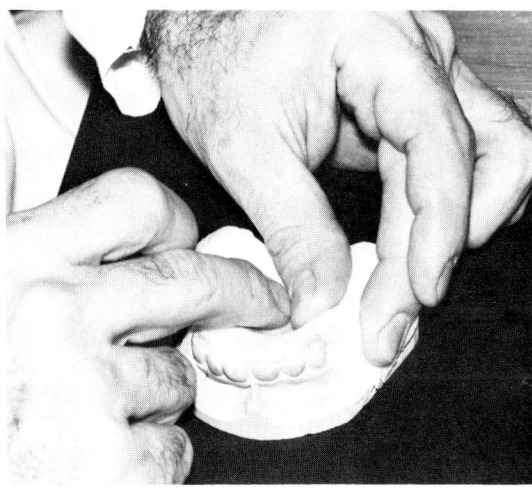

**Fig. 4-43.** Finger adaptation is continued until resin no longer rebounds from cast surface.

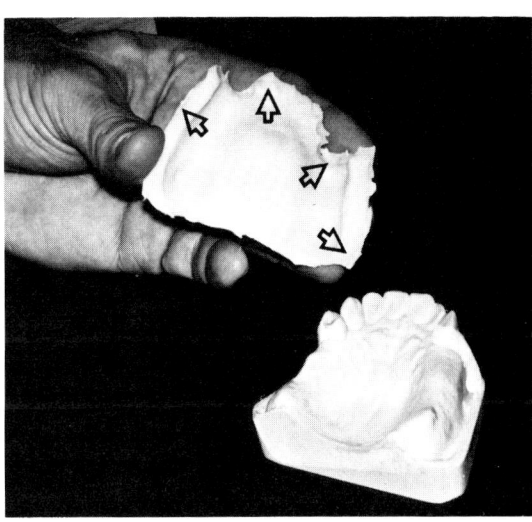

**Fig. 4-44.** Cured resin is removed from cast, and areas to be trimmed (arrows) are determined.

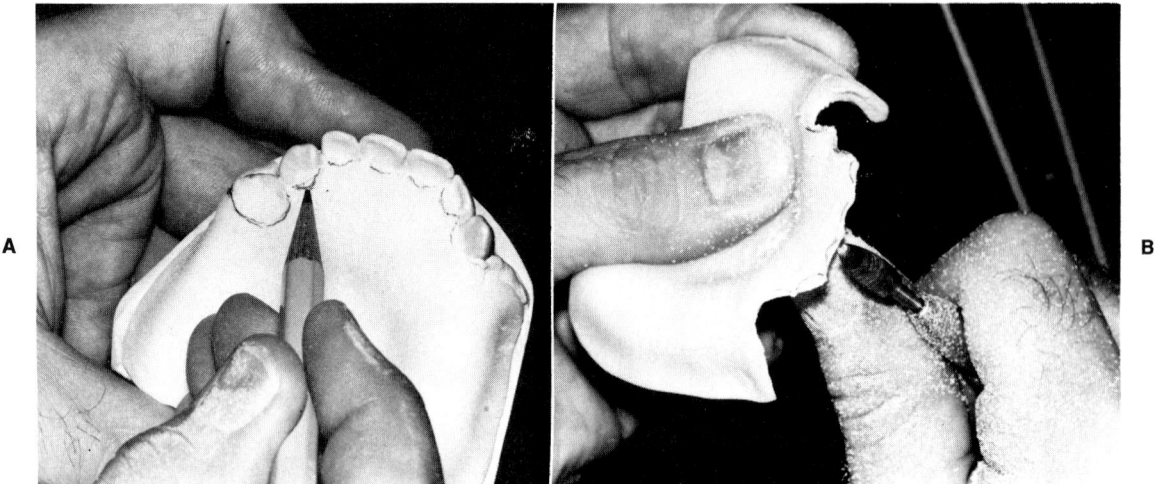

**Fig. 4-45. A,** Potential tooth interferences on lingual surfaces and cingulum areas of teeth are outlined. **B,** Carbide laboratory bur is used to reduce resin with pencil outline as guide.

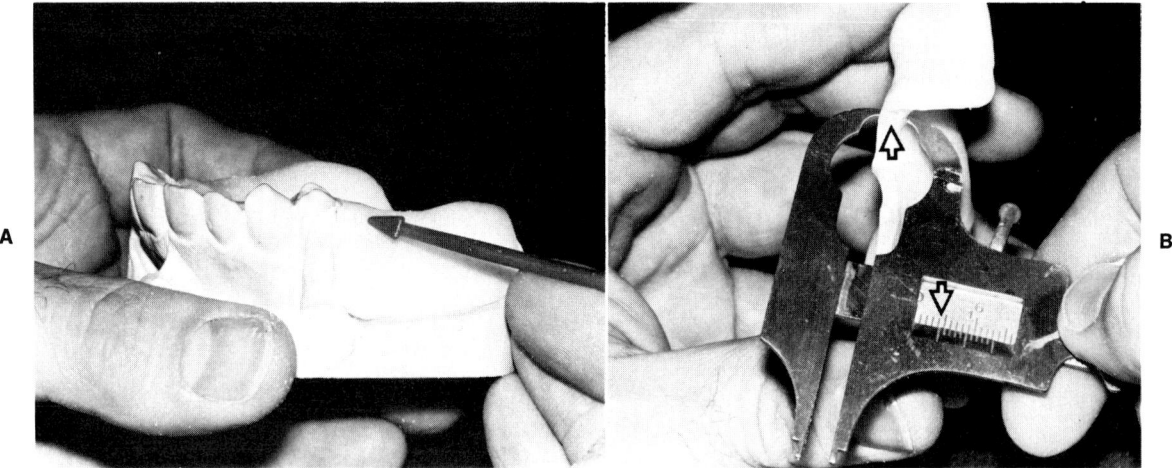

**Fig. 4-46. A,** Resin thickness over residual ridge should be evaluated for future placement of occlusion rim. **B,** Boley gauge will accurately measure amount of resin (arrows).

9. Replace the record base on the cast, and note any resin material that might interfere with the opposing teeth. Outline the lingual surfaces and cingulum areas of the teeth with a pencil. Trim the record base to the pencil outline with a tapered carbide bar (Fig. 4-45).

10. Determine the thickness of the record base over the residual ridge. The actual thickness can be easily measured with a Boley gauge (Fig. 4-46).

11. Evaluate the border thickness and adaptation to the cast (Fig. 4-47). After making the necessary corrections, the completed resin record base should be stored in water until needed by the dentist.

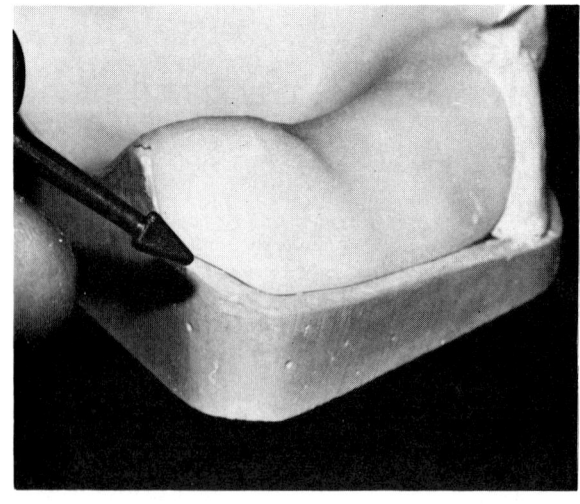

**Fig. 4-47.** Record base contour and adaptation are checked on cast. This resin record base is reasonably well adapted.

## PROBLEM AREAS

Several problems that can be encountered with this method, as well as probable causes and solutions, are described in Table 4-2.

1. *The completed record base cannot be removed from the cast.* Most commonly the undercuts have not been properly blocked out with baseplate wax, or the peripheral border has been extended into an undercut area. Block out severe undercuts with wax, and use rope caulk to confine the record base border from entering an undercut area. Use controlled pressure when adapting resin to avoid displacing the blockout material.

2. *Teeth on the cast are chipped or broken during removal of the record base.* The resin may enter undercut areas around and between the teeth. Control the extent of the resin base in these areas by flowing baseplate wax in the gingival crest and interproximal tooth areas.

3. *The completed record base fails to fit the cast.* When the resin has advanced beyond the dough stage, it will be difficult to achieve conformity between the record base and the cast. In its rubbery state the resin will have a tendency to pull away from the cast surface, thus preventing accurate adaptation. When adaptation of the resin has been initiated at the proper dough stage, its manipulation should be continued until no movement of the baseplate away from the cast is observed.

4. *The final record base has thick and thin areas.* Prominent areas of the cast, such as the ridge crest, may be too thin as a result of finger pressure, whereas inaccessible areas may be too thick. Control the initial thickness of the resin by rolling it on a board and then exercise light pressure over convex areas to maintain the optimal thickness.

### Wax-confined dough method

A method of making a record base with a wax form and autopolymerizing acrylic resin has been described by LaVere and Freda (1974). In their method, a thin mix of acrylic resin is placed into a hard baseplate wax form that has been previously adapted to the cast. The wax form is positioned on the cast to eventually provide an acrylic resin record base covered by the single thickness of baseplate wax. In the technique, the medium-hard baseplate wax used in the blockout of undercuts is incorporated into the resin record base. Some of the advantages cited for this technique are (1) increased stability of the record base because the wax blockout is an integral part, (2) no subsequent damage to the cast on removal, (3) use of the wax form controls the record base thickness, especially in the palatal portion, and (4) the wax form contributes to a neat and pleasing appearance overall.

**Table 4-2.** Finger-adapted dough method

| Problem | Probable cause | Solution |
|---|---|---|
| Record base unable to be removed from cast | Improper blockout of undercuts | Use wax to block out extensive undercuts; control extension of resin with rope caulk |
| Teeth chipped or broken during removal | Cingulum and interproximal tooth areas not blocked out with wax | Block out interproximal and gingival crest areas with baseplate wax |
| Failure of record base to fit cast | Finger adaptation not continued to polymerization stage | Actively adapt resin to cast until it no longer rebounds |
| | Resin beyond dough stage when adaptation was initiated | Adapt resin when in dough stage |
| Uneven thickness of record base | Excess pressure on convex areas | Apply light controlled pressure to convex or prominent areas of cast during adaptation |
| | Thickness of resin not controlled before application | Roll resin to optimum thickness; then adapt it to cast |

## PROCEDURE

1. Carefully examine the cast and determine all undercut areas (Fig. 4-48).
2. Flow baseplate wax into the gingival crevice and interproximal areas of the remaining teeth (Fig. 4-49).
3. Paint the cast surface with tinfoil substitute. Apply three coats, and allow them to dry. The third application should set for 10 minutes (Fig. 4-50).
4. Block out all tissue undercuts with medium-hard baseplate wax (Fig. 4-51).
5. Warm one layer of hard baseplate wax, and adapt it over the blocked out master cast to make the wax form. Reduce the wax so that it is about 2 mm short of the border reflection (Fig. 4-52). Chill the wax form and remove it from the cast.
6. Make a thin mix of autopolymerizing tray material using two parts polymer to one part monomer.
7. Place some of the resin mix in the borders of the cast and on the palate of the maxillary cast (Fig. 4-53).

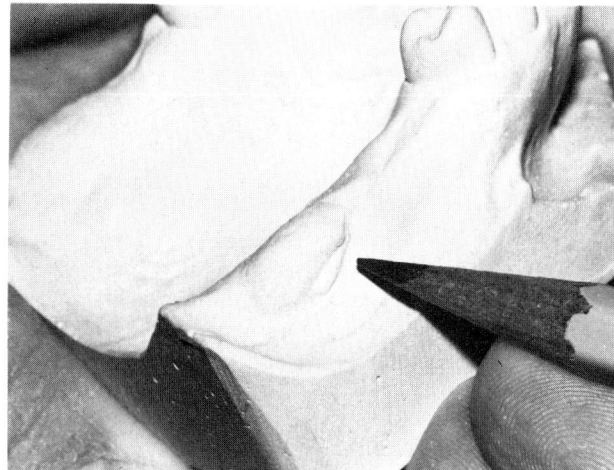

**Fig. 4-48.** Undercut areas are determined on cast.

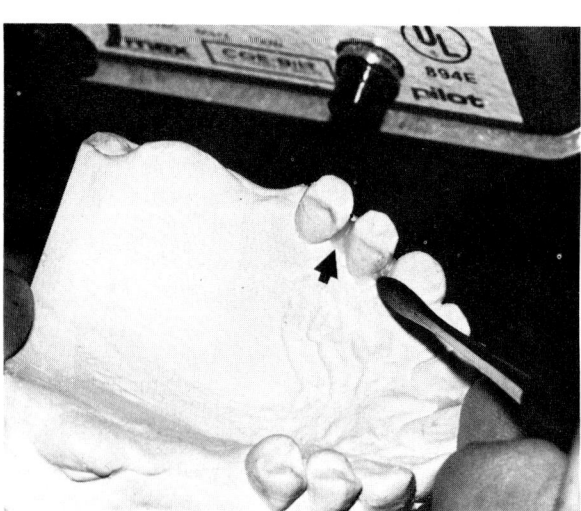

**Fig. 4-49.** Baseplate wax is added to tooth interproximal areas (arrow) to limit resin.

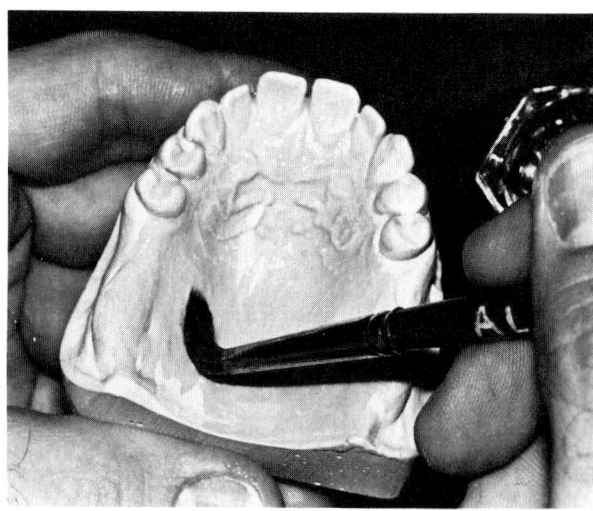

**Fig. 4-50.** Three coats of tinfoil substitute are applied to cast.

*Record bases and mounting casts* 93

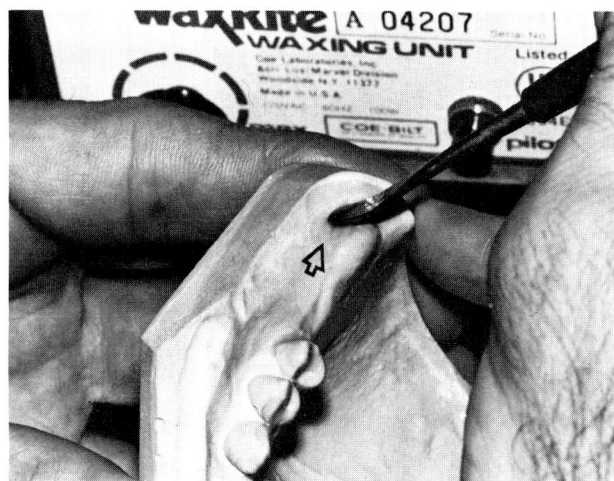

**Fig. 4-51.** Undercuts are blocked out with baseplate wax (arrow) prior to adaptation of wax form.

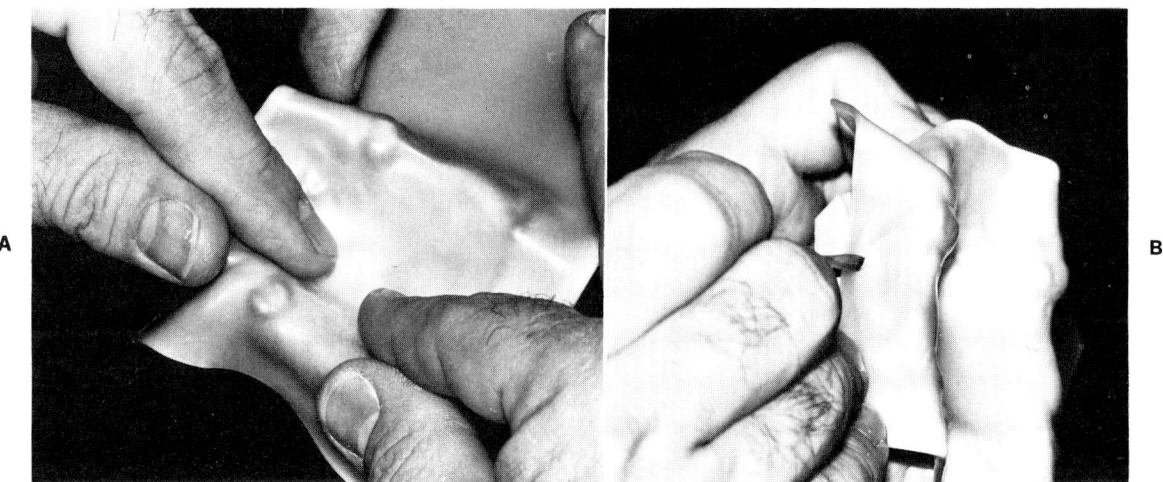

**Fig. 4-52. A,** One layer of hard baseplate wax is warmed and adapted over blocked out cast to make wax form. **B,** Wax form is trimmed 2 mm short of border reflection.

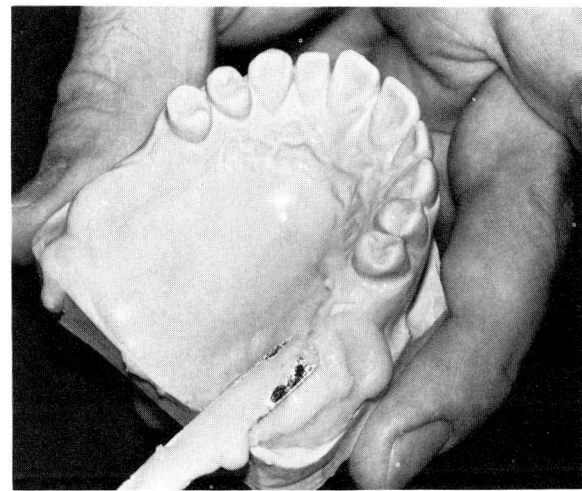

**Fig. 4-53.** Acrylic resin is mixed and placed into border reflections and palate to avoid air entrapment.

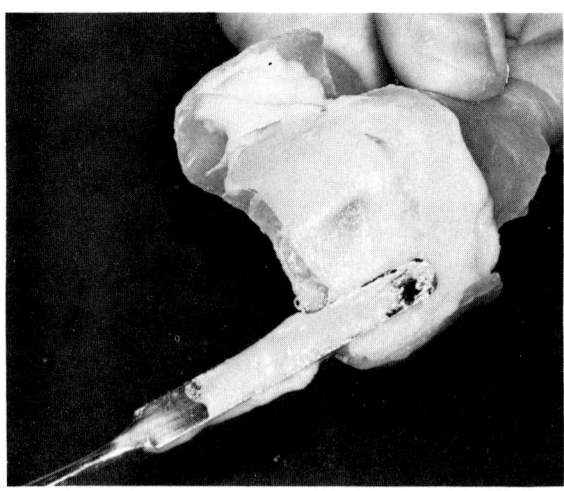

Fig. 4-54. Remainder of acrylic resin is loaded into wax form.

8. Pour the remainder of the mix into the wax form, and spread it evenly on the tissue surface (Fig. 4-54).

9. Invert the wax form, and carefully press the resin into place on the cast surface until it is about 1 to 2 mm thick. Mold the excess resin over the borders until it is approximately 2 mm thick over the wax around the baseplate border (Fig. 4-55).

10. Remove the excess resin from the teeth surfaces (Fig. 4-56).

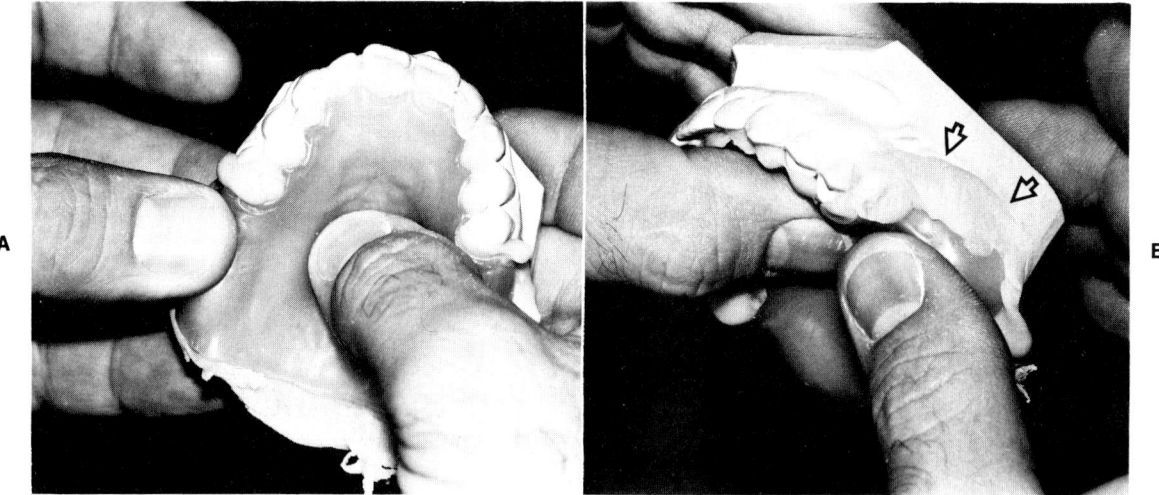

Fig. 4-55. **A,** Resin-loaded wax form is pressed into place, producing record base thickness of approximately 2 mm. **B,** Excess resin is molded over wax to establish borders (arrows).

Fig. 4-56. Excess resin is removed from teeth surfaces.

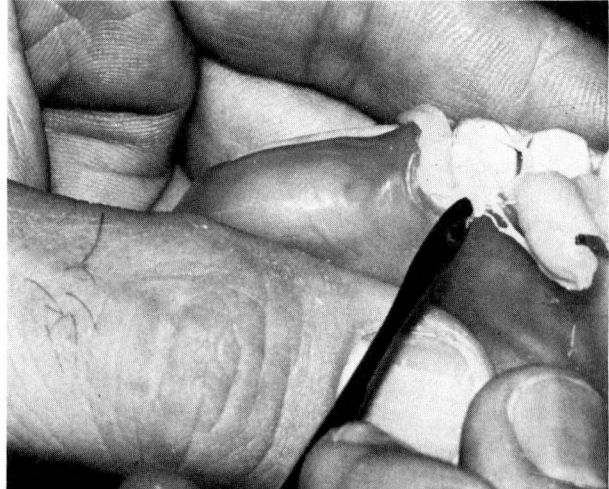

11. Cure the acrylic resin for 20 minutes in a pressure chamber with warm water at 20 psi (Fig. 4-57).

12. When cured, carefully remove the record base from the cast. The blockout wax should adhere to the resin surface, thus becoming an integral part of the record base (Fig. 4-58).

13. Smooth and lightly polish the resin border without overheating. The wax/resin record base should fit accurately and not abrade the cast on removal (Fig. 4-59). Fabricate wax occlusion rims on the record base.

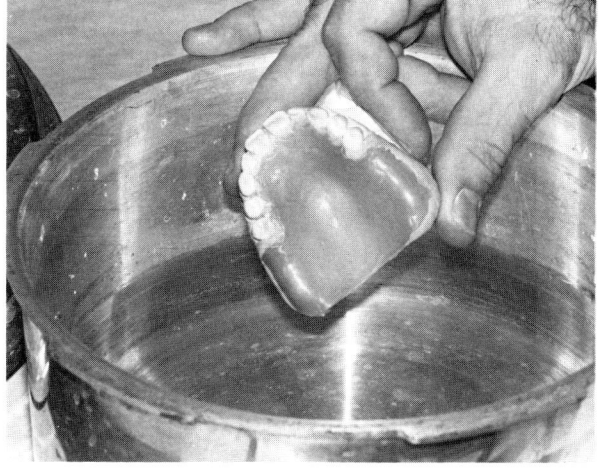

**Fig. 4-57.** Resin record base can be cured in pressure pot at 20 psi for 20 minutes.

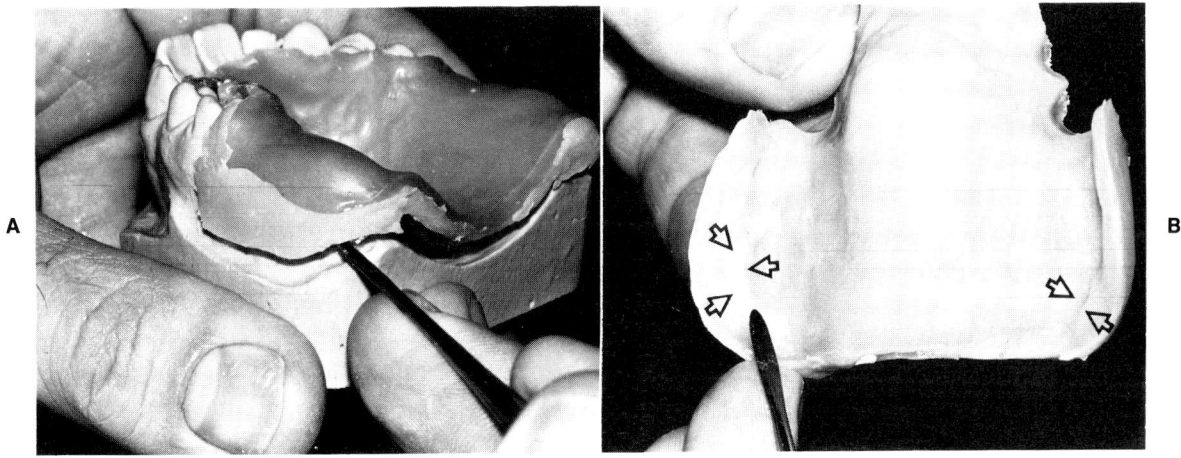

**Fig. 4-58. A,** Remove resin record base by gently prying on side opposite undercut. **B,** Blockout wax (arrows) should remain attached to inside of resin record base.

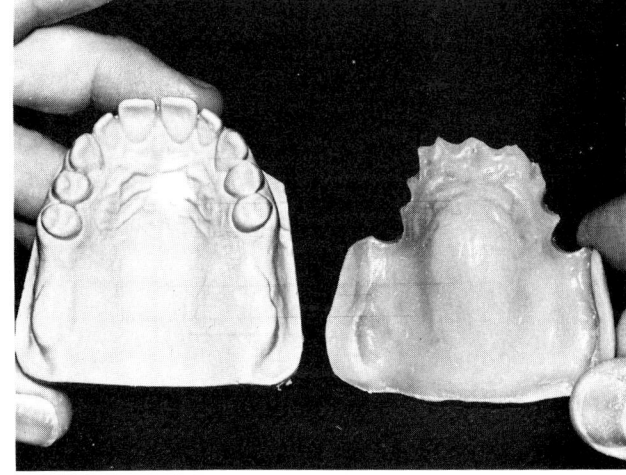

**Fig. 4-59.** Completed record base fits accurately and does not abrade cast on removal.

**Table 4-3.** Wax-confined dough method

| Problem | Probable cause | Solution |
|---|---|---|
| Record base too thin or thick | Wax form improperly seated on cast | Carefully seat wax form with resin to provide resin thickness of 1 to 2 mm |
| Excess resin on exterior wax surface of record base | Acrylic resin allowed to build up around wax border | Adapt resin carefully; remove any excess to ensure that wax exterior is free of resin |

### PROBLEM AREAS

Principal problems with this method are controlling the thickness of the acrylic resin and preventing excess resin from building up around the wax exterior surface of the record base (Table 4-3). When the wax form and resin are seated too firmly, excessive resin dough will be expressed, and the record base will be too thin. The record base will be too thick if the wax form and resin are inadequately seated on the cast surface. After seating the wax form, the excess resin at the border should be carefully adapted to provide optimal thickness. Excess resin should be removed to prevent possible interference with the occlusal relation (Fig. 4-60).

## SHELLAC RECORD BASES

Shellac continues to be one of the most commonly used materials for fabricating record bases. Shellac, acquired from the resinous exudate of the insect *Coccus lactis* is the base of this baseplate material (Greener et al., 1972). Other components such as powdered talc or mica may be incorporated as fillers to impart strength. Shellac is normally a brown resin, but it can be bleached, and an oil-soluble dye can be added to provide a more esthetic pink color. After heating the material to 60° to 70° C, it can be adapted to the cast by finger pressure. When overheated, the shellac will bubble and smoke, and the resultant black color is esthetically unacceptable. Although shellac record bases can be well adapted to casts, they are dimensionally unstable and frequently warp when rewarmed at mouth temperature due to release of stresses. Warpage can also be observed in the laboratory when making wax occlusion rims and setting denture teeth on the shellac record base.

Low cost and ease of handling are the principal advantages of shellac baseplates. They can be made in a minimal amount of time, and with proper ad-

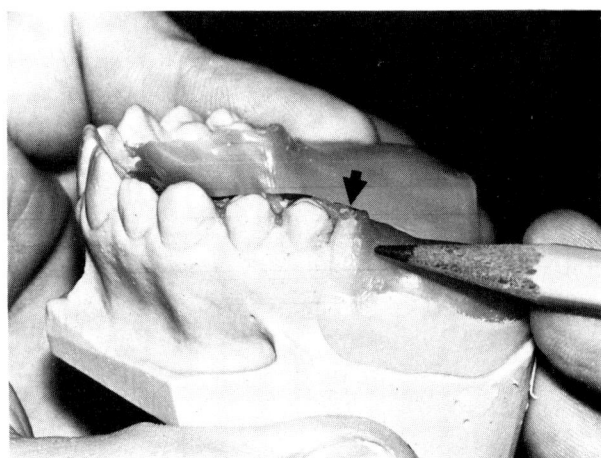

**Fig. 4-60.** Excess resin (arrow) can interfere with occlusal relation.

aptation and reinforcement serve adequately as recording bases. The chief disadvantage is that they easily warp when exposed to temperature change; however, they can be easily readapted for an accurate fit.

### PROCEDURE

1. Prevent the shellac material from sticking to the cast surface by soaking the cast in clear slurry water. Another alternative is to paint the cast surface with talc* (Fig. 4-61).
2. Block out severe undercuts with a mix of one part flour of pumice and one part plaster (Fig. 4-62).
3. Select the appropriate shaped shellac sheet, and, after warming it over a Bunsen burner flame, place it on the cast, and continue flaming the surface until it slumps on the cast (Fig. 4-63).

---

*Johnson's Baby Powder, Johnson & Johnson, New Brunswick, N.J., or equivalent.

Record bases and mounting casts 97

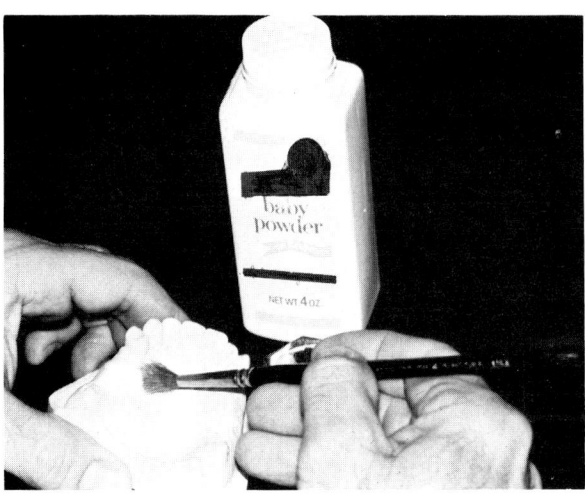

**Fig. 4-61.** Powdered talc is applied to cast surface as separator for shellac record base material.

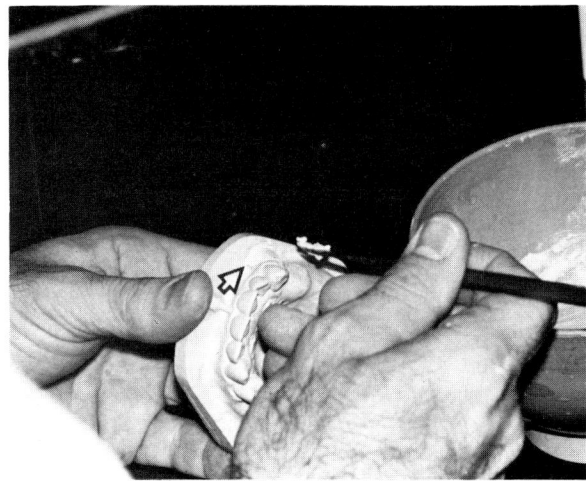

**Fig. 4-62.** Mixture of equal parts flour of pumice and plaster is used to blockout undercuts (arrow)

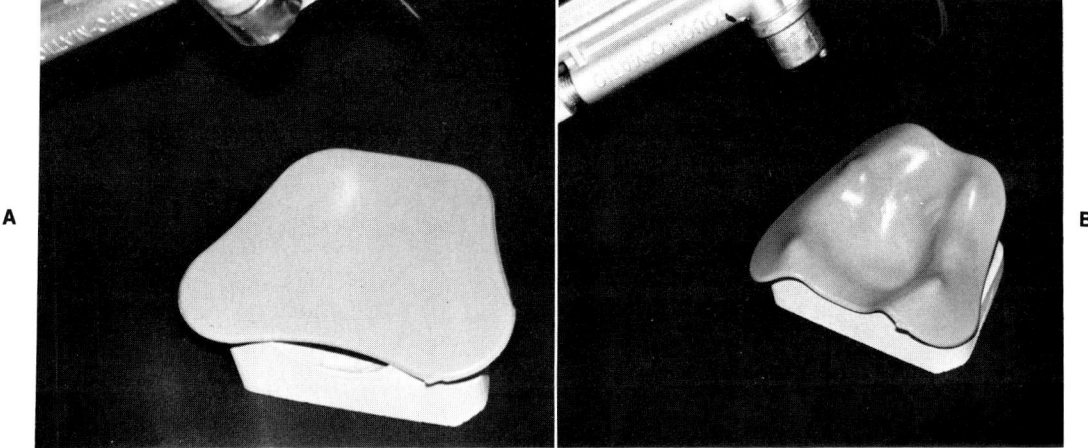

**Fig. 4-63. A,** Sheet of shellac is placed on cast and softened with brush flame from Bunsen burner. **B,** Baseplate material should be positioned to assure that all edentulous areas are covered.

4. Heat localized areas with an alcohol torch, and adapt the material with wet fingers (Fig. 4-64).

5. Remove the material from the cast while it is warm, trim it with scissors, and replace it on the cast. A No. 7 wax spatula can be used to reflect the trimmed edges back onto themselves to form a well-rounded border (Fig. 4-65).

6. Allow the shellac to cool, and remove it from the cast. Trim the borders with a lathe-mounted arbor band or stone, being careful to use light pressure, otherwise, the soft material will clog the trimmer (Fig. 4-66).

7. Remove the shellac material, and determine if there are any glossy areas, indicating lack of adaptation (Fig. 4-67). Soften these areas with the alcohol torch, and readapt the shellac.

8. Shellac record bases should be strengthened to resist warpage. Heavy-duty paper clips are a convenient source for this wire reinforcement (Fig. 4-68). Adapt the wire to the cast in the posterior palatal seal areas. Heat the wire, and embed it within the baseplate (Fig. 4-69). Cover the exposed wire with a piece of the shellac material, and then flame the surface to ensure a smooth transition (Fig. 4-70). For mandibular record bases, the reinforcing wire should be placed from first molar to first molar and lingual to the ridge crest.

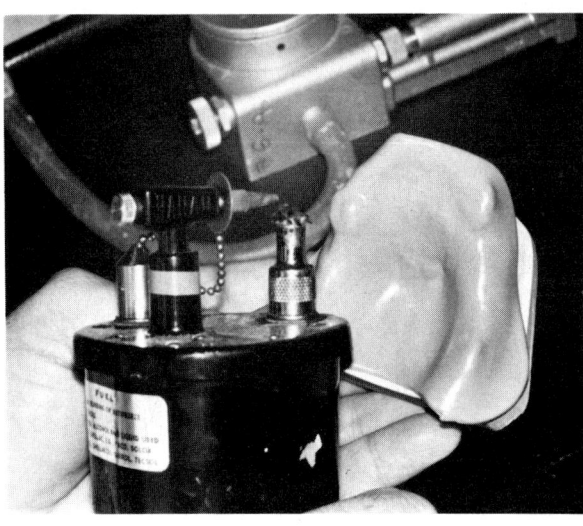

**Fig. 4-64.** Alcohol torch can be used to soften specific areas of shellac for adaptation.

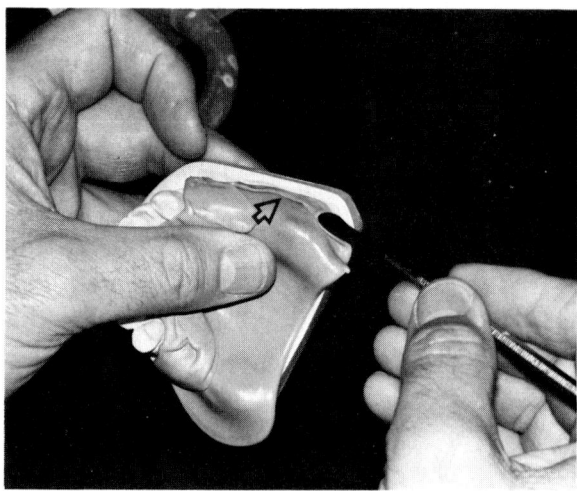

**Fig. 4-65.** Rounded borders (arrow) are formed by reflecting shellac back on itself.

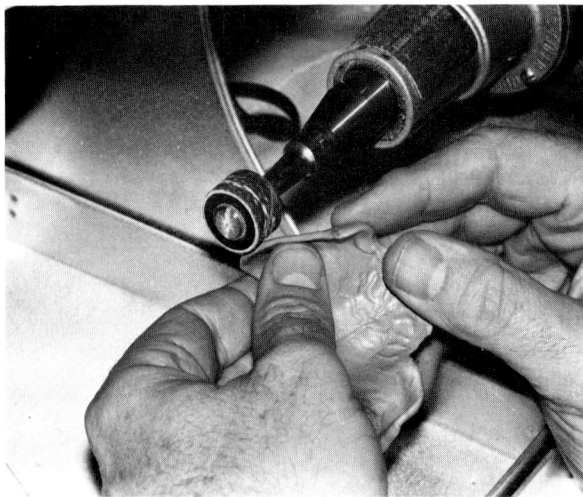

**Fig. 4-66.** Borders can be trimmed using lathe-mounted arbor band with light pressure. Heavy sustained pressure will clog arbor band.

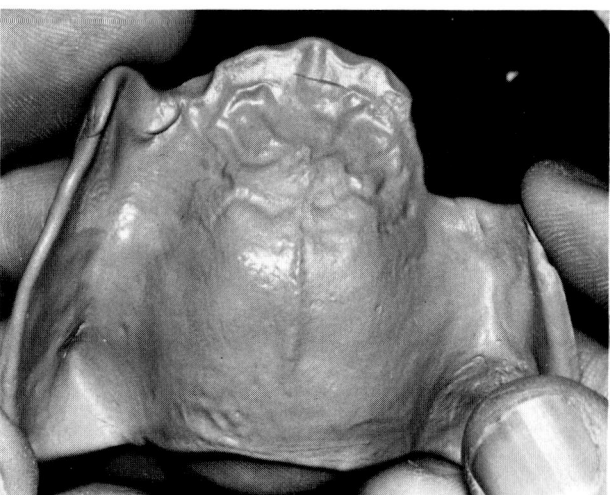

**Fig. 4-67.** Tissue surface is evaluated for adaptation. Any glossy areas should be heated and readapted.

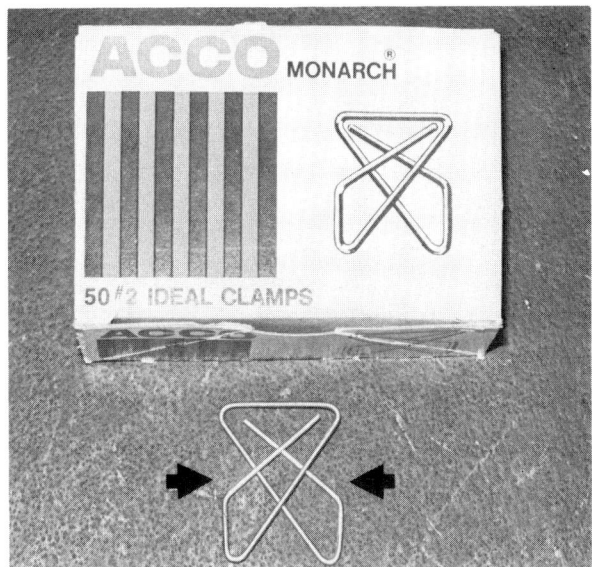

**Fig. 4-68.** Heavy-duty paper clips (arrows) are convenient for reinforcing shellac record bases.

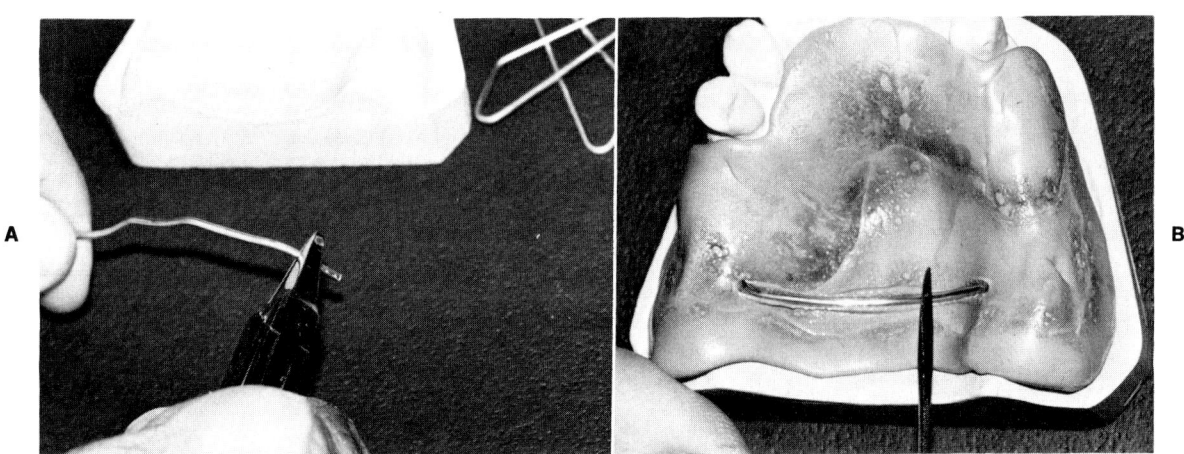

**Fig. 4-69. A,** Length of heavy-duty paper clip wire is adapted to cast across posterior palatal seal area. **B,** After heating wire, embed it into shellac material.

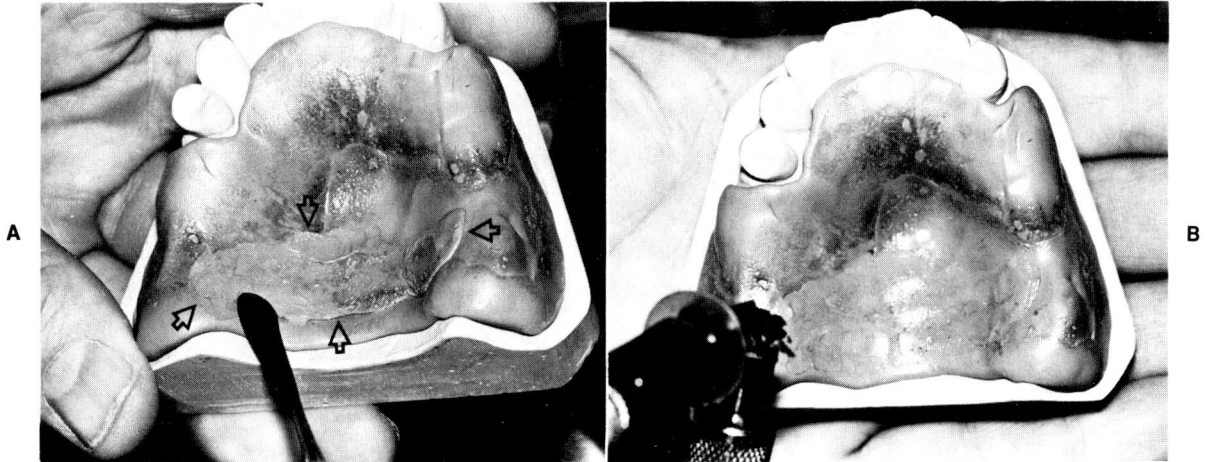

**Fig. 4-70. A,** Piece of shellac material (arrows) covers reinforcement wire. **B,** Surface is flamed to produce smooth transition of shellac material.

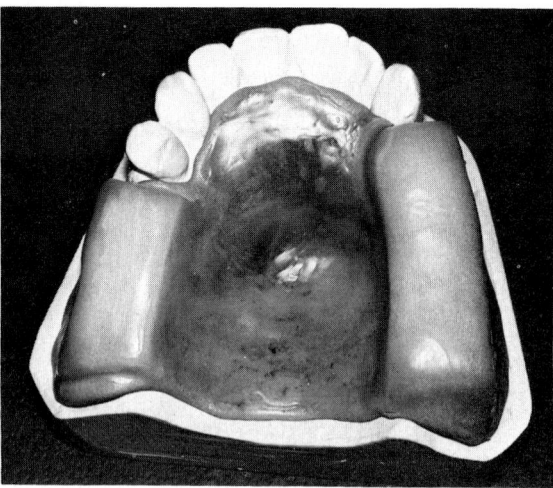

Fig. 4-71. After sealing wax occlusion rim to shellac record base, it is stored on cast to minimize warpage until needed.

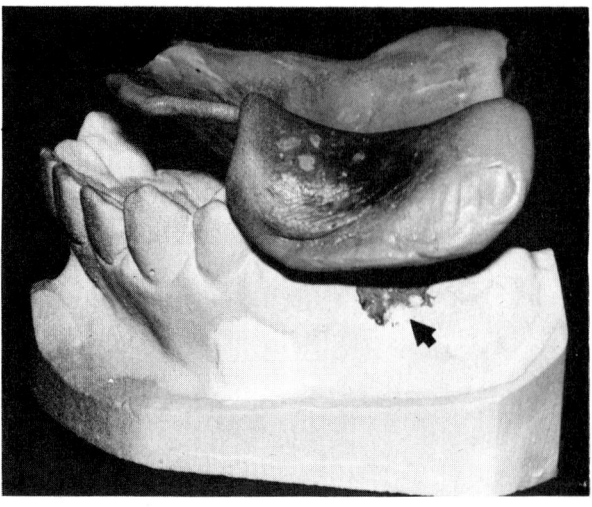

Fig. 4-72. Overheating of shellac may result in black, unesthetic color, and material can stick to cast surface (arrow).

9. Seal the wax occlusion rim to the shellac baseplate, and allow it to remain on the cast to minimize warpage before use (Fig. 4-71). Do not overheat the shellac material or adapt it to a dry cast because the molten shellac may penetrate the cast surface and adhere to the stone on cooling (Fig. 4-72). Attempts to remove the record base may result in a fracture of the stone surface.

## Stabilized shellac record bases

Numerous clinicians, including Fletcher (1951), Freese (1956), Jamieson (1956), Kapur and Yurkstas (1957), Hall (1958), and Malson (1964), have suggested various methods and materials for stabilizing shellac baseplates to compensate for their warpage. Most methods have recommended the employment of a second material such as metallic oxide–impression paste, elastomeric impression material, or autopolymerizing resin as a liner. The material is attached to the shellac surface to improve the adaptation and enhance rigidity. According to Jamieson (1956), a rigid, nonwarping baseplate is essential for the dentist to accurately record the maxillomandibular relationship.

## Record bases stabilized with zinc oxide–eugenol impression paste

Zinc oxide–eugenol impression paste used as a liner in the shellac baseplate will improve the adaptation and dimensional stability. Undercuts should be blocked out and tinfoil applied to the cast as a separator. It is essential to properly block out undercuts because the rigidity of the stabilized record base will prevent its removal from undercut areas. Ideally a thin layer of the zinc oxide–eugenol paste should be used as a liner to enhance adaptation to the cast and increase rigidity. If the lining paste is too thick, the interarch space required for taking records and setting tooth replacements may be compromised.

### PROCEDURE

1. Identify and block out undercut areas on the cast with a mix of equal parts of plaster and flour of pumice (Fig. 4-73).
2. Apply a layer of 0.001 inch (0.0025 cm) thickness tinfoil (Fig. 4-74). A modified pencil eraser and ball burnisher can be used to adapt the tinfoil in all areas of the cast (Fig. 4-75). Smooth any small folds on the cast surface with the large egg-shaped burnisher.

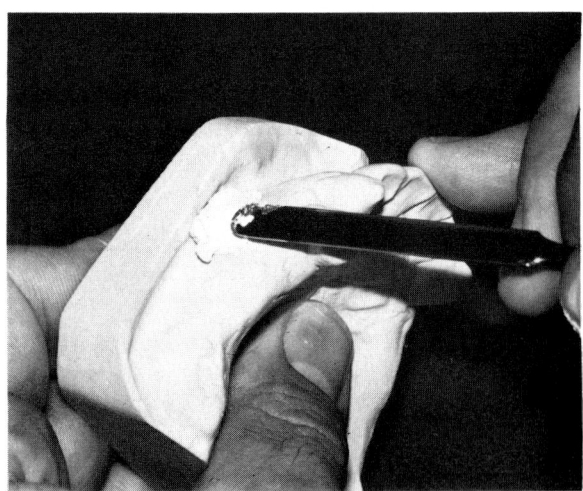

Fig. 4-73. Undercuts on cast are blocked out with mix of equal parts of plaster and pumice before adapting tinfoil.

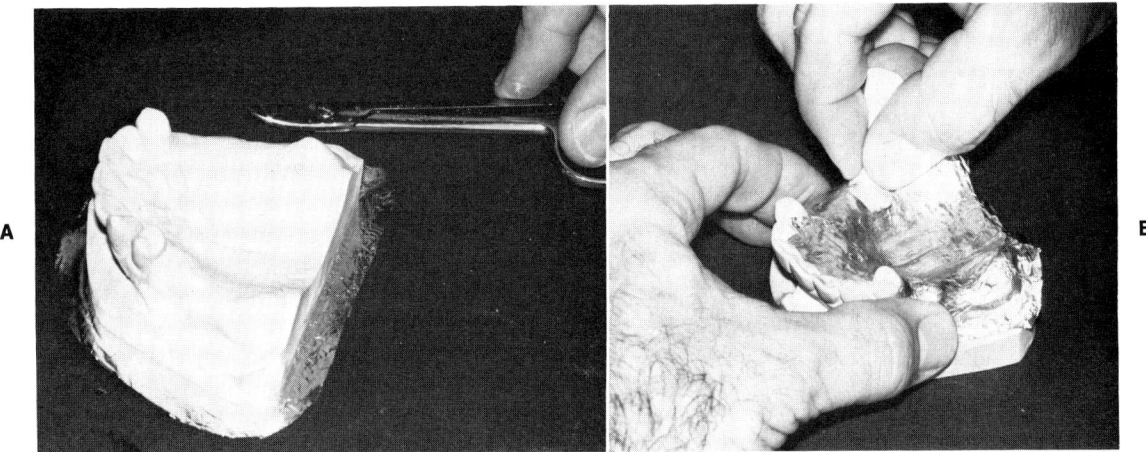

**Fig. 4-74. A,** Required amount of tinfoil needed to cover edentulous areas can be approximated by using base of cast as pattern. **B,** Adapt tinfoil to cast by burnishing with cotton.

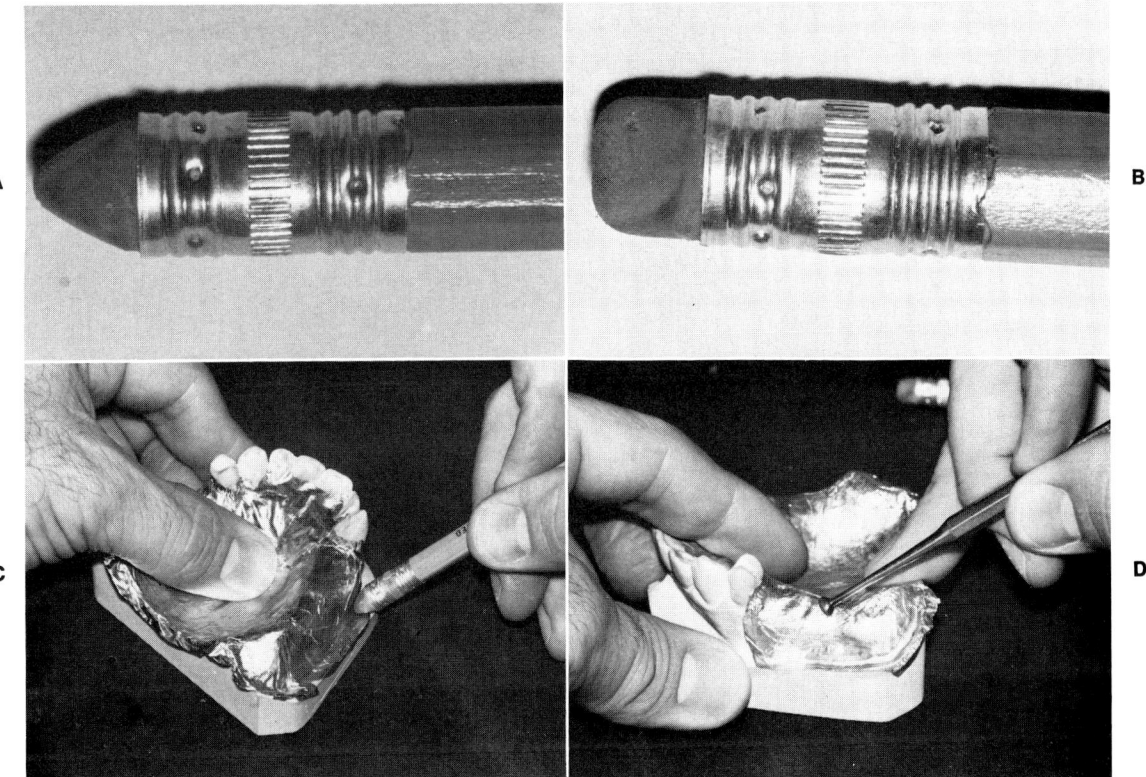

**Fig. 4-75. A,** Pencil eraser is shaped like wedge to adapt tinfoil to cast. This is particularly useful for adapting foil in border reflections of cast. **B,** Another view of rubber pencil eraser adaptor. **C,** Tinfoil is readily burnished into border areas of cast with wedge-shaped pencil eraser. **D,** Large egg-shaped burnisher is used to smooth any small folds of tinfoil on cast.

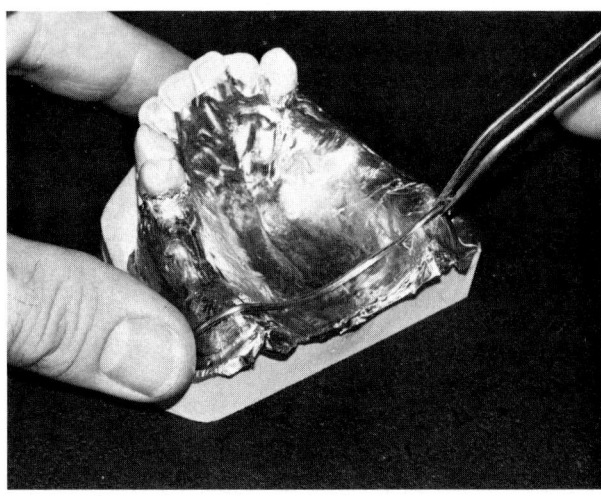

**Fig. 4-76.** Reinforcement wire is adapted across posterior extent of maxillary cast.

3. Adapt a reinforcing wire, and check the fit across the posterior palatal seal area (Fig. 4-76).

4. Adapt a shellac baseplate over the tinfoiled cast as previously described. Embed the reinforcing wire and smooth the surface (Fig. 4-77).

5. Remove the baseplate from the cast, and drill a hole in the palate with a No. 8 round bur (Fig. 4-78). The hole will serve as an escape vent for trapped air and excess impression paste.

6. Proportion and mix the zinc oxide–eugenol impression paste* according to the manufacturer's directions (Fig. 4-79).

---

*Opotow Standard Zoe impression paste, Teledyne Dental Products Co., Getz/Opotow Division, Elk Grove Village, Ill.; Luralite, Kerr Manufacturing Co., Romulus, Mich.; Coe-Flo, Coe Laboratories, Inc., Chicago, Ill., or equivalent.

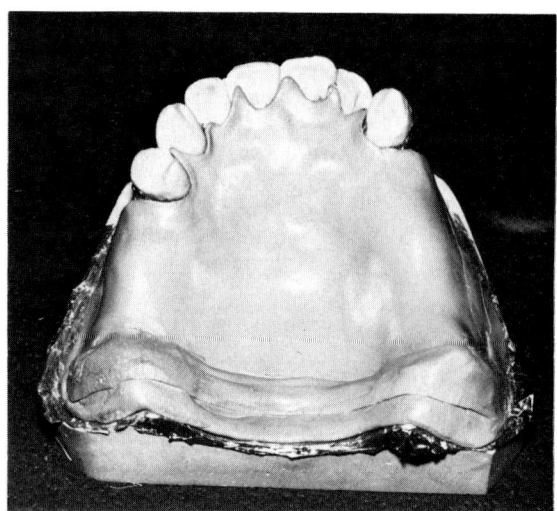

**Fig. 4-77.** After shellac baseplate is adapted, reinforcement wire is embedded and then covered with piece of shellac material.

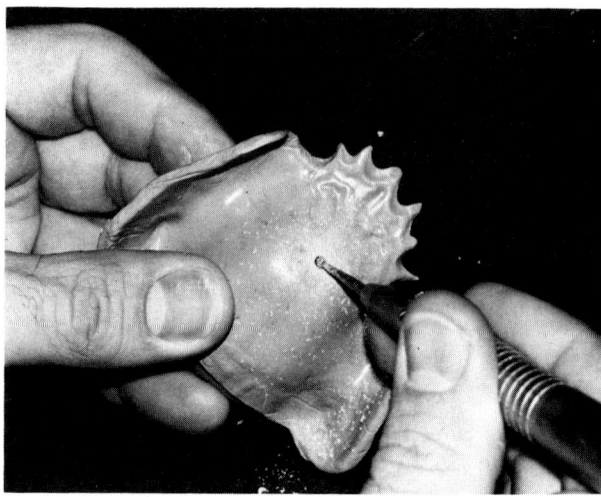

**Fig. 4-78.** Vent hole is drilled into palate with No. 8 round bur.

Record bases and mounting casts 103

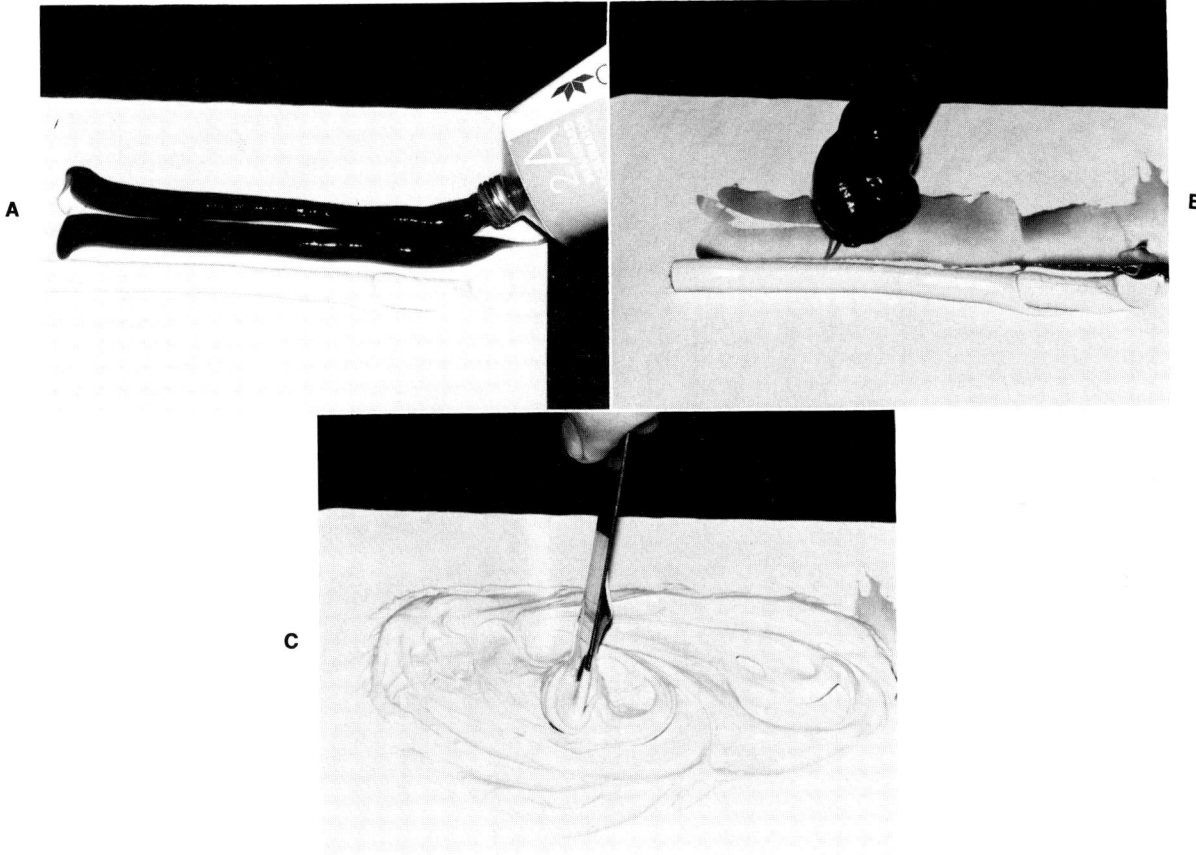

**Fig. 4-79. A,** Standard zinc oxide–eugenol impression paste is proportioned according to manufacturer's directions. **B,** Accelerator is blended with base material on mixing pad. **C,** Two components should be thoroughly mixed to produce uniform color devoid of any streaks.

7. Load the impression material onto the shellac baseplate, and spread it uniformly to cover the entire surface and the border areas. Cover the palatal portion of the cast with impression paste to minimize air entrapment. Seat the loaded baseplate on the tinfoiled cast in a manner that will provide a layer of impression material approximately 1 mm thick (Fig. 4-80).

8. Reflect the excess tinfoil at the border areas back onto the shellac before the impression material sets to ensure proper border thickness. Remove excess impression paste from the lingual areas of the teeth (Fig. 4-81).

9. After the impression material has set, remove the record base from the cast, and inspect the surface. The tinfoil usually adheres to the impression paste but may be peeled away if desired. Trim any excess material with a warm, sharp blade (Fig. 4-82). Store the final record base on the cast (Fig. 4-83).

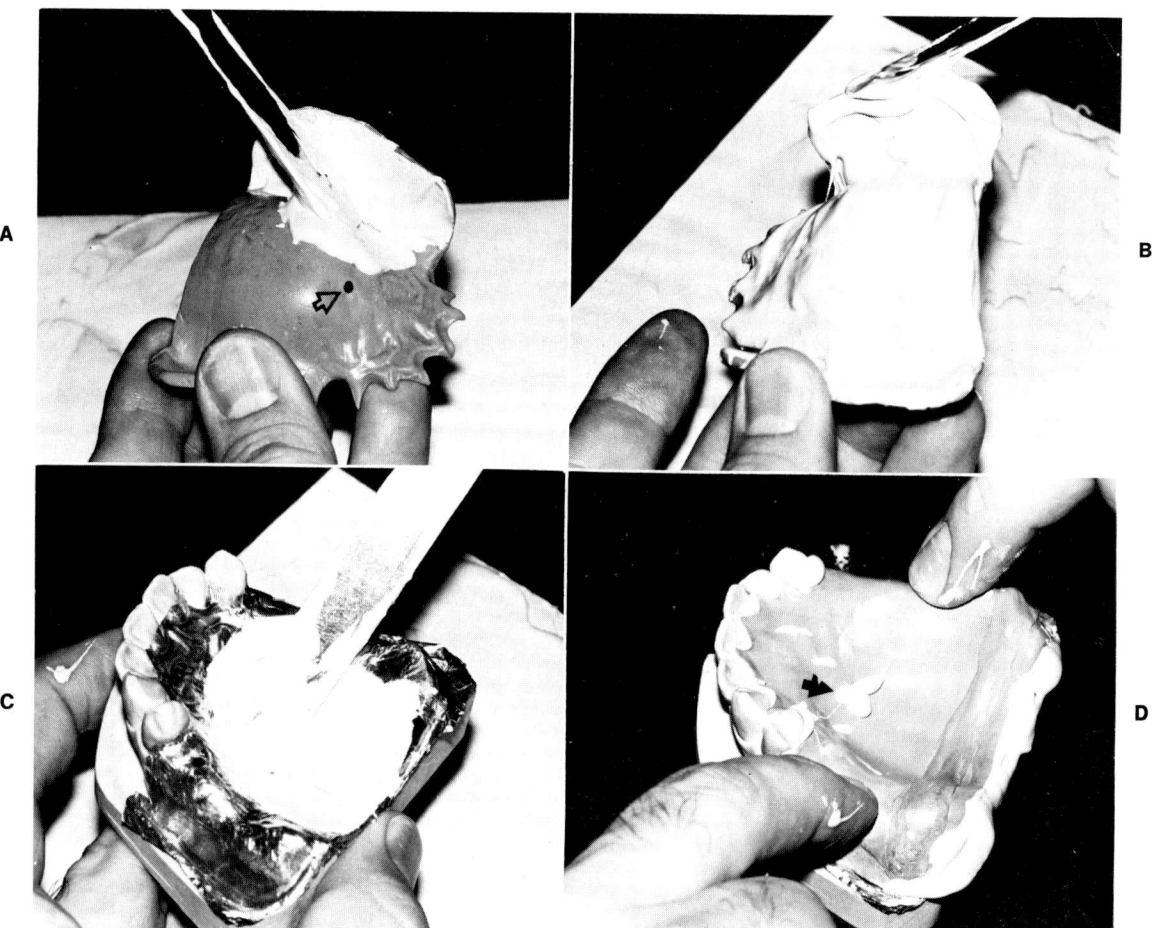

Fig. 4-80. **A,** Zinc oxide–eugenol impression paste is loaded in shellac record base. Note escape hole in palate (arrow) to vent excess impression paste and minimize voids. **B,** Spatula is used to cover entire tissue surface and borders with zinc oxide–eugenol impression material. **C,** Additional impression paste is placed on palatal portion of cast to minimize air entrapment. **D,** Loaded record base is carefully seated on tinfoiled cast to provide layer of impression paste of approximately 1 mm thickness. Note extrusion of excess impression material (arrow) through vent hole.

## Record bases and mounting casts    105

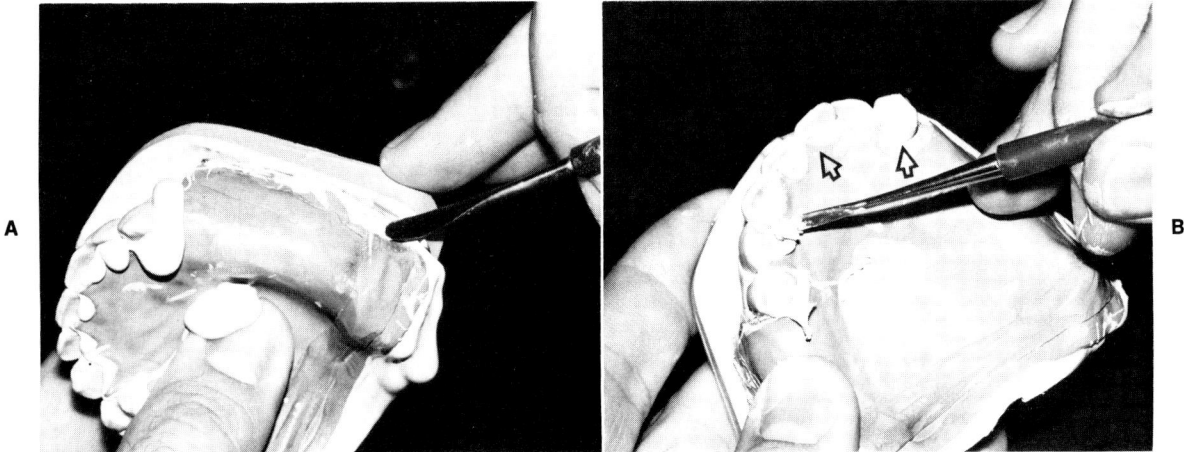

**Fig. 4-81. A,** Before impression material hardens, excess tinfoil is reflected back onto record base to establish proper border thickness. **B,** No. 7 spatula is used to remove excess impression paste from lingual tooth surfaces (arrows).

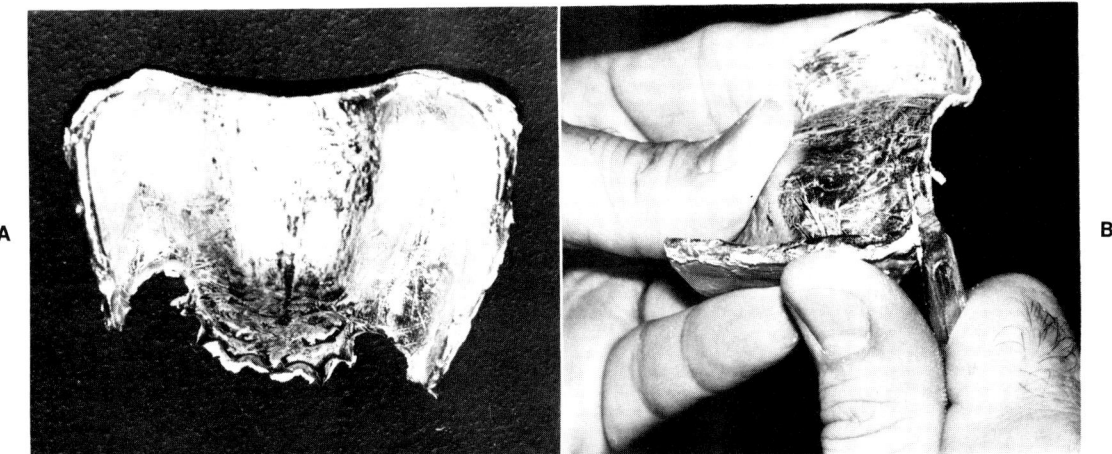

**Fig. 4-82. A,** Maxillary stabilized record base removed from cast. Tinfoil can be left in place or peeled away. **B,** Excess material can be trimmed with warm, sharp blade.

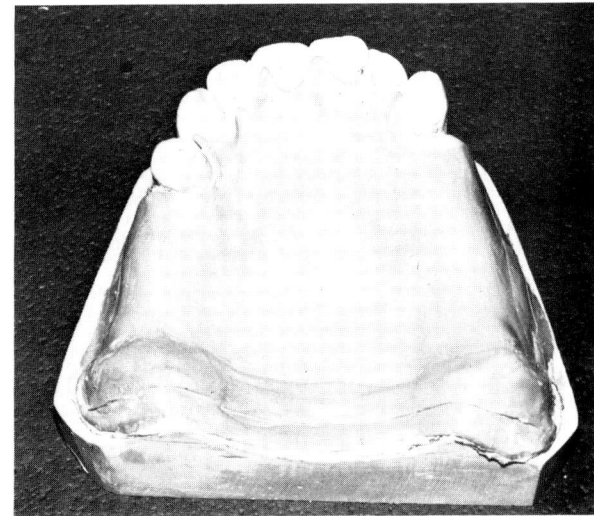

**Fig. 4-83.** Stabilized record base should be stored on cast until needed.

## PROBLEM AREAS

The record base will be difficult to remove and may damage the cast if the undercuts are not properly blocked out. Failure to place a vent hole or use sufficient impression paste may trap air, resulting in voids on the impression liner surface. Failure to seat the shellac baseplate completely may mean that it will be too thick. These problem areas can be prevented through proper blockout of undercuts, placement of an escape vent with an adequate amount of impression paste to impede void formation, and seating the baseplate on the cast to the extent that a thin layer of the impression paste is attained.

### Record bases stabilized with elastomeric impression material

Rubber base impression material has been advocated by Freese (1956), Hall (1958), and Malson (1964) to stabilize record bases. According to Greener et al. (1972), the basic material of polysulfide rubber is a polyfunctional mercaptan that can be polymerized by certain activators such as lead dioxide to produce a stable synthetic rubber. These materials accurately record the surface characteristics, while their intrinsic flexibility allows the material to be withdrawn from moderate undercut areas, thus minimizing the requirement for blockout of the cast. Severe undercuts may have to be blocked out because the rubber base liner is not thick enough to spring over the undercut. The major objections to the rubber base stabilization method include the possibility of making a record base that is too thick plus the additional expense attributed to material costs and laboratory fabrication time.

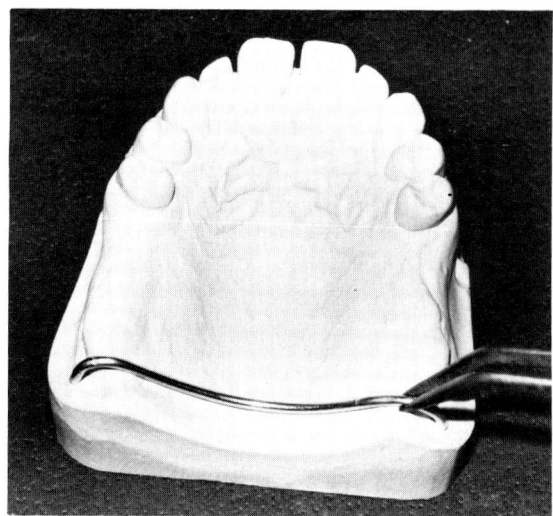

**Fig. 4-84.** Reinforcement wire is adapted to cast in posterior palatal seal area.

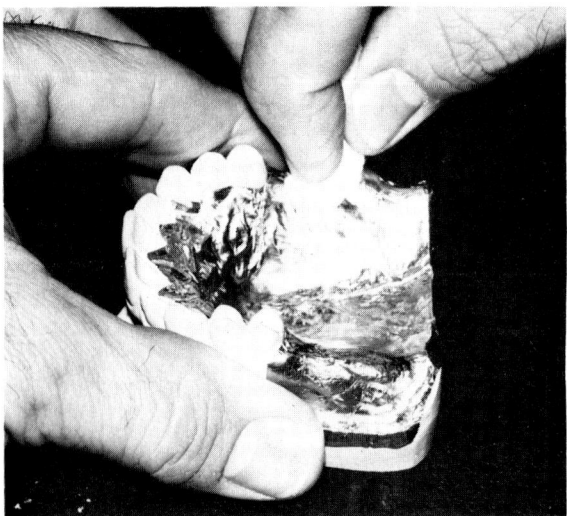

**Fig. 4-85.** Tinfoil (0.001 inch) is adapted to cast.

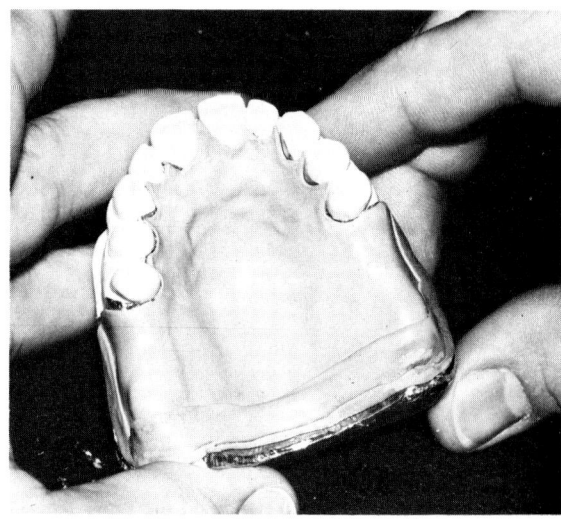

**Fig. 4-86.** Wire-reinforced shellac record base is adapted to tin-foiled cast.

## PROCEDURE

The technique for fabricating a record base stabilized with elastomeric impression material is similar to that described for zinc oxide–eugenol impression paste.

1. Adapt a reinforcement wire to the cast in the posterior palatal seal area (Fig. 4-84).
2. Apply tinfoil to the cast as previously described (Fig. 4-85).
3. Adapt a shellac baseplate, embed the reinforcing wire, and smooth the surface (Fig. 4-86).
4. Make a series of retention holes in the baseplate with a No. 8 round bur. Paint the tissue surface of the shellac baseplate with the recommended adhesive, and allow it to dry for 10 minutes (Fig. 4-87).
5. Proportion and mix the rubber base impression material* according to the manufacturer's recommendations.
6. Apply the impression material to the interior of the shellac baseplate and to the palatal portion of the cast (Fig. 4-88).

---

*Permlastic, Kerr Manufacturing Co., Romulus, Mich.; Coe-Flex, Coe Laboratories, Inc., Chicago, Ill., or equivalent.

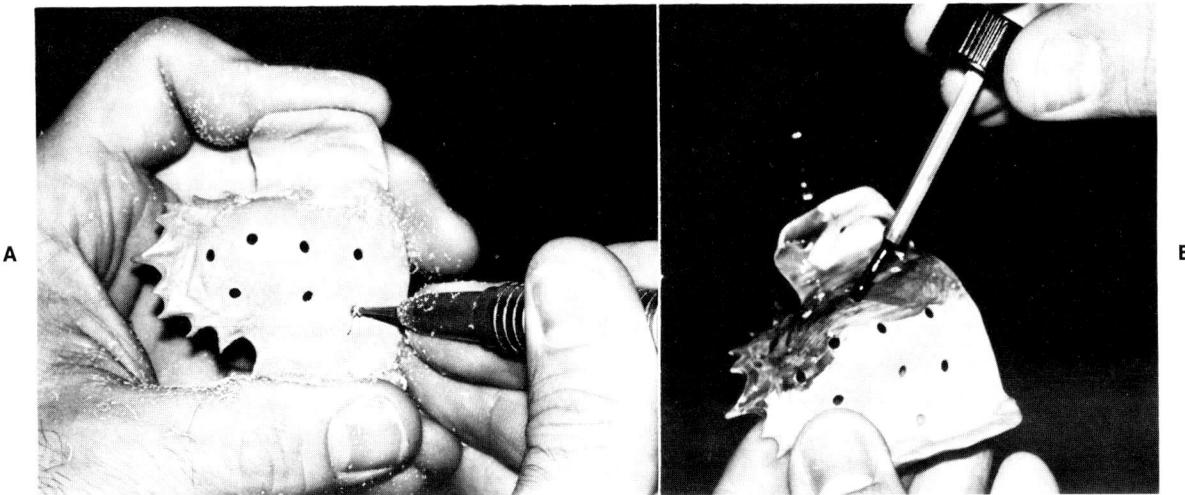

**Fig. 4-87. A,** Series of retention holes is made with No. 8 round bur. They will increase retention and serve as vents to minimize air entrapment. **B,** Adhesive is painted on shellac to increase adhesion to elastomeric impression material.

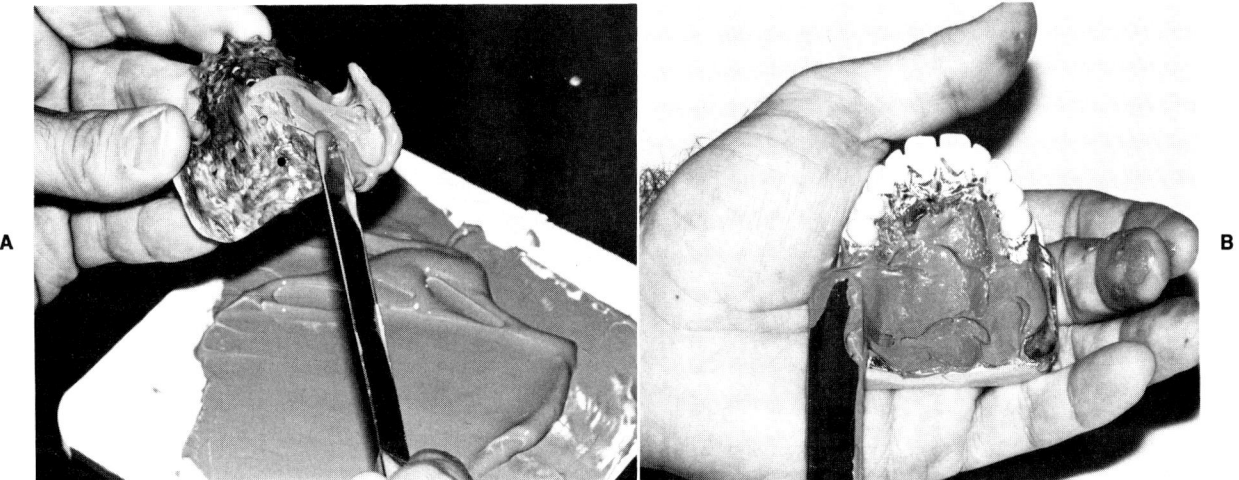

**Fig. 4-88. A,** After proportioning and mixing rubber base material according to manufacturer's recommendation, it is placed into shellac baseplate. **B,** Some impression material is placed on palatal area of cast to minimize voids.

**108** *Dental laboratory procedures: removable partial dentures*

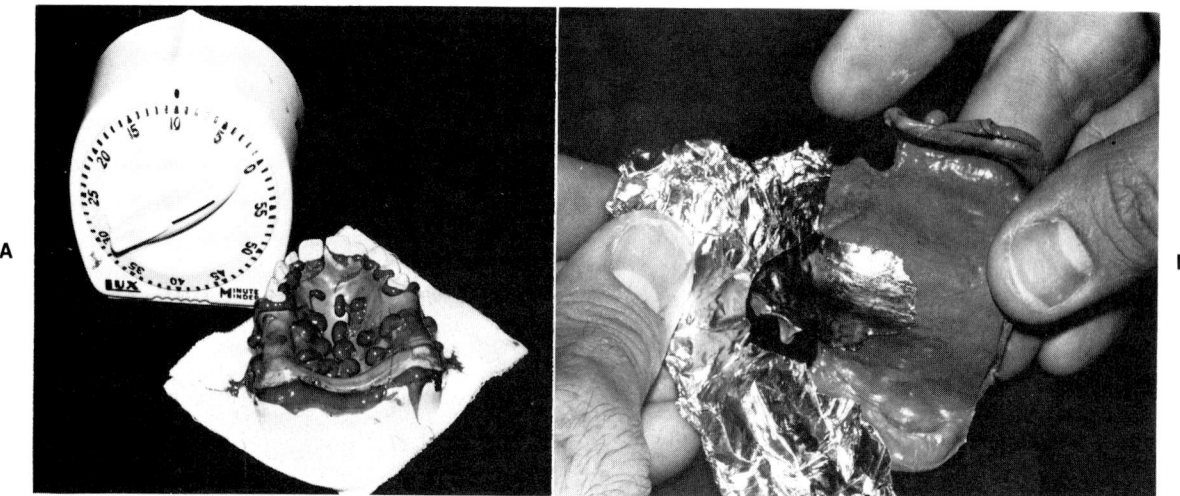

**Fig. 4-89. A,** After seating record base on cast with finger pressure, rubber should polymerize for minimum of 10 minutes. Note extrusions of impression material through perforations. **B,** Tinfoil can be peeled away from rubber surface.

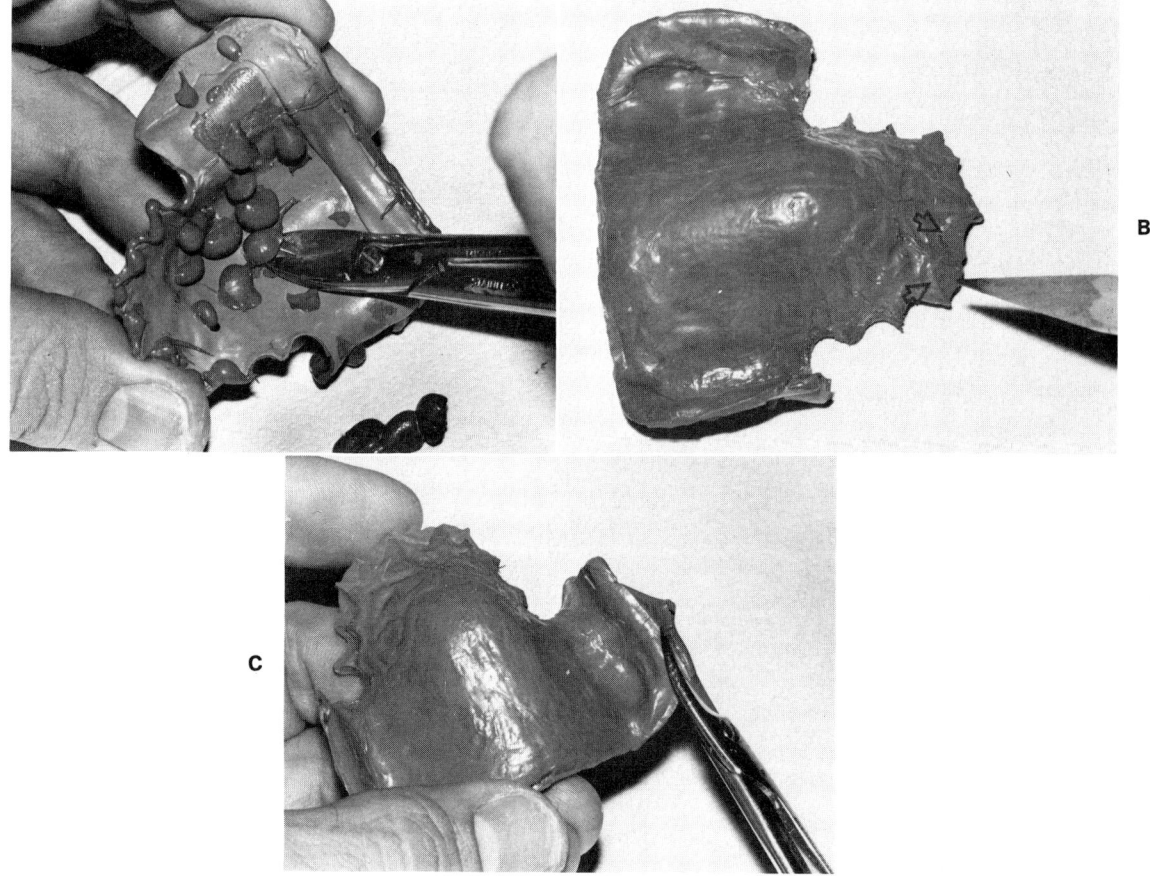

**Fig. 4-90. A,** Scissors are used to trim rubber impression material protruding through retention holes. **B,** Excess impression material on lingual tooth surfaces (arrows) must be removed to prevent occlusal interference. **C,** Borders are trimmed to maintain optimal thickness.

*Record bases and mounting casts* **109**

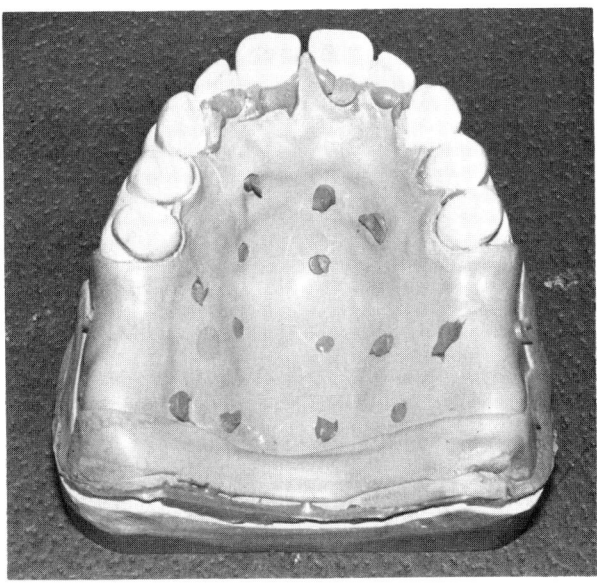

Fig. 4-91. Record bases stabilized with elastomeric impression material fit accurately and permit extension into moderate undercuts.

7. Seat the loaded baseplate carefully on the tinfoiled cast, and set the timer for 10 minutes. After the impression material has set, remove the record base from the cast, and peel the tinfoil away from the rubber (Fig. 4-89).

8. Trim the rubber impression material protruding through the retention holes and any excess material on the borders or over tooth surfaces that would interfere with normal closure (Fig. 4-90).

9. The stabilized record base should accurately fit the cast and be capable of removal over moderate undercuts (Fig. 4-91).

### Record bases stabilized with autopolymerizing resin

Shooshan (1953), Boos (1956), and Hall (1958) have advocated the stabilization of record bases with autopolymerizing acrylic resin. The cast must be properly blocked out with wax to facilitate removal of the record base without damage to the cast or record base. Lining the record base with the resin will enhance its rigidity and improve the fit. Disadvantages of this technique include the increased fabrication time and the prospect for distortion of the record base associated with the release of internal stresses in the acrylic resin lining material.

**PROCEDURE**

The procedures for fabricating a record base with autopolymerizing resin are similar to those described for stabilization with zinc oxide–eugenol impression paste.

1. Identify undercuts on the cast, including tooth interproximal areas, and ensure their blockout with baseplate wax. If the resin is allowed to flow into undercut areas, its rigidity will prevent the record base from being removed without possible damage to the cast or record base (Fig. 4-92).

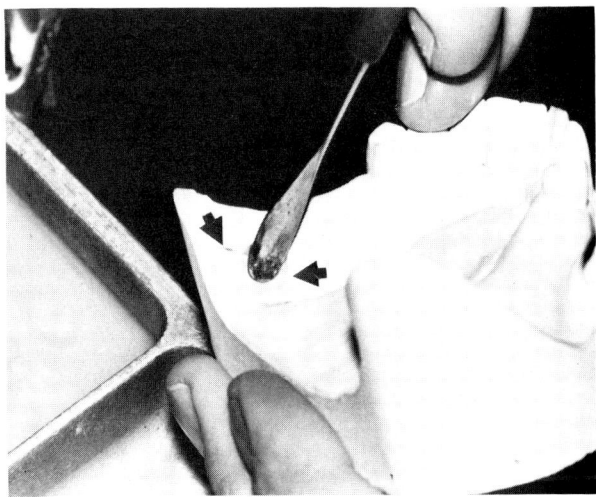

Fig. 4-92. Undercuts are identified and blocked out on cast with baseplate wax (arrows).

2. Apply a liberal coating of tinfoil substitute to the cast.

3. After adapting a shellac baseplate to the cast, trim 2 mm from the border reflection to accommodate the autopolymerizing resin border (Fig. 4-93).

4. Stabilize the shellac baseplate by embedding a curved piece of heavy-duty paper clip wire; then cover the wire with shellac material, and smooth the surface (Fig. 4-94).

5. Make two holes through the buccal and lingual slopes in the canine and molar areas with a No. 8 round bur. Place another vent hole in the palate when stabilizing a maxillary record base (Fig. 4-95).

6. Mix autopolymerizing acrylic resin, and apply it to the tissue surface of the shellac record base with a spatula (Fig. 4-96).

7. Seat the record base on the cast with enough pressure to assure a uniform (1 to 2 mm) thickness of acrylic resin. While the resin is soft, carefully remove any excess from the tooth surfaces with a No. 7 spatula (Fig. 4-97).

8. Allow the autopolymerizing resin to cure by covering the cast with a plaster bowl or placing it in a pressure pot at 20 psi.

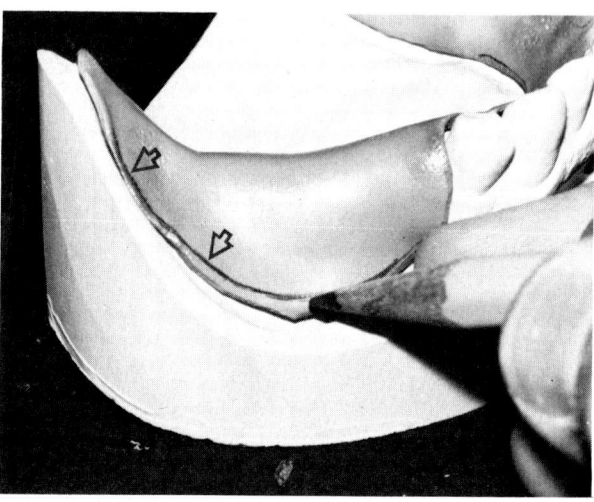

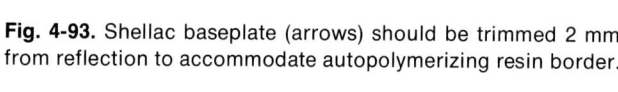

**Fig. 4-93.** Shellac baseplate (arrows) should be trimmed 2 mm from reflection to accommodate autopolymerizing resin border.

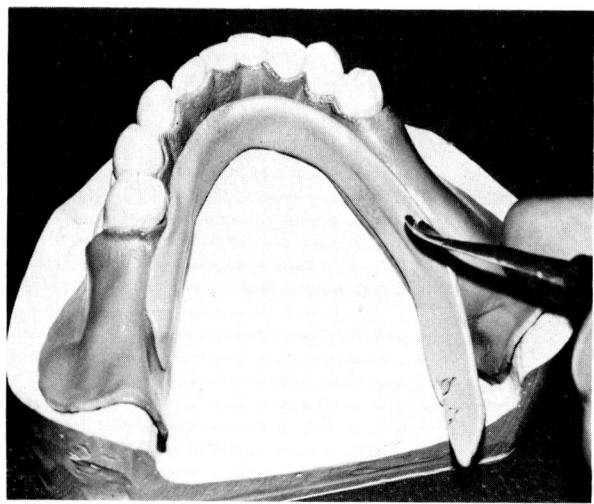

**Fig. 4-94.** Reinforcement wire is placed on lingual surface from first molar to first molar and covered with shellac material.

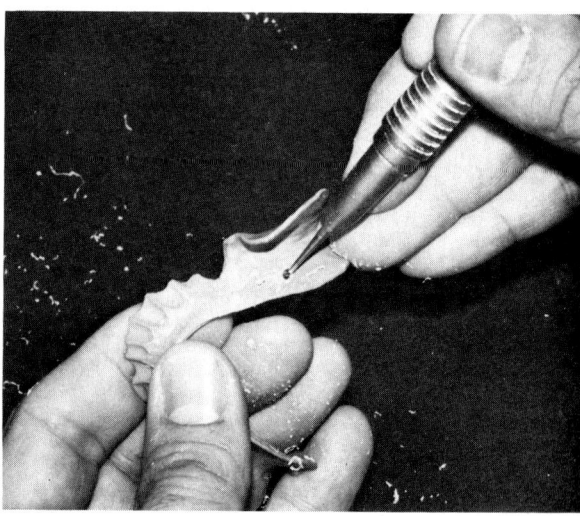

**Fig. 4-95.** Vent holes are placed in canine and molar areas with No. 8 round bur.

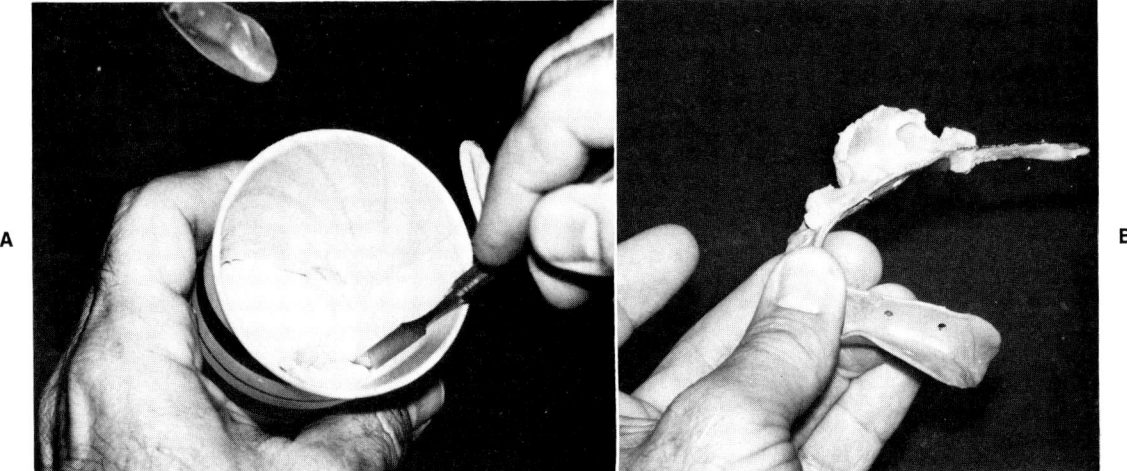

**Fig. 4-96. A,** Autopolymerizing acrylic resin is proportioned and mixed according to manufacturer's direction. **B,** Spatula is used to cover tissue surface with acrylic resin.

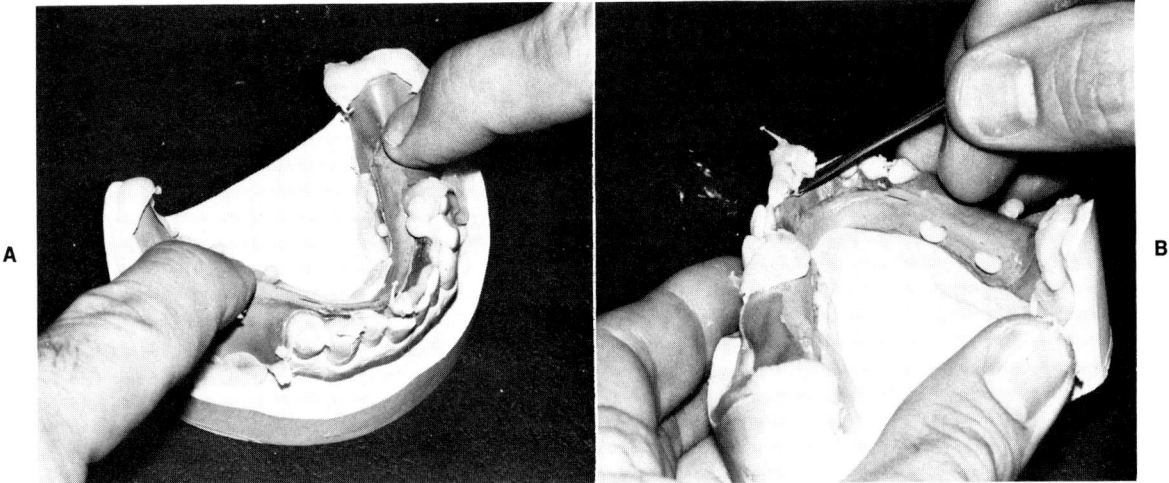

**Fig. 4-97. A,** Resin-filled shellac record base is carefully seated on cast. Optimal thickness is 1 to 2 mm of acrylic resin. **B,** Excess resin on tooth surfaces is removed with No. 7 spatula.

9. After curing, carefully remove the record base from the cast, and examine the tissue surface for any areas of excess resin. Trim the excess from the interproximal areas and borders with a carbide bur or arbor band (Fig. 4-98). Polish the record base borders with a slurry of water and flour of pumice (Fig. 4-99).

10. The acrylic resin–stabilized record base should be stored on the cast until ready for use (Fig. 4-100).

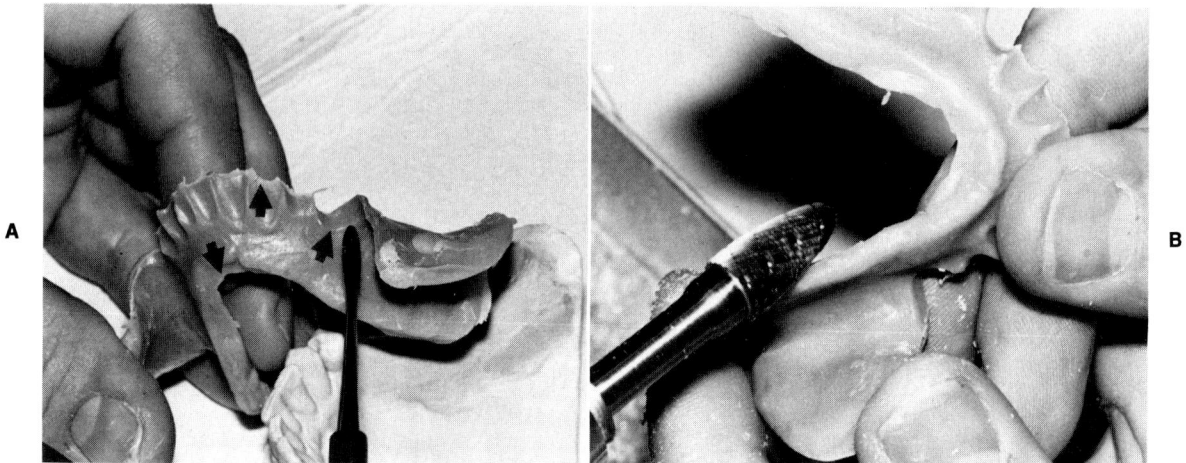

Fig. 4-98. **A,** Cured record base is examined for excess resin (arrows). **B,** Carbide bur is used to trim resin flash from record base borders.

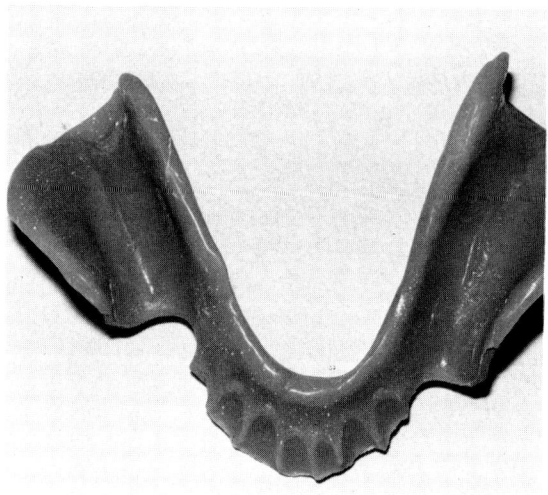

Fig. 4-99. Resin borders have been lightly polished with slurry of pumice and water.

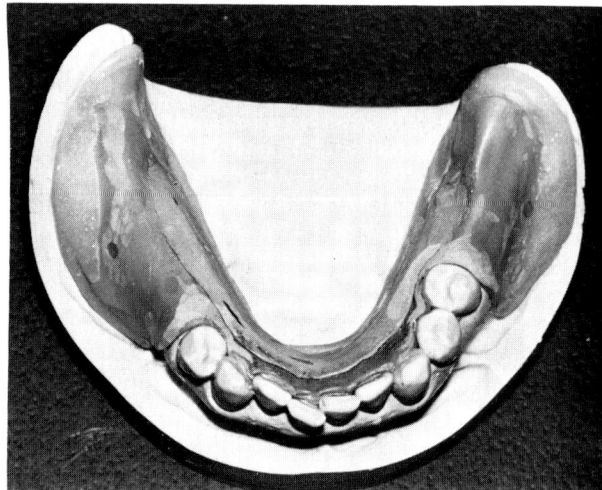

Fig. 4-100. Acrylic resin–stabilized record base should be stored on cast until needed.

**Table 4-4.** Shellac record base method

| Problem | Probable cause | Solution |
| --- | --- | --- |
| Teeth chipped or broken during removal | Interproximal and gingival tooth areas not blocked out with wax | Flow baseplate wax in gingival crest and interproximal areas to provide blockout |
| Record base removed from cast with difficulty | Insufficient blockout of undercuts | Block out undercuts with wax |
| | Shellac record base stuck to cast | Prevent overheating shellac record base during adaptation |
| | Failure to wet cast or apply talc before adaptation of shellac | Soak cast in slurry water, or apply talc before adapting shellac |
| Record base lacks rigidity | Record base too thin, and no wire reinforcement used | Add heavy-duty paper clip wire for reinforcement |
| Record base lacks uniform thickness | Stabilizing material addition too thick | Control flow of stabilizing material with adequate seating pressure |
| Void in stabilizing material | Insufficient stabilizing material, or trapping air due to failure to provide palatal vent hole | Provide vent hole in palate; use sufficient stabilizing material to eliminate voids |
| Failure of record base to fit cast | Warpage of record base by heat Distortion of record base by stabilizing material | Readapt shellac record base Remake record base |

**PROBLEM AREAS**

Failure to adequately block out interproximal tooth areas and tissue undercuts may result in chipping of the teeth and other critical parts of the cast or breakage of the record base (Table 4-4). It is also possible that the release of internal stresses in the acrylic resin may induce distortion of the shellac record base. When this occurs the shellac record base should be remade.

## VACUUM-ADAPTED THERMOPLASTIC RESIN RECORD BASES

Record bases can be rapidly and efficiently made by vacuum-molding thermoplastic resin on the cast. In this technique, a preformed resin sheet of 0.060 inch (0.15 cm) thickness is softened by an external heat source, and then drawn to the cast with a vacuum machine to produce a record base with reasonable adaptation and uniform thickness. According to Terry and Wahlberg (1966), the vacuum method provided more intimate adaptation of baseplate material to the cast when compared with a manual technique. A technique of fabricating resin record bases by vacuum molding has been described by Allred et al. (1968b). Principal advantages of the vacuum-adapting method are minimal construction time, simplicity of technique, uniformity of thickness, satisfactory rigidity provided that an adequate thickness of material is employed, reasonable adaptation to the cast, and an opportunity to use an assortment of materials for making record bases, impression trays, splints and mouth protectors. The disadvantages include the initial equipment cost, the problem in adapting the record base material to all portions of the cast and in particular any vestibular reflections, and the difficulty in forming a smooth rounded border of suitable thickness from only one thermoplastic resin sheet.

**114** *Dental laboratory procedures: removable partial dentures*

**PROCEDURE**

1. Examine the cast to determine that the sides are at right angles to the base to facilitate removal of the resin sheet (Fig. 4-101).

2. Block out any deep undercuts with a heat-stable blockout compound* to prevent cast breakage when removing the record base (Fig. 4-102). Because of the high temperatures involved, wax or any other blockout material affected by heat should not be used. Spray the blocked out cast with a lubricant* to keep the resin sheet from adhering to the stone surface (Fig. 4-103).

3. Although the configuration varies between manufacturers, the vacuum-adapting equipment† consists essentially of a heating element, holding frame for the resin sheet, and a vacuum motor (Fig. 4-104).

4. Place the blocked out cast on the vacuum plate, and confirm that the base of the cast is flat (Fig. 4-105).

5. Select an acrylic resin sheet‡ of the proper thickness (0.060 inch; 0.15 cm), and position it in the holding frame. The sheet should be carefully placed to ensure that all sides are firmly clasped for proper adaptation (Fig. 4-106).

---

*Omnidental blockout compound, Buffalo Dental Manufacturing Co., Brooklyn, N.Y.

---

*Omnilube Spray Silicone, Omnidental Corp., Chicago, Ill.
†Stalite Sta-Vac, Buffalo Dental Manufacturing Co., Brooklyn, N.Y., or equivalent.
‡Omnivac baseplate material, 0.060 inch, Buffalo Dental Manufacturing Co., Brooklyn, N.Y.

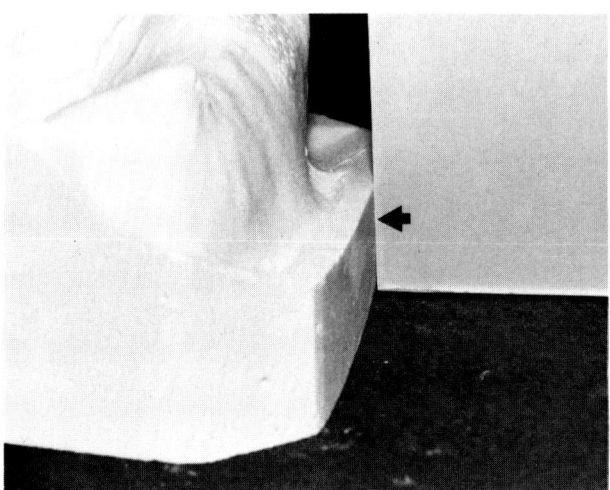

**Fig. 4-101.** Side of cast should be at right angle (arrow) to base to facilitate removal of resin sheet.

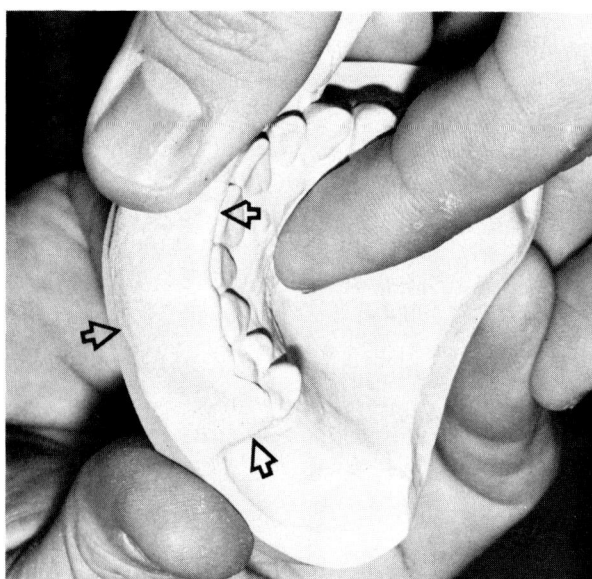

**Fig. 4-102.** Heat-stable blockout compound (arrows) is adapted to block out undercuts. It is carried up to labio incisal edge of remaining teeth for protection.

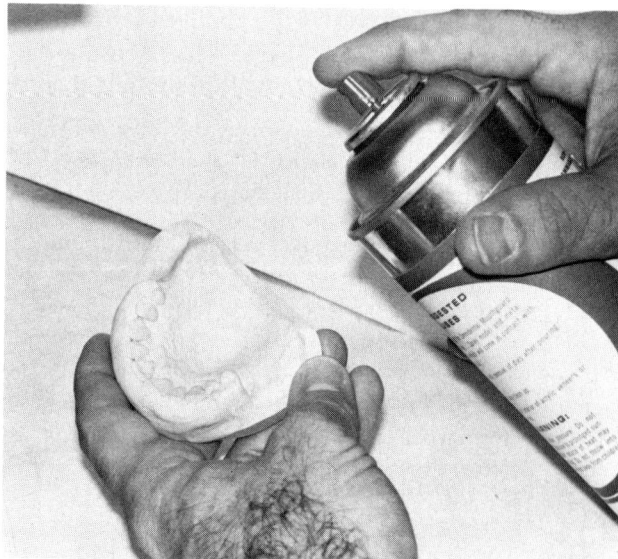

**Fig. 4-103.** Cast surface is sprayed with aerosol lubricant to prevent sticking of resin sheet.

*Record bases and mounting casts* **115**

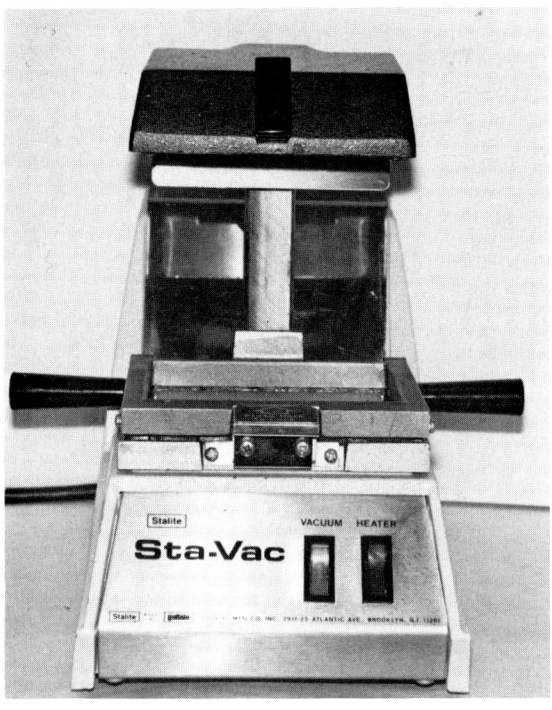

Fig. 4-104. Stalite Sta-Vac vacuum-adapting equipment.

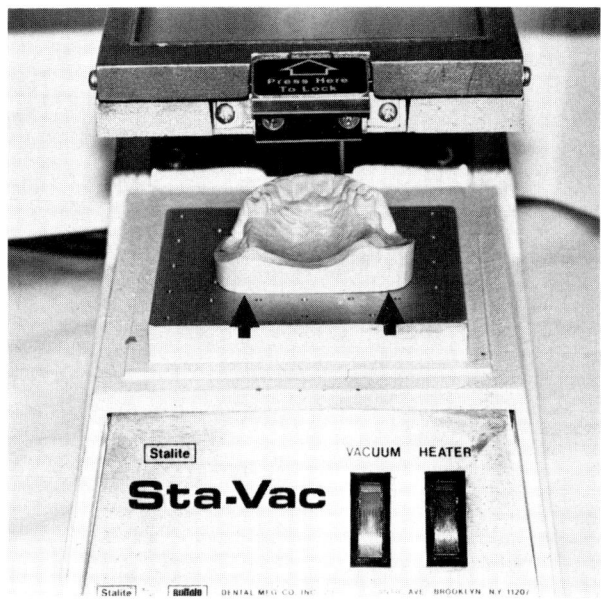

Fig. 4-105. Blocked out cast is positioned on vacuum plate (Sta-Vac). Note that cast base is flat (arrows).

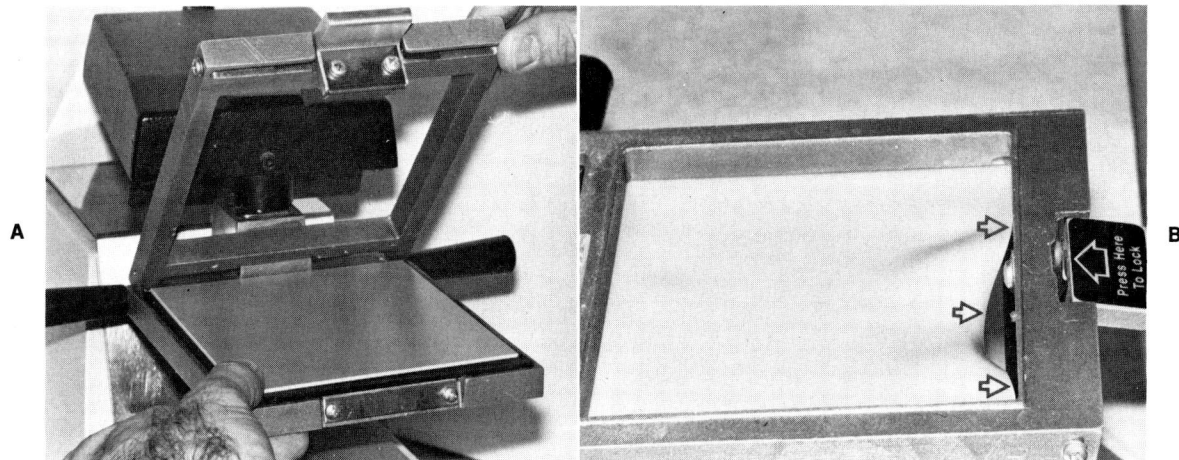

Fig. 4-106. A, Resin baseplate sheet (0.060 inch; 0.15 cm) is placed in holding frame. B, One side (arrows) of sheet has not been clasped by frame.

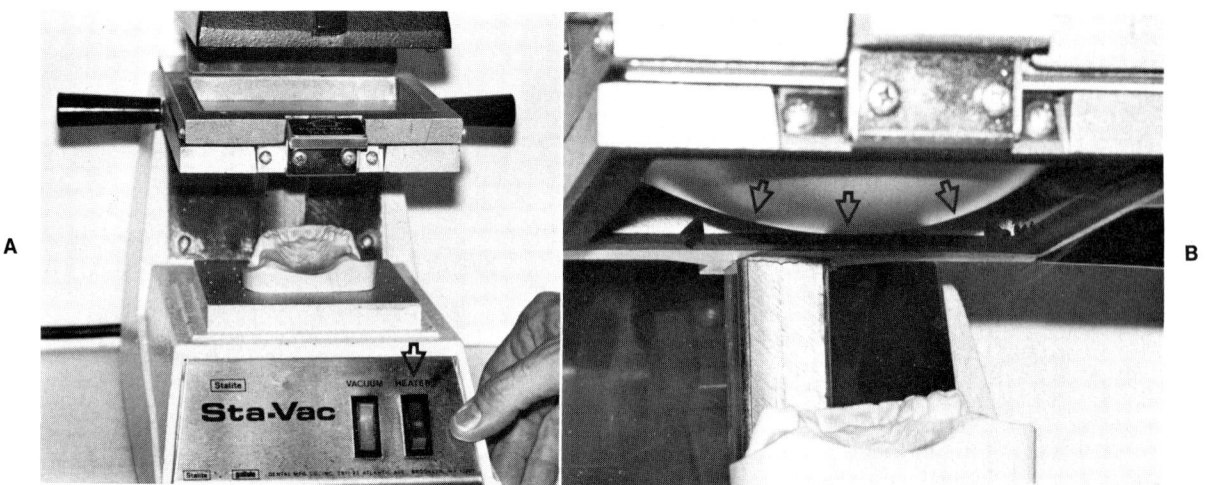

**Fig. 4-107. A,** After heating element is aligned over cast, heater switch (arrow) is activated. **B,** Resin baseplate material sags (arrows) as heat is generated from element.

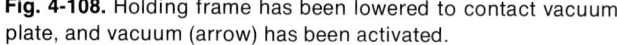

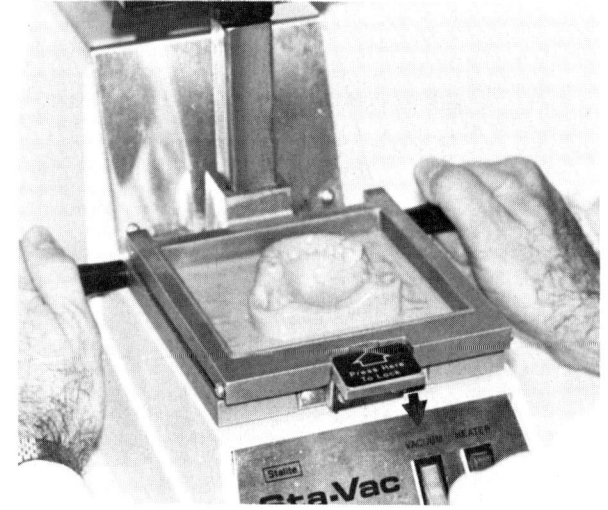

**Fig. 4-108.** Holding frame has been lowered to contact vacuum plate, and vacuum (arrow) has been activated.

6. Activate the heating element after aligning it over the cast. Heat the resin sheet, and watch for it to sag downward approximately ½ inch (1.3 cm) below the lower edge of the holding frame (Fig. 4-107). At this point, quickly lower the frame to contact the vacuum plate, and activate the vacuum motor. The heating element should be held over the cast for 15 seconds while adaptation is taking place (Fig. 4-108).

7. Turn the heating element off, and swing it out of the way. Continue vacuum adaptation for 30 seconds while manipulating the resin sheet with the fingers to improve accuracy of fit (Fig. 4-109).

8. Carefully remove the cast with the adapted resin sheet, and allow it to cool before trimming (Fig. 4-110). Cut the sheet with a carbide bur and strip away excess material from the cast periphery (Fig. 4-111).

*Record bases and mounting casts* 117

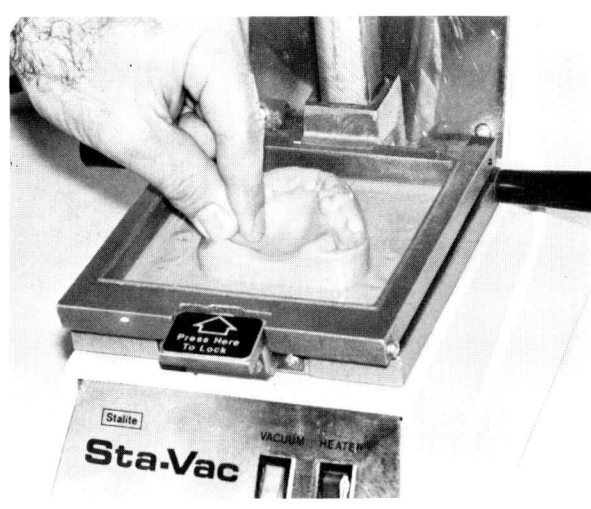

**Fig. 4-109.** Fit of resin sheet can be improved by finger adaption while resin cools. Care must be exercised because of heat of resin material.

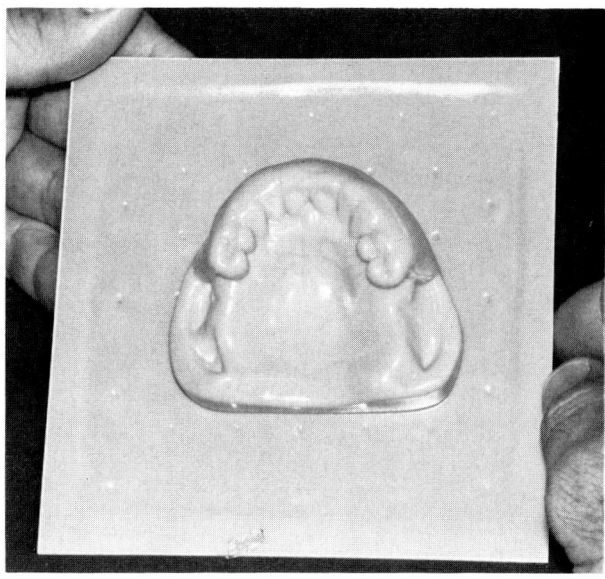

**Fig. 4-110.** Cast and resin sheet are carefully removed and allowed to cool before trimming.

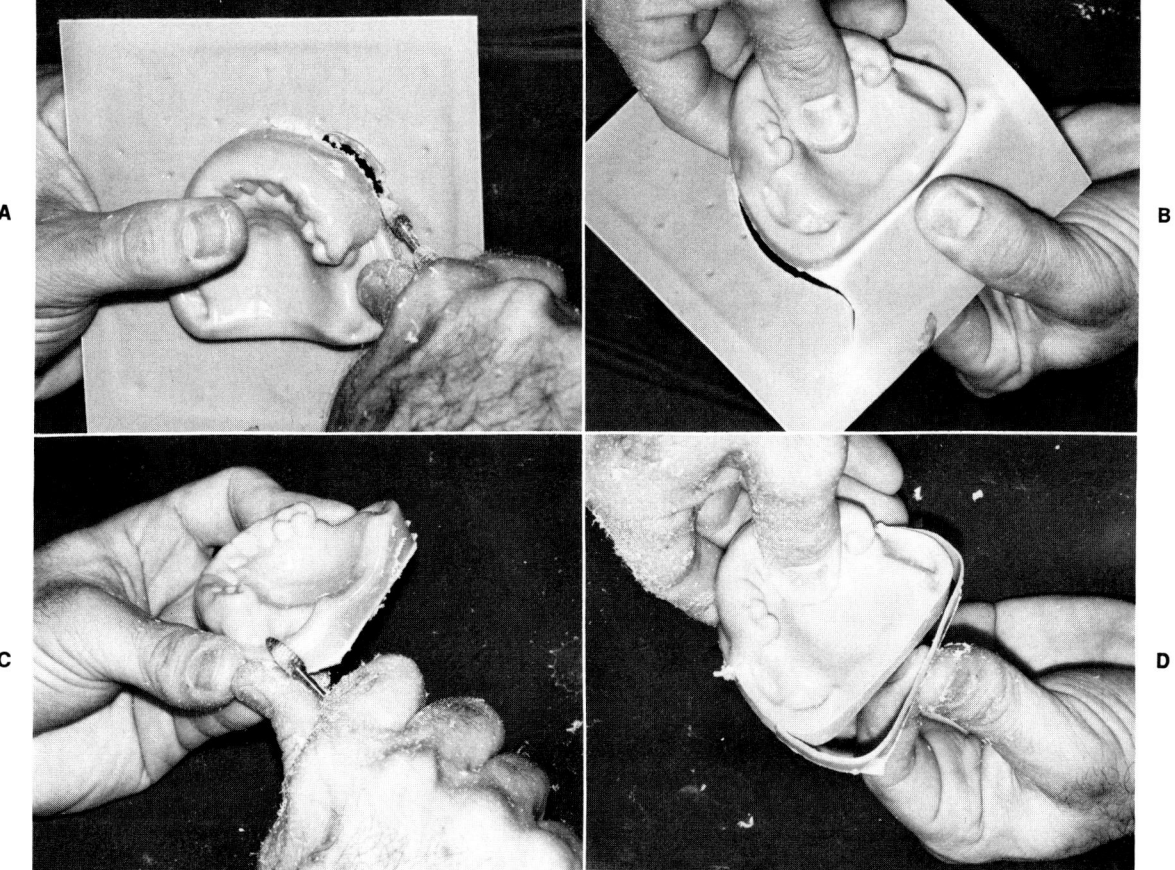

**Fig. 4-111. A,** Removal of adapted resin sheet from cast is initiated by cutting around periphery with carbide bur. **B,** Flat portion of sheet is separated from cast portion. **C,** Bur cut is made at junction of land area and side of cast. **D,** Cast resin borders can be stripped away.

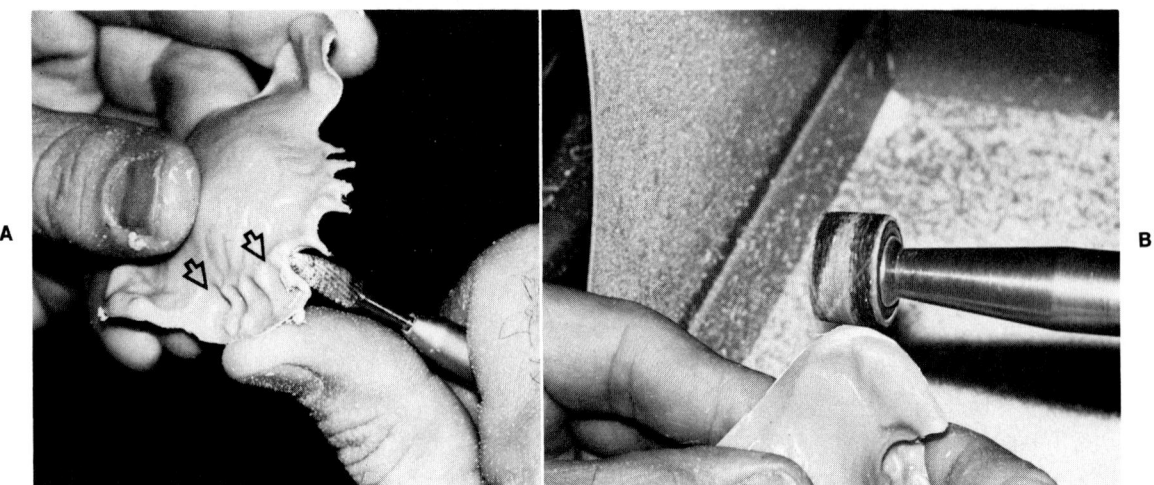

**Fig. 4-112. A,** Tapered carbide bur is used to trim away resin covering teeth (arrows). **B,** Additional finishing of borders can be accomplished with lathe-mounted arbor band.

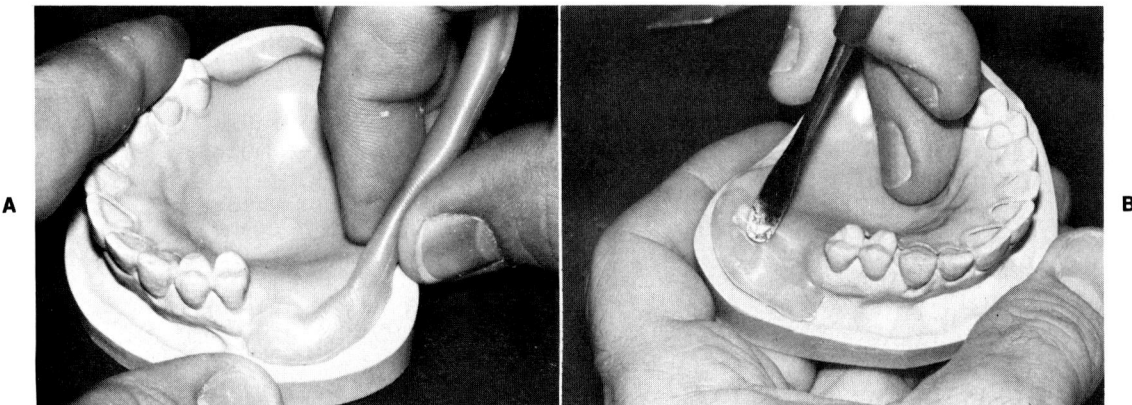

**Fig. 4-113. A,** Baseplate wax is added to resin sheet for proper border contour. **B,** Wax surface should be smooth and rounded for patient comfort.

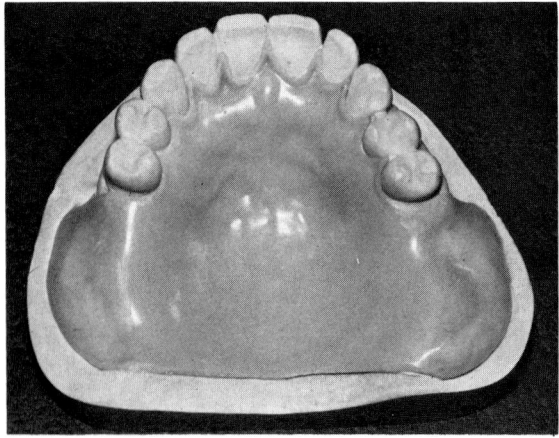

**Fig. 4-114.** Completed vacuum-adapted record base is stored on cast.

9. Remove the record base from the cast, and carefully trim away any material overlaying the cingulum tooth areas to prevent occlusal interference. Smooth the borders of the resin sheet with an arbor band (Fig. 4-112).

10. Increase the border thickness by adding baseplate wax. Flow the wax with a No. 7 spatula to provide a smooth transition of the two materials (Fig. 4-113). Heat areas that require additional adaptation, and mold them to the cast with a moistened finger. Store the record base on the cast (Fig. 4-114).

**Table 4-5.** Vacuum-adapted thermoplastic resin record base method

| Problem | Probable cause | Solution |
| --- | --- | --- |
| Record base removed from cast with difficulty | Insufficient blockout of undercuts | Block out undercuts with heat-stable blockout compound; spray cast with silicone lubricant |
| Teeth chipped or broken during removal | Labial tooth surfaces not blocked out | Carry blockout compound from undercut areas up to labioincisal edge of teeth |
| Record base borders not adapted into border reflections | Vestibular reflections of cast bridged by resin material | Readapt resin by heat and manual adaptation; develop proper border thickness by adding wax |
| Failure of record base to accurately | Insufficient softening of thermoplastic resin | Heat resin sheet until it sags properly |
| | Abbreviated vacuum molding | Continue vacuum molding for 30 seconds after heat is turned off; readapt deficient areas by manual adaptation |

### PROBLEM AREAS

Problems associated with the vacuum-adapted thermoplastic resin method are listed in Table 4-5. Insufficient blockout of undercuts may result in difficult removal of the record base and possible damage to the cast. In some instances, the resin sheet is not well adapted into the border reflections of the cast because of a bridging of the material over the deeper recesses. These deficiencies can usually be corrected by additional heating and manual adaptation. The manufacturer's directions for heating and vacuum-molding intervals should be carefully followed to enhance the adaptation to the cast. Proper thickness and contour of the record base border can be achieved by the addition of self-curing acrylic resin or wax to the thermoplastic material. The principal advantages of this method of record base construction are the simplicity and the minimal time requirement for fabrication.

### WAX RECORD BASES

Boucher et al. (1975) have described a method of fabricating record bases using hard baseplate wax. The record base can be easily and quickly adapted to the cast while providing optimum space for placement of the occlusion rim or replacement teeth. Unfortunately wax is known for an inherent lack of dimensional stability. Reinforcement with a heavy-duty paper clip wire will improve the stability, but the wax record base is still susceptible to warpage with temperature change. From a practical standpoint, the dentist may have to manually readapt the wax record base immediately prior to use to compensate for any dimensional change.

### PROCEDURE

1. Brush powdered talc on the cast surface to act as a separator and an adaptation indicator (Fig. 4-115).

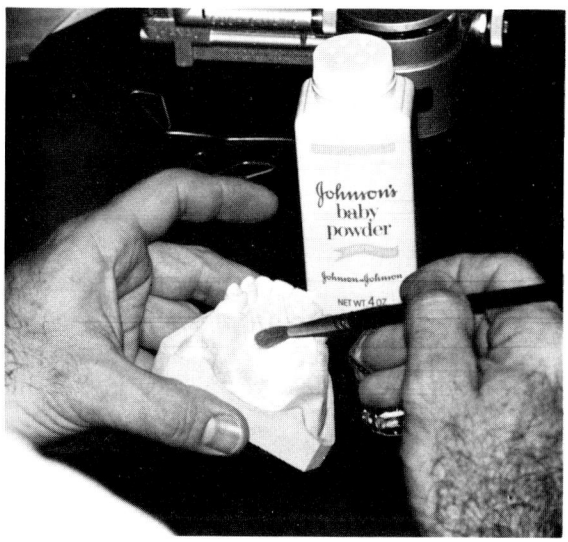

**Fig. 4-115.** Powdered talc is brushed onto cast surface as separator.

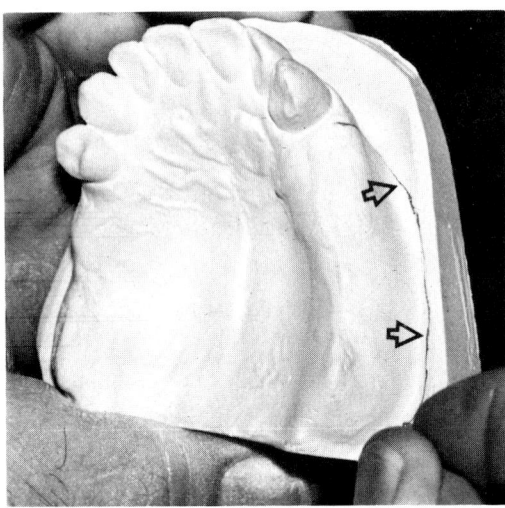

Fig. 4-116. Pencil outline (arrows) on edentulous area borders will facilitate trimming of adapted wax.

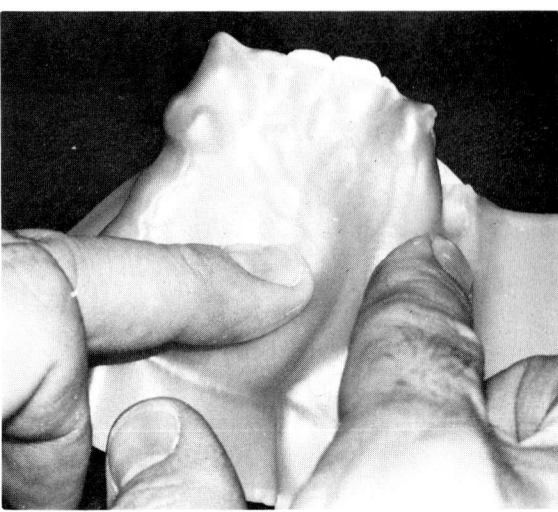

Fig. 4-117. Sheet of hard baseplate wax is softened and carefully adapted to cast. Intimate contact of wax and cast surface is desirable.

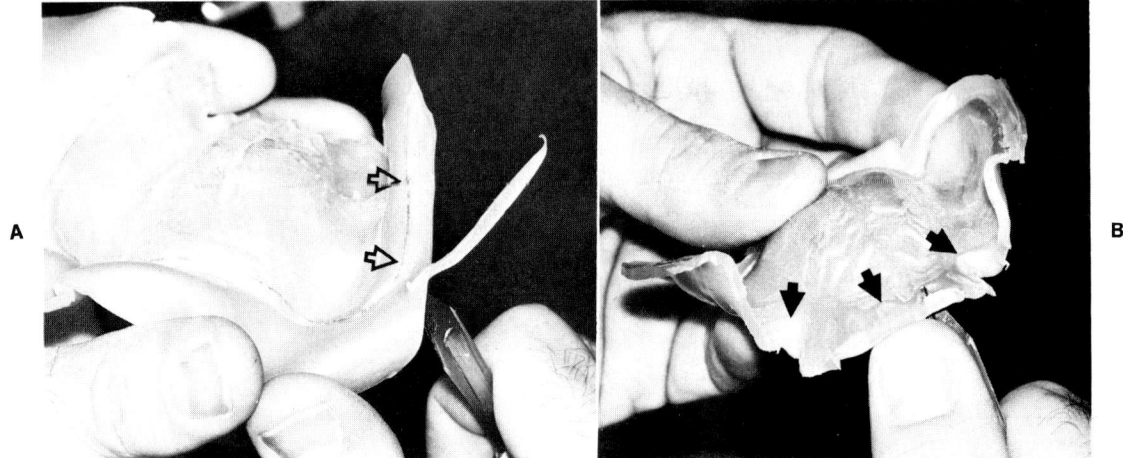

Fig. 4-118. **A,** Adapted wax is removed from cast and trimmed 3 mm beyond transferred pencil line (arrows). Extra wax will be reflected back onto wax base to create border contours. **B,** Wax is removed from cingulum and lingual aspect of teeth (arrows).

## WAX OCCLUSION RIMS

Although other materials may be employed, most occlusion rims are formed from baseplate wax. The wax can be warmed and rolled into the appropriate shape and sealed into place over the record base. Wax occlusion rims can also be formed by shaping the baseplate wax with a metal occlusion rim former,* or preformed wax rims can be purchased from several manufacturers (Fig. 4-125). In the early phases of partial denture construction, the wax rim and record base are employed to determine the existing occlusion. With this information, the dentist is then able to evaluate the arch relationship and plan for any tooth modifications to accommodate the removable partial denture. After the framework has been completed, the wax rim can be attached directly to the resin retention areas to serve as a stabilized record base for recording the maxillomandibular relationship and determining the proper position of the replacement teeth. The wax occlusion rim can be used to convey valuable information from the dentist to the dental laboratory technician. In addition to the arch relation, the occlusion rim can assist in the determination of the length and width of the replacement teeth, midline, occlusal plane, high and low lip lines, cuspid line, proper lip support, and the amount of vertical and horizontal overlap. The maxillomandibular relation must be transferred to the selected articulator accurately. Plaster of Paris can be used to mount casts, but ar-

---

*Bite Rim Former, Dentsply International, Inc., York, Pa.

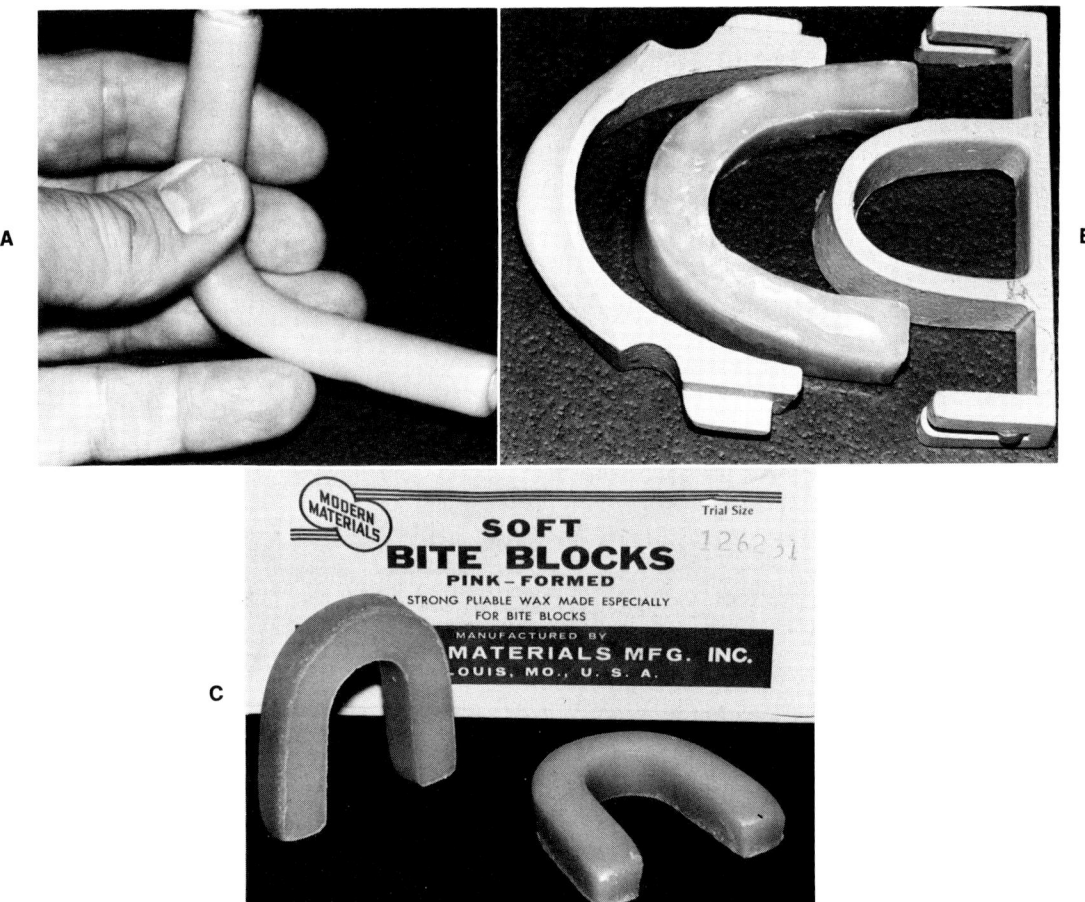

**Fig. 4-125. A,** Occlusion rims can be made from sheet of baseplate wax. Wax is softened and carefully rolled into homogeneous mass. It is important to heat wax thoroughly to avoid folds and air entrapment. **B,** Baseplate wax can be shaped into occlusion rim with metal occlusion rim former. Softened wax is molded into adjustable form to produce wax rim of desired width. **C,** Preformed wax occlusion rims of variable hardness are available from different manufacturers.

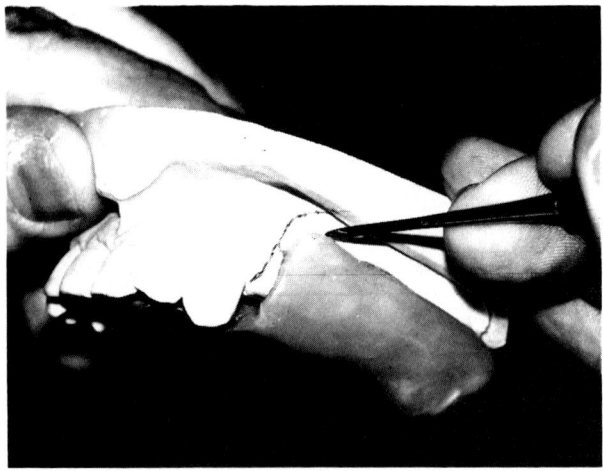

Fig. 4-122. When record base extends into undercut, wax should be warmed with alcohol torch. Record base is removed and replaced several times to assure its removal.

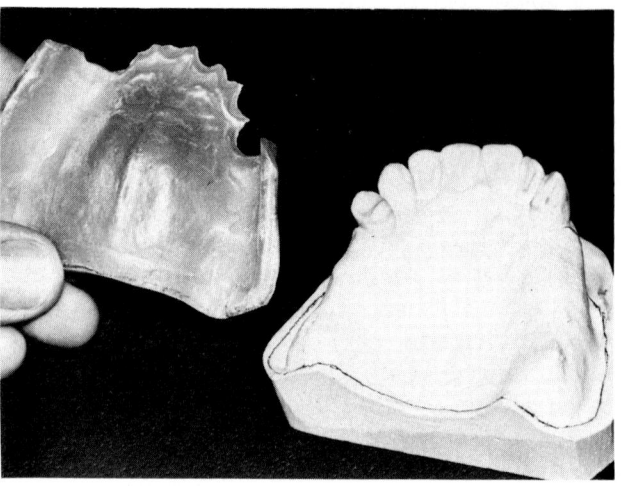

Fig. 4-123. Completed wax record base should be well adapted with smooth, properly contoured borders.

9. The wax should not be adapted into severe undercuts because there is no provision for their blockout with this method. This can be handled by warming the wax over any undercuts, then removing and inserting the record base several times to assure its removal (Fig. 4-122).

10. The wax record base should be well adapted with smooth borders that fill the vestibular reflection of the cast (Fig. 4-123). Store the finished wax record base on the cast, and readapt it as required (Fig. 4-124).

### PROBLEM AREAS

The main problem with the wax record base method is the lack of dimensional stability of the wax with subsequent warpage after fabrication. The wax can be readapted manually to correct this discrepancy prior to use (Table 4-6).

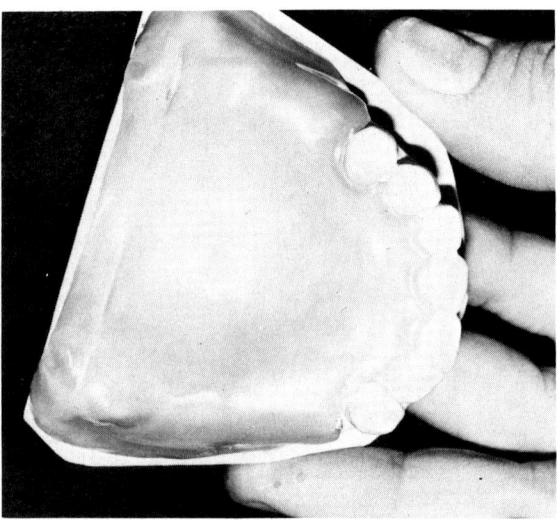

Fig. 4-124. It is convenient to store wax record base on cast and readapt it prior to use.

**Table 4-6.** Wax record base method

| Problem | Probable cause | Solution |
| --- | --- | --- |
| Failure of record base to accurately fit cast | Improper adaptation of wax to cast | Coat cast with talc; then adapt wax to attain intimate contact with cast surface |
| | Reinforcement wire not employed | Embed reinforcement wire to maintain dimensional stability and provide rigidity |
| | Warpage of wax record base after completion | Manually readapt wax record base |

8. Verify the adaptation of the record base by checking for smooth, talc-free areas on the wax tissue surface. Corrections can be made by reapplying talc to the cast, heating both sides of the wax, and then readapting it with the fingers (Fig. 4-121).

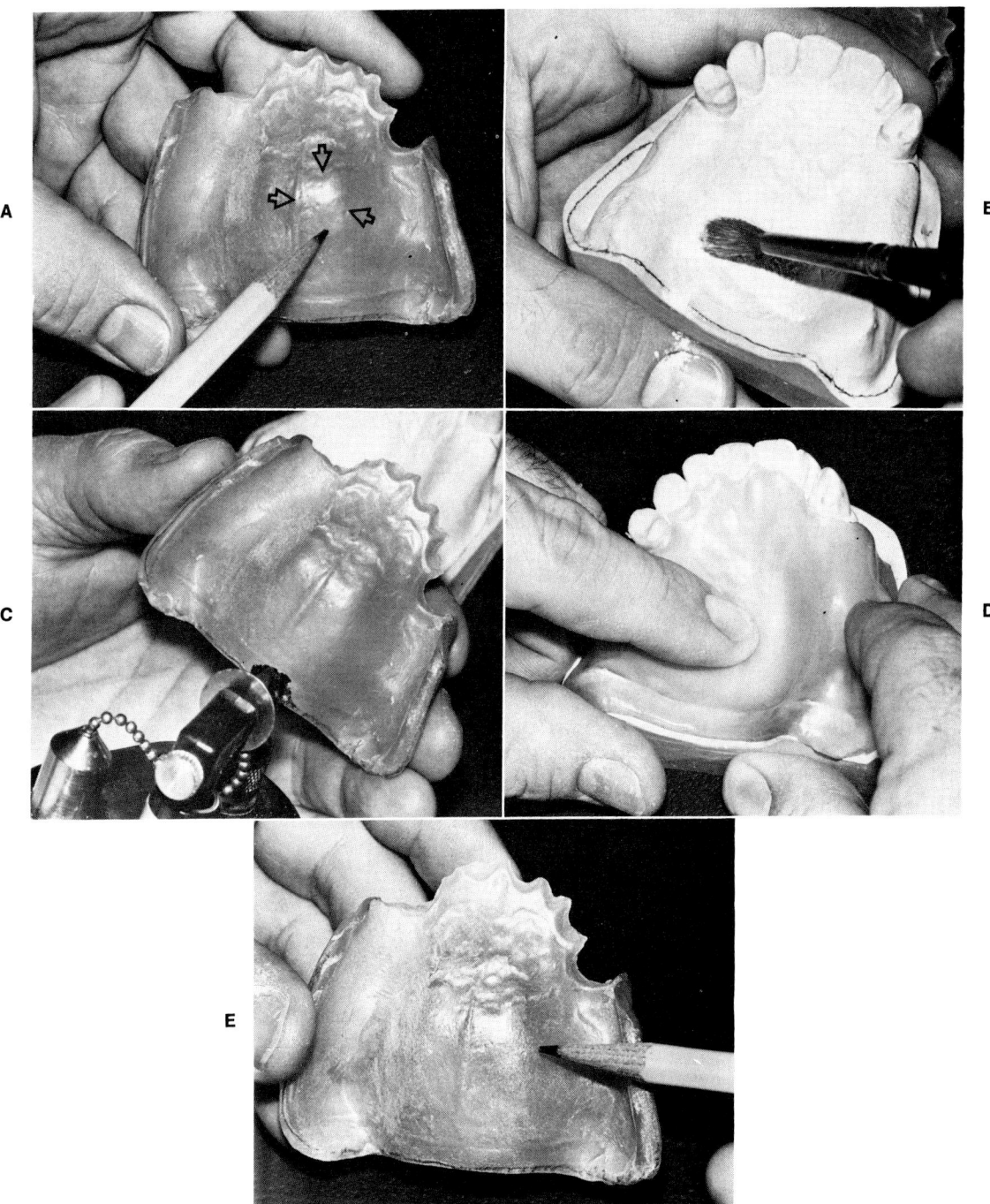

Fig. 4-121. **A**, Smooth, talc-free areas (arrows) on wax tissue surface indicate poor adaptation and need for correction. **B**, Talc is reapplied to cast surface in discrepancy area. **C**, Both sides of wax record base are heated with torch. **D**, Wax record base is replaced on cast and wax is readapted. **E**, Corrected wax record base is well adapted to cast.

2. Adapt a heavy-duty paper clip across the posterior extent of the maxillary cast about ⅛ inch (3 mm) anterior to the posterior border as described previously. For the mandibular record base, the wire should extend from first molar to first molar and be situated lingual to the ridge crest. The wire will be added to the baseplate wax for reinforcement and rigidity.

3. Use a pencil to outline the peripheral border on the cast to simplify subsequent wax trimming (Fig. 4-116).

4. Soften a sheet of hard baseplate wax, and carefully adapt it to the cast surface (Fig. 4-117).

5. Remove the wax, and trim it approximately 3 mm beyond the transferred pencil line in the border regions. Remove any wax from the maxillary tooth cingulum areas that might cause occlusal interference (Fig. 4-118).

6. Replace the wax on the cast, and fold the excess wax back onto itself to fill the vestibular reflection (Fig. 4-119). Add more wax if needed.

7. Heat the previously adapted reinforcement wire, and embed it in the wax record base. Flow additional wax over the wire, and smooth the surface (Fig. 4-120).

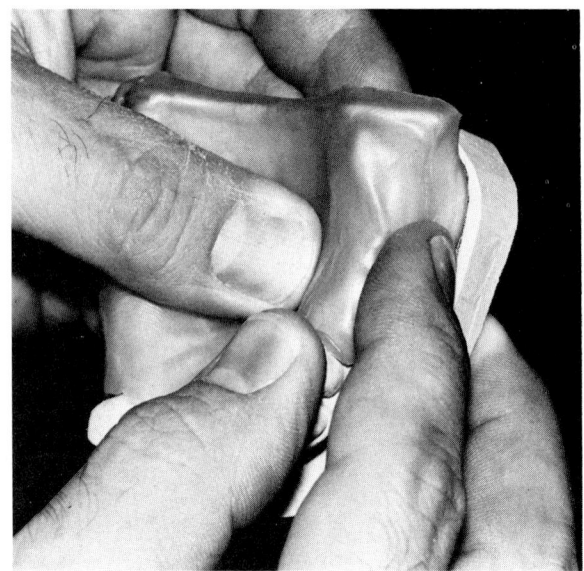

**Fig. 4-119.** Wax border thickness is evaluated, and proper contour is accomplished by adding wax as required.

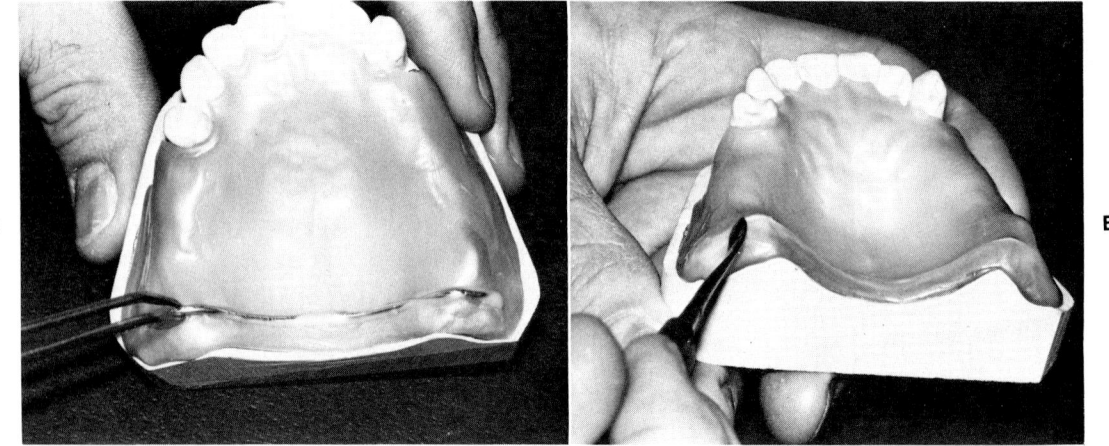

**Fig. 4-120. A,** Reinforcement wire is embedded into wax record base in posterior palatal seal area. **B,** Baseplate wax is flowed over reinforcement wire and finished to smooth surface.

Hudis, M. M.: Dental laboratory prosthodontics, Philadelphia, 1977, W. B. Saunders Co.

Keyworth, R. G.: Monson technic for full denture construction, J. Am. Dent. Assoc. **16:**130-162, Jan., 1929.

Martinelli, N.: Dental laboratory technology, ed. 2, St. Louis, 1975, The C. V. Mosby Co.

McCracken, W. L.: Auxiliary uses of cold curing acrylic resins in prosthetic dentistry, J. Am. Dent. Assoc. **47:**298-304, Sept., 1953.

McKevitt, F. H.: Finding lost prosthodontic terms, J. Prosthet. Dent. **7:**738-749, 1957.

Miller, E. L.: Removable partial prosthodontics, Baltimore, 1972, The Williams & Wilkins Co.

Morrow, R. M., Rudd, K. D., and Eissmann, H. F.: Dental laboratory procedures: Complete dentures, vol 1., St. Louis, 1980, The C. V. Mosby Co.

Peyton, F. A., Anthony, D. H., Asgar, K., Charbeneau, G. T., Craig, R. G., and Myers, G. E.: Restorative dental materials, ed. 2, St. Louis, 1964, The C. V. Mosby Co.

Ringsdorf, W. M.: Ideal baseplate, J. Am. Dent. Assoc. **50:**66-68, Jan., 1955.

Silverman, S. I.: The management of the trial denture base, Dent. Clin. North Am. **1:**231-243, 1957.

Sowter, J. B.: Dental laboratory technology: prosthodontic techniques, Chapel Hill, N.C., 1968, The University of North Carolina Press.

Wienski, J. C.: Stability of lower occlusion rims, Dent. Digest **65:**31, Jan., 1959.

Winkler, S.: Essentials of complete denture prosthodontics, Philadelphia, 1979, W. B. Saunders Co.

Woelfel, J. B., and Paffenbarger, G. E.: Stability of plastic impression trays, J. Am. Dent. Assoc. **63:**705-706, 1961.

Zuckerman, A.: Baseplate stability, Dent. Surv. **37:**594-595, 1961.

# CHAPTER 5

# SURVEY AND DESIGN

KENNETH D. RUDD, GEORGE KNIGHT, and KENNETH L. STEWART

**design** To plan and/or delineate by drawing the outline of a proposed prosthesis.
**survey line** a line produced on the various portions of a dental cast by a surveyor scriber or marker. It designates the greatest height of contour in relation to the orientation of the cast to the vertical scriber.
**surveying** The procedure of studying the relative parallelism or lack of parallelism of the teeth and associated structures so as to select a path of placement for a restoration that will encounter the least tooth or tissue interference and that will provide adequate and balanced retention; locating guiding plane surfaces to direct placement and removal of the restoration as well as to achieve the best appearance possible.
**surveyor** An instrument used to determine the relative parallelism of two or more surfaces of teeth or other portions of a cast of the dental arch.

Surveying and designing casts for removable partial dentures are important steps toward achieving a successful restoration. A well-executed design on the cast serves as a blueprint for fabrication of the removable partial denture, thus principles and methods for surveying and designing should be thoroughly understood. This chapter will deal with the principles of survey and design, components of removable partial dentures, and consideration of an effective method for designing casts. Using the described method, representative casts will be designed in accordance with the previously discussed principles.

## CLASSIFICATION OF REMOVABLE PARTIAL DENTURES

Several classifications for removable partial dentures have been described (Henderson and Steffel, 1977). Classifications have been based on functional requirements, distribution of missing teeth in the arch, and the type of support available for the prospective removable partial denture. Although no classification appears to be universally accepted, the Kennedy classification is often used to describe casts. As a result, it will be used throughout this text primarily to facilitate visualization of commonly occurring restorative situations in which removable partial dentures are often indicated. Further classification often aids recall of principles and design requirements for each class type and may suggest a typical or usual approach to that particular design. The classification is applicable to maxillary and mandibular casts.

### Class I (bilateral distal extension)

In Class I removable partial dentures, the abutment teeth are situated anterior to edentulous areas (Fig. 5-1). This type of denture receives support from soft tissue and the remaining teeth. The different nature of the available support requires careful consideration when designing a Class I removable partial denture.

#### *Principles for Class I removable partial dentures*
**KENNEDY CLASS I ARCHES**

The most posterior teeth on each side of the arch should be clasped. Following is the preferred order for clasping:

1. Distobuccal retention using a vertical projection clasp (T bar).
2. Mesiobuccal retention using an 18-gauge wrought wire clasp.
3. Mesiobuccal retention using a reverse circumferential clasp (approaching from the mesial aspect).

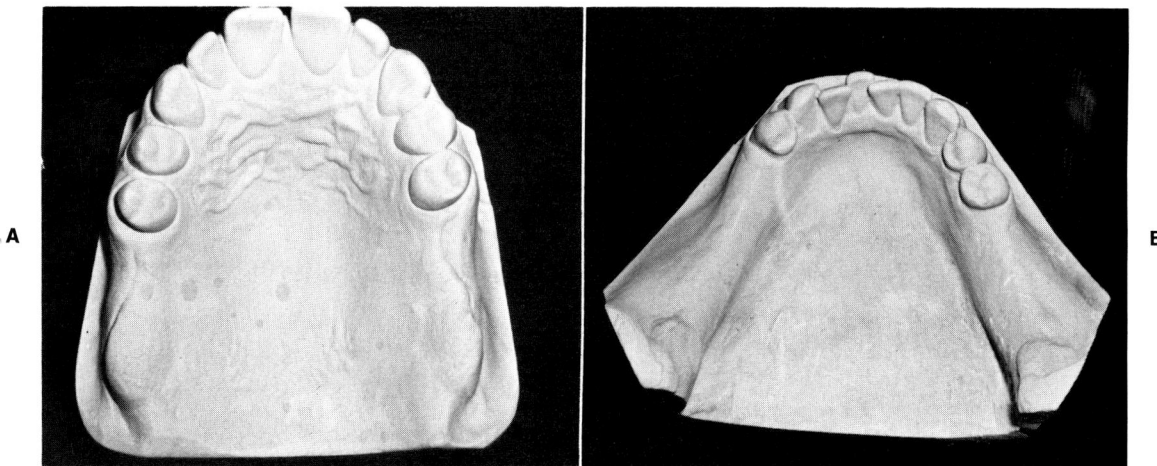

**Fig. 5-1.** Class I (bilateral distal extension) removable partial denture. **A,** Maxillary. **B,** Mandibular.

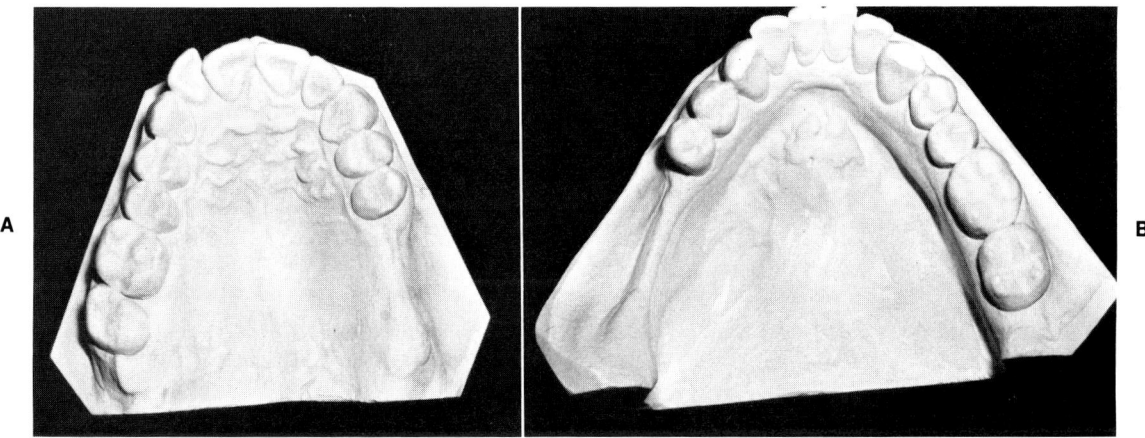

**Fig. 5-2.** Class II (unilateral distal extension) removable partial denture. **A,** Maxillary. **B,** Mandibular.

4. Lingual retention is seldom indicated due to shortness of clasp arms.

5. For all cast cobalt-chromium clasps, except on unusually large teeth, 0.010 inch of retention is sufficient. For wrought wire clasps, 0.020 inches may be used.

6. One clasp that is never indicated for Class I arches is a cast circumferential clasp engaging a mesiobuccal undercut on the posterior abutment tooth.

7. When bone loss has occurred around the posterior abutment tooth, double clasping on that side of the arch may be indicated. The clasping rules listed here still apply to the posterior tooth but the tooth anterior to it may be clasped in the most convenient manner.

## Class II (unilateral distal extension)

In Class II removable partial dentures, there is a distal extension base (free-end saddle) on one side only (Fig. 5-2). Support is received from teeth and soft tissue.

### Principles for Class II removable partial dentures

#### KENNEDY CLASS II ARCHES

1. All the rules that apply to clasping for Class I arches apply to the distal extension side.

2. For the dentulous side, if no modification space is present, two clasps should be used, one as far anteriorly as possible and one as posterior as possible. The location of the retentive area on each tooth, mesiobuccal or distobuccal, is not truly significant.

3. If a modification space exists on the dentulous side, the adjacent tooth should be clasped with the simplest clasp available, such as simple circlet clasps into a distobuccal undercut for the posterior abutment and mesiobuccal undercut for the anterior abutment tooth.

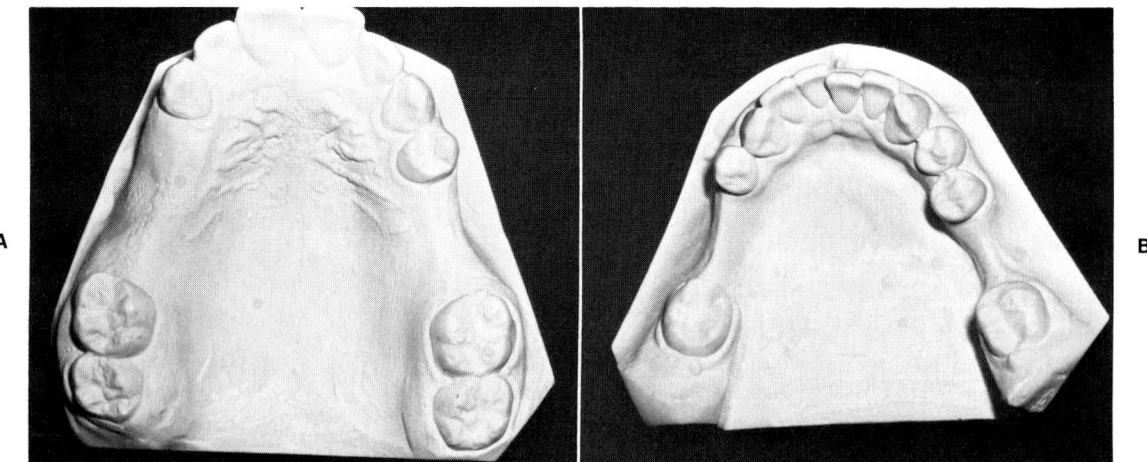

Fig. 5-3. Class III (all tooth-supported) removable partial denture. **A**, Maxillary. **B**, Mandibular.

## Class III

Edentulous areas are bounded anteriorly and posteriorly by abutments. Class III removable partial dentures are primarily supported by the natural teeth (Fig. 5-3). They may be unilateral or bilateral.

### Principles for Class III removable partial dentures
#### KENNEDY CLASS III ARCHES

1. If no modification space exists, the teeth adjacent to the edentulous space should be clasped as described for the dentulous side of a Class II, modification 1 arch. On the side where no space exists, clasping should be done with one clasp as far anteriorly as possible and one posteriorly positioned.

2. If a modification space does exist on the opposite side of the arch, all four abutment teeth adjacent to the edentulous spaces should be clasped with the simplest type of clasp available.

3. If one or both of the posterior abutment teeth are weak due to loss of bone, it may be advisable not to place retentive clasps on them but to place an occlusal rest for vertical support and nonretentive clasp arms for bracing against lateral movement.

## Class IV (anterior edentulous area)

Class IV removable partial dentures involve the placement of the anterior teeth, thus esthetics becomes a prime consideration (Fig. 5-4).

### Principles for Class IV removable partial dentures
#### KENNEDY CLASS IV ARCHES

1. The situation for movement around a fulcrum line is completely reversed when compared to Classes I and II arches. For this reason, the teeth

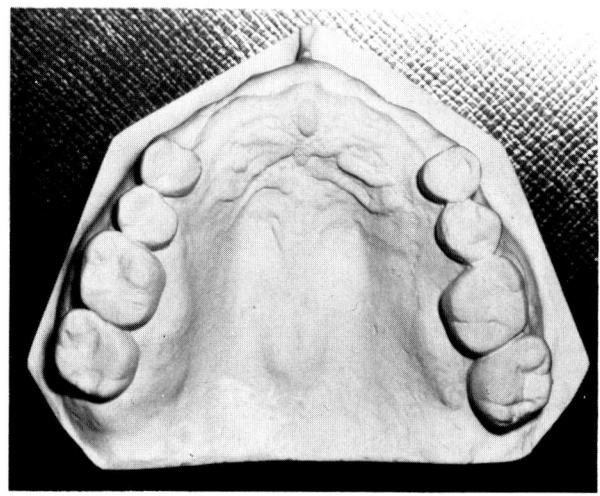

Fig. 5-4. Class IV (only anterior teeth missing) removable partial denture.

adjacent to the edentulous space should be clasped for retention with the retentive area located on the mesiobuccal surface of the most anterior teeth.

2. In addition, it is desirable to place another retentive clasp on each side of the arch as far posteriorly as possible, engaging a distobuccal retentive undercut. These clasps will act as indirect retainers in addition to being direct retainers.

Obviously many removable partial denture casts involve modifications of these classes. Missing teeth that are remote from basic classification areas are termed *modification areas* (Applegate, 1965) and may influence the design (Fig. 5-5). Although more elaborate classification systems exist, the Kennedy classification seems to fill most requirements, particularly since its inherent simplicity facilitates visual imagery.

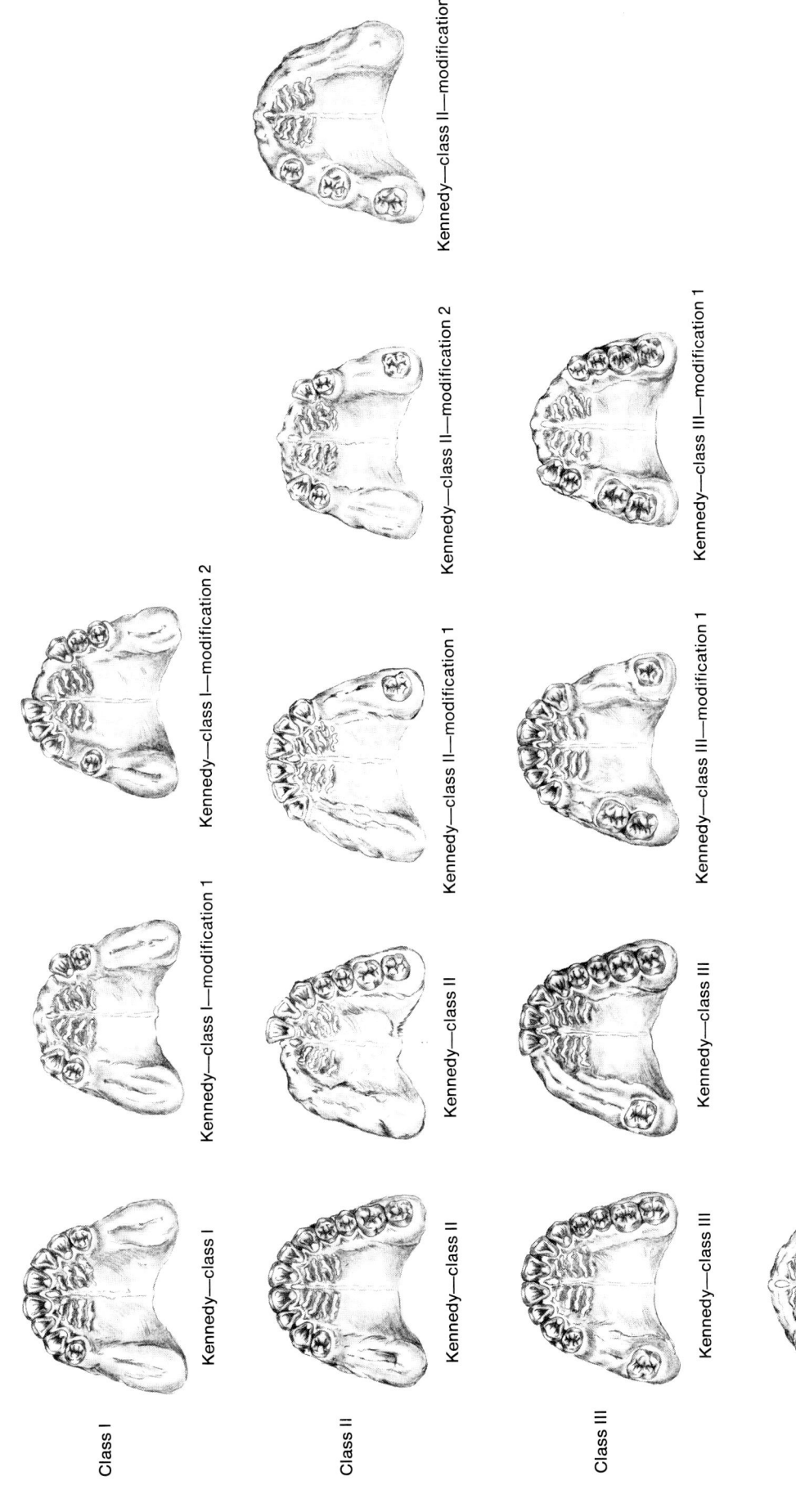

**Fig. 5-5.** Kennedy classification chart.

## MATERIALS FOR CAST FRAMEWORKS

Since the material used for a cast framework may affect design, a few generalizations on materials are appropriate here. Cast removable partial denture frameworks can be made from type IV gold alloys or from a variety of nonprecious alloys available for the purpose. Due to the cost of gold, its use for removable partial denture castings will continue to decline. If type IV gold is used, some changes should usually be made in the design, or more correctly, in the wax-up. Gold alloys may require slightly larger wax patterns than chromium alloys to compensate for the differences in physical properties of the two metals.

## REMOVABLE PARTIAL DENTURE COMPONENTS

The structural elements of a removable partial denture include clasps, major and minor connectors, the base of the removable partial denture, and the teeth. Proper design procedures require decisions concerning selection of the components that best meet the requirements of the particular patient. Thus from the practical standpoint, design involves selection of the clasps, major and minor connectors, the type of base, and the type of tooth replacement. To select components correctly, the designer should thoroughly understand the advantages and disadvantages of each removable partial denture component.

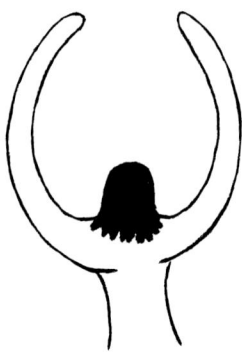

**Fig. 5-6.** At least one of the clasp arms terminates in undercut. If both clasp tips are in undercut, amount of undercut for each should be reduced. Rest (shaded area) contributes most of vertical support for partial denture.

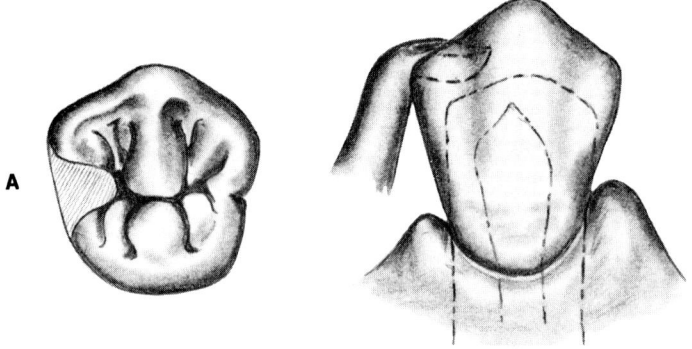
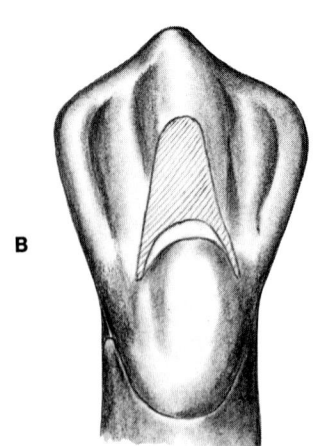
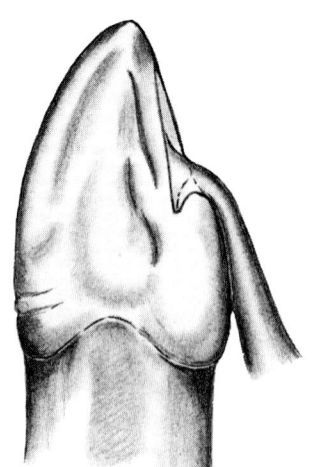
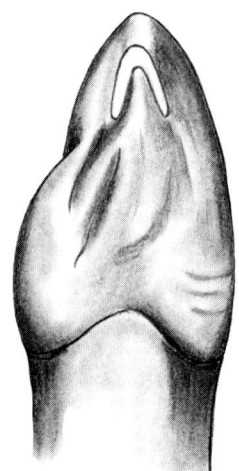
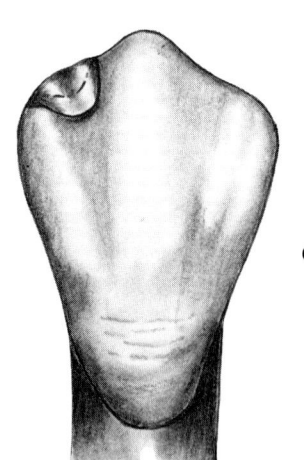

**Fig. 5-7. A,** Occlusal rest preparation (left), rest in place (right). **B,** Cingulum rest preparation (left), rest in place (right). **C,** Incisal rest preparation (left), rest fills in original contour of tooth (right).

## Clasps

A clasp is defined as an extracoronal direct retainer of a removable partial denture; the assembly usually consists of two arms joined by a body that may connect with a rest. At least one arm of a clasp must terminate in the cervical convergent area of the tooth encircled (Fig. 5-6). The functions of the clasp are to support, stabilize, and retain the removable partial denture. The rest projects onto the occlusal, lingual, or incisal surfaces of the tooth and provides support and some stability for the removable partial denture (Fig. 5-7). The body connects the rest and arms of the clasp to the minor connector (Fig. 5-8). The arms of the clasp may be further defined as the reciprocal arm and/or the retentive arm (Fig. 5-9). Clasp arms are further divided into a shoulder and a flexible clasp tip (Fig. 5-10). An approach arm may also be involved if the clasp is of the infrabulge type (Fig. 5-11). The approach arm extends from the removable partial denture frame-

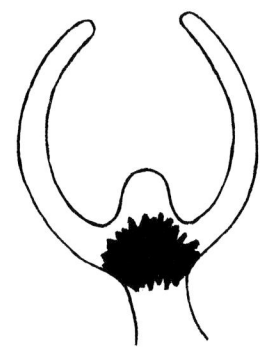

**Fig. 5-8.** Shaded part of clasp is body.

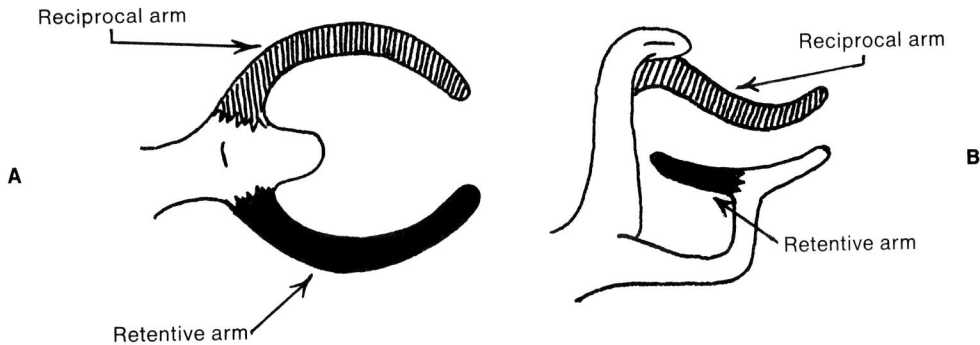

**Fig. 5-9.** Clasp arms may be either retentive or reciprocal. **A,** Suprabulge clasp. **B,** Infrabulge clasp.

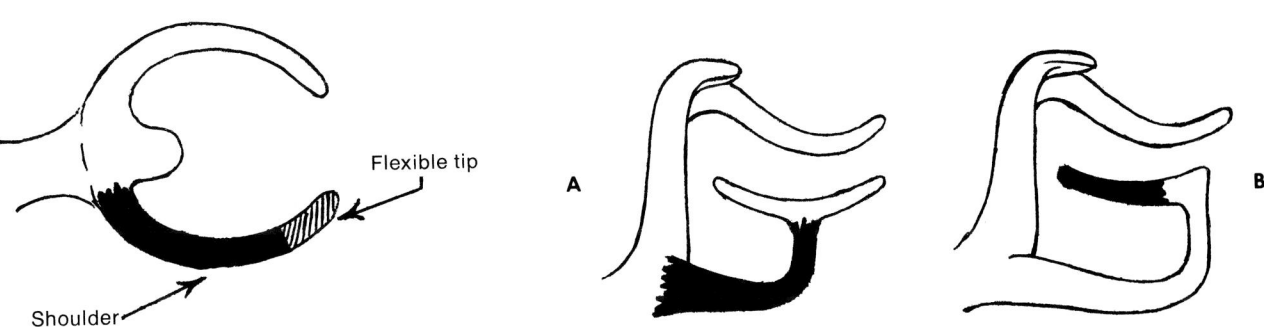

**Fig. 5-10.** Suprabulge clasp arm may be divided into two parts: shoulder and flexible tip.

**Fig. 5-11.** Infrabulge clasp arm has approach arm **(A)** and retentive tip **(B)**.

work to the clasp arm and approaches the undercut from below (Fig. 5-12). The retentive arm of the clasp is the flexible retentive tip that is placed in an undercut area on the tooth (Fig. 5-13). The reciprocating arm of the clasp is maintained above the survey line and provides lateral stability for the removable partial denture. Reciprocation is required for all clasps. The clasp shoulder is the rigid portion of the clasp arm and is always kept above the survey line (Fig. 5-14). The shoulder extends from the body of the clasp to the beginning of the flexible clasp tip. The shoulder provides bracing and stabilization against lateral forces.

### Requirements of clasps

1. Encirclement designed line.
2. Reciprocity that is provided by the so-called reciprocal arm of the clasp.
3. Passivity. When the clasp is in place on a tooth, it should be passive, exerting no force on the tooth whatsoever.
4. Retention should be obtained by the flexible clasp tip engaging in the undercut and not by the frictional retention gained by having the clasp adjusted to fit tightly against the surface of the tooth.

Clasps also may be classified as to the type of metal used in the clasp and the method of construction, such as cast gold or cobalt-chromium alloy or wrought wire. Clasps are also classified based on the direction of the approach to the undercut area on the tooth. For instance, a clasp may be a suprabulge clasp approaching the undercut from the suprabulge area or from the occlusal surface downward (Fig. 5-15). Suprabulge clasps are sometimes referred to as pull-type clasps.

### Suprabulge clasps

Circumferential clasps also called circlet clasps or Akers clasps or Class I clasps are suprabulge clasps. Circumferential clasps encircle more than 180 degrees of a tooth and contact the tooth throughout the length of the arms (Fig. 5-16). Again, circumferential clasps approach the undercut on the tooth from the suprabulge area or from the occlusal aspect of the tooth. Several types of this clasp class will be described.

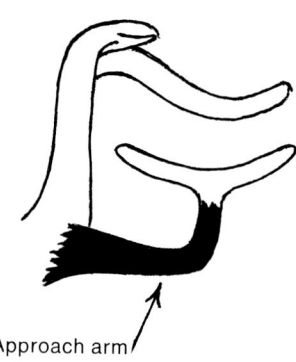

**Fig. 5-12.** Approach arm extends from denture base to infrabulge area of tooth.

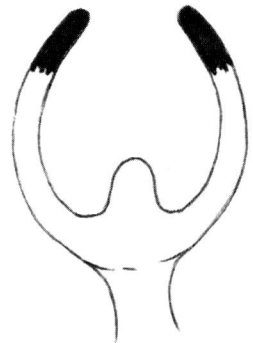

**Fig. 5-13.** Only retentive tip of clasp may be placed in undercut.

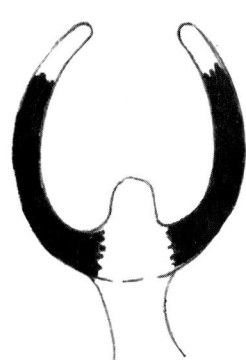

**Fig. 5-14.** Shoulder is too stiff to spring into undercut, so it must be kept on or above survey line.

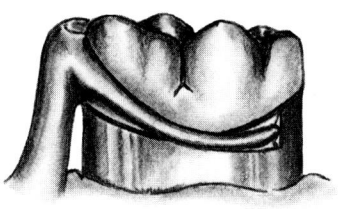

Fig. 5-15. Suprabulge clasp approaches retentive undercut from occlusal area of survey line.

## SIMPLE CIRCLET CLASP

The simple circlet clasp is also known as Akers clasp or Class I clasp (Fig. 5-17).

ADVANTAGES. Simple circlet clasps are easier to design and construct, possess outstanding bracing qualities, and are usually easy to repair if broken. They are also easier to adjust and have less tendency to collect food beneath the clasp. The simple circlet clasp provides excellent support, since its rigid shoulders are above the survey line and add their support to that of the occlusal rest.

DISADVANTAGES. The simple circlet clasp covers more of the tooth, which could contribute to caries. The clasp may not be esthetic on maxillary canines or premolar teeth, and it is usually not desirable to use simple circlet cast clasps on terminal abutments of unilateral and bilateral distal extension partial dentures. In addition, some authors report that the pull-type retention furnished by Class I–type clasps is not as effective as push-type obtained from infrabulge clasps.

INDICATIONS. Simple circlet cast clasps are used primarily in tooth-supported removable partial dentures (Classes III and IV) (Fig. 5-18).

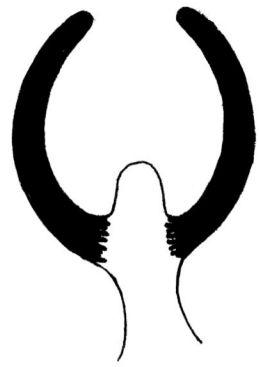

Fig. 5-16. Clasp must encircle tooth covering more than 180 degrees so tooth will be held into clasp.

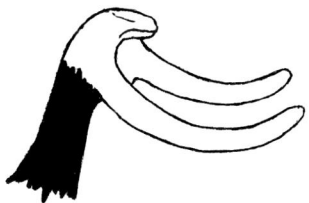

Fig. 5-17. This clasp goes by variety of names: circumferential, simple circlet, suprabulge, Akers, and Class I.

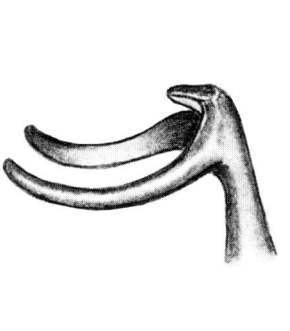

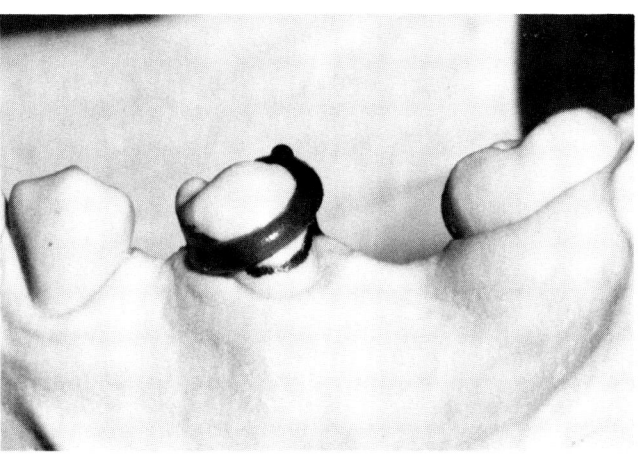

Fig. 5-18. Simple circlet clasp may be used on Classes III and IV partial dentures if desirable undercuts are located in favorable positions.

## REVERSE APPROACH CIRCLET CLASP

ADVANTAGES. Advantages of the reverse approach circlet clasps are similar to those for the simple circlet clasp except they may be used on distal extension partial dentures (Fig. 5-19).

DISADVANTAGES. Reverse approach circlet clasps require additional occlusal clearance to transmit the shoulder of the clasp through the embrasure.

INDICATIONS. This clasp can often be used in bilateral and unilateral distal extension partial dentures (Classes I and II) where deep tissue undercuts may preclude using the traditional infrabulge, or bar, clasp. The reverse circlet clasp may not be as esthetic, particularly when used on lower premolars, as an infrabulge clasp.

## CIRCLET C CLASP

This clasp is sometimes called a fish hook clasp (Fig. 5-20).

ADVANTAGES. Advantages of the circlet C clasp are essentially the same as the simple circlet clasp. It is, however, somewhat more difficult to construct.

DISADVANTAGES. This clasp is difficult to use on a tooth where the occlusogingival height is minimal.

INDICATIONS. Indications for the circlet C include mesially tilted molar teeth with the undercut located mesially and where tissue undercuts contraindicate an infrabulge clasp. This clasp is usually contraindicated in tilted molar teeth where space is not available for the transmission of the clasp shoulders. Although this clasp has disadvantages, it is

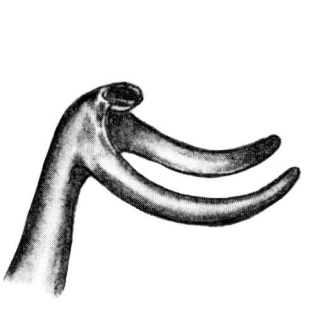
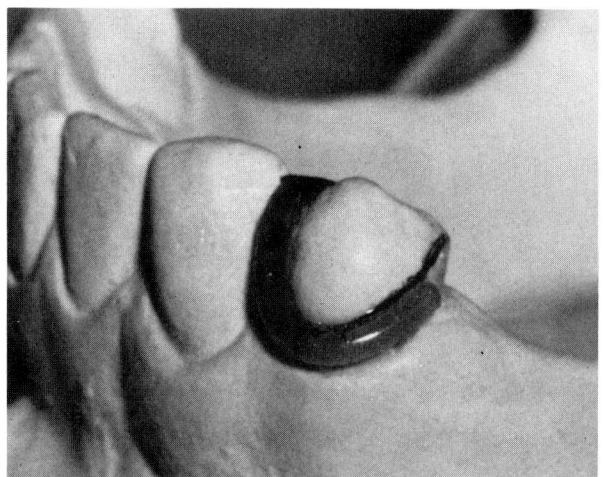

**Fig. 5-19.** Reverse approach circlet clasps may be used on Classes I and II partial dentures if there is sufficient clearance.

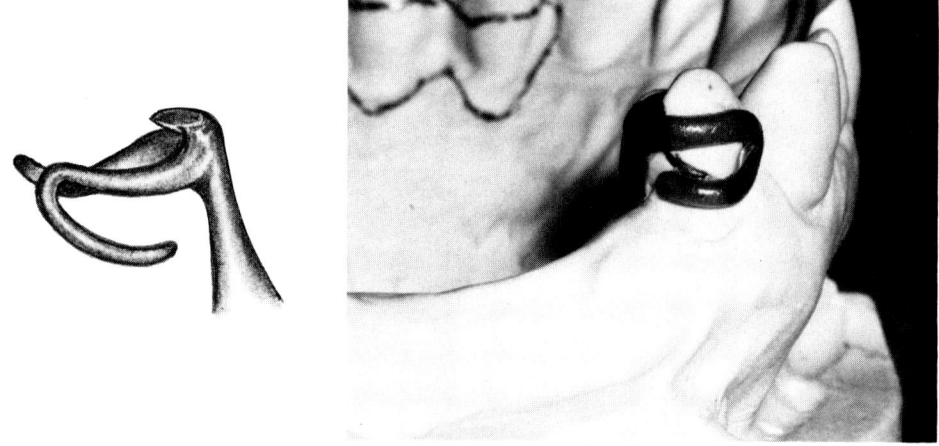

**Fig. 5-20.** Circlet C clasps may be used when bar-type clasps are contraindicated.

easier to construct, adjust, and maintain than a ring clasp.

### MULTIPLE CIRCLET CLASP

ADVANTAGES. This clasp can be used to provide additional support for weakened premolar teeth. It also permits use of adjacent retentive areas on approximating teeth (Fig. 5-21).

DISADVANTAGES. Disadvantages of this clasp are related to the difficulty in fabrication and the strength and rigidity of its minor connectors.

INDICATIONS. Multiple circlet clasps can be used where an abutment has compromised periodontal support. A removable partial denture and an adjoining tooth may be included. The clasp is most often used on premolar teeth or premolar/molar combinations.

### ONLAY CLASP

Onlay clasp arms extend from an occlusal onlay into an undercut that may be located mesially or distally. The retentive arm may arise from any point along the buccal or lingual margin of the onlay (Fig. 5-22).

ADVANTAGES. Advantages of the onlay clasp are that it permits a mesially tilted molar to be used to provide retention, plus the tilted molar's occlusion can often be improved by addition of the onlay. It is another method for approaching mesiofacial or mesiolingual undercuts on a tilted molar tooth.

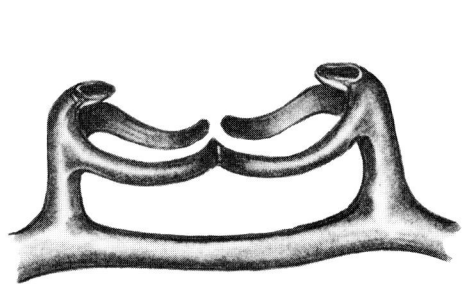
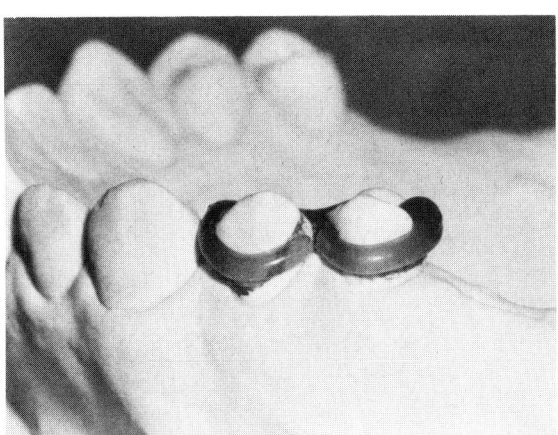

Fig. 5-21. Multiple circlet clasps are usually used to tie two premolars together.

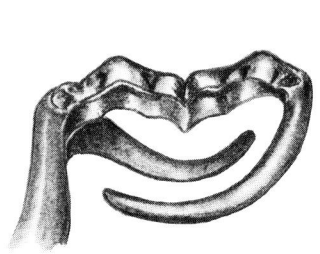
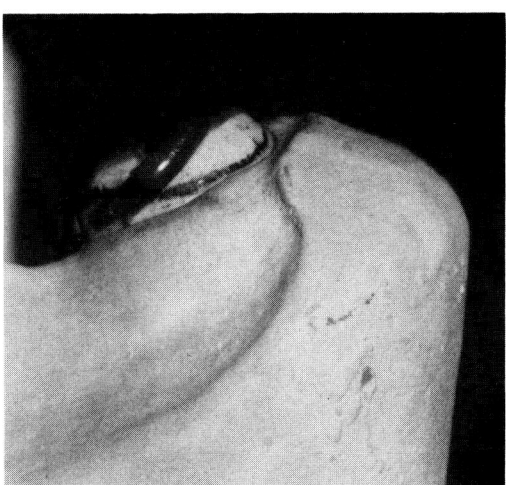

Fig. 5-22. Onlay clasps are used on tipped molars and may be used to correct plane of occlusion.

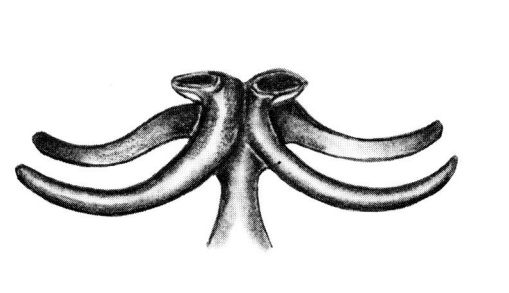
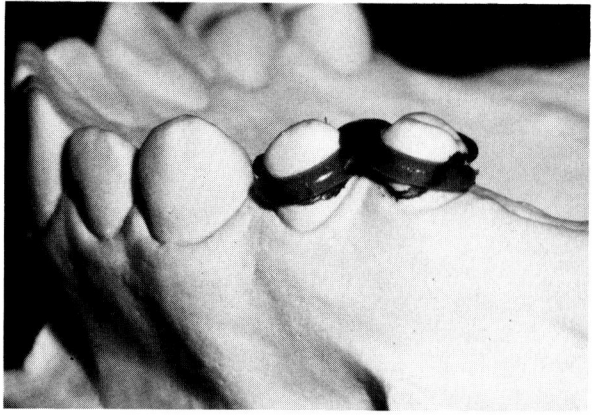

Fig. 5-23. Embrasure clasps are used most often on Class II partial dentures. It is usually more desirable to use two clasps more widely separated.

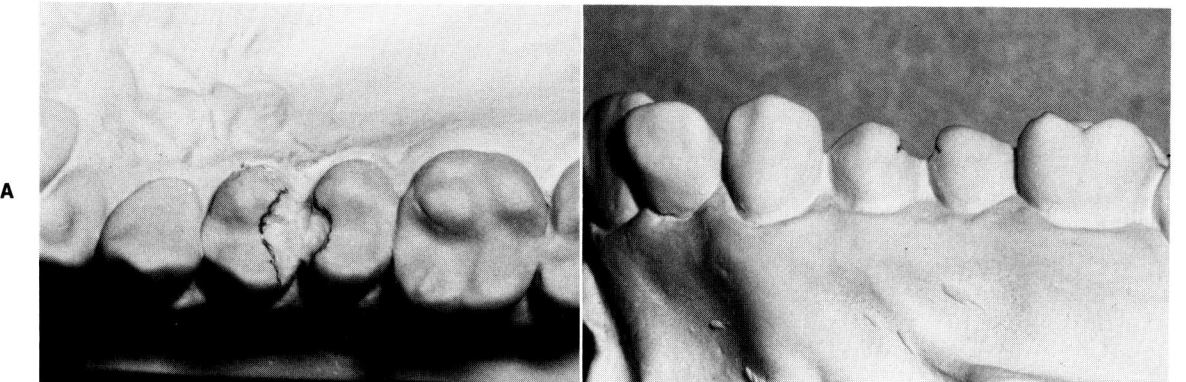

Fig. 5-24. Definite and adequate provisions must be made to transmit clasp across occlusal surface. **A,** Occlusal view of preparation. **B,** Facial view.

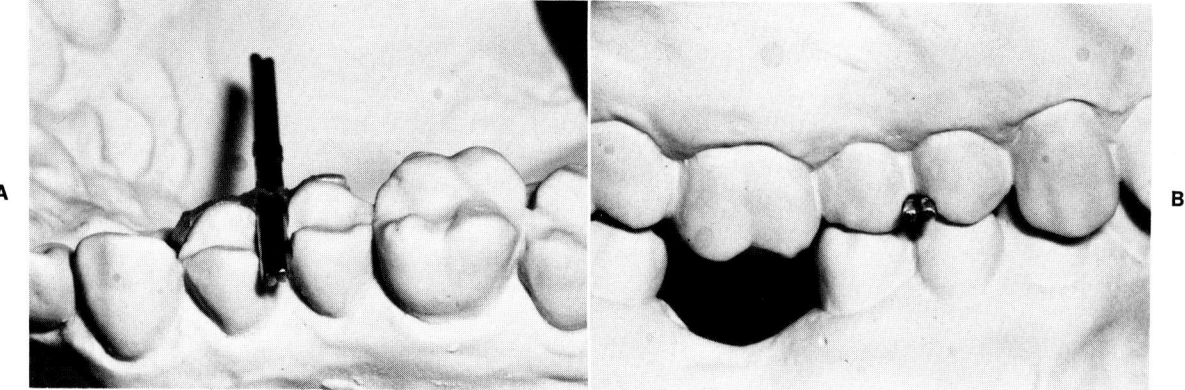

Fig. 5-25. Preparation should hold two 18-gauge wires side by side **(A)** and clear opposing occlusion with wires in place **(B)**.

DISADVANTAGES. It is more difficult to fit this clasp to the tooth because of the increased contact area. Thus the impression and resultant cast should be extremely accurate. These clasps usually require more fitting with disclosing wax at the time of try-in. Since the onlay clasp contacts the tooth over a large area, it could contribute to a caries problem if oral hygiene is not properly maintained.

### EMBRASURE CLASP

An embrasure clasp is used most often on premolar teeth (Fig. 5-23). The minor connector approaches the occlusal surfaces from the lingual embrasure, and the rests are on adjoining teeth. The mesial and distal rests are placed, and the shoulders of the clasp proceed through the buccal embrasure. One clasp arm proceeds distally into a distofacial undercut, and the other clasp arm proceeds mesially into a mesiofacial undercut.

ADVANTAGES. The embrasure clasp can be used for a distal extension partial denture where a deep tissue undercut contraindicates an infrabulge, or bar-type, clasp.

DISADVANTAGES. This clasp requires attention to proper rest preparations to prevent a wedging effect between approximating abutments. Adequate space must be provided in the buccal embrasure to transmit the clasp arms onto the buccal surfaces (Fig. 5-24). If this is not accomplished during mouth preparation, the clasp arms will interfere with the occlusion. If the arms are reduced at the time of insertion the clasp will be weakened and may break at the bucco-occlusal line angle. Depending on the patient's occlusion, it may be difficult to reduce the abutment teeth adequately to transmit a sufficiently thick clasp to prevent breakage. Overpreparation can result in mutilated teeth. A space equal to a double 18-gauge wire should be available to transmit this clasp (Fig. 5-25).

### Infrabulge clasps

Infrabulge clasps are also known as bar clasps, Roach clasps, push-type clasps, and Class II clasps (Fig. 5-26). Infrabulge clasps are defined as clasps whose arms are bar-type extensions from major connectors or from within the denture base; the arms pass adjacent to the soft tissues and approach the point of contact on the tooth in a cervico-occlusal direction. Bar clasps as a group are probably used most often on the terminal abutment of bilateral and unilateral distal extension partial dentures (Classes I and II). There are several types of bar clasps, most of which are identified by a corresponding letter of the alphabet, T clasp, modified T clasp, and I clasp.

### T CLASP

A T clasp is an infrabulge, or bar-type, clasp whose configuration resembles the letter T (Fig. 5-27). An approach arm contacts the tooth from the gingivo-occlusal direction and usually only one

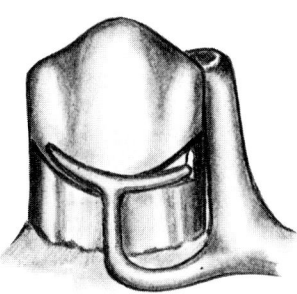

**Fig. 5-26.** Typical infrabulge clasp is also known as bar, Roach, push-type and Class II.

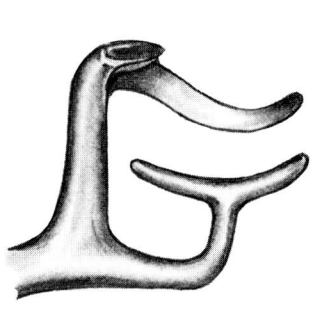
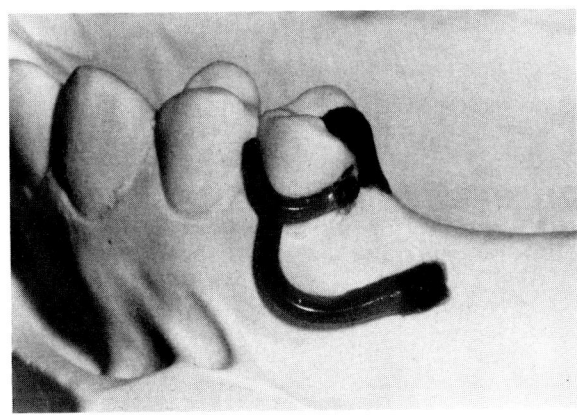

**Fig. 5-27.** T clasp in place on Class I partial denture. It may also be used on Class II partial denture.

arm of the T clasp, most often the distal arm, is placed in the undercut. The mesial arm of the T clasp provides bracing and is above the survey line.

ADVANTAGES. The T clasp is used on distal abutments of distal extension partial dentures. A properly designed T clasp has a stress-releasing capability that should be better tolerated by the abutment tooth. This clasp is used with mesial or distal rest and is often indicated for Classes I and II removable partial dentures.

DISADVANTAGES. The T clasp should not be used when soft tissue contours would result in placement of the approach arm in an undercut (Fig. 5-28). The T clasp may not be esthetic, particularly in the maxillary arch, provides minimal bracing, and is more difficult to fabricate and adjust.

### MODIFIED T CLASP

The modified T clasp is essentially a T clasp with one of the arms omitted, often the mesial arm (Fig. 5-29). The distal arm is usually retained and placed into a distofacial undercut. This particular clasp can be used on terminal abutments of the distal extension partial denture (Classes I and II).

ADVANTAGES. Advantages of the modified T clasp are essentially the same as the T clasp.

DISADVANTAGES. One disadvantage is that it is difficult to use where deep soft tissue undercuts are present. Also, as in the case of the T clasp, it may not be esthetic, particularly when used in the maxillary arch.

### I-BAR CLASP

I-bar clasps, as described by Kratochvil (1963, 1968) and Krol (1972, 1973), enjoy widespread use (Fig. 5-30). The clasp approaches the undercut from a gingival direction and does not cross the survey line once the removable partial denture is in position.

ADVANTAGES. Advantages of the I-bar clasp include favorable stress distribution to the abutment during functional movement of the denture base, minimal coverage of tooth and gingiva, and less interruption of natural tooth contours.

DISADVANTAGES. Disadvantages of the I-bar clasp are that it is somewhat more difficult to adjust and may not be as effective bracing as other infrabulge clasps.

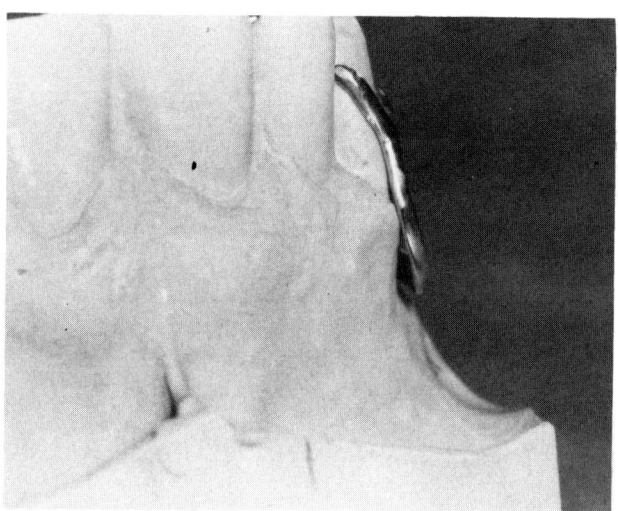

**Fig. 5-28.** This clasp should not be used unless approach arm can be against soft tissue.

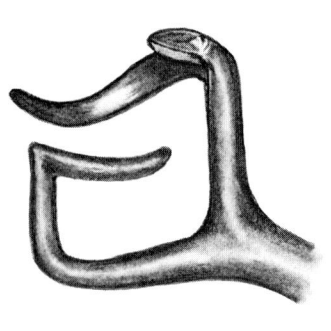
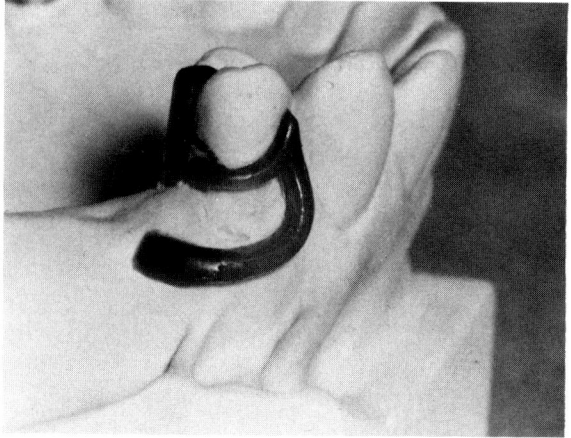

**Fig. 5-29.** Modified T clasp may be used as for T clasp, except that it is usually indicated for canines and premolars.

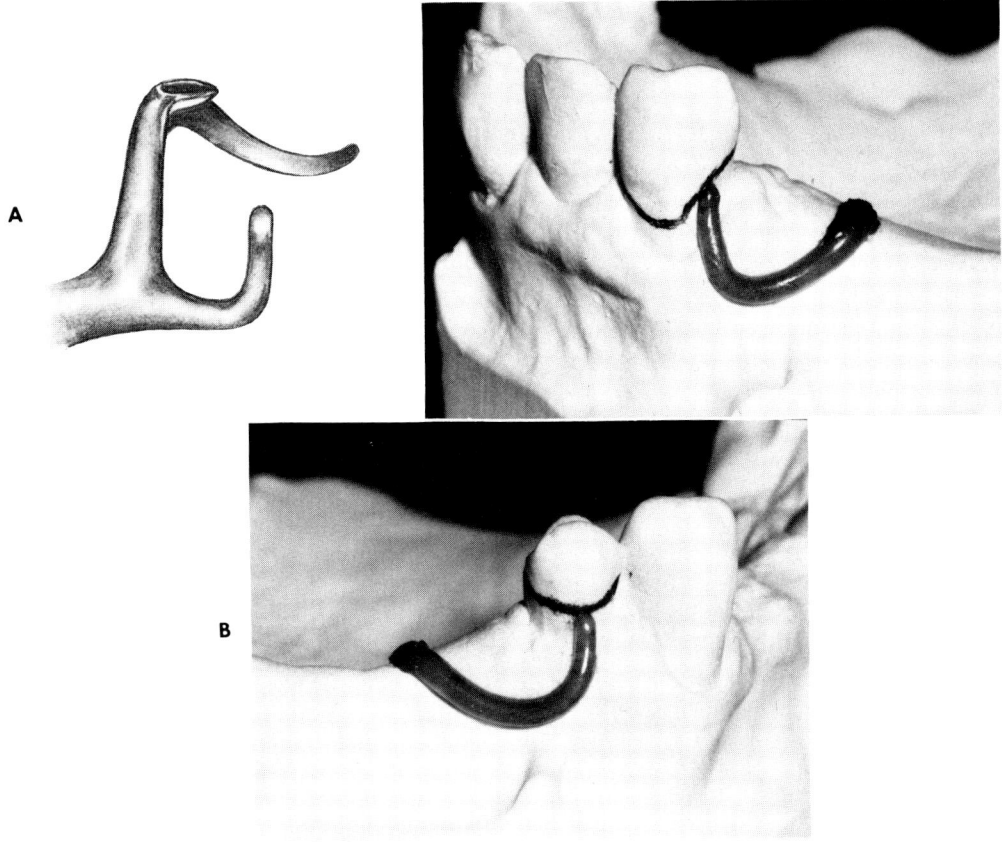

Fig. 5-30. **A**, I clasp is short stiff clasp usually used on canines for esthetics. **B**, I-bar clasp is much more desirable and, when used in conjunction with a clasping system, is very good for selected patients.

## WROUGHT WIRE CLASPS

Wrought wire clasps are made from precious and nonprecious alloys (Fig. 5-31). They are attached to connections by soldering, casting, or enclosing within the resin base.

ADVANTAGES. Wrought wire clasps have the advantage of increased flexibility. Since the clasp is round, the flexibility is equal in all directions. This may apply less stress to the abutment. Contact of the wrought wire clasp in the abutment tooth is less than a cast clasp of similar extension due to the contour of the wrought wire. Wrought wire has maximum strength for each cross-sectional area. A wrought wire clasp is usually easy to adjust should it become distorted and, because of its size, may be more esthetic than a cast clasp in a similar situation. The flexibility of the wrought wire clasp enables it to be used when a cast clasp may not be indicated. It can be used on terminal abutments of distal extension partial dentures and is usually placed in a mesiofacial undercut.

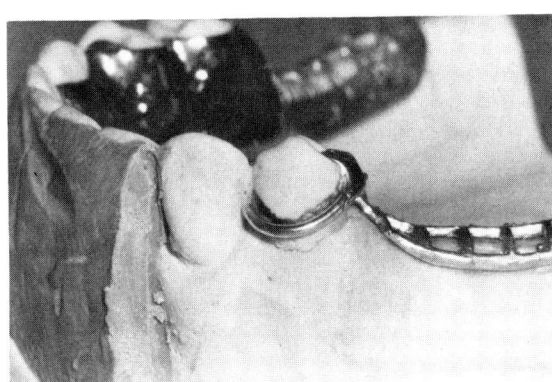

Fig. 5-31. Wrought wire clasps as rule may be placed into more undercut than cast clasp.

DISADVANTAGES. The wrought wire clasp is more time consuming to fabricate. It will provide less bracing than a comparable cast clasp, and there is a greater tendency for the patient to distort the wrought wire clasp, requiring more frequent adjustments. See Chapter 9 for a detailed discussion of the construction of wrought wire clasps.

### Other clasps

Other clasps that have been used for removable partial dentures include the ring clasp (Fig. 5-32), which has been recommended for mesially tilted lower molars. This clasp has seen decreasing use throughout the years due to the difficulty in fabricating the clasp and the extreme difficulty in adjusting the clasp should it become distorted. Generally, other more acceptable clasp designs satisfy this need. The mesiodistal clasp (Fig. 5-33) is another clasp that is used occasionally, primarily on maxillary anterior teeth. These clasps are used where some anterior retention is required. This clasp cannot be used if there is a distal extension base involved, and generally, other methods of retention are preferable. Other types of clasps that are rarely used are the U clasp, half and half (split) clasp, E clasp, and double I clasp (Fig. 5-34).

## Connectors

The partial denture clasps, base, and other structural units are joined by connectors. There are two types of connectors, major and minor.

### Major connectors

The principal function of the major connector is to unite the right and left sections of the partial denture framework. This connector then will permit stresses to be disturbed and provide bilateral stabilization. In certain instances, as in the case of the lingual plate or split lingual bar, a connector can provide indirect retention. Major connectors for the mandibular arch include the lingual bar, lingual plate, double lingual bar, and labial bar.

#### LINGUAL BAR

The lingual bar is used more often than any other major connector for mandibular removable partial dentures (Fig. 5-35). As a general rule, the lingual bar should be used unless another major connector is indicated. This occurs when additional indirect retention is required or where anterior teeth are weak and require additional support, in which case a lingual plate or a split lingual bar can be used. The lingual bar is particularly suited for Class III partial dentures.

DISADVANTAGES. The lingual bar is contraindicated in the presence of severe mandibular tori and where insufficient vertical space exists to accommodate the lingual bar. A minimum of 8 mm space is required, since the lingual bar is approximately 5 mm wide, and its upper edge should be no closer than 3 mm from the gingival margin of the lower anterior teeth. Structural requirements for the lingual bar include rigidity to permit distribution of stress, and no sharp notches or bends should be present that could concentrate stresses and result in an early failure of the prosthesis because of breakage.

#### LINGUAL PLATE

The lingual plate, also called the closed Kennedy bar, is a widely used major connector for mandibular removable partial dentures (Fig. 5-36).

ADVANTAGES. The lingual plate can be used where additional indirect retention is indicated. It is also indicated where the floor of the mouth is relatively high, and lingual bar cannot be used. The presence of lingual tori or severe lingual undercuts may also indicate the use of a lingual plate. Properly fitted lingual plates may also provide some splinting effect for mandibular anterior teeth whose periodon-

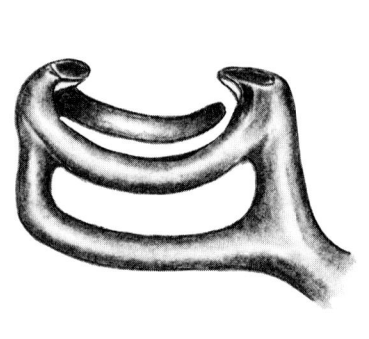
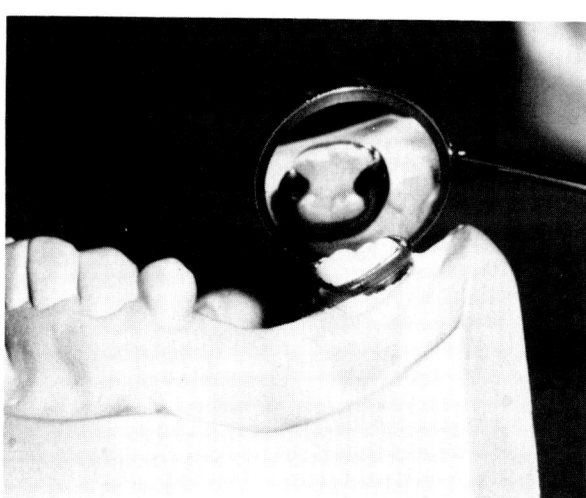

**Fig. 5-32.** Ring clasp is most beneficial when used on tipped molar.

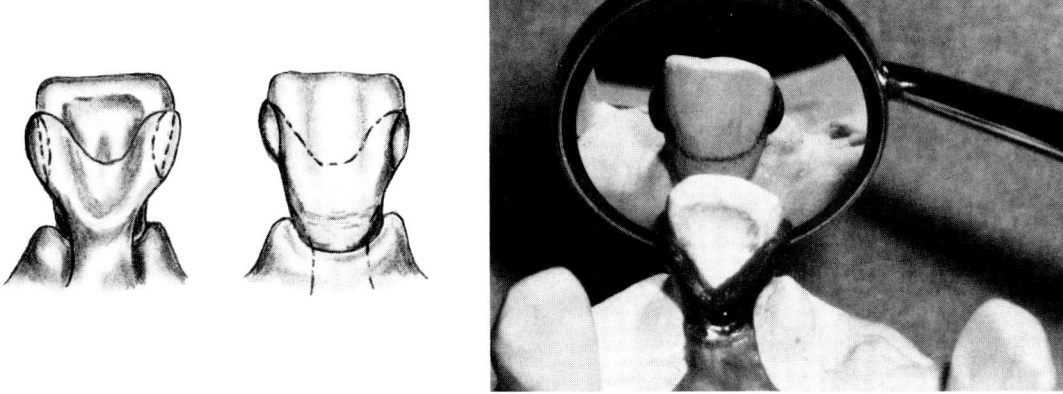

Fig. 5-33. Mesiodistal clasp is used very occasionally on maxillary centrals or canines.

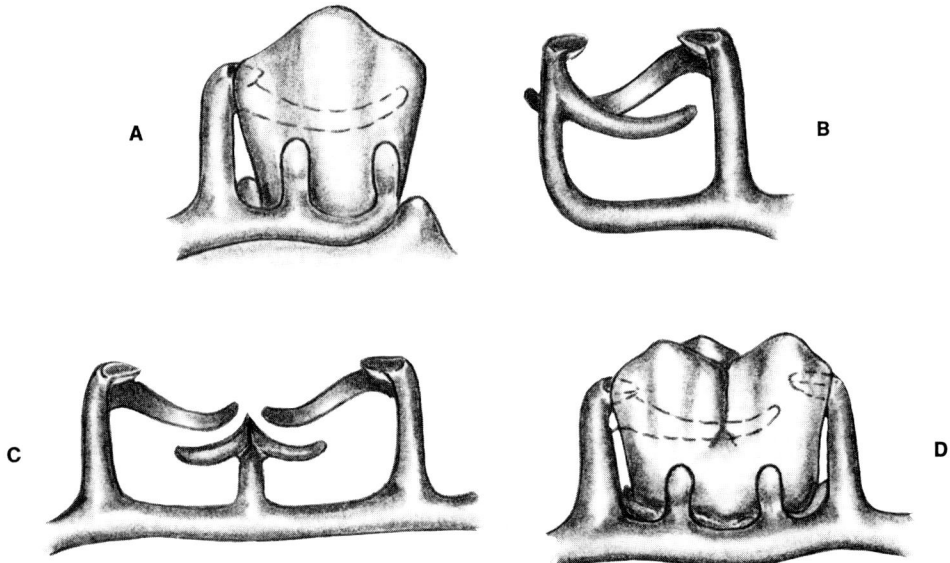

Fig. 5-34. **A,** U clasp. **B,** Half and half (split) clasp. **C,** E clasp. **D,** Double I clasp. These clasps are seldom, if ever, used in current laboratory procedures.

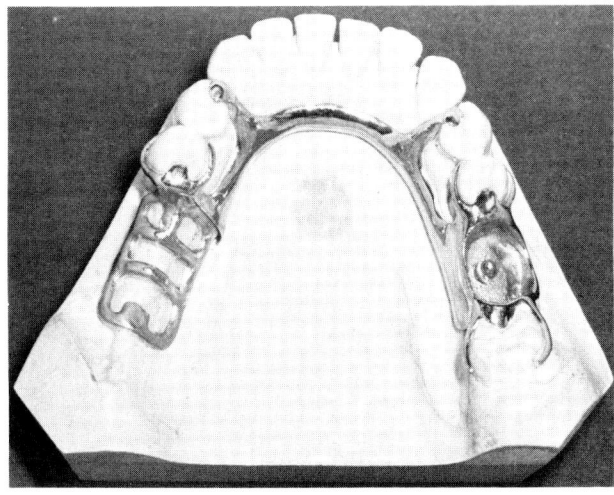

Fig. 5-35. Lingual bar.

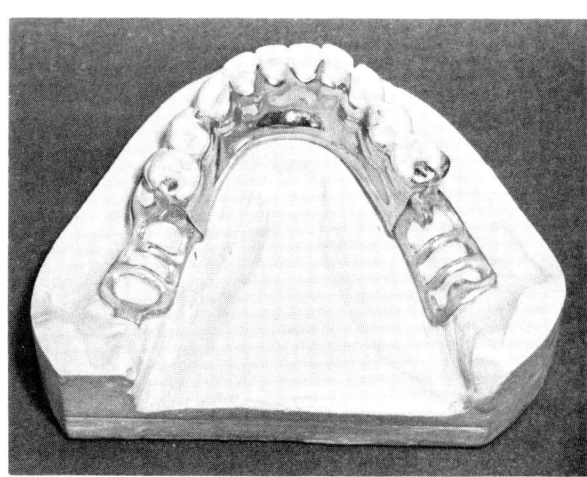

Fig. 5-36. Lingual plate.

tal support has been compromised. An additional advantage of the lingual plate over a lingual bar is the ability to add an anterior tooth to the removable partial denture should it be necessary. Lingual plates can be thin yet rigid due to the corrugation effect (Fig. 5-37).

DISADVANTAGES. The lingual plate should not be used in patients with poor oral hygiene or where anterior teeth are severely crowded or spaced. Spacers between the anterior teeth can produce esthetic problems when a lingual plate is used. It is also more difficult to fit a lingual plate accurately to prevent food impaction.

### DOUBLE LINGUAL BAR

ADVANTAGES. The double lingual bar, also called the Kennedy bar, is used primarily to provide additional support and stability for lower anterior teeth, yet provide access to the lingual surfaces for the natural cleansing effect of the tongue and certain foods. The double lingual bar or lingual plate may provide additional indirect retention, although it is not as effective as retention obtained with a well-designed rest.

DISADVANTAGES. Similar to the lingual plate, the double lingual bar is more difficult to fit accurately, and additional time and effort are needed to fit the casting at the time of the framework try-in (Fig. 5-38).

### LABIAL BAR

The labial bar is seldom used. When required, it is, however, about the only major connector that can be used. Where lower anterior and posterior teeth are severely inclined lingually, a labial bar may be indicated. In these situations it would be difficult, if not impossible, to place a lingual bar in contact with the lingual tissues. This occurs occasionally in some Class III malocclusions. Conceivably, a labial bar might be used where large lingual tori are present, and surgical intervention is contraindicated (Fig. 5-39).

DISADVANTAGES. A disadvantage of the labial bar is that its increased circumference makes construction of a bar with sufficient rigidity more difficult. Obviously, replacing anterior teeth with the use of a labial bar becomes an increasingly difficult technical problem.

## Maxillary major connectors

Maxillary major connectors include the palatal strap or bar, anterior-posterior palatal bar, horseshoe, closed horseshoe, and full palate.

### PALATAL BAR

The palatal bar, also called the single palatal bar and palatal strap, can be used in maxillary removable partial dentures, usually in tooth-supported partial dentures where the number of teeth to be

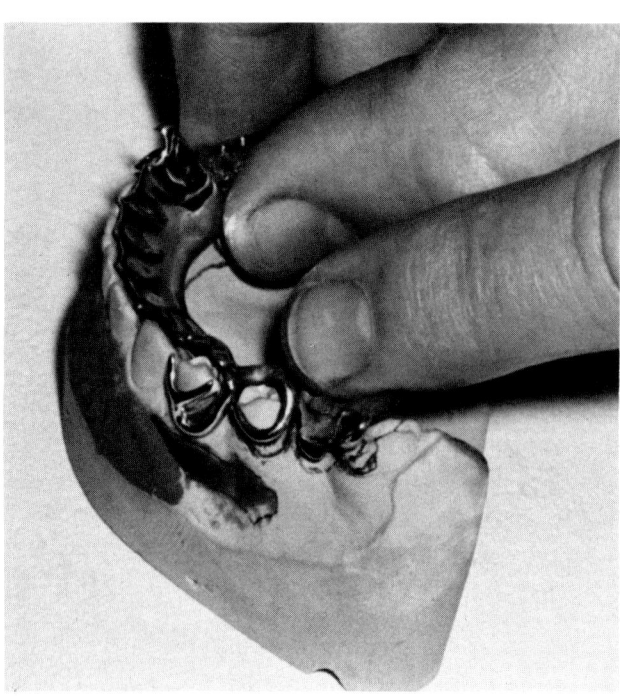

**Fig. 5-37.** Configuration of thin lingual plate makes it rigid.

replaced is not extensive (Class III) (Fig. 5-40). It can be used in a Class II partial denture where the denture base is relatively short, and when the force of the opposing occlusion is less, as when opposed by another removable partial denture. The single palatal bar or palatal strap is not indicated where anterior teeth must be replaced with the removable partial denture. Generally, the single palatal bar or strap should be for minimal tooth replacement found in a Class III partial denture.

## ANTERIOR-POSTERIOR PALATAL BAR

The anterior-posterior palatal bar (Fig. 5-41) is also referred to as the double palatal bar.

**ADVANTAGES.** The anterior-posterior palatal bar is a very strong design providing a closed ring that gives excellent strength. It can be used to replace long spans as Class II partial dentures. It can be used also where a prominent maxillary torus exists. The anterior-posterior palatal bar has an additional advantage in that it can provide access to palatal tis-

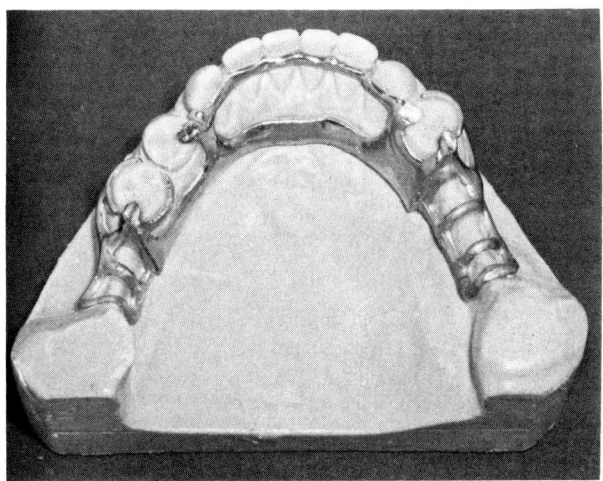

**Fig. 5-38.** Double lingual bar (Kennedy bar).

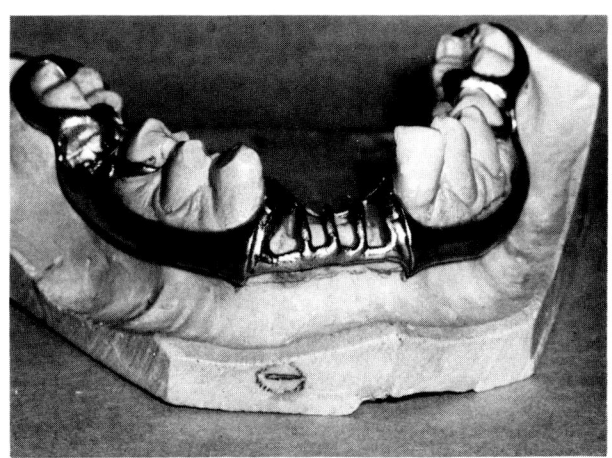

**Fig. 5-39.** Labial bar.

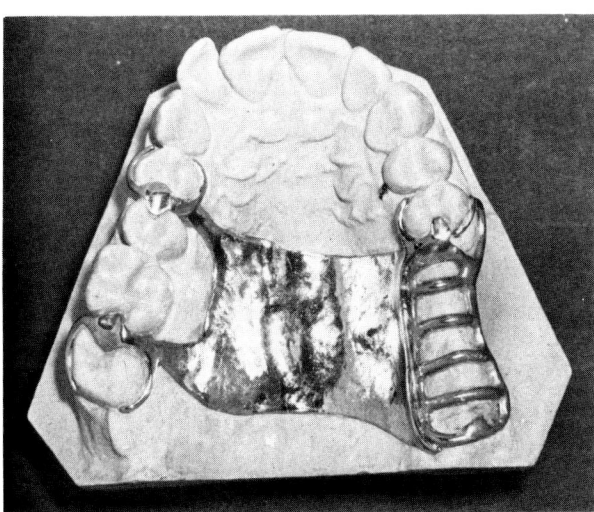

**Fig. 5-40.** Palatal bar or palatal strap.

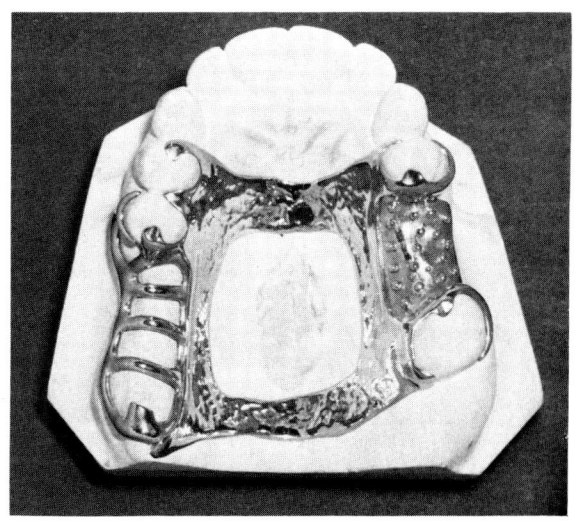

**Fig. 5-41.** Anterior-posterior palatal bar.

sues for the tongue. The anterior palatal bar can contact the anterior teeth as a lingual plate or be kept from the anterior teeth by 5 to 6 mm. The edges should be concealed in the valleys between the rugae (Fig. 5-42).

### HORSESHOE

The horseshoe is probably one of the most widely used and abused major connector designs (Fig. 5-43). One indication for the horseshoe design is where a torus exists and prevents the use of a strap or full palate. It also can be used to provide some splinting effect, and indirect retention is through the anterior lingual plate. The horseshoe is also recommended when anterior teeth are to be replaced, and where one side is tooth supported, and the opposite side has good soft tissue support. It is probably used more frequently for Class II removable partial denture designs. An additional indication is for the patient who cannot tolerate full coverage or a posterior strap because of hyperactive gag reflex.

DISADVANTAGES. The horseshoe connector must be rigid if flexing is to be avoided. Placing the design in more than one plane helps to achieve the desired rigidity.

### CLOSED HORSESHOE

Although the horseshoe major connector is usually flexible, the closed horseshoe is very rigid because the design completes a circle and is in more than one plane. It is used more frequently in Classes I and II removable partial denture designs. It is usually indicated for use when additional lateral bracing is needed and when a large torus palatinus is present.

DISADVANTAGE. The closed horseshoe connector may not be used for the patient who has a hyperactive gag reflex because the posterior location of its distal strap may not be tolerated (Fig. 5-44).

### FULL PALATE

The full palate is the strongest major connector to be used in the maxillary arch (Fig. 5-45). It is indicated where a maximum number of teeth are replaced, in the case of a bilateral distal extension (Class I) removable partial denture, and where masticatory forces will be quite heavy. This may occur when the maxillary removable partial denture is opposed by natural dentition in the mandibular arch. The full palate major connector can also be used where maximum bracing and splinting are required. This design also facilitates replacement of anterior teeth.

DISADVANTAGES. The primary disadvantage of the full palate connector is weight, and for those patients with hyperactive gag reflexes the full palate is contraindicated.

## Minor connectors

Minor connectors are those portions of the removable partial denture framework which connect the various components such as clasps to the major connector (Fig. 5-46). These are frequently referred to as tangs and struts.

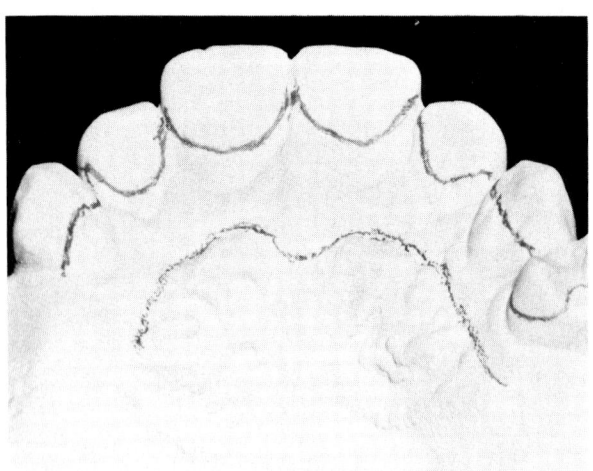

**Fig. 5-42.** Anterior portion designed to be concealed between valleys of rugae.

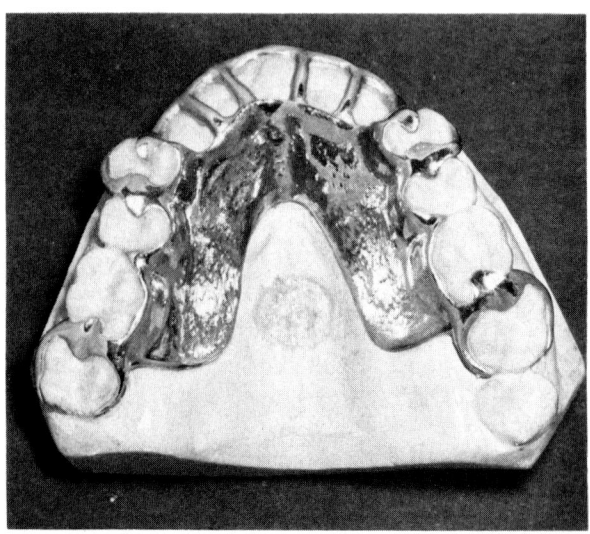

**Fig. 5-43.** Horseshoe.

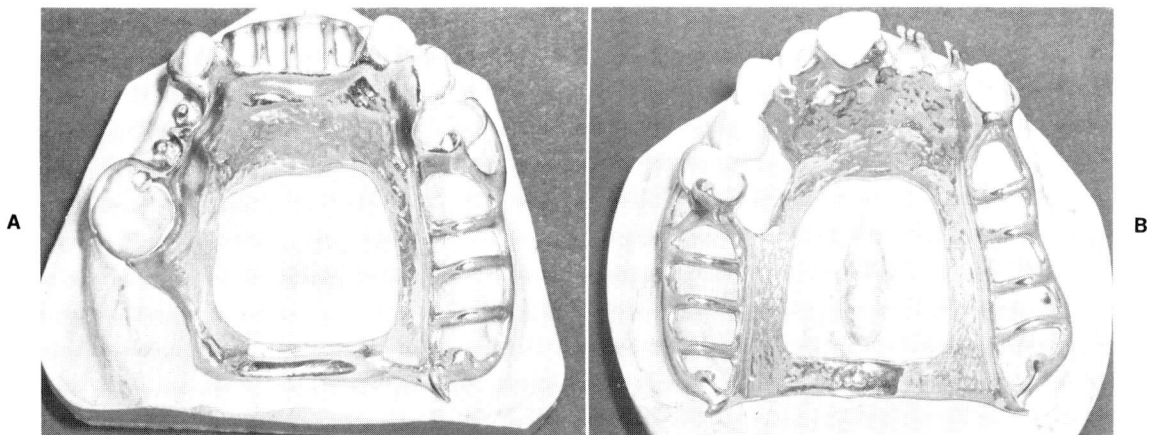

**Fig. 5-44. A,** Closed horseshoe is designed in two planes, which makes it more rigid. **B,** This major connector is often used when torus palatinus is present.

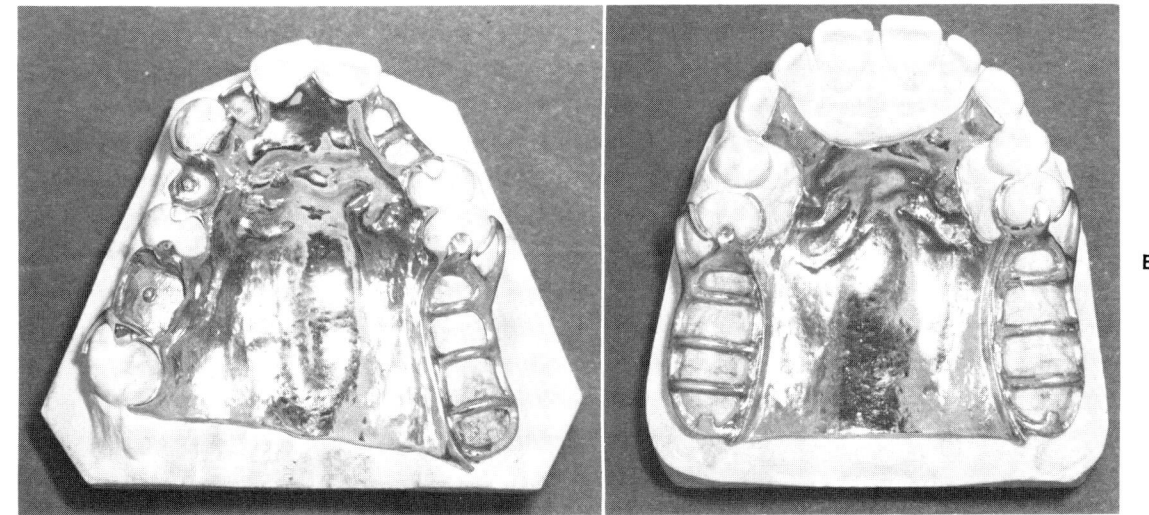

**Fig. 5-45. A,** Full palate. **B,** Modified full palate.

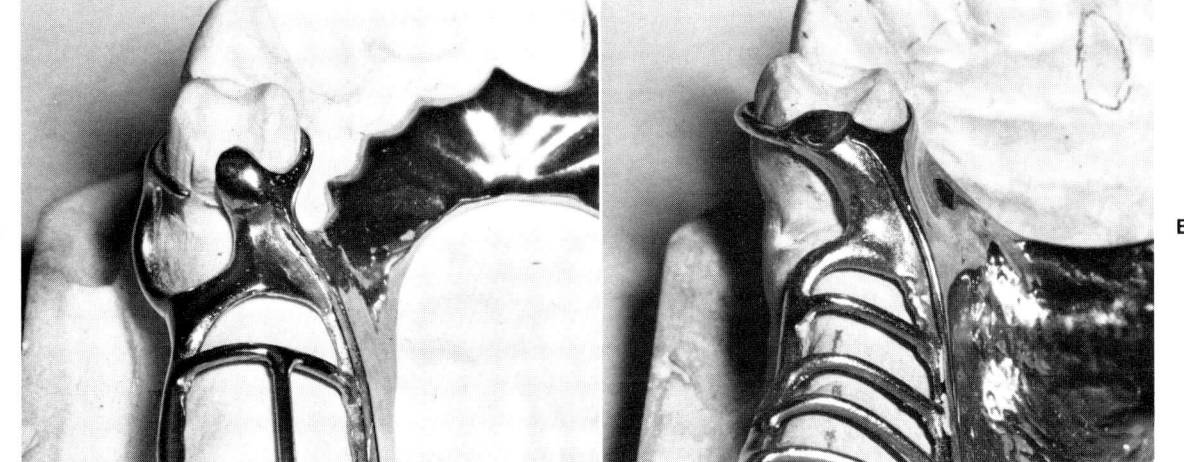

**Fig. 5-46.** Minor connector ties clasp and/or rest to major connector. **A,** Minor connector used with bar clasp on facial side. **B,** Minor connector used in conjunction with facial wire clasp.

## Denture bases

Two primary types of bases can be used for removable partial dentures. In the metal base (Fig. 5-47), the metal contacts the denture-supporting tissues, and in an acrylic resin base, the resin contacts the denture-supporting tissues (Fig. 5-48). If the possibility of a relining procedure is a primary concern, then acrylic resin bases are recommended. Where the removable partial denture is tooth supported and residual ridges are relatively well healed, a metal base may be used to good advantage, since it has been reported that the soft tissue response may be better than with resin. This may be related to the greater ease in keeping the metal clean, or it may be related to the thermal conductivity of the metal.

### Resin bases

The resin base is indicated when a reline may be necessary as ridge contours change and particularly in long-span distal extension replacements (Classes I or II). After surgical procedures, healing may result in ridge contour changes that are easier to compensate for with a resin base. Where severe resorption has occurred, the acrylic resin can compensate or "fill in" with less weight and improved esthetics.

### Metal bases

Metal bases may be used in some tooth-supported partial dentures where residual ridges are well healed and the ridge form is more stable. Metal bases are used where available denture space is severely limited and an acrylic resin base would be too thin.

### Denture base retention

Resin bases are retained on the framework through the use of open latticework or retention mesh (Fig. 5-49). Retention mesh and open latticework can be constructed over relief so when the acrylic resin is processed, the metal is enclosed within the plastic base (Fig. 5-50). A tissue stop is used in this situation to maintain framework position during compression molding of the denture base resin. Resin is retained on metal bases by beads, crystals, or nailheads (Fig. 5-51).

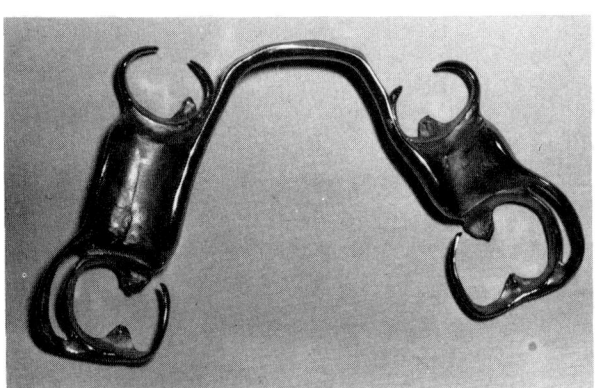

**Fig. 5-47.** All metal denture base.

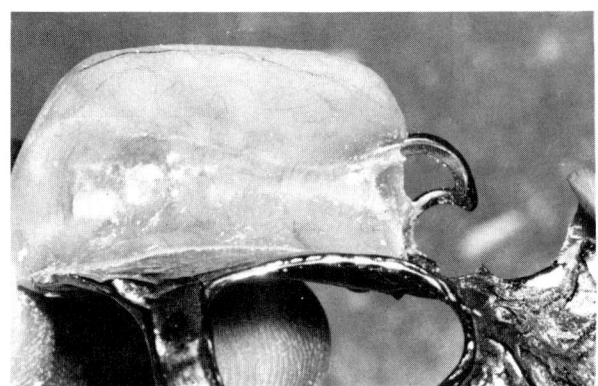

**Fig. 5-48.** Acrylic resin denture base.

Survey and design **151**

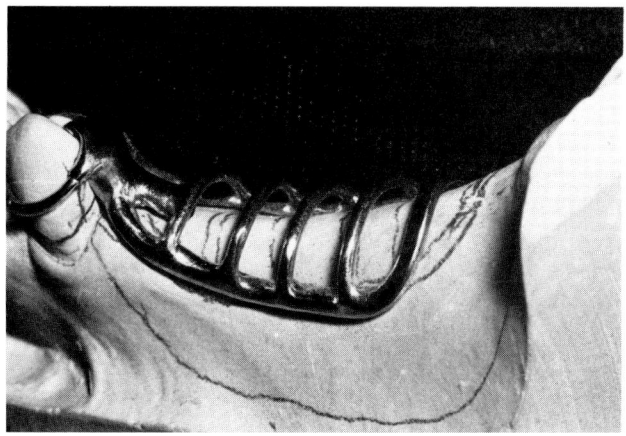

**Fig. 5-49.** Retention for acrylic resin denture base.

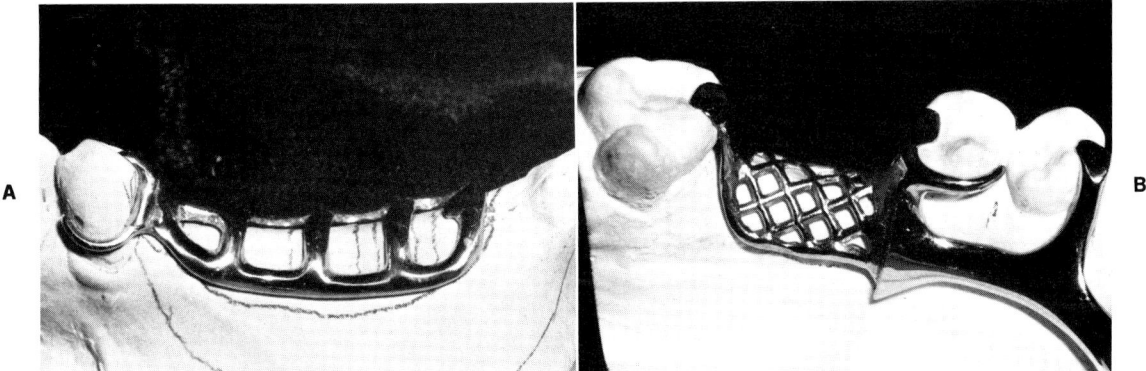

**Fig. 5-50.** Metal is designed to be completely surrounded by acrylic resin. **A,** Open retention. **B,** Lattice-work retention.

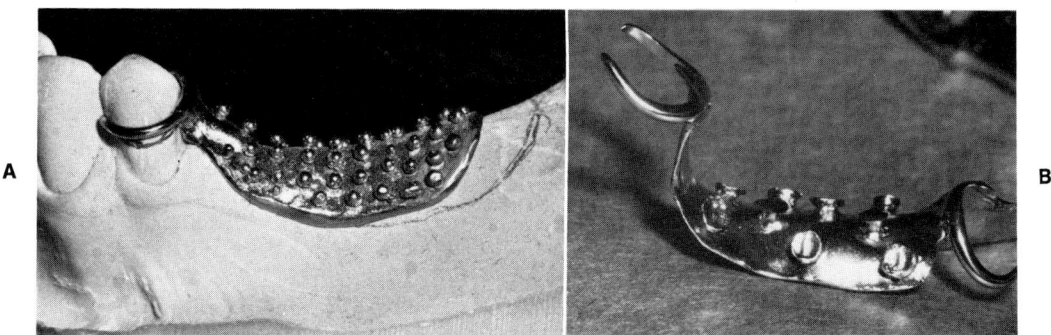

**Fig. 5-51.** Beads **(A)** and nailheads **(B)** retain acrylic resin on metal base. Resin does not go between metal and soft tissue.

## Anterior tooth replacement

Single anterior teeth are usually replaced with a fixed partial denture. It may be indicated, however, to replace a single tooth with a removable partial denture. This can occur when a fixed prosthesis is contraindicated for the patient. Multiple anterior tooth replacement with a removable partial denture may be indicated also where the span is too great or too much curve exists in the span to be supported adequately by a fixed partial denture. When canines are missing along with central and lateral incisors a removable partial denture may be indicated. A removable partial denture is often the method of choice for replacing missing anterior teeth where there has been a significant amount of anterior ridge resorption. In this case, it would be difficult to construct an esthetic fixed partial denture. The removable partial denture permits resin buildup of gingival contours to simulate appearance prior to resorption. There are essentially four methods for replacing missing anterior teeth with removable partial dentures: (1) facings (Steele's flat back), (2) tube teeth, (3) denture teeth processed on a denture base, and (4) reinforced acrylic pontic (Fig. 5-52). Each of these replacement methods has advantages and disadvantages. Methods for constructing these replacements are described in Chapter 18.

### Facings

Facings have been widely used for replacing single or multiple anterior teeth, particularly where minimal space is available (Fig. 5-53). The replace-

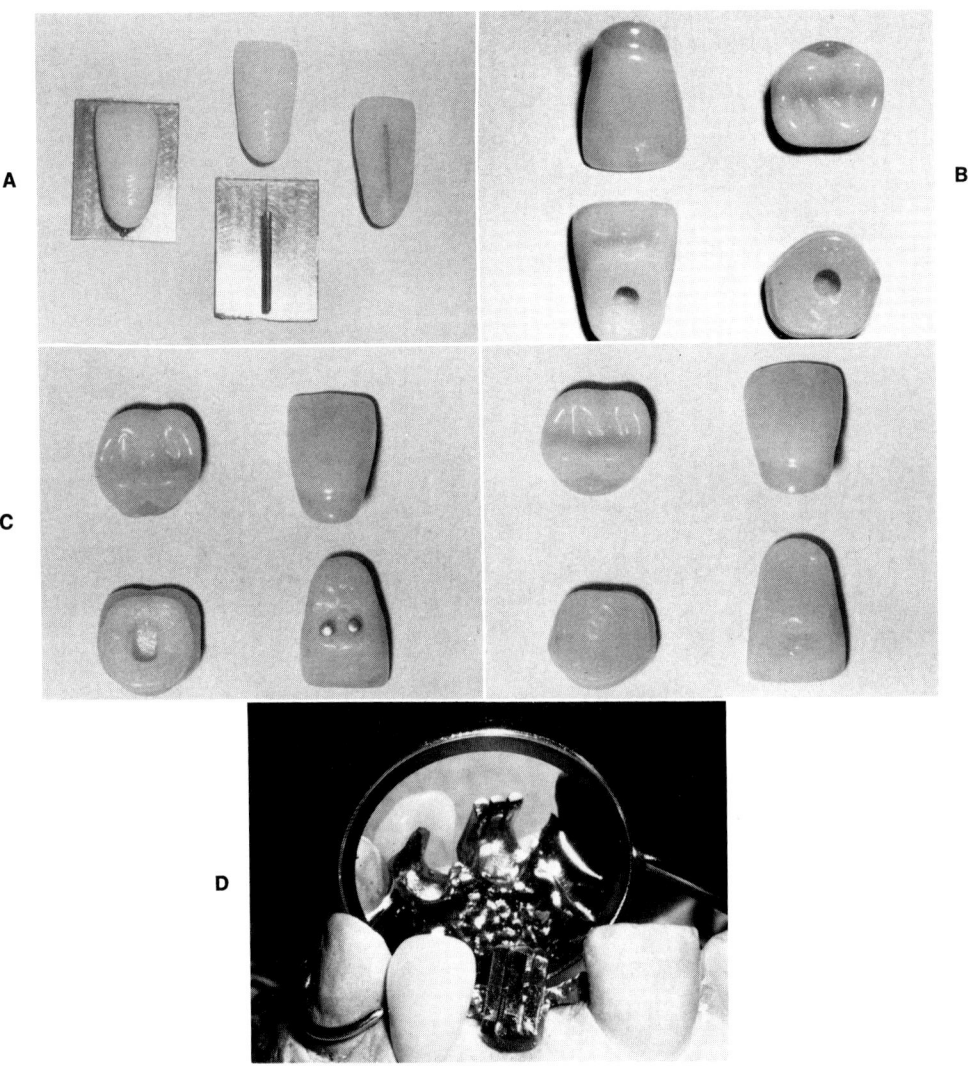

**Fig. 5-52. A,** Steele's flat back facings. **B,** Tube teeth. **C,** Porcelain denture teeth, (left) and plastic denture teeth (right). **D,** Reinforced acrylic pontic.

ment is very strong. Unfortunately, facings are often unesthetic due to their relative opacity when backed by metal. Facings should not be used where residual ridge resorption is severe, or the result may not be esthetic. Thus facings should be reserved for isolated single-tooth placements where space is minimal, residual ridges are well healed, and resorption is not severe. Disadvantages of facings include (1) poor esthetics, (2) difficulty in using them on a resorbed ridge, and (3) difficulty in relining should it be required.

### Tube teeth

Tube teeth are constructed by modifying resin or porcelain denture teeth (Fig. 5-54). A denture tooth is modified for adaptation to the ridge and occlusion. It is hollow ground to permit a portion of the casting to project into the tooth for retention. The tooth is waxed into position, the occlusion is checked, and the tooth is then removed from the wax-up. The completed wax-up is invested and cast. Following the framework try-in appointment, the tube tooth is cemented to the framework with autopolymerizing resin or conventional crown and bridge cement.

ADVANTAGES. Advantages of tube teeth include a wide variety of available denture teeth molds and shades, plus their use may eliminate the need for flasking and packing later.

DISADVANTAGES. A disadvantage of tube teeth is the difficulty in relining should it be required later. Although not a disadvantage, the casts must be mounted accurately in an articulator to permit reestablishment of occlusion. Tube teeth may be weakened by the recess, consequently they may fracture in service. Tube teeth are also more difficult to use where significant resorption has occurred. Tube teeth can be used for anterior and posterior replacements.

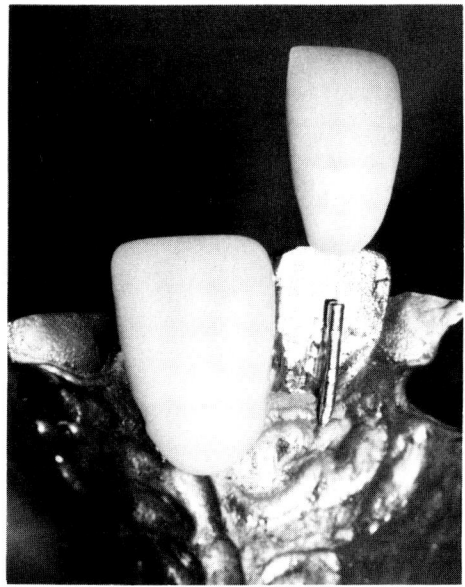

Fig. 5-53. Steele's facing on removable partial denture.

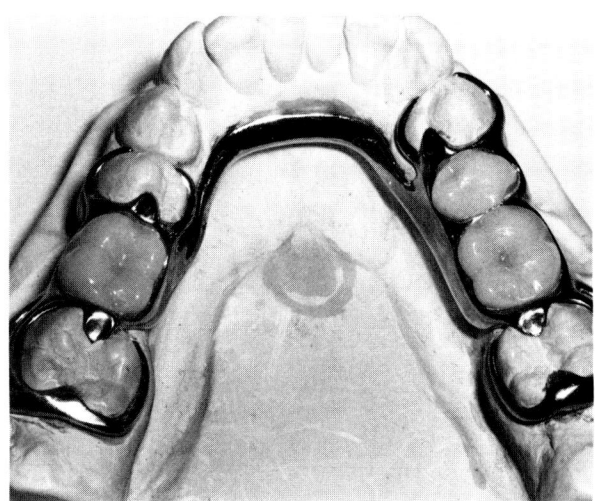

Fig. 5-54. Tube teeth on partial denture.

### Denture teeth

Usually the most esthetic multiple anterior replacement method for removable partial dentures is denture teeth on a denture base (Fig. 5-55). This is particularly true where significant change in ridge topography has occurred as a result of bone resorption.

ADVANTAGES. The wide variety of denture teeth molds and shades available also facilitate achievement of a satisfactory esthetic result. Additional advantages of this method include the ease of relining or rebasing if needed later and the ability to compensate for contour changes by addition of denture base resin that can simulate the original contour and color of the supporting tissues. The base resin can also be tinted and finished to satisfy particular color and texture requirements. An additional advantage of the denture tooth/denture base for anterior replacement includes the additional support provided by contact with the anterior residual ridge. This support may be more apparent than real; however, it can contribute to a more stable removable partial denture, particularly when overdenture-type abutments are used (Fig. 5-56). A secondary advantage is the occlusion that is transferred to acrylic resin rather than to metal as with facing replacements.

DISADVANTAGES. Disadvantages of denture teeth include the space requirement for the framework, resin, and teeth. The contraindications for this method are minimal denture space and inadequate thickness of the replacement to prevent breakage. It is also more difficult to use when replacing single teeth.

### Reinforced acrylic pontic (RAP)

Reinforced acrylic pontics are a significant advancement in anterior tooth replacement on removable partial dentures. They are similar to tube teeth in that acrylic resin teeth are adapted to the residual ridge and a casting fabricated to reinforce and harmonize with the tooth's position (Fig. 5-57). Construction of RAPs is discussed in Chapter 18. Pro-

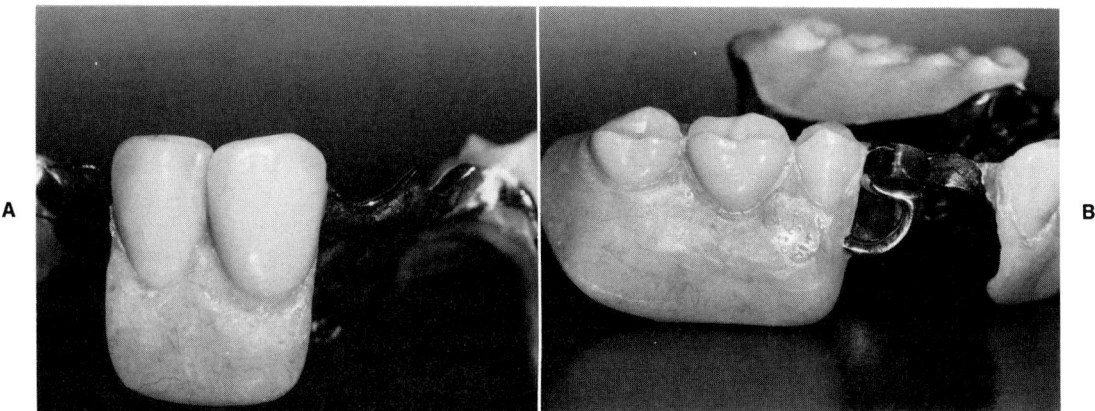

Fig. 5-55. Denture teeth processed on partial denture. **A,** Anterior teeth. **B,** Posterior segment.

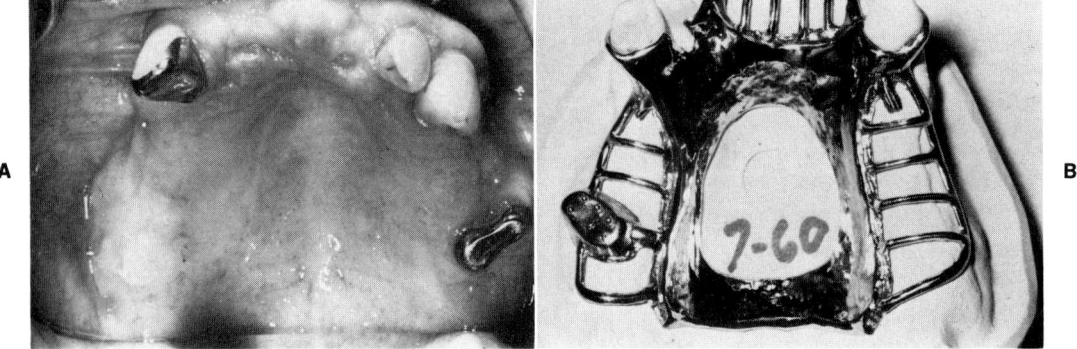

Fig. 5-56. Partial denture with denture teeth used for overdenture-type abutments. **A,** Molar overdenture abutment in mouth. **B,** Overlay abutment cover incorporated in metal casting.

jections are placed on the casting at strategic locations that will permit the acrylic resin denture tooth to be processed to the casting. The projections provide additional strength and result in a pontic that is acrylic resin, however, it is reinforced by the cast metal (Fig. 5-58).

ADVANTAGES. Advantages of RAPs include improved esthetics, since a variety of molds and shades are available for selection. When properly constructed, the replacement is strong and usually provides excellent service with minimal breakage, and RAPs can be used where space is minimal yet they give an adequately strong restoration.

DISADVANTAGES. RAPs are contraindicated where ridge resorption is severe, and where recent surgical procedures have been accomplished. In this situation, changes in ridge form subsequent to healing will result in a space developing beneath the replacement. Obviously, it is difficult to reline RAPs, and this type of replacement should not be used on inadequately healed ridges. It should be pointed out that facings on RAPs require additional clinical procedures. The RAP teeth should be evaluated in the mouth on a baseplate to develop the esthetic result of the replacement prior to the construction of the cast framework. Once the anterior teeth have been positioned in the mouth, they can be replaced on the cast, and a plastic or stone template can be constructed to preserve the arrangement. In this manner the positioning of the RAP tooth and the metal reinforcement can be coordinated. This additional clinical procedure is highly recommended to minimize improper location of tooth and metal reinforcement later.

### Posterior replacement

Methods available for replacing posterior teeth on a removable partial denture include resin and porcelain teeth processed to the denture base, tube teeth, metal pontics, metal pontics with resin facings, and metal occlusal teeth.

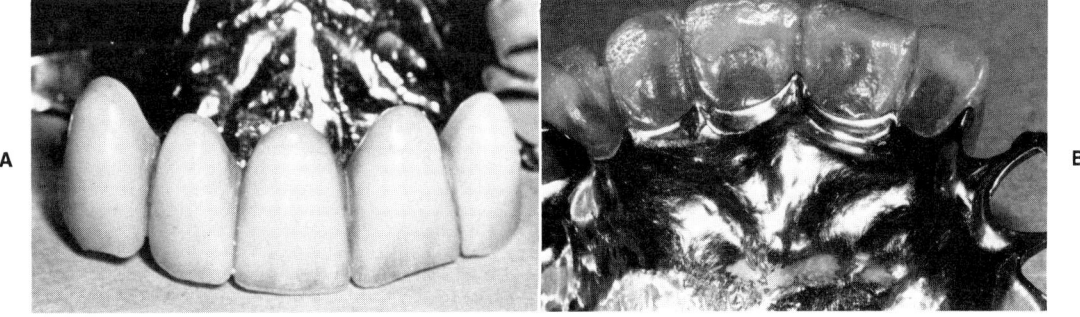

**Fig. 5-57.** Reinforced acrylic pontics on partial denture. **A,** Facial view. **B,** Lingual view.

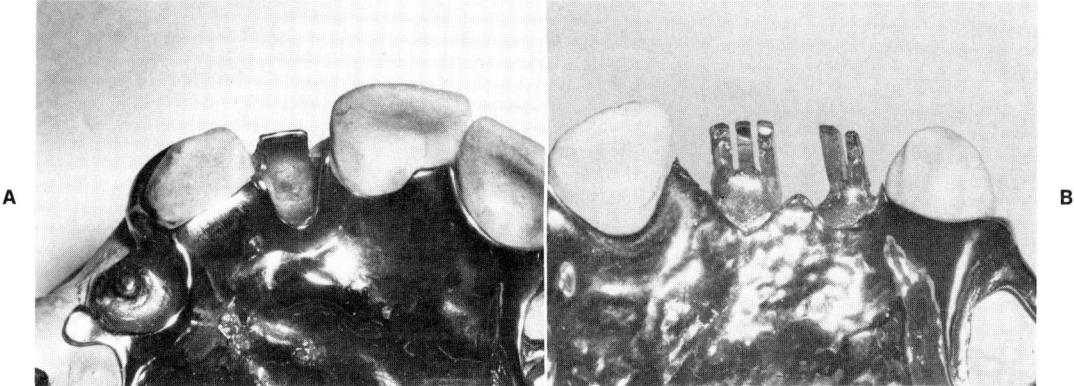

**Fig. 5-58.** Teeth are processed over metal projection on casting. **A,** Solid metal. **B,** Slotted metal.

## Resin or porcelain teeth processed to the denture base

Denture teeth processed to the resin base are most commonly used for replacing missing posterior teeth on a removable partial denture (Fig. 5-59).

ADVANTAGES. One advantage of resin or porcelain teeth processed to the denture base is the availability of a large number of molds and shades to meet the existing needs of the particular patient. Occlusion can be developed in resin or in porcelain as the situation requires, repairs can usually be completed easily, and rebasing and relining can be accomplished if needed. Resin denture teeth are usually used when opposing natural teeth, since porcelain teeth may produce pronounced wear on the opposing natural teeth and metal restorations. Porcelain teeth can be used when the opposing occlusion is a complete denture with porcelain teeth. The denture tooth adjacent to a rest should often be resin to prevent breakage, since adaptation to the minor connector usually requires grinding (Fig. 5-60).

## Metal occlusals on teeth

Denture teeth with metal occlusals can also be constructed for removable partial dentures and have significant advantages. Metal occlusal teeth can be easily harmonized to the patient's existing teeth, and gold occlusals can be used to oppose natural teeth and cast metal restorations in the opposing arch. In addition, metal occlusals provide

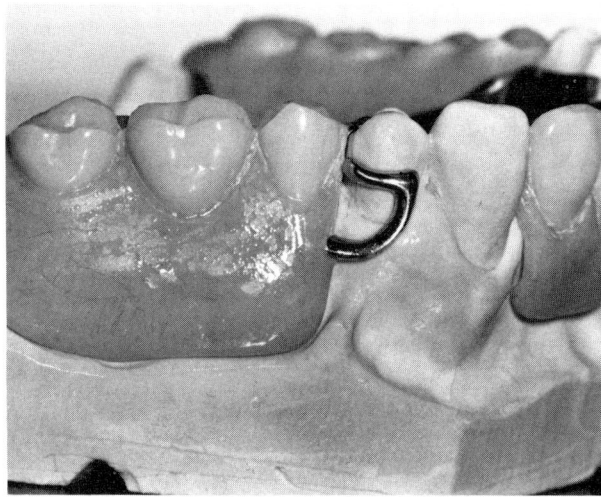

Fig. 5-59. Posterior replacements may be acrylic resin or porcelain denture teeth processed to denture base.

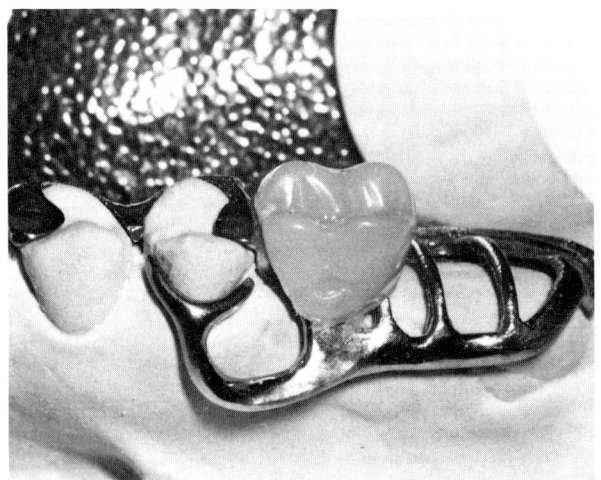

Fig. 5-60. Often, denture tooth next to minor connector must be ground considerably to fit contour. Plastic teeth are preferred for this area.

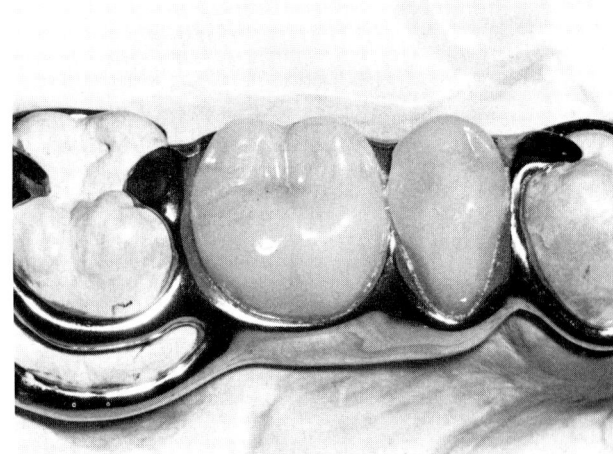

Fig. 5-61. Tube teeth may be used in posterior region.

strength for the removable partial denture. Their use is indicated particularly when the opposing occlusion is primarily cast gold restorations. Procedures for construction of metal occlusals are given in Chapter 6 of *Dental Laboratory Procedures: Complete Dentures* (Morrow et al., 1980).

### Tube teeth

Tube teeth can be used for replacement of premolar and molar teeth on a removable partial denture, particularly where space is minimal and residual ridges are relatively well healed and where residual ridge resorption is minimal (Fig. 5-61). The use of tube teeth entirely can eliminate the necessity for processing the framework later in a flask. This significantly reduces the possibility of the framework distortion during flasking, processing, and retrieval procedures. Similar to the case of anterior replacements, tube teeth should not be used where there has been significant change in ridge contour as a result of resorption and where recent surgery has been completed. Tissue shrinkage subsequent to surgery will inevitably produce a space between the partial denture and tissue that cannot be easily relined.

### Metal pontics

Metal pontics and metal pontics with resin facings can be used in the posterior arch where space is too narrow mesiodistally for a single denture tooth (Fig. 5-62). They may be used also if there is insufficient interarch space (Fig. 5-63). Where esthetics is critical, metal pontics can be constructed with a resin veneer.

DISADVANTAGES. Disadvantages for metal pontics are similar to those for tube teeth. It is difficult to reline metal pontics, and they may be quite heavy where significant residual ridge resorption has occurred. Occlusion on the metal pontic, in some situations, may produce wear of the opposing dentition. Metal pontics should be used where insufficient space exists to place a tube tooth or denture tooth.

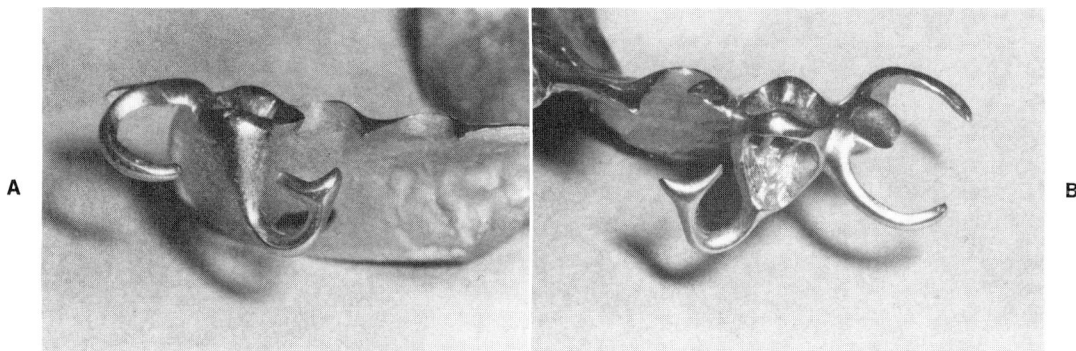

**Fig. 5-62. A,** Metal pontic is used when mesiodistal space is small and esthetics is not a problem. **B,** Plastic window may be used for esthetics.

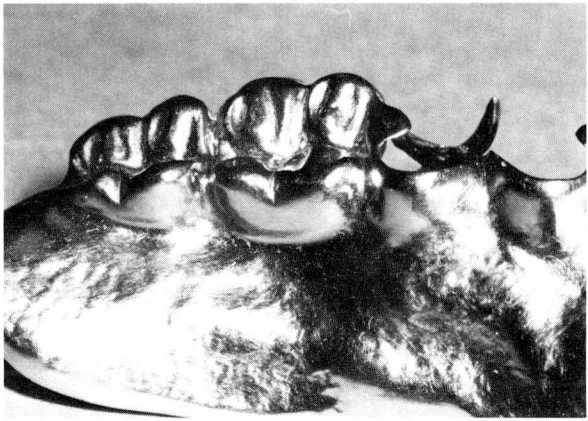

**Fig. 5-63.** When interarch distance is very small, all metal teeth may be used.

**158** *Dental laboratory procedures: removable partial dentures*

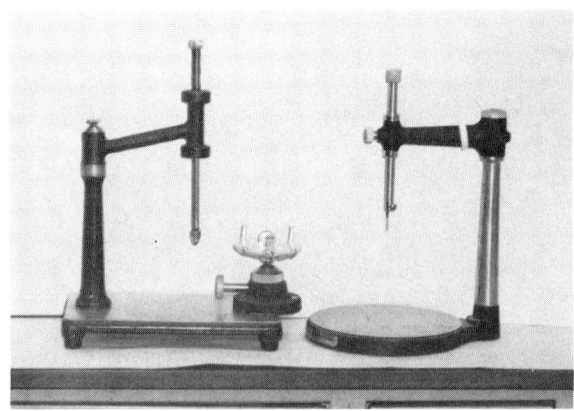

Fig. 5-64. Jelenko surveyor (left) and Ney surveyor (right).

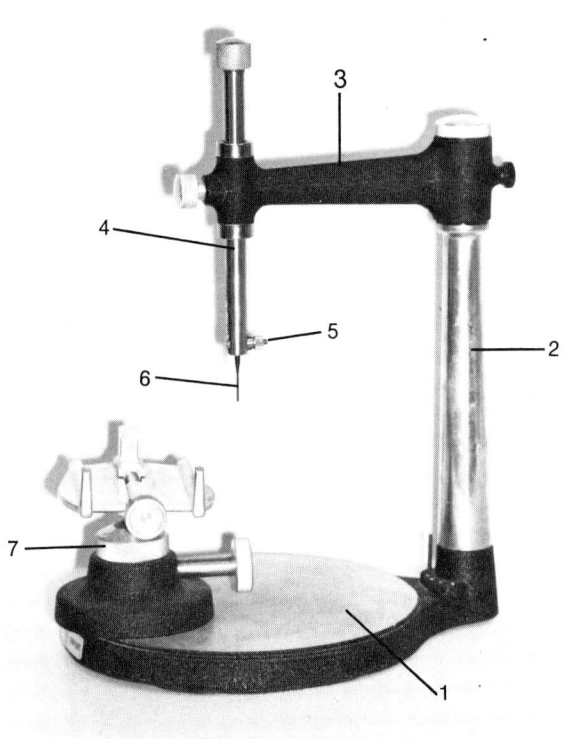

Fig. 5-65. Principal parts of typical surveyor: *1*, base or platform on which cast holder is moved; *2*, vertical column that supports superstructure is at right angle to base; *3*, horizontal arm extends at right angle from vertical column, from which surveying tool extends; *4*, surveying tool is capable of limited degree of movement in vertical plane; *5*, collet, or locking device, is designed to receive and hold interchangeable surveying instruments; *6*, surveying instrument (any of instruments shown in Fig. 5-66 may be used in this surveyor); and *7*, cast holder or surveying table to which cast is attached; ball-and-socket joint permits tilting cast, which can be locked in selected tilt.

## PRINCIPLES OF SURVEYING

Surveying is the procedure of studying the relative parallelism or lack of parallelism of the teeth and associated structures so as to select a path of placement for a restoration that will encounter the least tooth or tissue interference and that will provide adequate and balanced retention. Surveying also involves locating guiding plane surfaces to direct placement and removal of the restoration as well as to achieve the best appearance possible. The basic objectives of surveying are to locate and evaluate tooth and soft tissue undercuts on the cast and, based on this evaluation, select a path of insertion that will make optimal use of favorable undercuts while minimizing the effect of unfavorable undercuts. To do this a surveyor is used.

### Surveyor

A surveyor is a mechanical device that permits placement of the cast in a selected fixed position while the instrument is used to first analyze and then mark the undercuts on the cast. Surveyors are available from a number of different manufacturers. Probably the best known are the Ney* and Jelenko†

---

*Surveyor and parallelometer, The J. M. Ney Co., Bloomfield, Conn.
†Wills surveyor, J. F. Jelenko & Co., New Rochelle, N.Y.

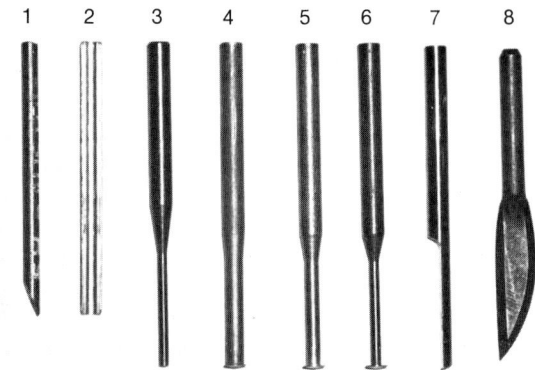

Fig. 5-66. Surveying instruments: *1*, carbon marker (5H drawing lead); *2*, shield to reinforce carbon marker to prevent breakage; *3*, analyzing rod; *4*, .010 undercut gauge; *5*, .020 undercut gauge; *6*, .030 undercut gauge; *7*, blockout trimmer; and *8*, wax trimmer.

surveyors (Fig. 5-64). A surveyor is composed of a platform or base, cast holder, and a vertical spindle or surveying tool that is maintained perpendicular to the base (Fig. 5-65). The spindle is designed to receive interchangeable surveying instruments, such as an analyzing rod, carbon marker, and various undercut gauges (Fig. 5-66). Since the surveyor spindle maintains a fixed position perpendicular to the horizontal plane, and the cast is held at the selected position on the cast table, lines placed on the cast with a carbon marker will have a fixed relationship to each other. Thus marks made on each tooth on the cast will also be correlated to each other and be considered when selecting the path of insertion.

## Surveying instruments

Instruments usually used in the surveyor include the analyzing rod, which is used to study and analyze undercuts on the cast, a carbon marker for placing marks on the cast once the path of insertion has been identified, a series of undercut gauges (usually .010, .020, and .030), which accurately measure the undercuts on individual teeth, and various wax carving instruments that are used during the blockout procedure (Chapter 6) (Fig. 5-67). The surveyor instrumentation can also include an attachment for securing a handpiece to the surveying instrument, in which case a bur placed in the handpiece can be

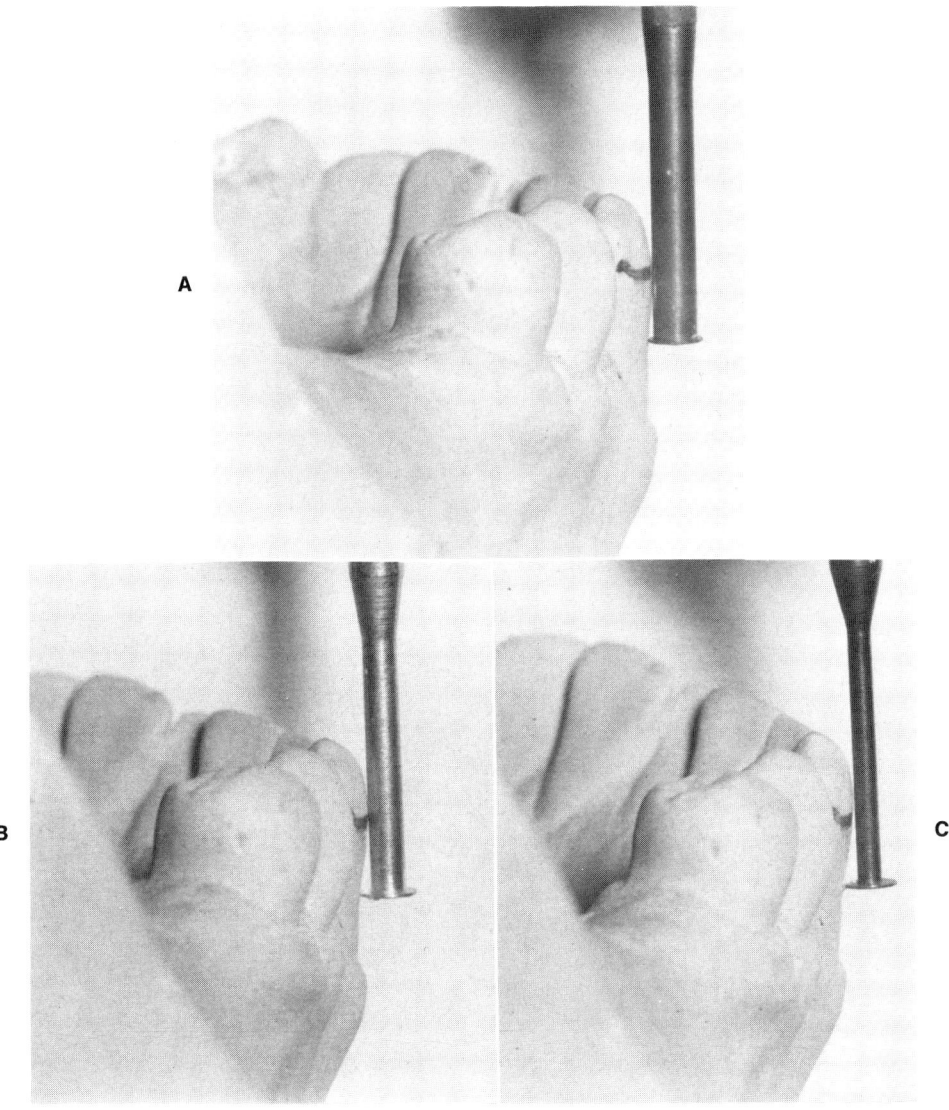

**Fig. 5-67.** Undercut gauges. **A**, .010. **B**, .020. **C**, .030.

used to mill metalic restorations to achieve parallel surfaces for guide planes (Fig. 5-68).

### Orientation of the cast

For purposes of description, it is convenient to select a standard cast orientation when describing placement of clasps and connectors. The standard position is for all casts to be considered as lower casts (Fig. 5-69). The position for description is from behind the cast or from the position of the tongue. Thus, when describing a clasp as being low on a given tooth, it means that the clasp is toward the gingiva, regardless of whether it is a mandibular or a maxillary cast. The standardized position minimizes confusion when describing placement of a clasp as being high or low. For instance, high on a maxillary cast might mean toward the gingiva whereas high on the mandibular cast might be toward incisal or occlusal surfaces. To further standardize descriptions, casts are oriented so that the anterior teeth are always toward the vertical member of the surveyor and away from the person making the survey. All references to the right side of the cast apply thus to the right side of the cast from this position; for instance, on mandibular casts the right side would be the actual right side of the lower arch (Fig. 5-70). For maxillary casts, however, the right side, when describing it on the surveyor, would be the maxillary left quadrant (Fig. 5-71). This is important when describing the tilt of a particular cast.

### Cast tilting

Tilting is simply changing the position of the cast, which thus changes the long axis of each tooth on the cast relative to the horizontal plane (Fig. 5-72). Obviously, changing the tilt also will change the position of the survey line in relation to the horizontal plane. More important, a change in tilt then changes the location and extent of any undercut area of the tooth (Fig. 5-73). Tilting is used to obtain the most advantageous path of insertion. Tilting may be used to increase desirable undercuts and to

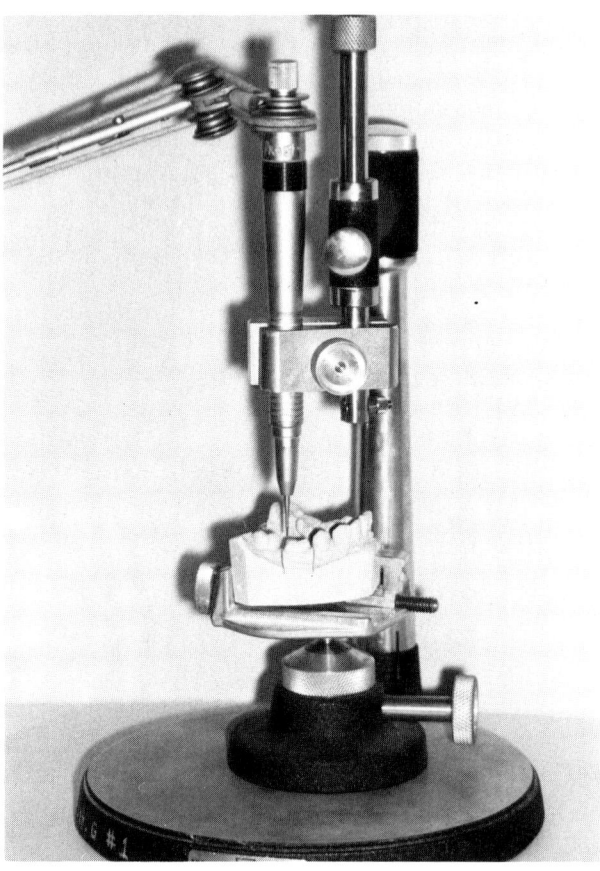

**Fig. 5-68.** Surveyor with handpiece held in place with handpiece attachment.

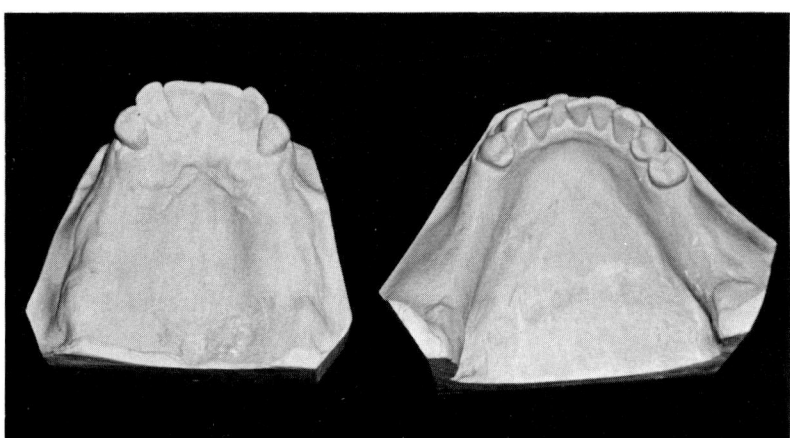

**Fig. 5-69.** All casts are considered as lower casts in standardized position to minimize confusion in describing partial denture.

*Survey and design* **161**

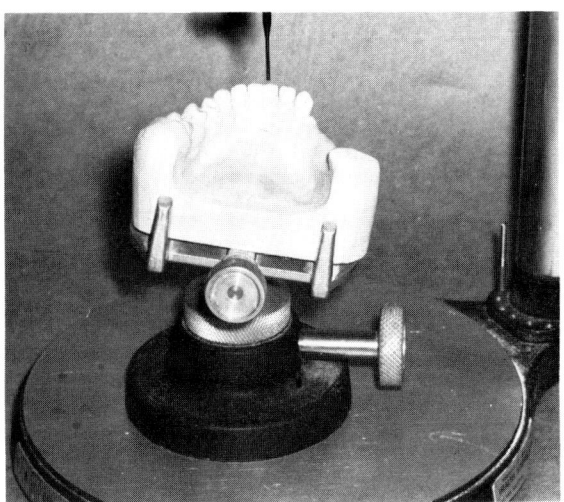

**Fig. 5-70.** Mandibular cast in position on surveying table and right side is actually right side of patient.

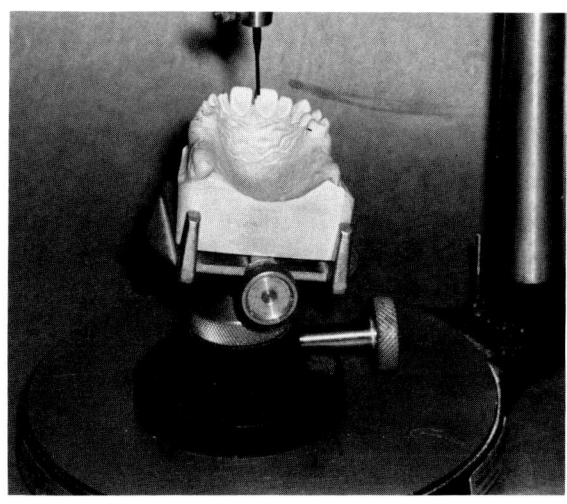

**Fig. 5-71.** Maxillary casts in position are different in that actual left side is considered right side at laboratory bench.

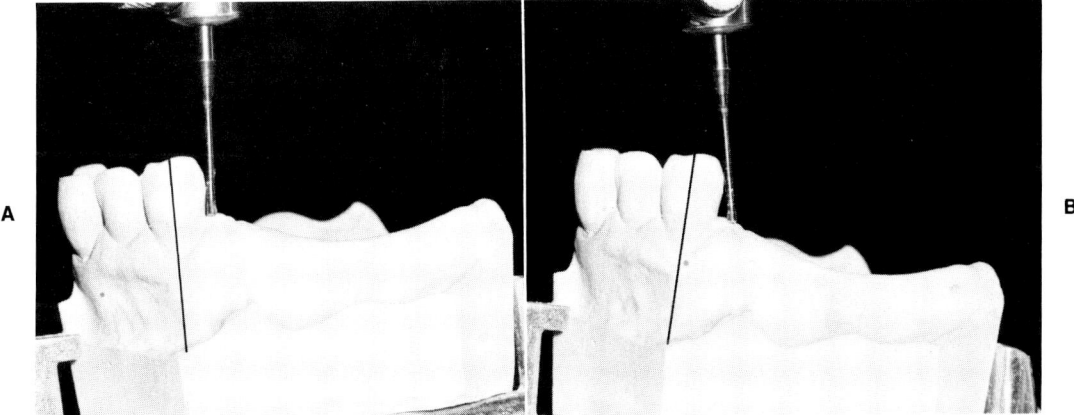

**Fig. 5-72.** Tilting changes long axis of tooth in relation to horizontal plane.

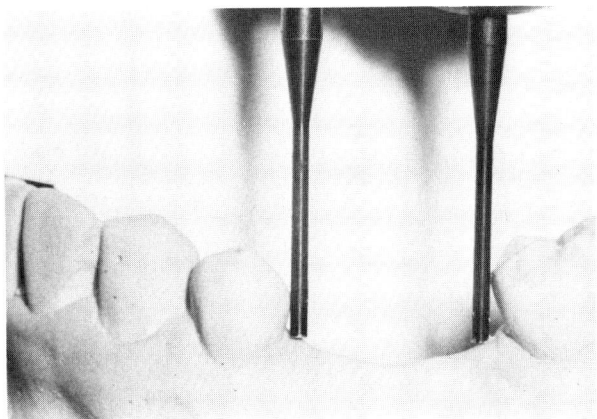

**Fig. 5-73.** Changing tilt changes undercut area on each tooth on cast.

decrease undesirable undercuts. Through tilting, it is possible to increase the undercuts on one side of the tooth while decreasing them on the other side of the tooth (Fig. 5-74). Thus it is important to remember that when tilting one must examine the effect of any tilt to establish a more desirable undercut on other teeth involved in the design. Although a given tilt may produce a very desirable undercut on one tooth, it may eliminate a desirable undercut on the opposite side of the arch (Fig. 5-75). Tilting can also be used to distribute available undercuts to produce more uniform retention throughout the available abutment teeth (Fig. 5-76). Tilting is also used to develop a path of insertion that will permit the most effective use of an anterior space for replacement. In fact, the presence of an edentulous anterior space on the removable partial denture sometimes dictates the final tilt to be selected. Tilting can also minimize unfavorable undercuts both on the teeth and soft tissue to facilitate better positioning of major and minor connectors and the base of the removable partial denture. It should be remembered that if a cast does not have usable undercuts, tilting in itself will not produce them.

### Basic cast tilts

The basic position or tilt of the cast on the surveyor should be the horizontal tilt, or, as some call

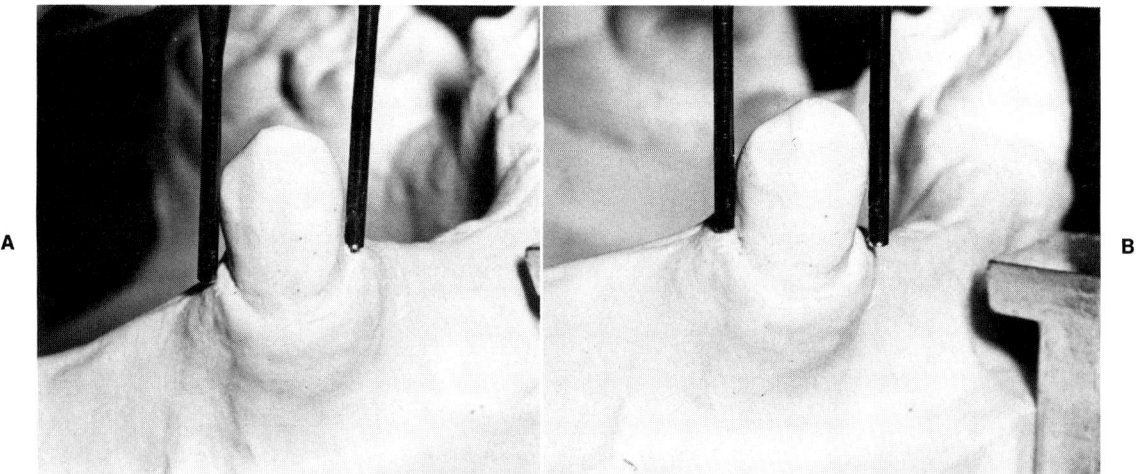

**Fig. 5-74.** By tilting, undercut area may be increased on one side of tooth and decreased on other side. **A,** Posterior tilt emphasizes distal undercut. **B,** When same cast is nearly horizontal, same tooth has mesial undercut.

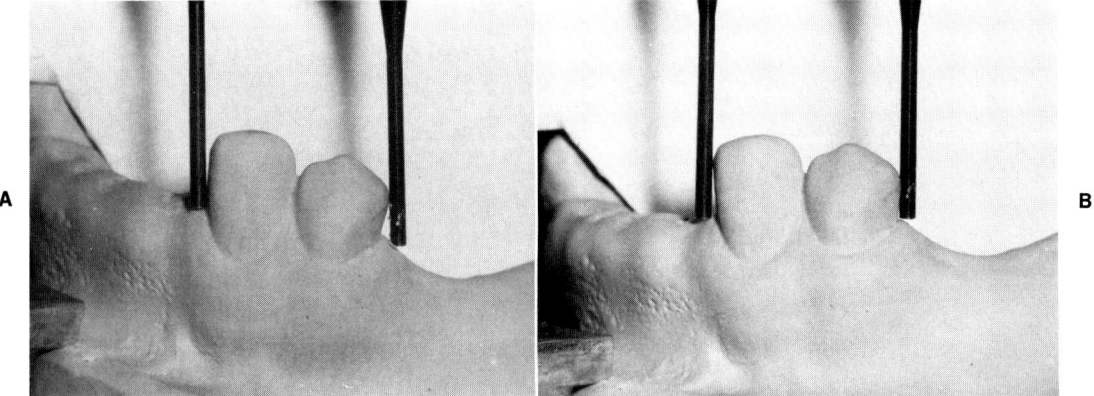

**Fig. 5-75.** Tilting may produce very desirable undercut on one tooth and eliminate all undercuts on another tooth. **A,** This tilt establishes good undercut on first premolar. **B,** Undercut is eliminated at this tilt.

Survey and design **163**

it, a zero tilt (Fig. 5-77). In the horizontal tilt, occlusal surfaces of the teeth are at or near parallelism to the horizontal plane. This is the standard reference position from which further tilts originate. The four basic tilts from the horizontal, or reference, position are (1) the anterior tilt, in which the anterior teeth are tilted downward (Fig. 5-78); (2) the posterior tilt, in which the posterior portion of the cast is tilted downward (Fig. 5-79); (3) the right lateral tilt, in which the right portion of the cast is tilted downward (Fig. 5-80); and (4) the left lateral tilt, in which the left portion of the cast is tilted downward (Fig.

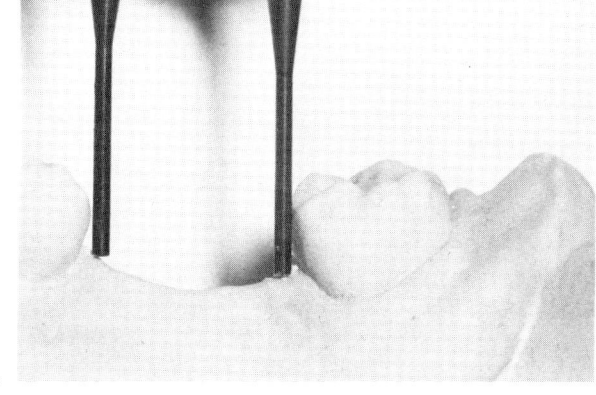

**Fig. 5-76.** Tilting can be used to equalize undercuts.

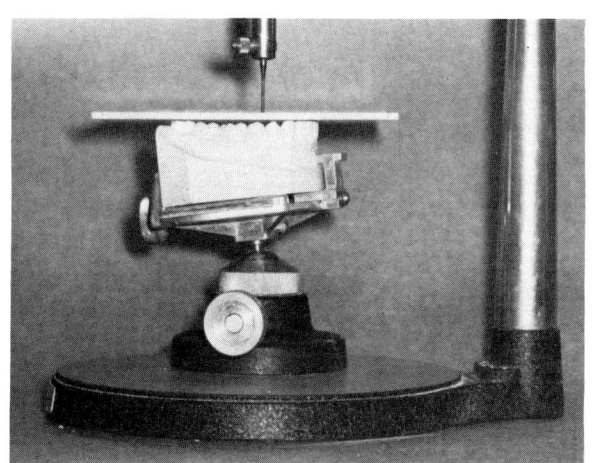

**Fig. 5-77.** Horizontal, or zero, tilt. Occlusal plane is parallel with floor.

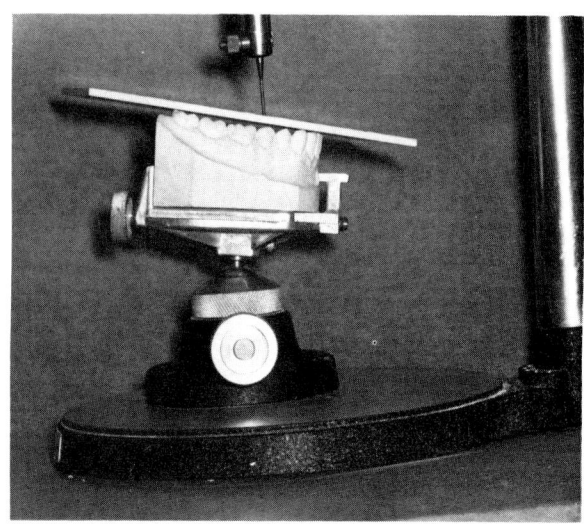

**Fig. 5-78.** Anterior tilt. Occlusal plane is lower in anterior region.

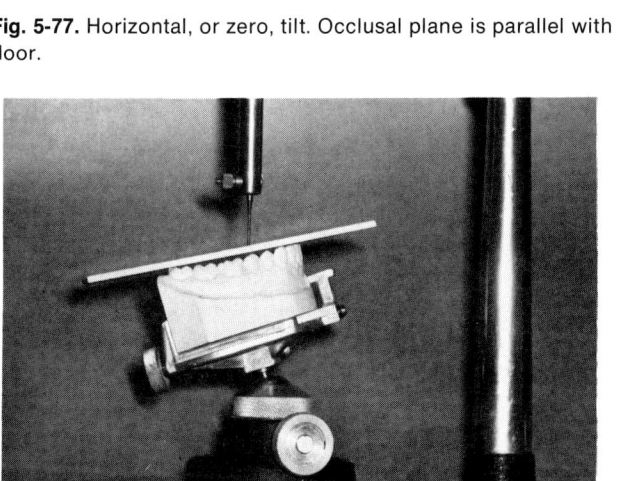

**Fig. 5-79.** Posterior tilt. Occlusal plane is lower in posterior region.

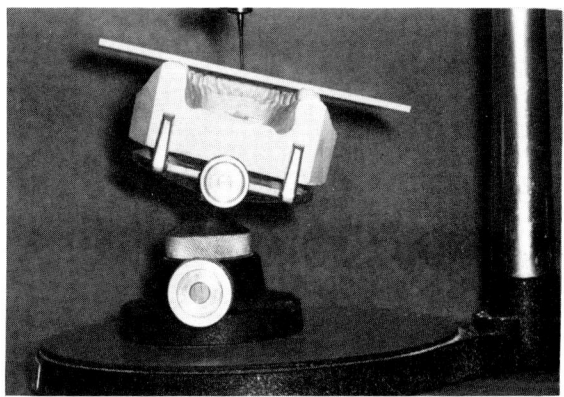

**Fig. 5-80.** Right lateral tilt. Occlusal plane is lower on right side.

5-81). Keep in mind that when using the right lateral tilt for a mandibular cast, the teeth on the right side will be tilted downward. However, a maxillary cast with a right tilt will mean that the left posterior teeth are tilted downward. Again, remember the standard orientation for descriptive purposes. The viewpoint in describing the basic position of tilt is always from the posterior aspect of the cast. The principle effects of tilting the cast on the undercuts are as follows: an anterior tilt will increase mesial undercuts on abutment teeth and residual ridges and decrease distal undercuts on teeth and residual ridges (Fig. 5-82). A posterior tilt will increase distal undercuts and conversely decrease mesial undercuts (Fig. 5-83). A right lateral tilt will increase undercuts on the buccal surfaces on that particular right side and will decrease buccal undercuts on the left side and increase undercuts on the lingual palatal surface on the left side (Fig. 5-84). A left lateral tilt will increase undercuts on the buccal surface of the left, or lowered, side and will decrease undercuts on the buccal surface of the right side. It will increase undercuts on the right lingual or palatal surface (Fig. 5-85). It must always be remembered when determining the most favorable tilt that the effect of the tilt on one particular tooth must always be considered throughout the entire cast. As a general rule, it is impossible to tilt a cast to create undercuts where no undercuts are present at a horizontal tilt. It is axiomatic that for most situations, the tilt to be selected will be at or near the horizontal tilt with minor modifications in one direction or another to optimize certain undercuts.

### Path of insertion

When a cast is tilted on the surveyor to make the most effective use of the available undercuts and after the effects of this tilt have been checked on all teeth and tissues involved in the removable partial denture, the path of insertion at this particular tilt will be indicated by the direction of the spindle in relationship to the tilt of the cast (Fig. 5-86). If, for instance, a straight horizontal tilt was selected for the design of the removable partial denture, the path of insertion as indicated by the spindle of the surveyor would be straight down. On the other hand, if the cast is tilted anteriorly and surveyed and designed for this tilt, the resultant path of insertion as indicated by the spindle will no longer be perpendicular to the occlusal plane. Instead, the path of insertion will traverse a path downward and anteriorly. Since the path of insertion indicates how the partial denture will be placed in the mouth, the terms must be converted as in Fig. 5-86, *C*.

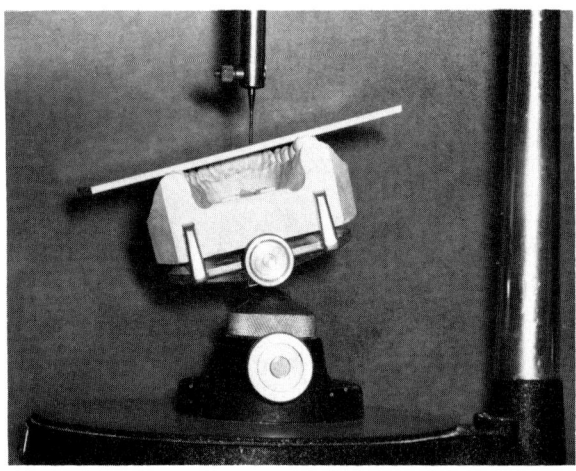

**Fig. 5-81.** Left lateral tilt. Occlusal plane is lower on left side.

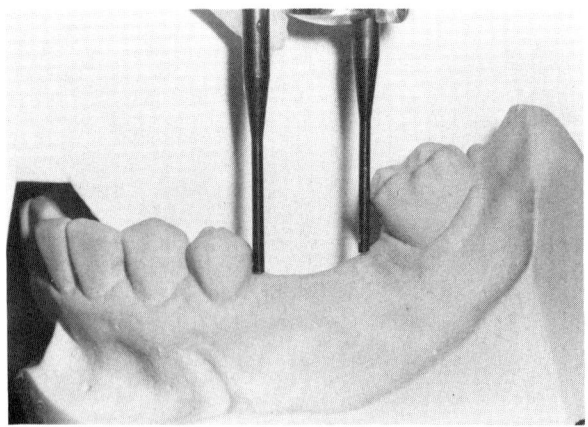

**Fig. 5-82.** Anterior tilt increases mesial undercuts and decreases distal undercuts.

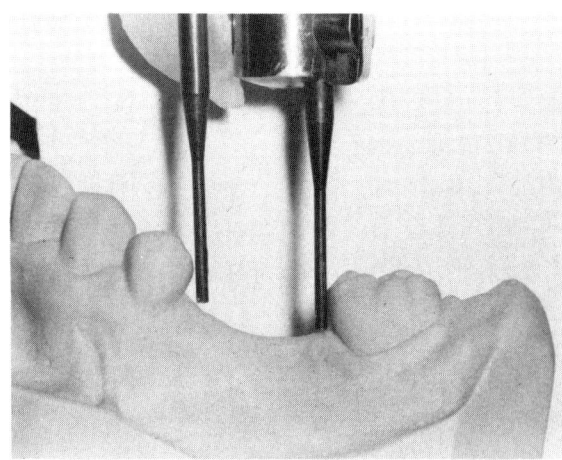

**Fig. 5-83.** Posterior tilt increases distal undercuts and decreases mesial undercuts.

Survey and design 165

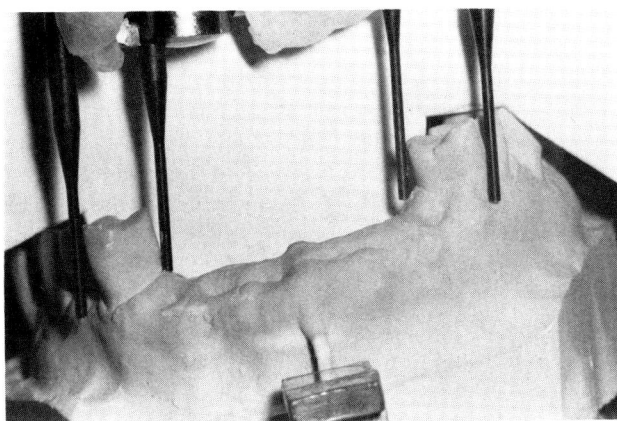

**Fig. 5-84.** Right lateral tilt will increase undercuts on buccal surfaces of teeth on right or low side and lingual surfaces of high side and will decrease undercuts on lingual surfaces of teeth on low side and buccal surfaces of high side.

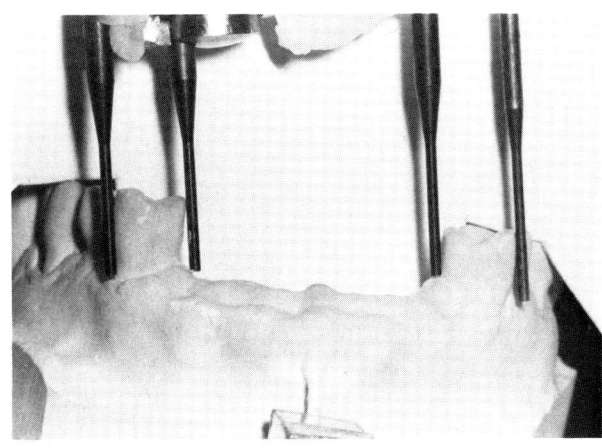

**Fig. 5-85.** Left lateral tilt will increase undercuts on buccal surfaces of teeth on left or low side and decrease those on lingual surfaces of low side. It will increase undercuts on lingual surfaces of teeth on high side and decrease buccal undercuts on that side.

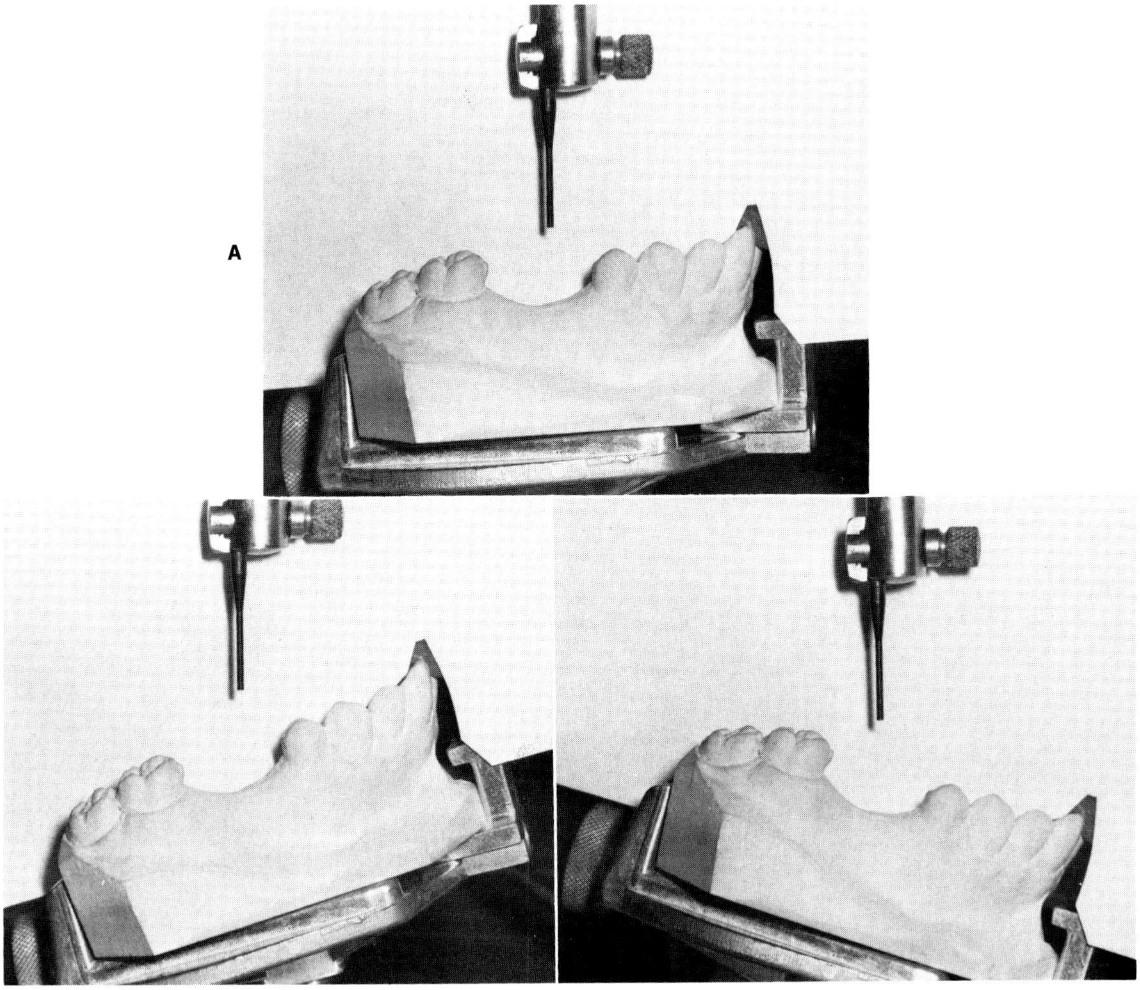

**Fig. 5-86.** Path of insertion in mouth is indicated by vertical spindle of surveyor in relation to occlusal plane of cast or tilt. **A,** Path of insertion is straight down for mandibular denture and straight up on maxillary denture. **B,** Path of insertion is upward and backward for maxillary denture and downward and backward for mandibular partial denture. **C,** Path of insertion is upward and forward for maxillary denture and downward and forward for mandibular partial denture.

**166** *Dental laboratory procedures: removable partial dentures*

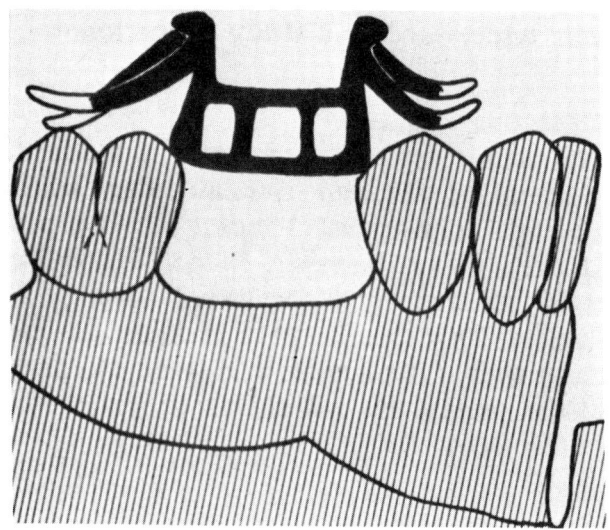

**Fig. 5-87.** Nonflexible portions of partial denture cannot spring into undercut.

### Undercuts

If almost any dentulous cast is placed on the surveying table and analyzed with a surveyor, undercuts will be found. Undercuts are classified as tooth undercuts or soft tissue undercuts. In addition, undercuts may also be classified as favorable undercuts or unfavorable undercuts. Since the removable partial denture is constructed of acrylic resin and cast metal, each of which is nonrigid, it is important to locate the undercuts on the cast so that rigid portions of the prosthesis will be kept clear of them (Fig. 5-87). It is equally important that favorable undercuts on the abutment teeth be located so that clasp tips can be extended into them to provide retention. When surveying a cast, the analyzing rod is used first to locate all undercuts, and, on the basis of this analysis, a tilt is selected that will produce a favorable path of insertion for the proposed prosthesis. The analyzing rod is then removed, and a car-

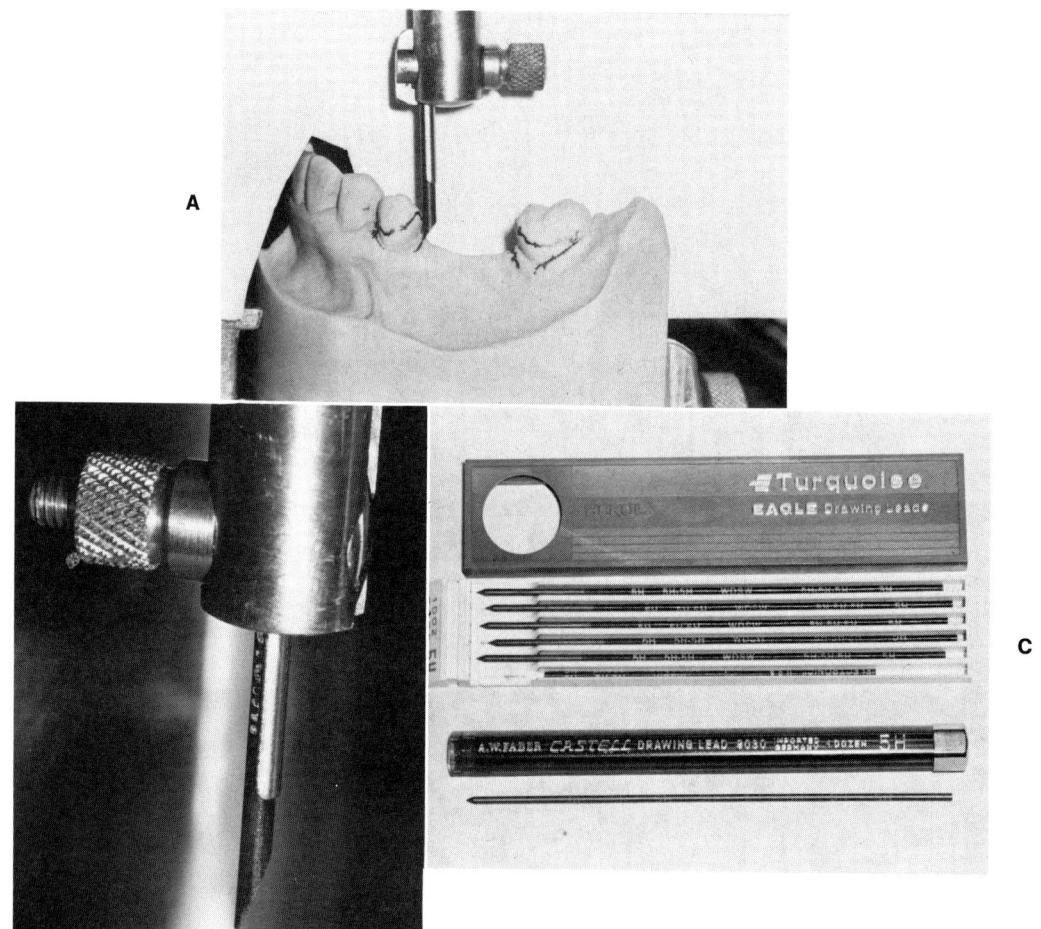

**Fig. 5-88. A,** Carbon marker rotated around tooth marks greatest diameter of tooth in any given position. This is known as survey line or neutral zone. **B,** Tip of carbon marker should be beveled as shown here. **C,** 5H drawing leads are excellent for this purpose.

bon marker is substituted in the surveyor spindle. Drawing leads* (5H) make good carbon markers and are less likely to break. While moving the surveyor table with the attached cast, a line can be placed on each tooth involved in the proposed design. The line on the tooth will indicate the greatest bulge of the tooth at the selected tilt (Fig. 5-88). The line will divide the tooth in a suprabulge area and an infrabulge area. Rigid portions of any clasp that is to be placed on the tooth must be kept above the survey line, whereas the flexible clasp tip is the only portion of the clasp that extends below the survey line. Thus, as previously stated, the survey line divides the tooth into a suprabulge, or nonundercut, area, and an infrabulge, or undercut, area. The design of most removable partial dentures is such that all rigid, or nonspringing, components of the partial denture framework are placed above the survey line, and only the flexible clasp tips are planned for placement below the survey line and into the right amount of undercut (Fig. 5-89). Correct placement of the flexible tip of the clasp is determined through the use of undercut gauges (Fig. 5-90). Desirable undercuts are those which are situated on the tooth so as to be effectively used with a clasp. Undesirable undercuts are those found on the abutment teeth which could interfere with the insertion and removal of the removable partial denture because of the particular contour of that tooth. Undesirable undercuts may occur when the tooth is malpositioned. Since undercuts can be significantly changed by tilting, it is important to understand what effect certain tilts will have on certain undercuts (Fig. 5-91).

---

*Eagle drawing leads, Berol Corp., Danbury, Conn.; Castell drawing leads, A. W. Farber-Castell Co., Newark, N.J.

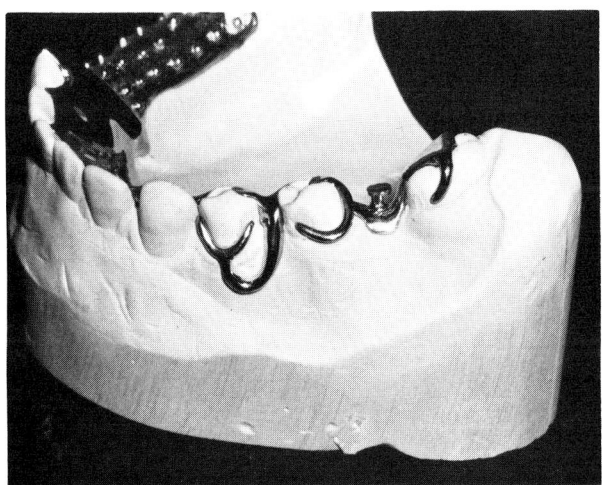

**Fig. 5-89.** Only flexible tip of clasp will spring into undercut.

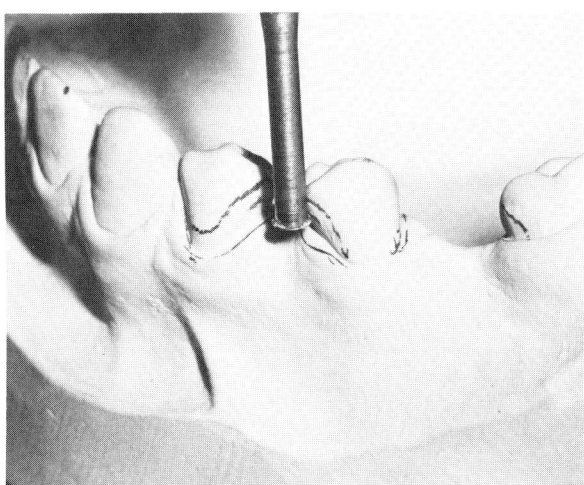

**Fig. 5-90.** Measured undercut locates bottom of tip of clasp.

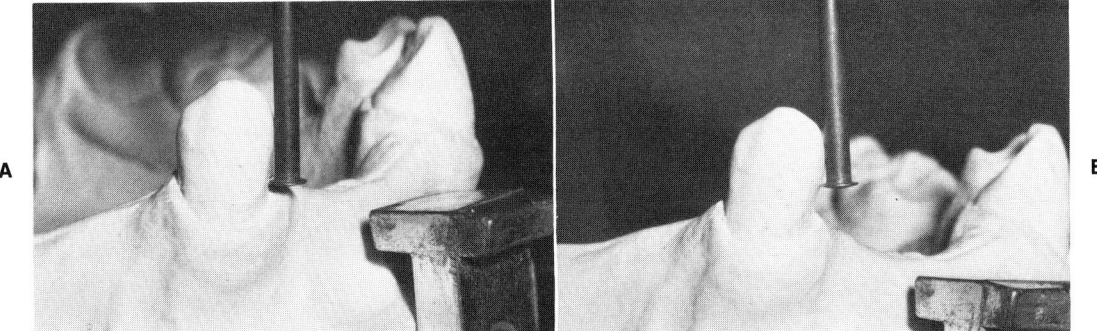

**Fig. 5-91.** Tilting may influence position of measured undercut considerably. **A,** Undercut is near gingival surface at this tilt. **B,** When tilt is changed slightly, same amount of undercut is near incisal surface.

Another type of undercut that must be dealt with when surveying and designing a removable partial denture is soft tissue undercuts. Soft tissue undercuts frequently affect the design of the removable partial denture; particularly when considering the use of the infrabulge, or bar-type, clasp. In this situation, a significant soft tissue undercut adjacent to a proposed abutment tooth for which a bar clasp is indicated may necessitate use of a different type of clasp (Fig. 5-92). Soft tissue undercuts also can affect the base of the removable partial denture. In this situation, the resin base may require modification before it can be put into place in the patient's mouth without scuffing the tissues and producing discomfort (Fig. 5-93). Other soft tissue undercuts, such as a maxillary torus or mandibular tori may also influence the selection of the major connector as previously discussed.

## Preserving the tilt through tripoding

Once a tilt has been selected for a given removable partial denture design, this tilt should be preserved, so that it can be reestablished accurately should the cast be removed from the survey table or should the survey table be inadvertently changed during the design procedure. This procedure is termed *tripoding*. Casts can be tripoded using several methods. Perhaps the most common method is to place the cast on the survey table at the desired tilt and, lowering the spindle of the surveyor with the analyzing rod in position, move the cast until three widely spaced points on the anatomical portion of the cast can be touched (Chapter 6). (Fig. 5-94). This must be done with the analyzing rod at one vertical height. In other words, one cannot touch the anterior portion of the cast at one height and then lower the analyzing rod or raise the analyzing rod to touch a position posteriorly. Three widely selected points are thus identified at the same vertical height. The analyzing rod is used to scratch the cast at three points, or it may be removed from the surveyor spindle and a carbon marker substituted. Using the carbon marker, a small line is made at the previously selected point approximately 3 mm long (Fig. 5-95). A mark is

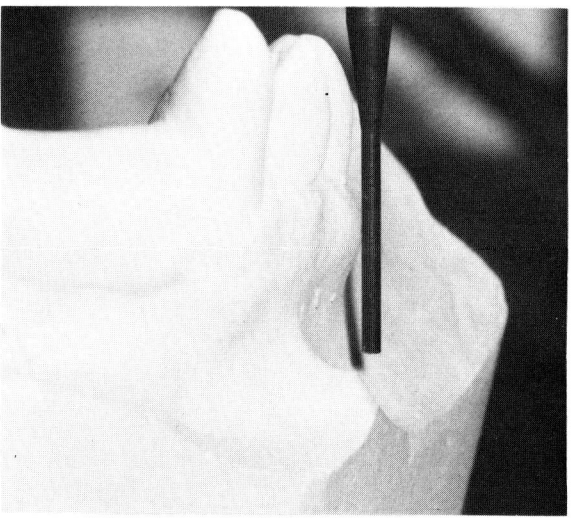

Fig. 5-92. Soft tissue undercut may preclude use of bar-type clasp.

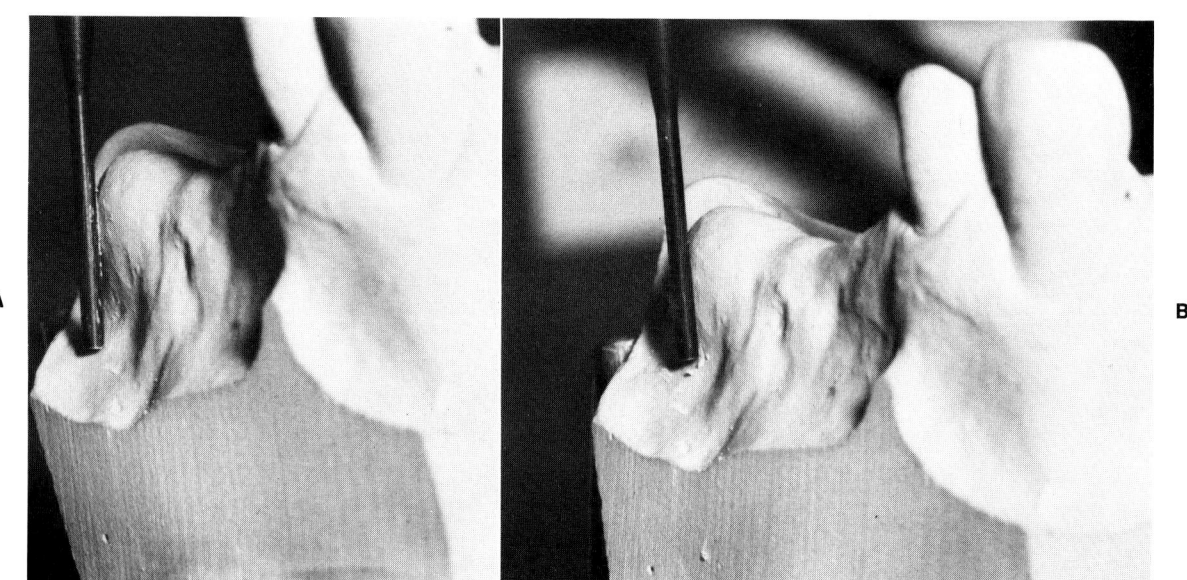

Fig. 5-93. Tilting may relieve soft tissue undercut in denture base area and permit partial denture to seat without injury to tissue. **A,** At this tilt, undercut is large. **B,** Slightly different tilt can eliminate undercut.

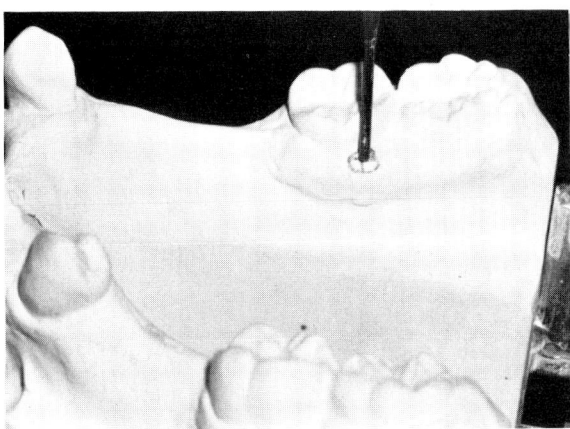

**Fig. 5-94.** When tilt is finally determined, cast should be tripoded so it may be removed from surveying table and replaced at subsequent time in exact same position.

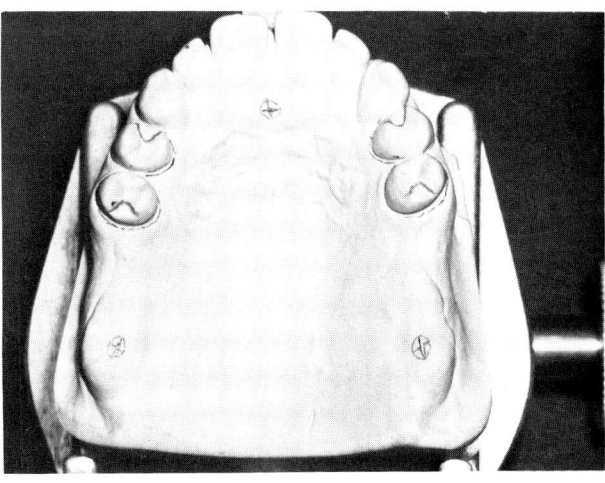

**Fig. 5-95.** Three widely separated tripod marks on cast.

made across this line with a pencil, and the resultant cross can be further circled to identify the area of the tripoding. The tripod should be on the cast incident to designing the partial denture. The cast tripoded in this manner can be removed from the cast holder. Cast position can also be tripoded by making lines on the base of the cast with the surveyor and a carbon marker after the tilt has been selected (Fig. 5-96). This method has the disadvantage of smudging the lines during handling of the cast.

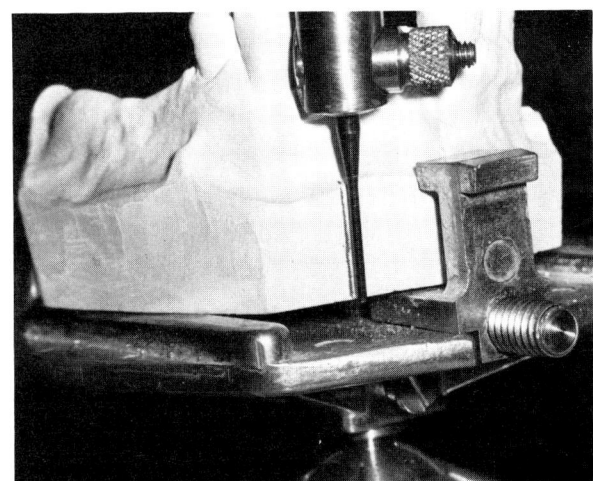

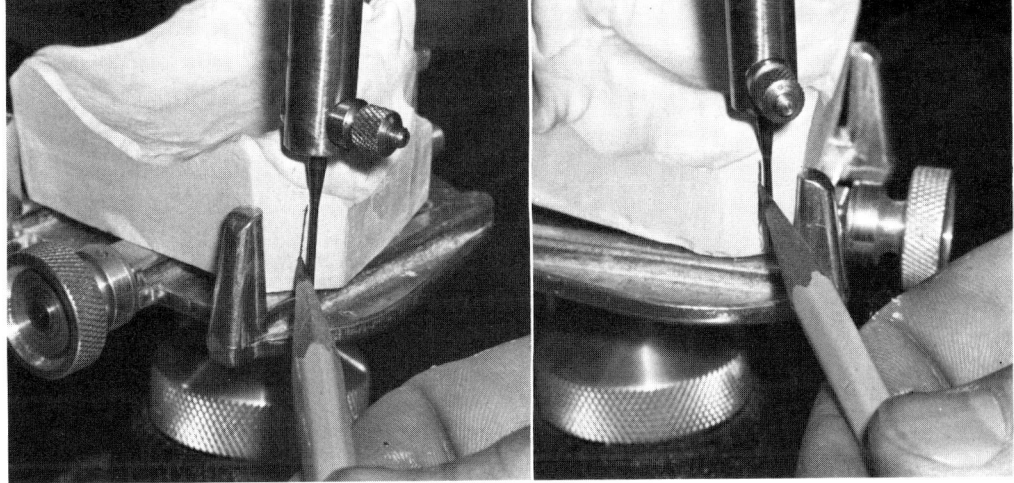

**Fig. 5-96.** Cast may also be tripoded by making vertical marks on cast. **A,** Anterior mark. **B,** Right posterior mark. **C,** Left posterior mark.

## PROCEDURE FOR DESIGN OF DIAGNOSTIC CASTS FOR REMOVABLE PARTIAL DENTURES

The dentist who initiates making a removable partial denture prosthesis is responsible for the design of the restoration. This is not, and should not be, the responsibility of the dental laboratory. This procedure is presented as a guide for the dentist. It advocates the use of diagnostic casts as an aid and guide in diagnosis and treatment planning as well as the actual mouth preparation. Completely designed diagnostic casts represent probably the best prescription to the dental laboratory. The dental laboratory is responsible for the technical fabrication of the restoration as prescribed by the dentist.

### Armamentarium (Fig. 5-97)

1. Surveyor, complete with cast holder, analyzing tool or stylus, and surveyor carbon marker
2. Ney undercut gauges: .010, .020, and .030
3. Crayon-type pencils, Venus Unique No. 1211 (red and blue) and Venus Unique No. 1212 (brown)
4. Lead pencil: 4H or 5H

### Color code (Fig. 5-98)

1. Red—areas to be ground, prepared, or recontoured
2. Blue—acrylic resin denture base
3. Brown—metal (framework or denture base)
4. Black—survey line and tissue undercut areas

#### PROCEDURE

1. Carefully examine the occluded diagnostic casts (Fig. 5-99).
   a. Locate the rest spaces to be prepared. Indicate these areas by a mark on the base or capital portion of the diagnostic casts and not on the cast teeth (Fig. 5-100). Ensure adequate rest spaces. Indicate in red crayon any cuspal relief required to give additional rest clearance (Fig. 5-101).
   b. Examine the lingual aspect of the occluded casts to assure adequate space for proposed lingual rests and indirect retainers. Draw a pencil line on the lingual surface of the upper anterior teeth, using the occluded lower anteriors as a guide, to determine the gingivo-occlusal limits of any proposed rests or indirect retainers (Fig. 5-102).

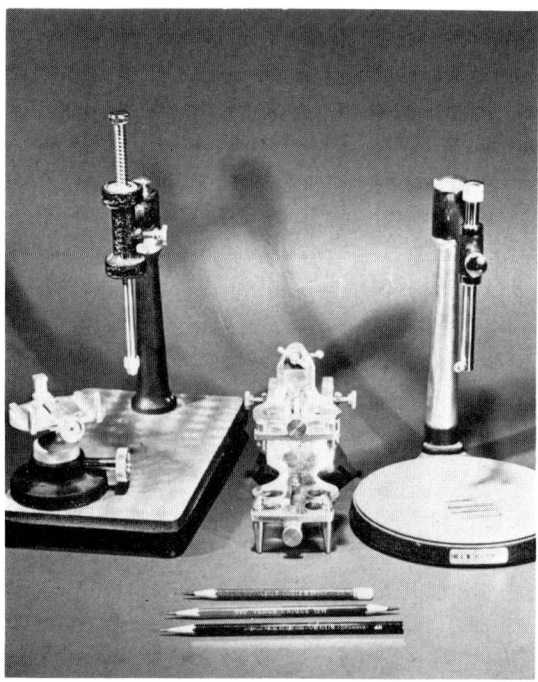

**Fig. 5-97.** Instruments required for surveying cast.

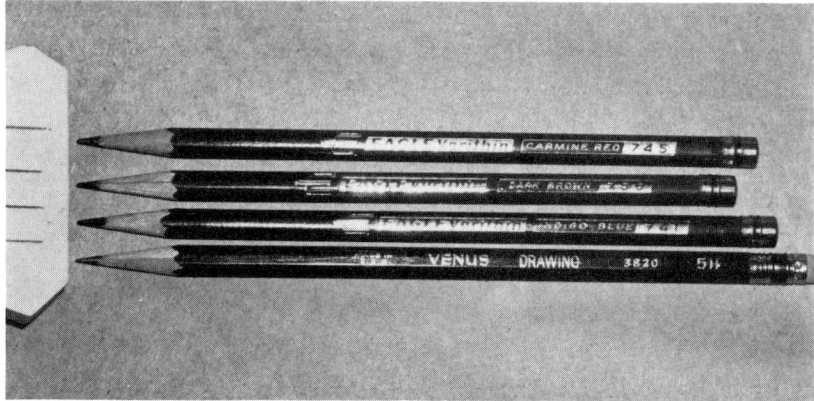

**Fig. 5-98.** Color code is used to indicate different material or procedures to be used in fabrication of partial denture. Red—areas to be ground. Blue—acrylic resin denture base. Brown—metal. Black—survey line and undercuts.

*Survey and design* **171**

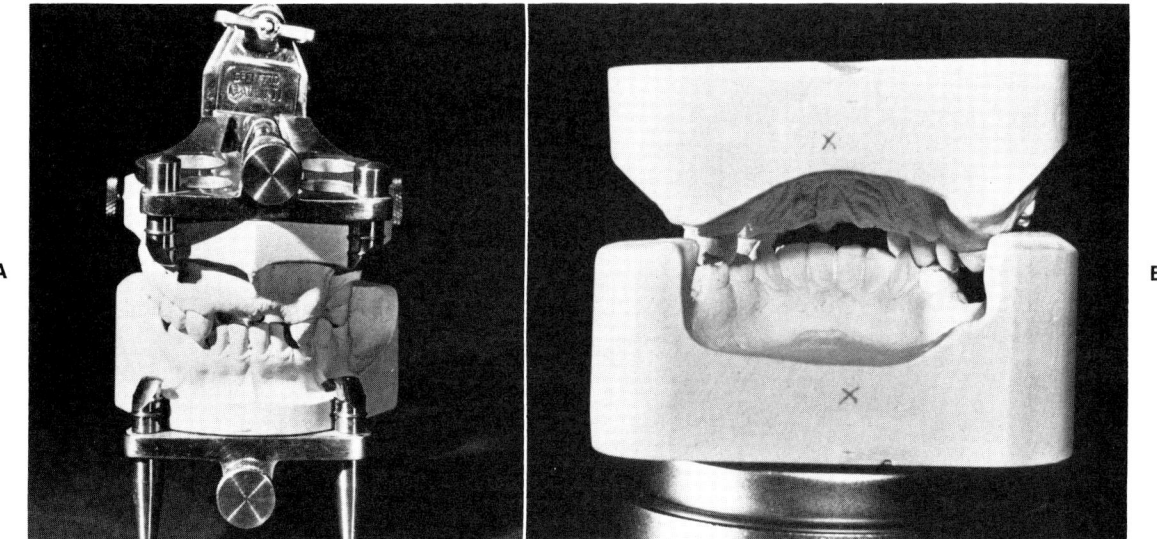

**Fig. 5-99.** Examine occluded casts carefully. **A,** Facial surface. **B,** Lingual area.

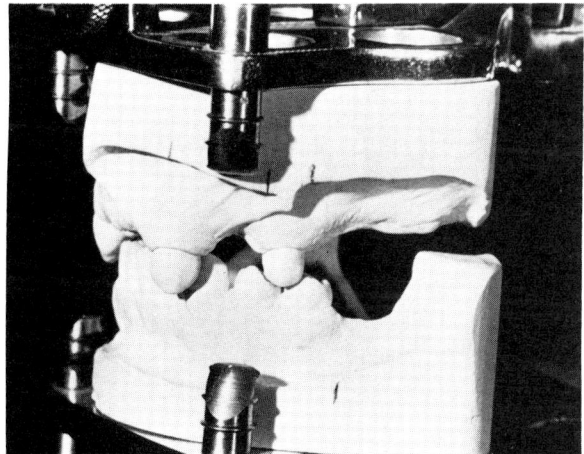

**Fig. 5-100.** Indicate desired rest areas by drawing short line on base of cast.

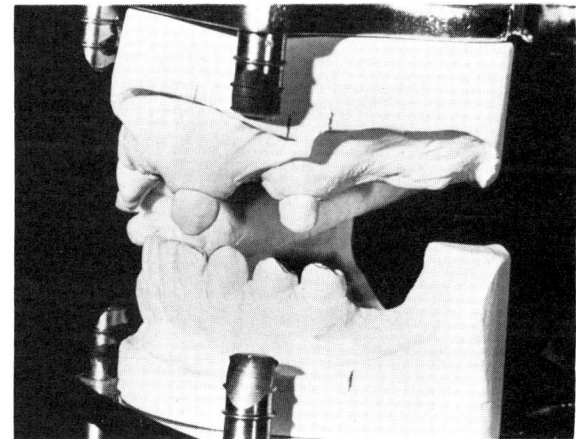

**Fig. 5-101.** Indicate rest areas and cuspal relief by marking in red.

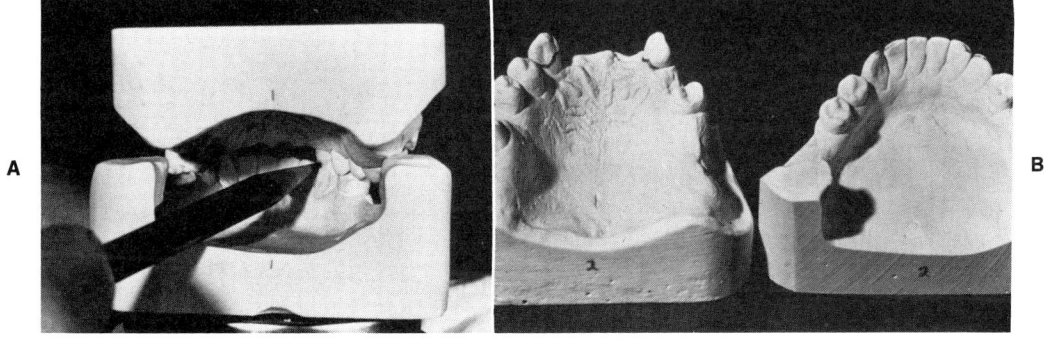

**Fig. 5-102. A,** Draw pencil line on upper anterior teeth using lower anterior teeth as guide. **B,** Pencil line indicates how far metal can go onto anterior teeth without causing interferences.

c. If tube teeth, facings, or metal pontics are required, indicate so with a pencil using the following symbols: tube teeth, T; facings, F; metal pontic, M; metal pontic with an acrylic resin window, M/AC; reinforced acrylic pontic, RAP. For denture teeth in an acrylic resin denture base, outline the denture base area with a blue pencil. Draw each symbol on the soft tissue or art portion of the diagnositc cast adjacent to the area indicated (Fig. 5-103).

2. Place the cast on a surveyor cast holder at a level or horizontal tilt (Fig. 5-104). Examine the teeth to be clasped with an analyzing tool of the surveyor to determine the location of usable undercuts, as well as the shape and contour of the proposed abutment teeth. If the shape and contour of these teeth necessitates recontouring, indicate the location and extent of the proposed alteration with a red crayon pencil (Fig. 5-105). Check the minor connectors or strut areas at this time. Determine the most favorable tilt (if required) that will permit convenient and proper placement of clasps, minor connectors, anterior teeth, and denture base areas (Fig. 5-106).

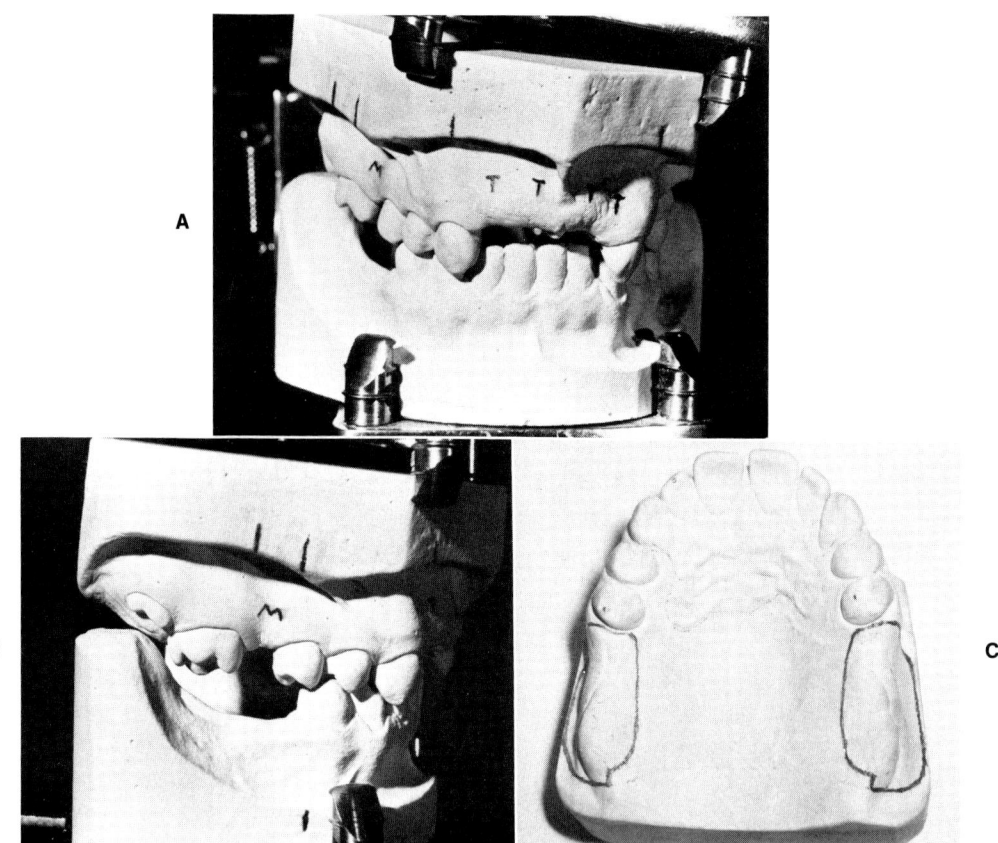

Fig. 5-103. Mark symbol for replacement tooth directly on art portion of diagnostic cast. **A,** "T" for tube teeth or "F" for facings. **B,** "M" for metal pontic or "M/AC" for metal pontic with an acrylic resin window. **C,** Denture base outlined in blue means denture teeth in acrylic resin.

*Survey and design* **173**

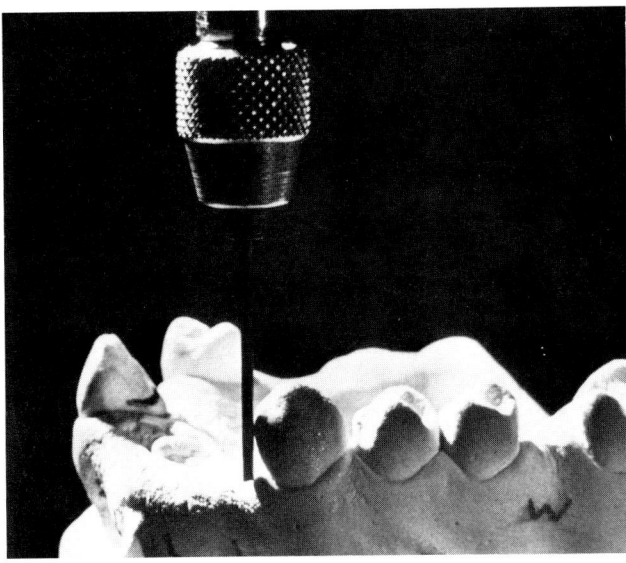

**Fig. 5-104.** Start surveying procedure by placing cast on surveying table with occlusal plane horizontal (parallel to tabletop) and use metal analyzing rod in surveyor.

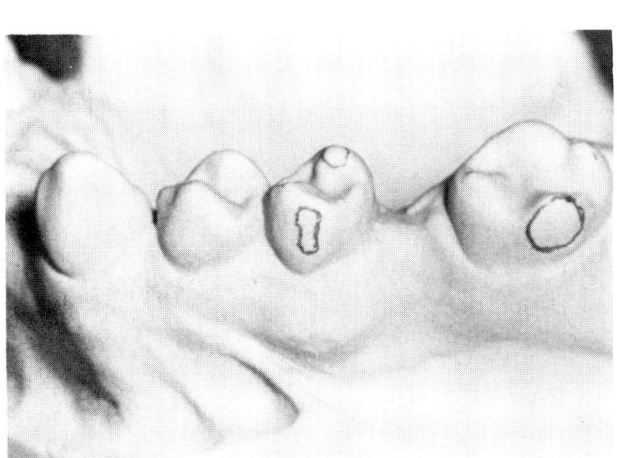

**Fig. 5-105.** If teeth will require recontouring, outline in red exact location and extent of proposed alteration.

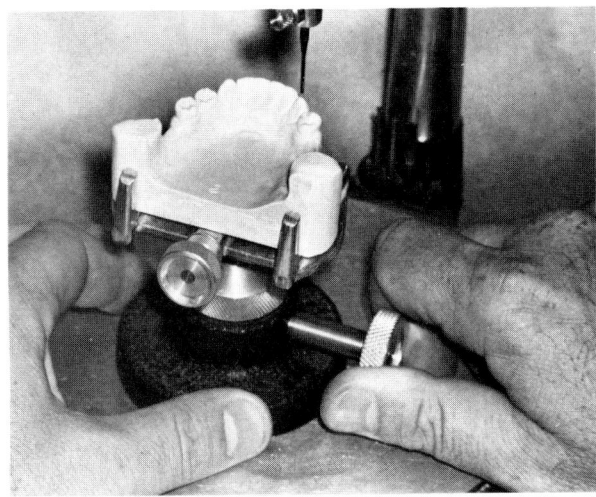

**Fig. 5-106.** When most favorable tilt is determined, lock survey table securely so it will not change positions during subsequent procedures.

3. Tripod the diagnostic cast (Fig. 5-107).
4. Remove the cast from the cast holder (Fig. 5-108) (optional).
   a. With a red crayon pencil, draw the extent of the rest areas that are to be prepared in the mouth (Fig. 5-109).
   b. Outline the complete denture base areas with a crayon pencil. Blue crayon pencil indicates acrylic resin denture base areas. Brown crayon pencil indicates metal denture base areas (Fig. 5-110).
   c. With a brown crayon pencil, outline the extent of the framework design to harmonize and join the major connectors, rest areas, indirect retainers, and denture base areas (Fig. 5-111).
5. Remount the cast on the cast holder in the same relation as in step 3, and draw the survey line on the abutment teeth as well as other teeth that will be involved in the design of the restoration (Fig. 5-112).

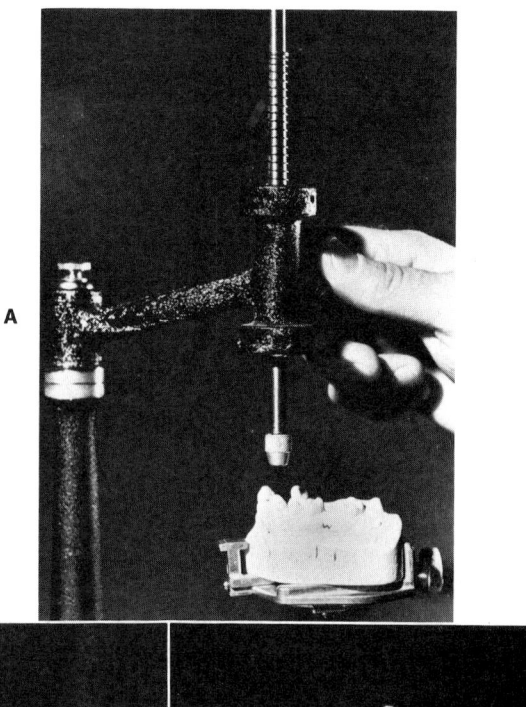
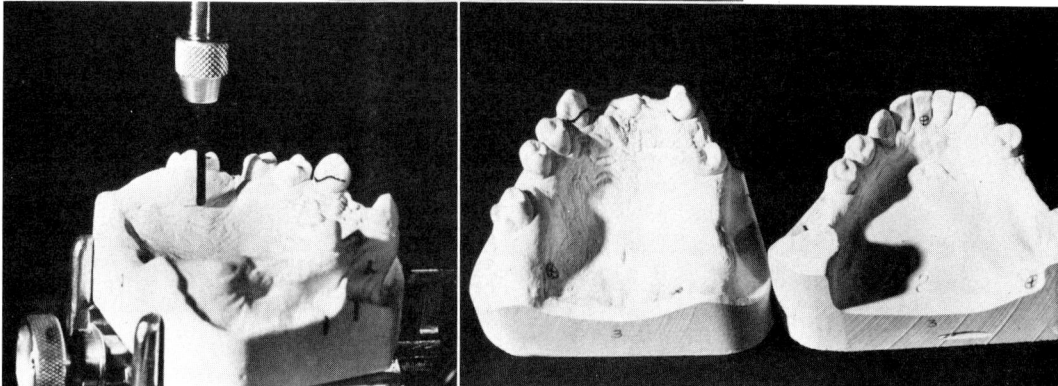

**Fig. 5-107.** Tripod by marking three widely separated points on cast at same vertical height. **A,** Lock vertical arm of surveyor. **B,** Mark three widely separated points on cast. **C,** Cross these marks with another mark, and circle area marked.

*Survey and design* **175**

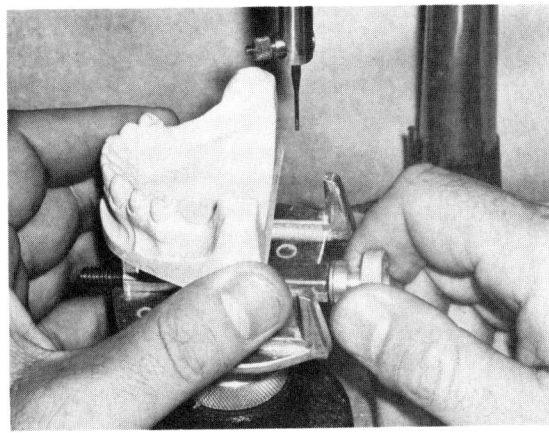

**Fig. 5-108.** If it is more convenient, cast may now be removed from surveying table. It can be replaced at any time in exactly same position by aligning tripod marks.

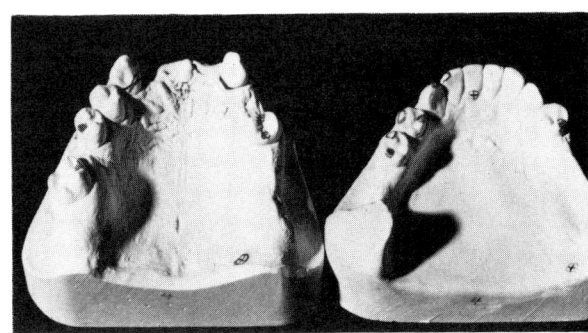

**Fig. 5-109.** Use red pencil and draw rest areas that are to be prepared in mouth. Try to mark exact shape and depth of rest. Make rest solid red.

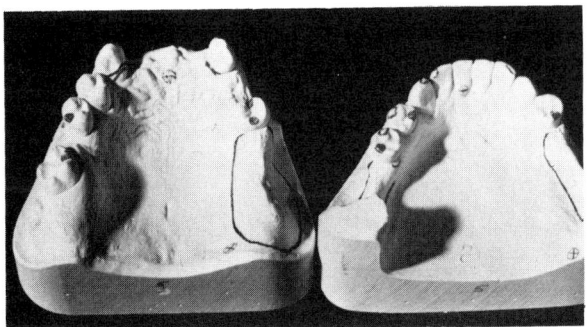

**Fig. 5-110.** Outline denture base area with crayon pencil. Use blue for acrylic resin and brown for metal base (Figs. 5-47 and 5-48).

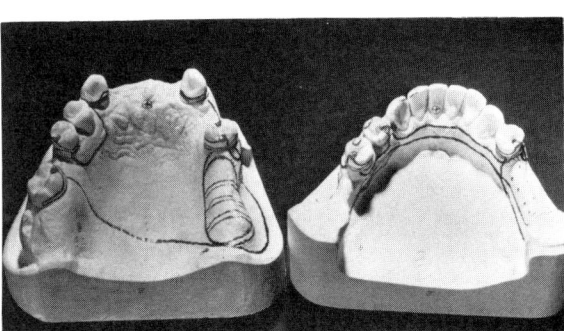

**Fig. 5-111.** Use brown crayon pencil to outline major connector and acrylic retention area of denture base. Major connector joins rests, indirect retainers, and denture base areas.

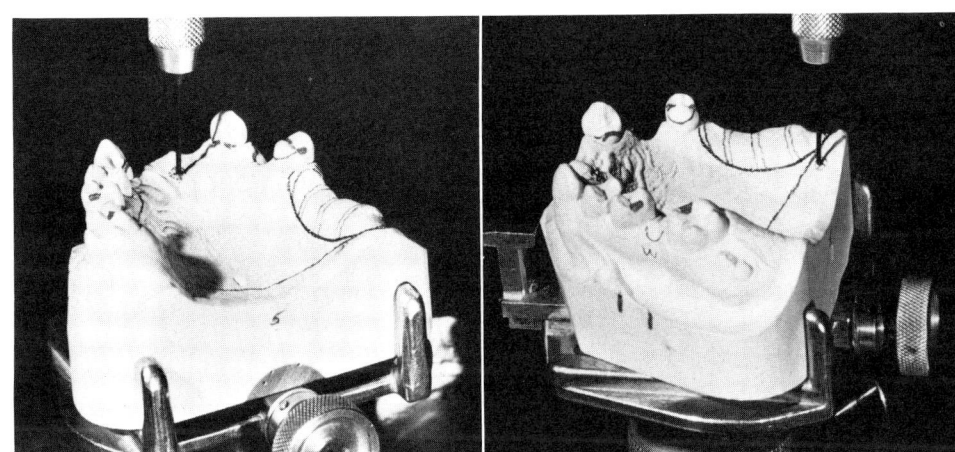

**Fig. 5-112.** If cast has been removed from surveyor table, remount it in same relation as in step 3 of text. Align three marks in horizontal plane as accurately as possible by eye. **A,** Touch center of one of tripod marks with analyzing rod, and lock vertical arm. **B,** Slide base so stylus points to one of other marks. Then slide base so stylus points to third mark. If stylus points above or below last two points, loosen universal joint on cast holder and tilt cast in direction that will more nearly align marks. Reset stylus to first tripod mark, and check others again. Continue until all three tripod marks can be touched by stylus when vertical arm is locked in place.

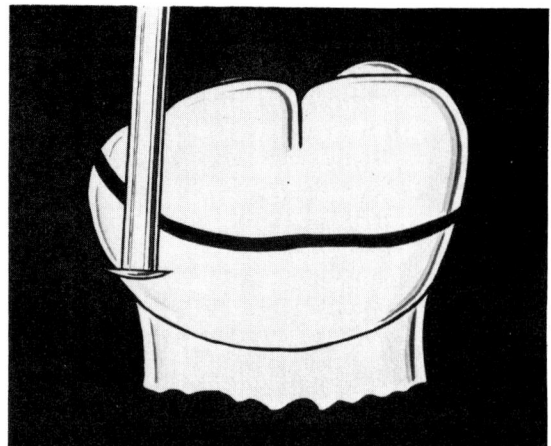

**Fig. 5-113.** Replace carbon marker with proper undercut gauge.

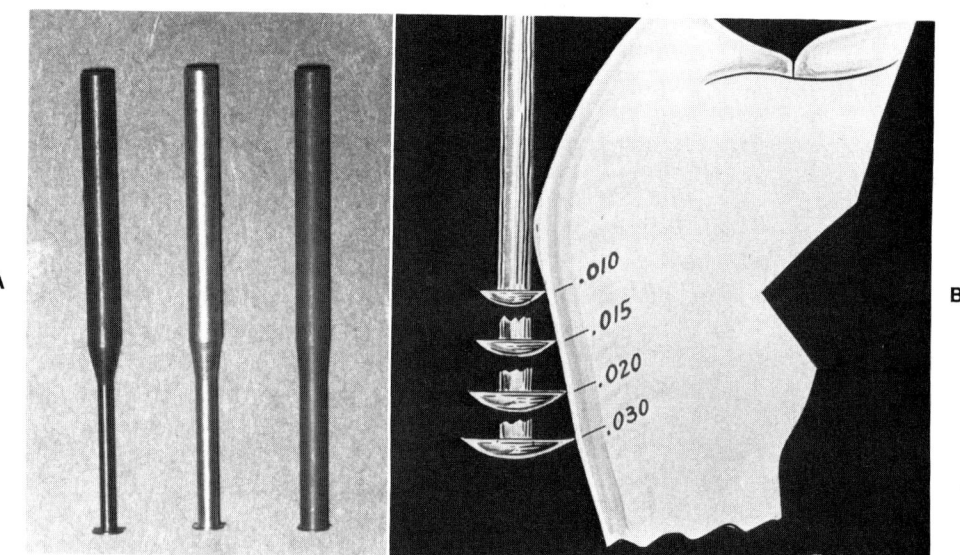

**Fig. 5-114. A,** Undercut gauges: .030, .020, and .010 (left to right). **B,** Drawing of gauges in use.

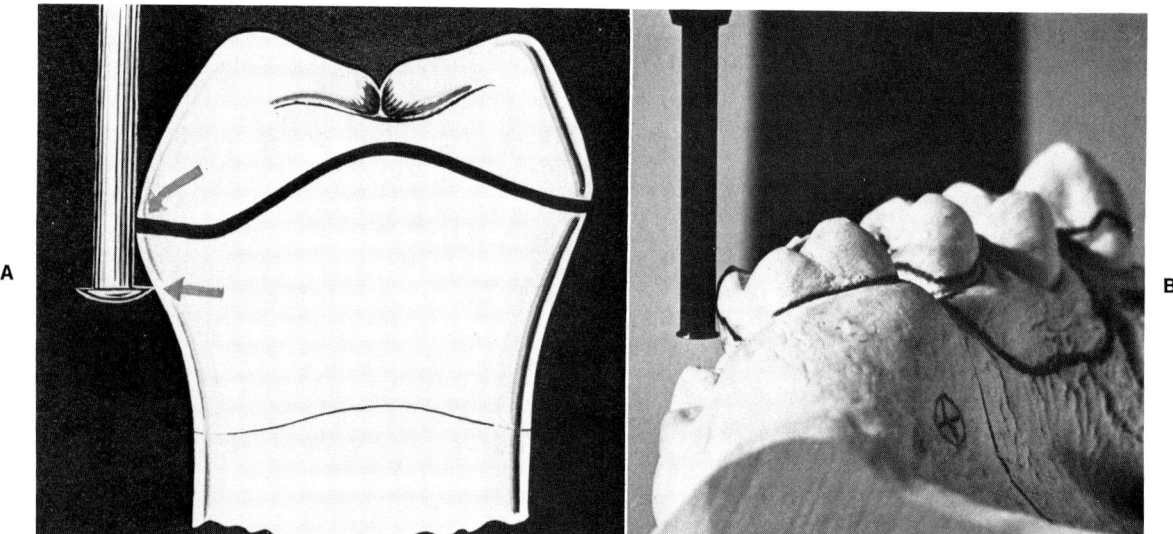

**Fig. 5-115. A,** With undercut gauge in vertical arm of surveyor, move cast so shank of gauge touches tooth on cast at survey line (top arrow). Raise spindle of surveyor until measuring edge of undercut gauge touches tooth on cast (bottom arrow). **B,** .010 Undercut gauge in use.

a. Replace the carbon marker in the surveyor with the .010, .020, or .030 Ney undercut gauge* as the undercut condition, length, and size of the clasp arm indicate (Fig. 5-113). NOTE: With chromium-cobalt castings, the .010 gauge will suffice for short clasp arms, the .020 gauge will suffice for long clasp arms, and the .030 gauge will be used for *extremely* long flexible clasp arms fabricated of wrought wire (Fig. 5-114). Gold alloy castings accommodate slightly more undercut than the chromium-cobalt alloy castings. Place the gauge on the desired retentive undercut area so that the head and shank of the undercut gauge touch the tooth simultaneously (Fig. 5-115). Mark this spot with a pencil (Fig. 5-116). Verify the accuracy of this mark with the head of the undercut gauge (Fig. 5-117). This mark will represent the gingival edge of the clasp tip that will engage the undercut (Fig. 5-118).

*The J. M. Ney Co., Bloomfield, Conn.

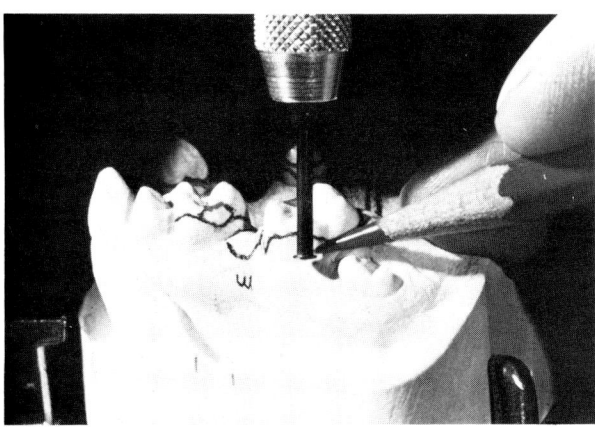

**Fig. 5-116.** Mark spot on tooth touched with undercut gauge with red pencil. This is amount of measured undercut.

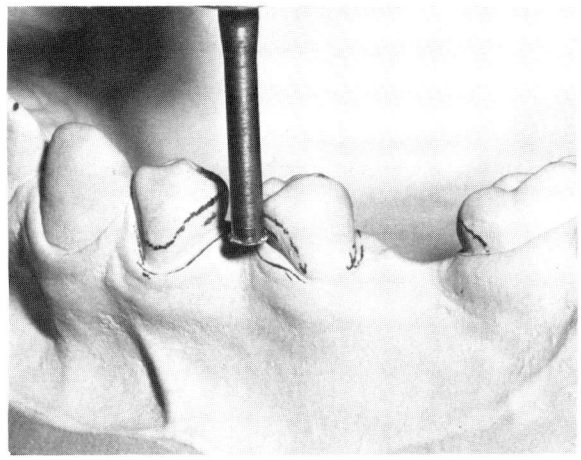

**Fig. 5-117.** Verify this mark by touching it again with gauge.

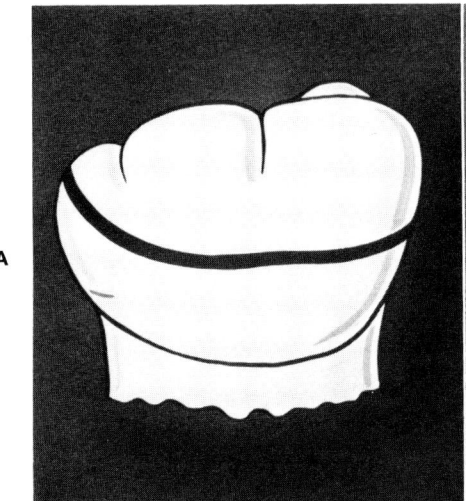

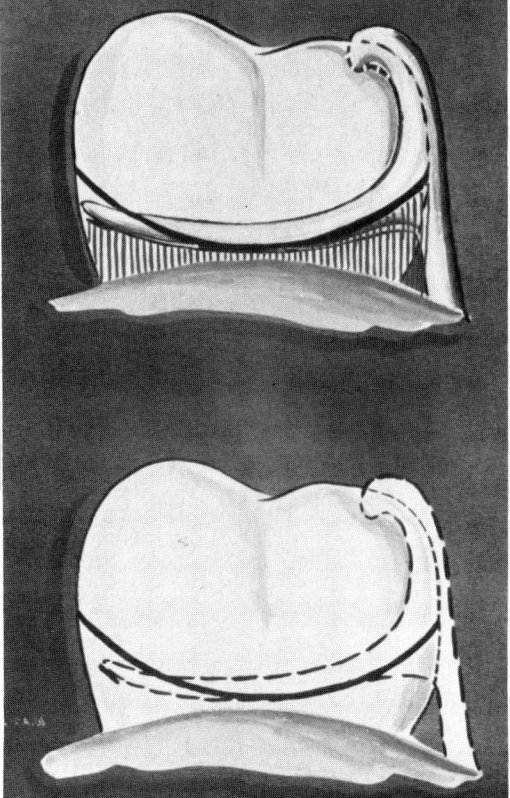

**Fig. 5-118. A,** This mark will position bottom edge of tip of clasp. **B,** Sketch of clasp shows position.

**178** *Dental laboratory procedures: removable partial dentures*

b. With the brown crayon pencil, draw the clasp arms with a *double* line so that the occlusogingival portions of the clasp arms will be indicated to the laboratory (Fig. 5-119). NOTE: Keep the clasp arms gingivally as far as possible on the clinical crown in harmony with the position and location of the survey line and the depth of the undercut to be engaged by the clasp tip.
c. Indicate the position and extent of undesirable tissue undercuts that may interfere with the insertion of the restoration (Fig. 5-120).

6. The design should now be completed (Fig. 5-121).

### ALTERNATE PROCEDURE

After preparations and recontouring have been accomplished in the mouth, the master impression is made, and the cast is poured with artificial stone. Using the master cast as a reference, grind or scrape the diagnostic cast to approximate the alterations that appear on the master cast. After this is accomplished, make the necessary correction of the design on the diagnostic cast to conform to the preparations that have been made in the mouth. No markings, oil, grease, powder, or design should be made on the master cast. Most casts may be designed in several ways, and, if the principles are followed, one will work about as well as another (Fig. 5-122).

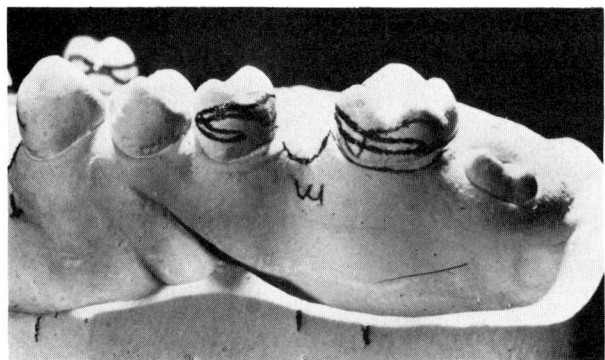

**Fig. 5-119.** With brown pencil, draw clasp arm on each tooth to be clasped using double line so occlusal and gingival portions of clasp arms will be indicated.

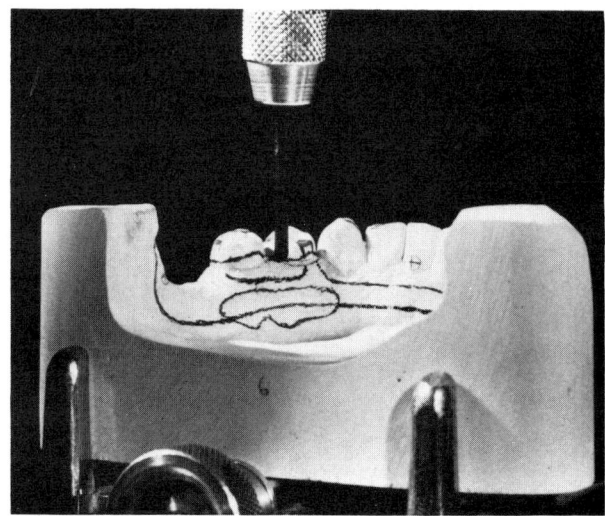

**Fig. 5-120.** Outline with black pencil, position and extent of undesirable tissue undercuts that may interfere with seating of partial denture.

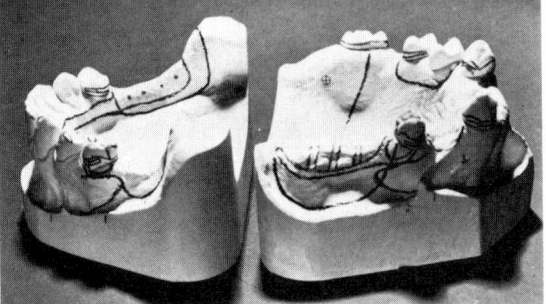

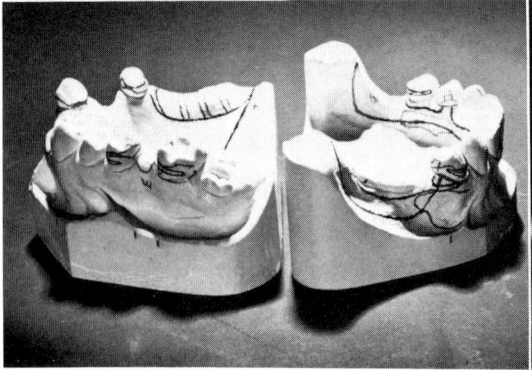

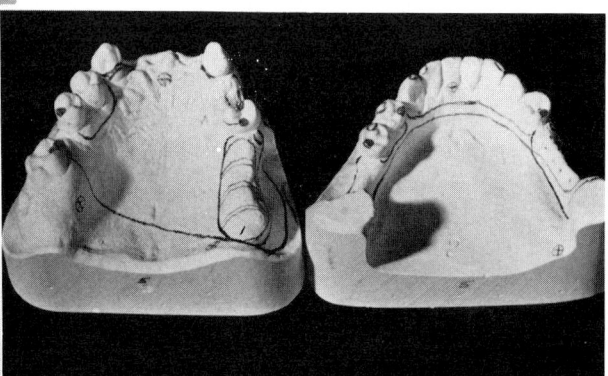

**Fig. 5-121.** Completely designed diagnostic casts. **A,** Left side. **B,** Right side. **C,** Occlusal view.

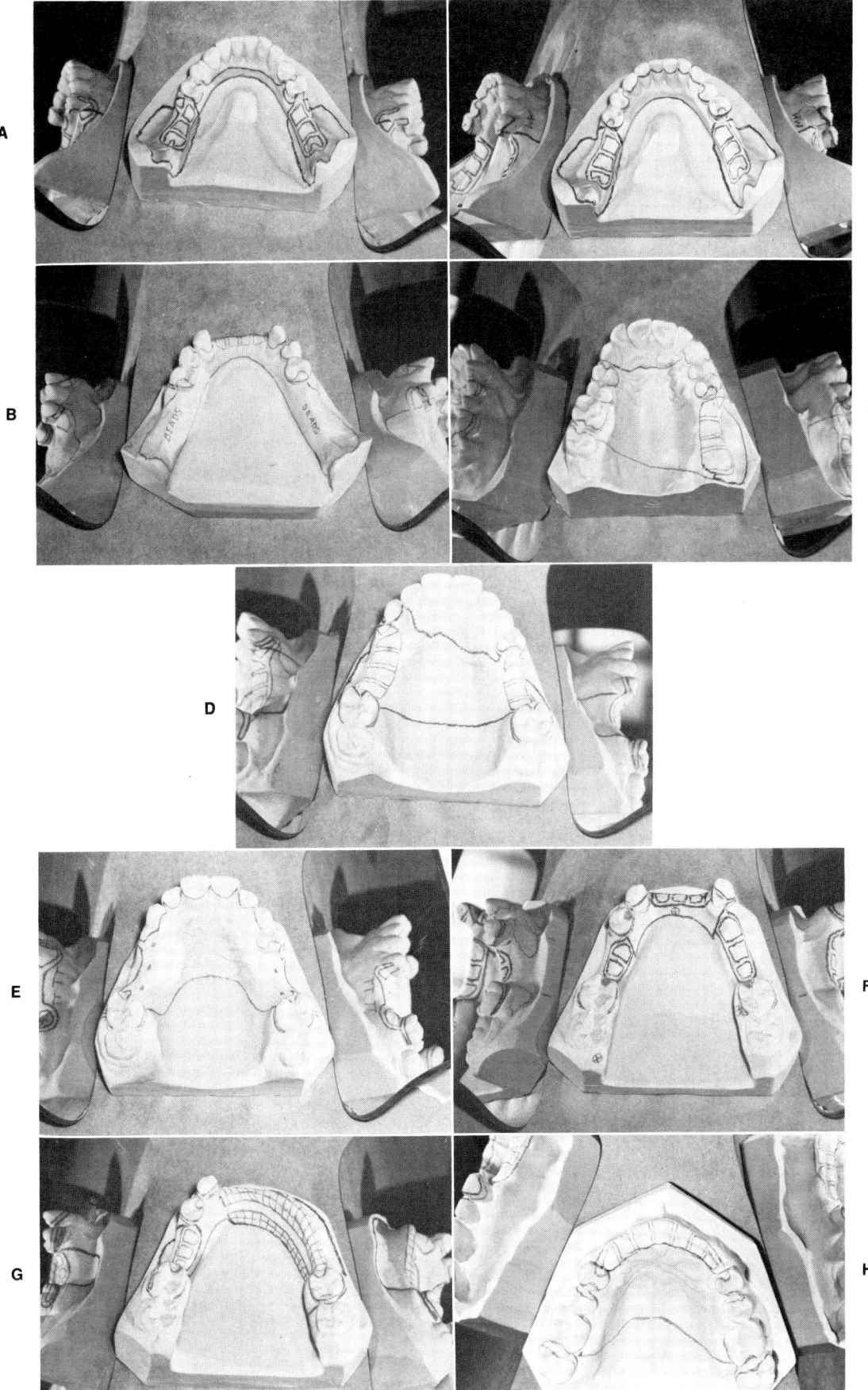

**Fig. 5-122.** Some typical designs for various classifications of removable partial dentures. **A,** Class I with I-bar clasp (left) and with wire clasps (right). **B,** Class I, modification 1. **C,** Class II. **D,** Class III with palatal strap. **E,** Class III with horseshoe. **F,** Class III with lingual plate. **G,** Class II, modification 1. **H,** Class IV.

## SUMMARY

In this chapter, the multitude of factors and principles involved in designing removable partial dentures were considered and a systematic method for designing diagnostic casts described. A thoroughly planned and well-executed design provides a blueprint for the proposed prosthesis.

## REFERENCES

Applegate, O. C.: Essentials of removable partial denture prostheses, Philadelphia, 1965, W. B. Saunders Co.

Henderson, D., and Steffel, V. L.: McCracken's removable partial prosthodontics, ed. 5, St. Louis, 1977, The C. V. Mosby Co.

Kratochavil, F. J.: Influence of occlusal rest position and clasp design on movement of abutment teeth, J. Prosthet. Dent. **13:**114-124, 1963.

Kratochavil, F. J.: The removable prosthodontics partial denture syllabus, Los Angeles, 1968, The University of California at Los Angeles, School of Dentistry.

Krol, A. J.: Removable partial design: an outline syllabus, San Francisco, 1972, University of the Pacific School of Dentistry.

Krol, A. J.: Clasp design for extension-base removable partial dentures, J. Prosthet. Dent. **29:**408-415, 1973.

Morrow, R. M., Rudd, K. D., and Eissmann, H. F.: Dental laboratory procedures: complete dentures, St. Louis, 1980, The C. V. Mosby Co.

## BIBLIOGRAPHY

Air Force Manual 160-29: Dental laboratory technicians manual, United States Air Force, Washington, D.C., 1959, U.S. Government Printing Office.

Air Force Manual 162-6: Dental laboratory technology, United States Air Force, Washington, D.C., 1975, U.S. Government Printing Office.

Fundamentals of survey and design: School of Aviation Medicine, United States Air Force, Washington, D.C., 1956, U.S. Government Printing Office.

Removable partial denture laboratory manual, San Antonio, 1979-1980, The University of Texas Health Science Center at San Antonio, Dental School.

Sowter, J. B.: Dental laboratory technology: prosthodontic techniques, Chapel Hill, N.C., 1968, The University of North Carolina Press.

# CHAPTER 6

# DESIGN TRANSFER, BLOCKOUT, RELIEF, AND BEADING

KENNETH D. RUDD, ROBERT M. MORROW, and GEORGE KNIGHT

**beading** Scoring a cast with a sharp instrument or bur in any desired area to provide a seal between the finished prosthesis and the soft tissue.

**blockout (wax out)** Elimination of undesirable undercut areas on a cast to be used in the fabrication of a removable partial denture.

**design transfer** Conveying the outline of the proposed prosthesis from the diagnostic cast to the master cast.

**relieve** The procedure of placing sheet wax in strategic areas on a master cast to be duplicated so that a refractory cast can be made. The purpose of relieving the master cast with wax is to provide space between certain components of the framework and the adjacent oral structures, such as the minor connector to which the denture base will be attached.

Designed diagnostic casts should accompany the master casts to the dental laboratory. The casts should be packed carefully to minimize the possibility of breakage in transit. If designed casts are not provided by the dentist, the laboratory technician will design the master casts to the best of his ability using the available information. Preferably, designed diagnostic casts will accompany the master casts together with a properly executed work order (Chapter 4). Using the designed casts and work order, the laboratory technician will examine the design and casts, consult with the dentist if needed, and then transfer the design of the metal framework to the master casts. In this chapter, the methods used to transfer the design and prepare the master cast for duplication will be described.

## DESIGN TRANSFER

If designed diagnostic casts accompany the master casts to the laboratory, the metallic portion of the design on the diagnostic casts will be transferred to the master cast (Fig. 6-1). If designed diagnostic casts are not supplied by the dentist, the laboratory technician will design the master casts to the best of his ability, using the available facts (Chapter 4).

### PROCEDURE

1. Examine the master casts to determine acceptability. If acceptable, the casts should be examined for nodules that must be removed (Fig. 6-2). If large nodules appear in critical areas such as rest preparations, new master casts should be requested.

2. Remount the diagnostic casts on the surveying table by aligning the tripod marks (Fig. 6-3). Tripoding is discussed in Chapter 4.

3. Choose new tripod marks that can be touched by the stylus when it is locked in one position. The new marks should be easily located on the master cast (Fig. 6-4). Marks should be placed on tooth landmarks that are easily and accurately located on both the diagnostic cast and master cast.

4. Place three widely separated marks on the diagnostic casts (Fig. 6-5).

5. Mark three spots on the master cast in exactly the same place as on the diagnostic casts (Fig. 6-6).

6. Tripod the master cast using these three marks

**182** *Dental laboratory procedures: removable partial dentures*

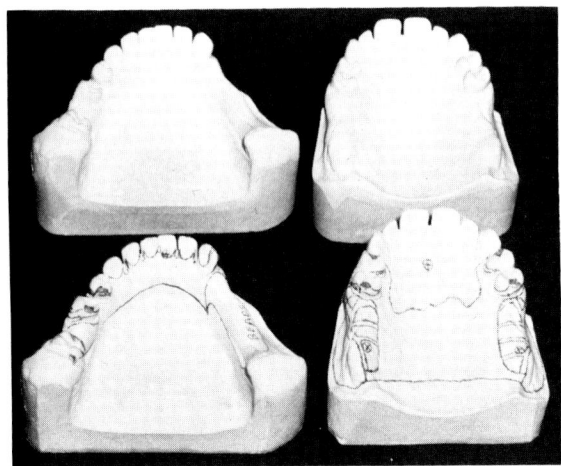

**Fig. 6-1.** Designed diagnostic cast and master casts.

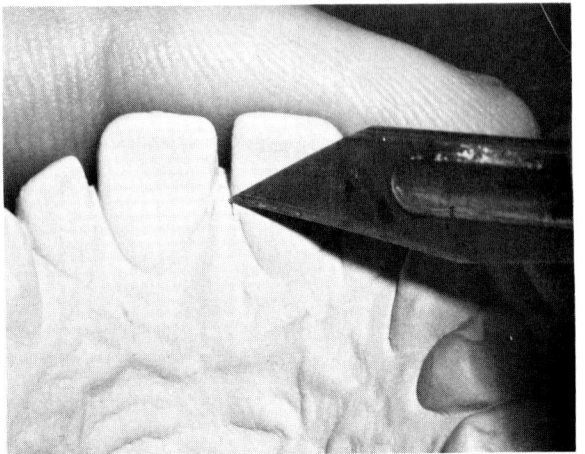

**Fig. 6-2.** Pick casts clean by removing nodules.

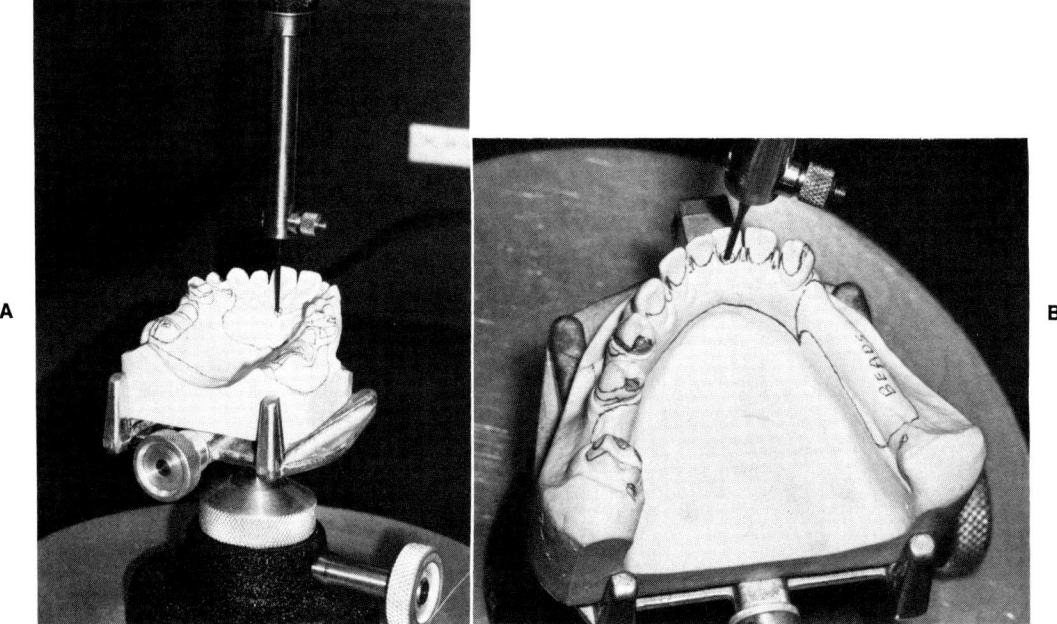

**Fig. 6-3.** Diagnostic cast is mounted on surveying table by aligning tripod marks. **A**, Maxillary cast. **B**, Mandibular cast.

## Design transfer, blockout, relief, and beading 183

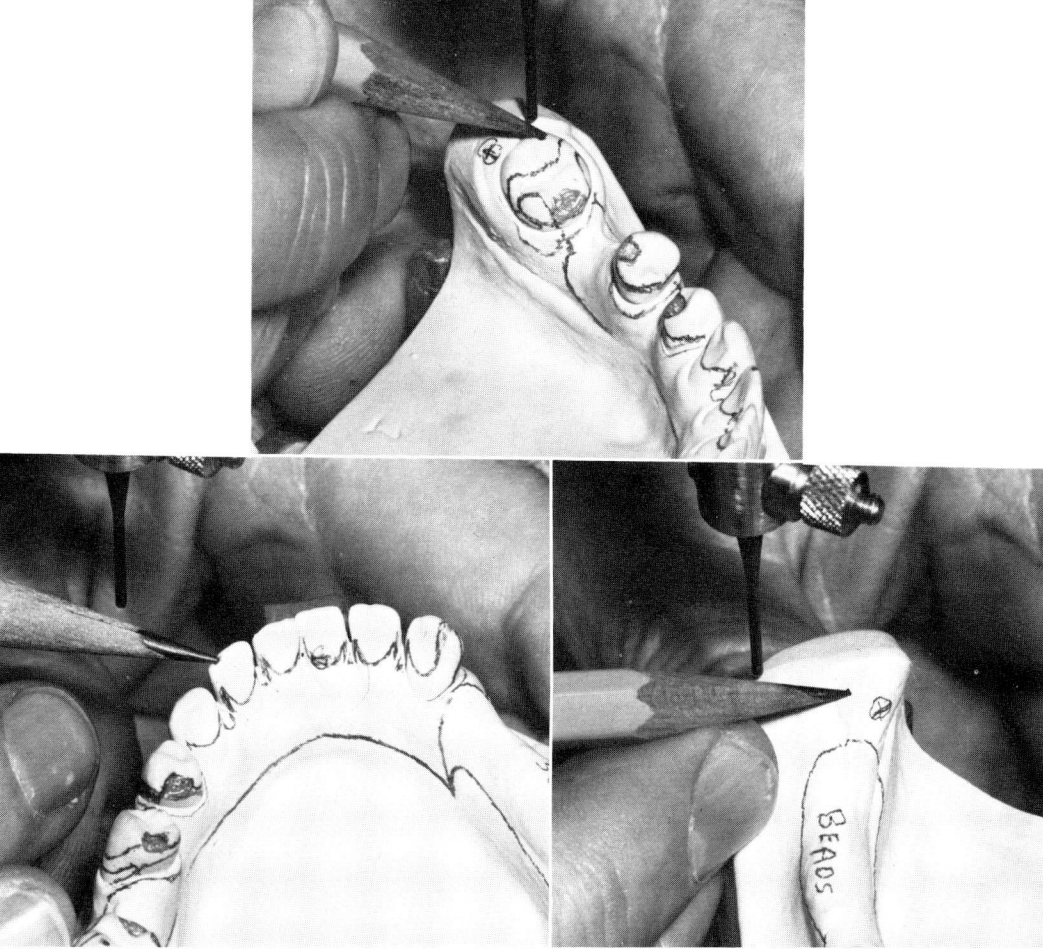

**Fig. 6-4.** Use stylus in locked vertical arm to locate three new marks on teeth or nonmovable soft tissue of diagnostic cast.

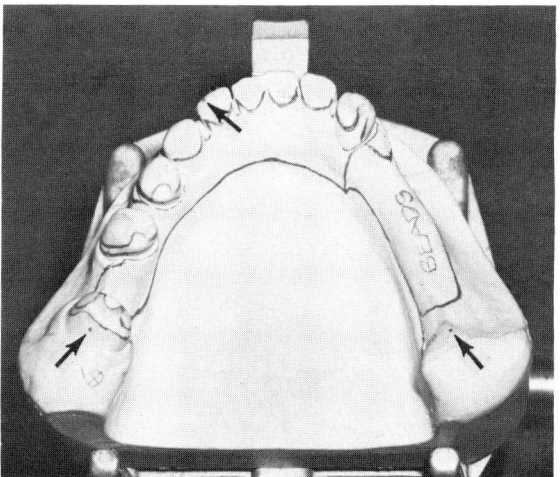

**Fig. 6-5.** Three new marks located on diagnostic cast.

**184** *Dental laboratory procedures: removable partial dentures*

(Fig. 6-7). Since tripod marks are the same on both casts, the master cast will be tripoded in the same plane as the diagnostic cast. Two planes parallel to the same plane are parallel to each other.

7. Using the carbon marker in the surveyor, mark survey lines on the master cast. Survey lines should be marked on all teeth that will be contacted by metal (Fig. 6-8). Soft tissue undercuts near teeth should also be marked (Fig. 6-9).

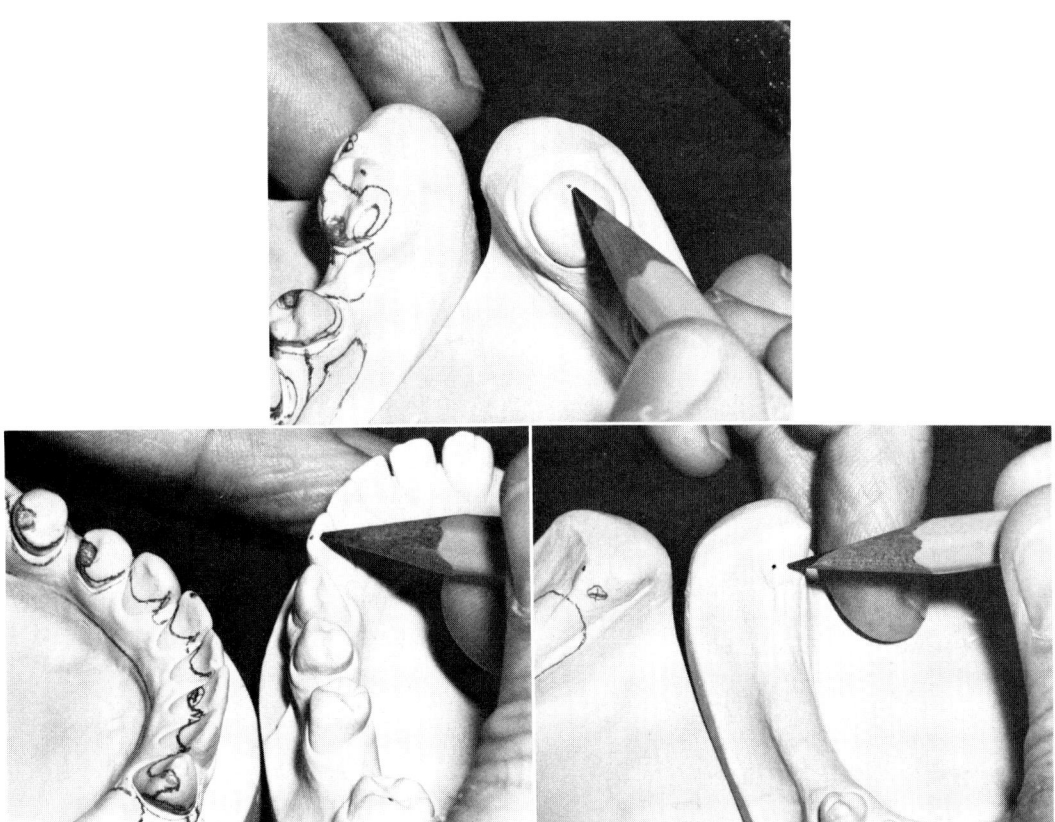

**Fig. 6-6.** Spots marked on master cast in same place as on diagnostic cast.

### Design transfer, blockout, relief, and beading 185

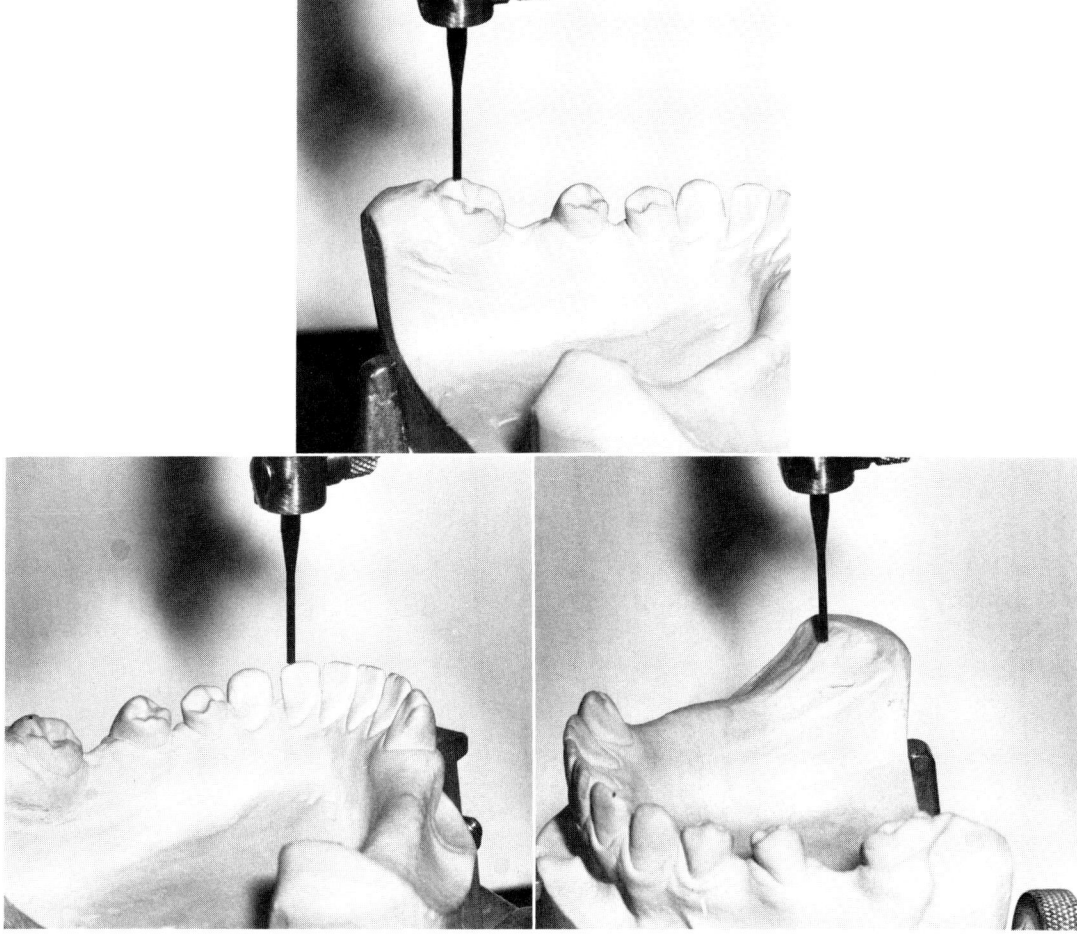

**Fig. 6-7.** Using three new spots on master cast, tripod master cast.

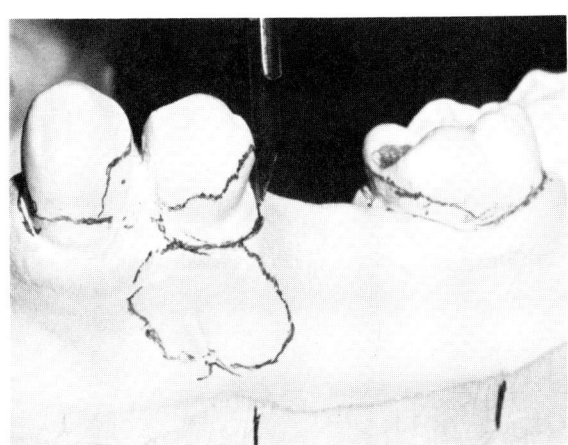

**Fig. 6-8.** Survey lines are placed on all teeth that will be contacted by metal.

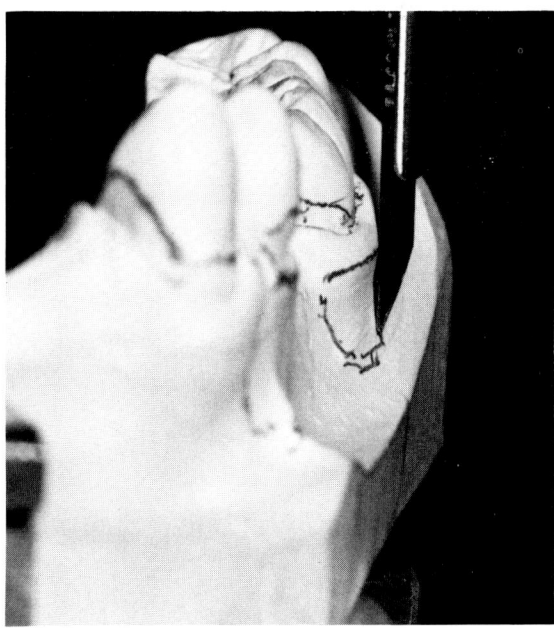

**Fig. 6-9.** Soft tissue undercuts also are surveyed and marked.

8. Retentive undercuts are marked on the master cast in red to locate the tips of the retentive clasps. Short clasp arms such as circlet clasps on premolars require 0.010- to 0.015-inch retentive undercuts, whereas long clasp arms such as bar clasps and circlet clasps on molars require 0.015- to 0.020-inch retentive undercuts (Fig. 6-10).

9. Rests are marked on the master cast in red to unmistakably identify them for the person waxing the framework (Fig. 6-11).

10. Using the diagnostic cast as a guide, draw the metallic portion of the design on the master cast with a brown pencil and resin finish lines with blue pencil (Fig. 6-12).

11. The design on the master cast should be the same as the design on the diagnostic cast (Fig. 6-13).

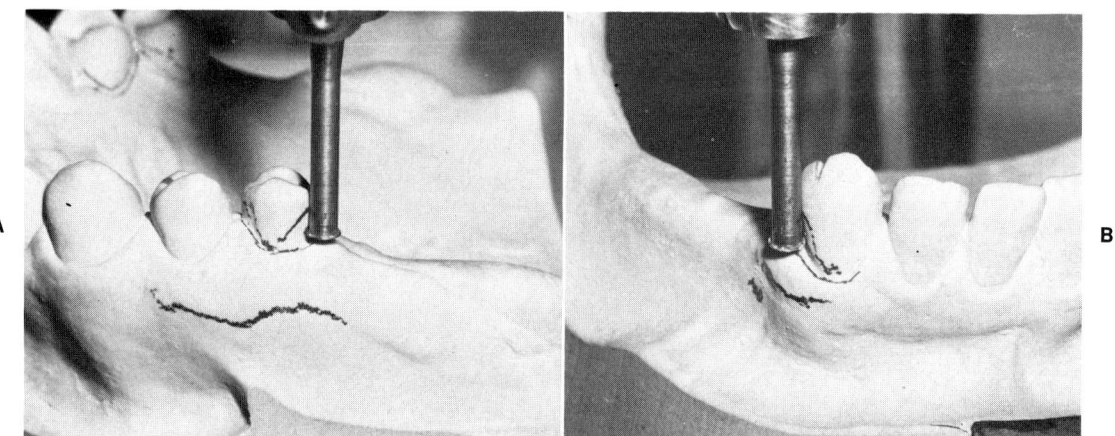

**Fig. 6-10.** Retentive undercuts are marked on casts. **A,** Maxillary second premolar. **B,** Mandibular canine.

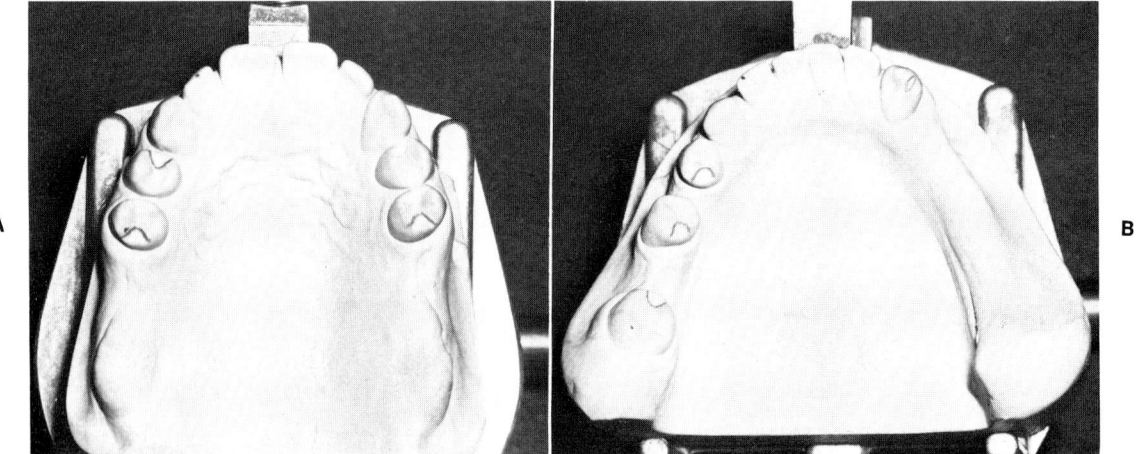

**Fig. 6-11.** Rests are marked in red. **A,** Maxillary. **B,** Mandibular.

## Design transfer, blockout, relief, and beading    187

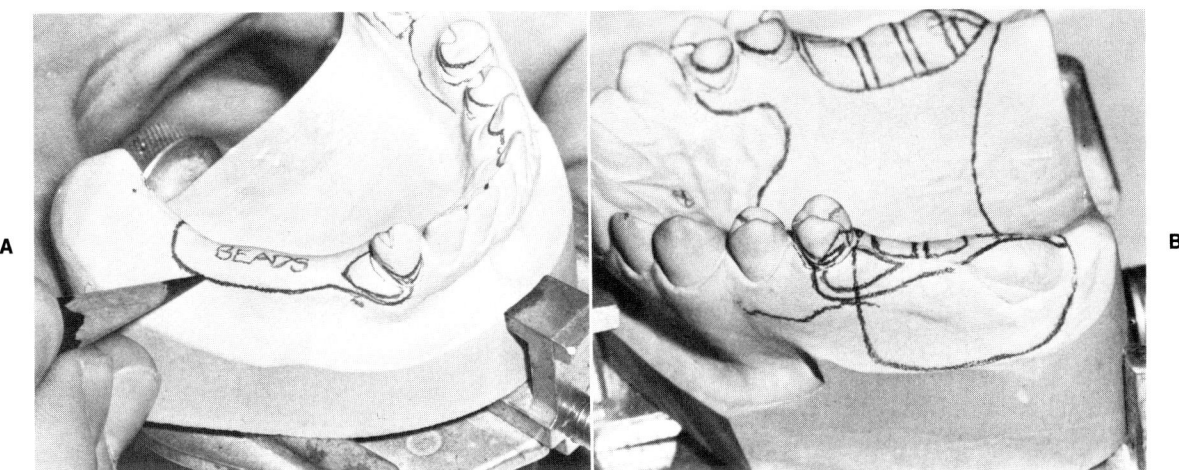

**Fig. 6-12. A,** Metallic outline is drawn on master cast using brown pencil. **B,** Finish lines are marked in blue.

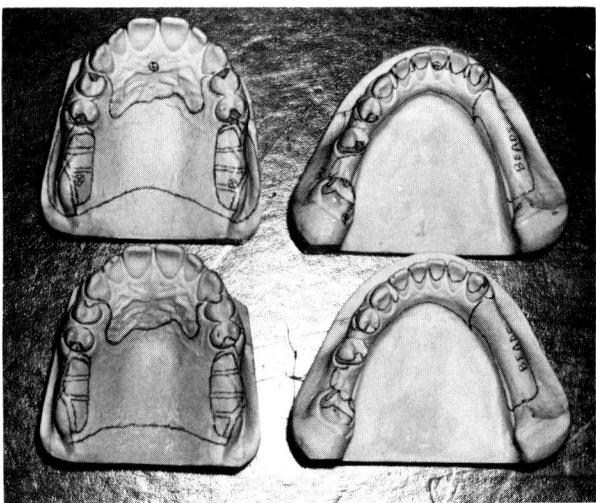

**Fig. 6-13.** Completed transfer of metal outline on master cast should be like design on diagnostic cast.

## BLOCKOUT AND DUPLICATION
### Preparing the casts for duplication

Casts are blocked out to eliminate undercut areas on the master cast that will be crossed by rigid parts of the partial denture. All parts of the framework, except the retentive clasp tips, are nonflexible and will not spring into an undercut. Additional areas to be blocked out or relieved are those not directly involved, but which are eliminated for convenience, such as (1) ledges on which clasp patterns will be placed, (2) beneath connectors to avoid soft tissue impingement, and (3) to provide for later attachment of the denture base to the framework.

Types of blockout may be classified as parallel, shaped (ledging), arbitrary, and relief. Parallel blockout is made by using different styli in the surveyor to establish 0-degree, 2-degree, or 6-degree taper in the blockout wax (Fig. 6-14). This blockout extends from the survey line to the gingiva (Fig. 6-15). A very good blockout tool combining a 0-degree taper and 2-degree taper and used as a wax trimming tool can be made that is superior to the

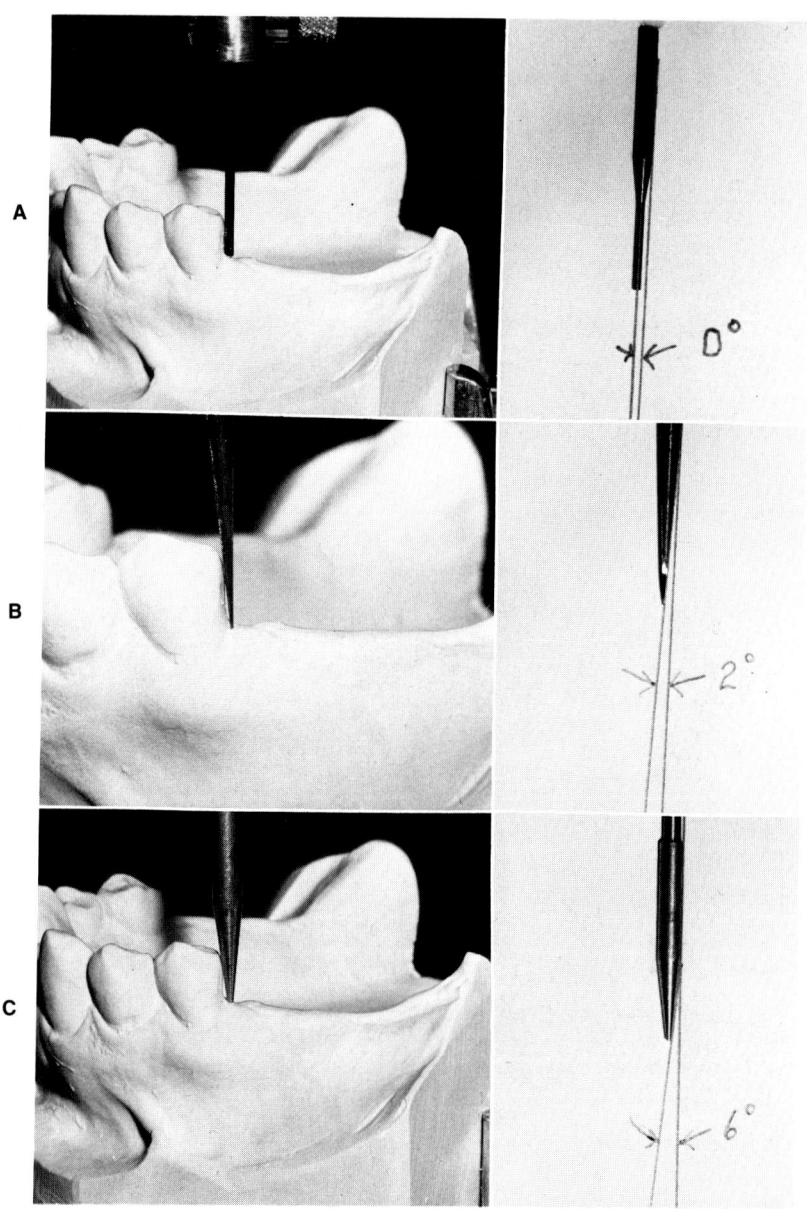

Fig. 6-14. Parallel blockout. **A**, Zero-degree taper. **B**, Two-degree taper. **C**, Six-degree taper.

tools currently available on the market. The plans for such a tool are shown in Fig. 6-16. It is used for proximal surfaces that are to be used as guiding planes, beneath minor connectors, in soft tissue undercuts that are to be crossed by rigid connectors, in deep interproximal spaces that are to be covered, and in undercut areas on teeth that are to be crossed by the approach arms of bar clasps (Fig. 6-17).

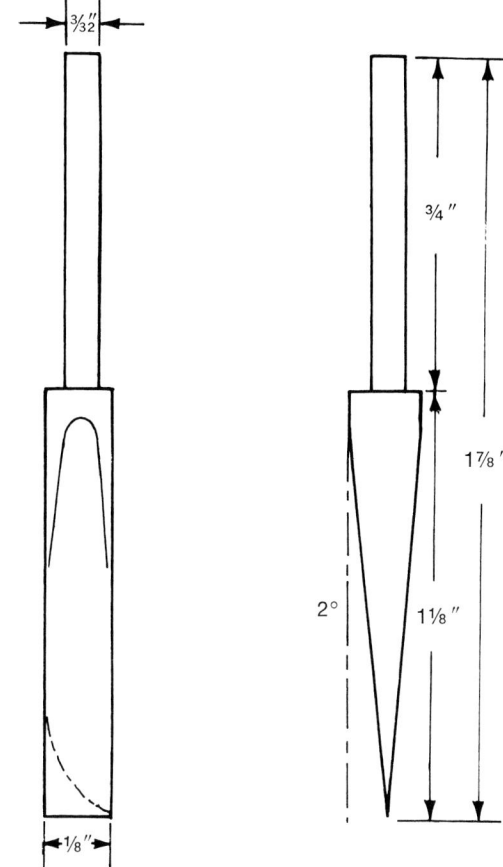

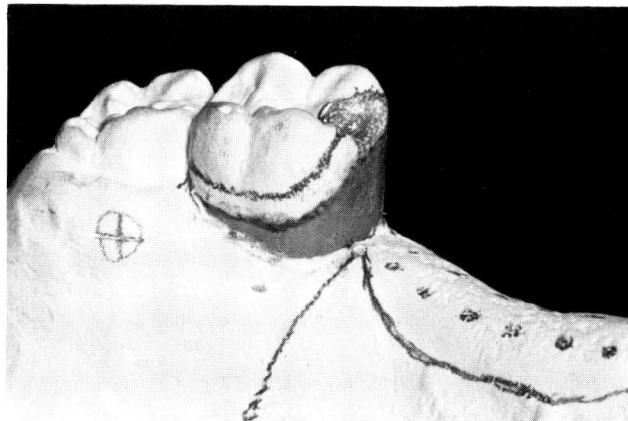

**Fig. 6-15.** Parallel blockout extends from survey line to gingiva.

**Fig. 6-16.** Machinists drawing for excellent blockout tool.

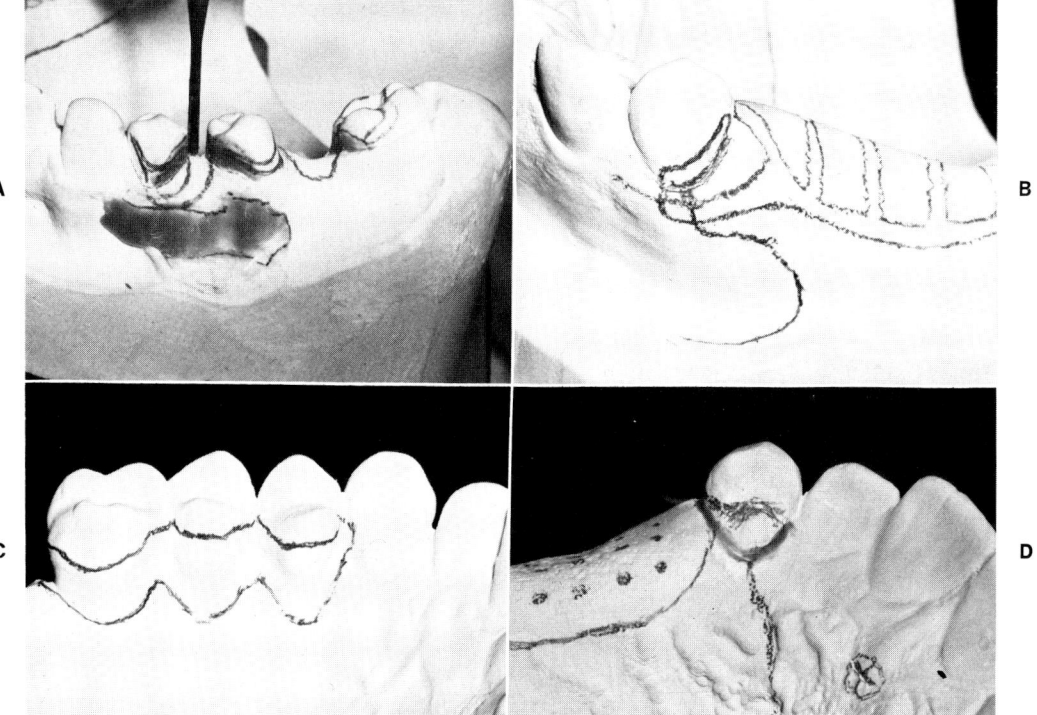

**Fig. 6-17.** Parallel blockout is used beneath minor connectors **(A)**, on soft tissue undercuts that may be crossed by rigid connectors **(B)**, in deep interproximal spaces **(C)**, and in undercut areas on teeth that will be crossed by clasp arm. **(D)**.

Shaped blockout or ledging is used on buccal or lingual surfaces to facilitate accurate placement of plastic or wax patterns for clasp arms. The blockout wax may be placed in the undercut and trimmed flush with the survey line using the proper stylus or wax trimmer (Fig. 6-18). The wax should be placed and trimmed carefully so that the tooth on the cast is not scraped or marred. If some of the stone is scraped from the tooth with the stylus or wax carver, the framework will fit too tightly or may not go into place in the mouth (Fig. 6-19). Consequently, a round stylus is recommended rather than a knife-shaped stylus.

Ledging may be only in the area of the tip of the clasp; this is the most desirable method (Fig. 6-20). It permits more flexibility in the waxing procedure, and, if the refractory cast is well made, there is no difficulty in placing the bracing portion of the clasp. Some technicians prefer to build up the ledge so it can be used as a guide for positioning the entire length of the clasp on the tooth (Fig. 6-21). In this method, the wax must be placed very accurately, since the ledge cannot be changed on the refractory cast if improperly placed.

Arbitrary blockout is used in less critical areas to prevent the encroachment of metal on the soft tissues and to facilitate withdrawal of the blocked out cast from the duplicating material. It is used for all gingival crevices, spaces between the teeth when they are not in the design, for gross tissue undercuts below areas involved in the design of the framework, and in tooth or tissue undercuts not involved in the design but that would complicate the duplication procedure (Fig. 6-22).

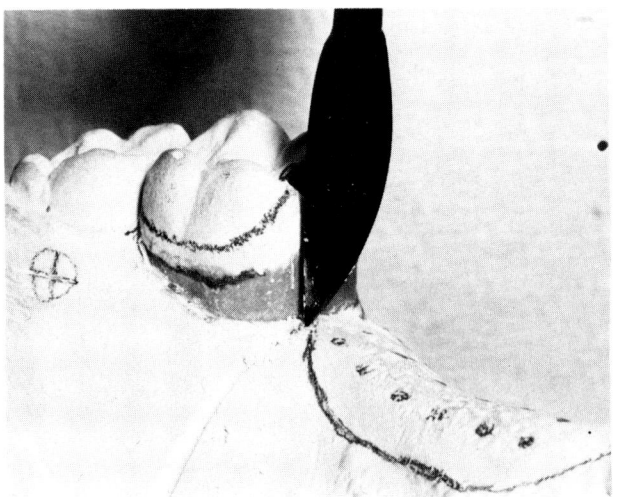

Fig. 6-18. Blockout trimmed flush on tooth.

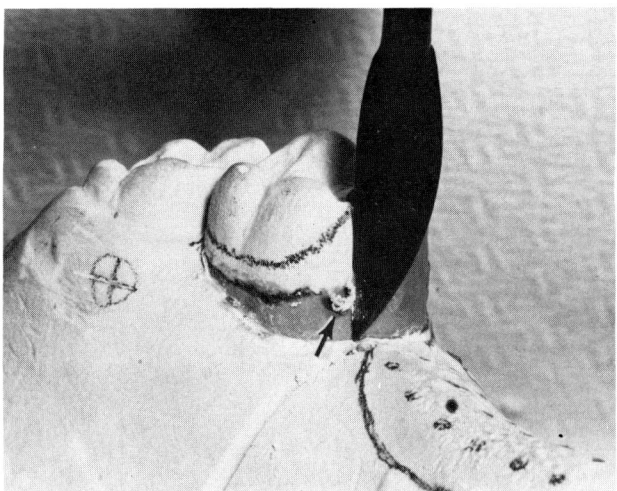

Fig. 6-19. This is not satisfactory blockout because some stone has been removed from cast.

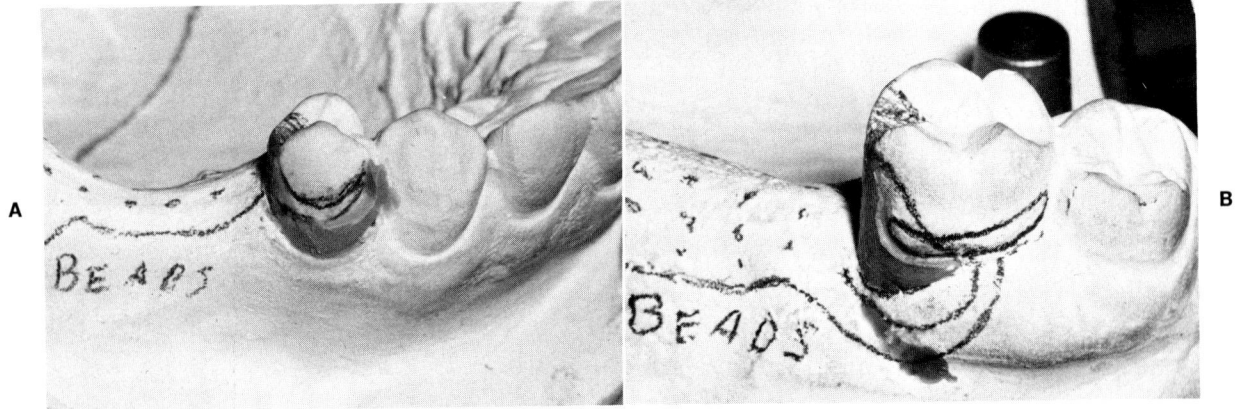

Fig. 6-20. Preferred method for ledging is to ledge for tip of clasp only. A, Ledging for circlet-type clasp. B, Ledging for bar-type clasp.

Relief may not be required under the portion of the metal framework used to cover the edentulous area when the residual ridge is well healed. Several advantages occur when relief is not used. It eliminates one step and the chance for an error. If there is no relief, there is no chance for the wax to be deformed during the duplicating process. Also there is no need for a conventional internal finish line, which, if not done precisely, is unsatisfactory. Relief is not used for complete denture bases, bead or nailhead retention, or open retention where the outer support is against the cast (Fig. 6-26).

Beading on the borders of the maxillary major connectors serves to prevent food particles from collecting beneath the framework and producing discomfort for the patient. The beading is also used by the dentist to indicate if the partial denture fits snugly against the palate. Beading is accomplished with a small spoon excavator by scraping the cast along the anterior and posterior borders of the major connector. Beading depth should not exceed 1 mm, and it should fade out as the gingival margins are approached or as a prominent area in the midline of the palate is approached (Fig. 6-27).

### PROCEDURE

1. Use a Roach carver or a No. 7 spatula to flow blockout wax below the survey line on each tooth that is to be contacted by the metal framework. Use enough wax to eliminate all of the undercuts. Also block out soft tissue undercuts. Blockout wax* may be purchased or may be made easily in the laboratory (Fig. 6-28).

*Formula for blockout wax*
$4\frac{1}{2}$ Sheets baseplate wax
$4\frac{1}{2}$ Sticks gutta-percha
3 Sticks sticky wax
$\frac{1}{2}$ Teaspoon kaolin† (powder)
$\frac{1}{2}$ Tube lipstick

---

*Ney undercut wax, The J. M. Ney Co., Bloomfield, Conn.
†Mallinckrodt, Inc., St. Louis, Mo.

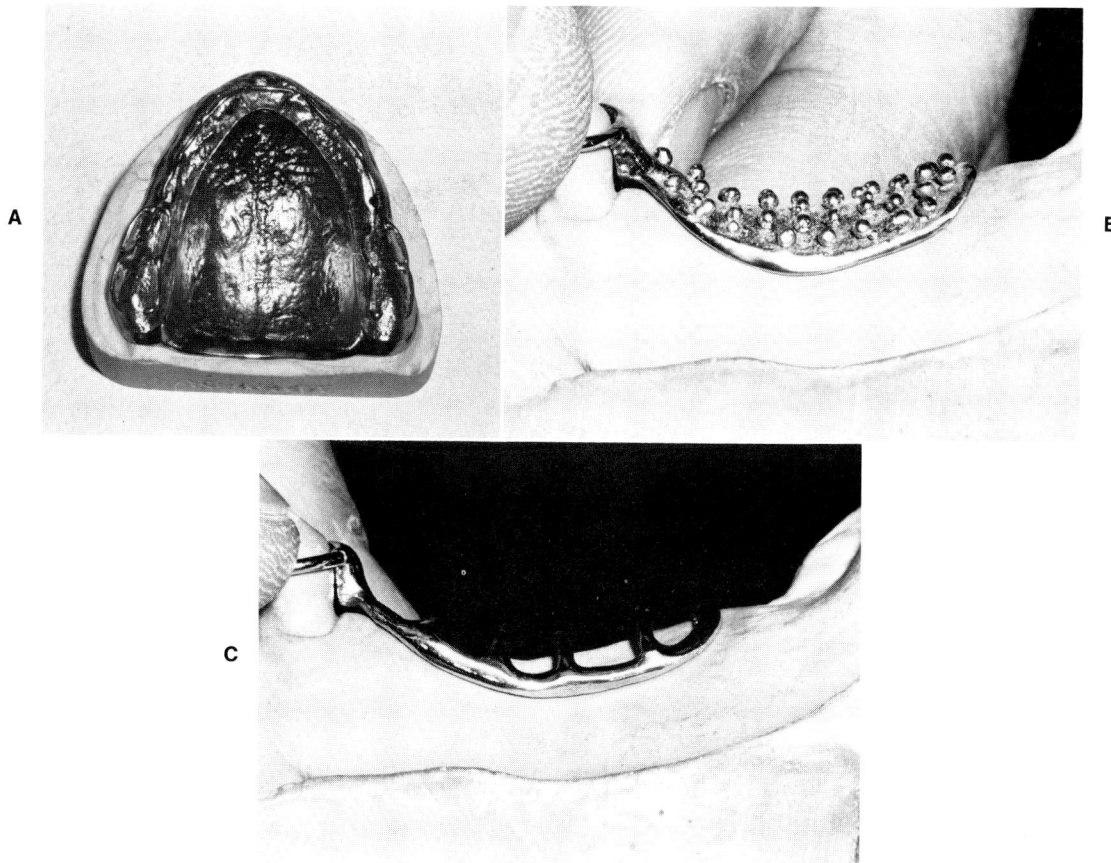

Fig. 6-26. Relief is not used for metal complete denture bases (A), bead or nailhead retention (B), and open retention when outer support is against cast (C).

Design transfer, blockout, relief, and beading 193

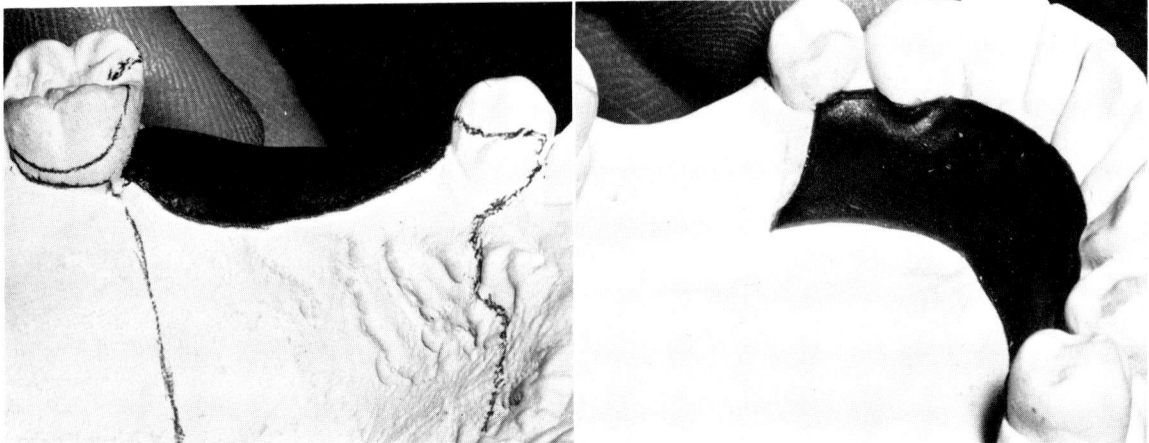

**Fig. 6-24.** Relief is adapted to both the maxillary and mandibular casts to form internal finish lines.

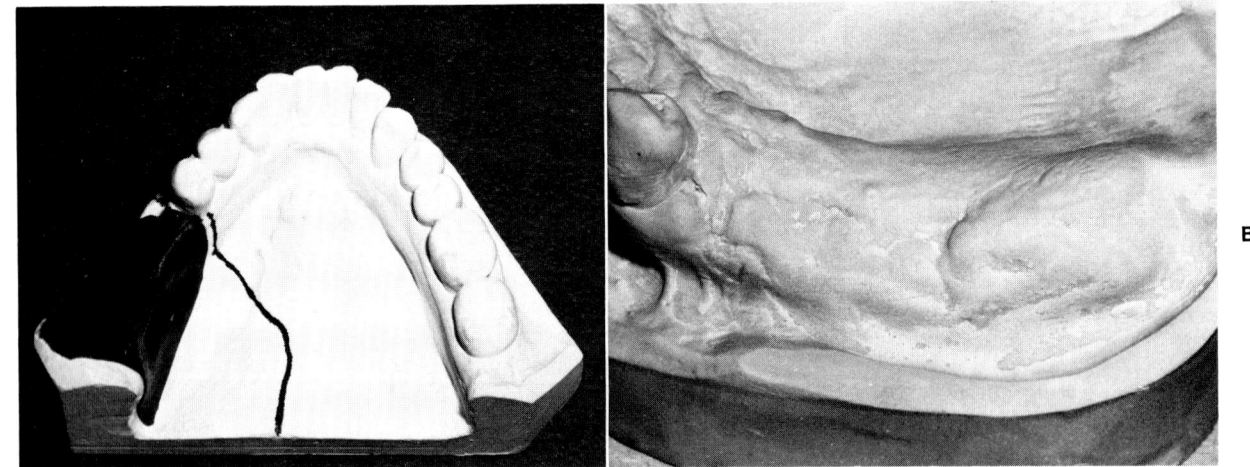

**Fig. 6-25.** Relief is usually required when altered cast impression procedure will be used **(A)** and ridge to be covered by denture base is not well healed **(B).**

Relief is used to create a space between the framework and the cast or soft tissue. It is usually used beneath lingual bars and in other areas where major connectors will contact thin soft tissue such as maxillary and mandibular tori (Fig. 6-23). If the sheet wax is cut in a curved form, it is easier to adapt to the lingual bar area. Relief is also used beneath framework extensions, in edentulous areas to provide for attachment of denture bases, and to form internal finish lines (Fig. 6-24).

Not all techniques require relief under the metal framework. This usually depends on the condition of the residual ridge to be covered by the denture base and by the impression technique that will be used. The dentist should specify whether or not relief is needed beneath the framework. If the altered cast technique is to be used in making the impression, relief must be placed under the denture base area of the framework (Fig. 6-25). It is also used when the ridge to be covered is not well healed. When residual ridges are not well healed, changes in ridge contour can be expected after the partial denture is delivered, thus often necessitating a rebase or reline.

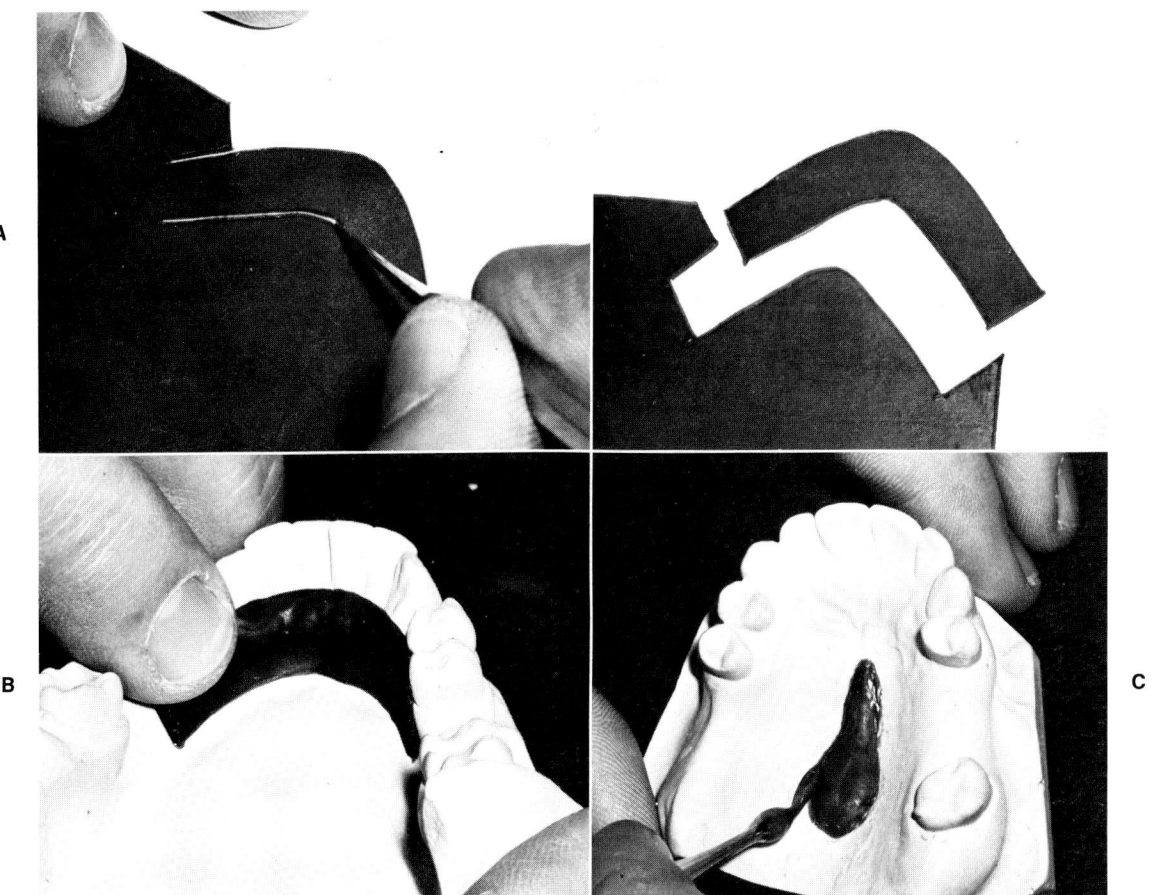

**Fig. 6-23.** Relief is used to create space between framework and cast or soft tissue. **A,** Relief cut in curved form. **B,** This shape makes it easier to adapt to cast for lingual bar. **C,** Relief is used over tori or other tender areas.

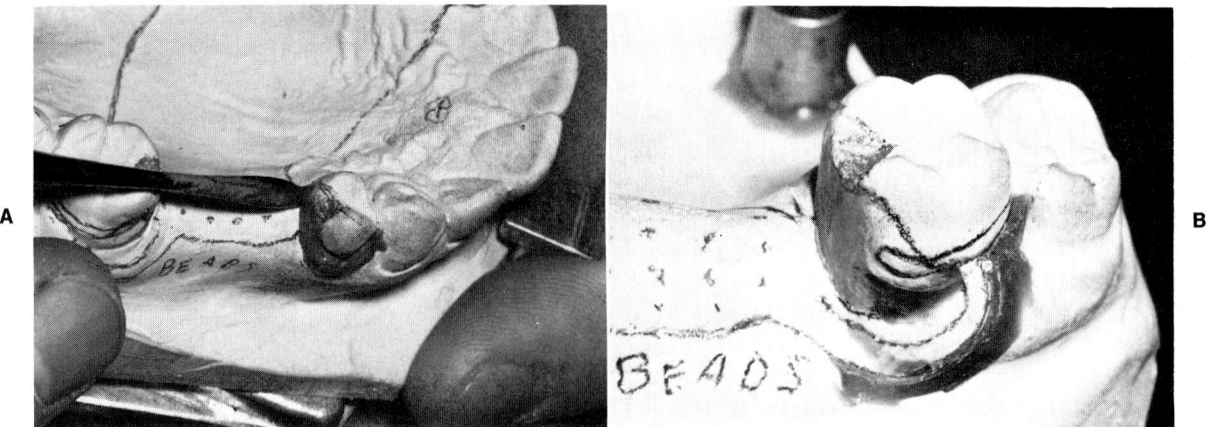

**Fig. 6-21.** Ledging can be built up to serve as guide for placing entire length of clasp. **A,** Procedure for circlet clasp. **B,** Procedure for bar clasp.

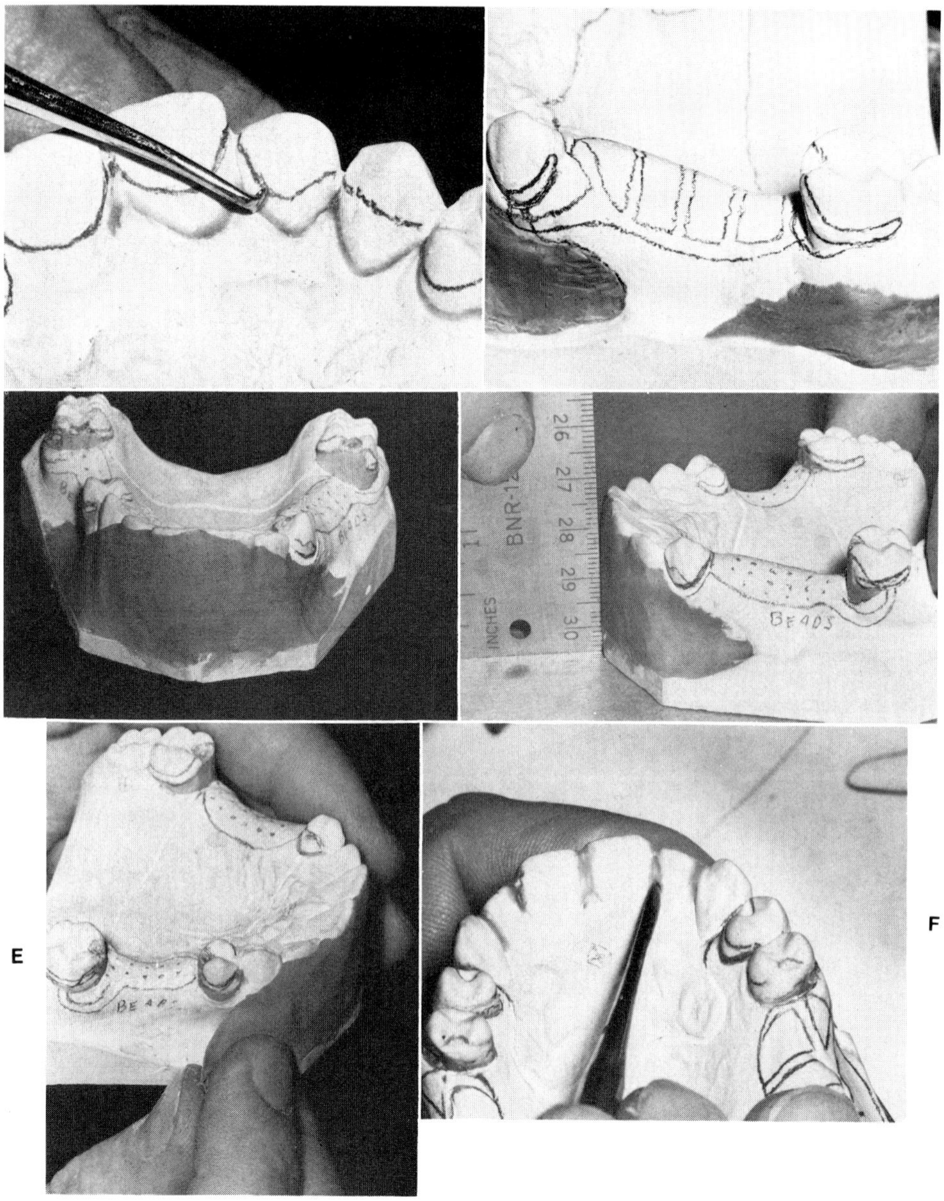

**Fig. 6-22.** Arbitrary blockout with wax. **A,** All gingivae crevices. Discoid carver is good to remove excess wax. **B,** Gross undercuts below design. **C** to **E,** Areas that would complicate duplication. Plasticine may be used also for **B** and **C. F,** Gross spaces between teeth.

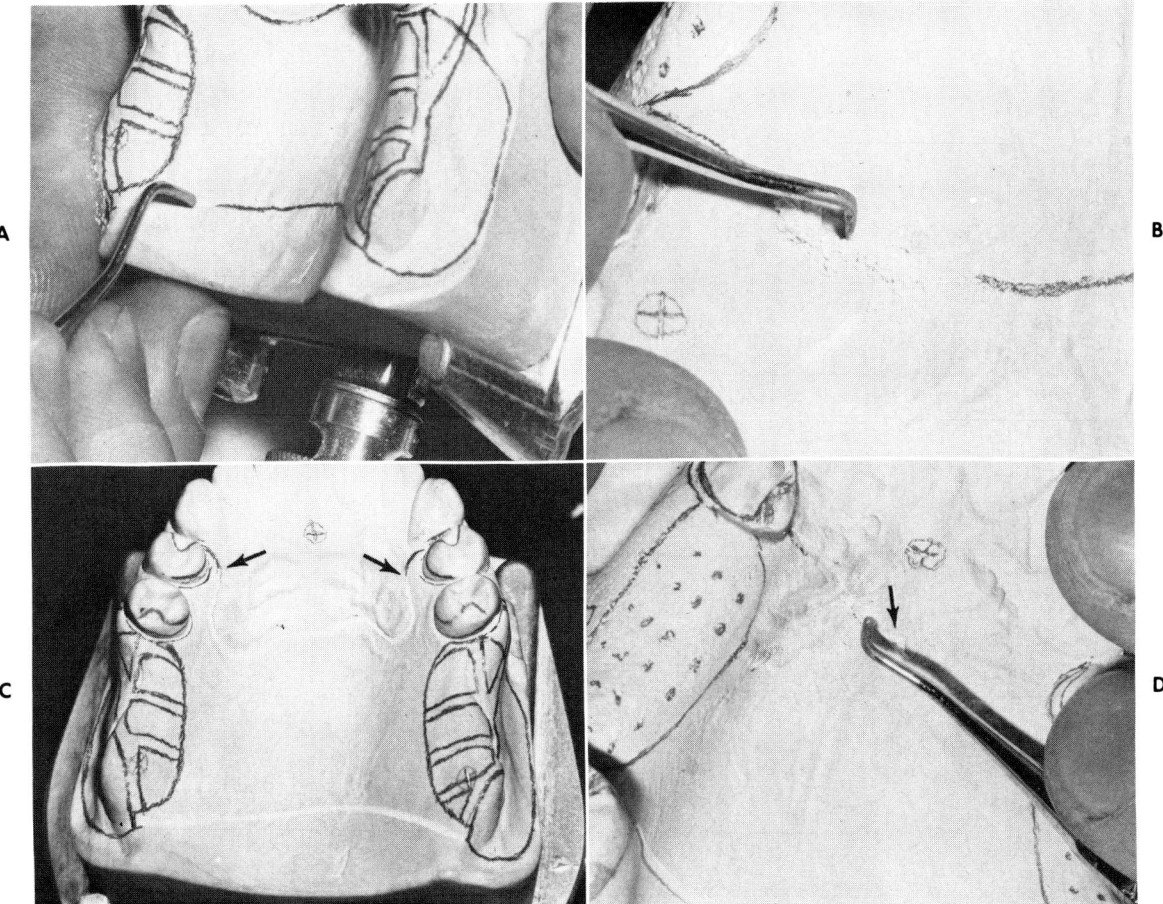

**Fig. 6-27.** Beading palate. **A,** Using small spoon excavator. **B,** Using cleoid instrument being careful to not make it too deep. Maximum depth should be about 1 mm. This is preferred method. **C,** Beading fades out as it approaches gingiva. **D,** Beading fades out as it approaches torus.

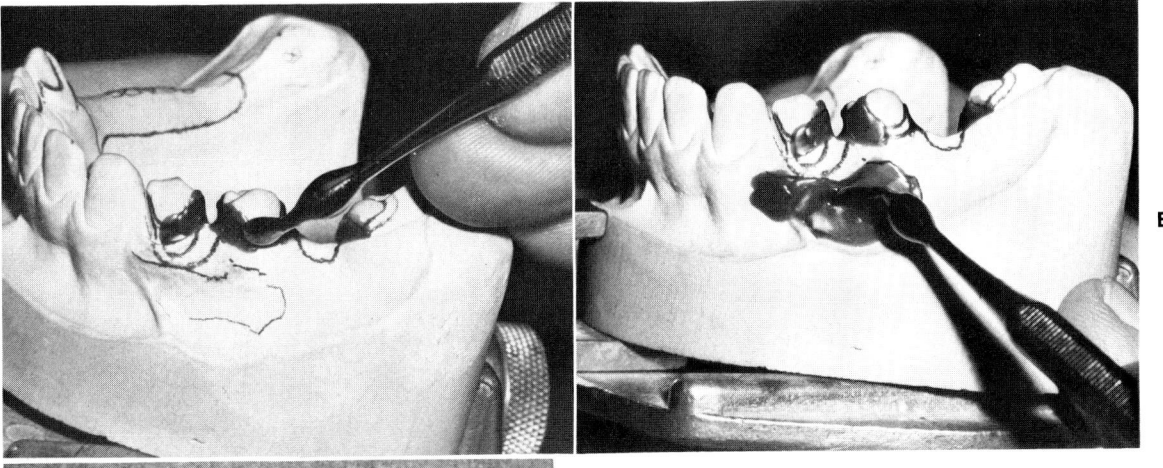

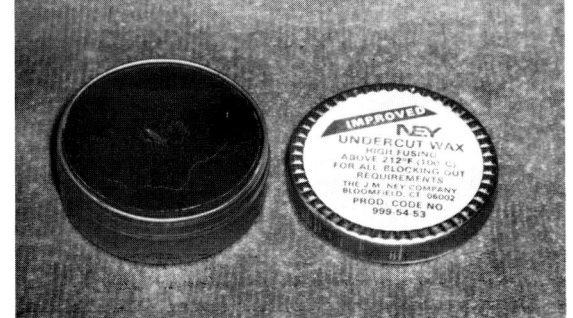

**Fig. 6-28. A,** Flow blockout wax below survey line on each tooth that is to be contacted with metal. Make certain that all undercuts are eliminated. **B,** Flow blockout wax into soft tissue undercuts that are to be blocked out. **C,** Blockout wax can be purchased or made in laboratory.

It is very important to use the following sequence when mixing:
1. Melt the gutta-percha to a pasty consistency*
2. Sticky wax
3. Kaolin
4. Baseplate wax
5. Coloring (red lipstick or carpenter blue chalk)

---

*Melt, combine, and blend the ingredients in each step thoroughly before adding the next ingredient. When all are combined, remove from the fire, immerse in water, and continue stirring until mixture cools considerably to the point where it can be poured into containers for storage; otherwise, the ingredients will separate. A good container is a small unwaxed paper cup or a small jar.

2. Insert the analyzing rod in the vertical arm of the surveyor (Fig. 6-29). This rod is preferred over the wax trimmer or the wax knife because there is less chance of scraping the cast.

3. The analyzing rod will work more easily if it is warmed slightly with an alcohol torch (Fig. 6-30).

4. Keep removing wax until the surveying line is visible all around the tooth (Fig. 6-31).

5. With the knife end of a Roach carver, remove the wax forming a ledge for the retentive tip of the clasp. Carve the wax so it creates a sharp definite ledge that tapers out at the survey line. The shape must follow the contour of the intended clasp arm (Fig. 6-32) and serves to position the wax or plastic pattern of the clasp arm in the refractory cast.

OPTIONAL LEDGING. Some prefer to ledge the entire

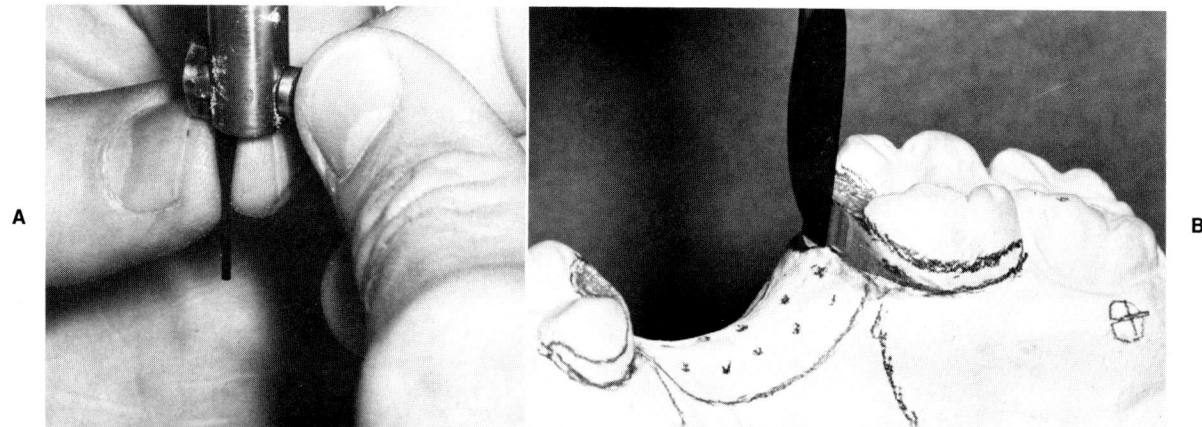

**Fig. 6-29. A,** Analyzing rod inserted into surveyor ready for trimming wax. **B,** Wax knife can easily scrape cast; use caution.

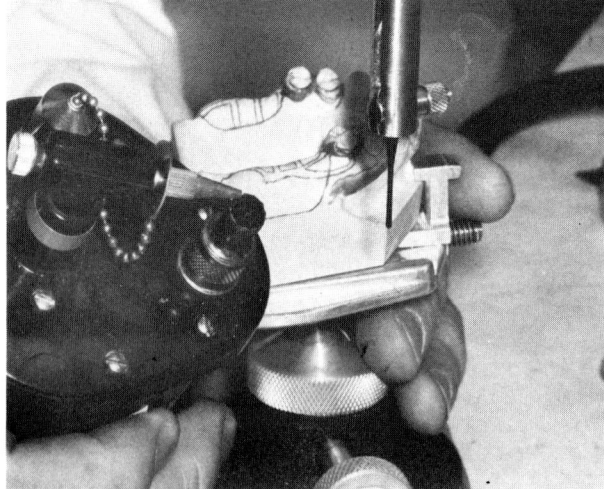

**Fig. 6-30.** Warm analyzing rod with flame, and it works much more easily.

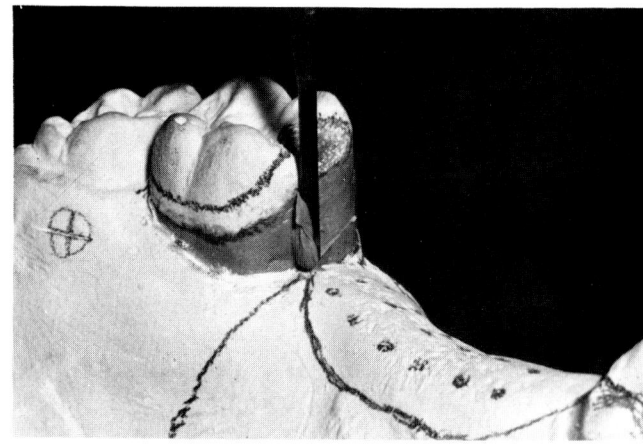

**Fig. 6-31.** Remove wax until survey line is visible all around tooth.

length of the clasp arm. If this ledging system is followed, it severely limits the positioning of the clasp arm by the person who waxes the partial framework because he must follow the ledging. If the ledging is wrong, it cannot be corrected accurately without making another refractory cast. This may be an advantage if the person who does the ledging is very skilled and is able to place the ledging perfectly every time. Then, the person who waxes depends on him for positioning the clasp arms (Fig. 6-33).

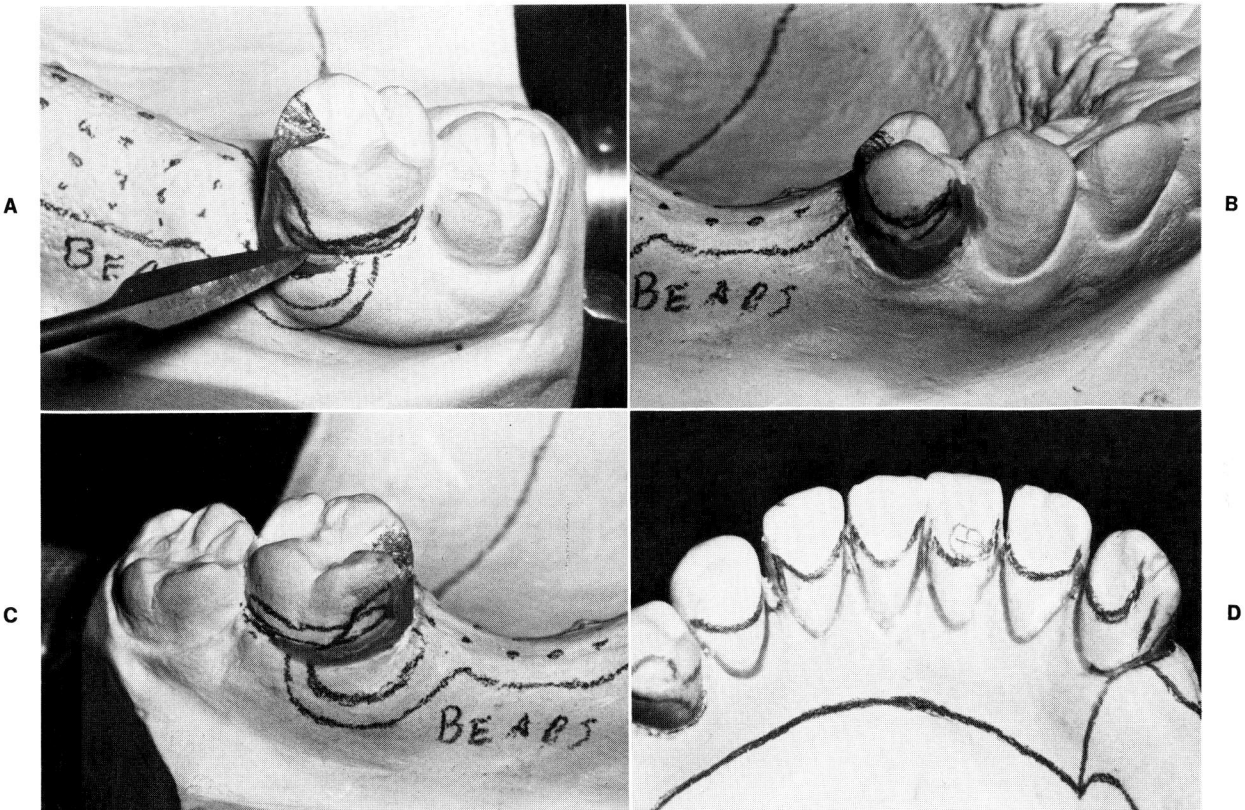

Fig. 6-32. **A,** Ledging is carved with Roach carver, depending on shape of clasp arm to be used. **B,** Ledging for circlet clasp arm. **C,** Ledging for bar clasp arm. **D,** Gingival crevice filled with blockout wax and trimmed with cleoid carver.

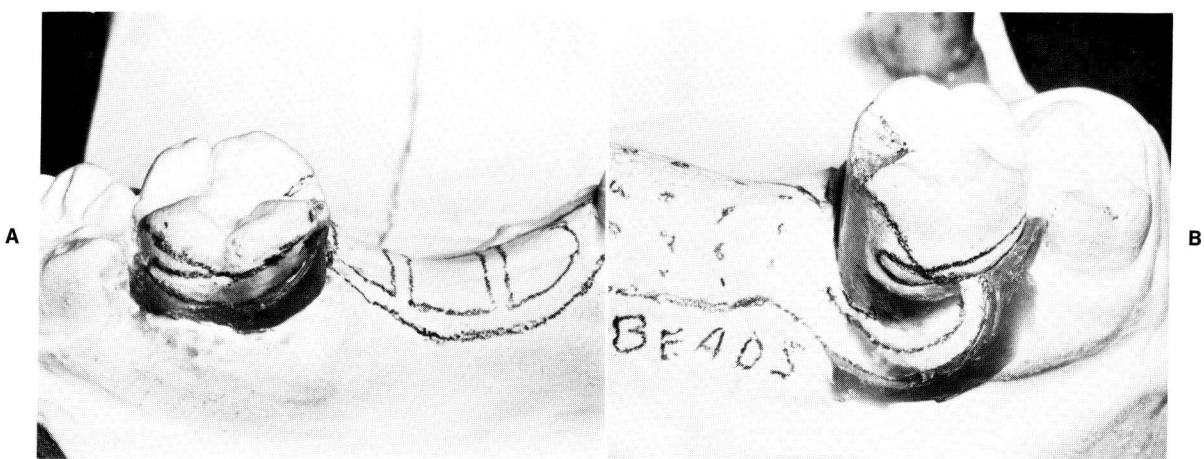

Fig. 6-33. Ledging may be placed along entire clasp arm; however, this requires much more accuracy. **A,** Full-arm ledging for circlet cast clasp or wire clasp. **B,** Full-arm ledging for a bar-type clasp.

6. If relief over the edentulous areas is not to be used, go directly to step 9. Adapt a piece of 22-gauge adhesive wax over the edentulous ridges.

7. The lingual portion of the relief wax may serve as an internal finish line and should be positioned and trimmed very precisely. In the palate, it should follow the contour of the ridge, allowing sufficient room for setting the teeth (Fig. 6-34). Pencil erasers may be shaped and used as an aid to adapt the relief wax (Fig. 6-35). Relief on the lingual side of the maxillary cast is trimmed precisely to serve as an internal finish line (Fig. 6-36). Relief on the lingual side of the mandibular cast is used for an internal finish line on lingual bars and some other designs (Fig. 6-37). The relief wax should blend in with the blockout wax to form a smooth even joint.

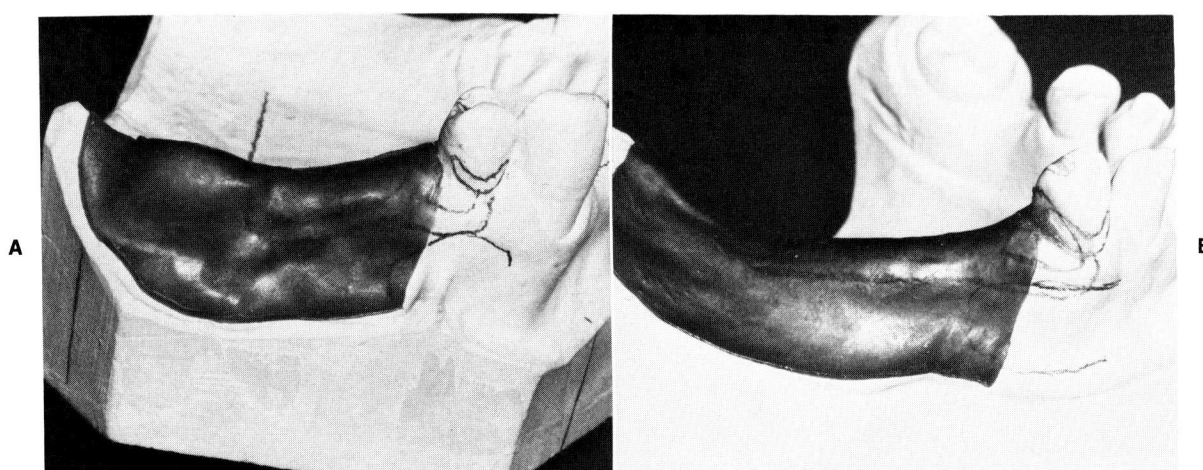

**Fig. 6-34. A,** Relief should cover more than penciled outline drawn on endentulous areas of cast on facial surface and entire tuberosity on maxillary cast. **B,** Relief should cover retromolar pad on mandibular cast.

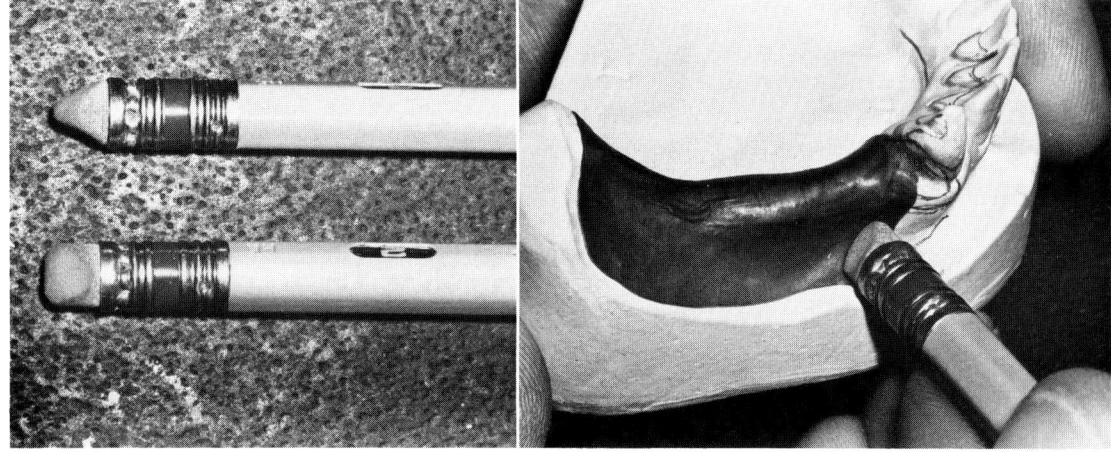

**Fig. 6-35.** Pencil erasers may be shaped and used to adapt relief wax.

Design transfer, blockout, relief, and beading **199**

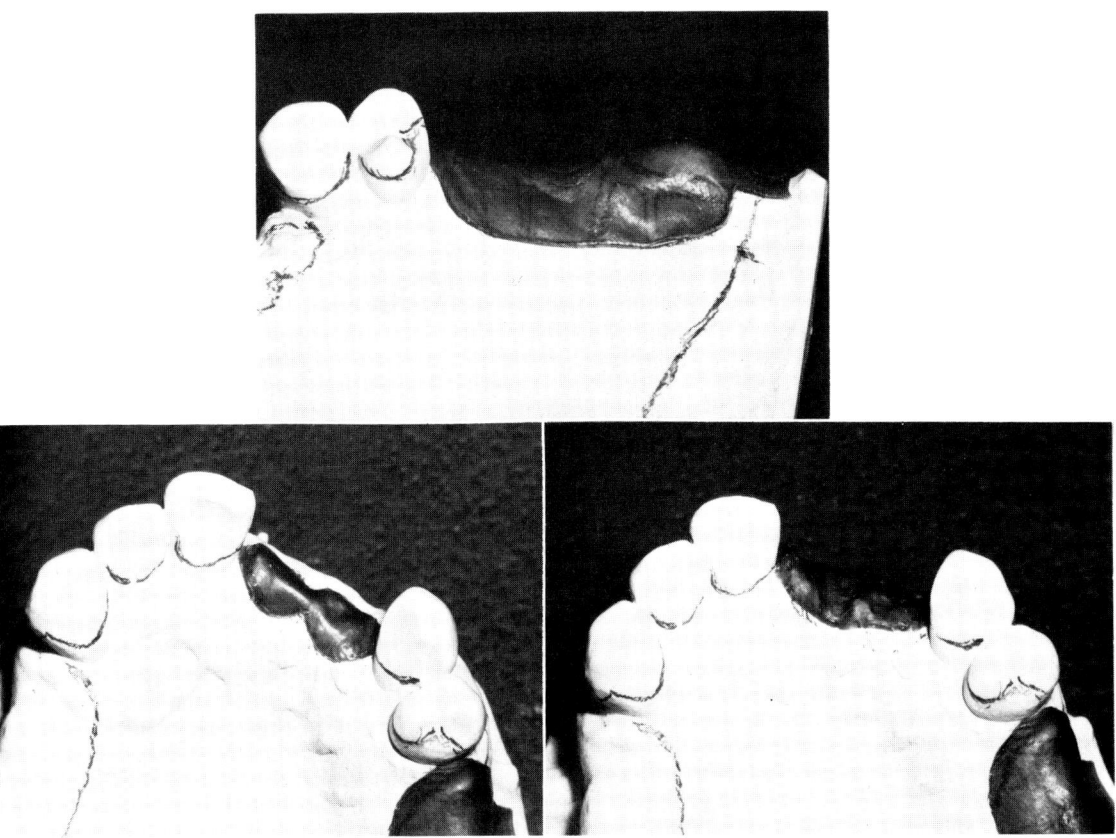

**Fig. 6-36.** Relief wax is trimmed precisely in lingual region of maxillary cast to serve as internal finish line and in certain types of relief in anterior portion.

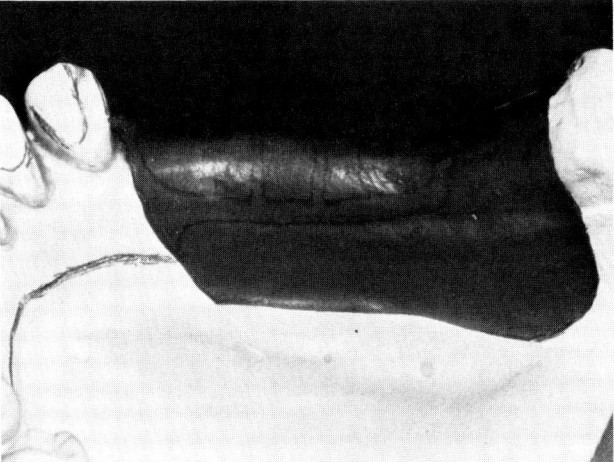

**Fig. 6-37.** Relief wax is placed to form internal finish line at lingual bar and all along lingual flange in some designs.

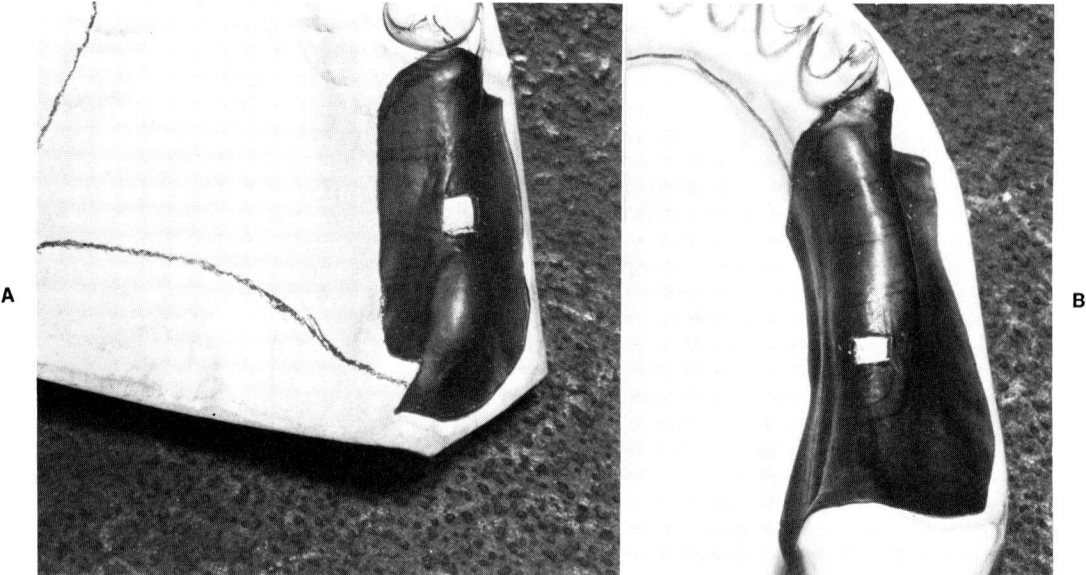

**Fig. 6-38.** Cut out 2 × 3-inch (5 × 7.5-cm) square of relief wax to serve as tissue stop. **A,** Stop cut for maxillary cast. **B,** Stop cut for mandibular cast.

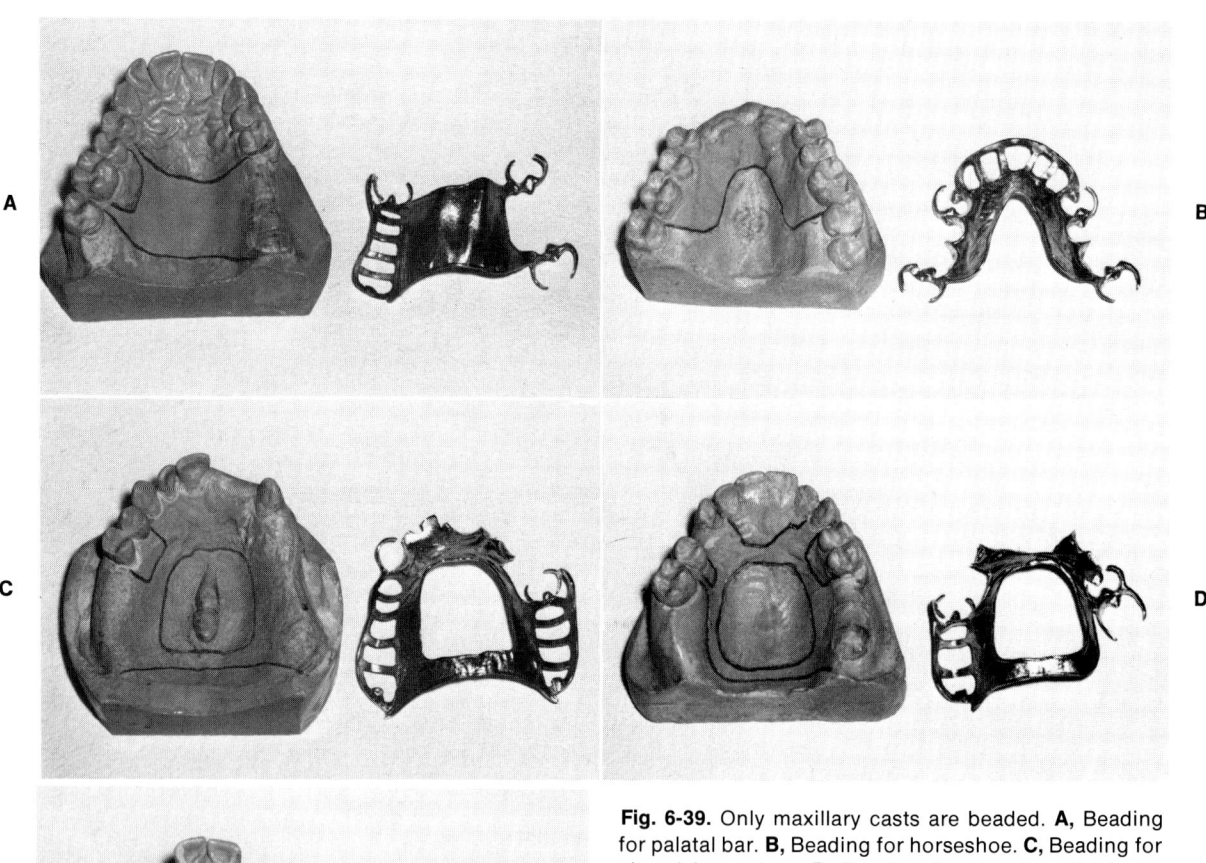

**Fig. 6-39.** Only maxillary casts are beaded. **A,** Beading for palatal bar. **B,** Beading for horseshoe. **C,** Beading for closed horseshoe. **D,** Beading for double palatal bar. **E,** Beading for full palate.

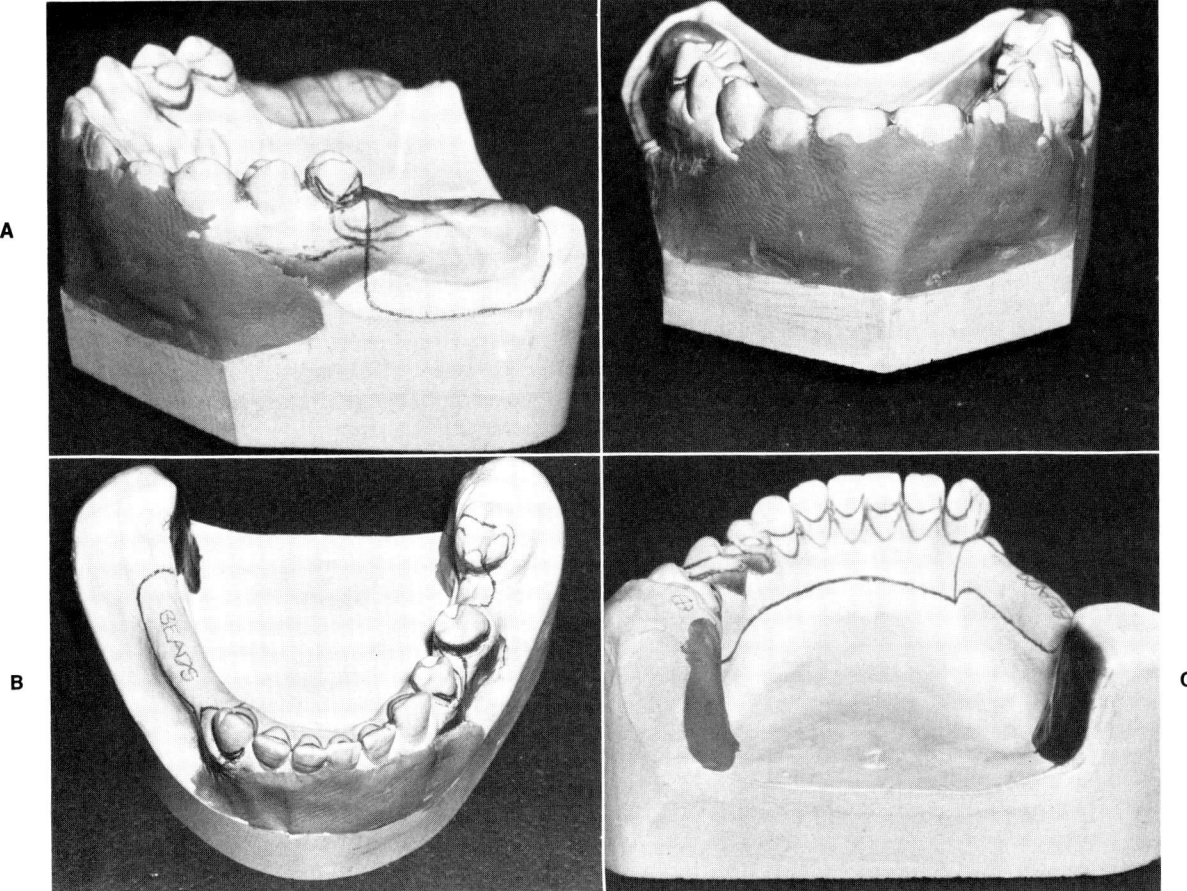

**Fig. 6-40.** Gross soft tissue undercuts labial and buccal to remaining teeth are arbitrarily blocked out with Plasticine or scrap wax. **A,** Maxillary cast. **B,** Facial view of mandibular cast. **C,** Lingual view of mandibular cast. NOTE: Make sure that arbitrary blockout does not touch any part of design.

8. Cut out a 2 × 3-mm square of relief wax over the most posterior cross strut of the latticework (Fig. 6-38). This will serve as a tissue stop.

9. Bead the maxillary cast with a spoon excavator. All borders ending on soft tissue should be beaded. The depth of the bead should not exceed 1 mm and should fade out as it approaches the gingival margin or a torus (Fig. 6-39).

10. Use Plasticine or scrap wax to arbitrarily block out gross tissue undercuts that are labial and buccal to the remaining teeth (Fig. 6-40). Make certain the arbitrary blockout does not contact any area of the design.

11. The relief, blockout, and beading are now complete, and the casts are ready for duplication (Fig. 6-41).

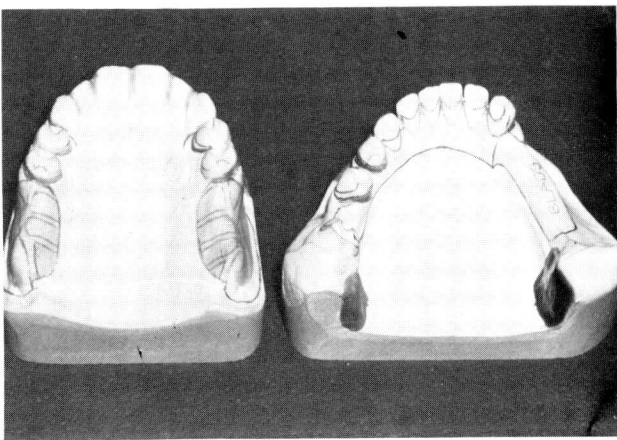

**Fig. 6-41.** Maxillary and mandibular casts are ready for duplication.

**Table 6-1.** Design transfer, blockout, relief, and beading of the master cast

| Problem | Probable cause | Solution |
|---|---|---|
| Complete framework fits too tightly, will not seat | Blockout not completed properly, permitting rigid part of framework to be placed in undercut | Carefully block out all undesirable undercuts |
| | Tooth on cast marred by stylus when trimming blockout wax | Use round stylus to trim wax, thus preventing damage to tooth or cast |
| Framework is too retentive | Ledging placed incorrectly into deep undercut | Check undercut accurately with gauge; trim ledging at correct level |
| Hydrocolloid mold torn when master cast removed | Inadequate blockout of undesirable undercuts on master cast | Block out undesirable undercuts to permit easier withdrawal of cast from duplicatng material |
| Lingual bar of framework impinges on lingual tissues | Relief wax not placed on cast in region of lingual bar | Reline master cast with wax to avoid impingement |
| Framework beading blanches tissue when inserted | Beading on cast too deep | Bead cast lightly to avoid blanching |

## PROBLEM AREAS

The principal problems associated with blockout, relief, and beading are associated with failure to identify and obturate undesirable undercuts, inaccurate placement of blockout wax, overrelieving or underrelieving the cast, and improperly beading the cast too deeply or too shallowly (Table 6-1).

## SUMMARY

In this chapter, the procedures for transferring the partial denture design to the master cast, and blockout, relief, and beading of the master cast were described. These procedures are prerequisites for obtaining an acceptable refractory cast.

## BIBLIOGRAPHY

Air Force Manual 160-29: Dental laboratory technicians manual, United States Air Force, Washington, D.C., 1959, U.S. Government Printing Office.

Air Force Manual 162-6: Dental laboratory technology, United States Air Force, Washington, D.C., 1975, U.S. Government Printing Office.

Sowter, J. B.: Dental laboratory technology: prosthodontic technique, Chapel Hill, N.C., 1968, The University of North Carolina.

Stewart, K. L., and Kuebker, W.: Removable partial denture laboratory manual, San Antonio, 1979, The University of Texas Health Science Center at San Antonio.

Zarb, G. A., Bergman, B., Clayton, J. A., and MacKay, H. F.: Prosthodontic treatment for partially edentulous patients, St. Louis, 1978, The C. V. Mosby Co.

## CHAPTER 7

# DUPLICATION AND REFRACTORY CASTS

KENNETH D. RUDD, ROBERT M. MORROW, and GEORGE KNIGHT

**duplication** The procedure of accurately reproducing a cast.
**refractory cast** A cast made of materials that will withstand high temperatures without disintegrating and, when used in partial denture casting techniques, has expansion to compensate for metal shrinkage.

Prepared master casts are duplicated to produce an exact copy of the master cast in investment material. This cast is called the refractory cast because it contains ceramic material that permits it to withstand burnout temperatures of about 1300° F (704° C). The framework pattern is formed on the refractory cast using wax and plastic. After the framework wax-up is complete, it is invested, burned out, and cast to produce the metal framework.

## REVERSIBLE HYDROCOLLOID (AGAR) MOLDS

Reversible hydrocolloid (agar) is used most often to make the mold for duplication. Since this material is heat reversible, it may be reused many times. Alginate irreversible hydrocolloid may also be used by increasing the volume of water to three times the volume used for a regular impression. The thin alginate mix can be poured into a duplicating flask (Fig. 7-1). Alginate is as accurate as the agar hydrocolloid; however, it is much more expensive for volume duplication, since it is not reversible and only one duplicate can be made from each mix. Reversible hydrocolloid also seems to produce a smoother cast surface with some investment materials. Another material used for duplicating is a reversible plastic gel, which is basically polyvinyl chloride.

Agar hydrocolloid is prepared by grinding or chopping the colloid into small pieces and heating it until it liquefies at 212° F (100° C). The melted colloid can be stored for a few days in a hydrocolloid storage unit at 135° to 140° F (57° to 60° C). The material may be reused a number of times to make duplicate casts. After each use, it should be washed under cool water to remove all traces of stone and investment, cut into small pieces, and stored in a closed container to prevent loss of water. If the material is permitted to dry out, it cannot be used again.

A duplicating flask* will be used to support the cast and confine the hydrocolloid, since it aids in controlling shrinkage. It is a simple design, consisting of three pieces: the base, the body, and the reservoir ring (Fig. 7-2). Two holes in the top surface of the body permit air to escape as the duplicating material fills the flask.

### PROCEDURE

1. The master cast must be thoroughly soaked in clear slurry water. A minimum of 30 minutes soaking is usually required. NOTE: It is a good idea to stand the cast on end as it soaks (Fig. 7-3). As the cast becomes wet, it changes color. When the color in the entire cast has changed, it is an indication that the cast is thoroughly soaked (Fig. 7-4). If a cast is completely submerged in water, it will require 5 to 8 hours to soak all the way through.

---
*Duplicating flask, Ticonium Co., Albany, N.Y.

**204** *Dental laboratory procedures: removable partial dentures*

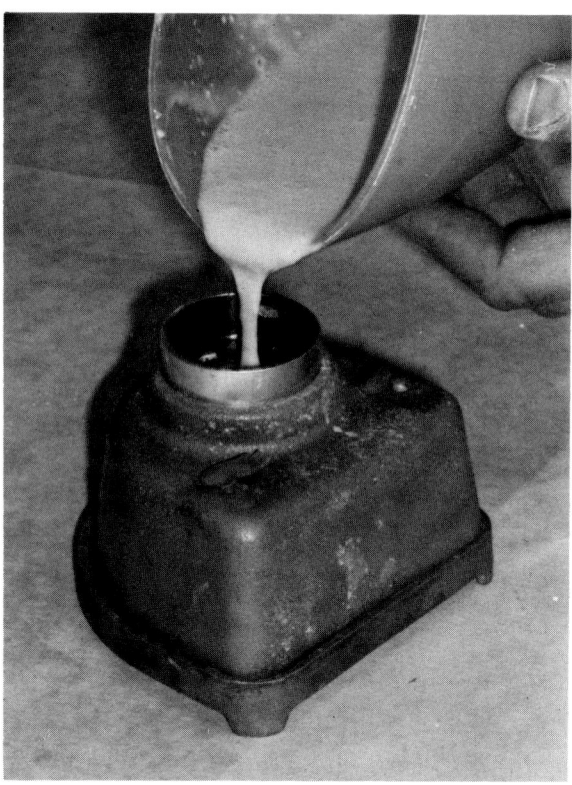

2. Place the cast on the base of the duplicating flask to make sure that space around and above the cast is sufficient for the duplicating material. There should be at least ¼-inch (0.63-cm) clearance in all directions (Fig. 7-5). If there is not enough space, the cast must be trimmed or a larger flask used (Fig. 7-6).

**Fig. 7-1.** Alginate may be mixed thin enough to pour and still make accurate duplication.

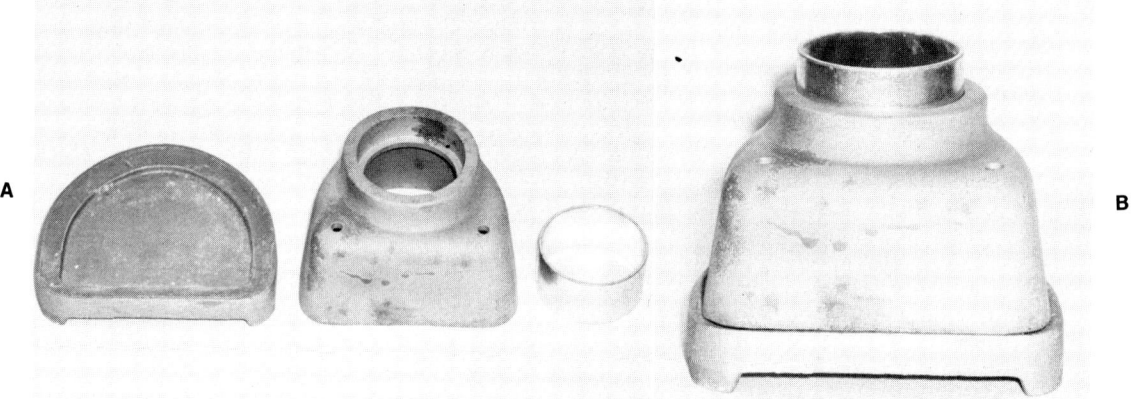

**Fig. 7-2.** Ticonium duplicating flask is used because of its simple design and reliability in controlling shrinkage. **A,** Exploded view. **B,** Assembled.

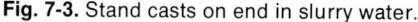

**Fig. 7-3.** Stand casts on end in slurry water.

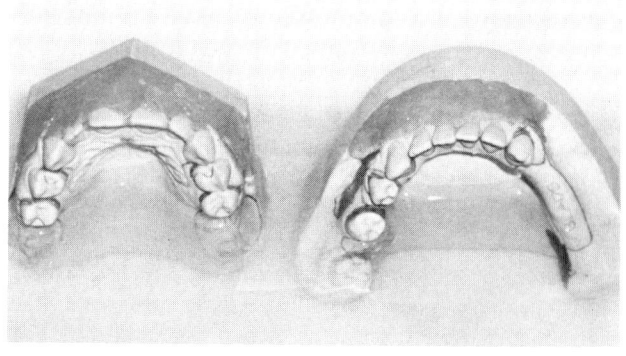

## Duplication and refractory casts 205

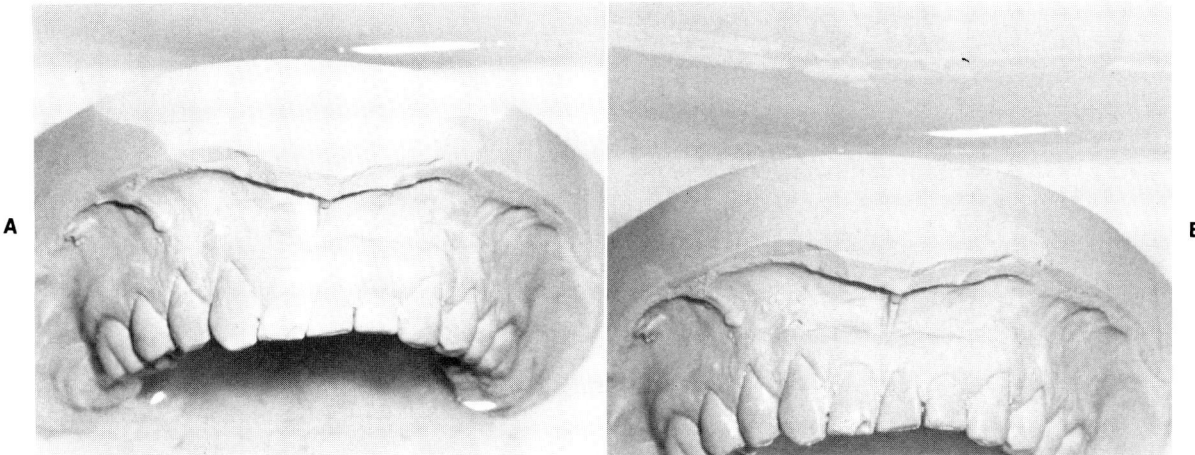

**Fig. 7-4. A,** As cast soaks, wet part changes to slightly darker color. **B,** When entire cast is soaked, it will be darker in color, indicating that it is wet completely through.

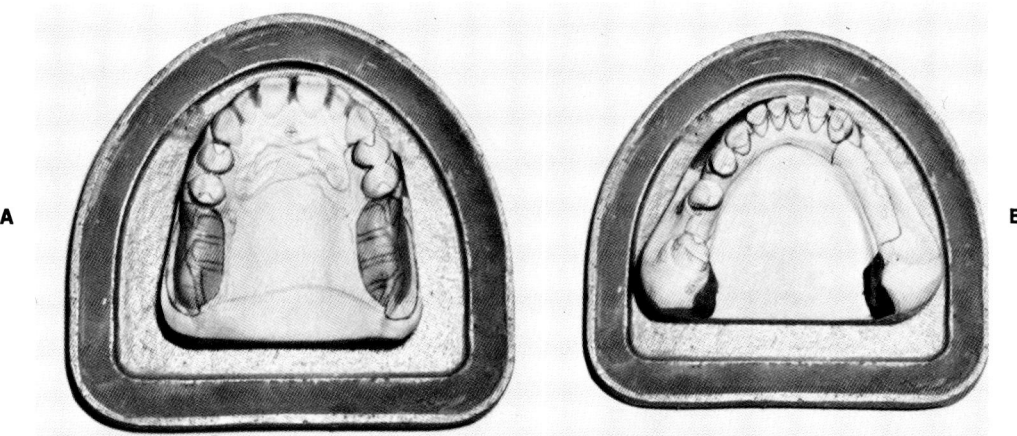

**Fig. 7-5.** There should be at least ¼-inch (0.63-cm) clearance around cast in all directions. **A,** Place cast on base to see if clearance on sides is adequate. **B,** Flask too small.

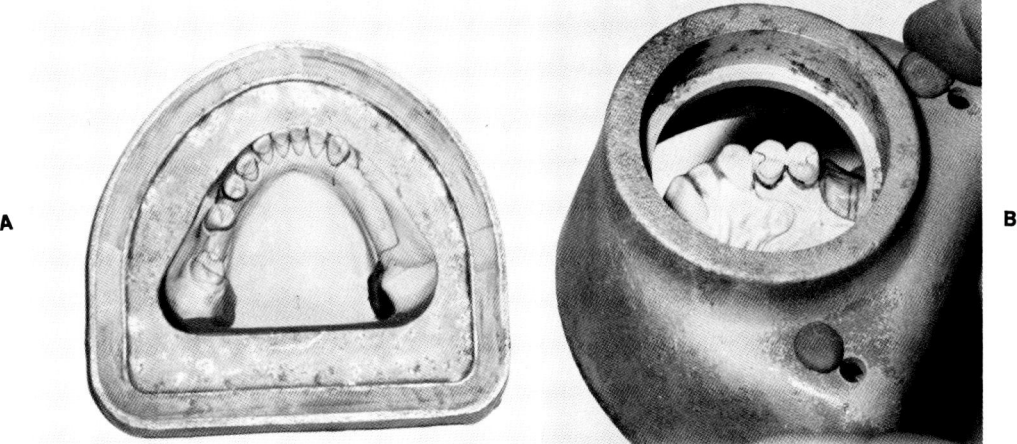

**Fig. 7-6. A,** Larger flask used. **B,** Place body of flask over cast to see if teeth clear top by at least ¼ inch (0.63 cm).

3. Center the cast on the base of the flask, and secure it with three small pieces of modeling clay (Plasticine) (Fig. 7-7).

4. Make sure the outer rim of the flask base is filled with modeling clay (Fig. 7-8), and seat the body of the flask firmly into this rim (Fig. 7-9). This acts as a seal and prevents the hydrocolloid from escaping. It also acts as an insulating area when the flask is being cooled slowly.

5. Place the reservoir ring in the body of the flask (Fig. 7-10).

6. Place a small ball of modeling clay adjacent to but not over the two vent holes in the top surface of the body of the flask (Fig. 7-11). These will be used to close the holes when the duplicating material has filled the flask, and the air has escaped.

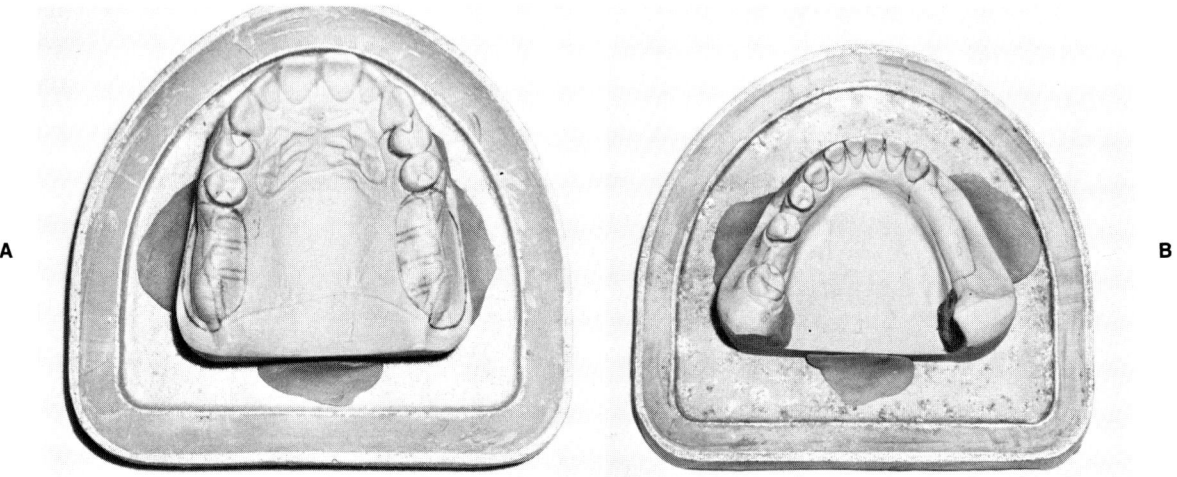

**Fig. 7-7.** Cast centered on base of flask and secured with three pieces of modeling clay. **A,** Maxillary cast. **B,** Mandibular cast.

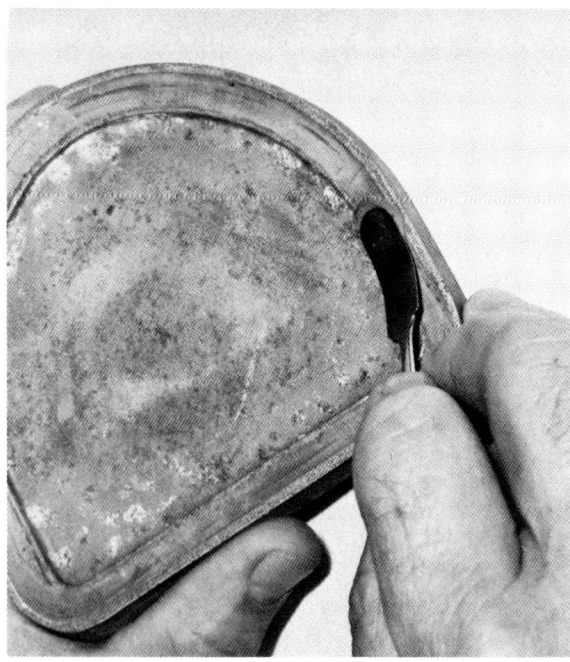

**Fig. 7-8.** Outer rim of flask base must be filled with modeling clay.

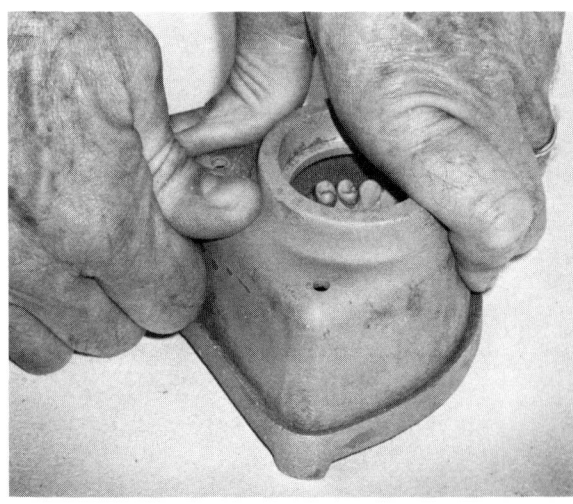

**Fig. 7-9.** Seat body firmly into rim of base.

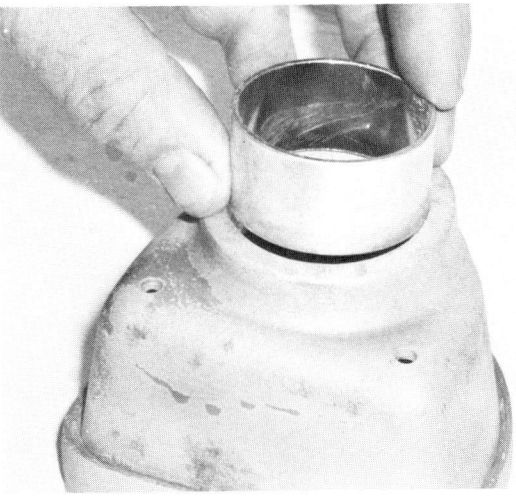

**Fig. 7-10.** Reservoir ring is placed in flange on top of body of flask.

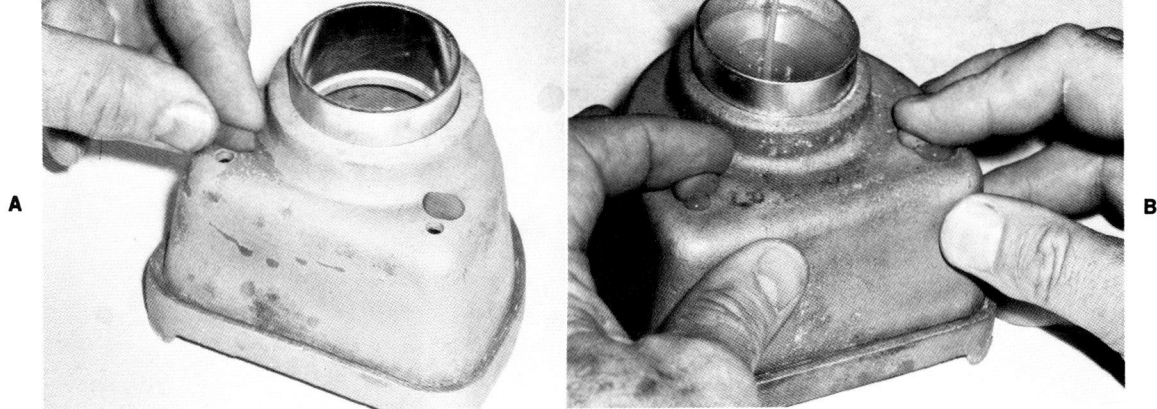

**Fig. 7-11.** Small balls of modeling clay are placed on body of flask next to vent holes. **A,** Balls of modeling clay in place. **B,** Balls of clay placed over holes as agar starts to come through them.

**208** *Dental laboratory procedures: removable partial dentures*

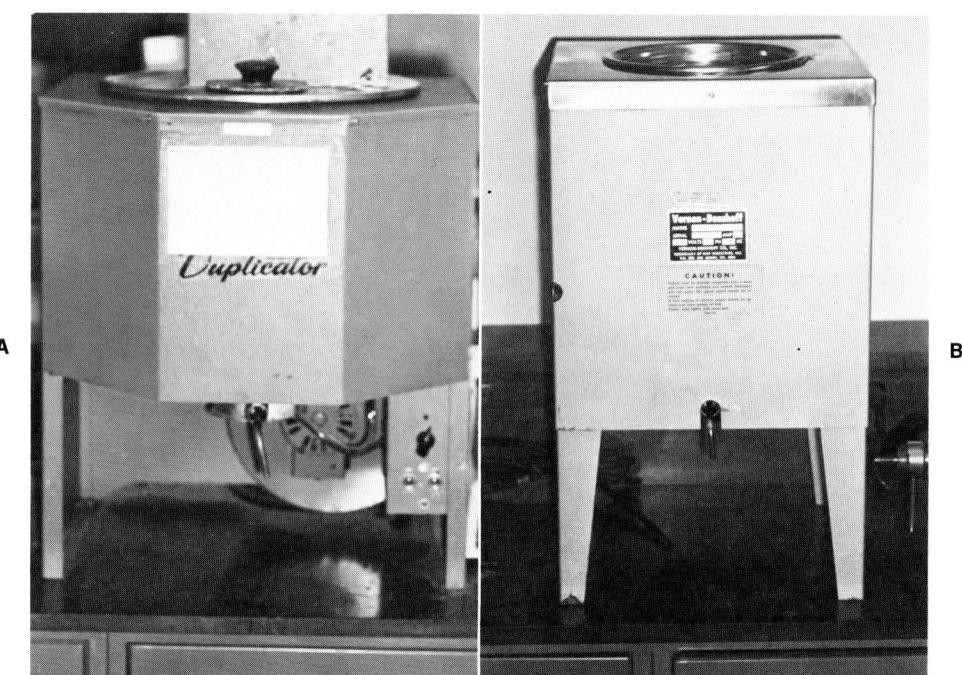

**Fig. 7-12.** Storage unit containing prepared duplicating material ready to use at 135° to 140° F (57° to 60° C). **A,** This Austenal unit breaks material down, then stores it. **B,** This Ticonium unit stores only. Material must be prepared, then poured into unit for storage.

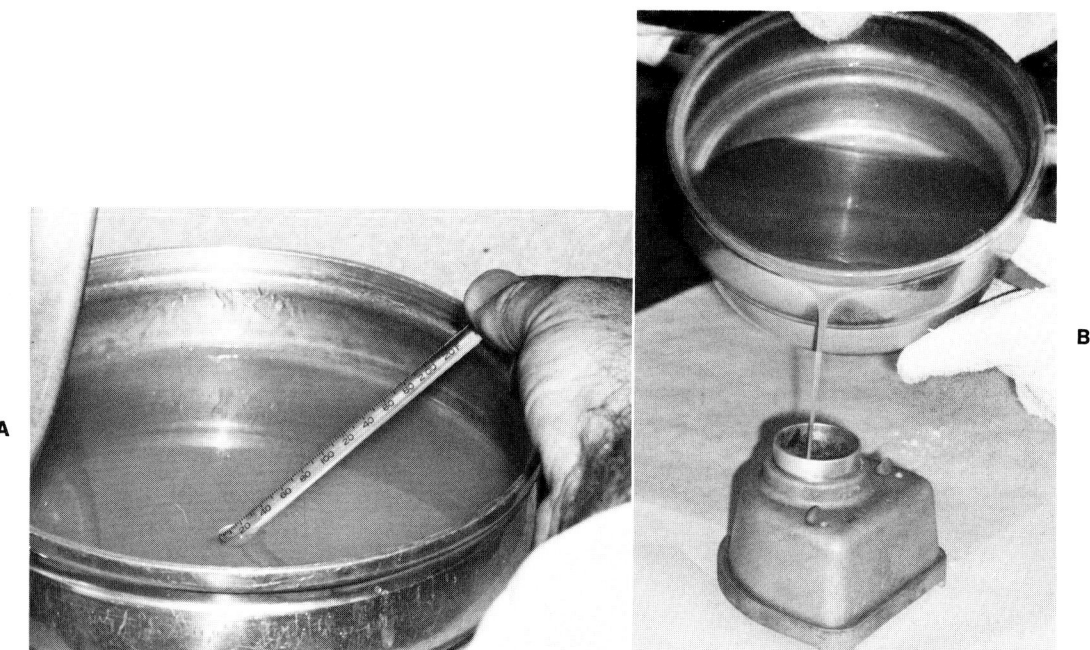

**Fig. 7-13. A,** Temperature of agar in double boiler must not exceed 140° F (60° C) when poured. **B,** Agar will reach about 190° F (88° C) when it is broken down, so it must be cooled before pouring.

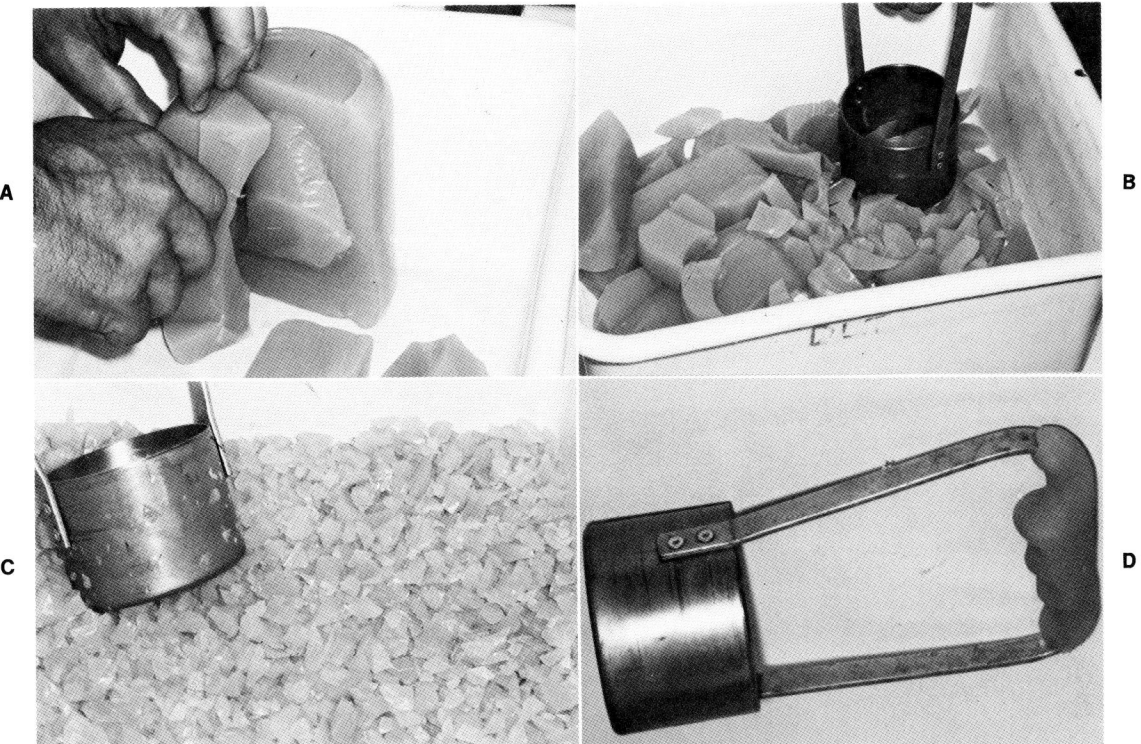

**Fig. 7-14.** Both old and new agar must be chopped or mashed to fine consistency before it is heated. It may be ground in electric or handpowered food grinder. **A,** Cut into small pieces. **B,** Chop into small pieces. **C,** Reduce all material to fine pieces. **D,** Chopper can be made by riveting handle to large stainless steel casting ring.

7. Check the temperature of the duplicating material in the storage unit (Fig. 7-12) or the double boiler (Fig. 7-13), depending on which is used. If a storage unit is used, directions for use will be included with the unit. NOTE: When using a double boiler to liquefy the agar hydrocolloid, allow sufficient time because it takes about 2 hours and 30 minutes to get it ready for duplication. Be sure the agar is chopped finely. A chopper may be made easily by riveting a handle to a large stainless steel casting ring (Fig. 7-14). Fill the top of the double boiler with agar (Fig. 7-15) and the bottom of the boiler with water (Fig. 7-16). Put the boiler together, place it on a fire, and boil the water (Fig. 7-17). It will require about 1 hour and 30 minutes for all of the agar to liquefy. Remove the boiler from the fire, and allow the agar to cool for about 1 hour, until it reaches between 135° to 140° F (57° to 60° C). It is now ready to pour into the flask. *Caution:* Agar hydrocolloid cannot be heated in a pan directly over a heat source because it will burn and cannot be used.

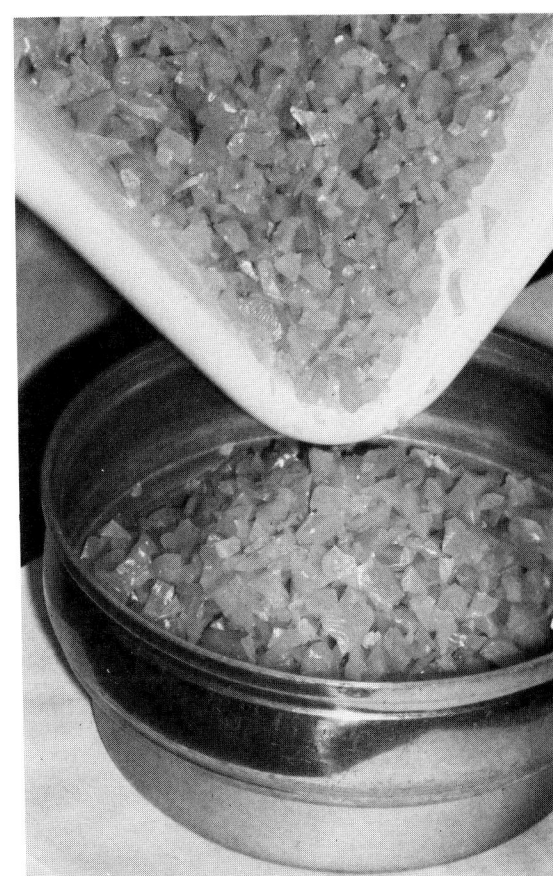

**Fig. 7-15.** Agar in top portion of double boiler.

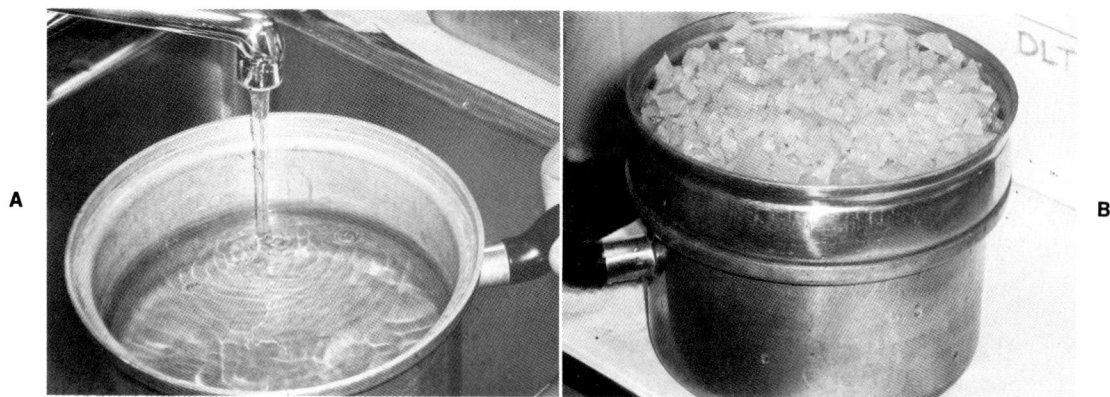

**Fig. 7-16. A,** Water in bottom half. **B,** Use good amount of water but allow for top part of double boiler to seat in bottom half.

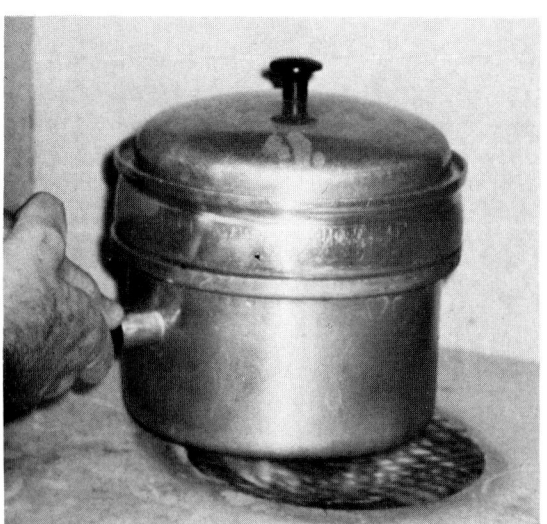

**Fig. 7-17.** Filled double boiler placed on fire and permitted to boil.

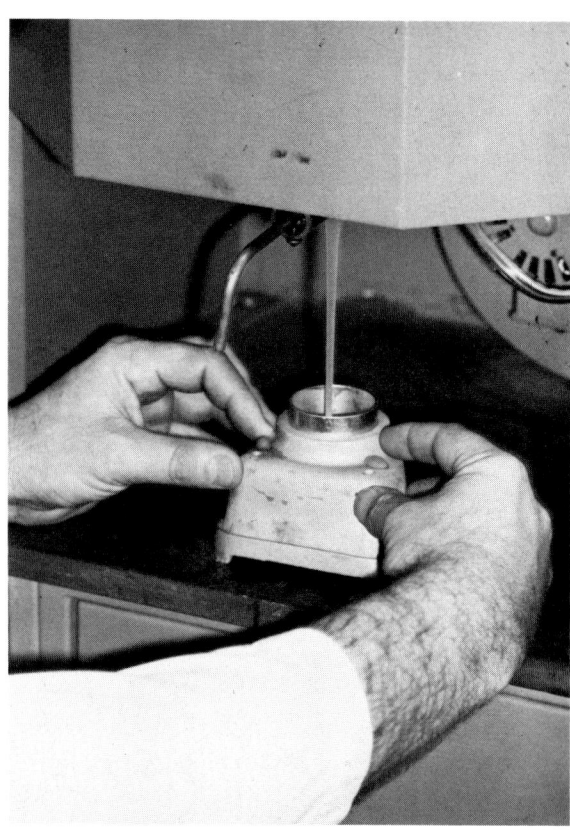

**Fig. 7-18.** When agar is kept in storage unit, it is ready to use any time of day. Flask is centered under pouring spout and valve turned on until stream is about diameter of lead pencil.

8. Fill the duplicating flask with agar hydrocolloid duplicating material. If the storage unit is used, center the duplicating flask under the pouring spout, and open the valve. A stream the diameter of a lead pencil is desired (Fig. 7-18). When using the double boiler, pour from it slowly so the stream is the diameter of pencil lead (Fig. 7-19).

9. Continue to fill the flask until the agar starts to run out of the holes on top of the flask. Block the holes with modeling plastic (Fig. 7-20) until the flask and reservoir are completely filled (Fig. 7-21).

10. Cool the duplicating material in the flask in an exacting manner. It should be placed on a tray of cool running tap water (Fig. 7-22). The water should contact only the base of the flask (Fig. 7-23). Cooling the base of the flask causes the hydrocolloid to shrink in the direction of the lower temperature or

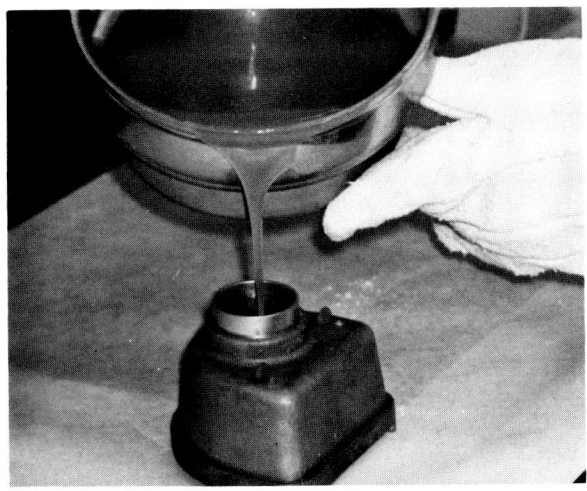

**Fig. 7-19.** When double boiler is used, care must be taken to pour agar slowly so flask does not fill too rapidly.

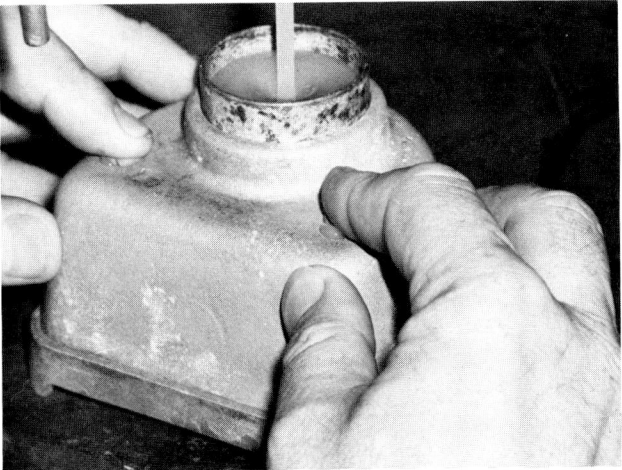

**Fig. 7-20.** Block holes in flask with modeling plastic when agar starts to flow out. Then continue to fill flask.

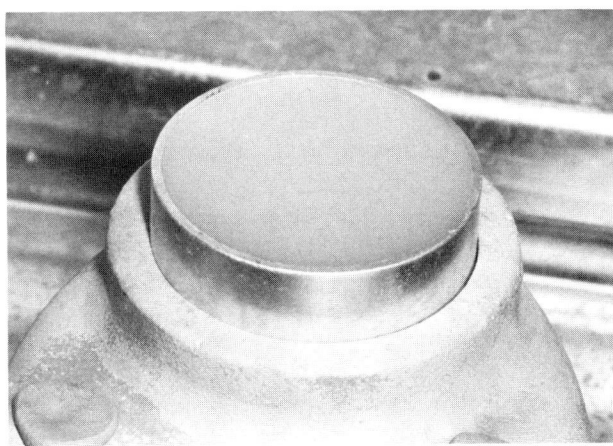

**Fig. 7-21.** Duplicating flask completely filled with agar.

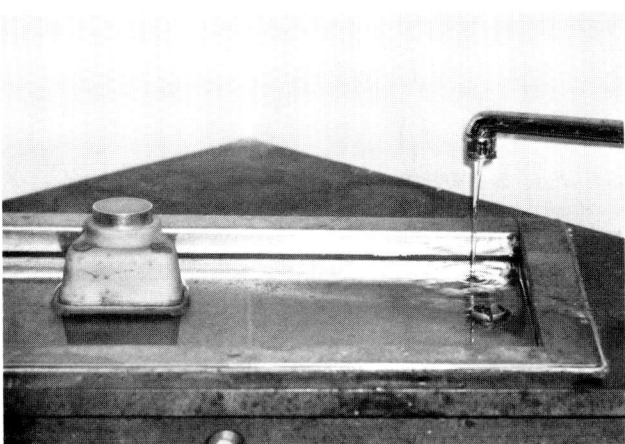

**Fig. 7-22.** Tray of running tap water. Tray is constructed so water level will not be higher than base of duplicating flask.

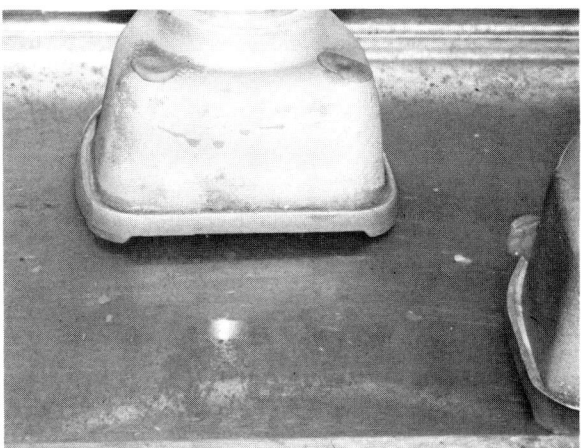

**Fig. 7-23.** Running tap water contacts only base of flask.

toward the cast, thus causing it to adapt more closely to the cast. The reservoir ring supplies the additional material needed to compensate for the shrinkage. Leave the flask in the water for at least 45 minutes to cool it completely. A cross section of the cooled agar in the reservoir shows how much it has shrunk on cooling (Fig. 7-24). NOTE: The flask should not be cooled in ice water because this makes it too cold and causes distortion.

11. Remove the flask from the water and remove the reservoir ring (Fig. 7-25). Use a sharp knife, and trim the hydrocolloid flush with the top of the flask (Fig. 7-26).

12. Invert the flask, and gently twist and remove the base of the flask (Fig. 7-27).

13. If the modeling plastic retentions were not removed with the base, they should be removed now (Fig. 7-28).

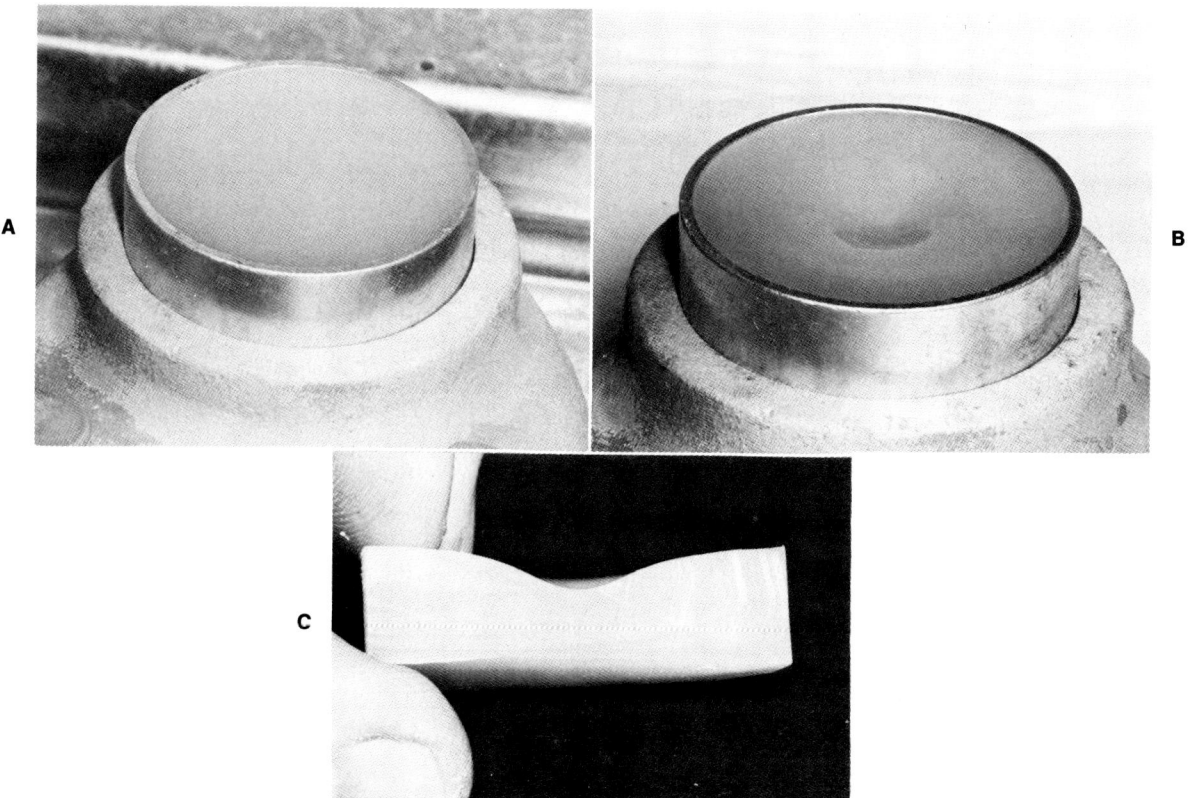

Fig. 7-24. Additional material is fed into body of flask from reservoir as hydrocolloid cools. **A,** Freshly filled reservoir. **B,** Same reservoir after it has cooled. **C,** Cross section of agar removed from reservoir after cooling.

Duplication and refractory casts    **213**

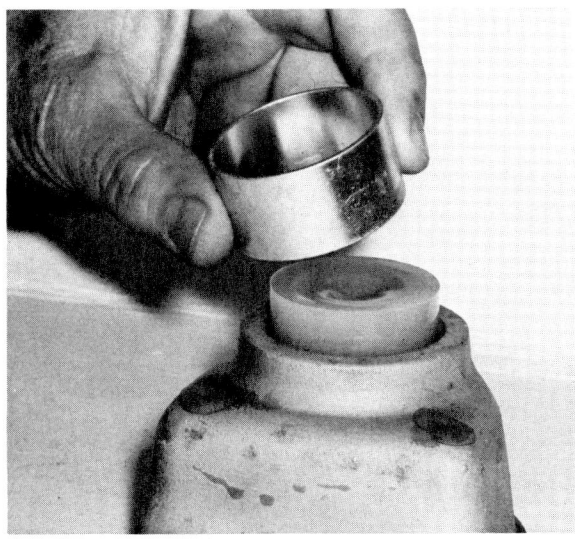

Fig. 7-25. Reservoir ring removed from flask after it has cooled.

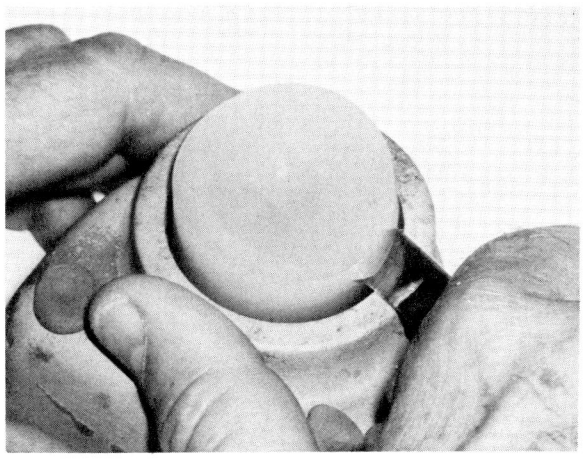

Fig. 7-26. Sharp knife is used to trim hydrocolloid flush with top of flask.

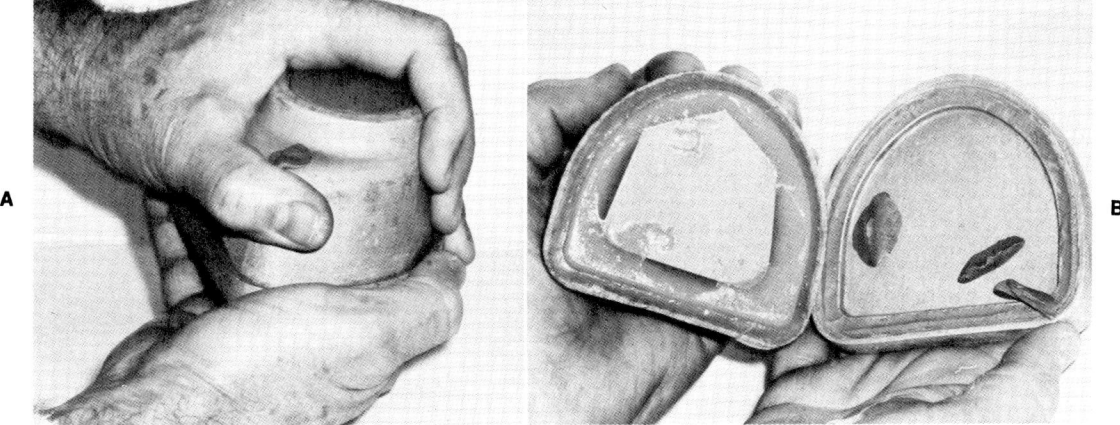

Fig. 7-27. **A,** Gently twist base, and remove it from flask. **B,** Base removed.

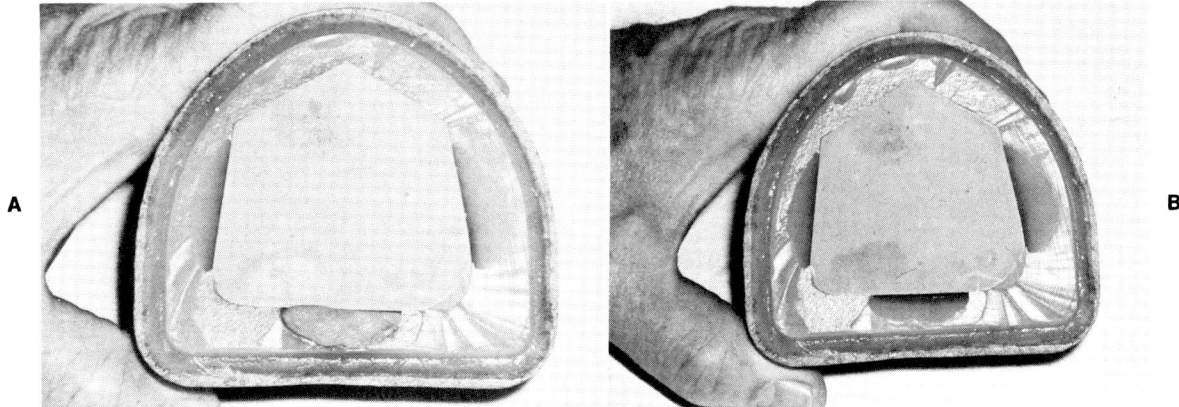

Fig. 7-28. **A,** Modeling plastic retentions often remain in duplication. **B,** Modeling plastic wedges removed.

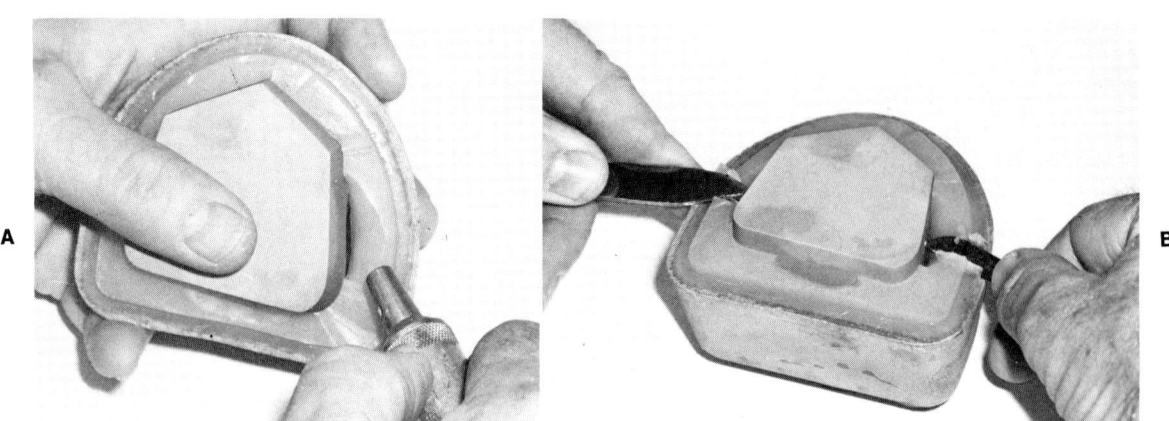

Fig. 7-29. **A,** Blow air to loosen, and remove cast from mold. **B,** Removing cast from flask with knife.

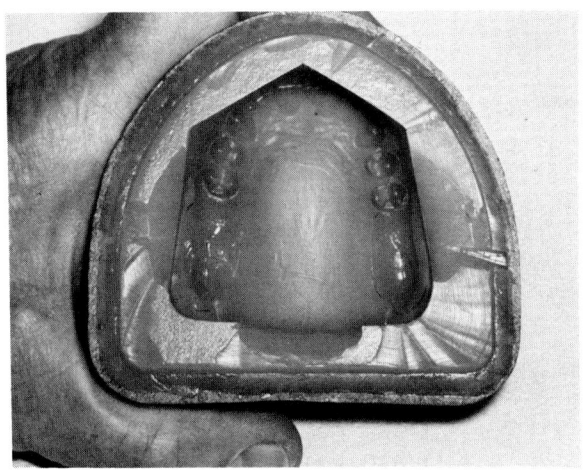

Fig. 7-30. Hydrocolloid mold ready to be filled with investment.

14. Insert the tips of two knives in the depression on each side of the cast made by the small mounds of modeling clay that held the cast. Pry upward using a swift action and equal pressure on both knives. NOTE: The cast may be loosened first with gentle blasts of air around the borders of the cast base (Fig. 7-29).

15. After the cast is removed, examine the hydrocolloid carefully for tears or voids. Tears may indicate that the hydrocolloid is old or spoiled and needs replacing. If it is acceptable, pour it immediately (Fig. 7-30).

## INVESTMENT CAST

Most gold alloys are cast into gypsum-bound silica investment. Cobalt-chromium alloys that solidify at a temperature of about 1300° C also use a gypsum binder. Ticonium 100* is an example of these metals. Other cobalt-chromium alloys that have solidifying temperatures above 1300° C, such as Vitallium,† must use a binder other than gypsum, such as organic and inorganic silicates and phosphates. These are usually referred to as phosphate-bound investments, and they are also used with high-fusing gold and other alloys to which porcelain is fused.

All investment or refractory casts abrade easily and must be handled carefully to preserve the accuracy of their surfaces.

Investments vary considerably in the manner in which they obtain their expansion. The water-powder ratio is very critical, and the manufacturer's directions should be followed precisely.

In this book, the procedure for making a low–gold content alloy‡ casting will be discussed. Most cobalt-chromium alloys are controlled by franchises. Each company has a system of compatible materials and equipment, as well as detailed instructions for their use. For best results their recommended techniques should be kept pure and should not consist of a mixture of different manufacturer's materials and techniques.

One of the cobalt-chromium franchises was Durallium. J. F. Jelenko & Company purchased the Durallium Company in 1971. At that time the company's alloys, materials, and equipment were made

---

*Ticonium 100, Ticonium Co., Albany, N.Y.
†Vitallium, Howmedica, Inc., Chicago, Ill.
‡Jelenko alloy, J. F. Jelenko & Co., New Rochelle, N.Y.

available under the Jelenko name to all dentists and laboratories.

They presently market two alloys; JD and LG. JD is similar both physically and chemically to some of the popular franchised alloys, whereas LG relates closer to the handling properties of gold and is an exclusive with Jelenko. In addition, they supply a complete line of investment, abrasives, materials, and equipment necessary to fabricate partial dentures of these alloys.

### PROCEDURE

1. Pour the investment into the mold immediately. Use a good-quality model investment for gold* (Fig. 7-31).

---

*Gray Investment, The Ransom & Randolph Co., Toledo, Ohio

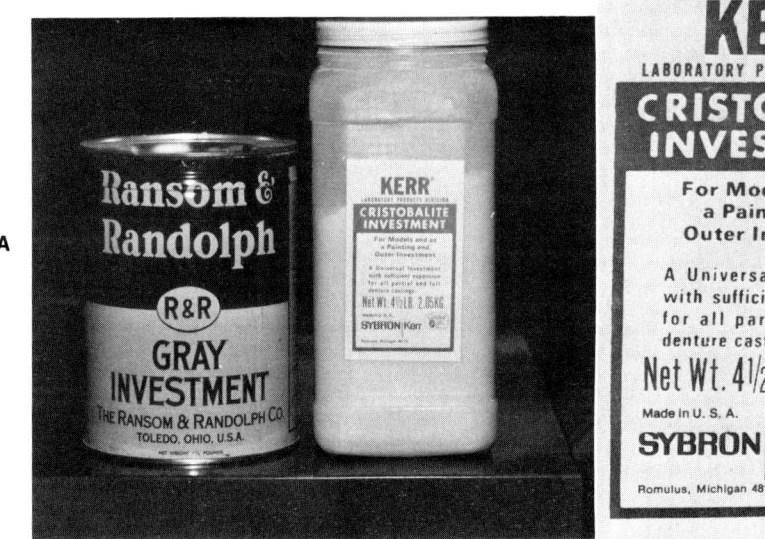
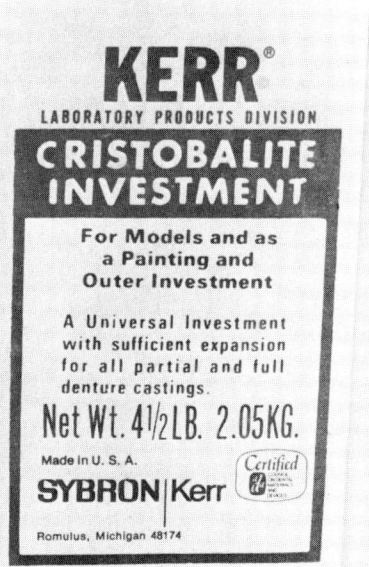

**Fig. 7-31. A,** Use a high-quality model investment to vibrate into mold. **B,** Typical model investment. **C,** Follow manufacturer's directions for water-powder ratio.

2. The water-powder ratio for christobalite* investment for models is thirty-one parts water to one hundred parts powder by weight. It must be weighed accurately with good scales such as the triple beam balance† (Fig. 7-32). For most casts, 200 gm of investment is enough. Be sure to follow the manufacturer's recommendations for the water-powder ratio, and use accurate scales.

---

*Cristobalite Model Investment, Kerr Manufacturing Co., Romulus, Mich.
†Triple beam balance, Ohaus Scale Corp., Florham Park, N.J.

3. Add the powder to the water. Mechanical-vacuum mixing for 30 seconds is preferred for the cast (Fig. 7-33). If mixing by hand, spatulate for 60 seconds. The outer investment should not be vacuumed.

4. Mechanical vibration is needed because the mix will be thick. Add very small portions of the mix to each tooth that will be clasped first, then add to one posterior extension of the mold (Fig. 7-34). Observe the flow of the mix across the surface of the mold and into each tooth impression. Make sure that air is not trapped in tooth impression. Continue

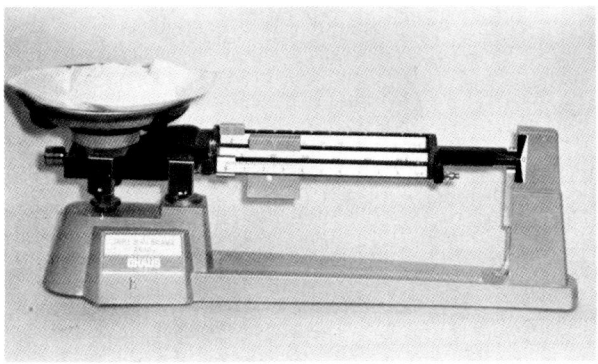

**Fig. 7-32.** Measure water and weigh powder very accurately. It is essential to have good scales as illustrated.

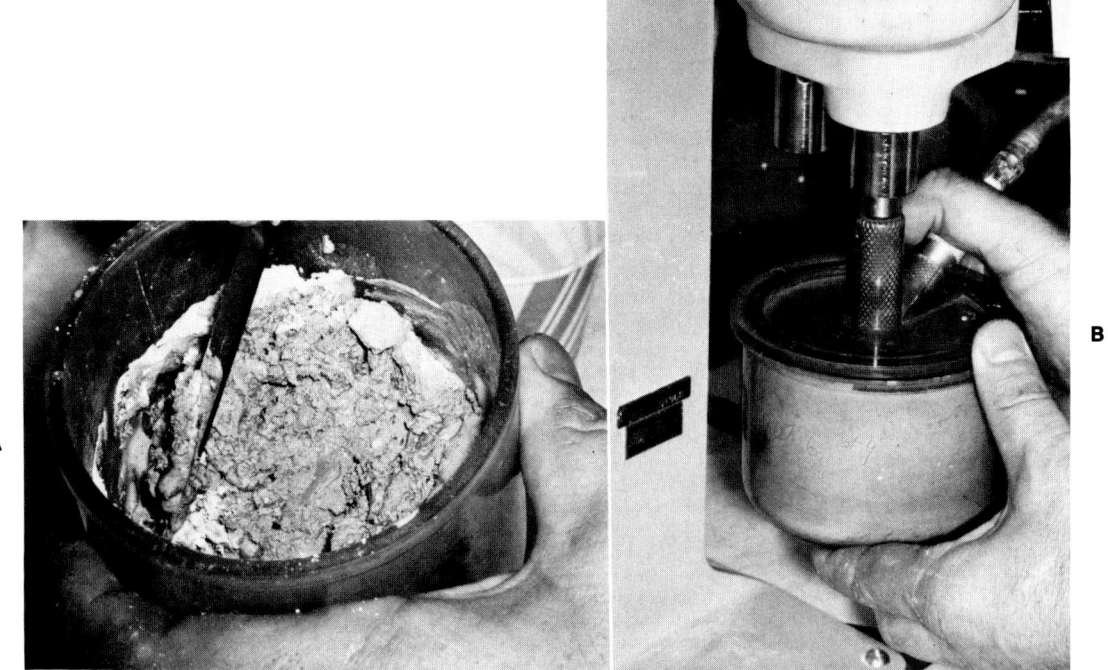

**Fig. 7-33. A,** Add powder to water, and mix with spatula until investment is wet. **B,** Vacuumed mechanical mix of investment is preferred for cast.

until the mold is filled (Fig. 7-35). The investment should not be vibrated into the mold from one position only, as with an impression, because the salts are vibrated out of the investment and collect in concentrated areas, making refractory cast inaccurate. Do not allow the investment to extend to the sides of the flask, since this restrains the setting expansion and causes distortion (Fig. 7-36).

5. Permit the investment to set for 1 hour, then separate it from the duplicating material very carefully.

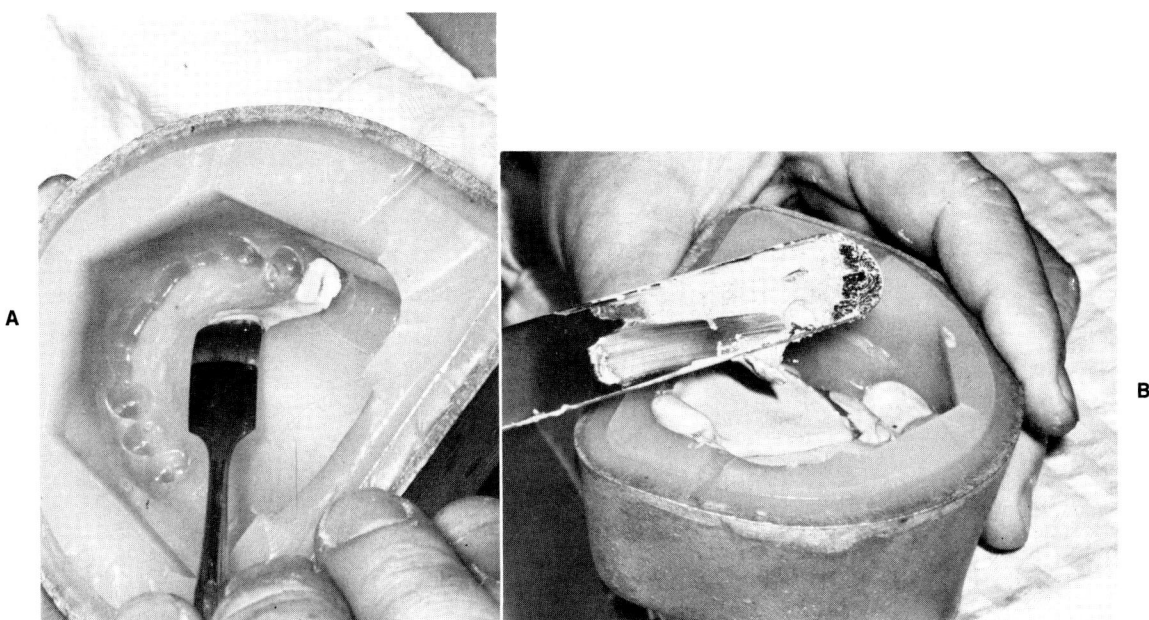

**Fig. 7-34.** Investment is vibrated into mold in small increments. **A,** First, vibrate very small amount into each tooth that is to be clasped. **B,** Second, vibrate investment into remaining teeth and continue until mold is filled.

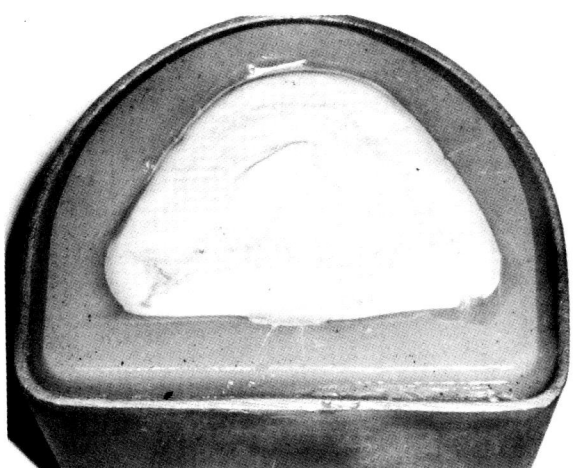

**Fig. 7-35.** Mold is properly filled with investment mix.

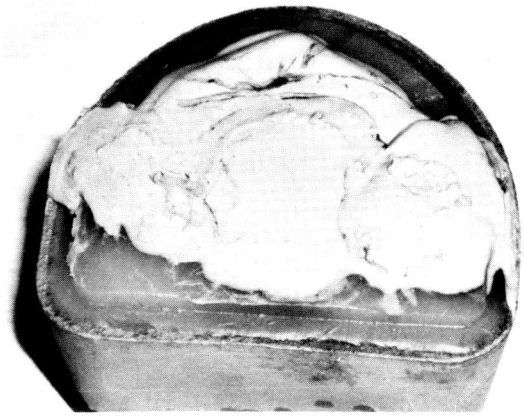

**Fig. 7-36.** This mold is overfilled, and investment touching sides of flask may restrict expansion and cause significant distortion in refractory cast.

6. Do not pry the cast from the mold. Remove the hydrocolloid with the cast from the body of the duplicating flask in one piece. This may be accomplished by inserting a knife blade through the duplicating material in the reservoir until it rests on the internal lip of the reservoir, then rotate the knife blade horizontally to free the duplicating material in the reservoir (Fig. 7-37). Place the thumbs in the reservoir, and apply pressure to the hydrocolloid (Fig. 7-38). Cut the hydrocolloid very carefully in four or five places, and use extreme caution when peeling it from the refractory cast (Fig. 7-39). Do not mar the cast. Do not touch the anatomic portion of the refractory cast at this time because it will be very soft.

7. It may be necessary to trim the base to make it fit the casting ring (Fig. 7-40). Trimming may be done in several ways, but, no matter how it is trimmed, the surface of the cast should be handled very carefully.

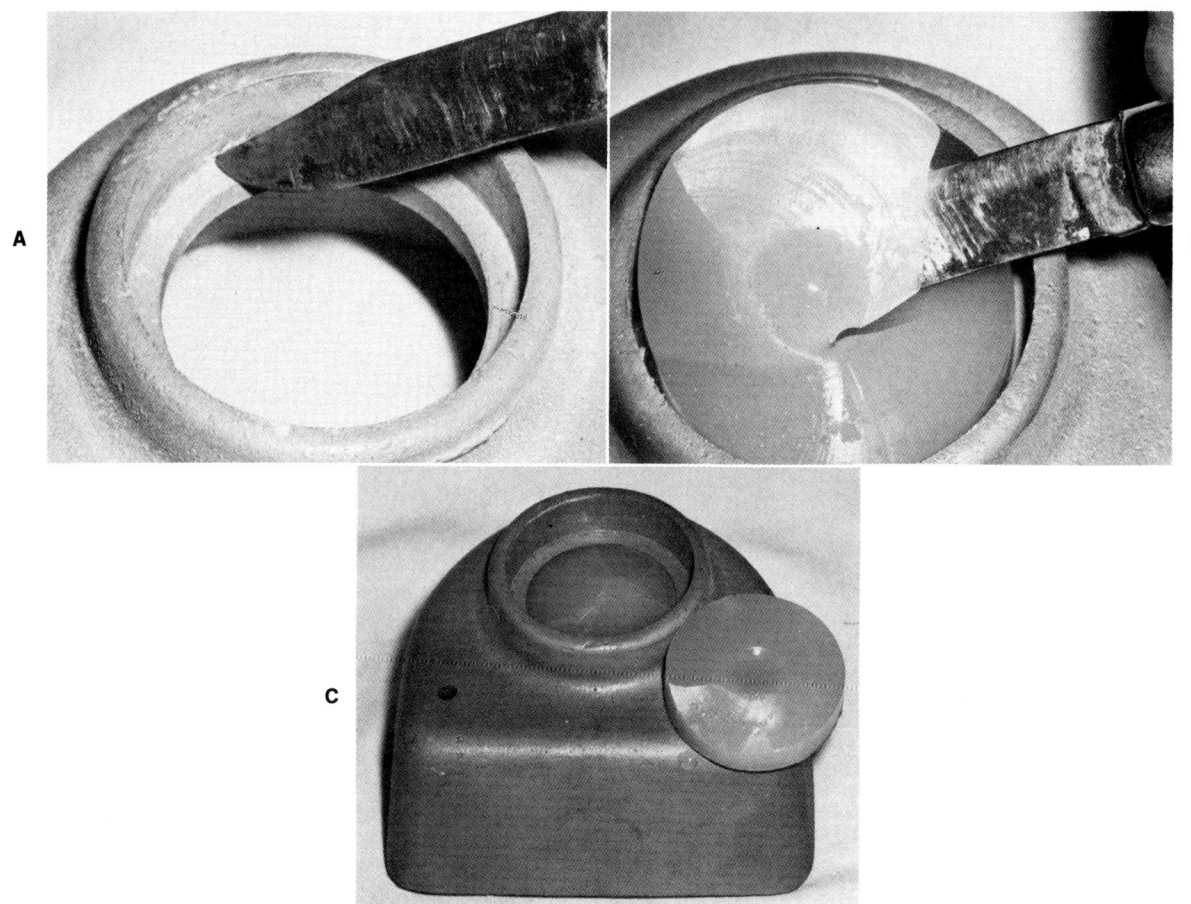

**Fig. 7-37. A,** Knife blade is placed on inside lip of spout to guide it in removing agar. **B,** Knife is turned in complete circle. **C,** Agar in neck is removed.

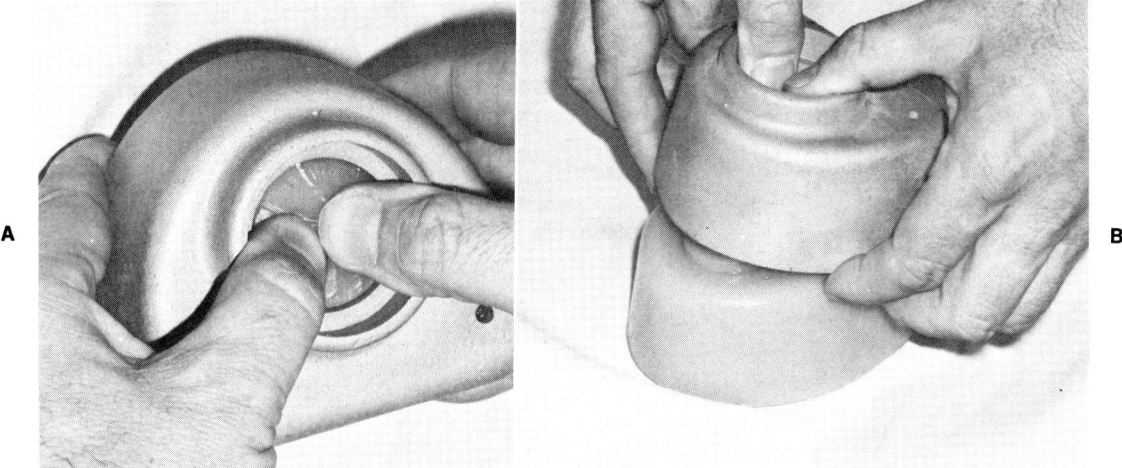

**Fig. 7-38.** Push duplicating material and cast from body of flask by inserting thumbs in reservoir and applying pressure to hydrocolloid. **A,** Hold flask in this manner when applying pressure. **B,** Hydrocolloid and refractory cast removed in one piece.

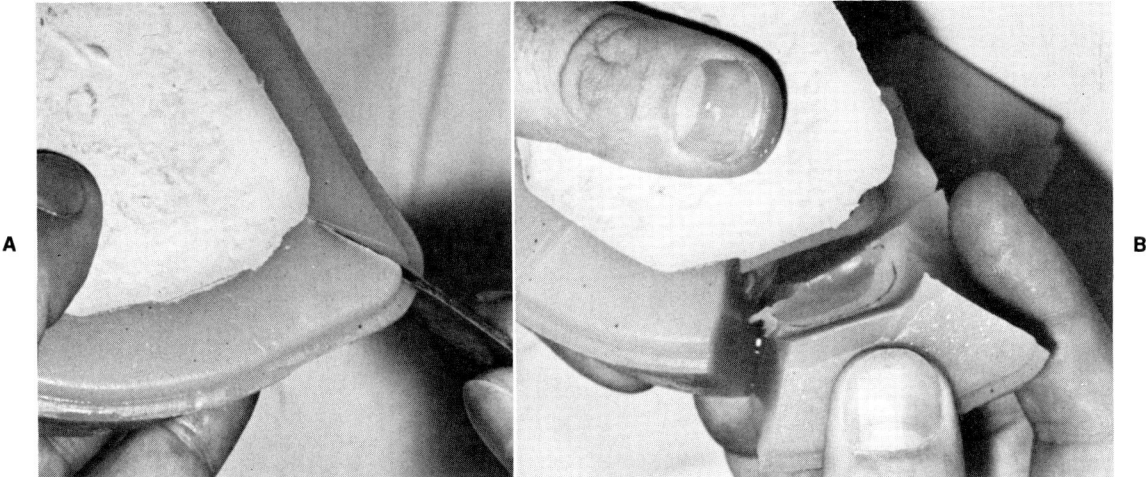

**Fig. 7-39. A,** Cut agar in four or five sections. (Do not touch cast.) **B,** Peel hydrocolloid carefully from refractory cast, making certain that none remains on cast.

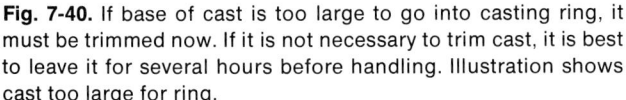

**Fig. 7-40.** If base of cast is too large to go into casting ring, it must be trimmed now. If it is not necessary to trim cast, it is best to leave it for several hours before handling. Illustration shows cast too large for ring.

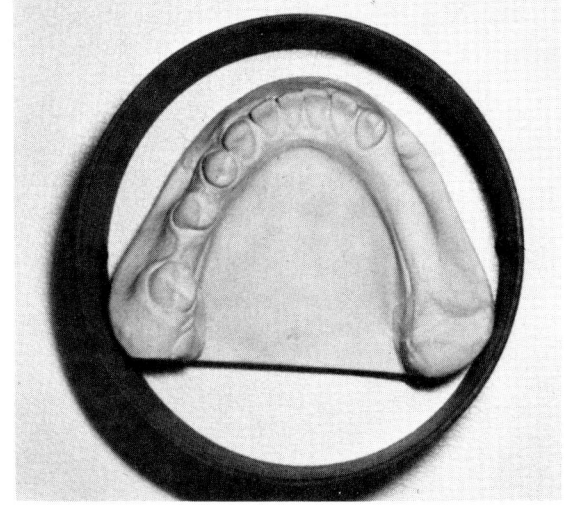

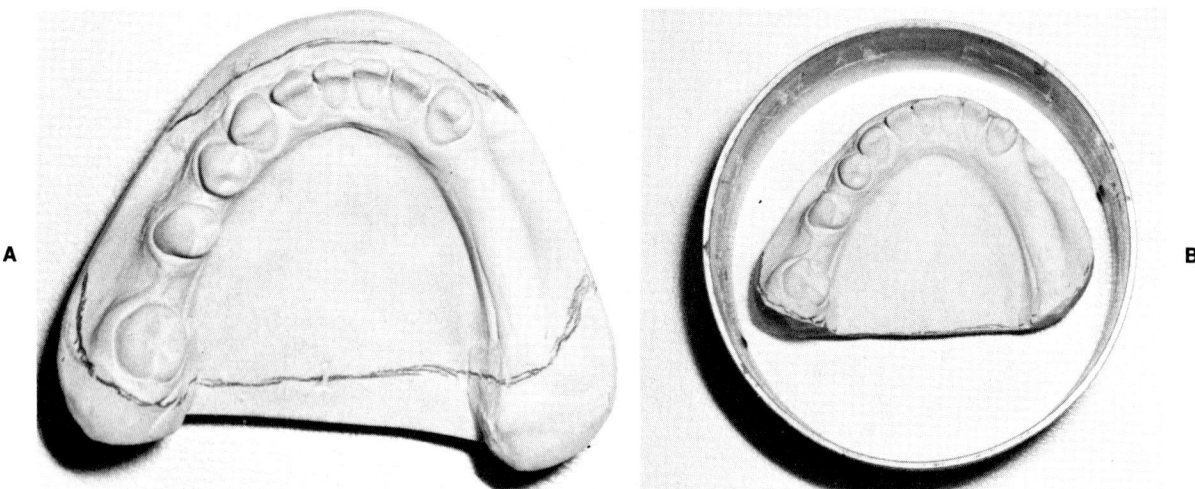

**Fig. 7-41. A,** Line is sketched on cast to act as guide when trimming to size with Bard-Parker knife. **B,** Trimmed cast fits ring.

a. *Preferred method.* If trimming is necessary, shape the cast immediately after the hydrocolloid has been removed from it. It is still very friable and can be trimmed easily with a Bard-Parker knife. *Caution:* Since the cast is relatively soft, the teeth and soft tissue area to be contacted by the metal framework should not be touched because they can be abraded very easily. Scribe line on the cast ¼ inch (0.63 cm) outside the posterior and lateral limits of the extent of the framework, and trim the cast to that point (Fig. 7-41).

b. *Alternate method.* When the cast is still wet, shape it carefully on the model trimmer. The danger here is that water from the model trimmer may wash away some of the surface of the still soft cast, and the splatter from the grinding will be difficult, if not impossible, to remove without damage to the cast.

c. *Alternate method.* Permit the cast to dry thoroughly, then shape it with a grinding wheel on a lathe. In this method, it is difficult to remove the debris from grinding that collects on the surface of the cast without damage to the surface. In addition, the vibration of the grinding wheel may damage the cast as it cuts.

If possible, it is best to avoid touching the anatomic portion of the cast until after it is treated with wax or sealed with model spray. In reality, it is usually necessary to remove some imperfections before the cast is treated; however, contact should be very minimal and

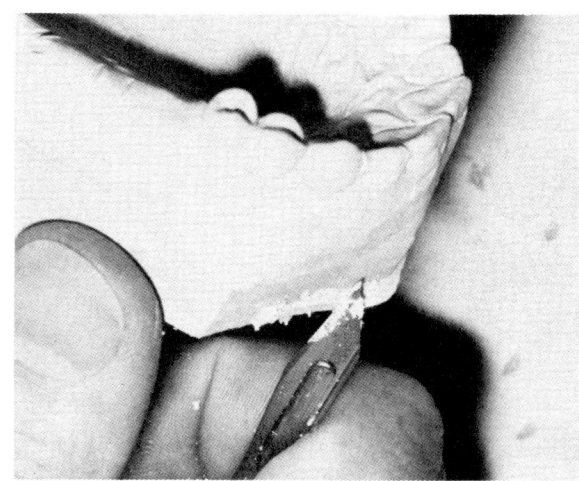

**Fig. 7-42.** Very carefully remove any imperfections with knife or instrument. Note position of hands so that contact with teeth and soft tissue areas of cast is avoided.

should avoid as much as possible the eventual outline of the metal framework (Fig. 7-42). NOTE: Do not wash the cast with water or slurry water. It is best to use gentle blasts of air to remove any debris from the cast (Fig. 7-43).

8. Save the reversible hydrocolloid, and wash it to remove all traces of investment (Fig. 7-44).

9. Cut the hydrocolloid into small pieces, and place it in a closed container or plastic bag to prevent it from drying out (Fig. 7-45).

## Duplication and refractory casts  221

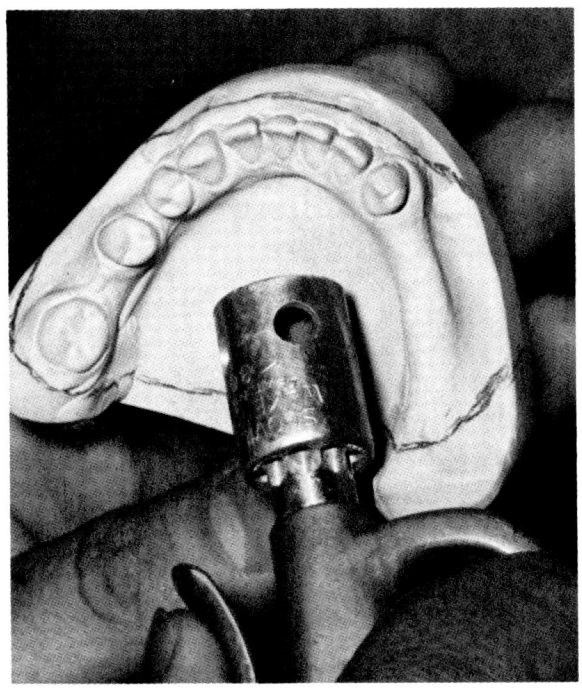

**Fig. 7-43.** Use gentle blasts of air to remove debris from cast. Do not wash it in tap water or slurry water.

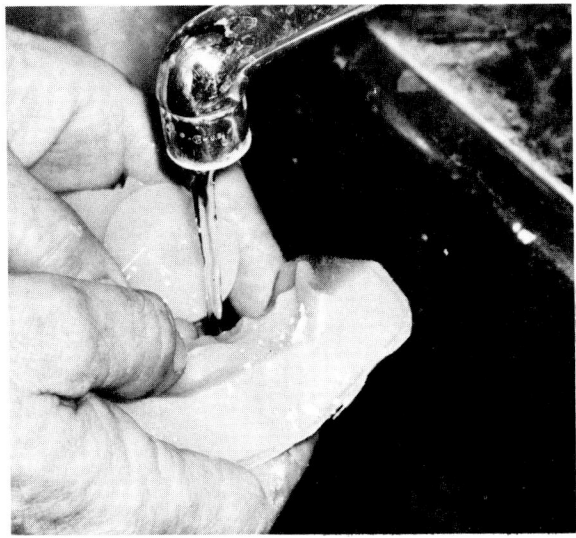

**Fig. 7-44.** Wash reversible hydrocolloid to remove all traces of investment.

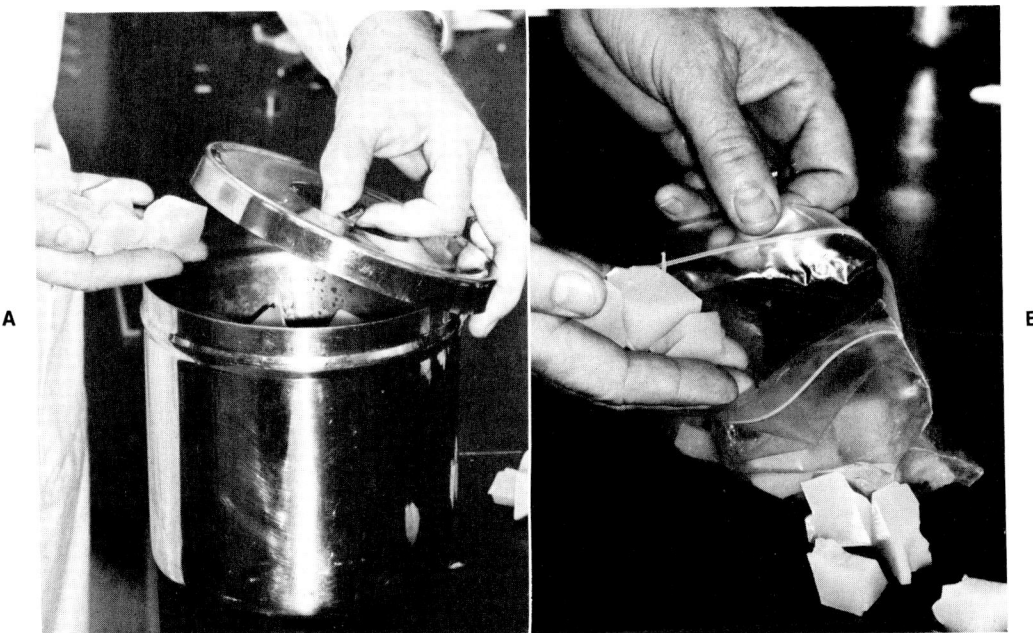

**Fig. 7-45.** Cut hydrocolloid into small pieces, and store it in closed container **(A)** or plastic bag **(B)**.

10. The trimmed and cleaned cast is ready for treating with wax or model spray (Fig. 7-46).

### PROBLEM AREAS

The principal problems associated with duplication and pouring the refractory cast are related to improper temperature control of the duplicating material, using duplicating material too long, improper cooling procedures, incorrect water-powder ratio for the investment material, and abrading the refractory cast (Table 7-1). Careful attention during each phase of the duplication and pouring procedures will significantly reduce errors and maintain accuracy.

### Treating the refractory cast

The surface of the refractory cast is treated by one of two methods that will be described separately. When the casts are treated with either model spray or wax, the surface is hardened to make it less susceptible to abrasion, assure a smooth dense surface on which to wax the framework, eliminate soaking

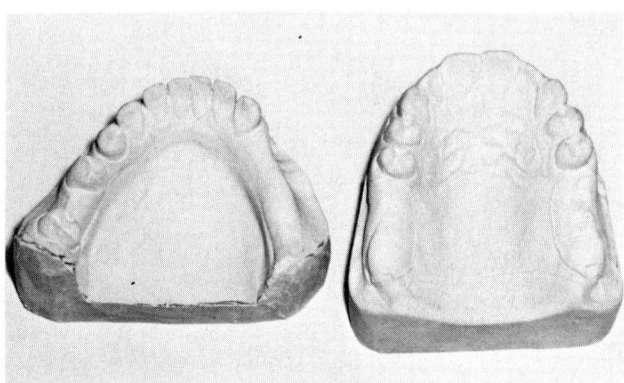

**Fig. 7-46.** Trimmed cast ready for treating with wax or model spray.

**Table 7-1.** Duplication and refractory casts

| Problem | Probable cause | Solution |
| --- | --- | --- |
| Blockout and relief wax melted by reversible hydrocolloid | Reversible hydrocolloid too hot | Cool liquefied reversible hydrocolloid to approximately 135° F (57° C) before duplicating |
| Hydrocolloid mold damaged during master cast retrieval | Master cast blockout inadequate | Block out undesirable undercuts to permit removal of master cast from mold |
| Metal frameworks do not fit master cast | Reversible hydrocolloid duplicating material used too long | Record duplications from each batch of hydrocolloid; change to new material at predetermined intervals; make test casting to check duplication accuracy |
|  | Mold cooled improperly | Cool mold in water bath as directed; do not chill in ice water |
|  | Incorrect water-powder ratio used for investment cast | Follow manufacturer's recommendations for water-powder ratio; coordinate with alloy used |
|  | Refractory cast abraded by handling | Take care to avoid unnecessary finger contact with cast |

the refractory cast prior to applying the paint-on layer of investment, and drive excess moisture from the cast.

### Model spray
**PROCEDURE**

1. Immediately on removing the hydrocolloid from the refractory cast, remove the surface moisture with a gentle blast of air, and spray the anatomic portion of the cast (Fig. 7-47) with model spray.* Two even light coats are essential. Allow 2 or 3 minutes drying time between coats.

2. In a few minutes, the spray will dry on the refractory casts, and they can be shaped to size on a model trimmer with water and a fine-cut wheel. Cleaning the casts by rinsing them lightly in water will not have any effects on them (Fig. 7-48).

---

*J. F. Jelenko & Co., New Rochelle, N.Y.

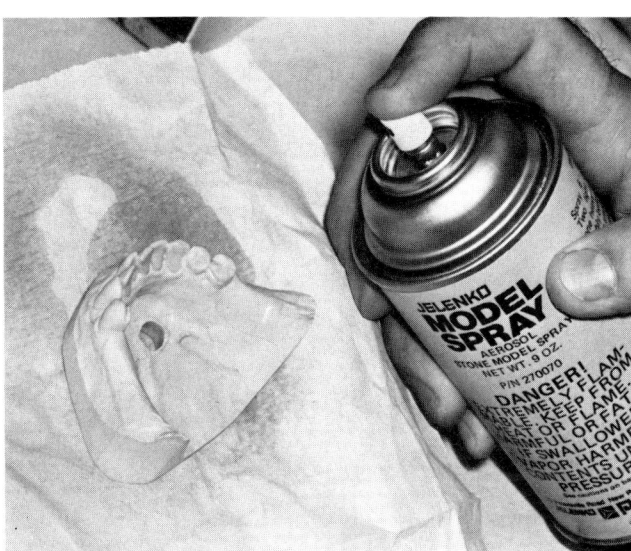

**Fig. 7-47.** For model spray procedure, cast is dried with gentle blast of air and sprayed with two coats of model spray.

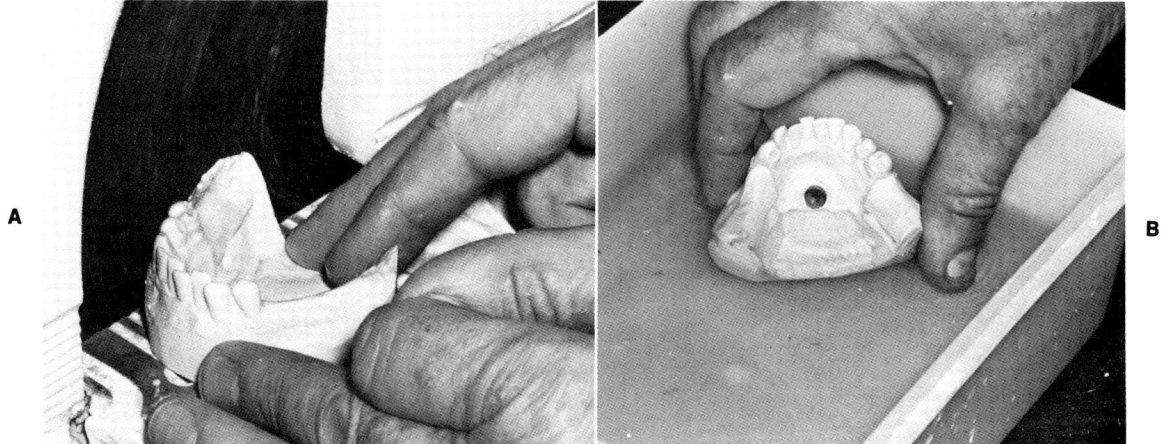

**Fig. 7-48. A,** After cast is coated with model spray, it may be ground to shape and size on model trimmer. **B,** Cast may be rinsed in water lightly without damage to cast.

3. Do not trim the cast closer than ¼ inch (0.63 cm) to the proposed framework. There must be a minimum of ¼-inch clearance between the sides of the cast and the ring (Fig. 7-49).

4. Casts are placed in a drying oven at a temperature between 180° and 200° F (82° and 93.5° C) for a period of 2 to 3 hours, depending on the amount of material in the oven (Fig. 7-50).

5. Remove the casts from the oven one at a time, and spray them completely (top and bottom) while warm (Fig. 7-51). NOTE: If the spray is applied too generously, it may form an undesirable coating on the surface of the cast, and if it is not applied evenly, it may leave an uneven film on the cast. When spray is used on the casts, they must not be dipped in wax at any time.

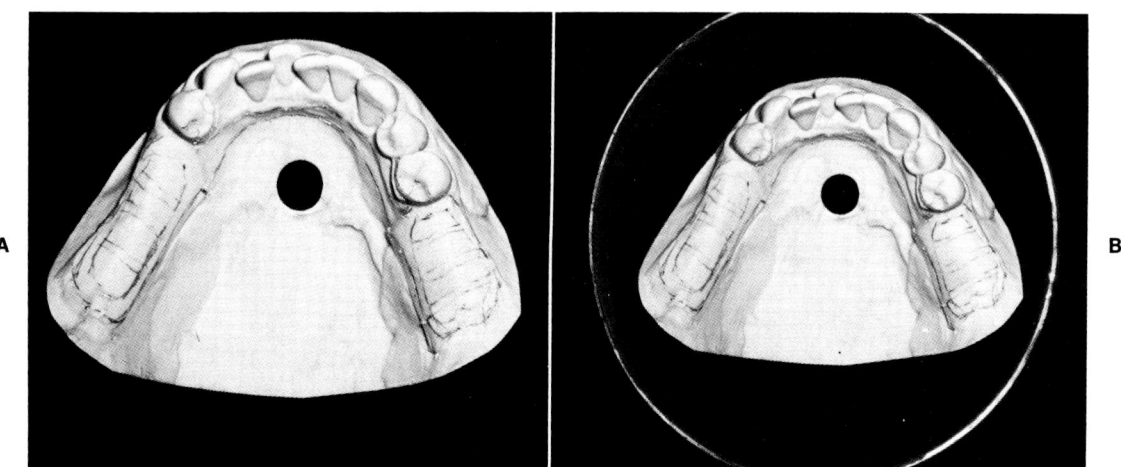

**Fig. 7-49. A,** Cast is trimmed to within ¼ inch (0.63 cm) of proposed framework. **B,** Cast should clear sides of casting ring by ¼ (0.63 cm).

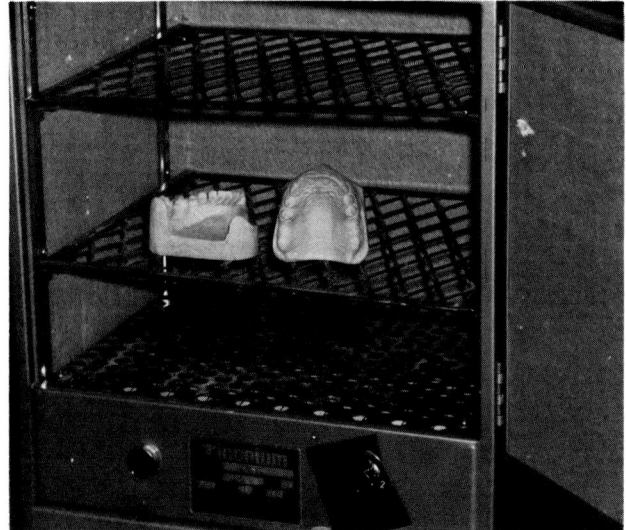

**Fig. 7-50.** Casts are permitted to dry in drying oven for period of 2 to 3 hours in temperature, ranging between 180° to 200° F (82° to 93.5° C).

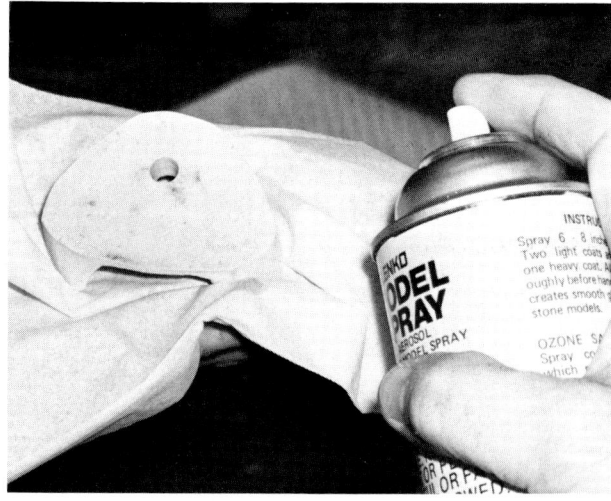

**Fig. 7-51.** Cast is sprayed again while it is still warm. Be sure entire cast is covered with thin coating of spray.

## Wax

**PROCEDURE**

1. Immediately on removal of the refractory cast from the hydrocolloid, trim it with a Bard-Parker knife if necessary (Fig. 7-52). Be careful not to touch the surface of the cast that will be covered by the framework.

2. Do not trim the cast closer than 1/4 inch to the proposed framework. There must be a minimum of 1/4-inch clearance between the sides of the cast and the ring (Fig. 7-53).

3. Place the casts in a drying oven for 2 to 3 hours. The temperature of the oven should be between 180° and 200° F (Fig. 7-54).

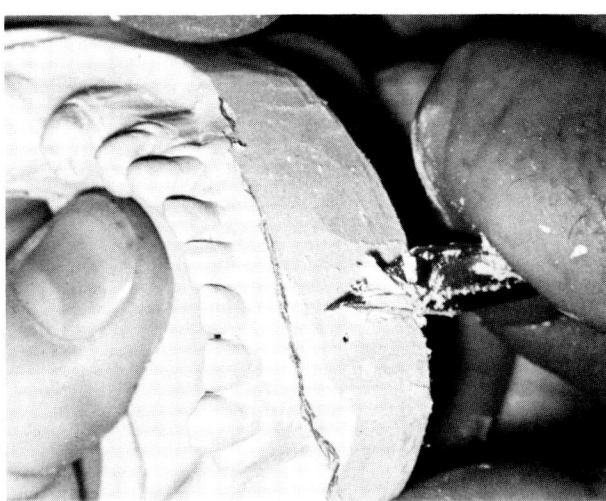

**Fig. 7-52.** For wax dipping procedure, cast is trimmed with sharp Bard-Parker knife. Do not touch surface of cast that will be covered by framework.

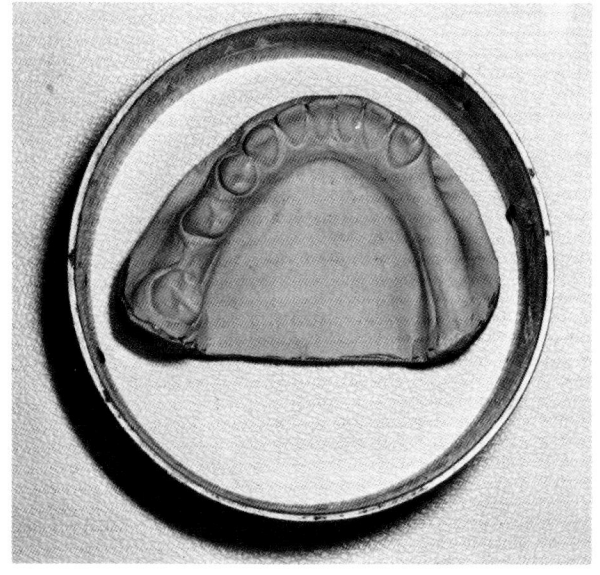

**Fig. 7-53.** There must be at least 1/4-inch (0.63-cm) clearance between cast and ring.

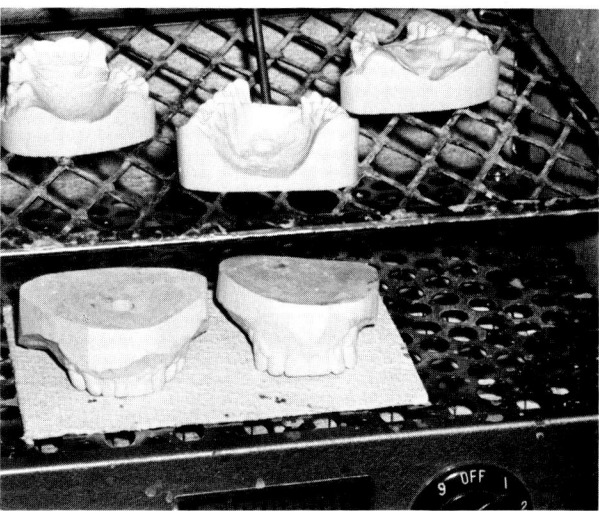

**Fig. 7-54.** Casts in drying oven for 2 to 3 hours at 180° F (82° C).

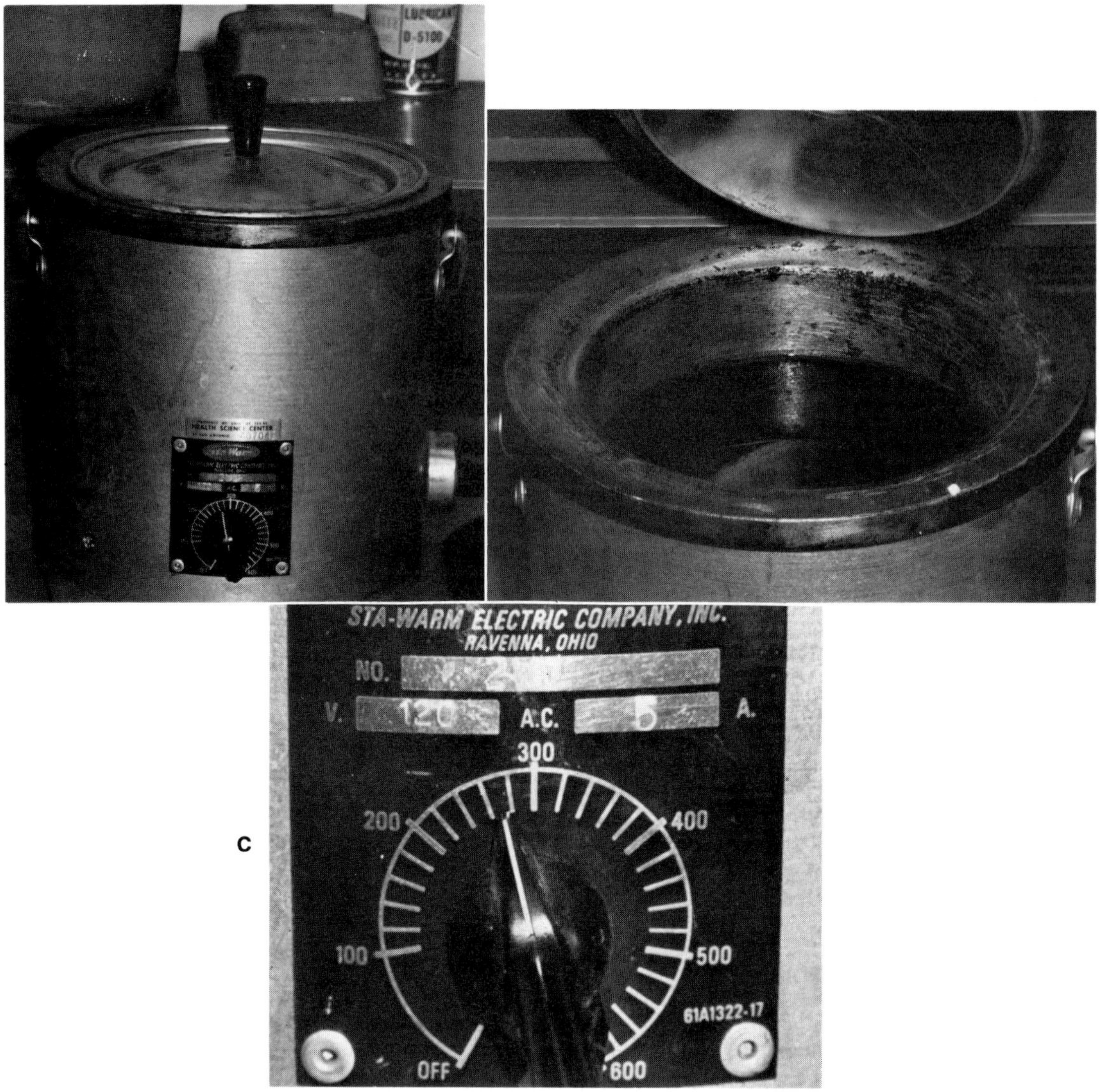

**226** *Dental laboratory procedures: removable partial dentures*

**Fig. 7-55. A,** Wax pot. **B,** Melted beeswax in pot. **C,** Melted beeswax in wax pot should be held between 280° to 300° F (130° to 149° C).

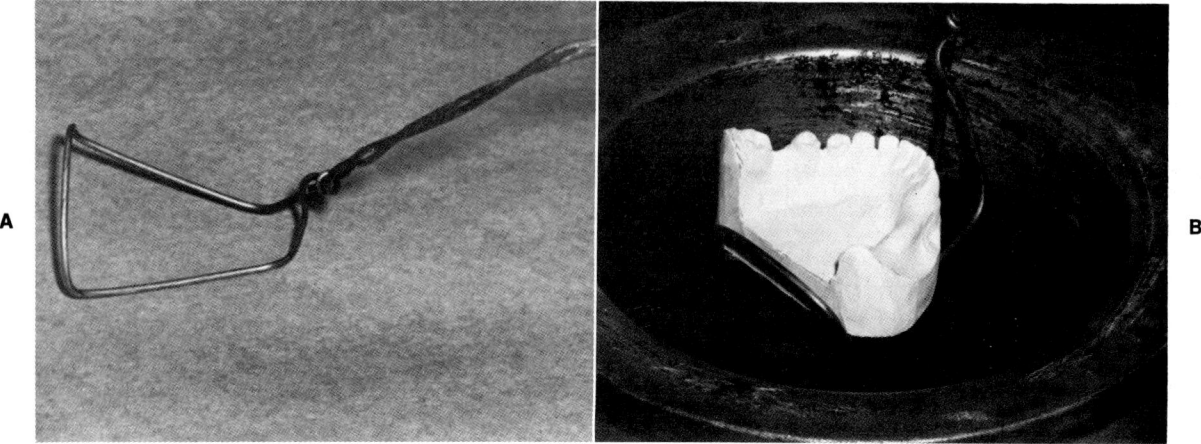

**Fig. 7-56. A,** Suitable holder for dipping cast may be made from wire coat hanger. **B,** Using wire holder cast is immersed in hot beeswax.

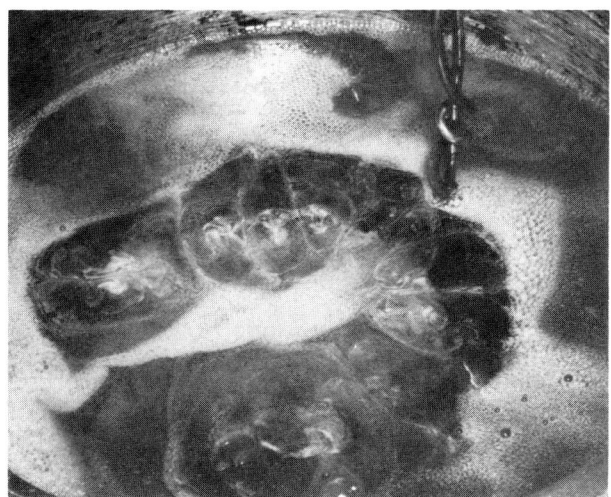

Fig. 7-57. Cast remains in wax for 15 seconds after it starts to foam.

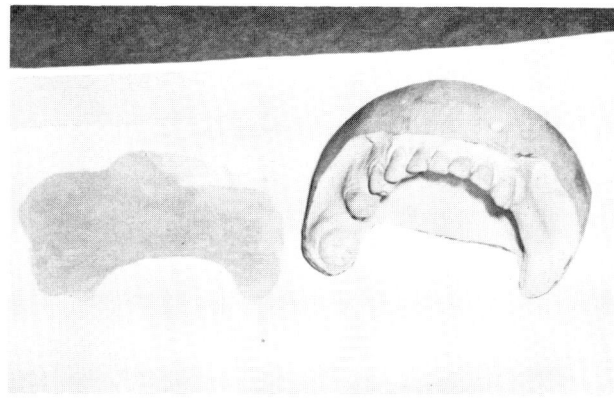

Fig. 7-58. Stand cast on end to drain when it is removed from hot wax. Move the cast frequently to prevent wax from building up as it drains.

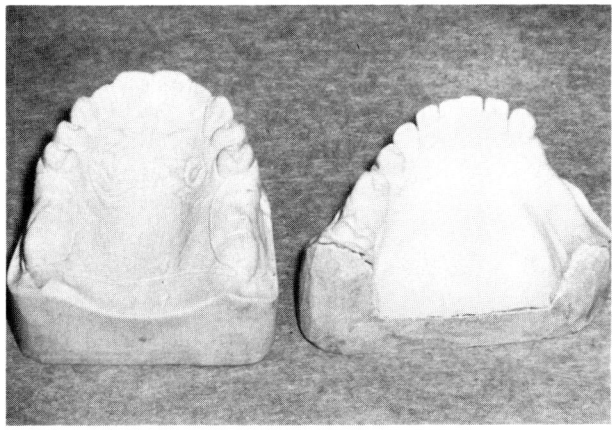

Fig. 7-59. Casts ready for transfer of design from master casts.

4. Refined beeswax is heated in a wax pot to a temperature of 280° to 300° F (138° to 149° C). Do not overheat the beeswax. The temperature is correct when the beeswax just begins to smoke (Fig. 7-55).

5. Using a cradle made of a coat hanger, or some other suitable holder, immerse the cast in the beeswax (Fig. 7-56). The wax will begin to foam after a few seconds. Let the cast remain in the pot for 15 seconds after the foaming begins (Fig. 7-57).

6. Remove the cast, and stand it on end on absorbent paper to drain off the excess wax (Fig. 7-58). Change the position of the cast frequently to prevent wax from collecting at the base of the cast.

7. When the cast has cooled, it is ready for design transfer from the master cast, and the framework is ready for waxing (Fig. 7-59).

## SUMMARY

In this chapter the procedures for making duplications and refractory casts were described. Although irreversible hydrocolloids are accurate enough for duplicating, the reversible hydrocolloids are usually used more extensively because they are less expensive. Step-by-step procedures for making molds and investment casts, as well as details for treating investment casts are helpful in maintaining accuracy in fabrication.

### BIBLIOGRAPHY

Air Force Manual 160-29: Dental laboratory technicians manual, United States Air Force, Washington, D.C., 1959, U.S. Government Printing Office.

Air Force Manual 162-6: Dental laboratory technology, United States Air Force, Washington, D.C., 1975, U.S. Government Printing Office.

Lanier, B. R., Rudd, K. D., and Strunk, R. R.: Making chromium-cobalt removable partial dentures: a modified technique, J. Prosthet. Dent. 25:197-205, Feb., 1971.

Martinelli, N.: Dental laboratory technology, ed. 2, St. Louis, 1975, The C. V. Mosby Co.

Sowter, J. B.: Dental laboratory technology: prosthodontic techniques, Chapel Hill, N.C., 1968, The University of North Carolina Press.

Zarb, G. A., Bergman, B., Clayton, J. A., and MacKay, H. F.: Prosthodontic treatment of partially edentulous patients, St. Louis, 1978, The C. V. Mosby Co.

# CHAPTER 8

# WAXING AND SPRUING

KENNETH D. RUDD, ROBERT M. MORROW, and GEORGE KNIGHT

**waxing** Contouring wax, and preformed wax or plastic patterns, to form the pattern for a removable partial denture framework.

**spruing** Attaching wax, metal, or plastic forms to the wax pattern to provide an entrance to the mold space and to serve as a reservoir of metal during the casting procedure.

After the master cast is duplicated to make a refractory cast, it is necessary to transfer the design to the refractory cast and complete the wax pattern. In this chapter, waxing and spruing procedures for removable partial dentures will be discussed.

## DESIGN TRANSFER

The outline of the framework can be transferred from the master cast to the refractory cast and positioned quite accurately without using a surveyor. The relief, blockout, and beading can be easily seen on the refractory cast. The ledges reproduced from the blockout permit outlines of the clasps to be drawn exactly as they are on the master cast. When drawing on a refractory cast, always use a wax pencil, never a graphite pencil. Any color wax pencil is acceptable, although brown is usually preferred. The outline of the major connectors on the maxillary cast can be drawn easily by following the beads (Fig. 8-1), and the major connectors on the mandibular cast can be outlined by following visible landmarks (Fig. 8-2). The rest of the outline can be approximated by following the design on the master cast (Fig. 8-3). When outlining the lingual plating, whether it is on the anterior or posterior teeth, it is crucial to draw the superior margin of the plate occlusal to the survey line, which is where the blockout wax ended on the master cast. This area can be seen on the refractory cast. If this is not done and the design is made over an area that had been blocked out, there will be a space between the metal and the tooth when the casting is completed. Such a space is undesirable because it permits food to collect and work its way under the partial framework. Therefore the designs of the metal outline on both the master cast and the refractory cast should be identical (Fig. 8-4). The brown wax pencil outline will be helpful in establishing the margins of the forms during the waxing procedure.

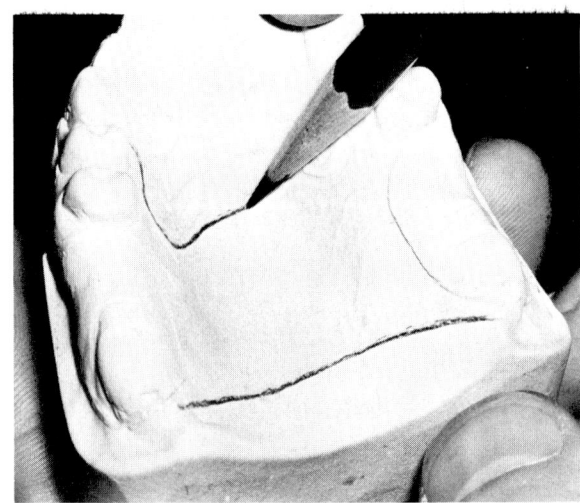

**Fig. 8-1.** Brown wax pencil is used to draw outline of major connectors in palate of maxillary refractory cast by following beading.

*Waxing and spruing* **229**

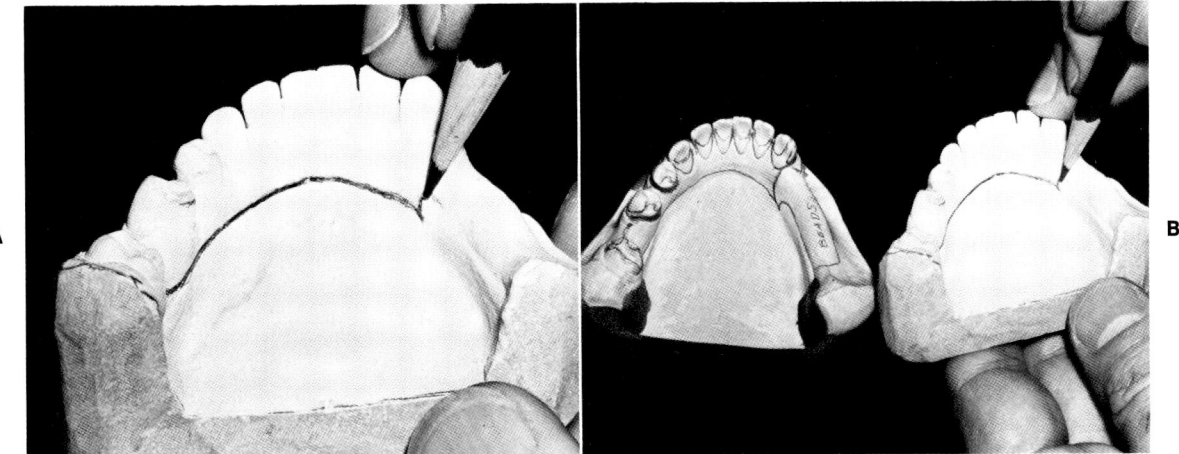

**Fig. 8-2.** Brown wax outline of mandibular major connector is drawn on the refractory cast by following landmarks on casts **(A)** and design on master cast **(B)**.

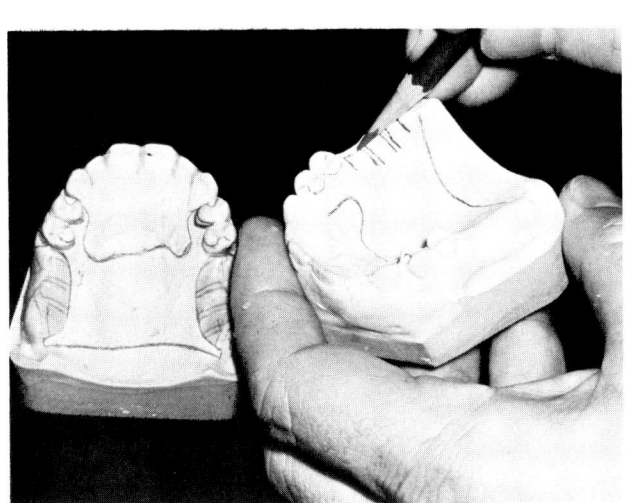

**Fig. 8-3.** Complete outline on maxillary refractory cast by following design on master cast.

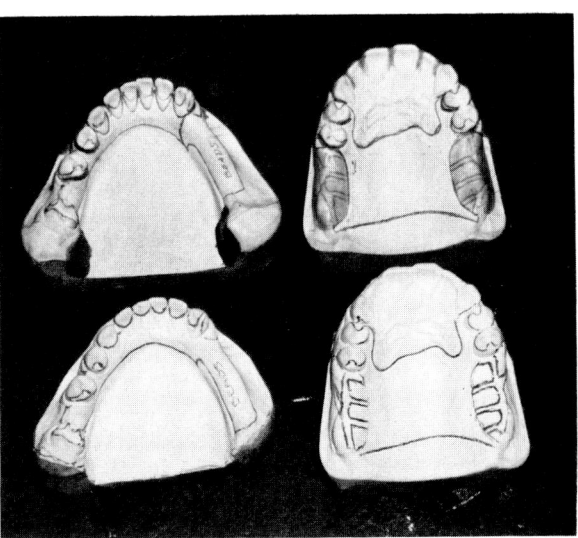

**Fig. 8-4.** Design of metal is accurately transferred to refractory casts.

## WAXING THE FRAMEWORK

Both wax and plastic patterns can be purchased in a large variety of shapes, sizes, and thicknesses (Fig. 8-5). When waxing the framework for a gold casting, the patterns should be slightly heavier than those used for cobalt-chromium castings. Following are some examples of gauges for gold castings:

1. Full palate, 26 gauge
2. Palatal strap, 22 gauge
3. Horseshoe and double palatal bar, 24 gauge
4. Lingual plating, 6-gauge half-pear shape with 28-gauge wax adapted over it and extending onto the teeth
5. Lingual bar, 6-gauge half-pear shape reinforced with a layer of 28-gauge wax

Gauge wax sheets are available with adhesive backs and in various colors. The green nonadhesive and the yellow adhesive sheets are soft waxes, whereas the pink is a harder wax. Gauge plastic sheets come with either a smooth surface or a stippled surface. Generally, it is easier to make lingual platings on both the anterior and posterior teeth with wax rather than plastic.

In adapting these various shapes to the refractory cast, care must be taken not to stretch and thin the pattern as it is being positioned on the cast. One of the most frequent causes of incomplete castings, particularly of palatal major connectors, is that the sheet of wax or plastic was stretched so thin that the metal could not flow completely during the casting procedure. Waxing the maxillary and mandibular casts will be described separately, since each cast is waxed individually before beginning the next.

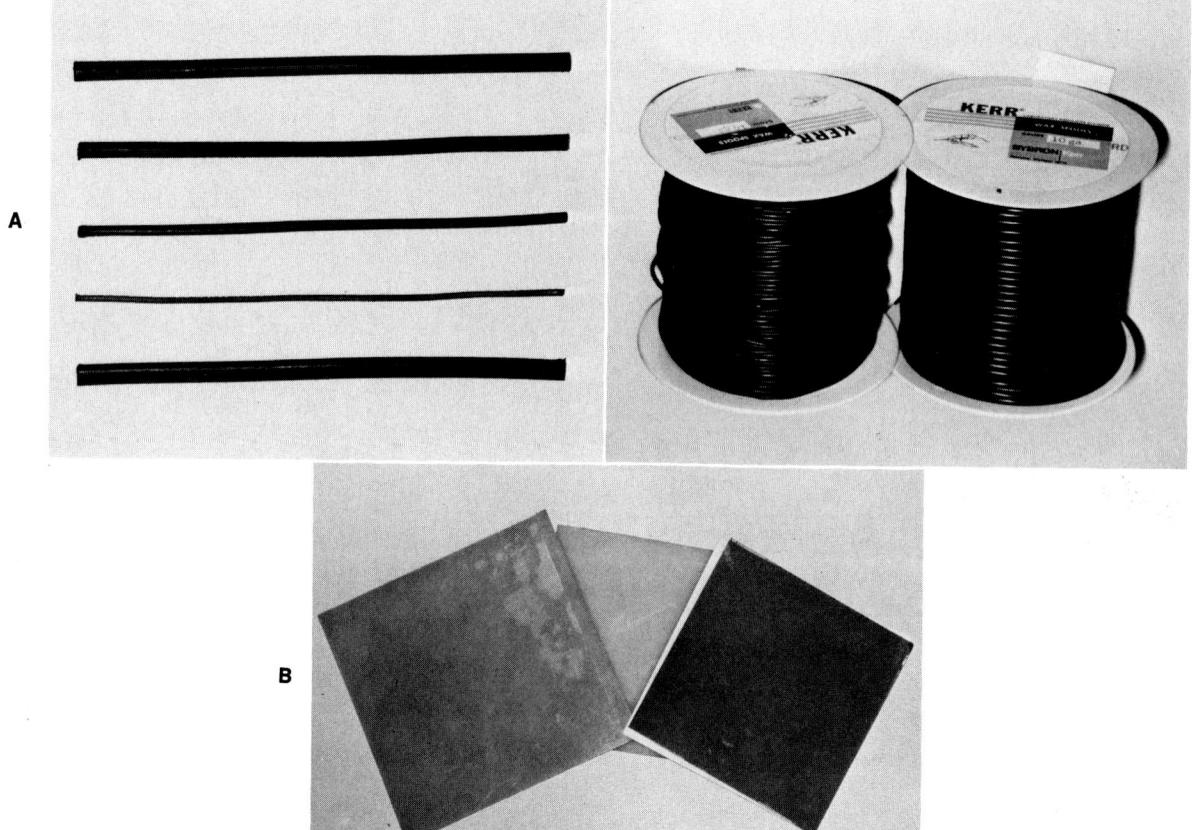

**Fig. 8-5.** Wax and plastic patterns are available in wide variety of shapes, sizes, and thicknesses. **A,** Wax shapes in short lengths (left) and on spools (right). **B,** Wax sheets. **C,** Plastic shapes. **D,** Plastic sheets.

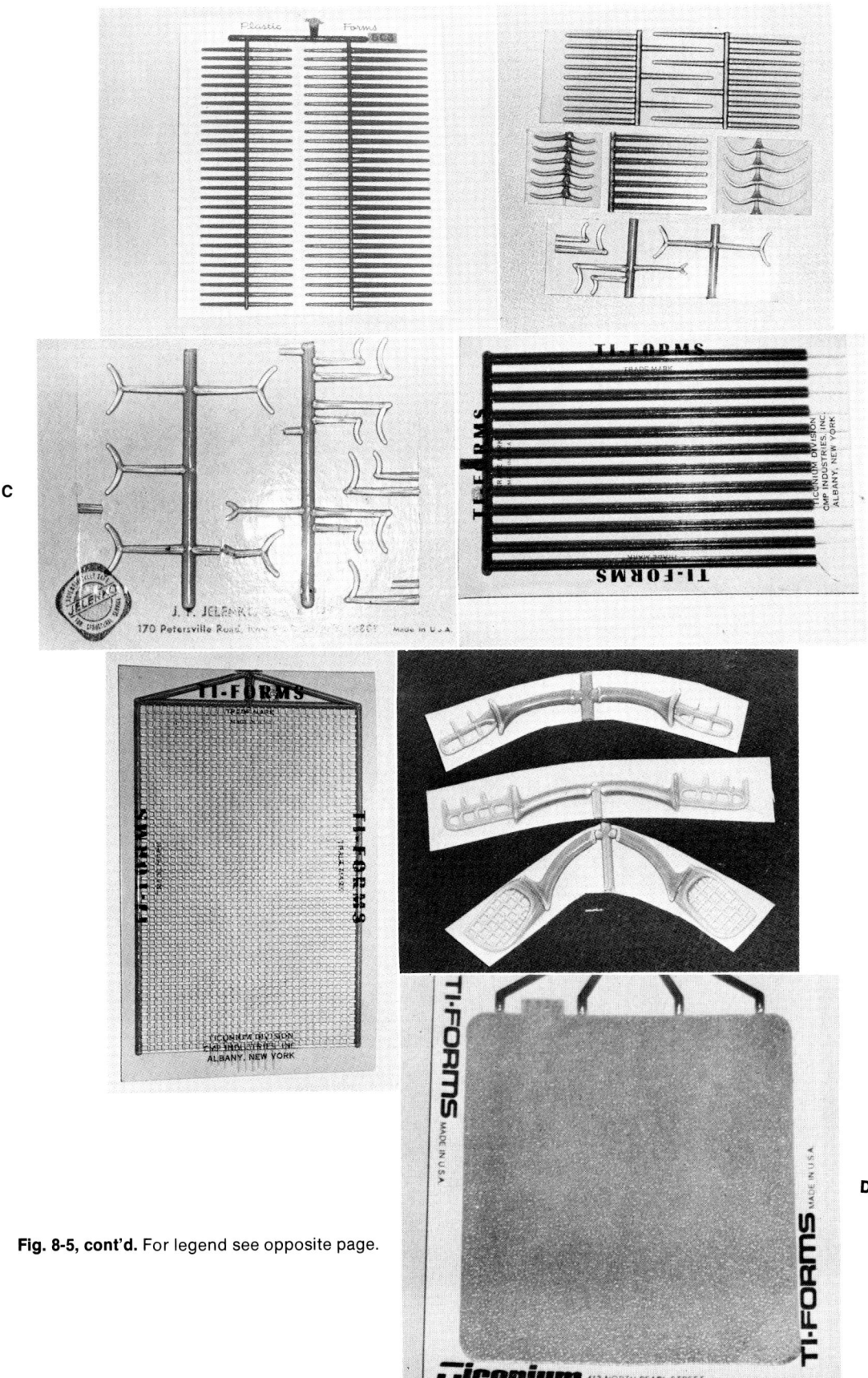

**Fig. 8-5, cont'd.** For legend see opposite page.

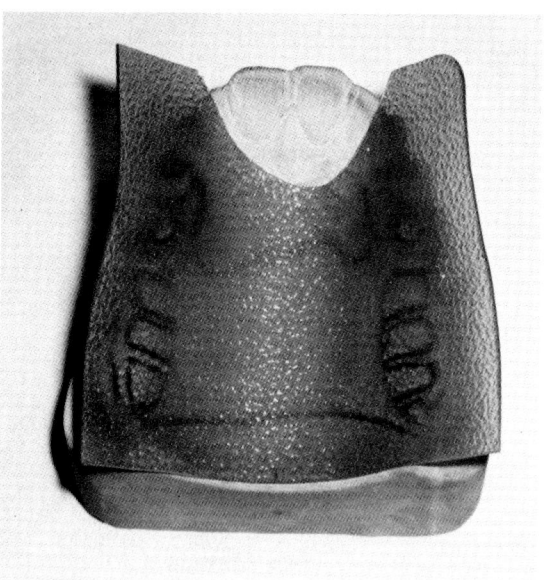

**Fig. 8-6.** Roughly cut sheet of plastic or wax to shape of major connector outline on cast, and adapt it gently to cast.

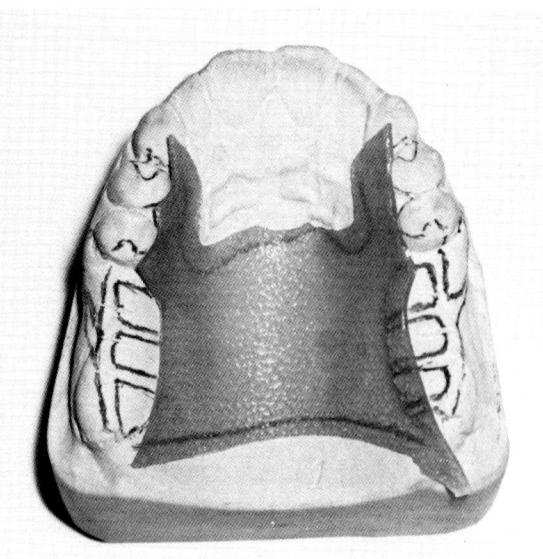

**Fig. 8-7.** Remove sheet, and trim it so it is just short of brown pencil outline of major connector. This plastic is overextended and should be trimmed more.

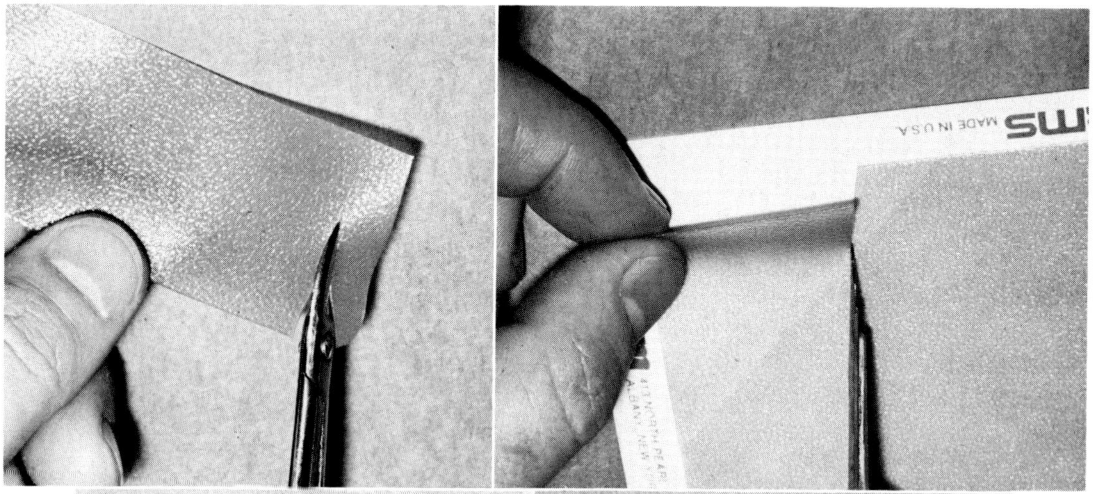

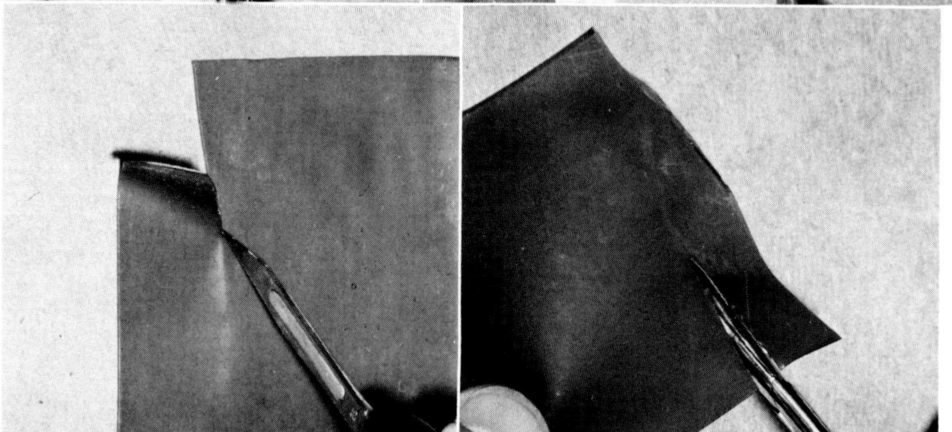

**Fig. 8-8. A,** Plastic sheets can be trimmed with scissors (left) or knife (right). **B,** Wax sheets can be trimmed with warmed knife or Roach carver (left), or scissors (right).

# Waxing and spruing

## WAXING THE MAXILLARY CAST
### PROCEDURE

1. Cut one thickness of sheet casting wax or plastic to the approximate outline of the major connector (Fig. 8-6). NOTE: Do not wax or seal the sheet in place until step 2 is completed. Stop it just short of the beading or brown pencil outline (Fig. 8-7). Both plastic and wax sheets may be trimmed with scissors or a somewhat dull Roach carver that has been heated (Fig. 8-8). *Caution:* Care should be taken not to mar the cast in the process. If the lingual surface of the teeth is to be plated, extend the sheet of wax or plastic to the brown pencil line, stopping it just short of the line (Fig. 8-9). This permits the remaining distance to be filled in by flowing wax in the area. If relief has been used on the master cast, the major connector butts up against the ridge created by the relief. When no relief was used, the sheet may cover the ridge, depending on the design.

2. Before the sheet is sealed in place, flow soft blue casting wax into the beading and all along the anterior and posterior borders of the major connectors. This wax should be thin, not more than 1 mm in thickness, and serve as a reinforcement to the major connector. It also permits some leeway in finishing. A thin layer of soft wax may also be crisscrossed in the palate for reinforcing (Fig. 8-10). The wax is flowed on the cast rather than onto the surface of the sheet because it is easier to make a smooth surface, especially if a plastic sheet is being used.

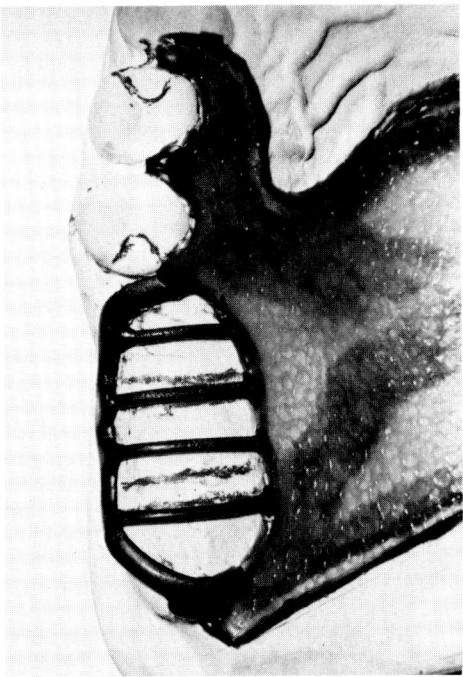

**Fig. 8-9.** Extend plastic or wax sheet up onto lingual surface of teeth that are to be plated, stopping it just short of brown line. Then flow blue casting wax on edge to seal it to cast.

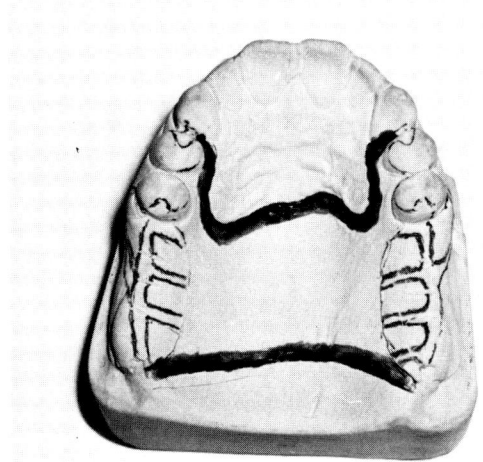 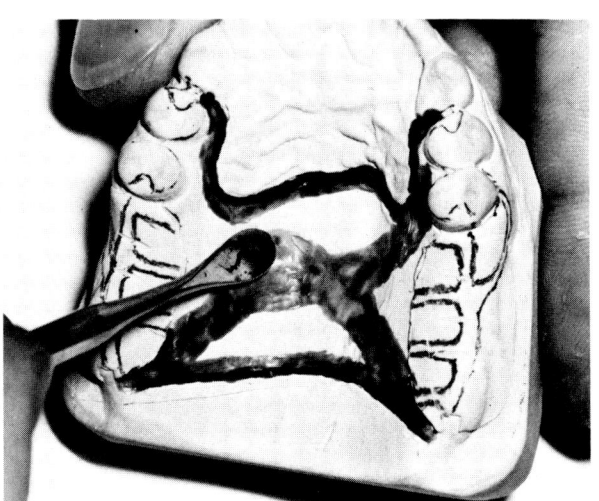

**Fig. 8-10. A,** Blue casting wax is flowed into beading where it should be about 1 mm thick and taper out as it goes away from bead. Width should be between 2 and 3 mm. **B,** Thin layer of wax may also be flowed across palate for reinforcement.

3. Paint the cast with tacky liquid.* Keep it within the confines of the brown outline and away from the blue casting wax that was flowed into the beading (Fig. 8-11).

*Tacky liquid may be made by dissolving plastic pattern scrap in acetone, or it may be purchased (Ti-Seal, Ticonium Co., Albany, N.Y.)

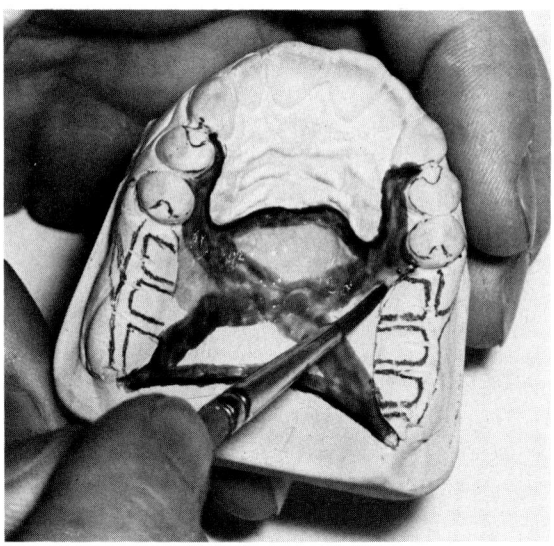

**Fig. 8-11.** Tacky liquid is painted on refractory cast within borders of brown outline. It should not be painted on blue wax. This can be used on plastic and wax alike and holds sheet securely in place.

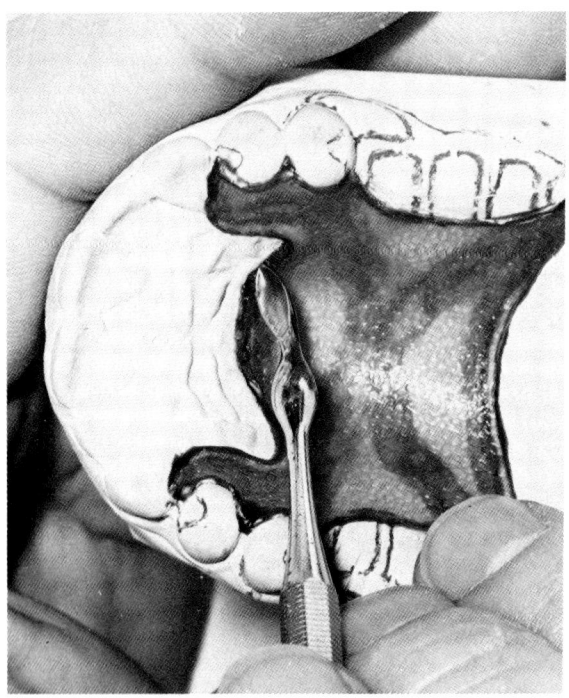

**Fig. 8-12.** Use spoon end of Roach carver to flow soft blue casting wax between sheet and brown line. This also seals it in place.

4. Flow soft blue casting wax along the borders of the plastic sheet to seal it in place and fill in between the sheet and the brown line (Fig. 8-12). Finish the wax to a thin edge when it goes onto the teeth, and leave it slightly rounded on the border of the major connector (Fig. 8-13).

5. Add wax for the denture base, which will be used to retain the pink plastic and the denture teeth. Different procedures are required, depending on whether the denture base area on the master cast was relieved or not. There are four main types of retention: (1) beads or nailheads, (2) open retention without relief, (3) open retention or mesh with relief, and (4) all metal base with or without tube teeth, without relief. Of course, the retention originally called for on the designed diagnostic cast or the master cast is the one that must be used. Quite often there may be a combination of two or more on the same partial denture.

   a. Bead or nailhead retention is made by extending the sheet wax or plastic for the major connector over the edentulous area to the outside brown pencil line. If the cast is not too large, this is usually done as a part of the major connector without splicing. However, splicing is no problem, and some individuals prefer to

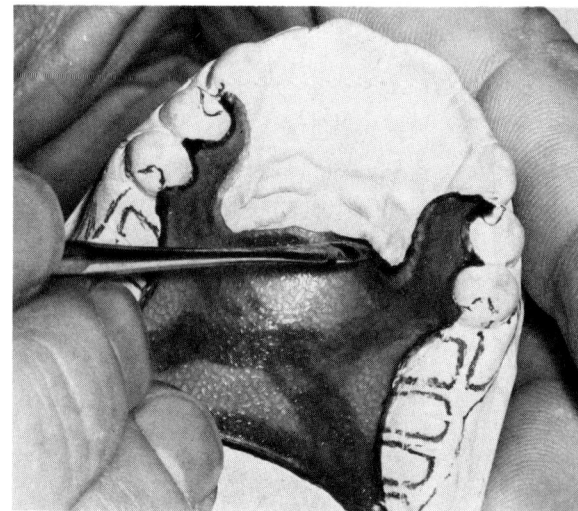

**Fig. 8-13.** Wax is finished to thin edge where it contacts tooth and is slightly rounded on borders of major connector.

add the denture base area separately (Fig. 8-14). The beads or nailheads will be added later.

b. Open retention without relief is made by using a 12- or 14-gauge half-round wax shape and adapting it to the cast to form the outer strut of the retention. It may be placed either flat side against the cast or away from the cast. Wax the strut in place at either end (Fig. 8-15), and use 16- or 18-gauge round wax for the cross struts.

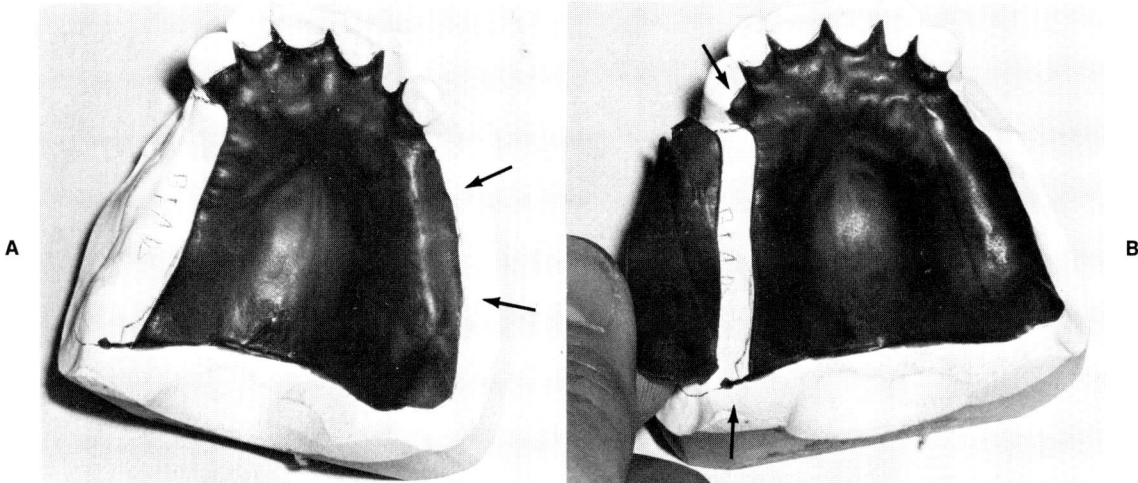

**Fig. 8-14.** Denture base coverage for beading or nailhead retention is extension of major connectors. **A,** Sheet forming major connector may continue across crest of ridge to brown line. **B,** Major connector may stop at some point on lingual aspect of ridge and remainder of area covered by splicing part of sheet to it.

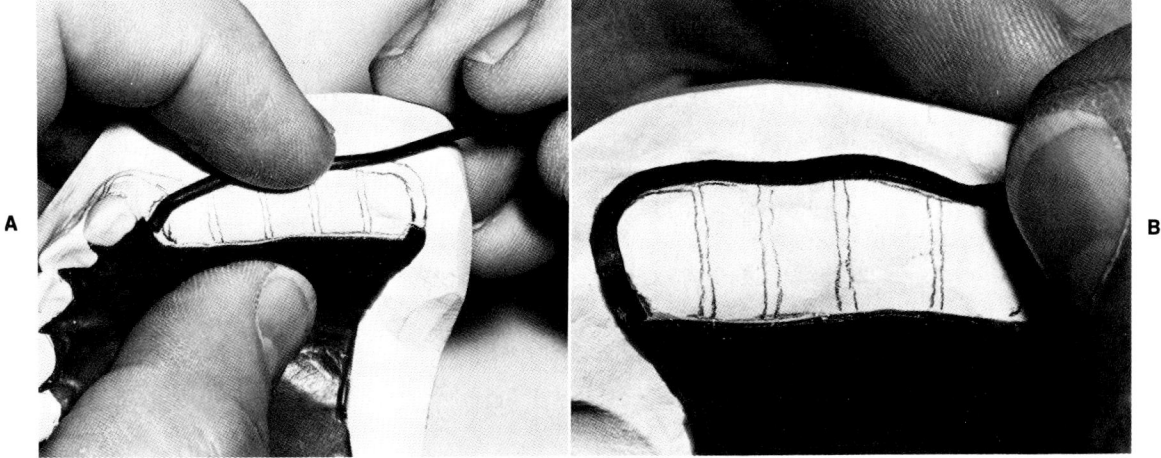

**Fig. 8-15.** Open retention without relief is made by using 12- or 14-gauge half-round wax for outer strut. **A,** Half-round wax placed with flat side against cast and sealed at both ends. **B,** Half-round wax placed with flat side away from cast and sealed. Flat side against cast is preferred.

Seal them at each end, but do not force them down against the cast (Fig. 8-16).

c. Open retention with relief on the master cast is made somewhat differently than that in step b. In this type of retention, the outer strut must be kept on the relief. Use 12- or 14-gauge half-round wax, and adapt it over the brown pencil outline for the outer strut with the flat surface against the cast. Seal it in place (Fig. 8-17). Use 16- or 18-gauge round wax for the cross struts. Keep the cross struts on the cast, and butt them against the inside edge of the center strut. Extend them across the ridge to overlap the major connector slightly. If provision was made for a tissue stop in the relief wax, be sure that a cross strut crosses this area and the area is filled with wax. The major connector will be butted against the relief. Seal them at both ends, making the end that overlaps the outer strut slightly more prominent (Fig. 8-18).

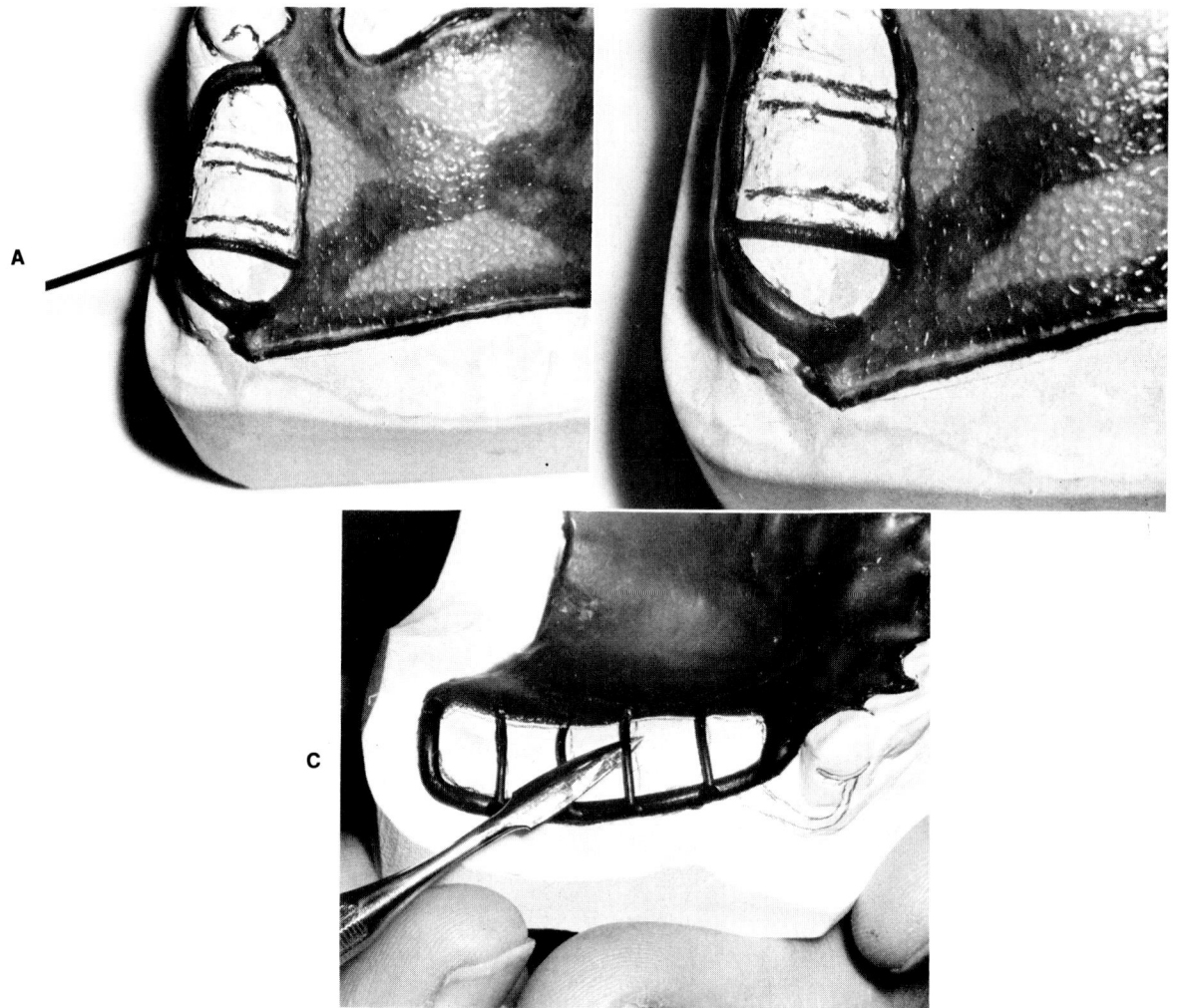

**Fig. 8-16. A,** Sixteen- or eighteen-gauge round wax is used for cross strut and is placed from major connector to outer strut. NOTE: Round wax is placed on top of major connector and outer strut. **B,** Cross strut is sealed at both ends with bead of wax. **C,** Leave space between cross strut and cast.

*Waxing and spruing* **237**

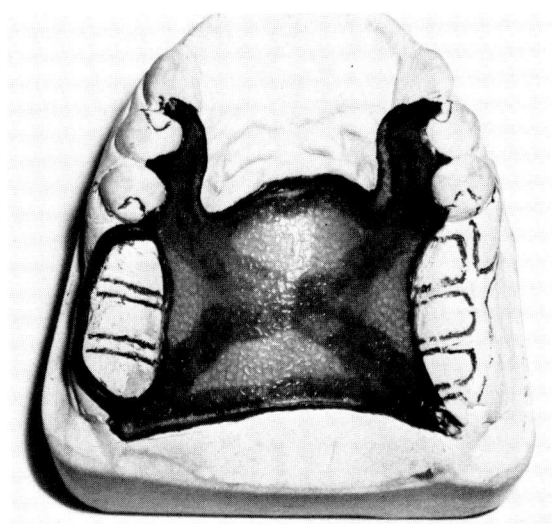

**Fig. 8-17.** When relief is used on ridge, 12-gauge half-round wax is adapted over brown pencil outline of outer strut with flat side against cast and sealed in place.

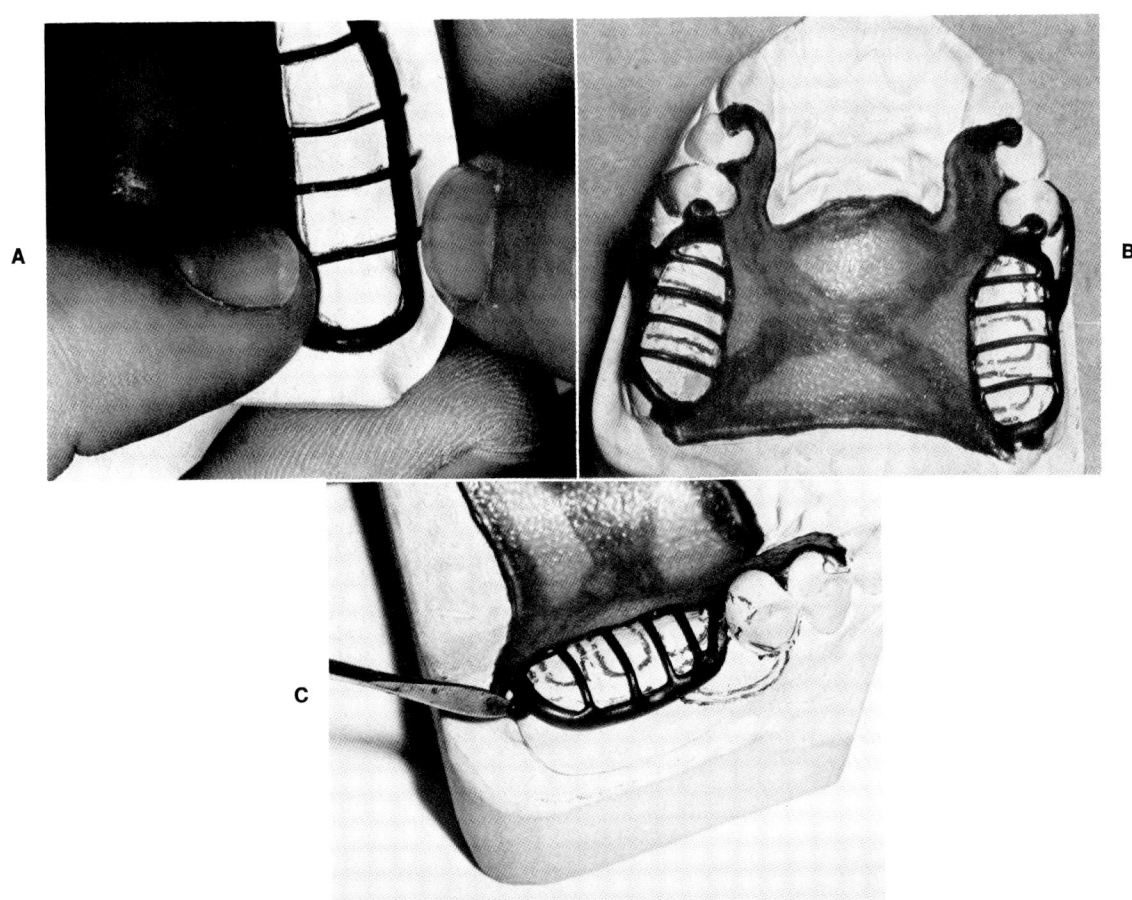

**Fig. 8-18.** Eighteen-gauge round wax adapted on cast to form cross struts. **A,** Cross struts extend from outer strut to overlap major connector slightly. **B,** Struts are sealed in place with soft blue wax. NOTE: Seal on outer strut is larger than on major connector. **C,** If provision is made in relief for tissue stop, this area is filled with wax and attached to strut.

Adapt mesh directly to the cast, making sure that it is on the relief. It should overlap the major connector slightly and fill in the brown pencil outline (Fig. 8-19). Seal the mesh in place in several places, taking care to seal it smoothly to the major connector (Fig. 8-20).

d. Relief cannot be used in the edentulous area when the denture base is to be all metal either with or without tube teeth. Adapt 16- or 18-gauge round wax to the brown pencil line on the buccal flange of the denture base, and seal it in place. Flow soft blue wax all along the inside edge of the round wax to tack it to the cast. Adapt the major connector sheet wax over the ridge and the wax on the peripheral outline as in step b. Seal it carefully to the wax in the peripheral border to form a rounded edge. The most accurate way to grind in tube teeth, whether they are porcelain or plastic and whether they are anterior or posterior, is to grind them in on the mounted master casts (Fig. 8-21). When they are ground in accurately (Fig. 8-22), make a transfer splint of dental stone (Fig. 8-23), and transfer them to the refractory cast (Fig. 8-24). Lubricate the exposed portion of the tube teeth well with a separating medium,* then flow inlay wax

---

*Die Lube, J. F. Jelenko & Co., New Rochelle, N.Y.

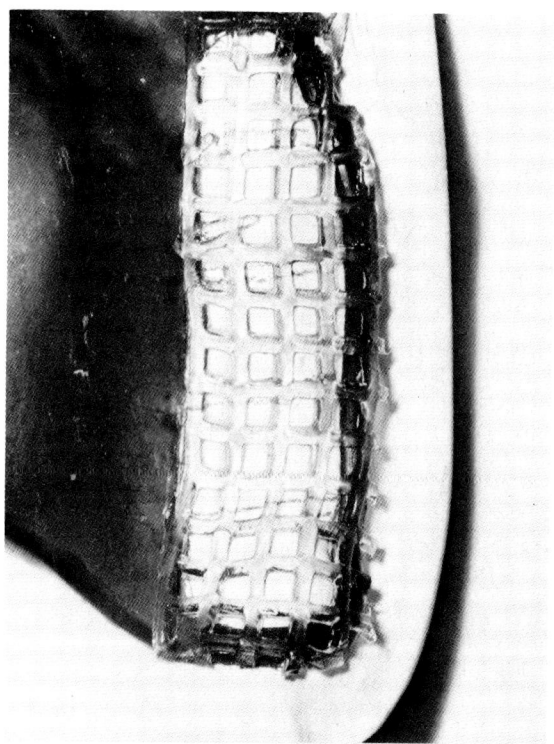

Fig. 8-19. Mesh adapted directly to cast, slightly overlapping major connector and outer strut.

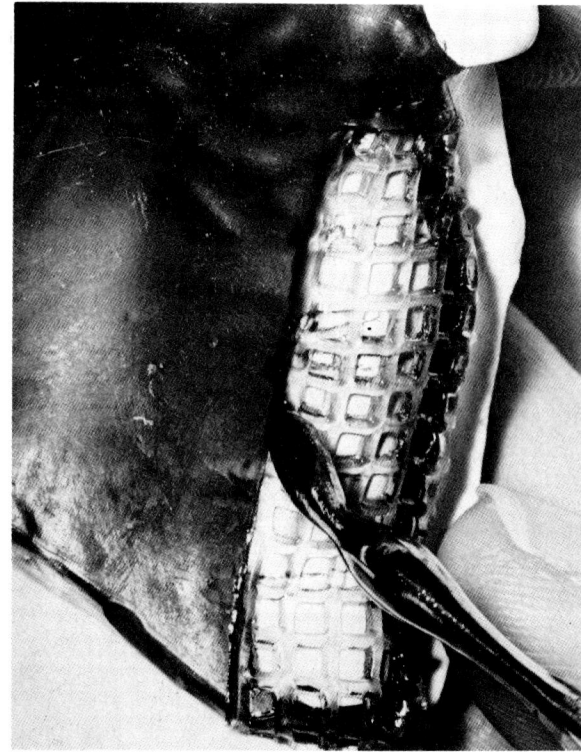

Fig. 8-20. Mesh is sealed in place with soft blue wax and sealed carefully and smoothly where it is attached to major connector.

*Waxing and spruing* **239**

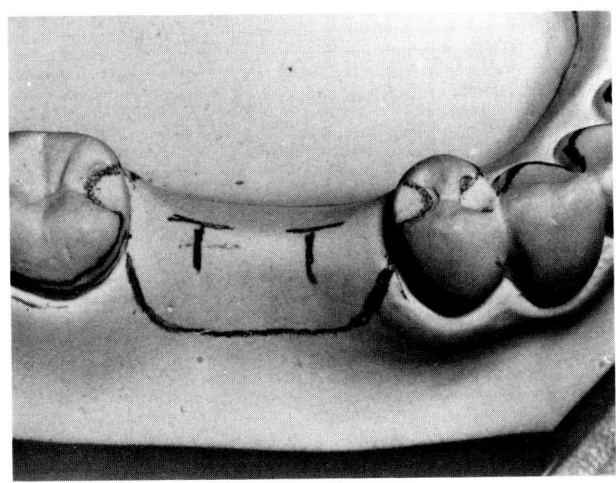

**Fig. 8-21.** Tube teeth are ground in on master casts mounted in articulator.

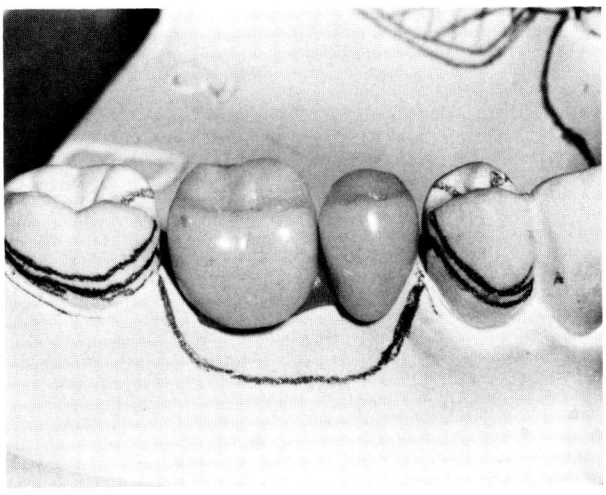

**Fig. 8-22.** Posterior tube teeth ground in.

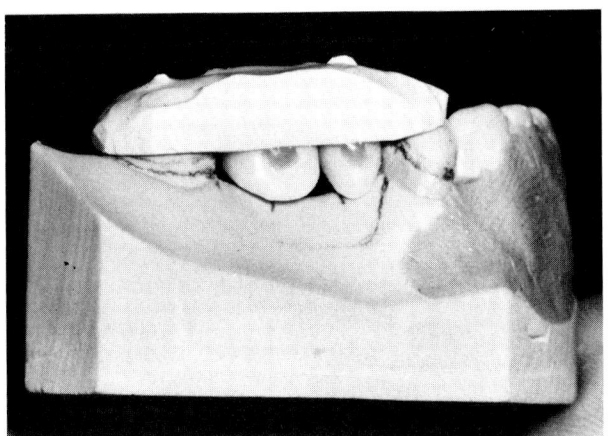

**Fig. 8-23.** Transfer splint made for tube teeth. *Caution:* Be sure to lubricate master cast well before applying stone for transfer splint.

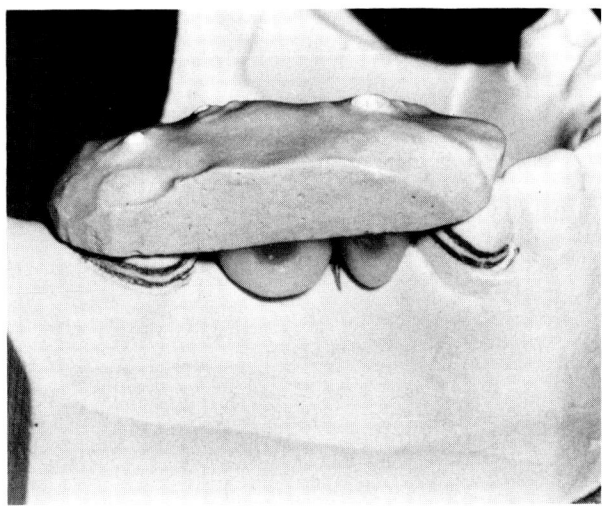

**Fig. 8-24.** Transfer splint in place on refractory cast.

**240** *Dental laboratory procedures: removable partial dentures*

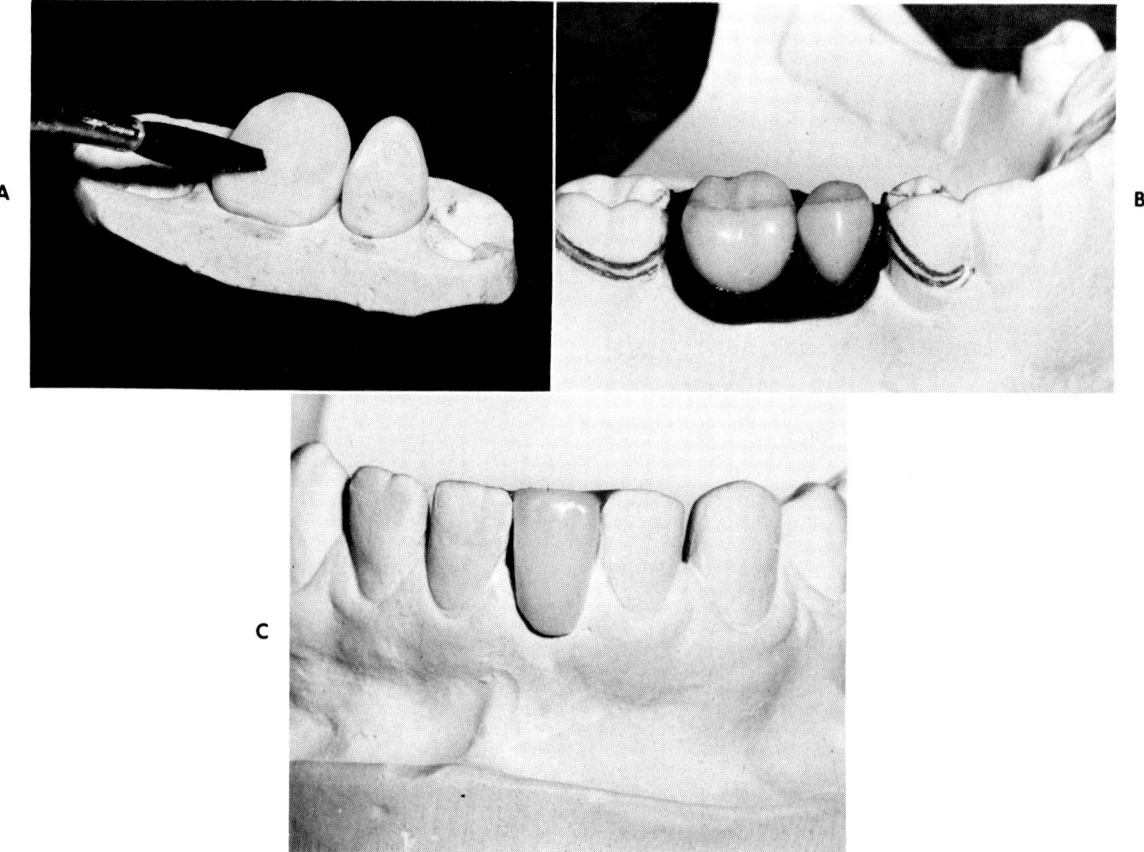

**Fig. 8-25. A,** Exposed portion of teeth is lubricated with separating medium. **B,** Inlay wax flowed around teeth. **C,** Anterior tube teeth waxed in place. Note difference in waxing technique, since anterior tube teeth are usually butted against ridge.

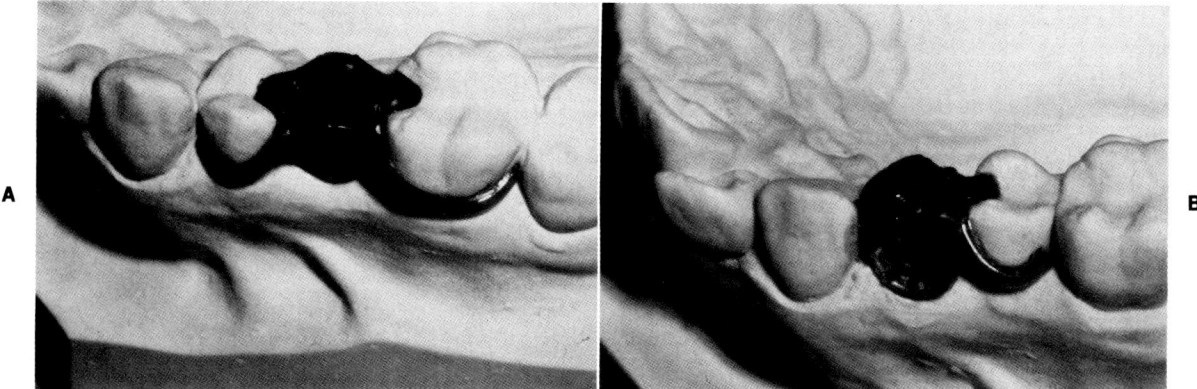

**Fig. 8-26. A,** Wax tooth carved directly on denture base for solid metal tooth. **B,** Tooth carved with window to receive tooth-colored plastic after casting is made.

around them to make a box and hold them in place. Anterior tube teeth and first premolars are usually butted against the soft tissue on the ridge. Note the different waxing procedure for the anterior teeth (Fig. 8-25).

Sometimes there is not enough space for plastic or porcelain teeth on the denture base, and the teeth are carved directly in the denture base and cast in metal or metal with a tooth-colored plastic window on the facial surface (Fig. 8-26).

6. Select the proper plastic clasp forms. Remove them from the cardboard holder with a quick snap to prevent them from distorting, and pass them very quickly through a flame to remove the flash on the pattern (Fig. 8-27). Dampen the tissue side of the

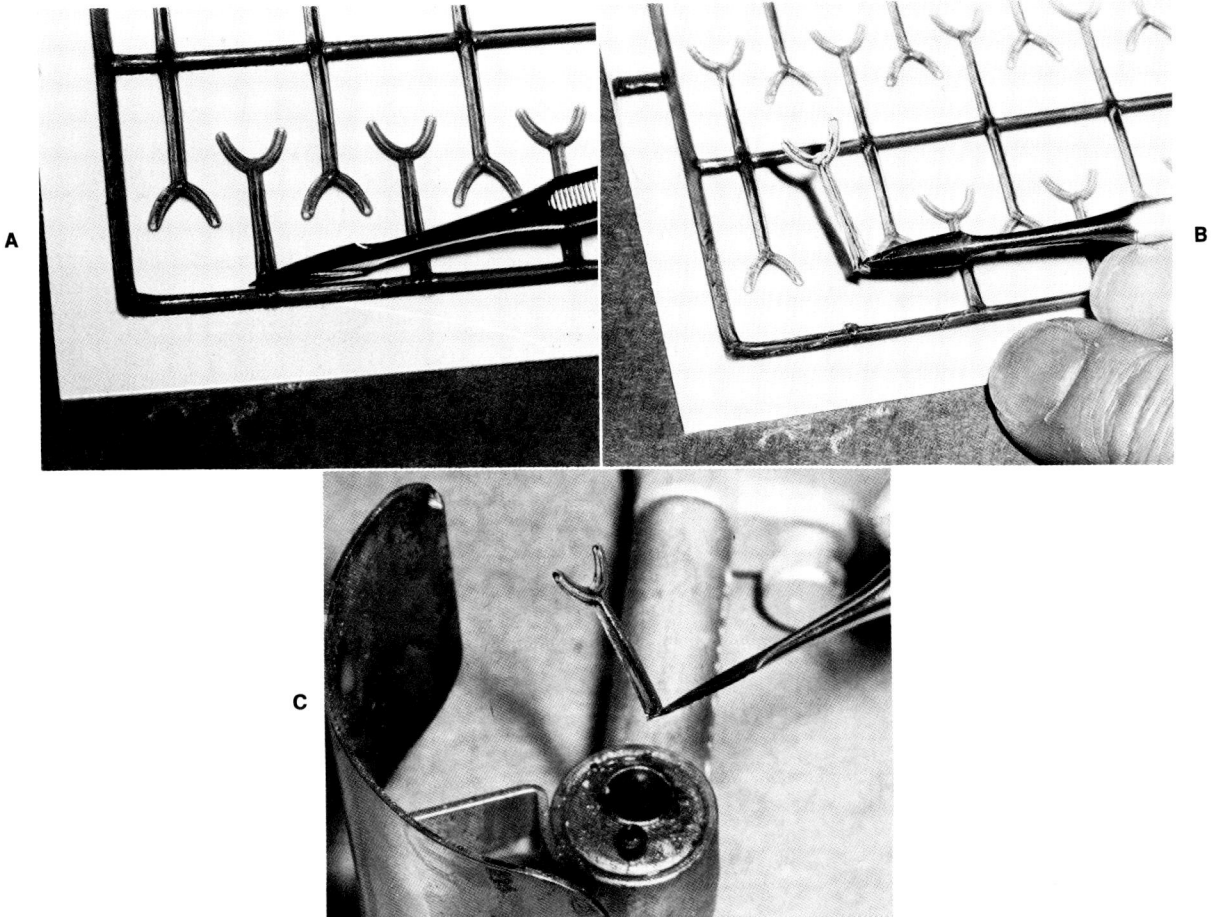

**Fig. 8-27.** Plastic clasp form is removed from cardboard holder with Roach carver blade with quick motion (**A** and **B**) and passed very quickly through flame to remove flash on plastic pattern (**C**).

plastic form with tacky liquid. Adapt the form to the tooth surface over the clasp outline and be guided by the ledging (Fig. 8-28). Position the tip of the clasp first and then the body and shoulder of the clasp. Cut off the excess length at the minor connector area by warming the tip of a knife blade and very carefully cutting the plastic (Fig. 8-29). The bar clasp should be attached and thickened where a cross strut attaches to the outer strut. This will aid in providing space for the flow of metal to the bar clasp during the casting procedure (Fig. 8-30).

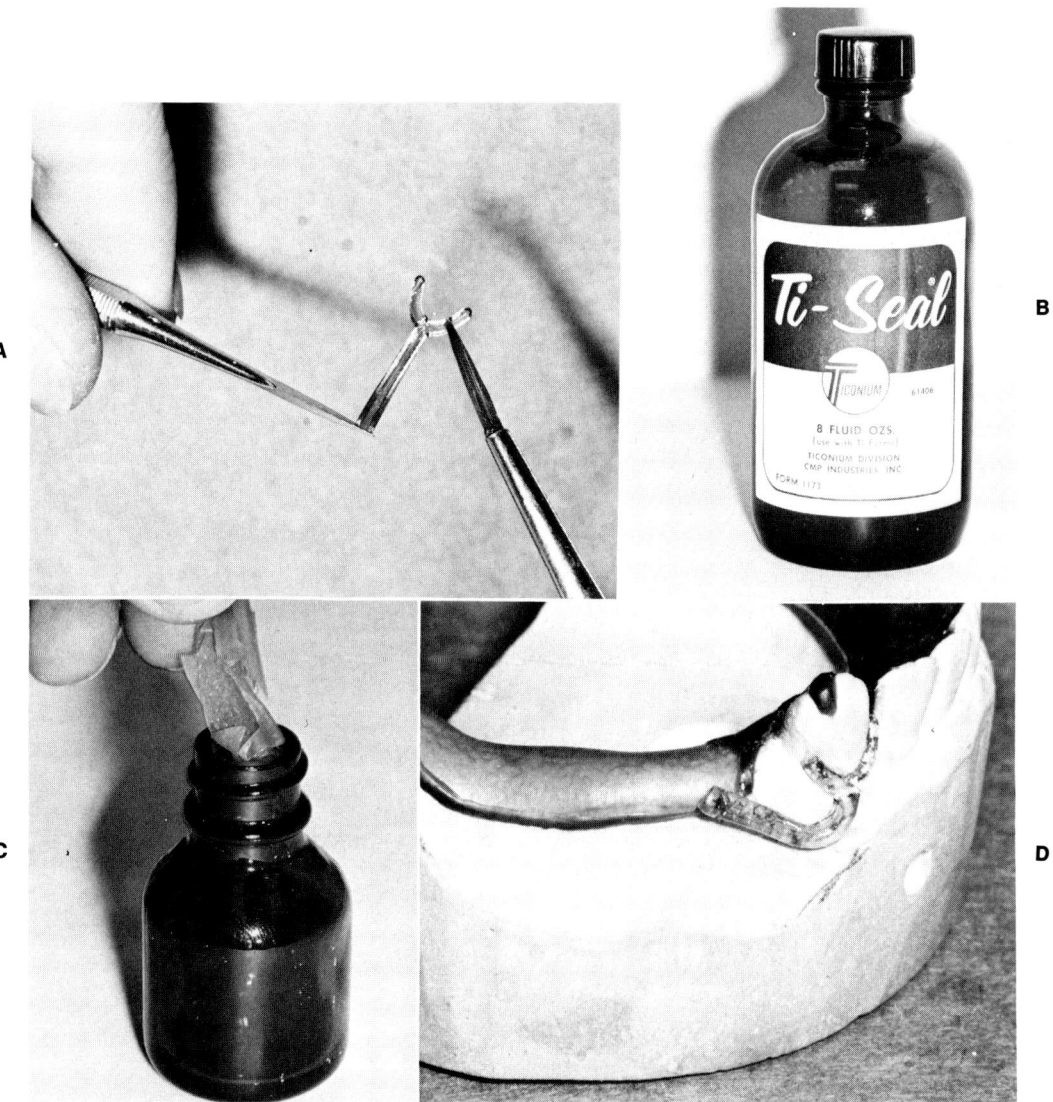

Fig. 8-28. **A,** Tacky liquid painted on flat side of plastic clasp form. **B,** Ti-Seal is prepared tacky liquid. **C,** Tacky liquid may be made by dissolving scrap plastic forms in acetone. **D,** Form in place on tooth.

*Waxing and spruing* **243**

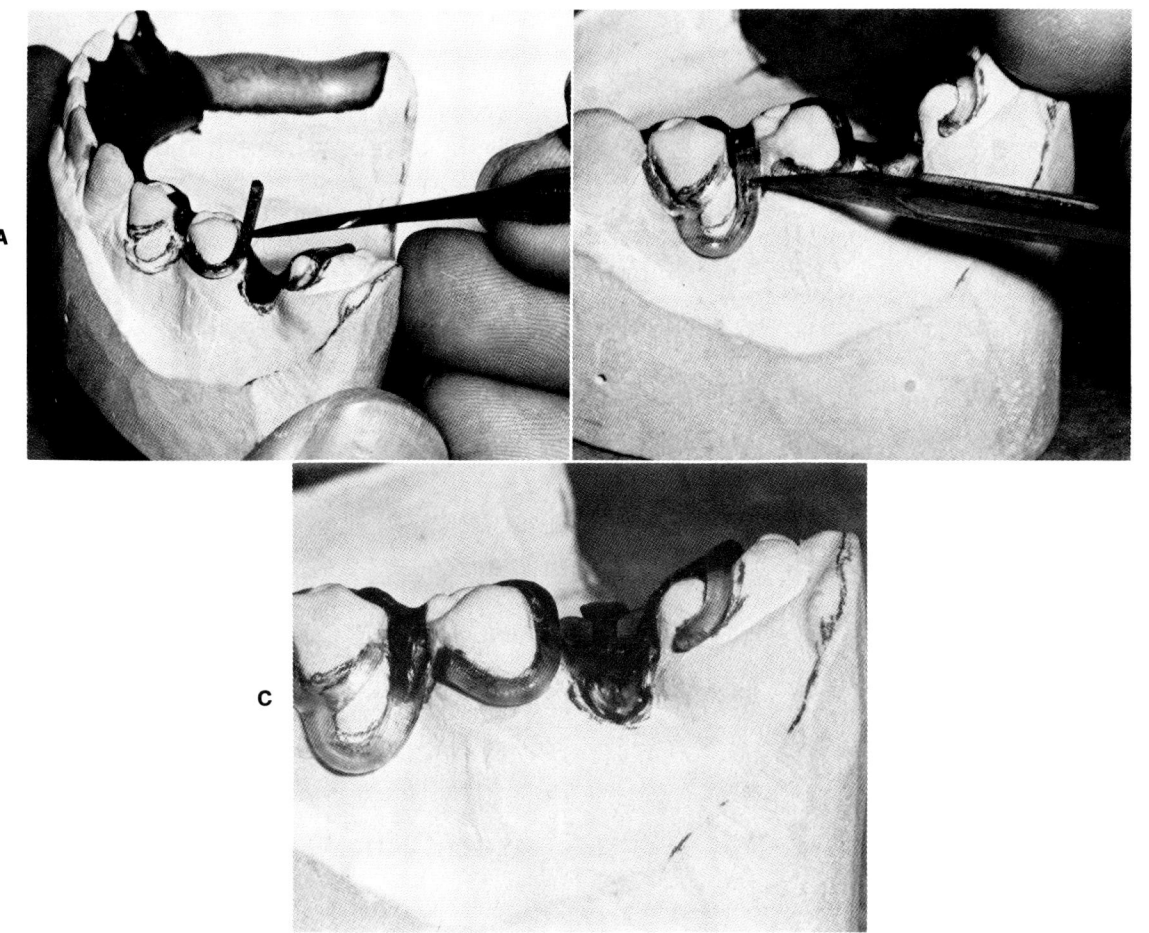

**Fig. 8-29.** Excess length of clasp arm is removed by warmed knife blade. *Caution:* Be careful not to mar cast. **A,** Excess of circlet clasp removed. **B,** Excess of bar clasp removed. **C,** Clasps sealed in place.

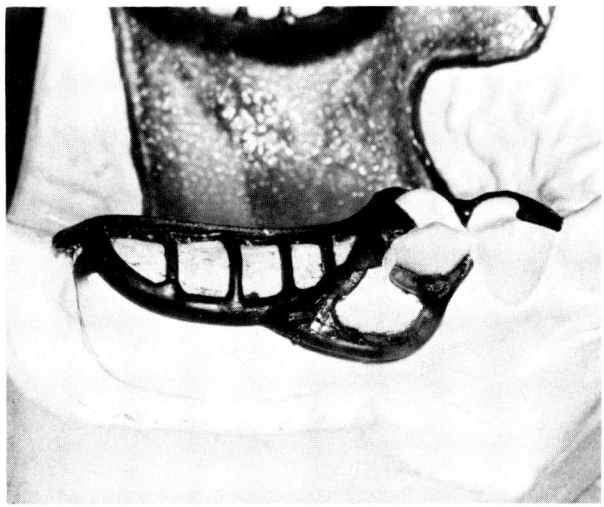

**Fig. 8-30.** Bar clasp is attached where cross strut attaches to outer strut, and area is then reinforced.

7. Flow soft casting wax into the occlusal rest seats to a thickness of 1 to 1.5 mm. The surface should be slightly concave (Fig. 8-31). Continue waxing over the marginal ridges, and develop the minor connectors on the proximal surfaces. Keep the greatest bulk of the minor connector toward the lingual surface, since this will make the problem of positioning the artificial teeth much easier. The minor connectors should be waxed broadly buccolingually but narrowly mesiodistally. Wax at the proximal surface of the marginal ridge should be at least 1.5 mm thick (Fig. 8-32).

8. Develop the external finish lines on the lingual slope of the palate adjacent to the edentulous spaces. These finish lines form the junction between the acrylic resin and the metal. The finish line must be sharp and definite and should be undercut to aid in locking the resin securely in position (Fig. 8-33).

Adapt 12-gauge half-round wax to the palatal major connector with its flat side up. The wax should extend from the top of the minor connector, beginning at the lingual extent of the rest seat and continuing to the posterior edge of the major connector. It should be positioned lingually enough to permit setting the maxillary teeth but not enough to create a large space that must be filled with acrylic resin (Fig. 8-34).

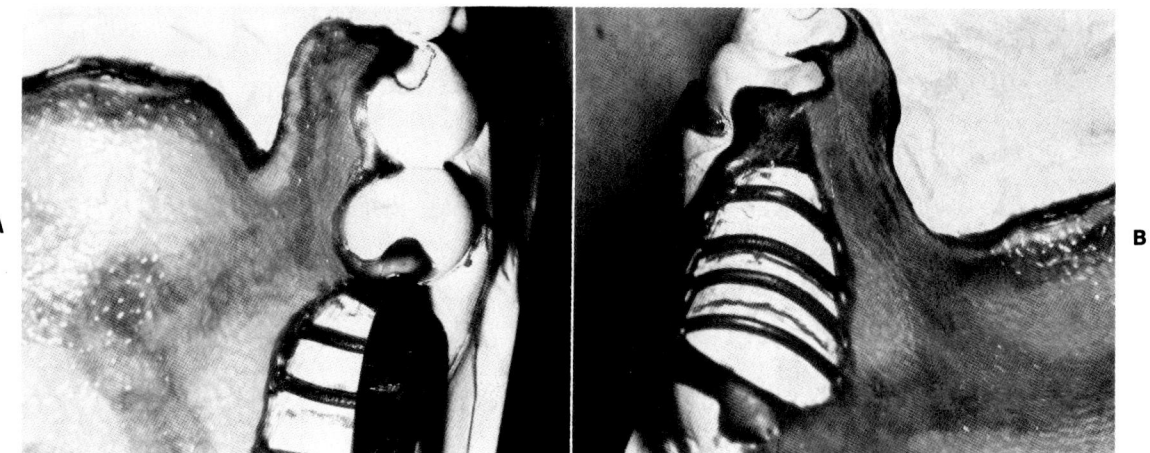

**Fig. 8-31. A,** Rest waxed to depth of 1 to 1.5 mm. **B,** Rest made slightly concave on occlusal surface.

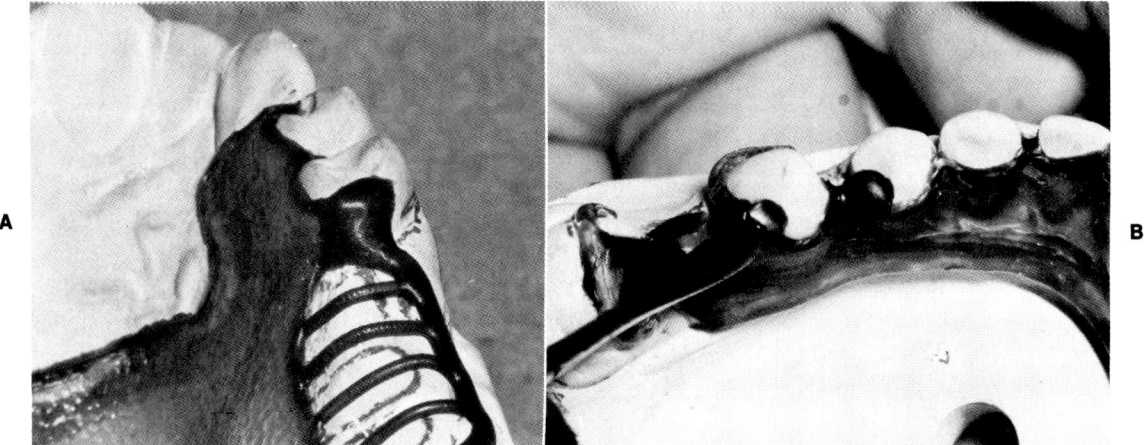

**Fig. 8-32. A,** Minor connector broadly waxed buccolingually with greatest bulk toward lingual aspect. **B,** Wax at proximal edge of marginal ridge is built up to thickness of about 1.5 mm and incorporates ends of plastic clasp pattern smoothly.

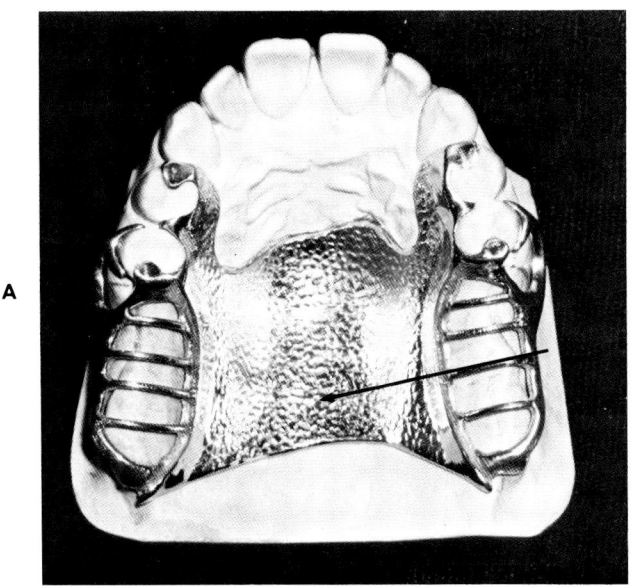
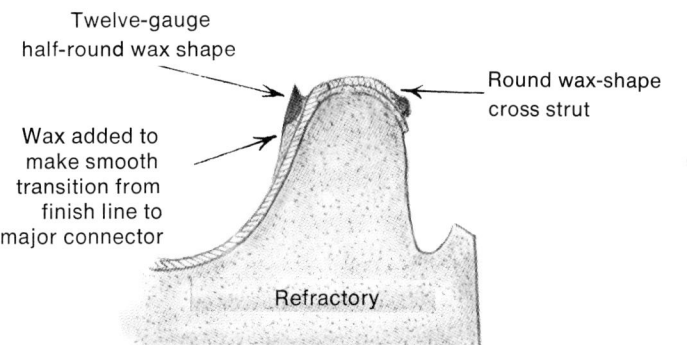

**Fig. 8-33. A,** Maxillary partial denture showing area (arrow) of which cross section will be drawn. **B,** Cross section of area indicated by arrow. NOTE: Undercut will lock acrylic resin in place.

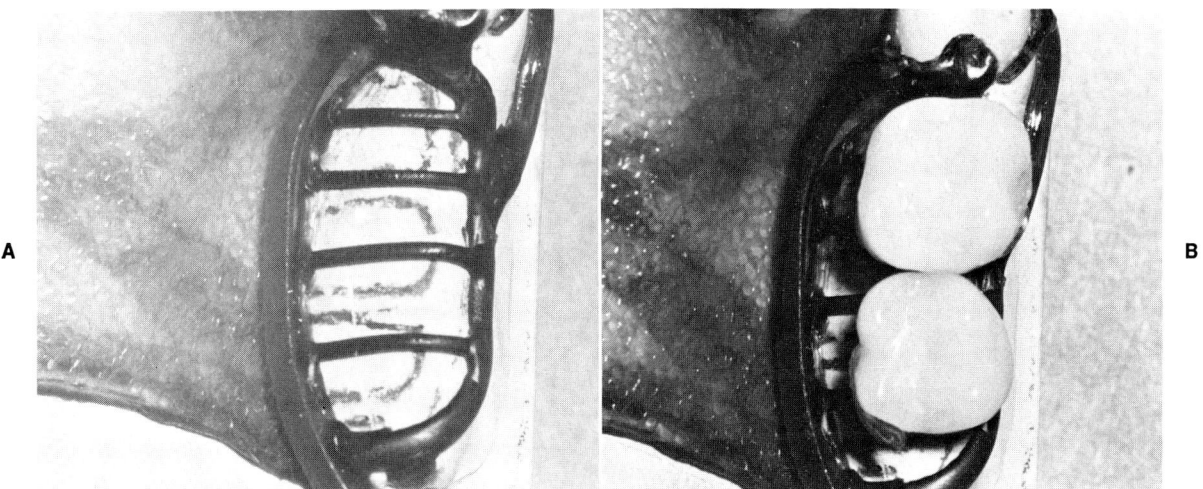

**Fig. 8-34. A,** Twelve-gauge half-round wax adapted flat side up from top of minor connector to distal side of major connector. **B,** Finish line is positioned to permit setting teeth.

Flow soft casting wax between the 12-gauge half-round wax and the sheet forming the major connector to make a smooth continuous surface (Fig. 8-35). The side of the half-round wax facing the edentulous ridge is burnished slightly to accentuate the V shape of the finish line undercut (Fig. 8-36).

9. After the finish lines are completed, it is time to add the beads or nailhead retention, depending on the design. Paint the surface of the sheet covering the edentulous ridge with tacky liquid, and position large beads of acrylic resin polymer* on this sticky surface (Fig. 8-37). The beads will eventually be cast in metal and will provide the retention necessary for the acrylic resin denture base.

---

*Retention beads for metal casting, Kay Cee Dental Manufacturing Co., Kansas City, Mo.

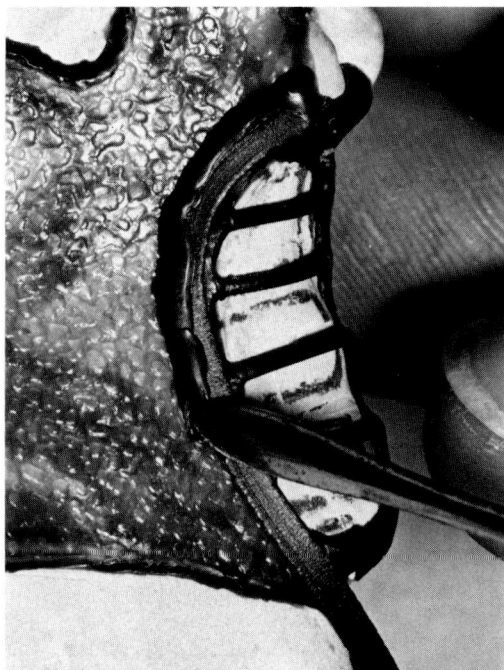

Fig. 8-35. Soft blue wax is flowed along 12-gauge half-round wax and then smoothed to form continuous surface. Do not flame wax because it is so soft it will melt and dull sharp edge.

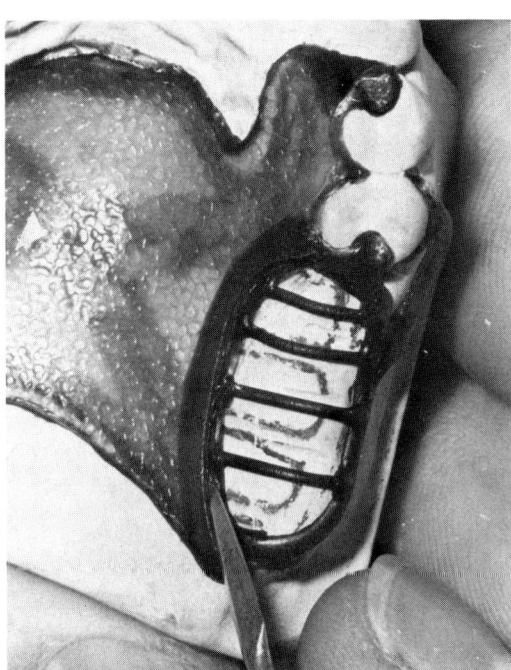

Fig. 8-36. Burnish V side of finish line to accentuate it.

*Waxing and spruing* **247**

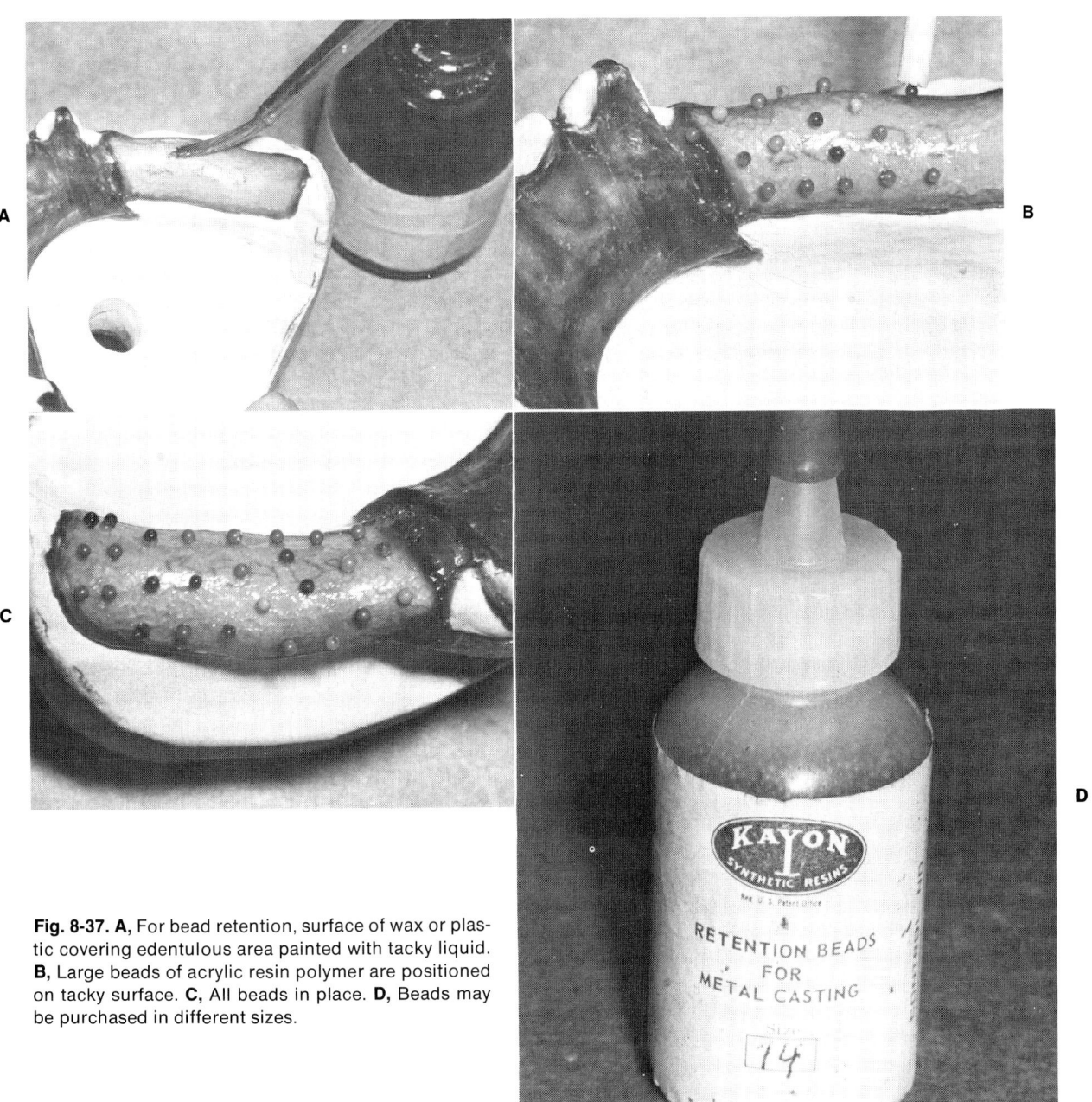

**Fig. 8-37. A,** For bead retention, surface of wax or plastic covering edentulous area painted with tacky liquid. **B,** Large beads of acrylic resin polymer are positioned on tacky surface. **C,** All beads in place. **D,** Beads may be purchased in different sizes.

**248** *Dental laboratory procedures: removable partial dentures*

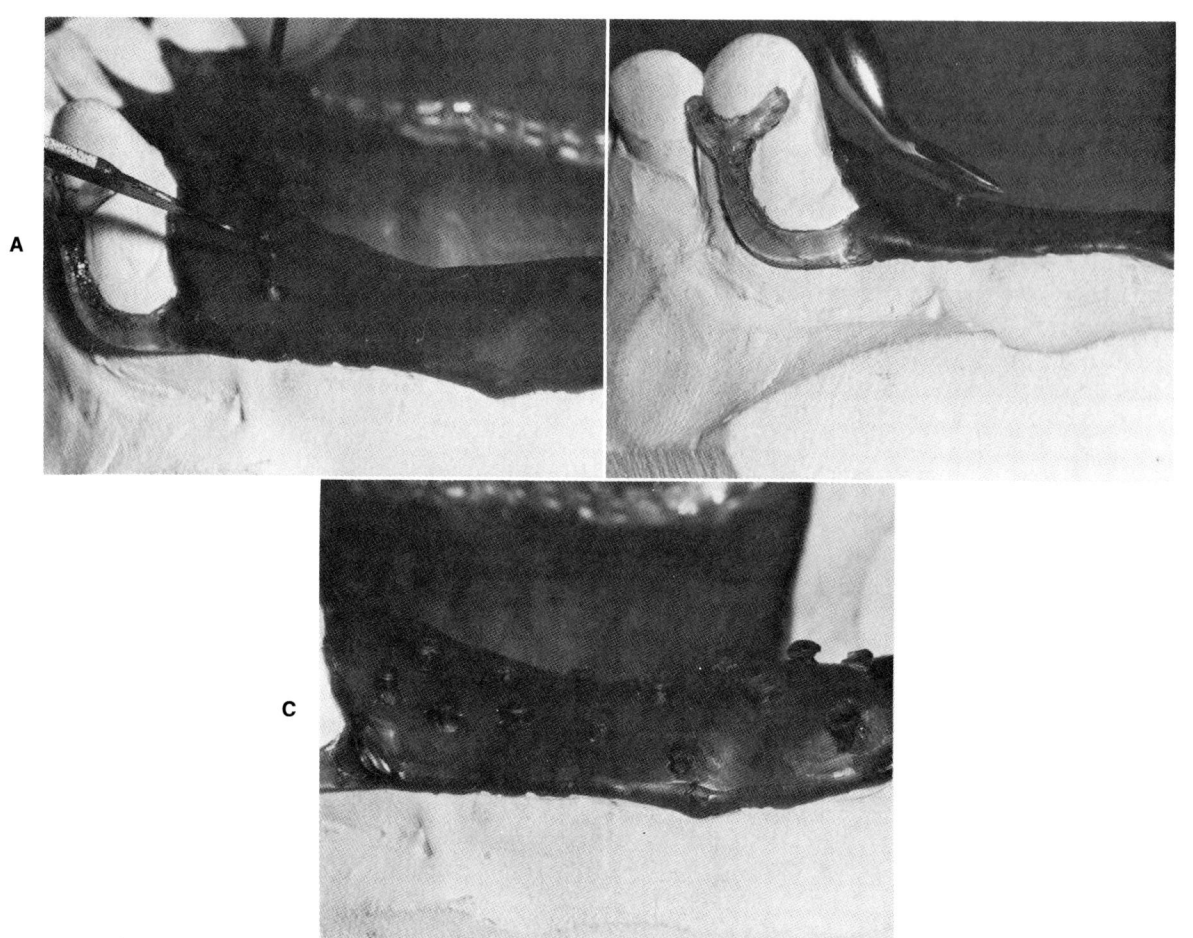

**Fig. 8-38. A,** For nailhead retention, eighteen-gauge round wax is attached to wax sheet and cut to about 2 mm in length with warmed knife blade. **B,** With warm instrument, flatten 18-gauge wax to form head. **C,** Complete nailhead waxed.

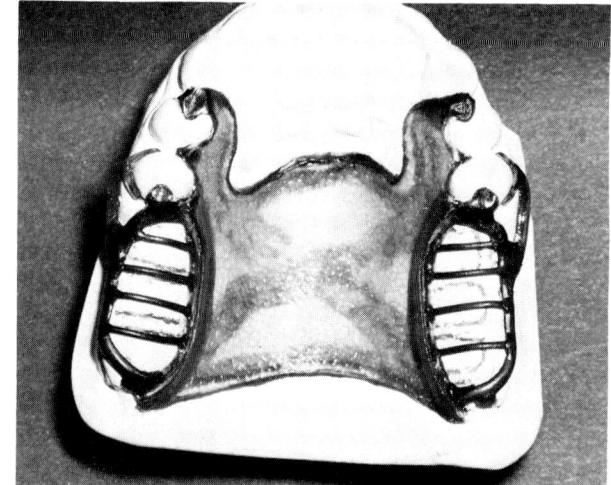

**Fig. 8-39.** Maxillary wax-up complete.

Retention can also be made with wax in the form of nailheads. Attach short pieces of 18-gauge round wax to the surface of the wax covering the edentulous area by softening the sheet wax and pushing the 18-gauge wax into it. When it hardens cut the wax off so it is about 2 mm long. When all are in place, mash the top with a slightly warmed instrument to form the retention head (Fig. 8-38).

10. Now smooth the entire surface. Irregularities, pits, and waves are much more easily removed in wax than they are in metal. A soft cloth may be used to smooth the wax. The principal reason for using soft casting wax to develop the framework instead of hard inlay wax is the ease with which it can be smoothed. Avoid thinning the wax during this procedure. The wax-up is complete (Fig. 8-39).

## WAXING THE MANDIBULAR CAST

Study the framework design that was transferred from the master cast. The most critical point of the transfer is the lingual bar. The superior margin of the bar must not be placed closer than 3 mm to the gingival margin of the teeth. Also, it must not be so low that the inferior border will interfere with the frenum when the tongue is raised. The position of the clasps and rests is determined by the rest seat preparations and by the ledges created during the blockout procedure.

### PROCEDURE

1. Using a fine-point brush, the entire design outline may be painted with a light coat of tacky liquid. This will aid in keeping the wax and plastic forms securely attached to the refractory cast. Do not use an excess of tacky liquid or allow it to flow outside the design outline, since it may produce a "flash" on the metal casting and complicate the polishing procedure (Fig. 8-40).

2. The major connector on the mandibular cast may be a lingual bar, a double lingual bar, or a lingual plate. The basis for all of these is a 6-gauge pear-shaped form made of wax or plastic (Fig. 8-41).

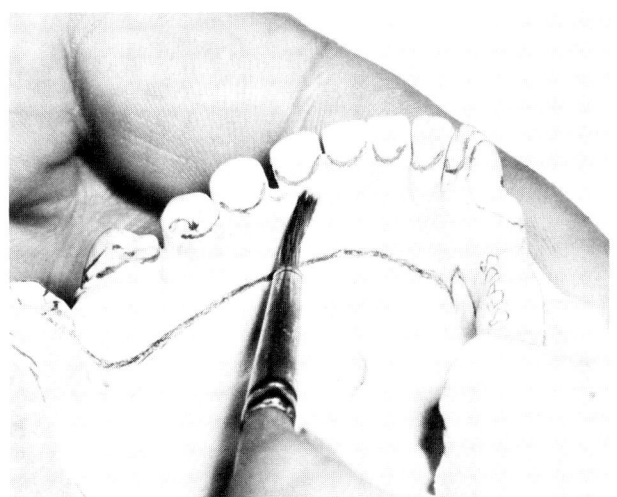

Fig. 8-40. Tacky liquid painted within entire design outline on mandibular refractory cast.

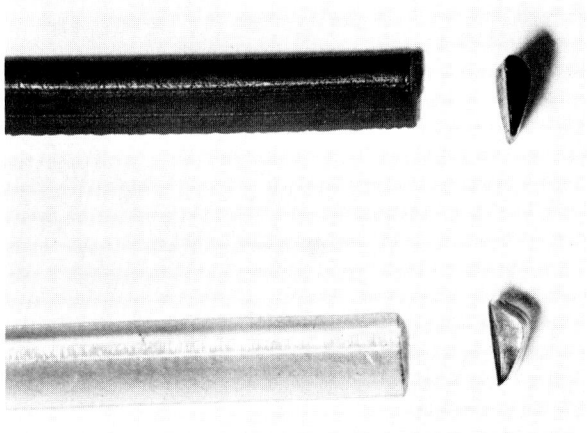

Fig. 8-41. Six-gauge pear-shaped form is applied in wax or plastic to form lingual bar. Cross section of wax (top) and plastic (bottom).

Starting at the finish line on one side, adapt the lingual bar around the lingual surface to the finish line on the other side. If any doubt exists, seal the margins of the lingual bar to the cast with wax. Position the pear-shaped form so that the bulky part makes up the lower part of the bar (Fig. 8-42).

When a double lingual bar is required, use a 12-gauge half-round wax shape as a basis, position it over the pencil outline, and fill in the contours with wax. Trim it carefully to form a contour around the anterior teeth (Fig. 8-43).

In making a lingual plate, 28- or 26-gauge wax is

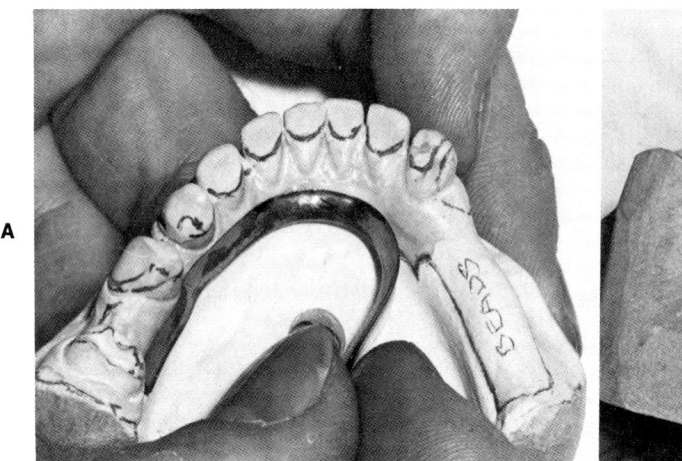
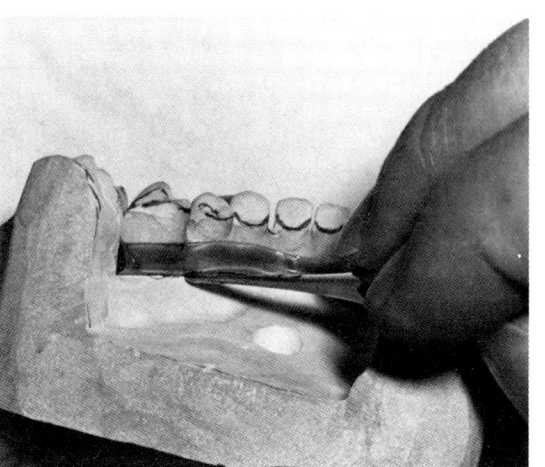

**Fig. 8-42. A,** Lingual bar adapted to refractory cast. **B,** Seal it with hot instrument. NOTE: Bulk of wax shape is at bottom.

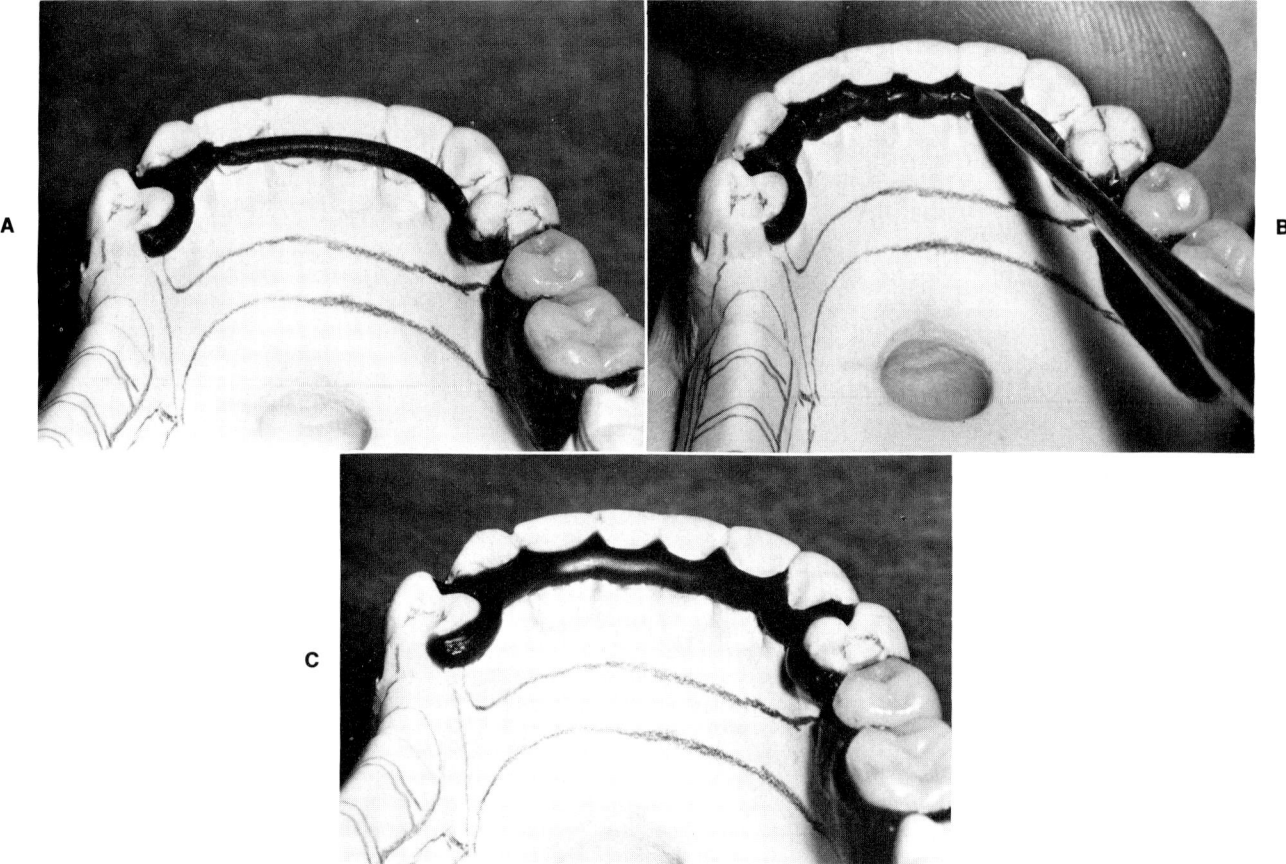

**Fig. 8-43. A,** For upper part of double lingual bar, 12-gauge half-round wax is adapted to outline. **B,** Soft blue wax is flowed around wax to fill in outline. **C,** Wax has been trimmed to shape.

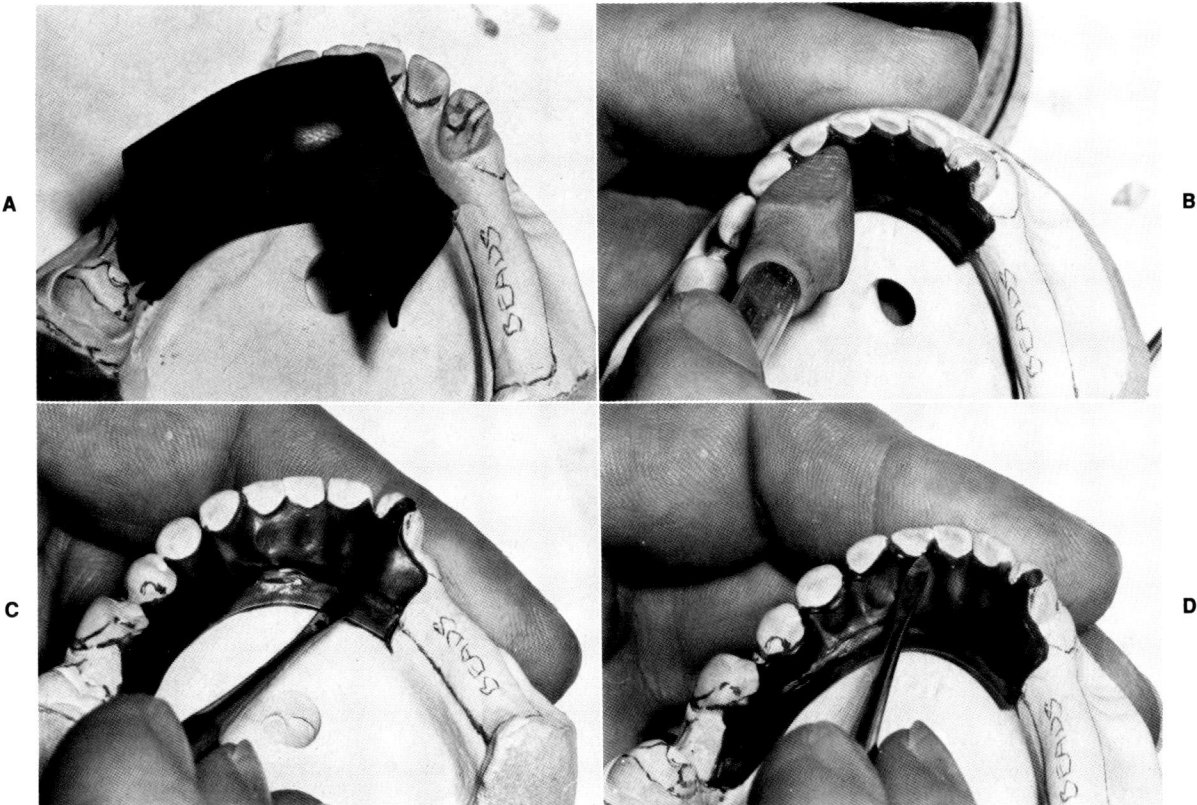

**Fig. 8-44. A,** Twenty-eight gauge wax adapted over lingual bar and onto anterior teeth. **B,** Contour it around anterior teeth with instrument or shaped pencil eraser. **C,** Wax is scalloped at superior border and blended with lingual bar. **D,** Wax sealed to cast using hot wax instrument.

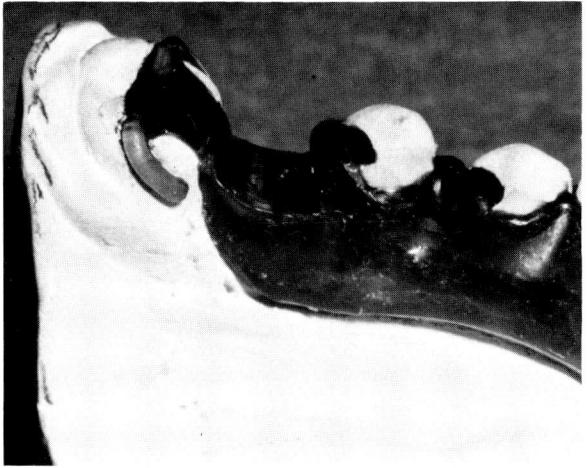

**Fig. 8-45.** Minor connector is blended into lingual bar.

adapted over the lingual bar and on the lingual surface of the anterior teeth to the brown pencil line. Contour it around the teeth, being careful not to stretch it too thin. Scallop the wax at the superior border to follow the brown pencil outline, and seal it in place (Fig. 8-44).

3. Adapt wax or plastic to the denture base as described in step 5 of the procedure for waxing a maxillary cast.

4. Select proper plastic forms and adapt them to the cast as described in step 6 of the procedure for waxing the maxillary casting.

5. Make the occlusal rests and minor connectors as described in step 7 of the procedure for waxing the maxillary cast. The junction of the minor connector and the lingual bar should be smooth and rounded (Fig. 8-45).

**252** *Dental laboratory procedures: removable partial dentures*

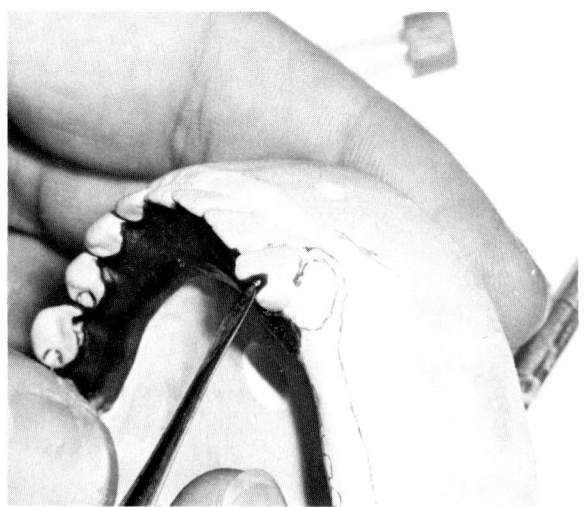

**Fig. 8-46.** Incisal rest is placed by freehand waxing.

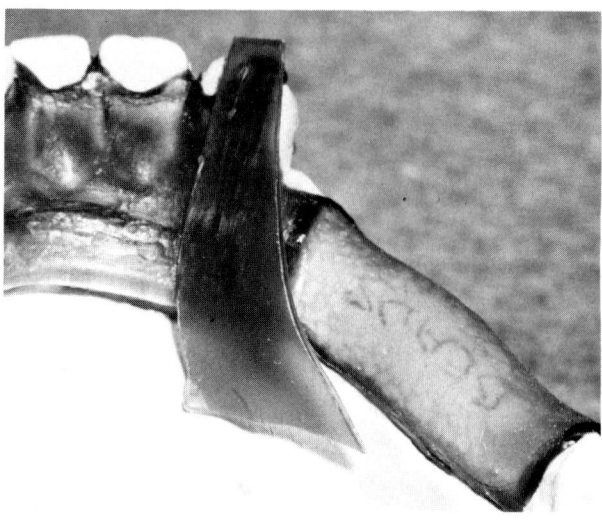

**Fig. 8-47.** Small piece of 28-gauge green casting wax burnished to lingual bar to form finish line. Wax is generally shaped to blue pencil outline.

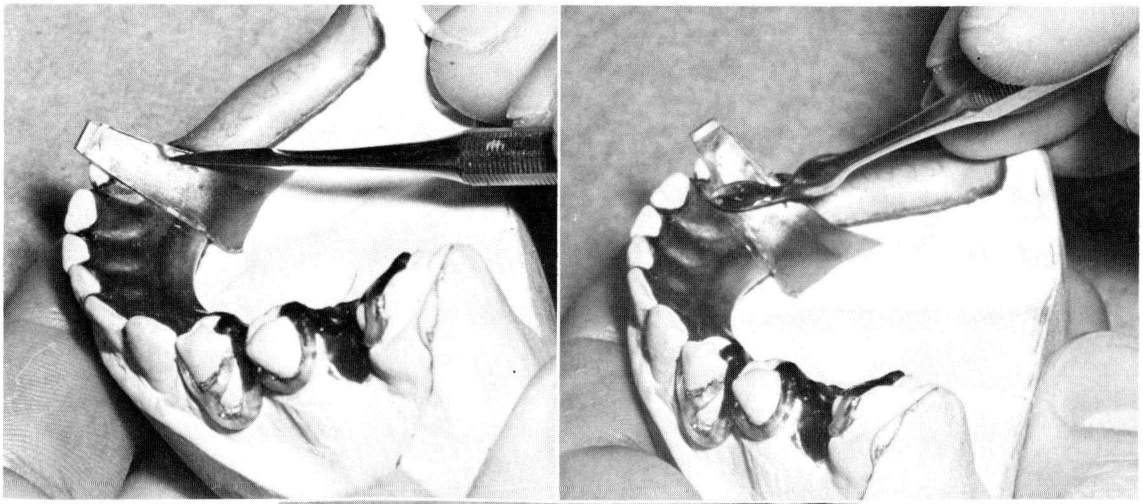

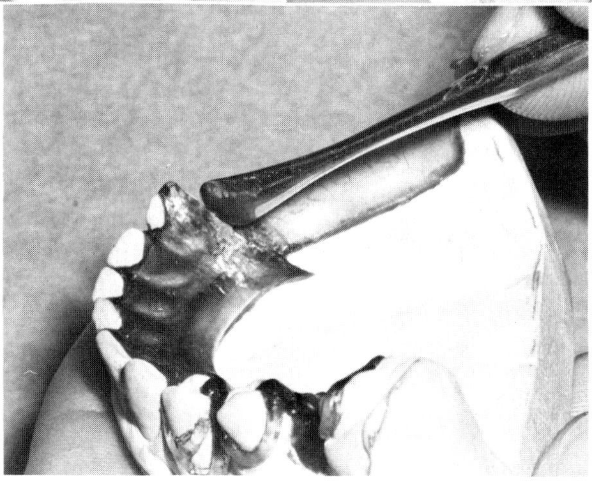

**Fig. 8-48. A,** Excess wax trimmed with warm Roach carver knife. **B,** Wax is burnished and sealed in place. **C,** Edge of finish line can be shaped with hot spatula.

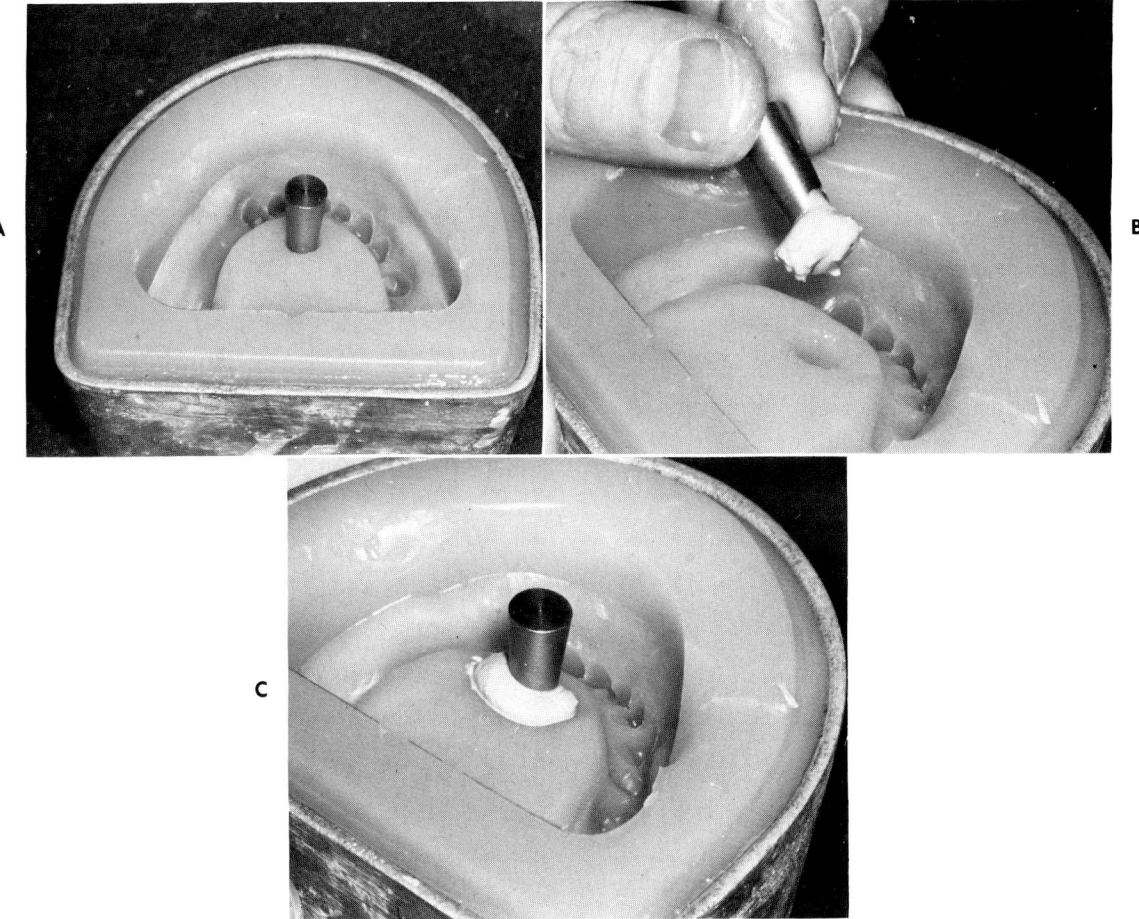

**Fig. 8-54. A,** Medium sprue cone B in place in duplicating hydrocolloid mold. Hole was made by sprue cone A on master cast. **B,** Some investment on top of sprue cone B before it is placed in hole will help hold it in place when remainder of investment is vibrated into mold. **C,** Sprue cone B seated in mold with investment holding it in place.

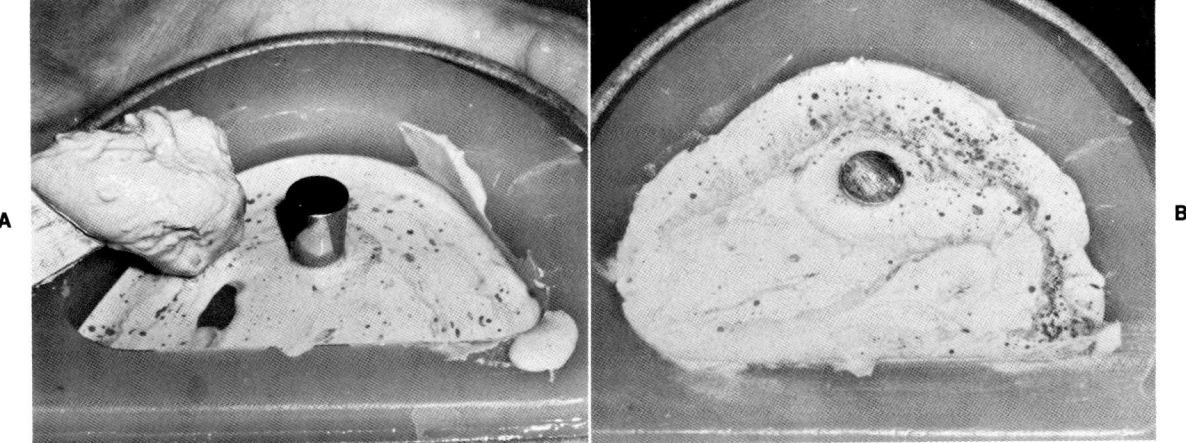

**Fig. 8-55. A,** Medium sprue cone B is left in place while investment is vibrated into mold. **B,** Mold is filled with investment to extent that sprue cone B is not covered.

**258** *Dental laboratory procedures: removable partial dentures*

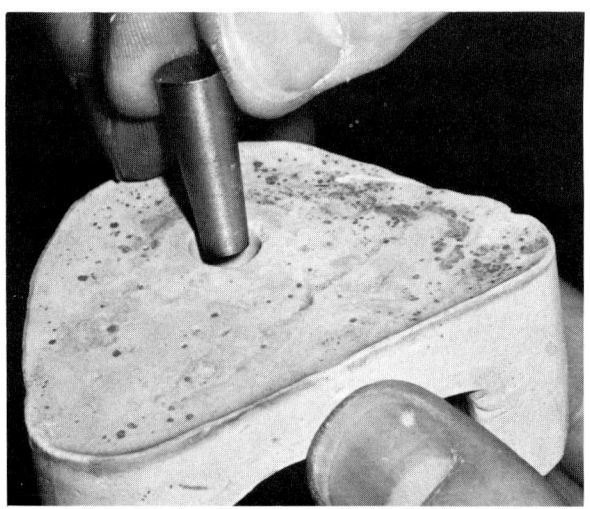

**Fig. 8-56.** After investment sets and is separated from mold, medium sprue cone B is removed from refractory cast.

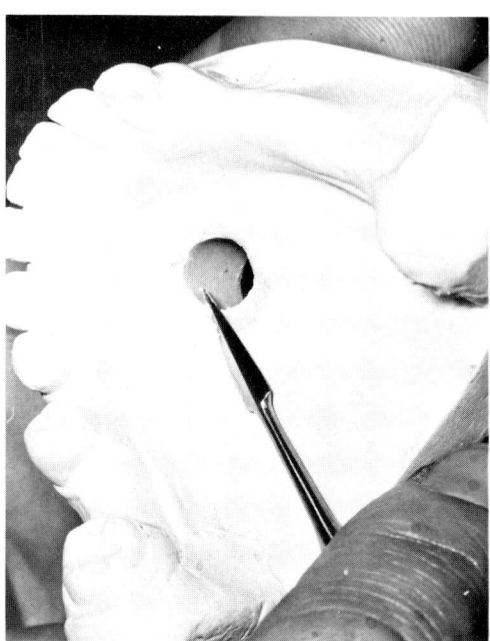

**Fig. 8-57.** Flash is trimmed even with surface of refractory cast.

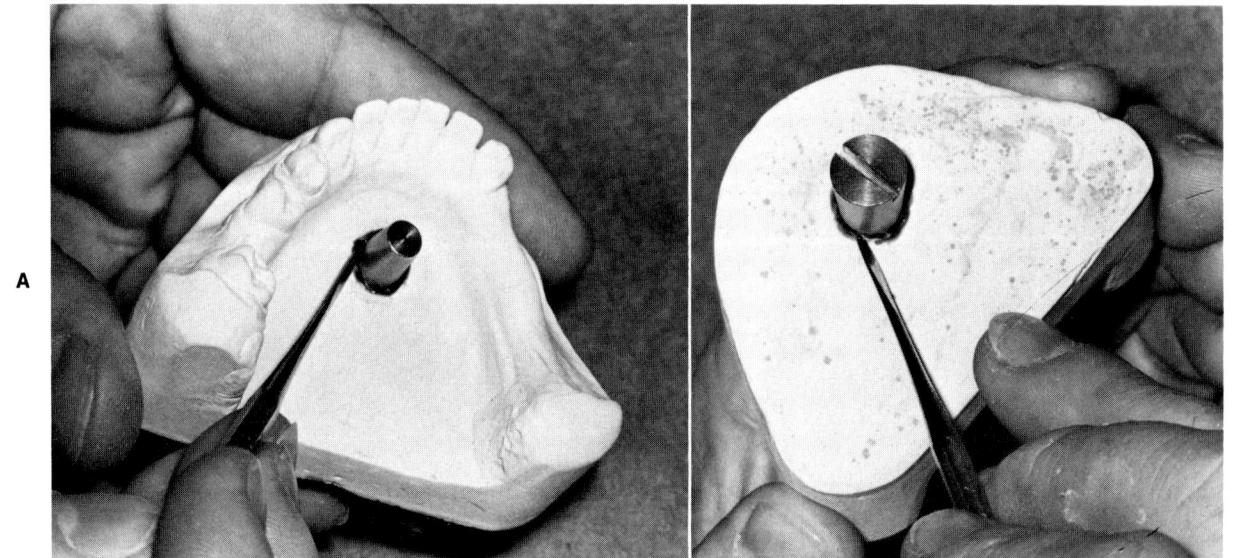

**Fig. 8-58. A,** Longest sprue cone C is waxed into place in hole in cast. **B,** Slot in sprue former facilitates its removal from investment.

mold, the medium sprue cone is removed from the refractory cast (Fig. 8-56). If the investment flash shows around the hole, smooth it off even with the surface of the cast (Fig. 8-57). Place the longest sprue cone in the hole, and wax it in place. NOTE: The long sprue cone has a slot in it, making it easier to remove from the investment (Fig. 8-58). Sprue leads are attached directly to this metal sprue cone using the overjet principle (Fig. 8-59). The sprue cone can be used to position the refractory cast in the investment (Fig. 8-60). After the investment has set, a coin or a screwdriver may be used to remove

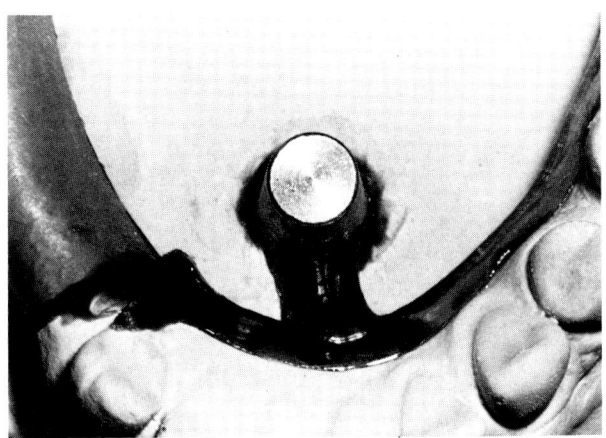

**Fig. 8-59.** Sprue leads are attached directly to metal sprue cone using overjet principle.

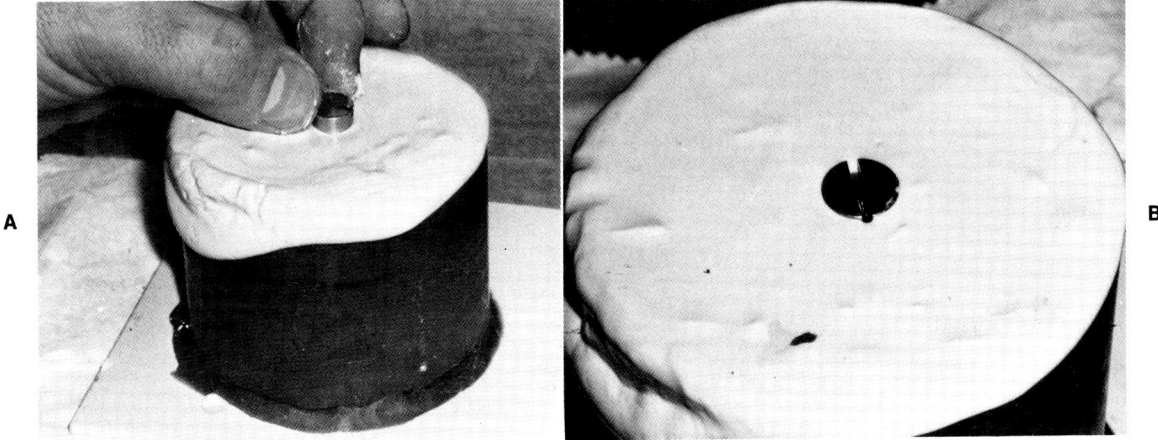

**Fig. 8-60. A,** Sprue cone is used to position refractory cast in investment in casting ring. **B,** Investment should not cover sprue cone.

the sprue cone from the investment. Smooth the investment, and make it level with the metal ring (Fig. 8-61). If desired, the hole may be enlarged somewhat (Fig. 8-62).

3. Soften half a sheet of baseplate wax. Lay a straight handpiece fissure bur on the edge of the wax, and roll the wax in a rod large enough to just pass through the hole in the base of the cast (Fig. 8-63). Push the wax rod through the base of the refractory cast until it protrudes from the other side

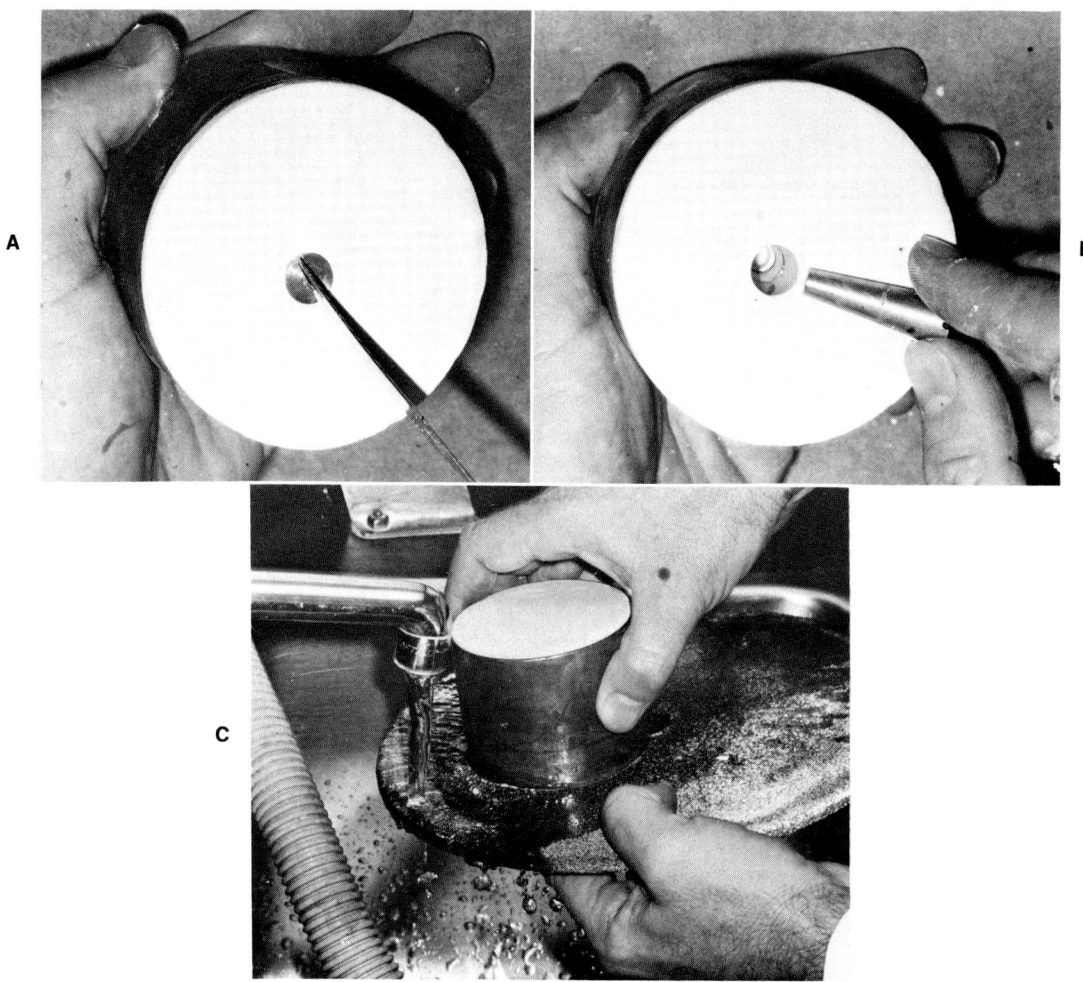

**Fig. 8-61. A,** Screwdriver or instrument is used to loosen sprue cone so it may be removed from investment. **B,** Sprue hole made by cone. **C,** Surface is made flush with casting ring by rubbing it over rough surface such as grinding plate of cast trimmer. Water helps to keep surface clean.

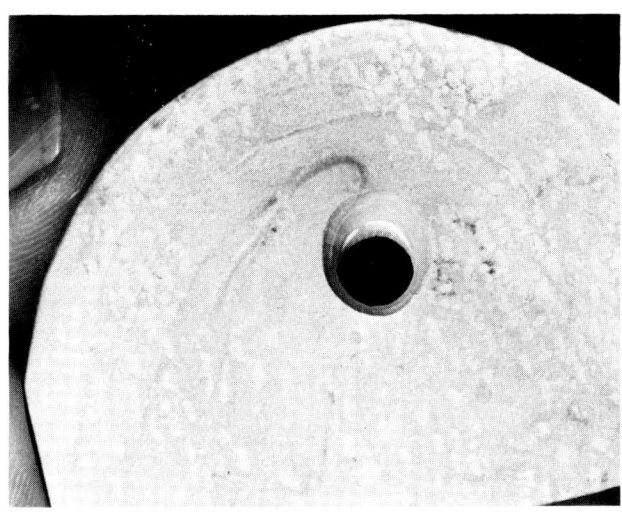

**Fig. 8-62.** Hole may be enlarged if necessary, but should be avoided if possible.

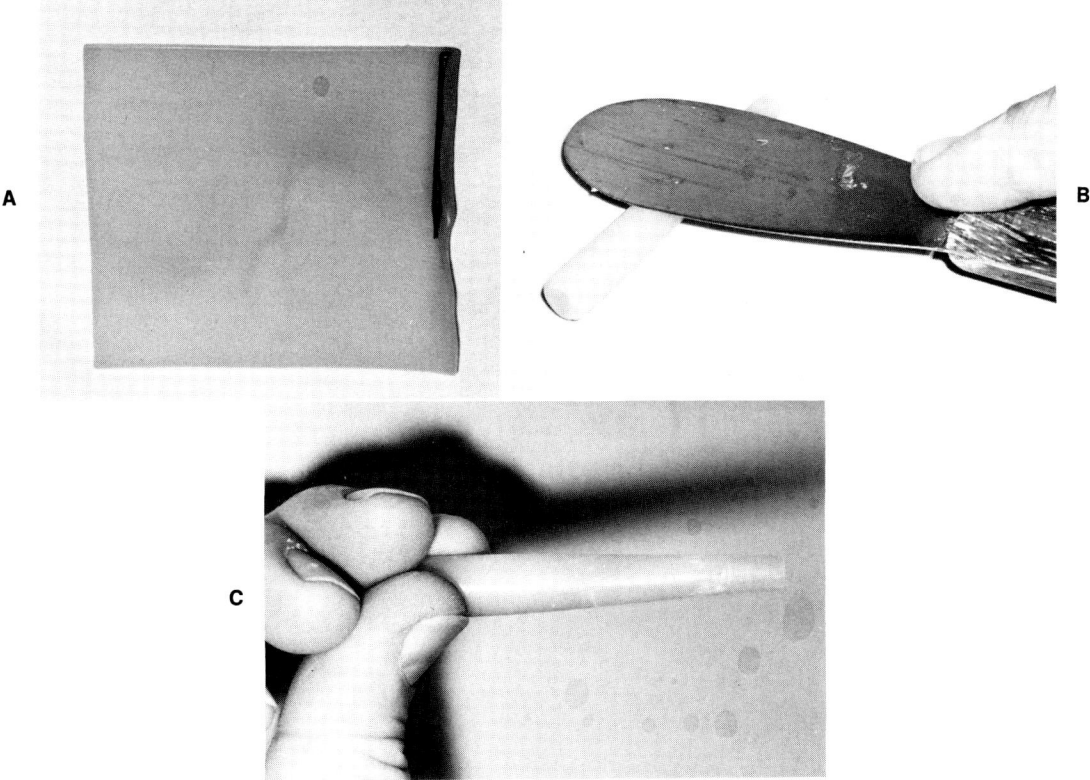

**Fig. 8-63. A,** Straight handpiece fissure bur is laid on edge of half sheet of softened baseplate wax, **B,** Wax is rolled around it to form rod large enough to just pass through hole in cast. **C,** Wax sprue cone completed.

about 10 mm. Seal the rod to the cast with wax on both sides of the cast (Fig. 8-64). The rod protruding through the bottom of the cast will act as a handle during the investment procedure. The fissure bur provides reinforcement for the wax handle and will be removed after the investing is completed.

4. Use 8- or 10-gauge round wax for sprue leads on mandibular casts, and lay them directly on the surface of the cast. Attach one end to the central sprue and the other to the bottom edge of the major connector. Usually one sprue to the center of the lingual bar is enough. Some, however, prefer three or more sprues attached to the bottom edge of the lingual bar near each finish line and occasionally to the denture base retention. Be careful not to involve the margins of the external finish lines (Fig. 8-65). When distal clasps are separated from the lingual bar by mesh or open retention, it may be desirable to run an auxiliary lead to them. An auxiliary lead is usually made of 14-gauge round sprue wax and is attached to the central sprue on the same level as the main sprues. It should run as straight as possible and attach to the minor connector on the molar just below the occlusal rest or to the distal portion of the denture base retention, if one was used (Fig. 8-66).

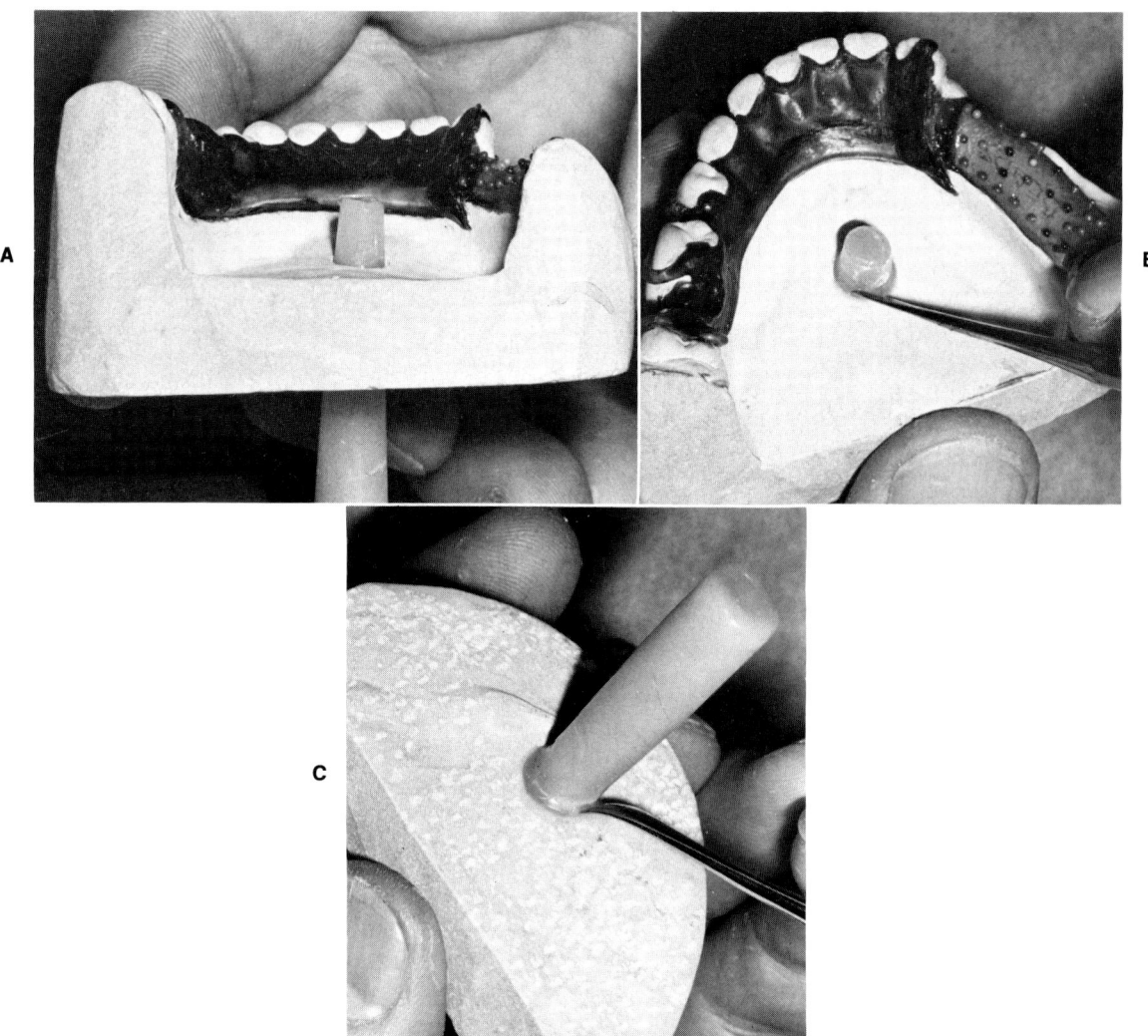

**Fig. 8-64. A,** Wax rod is pushed through hole until it extends about 10 mm on pattern side of cast. **B,** Wax rod is sealed to cast on pattern side. **C,** Wax rod is sealed to bottom of cast.

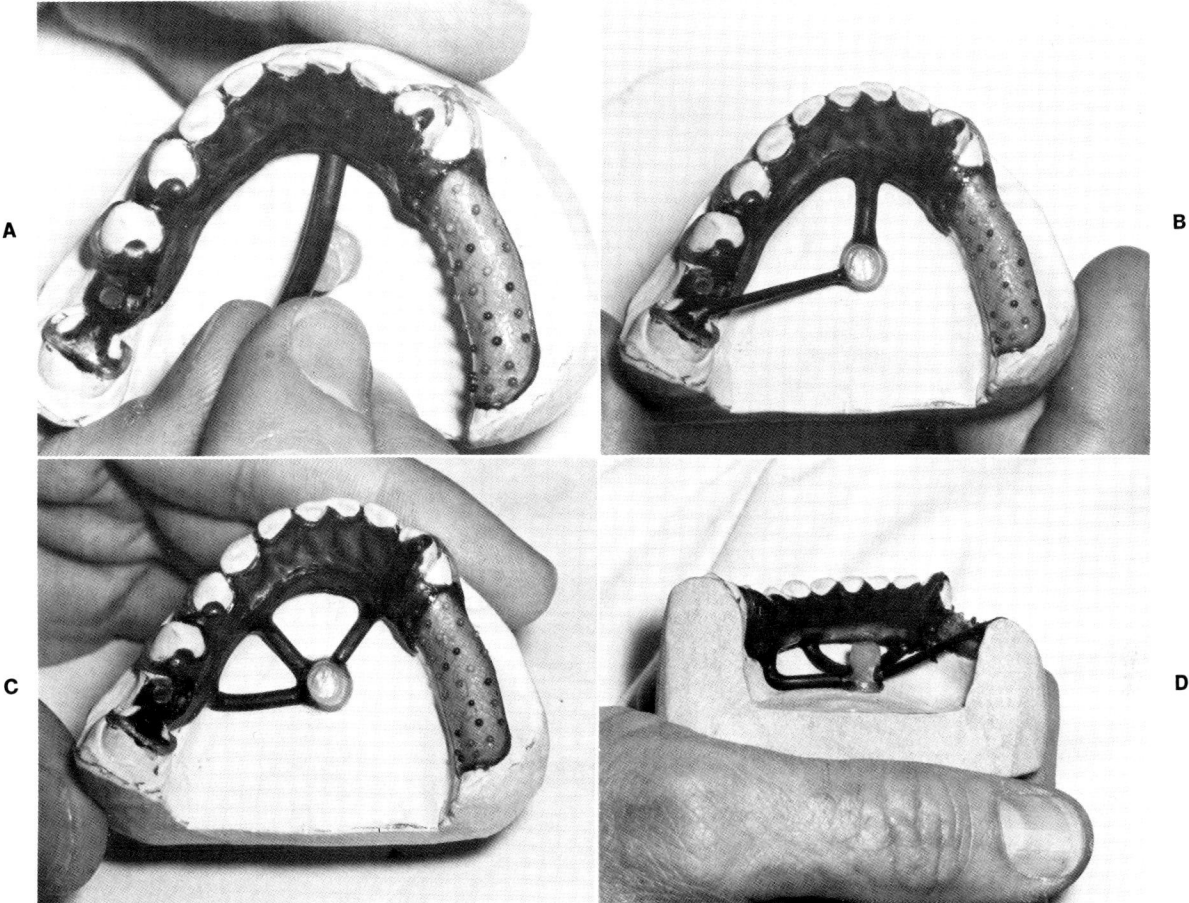

**Fig. 8-65. A,** Sprue leads are positioned directly on mandibular cast and sealed at both ends. **B,** Some prefer single main sprue lead with auxiliary lead. **C,** Others prefer three sprues. **D,** Note that they are all attached to central sprue at same height, and joint at each end is well rounded.

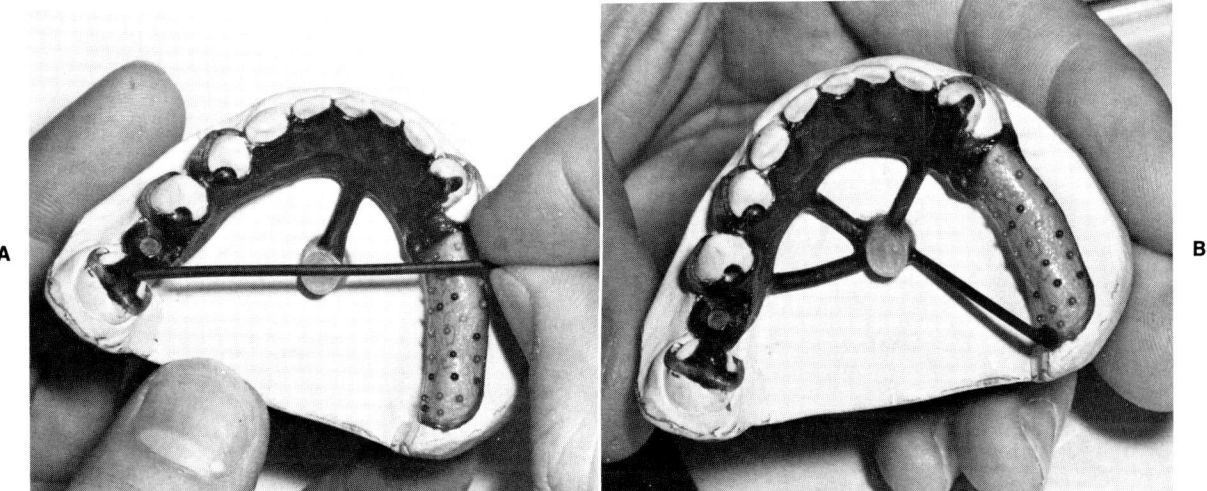

**Fig. 8-66. A,** Fourteen-gauge round wax is used for auxiliary sprues on molar clasp that are separated from lingual bar by thin section. **B,** Auxiliary sprues are attached to central sprue at same level as main sprues, and joints are well rounded.

Six-gauge half-round wax is most often used for sprue leads when spruing maxillary cast wax-ups that lend themselves to this procedure. The wax rod is made and placed as described in step 3 (Fig. 8-67). Wax-ups on maxillary casts may also be sprued using the wax rod and overjet principle as in the mandibular cast but approaching it from above rather than through the cast.

Another method uses a homemade wax sprue former in a direct overhead approach. Attach 10-gauge sprue leads to the wax patterns, and fasten them together over the center of the wax-up (Fig. 8-68). Pour melted baseplate wax into a dappen dish or similar shaped container (Fig. 8-69). When the baseplate wax sets, remove it from the dappen dish, and smooth the flat side with a hot spatula (Fig. 8-70). Seal the homemade wax spur former to the sprue leads, making a smooth joint (Fig. 8-71), and adjust the height of the cast and sprue former to the length of the investing ring.

Maxillary casts may also be sprued from the distal aspect at the level of the major connector. A piece of baseplate wax may be used to attach the main sprue former to the major connector. This usually requires a longer investing ring than the other methods.

5. Reinforce and smooth all junctions between the sprues and the framework patterns, and they are ready for investing (Fig. 8-72).

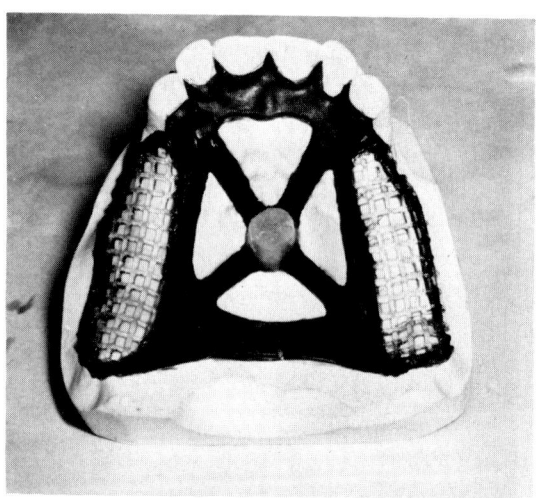

**Fig. 8-67.** Wax rod is sealed in place on maxillary cast as it was on mandibular cast and sprued with 6-gauge half-round leads, if shape of major connector permits this form of spruing.

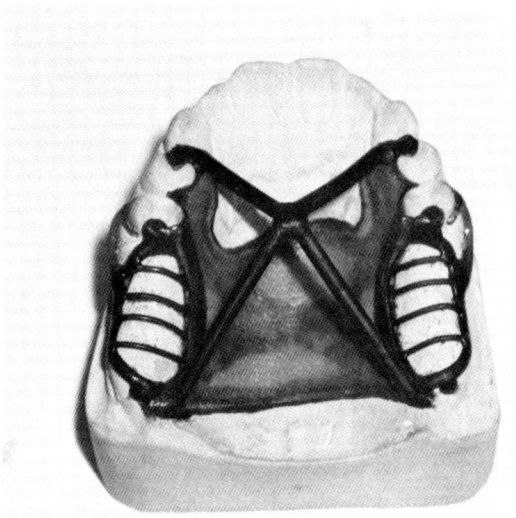

**Fig. 8-68.** When maxillary wax-ups are sprued from above, 10-gauge round wax leads are used and fastened together over center of wax-up.

## Waxing and spruing

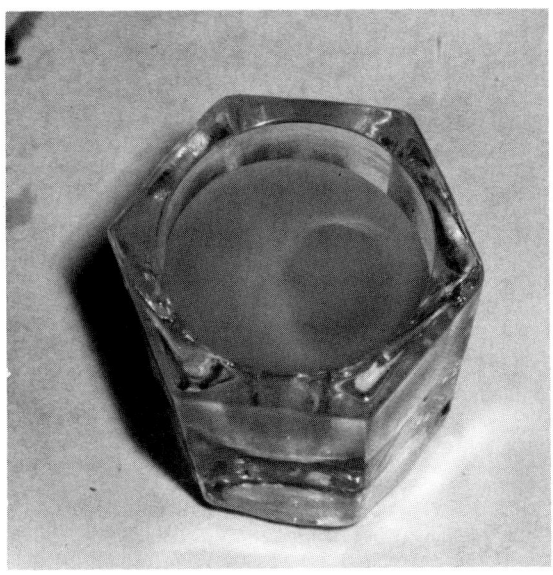

**Fig. 8-69.** Melted baseplate wax is poured into dappen dish to make wax sprue former.

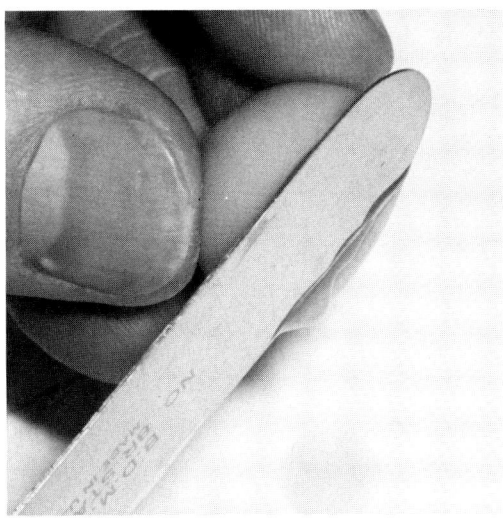

**Fig. 8-70.** When wax is hard, remove it, and smooth flat side with hot spatula.

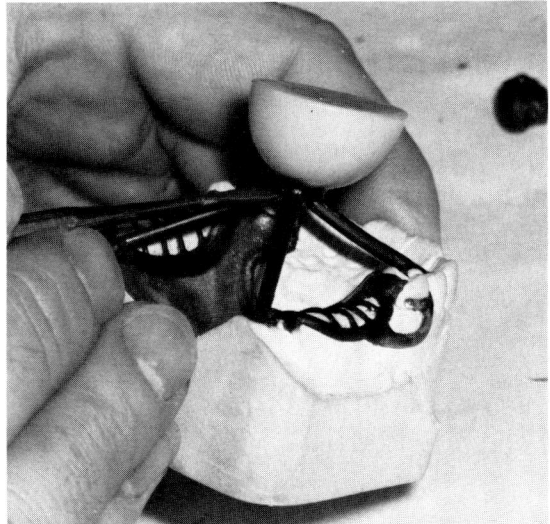

**Fig. 8-71.** Adjust height of sprue leads so base of cast will be approximately 8 mm from one end of investing ring when wax crucible former is flush with other end. Seal sprue former in place.

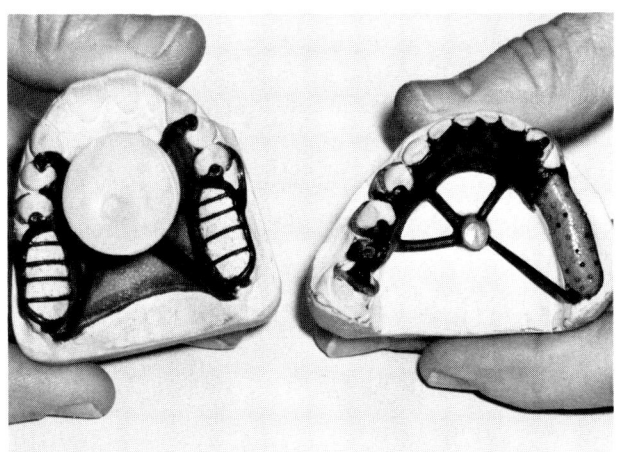

**Fig. 8-72.** Wax-ups ready for investing.

**Table 8-2.** Spruing

| Problem | Probable cause | Solution |
| --- | --- | --- |
| Small particles of investment in casting | Sprue leads not joined to main sprue on wax pattern properly | Attach sprue leads with smooth rounded amount of wax so no sharp edges of investment remain after burnout |
| | Sprue hole was enlarged by cutting with knife, leaving roughened surface for metal to flow over | Make original sprue former smooth and large enough to hold metal without having to cut it; this leaves smooth glazed surface |
| Metal spilled when casting | Sprue hole is too small for bulk of metal | Make sprue hole large enough to accommodate twice the amount of metal required for casting |
| | Sprue leads broken during investing procedure | Attach sprue leads smoothly and firmly at both ends, and do not vibrate excessively |
| Porosity in casting | Improper spruing procedure | Always run sprue lead directly to bulky part of pattern; never try to reach thick section through thin section |

## PROBLEM AREAS

The principal problems associated with spruing include incorporation of the investment in the casting, metal spillage when casting, and porosity in the cast framework (Table 8-2). Controlling the angulation of the sprues, eliminating sharp edges of investment, using a smooth sprue former, firmly attaching the sprues to the pattern, and spruing directly to bulky parts of the pattern can significantly reduce problems.

## SUMMARY

In this chapter methods for waxing and spruing a removable partial denture framework pattern was described. Potential problem areas, as well as solutions, were also presented.

### BIBLIOGRAPHY

Air Force Manual 160-29: Dental laboratory technicians manual, United States Air Force, Washington, D.C., 1959, U.S. Government Printing Office.

Air Force Manual 162-6: Dental laboratory technology, United States Air Force, Washington, D.C., 1975, U.S. Government Printing Office.

Sowter, J. B.: Dental laboroatory technology: prosthodontic techniques, Chapel Hill, N.C., 1968, The University of North Carolina Press.

# CHAPTER 9

# WROUGHT WIRE CLASPS

JAMES S. BRUDVIK

## DEFINITION

Wrought wire clasp arms can be constructed in any configuration to be compatible with any design concept. Except in the case of certain temporary appliances, these arms are used only for the retentive portion of the clasp assembly. The nonretentive (bracing) component is either cast metal or, in some cases, resin.

## DESCRIPTION

The classic configuration is the circumferential form, which originates in an edentulous space and passes either anterior or posterior to engage opposite facial retentive areas. This clasp has been used throughout the modern history of dentistry. More recently, wrought alloys have been used in infrabulge clasp forms as well. Gold alloy wires have been considered the clasps of choice, but the recent rise of precious metal costs, coupled with improved cobalt-chromium-nickel and stainless steel alloys have greatly reduced their use.

Wire retentive arms are most often 18 or 19 gauge. Certain nonprecious alloys are used in the 20-gauge size for extremely short arms to gain adequate flexibility. Some manufacturers provide wires in half-round shapes, as well as the more common round form.

The circumferential wire clasp is ideally placed so that only the terminal third lies in the infrabulge area. The proximal two thirds should lie at or above the height of the contour (Fig. 9-1). Teeth that have not been properly prepared or that have bizarre

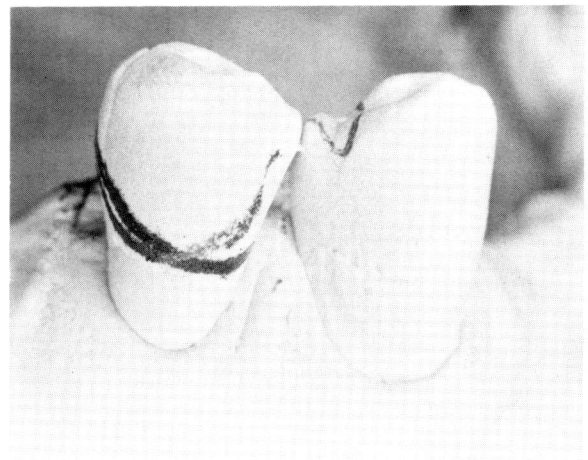

**Fig. 9-1.** Ideal circumferential clasp relation to height of contour. Terminal third extends into undercut and proximal two thirds are at or above line.

contours may not allow circumferential clasp placement above the height of the contour. Rather than place the entire clasp arm into infrabulge contact, the proximal two thirds may have to stand slightly away from the tooth (Fig. 9-2).

The depth of the undercut used varies with clinical preference and the gauge and alloy used for the clasp; 18-gauge gold alloy wires perform well clinically when the terminal third is placed into an undercut of up to 0.015 inch. Wrought clasp arms placed into greater degrees of undercut tend to distort with use unless the clasp length is increased beyond normal limits.

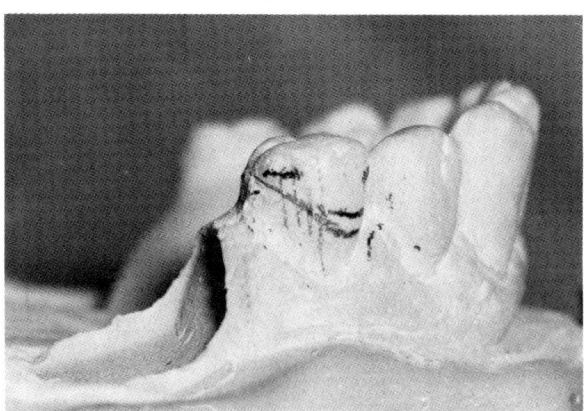

**Fig. 9-2.** If abutment tooth is poorly contoured, proximal two thirds may have to be positioned slightly away from tooth.

## MATERIALS
### Precious metal alloys

***Gold.*** A variety of precious metal wires are available for construction of retentive clasp arms. The American Dental Association (ADA) Specification No. 7 gives two divisions of wire based on precious metal content. High precious metal content, those with 75% or higher gold and platinum groups are called type I, and those with 65% or higher gold and platinum group content are called type II. These wires are available in gauges from 16 to 21; 18-gauge clasp wires are by far the most commonly used size. Precious metal wires come from the manufacturer fully annealed. If excessive recontouring is necessary, as in the situation where an error has been made, the formed clasp can be annealed to relieve work hardness by quenching from the manufacturer's indicated annealing temperature. Heat hardening will occur automatically by allowing the clasp to air cool after soldering. Platinum-gold-palladium and platinum-iridium wires are not considered to be effected by heat-hardening treatment because they contain no cooper. Adequate research findings are available to indicate that the best dental wires will contain enough platinum and palladium to preserve fine grain structure during all heating operations. Care must always be taken that no precious alloyed wire be heated above its recrystallization temperature.

***Platinum-gold-palladium (PGP).*** The PGP wire may be considered the finest precious metal clasp wire. Its composition, platinum, 40% to 50%, gold, 25% to 30%, and palladium 25% to 30%, make it more expensive than other dental wires. It meets the type I, ADA specification with a tensile strength above 136,000 psi and a fusion temperature range of 2730° to 2790° F (1499° to 1532° C).

This high-fusion temperature allows (PGP) to be used in those situations where chrome or type IV gold alloy partial denture frameworks are cast to the preformed wire.

### Nonprecious metal alloys

***Stainless steel.*** Stainless steel wire (18-8) has been used as a clasp wire as well for orthodonic appliances. This alloy is a steel with approximately 18% chromium and 8% nickel. It is corrosive resistant in its original state, but the heat generated in soldering can effect its resistance. The solders used with stainless steel wires must be in the range of 10 carat so that their melting temperature will not be high enough to anneal the wires. These solders will corrode because they are cathodic to the stainless steel.

Generally 18-8 stainless steel is not a good material for other than temporary dental prostheses. It performs best where it is attached to the appliance by resin only.

***Nickel-chromium.*** Nickel-chromium alloys are approximately 80% nickel and 20% chromium. They have high corrosion resistance and do not soften greatly during soldering. The same potential for corrosion problems associated with soldering exists here as with the stainless steel wire, but a higher soldering temperature can be used; 450-fine solder gives a stronger joint than lower carat solder.

***Cobalt-chromium.*** Cobalt-chromium alloys are among the most common nonprecious wrought alloys for use with removable partial dentures. They have a composition of roughly 50% cobalt, 20% chromium and 15% nickel. Alloys of this type were originally designed for watch springs, and their excellent properties make them ideal for retentive clasp arms. The heat treatment of these wires that occurs when they are soldered to a framework with electric soldering and allowed to cool in air gives a result quite similar to that recommended as ideal (900° F; 482° C for 3 minutes and cooled in air). They are used with apparent equal success in the same situations in which precious metal wires may be used.

## ARMAMENTARIUM

There is a variety of wire-bending pliers available to the dental profession. The majority have been designed for use in orthodontics. The basic instruments will include the following (Fig. 9-3):
1. Gordon contouring plier
2. Three-prong clasp-adjusting plier
3. Wire-binding plier (three-groove)
4. Wire-cutter with vinyl inserts

# Wrought wire clasps

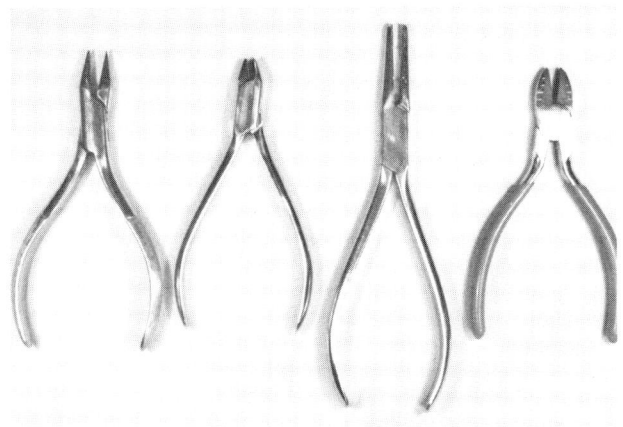

**Fig. 9-3.** Basic wire-contouring pliers (left to right): Gordon contouring plier, three-prong clasp-adjusting plier, three-groove wire-bending plier, and wire cutter with vinyl inserts.

With this group of pliers, or ones of similar shapes and functions, retentive clasps arms of any type can be contoured. An electric soldering machine* will be used to solder wire clasp arms to partial denture frameworks (Fig. 9-4).

## WIRE SELECTION

The alloy and the gauge of the wire clasp should come from the prescription. When this information is not available, the following guidelines can be used:

1. Nonprecious wires are generally more rigid than precious wires. To gain the same clasp flexibility, the nonprecious wire is used one gauge size smaller. For circumferential clasp arms on molars and large premolars, 18-gauge PGP (or similar wire), and 19-gauge cobalt-chromium† give approximately the same retentive properties.

2. When the active clasp length falls below 8 mm, the gauge selected must be reduced, or the clasp will be too rigid if the same degree of undercut is engaged. In this case, 19-gauge PGP or 20-gauge cobalt-chromium is indicated.

3. For long infrabulge clasp arms, a change in the other direction must be made. With an active clasp length of more than 12 mm, 17-gauge PGP or 18-gauge cobalt-chromium wire should be used.

NOTE: Active clasp length refers to the portion of the wire that is expected to flex. It is measured from where the clasp exits from the resin or metal at the minor connector.

*Torit model 21A, The Torit Corp., St. Paul, Minn., or equivalent.
†Ti-Wire, Ticonium Co., Albany, N.Y., or equivalent.

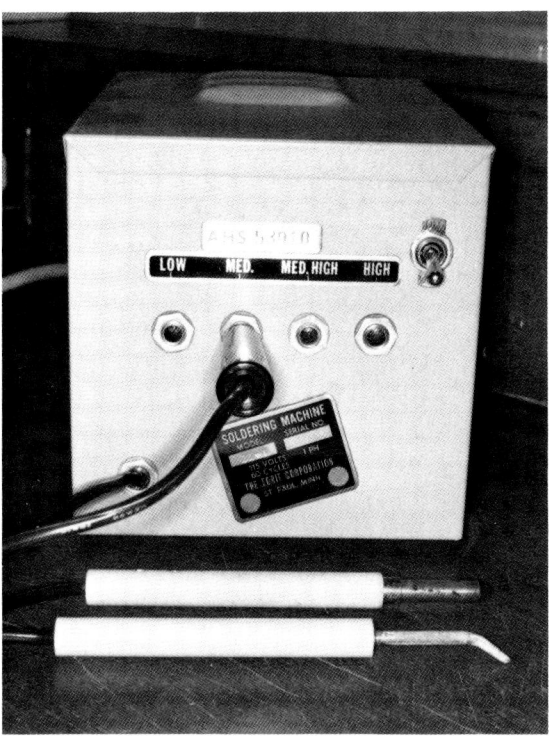

**Fig. 9-4.** Torit Model 21-A is used to solder wires to removable partial denture frameworks.

## CONSTRUCTION TECHNIQUES

Contouring the clasp form requires the development of a strong sense of spacial relationships. This development is always individual and comes only with practice. The following basic principles will form a basis for developing personal techniques:

1. *Hold* the wire with a plier, and *bend* it with finger pressure.

2. Bend the wire to a curve that conforms to the tooth contour. Then move it along the tooth until a position is found where the contour of the tooth and wire match. Mark the wire extending past the tip of the clasp, as indicated on the cast by a pencil line, with a wax pencil, and cut it with a disk or plier.

3. Do not attempt to start at the clasp tip and work back to the body of the clasp. This is much more difficult and frustrating than the approach described in step 2.

4. Do not hold the wire so tightly that the plier break dents the wire. With those pliers having both a round and a square beak, the wire must always be bent against the round beak.

5. Do not use three-pronged pliers to bend clasps in the area where they are expected to flex. They will invariably nick the wire. Their use should be restricted to bends made in the nonflexing areas within the resin.

## Clasp contouring

Before clasp contouring can begin, the position of the clasp arm must be drawn on the master cast. It is a definite advantage to draw this line in a color dramatically different from the one used for the design outline of the remainder of the appliance (Fig. 9-5). Red is used in many laboratories for frame design and blue for wire clasp arms.

***Circumferential clasp arms.*** When the tooth is ideally contoured, the blue line will lay on or above the height of contour for two thirds of its length. (This height of contour line is put on the cast by the surveyor lead at the selected path of insertion before the design is transferred.) The terminal third of the line will be in the undercut area to a depth of 0.010 to 0.015 inches. A wire clasp adapted to this blue line in an ideally contoured tooth will be curved in *one plane only* (Fig. 9-6). The addition of bends in the wire in additional planes is *always* considered a compromise because each additional bend increases the rigidity of the clasp.

When the tooth is not ideally contoured, it may not be possible to keep the proximal two thirds at or above the height of contour and maintain a contour in one plane while keeping this clasp in contact with the tooth throughout its length. Where a steep undercut exists at the proximal line angle, it is preferable to have the proximal two thirds of the clasp actually stand away from the tooth than to try to keep the wire above the height of contour, which invariably will bring additional bends to the wire and place it at the marginal ridge area. Wires placed this high on the proximal surface often interfere with occlusal relationships and may actually come into occlusion with opposing structures themselves.

1. Place the designed master cast on the workbench with the tooth to be clasped facing the operator. Hold the selected wire with one of the two pronged pliers near its end. The thumb and forefinger on the opposite hand should be used to curve the wire away from the operator (Fig. 9-7). This first bend actually forms the basic curve of the wire. Remove the plier, and lay the wire against the blue line. At this point, evaluate the basic curve. This curve may be too sharp, not sharp enough, or in harmony with the curve of the tooth. If care is taken, this first try is almost always too shallow and will require additional bending in the same plane to bring it into harmony. This is preferable to overbending and should become a habitual approach.

2. When the basic curve is established, move the wire forward and backward along the blue line until a segment of the curve that corresponds to the tooth curvature is found.

3. Transfer the tip of the clasp arm to the wire from the blue line drawing. This marking is best done with a wax pencil (Fig. 9-8). Cut off the excess wire beyond this point. It is preferable to cut the excess wire with a disk on a high-speed lathe. Wire cutters actually crimp the wire somewhat in cutting it and leave a tip that requires further contouring. The disk cut leaves a square cut at right angles to the wire surface that requires only a rounding of the edge to complete the clasp tip.

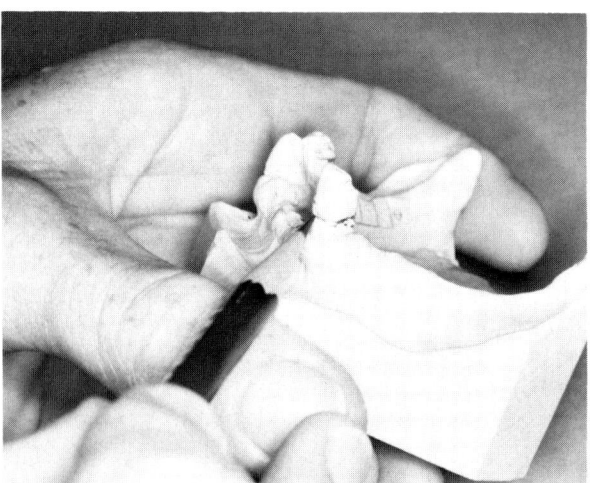

Fig. 9-5. Wire clasp arm is drawn on master cast with different color than is used for remainder of design.

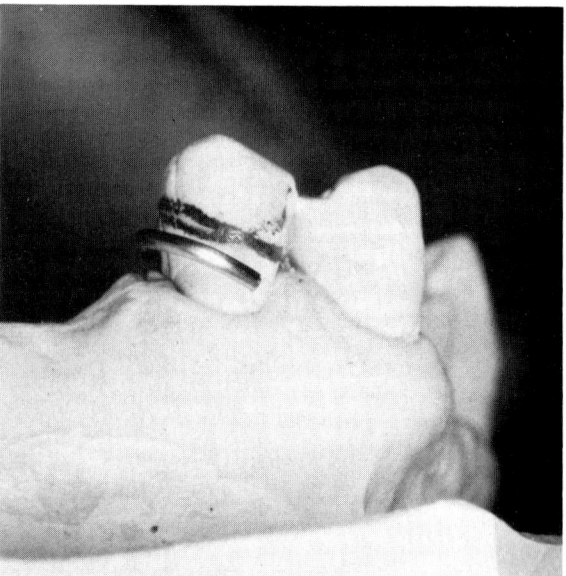

Fig. 9-6. Ideal wire clasp arm is curved in one plane only.

4. Estimate the amount of proximal wire needed to reach the soldering spot, and cut the wire again slightly beyond this length (¼ inch; 0.63 cm) (Fig. 9-9).

5. With the tip completed, the bend at the line angle can be accomplished. This bend will carry the base of the clasp wire to the minor connector and into the edentulous space where it will be electro-soldered to the retentive mesh or bead retentive area. Since this bend is usually within the area that will be resin in the final appliance, it is not as critical as the basic clasp curve. The bend should place the wire as close as possible to the minor connector without requiring an additional bend. Make the bend at the proximal line angle by first marking the wire at the spot where the wire will enter the resin or touch metal of the minor connector (Fig. 9-10).

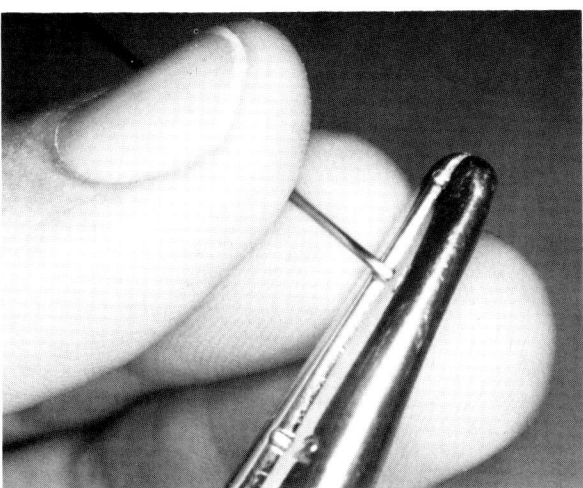

**Fig. 9-7.** Wire should be bent away from operator and toward round beak of plier.

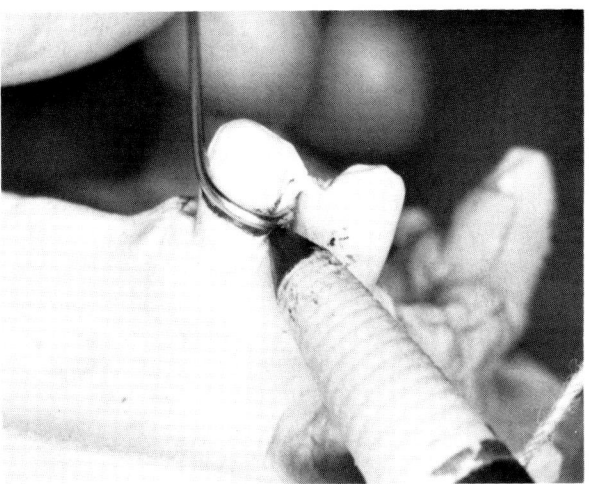

**Fig. 9-8.** Tip of designed clasp length is marked with wax pencil and excess cut off with disk.

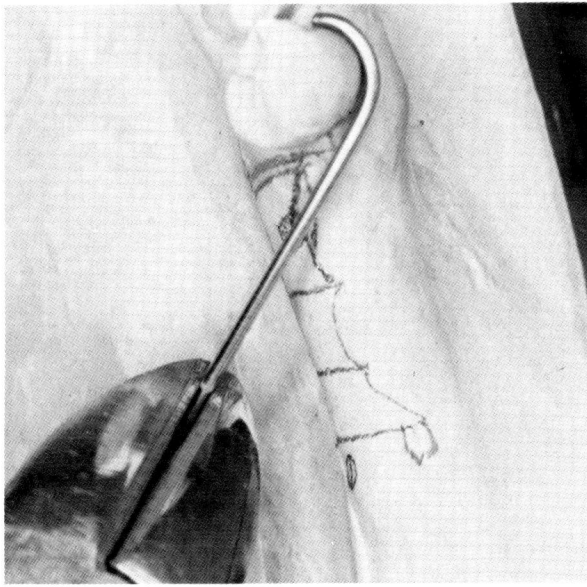

**Fig. 9-9.** Before cutting wire, ¼ inch (0.63 cm) should be added to estimated length of any clasp.

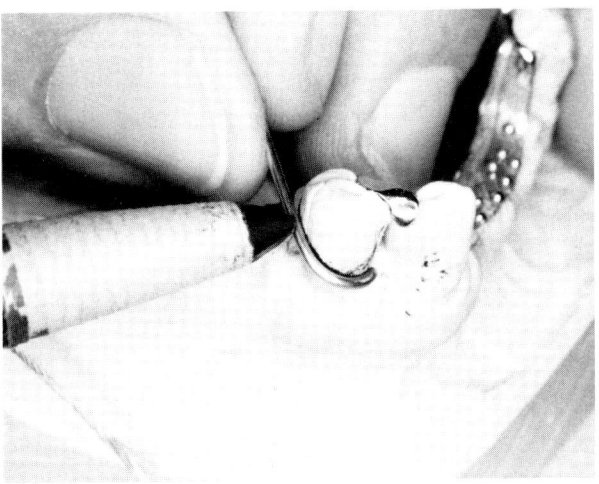

**Fig. 9-10.** Bend at proximal angle is marked with wax pencil.

6. With the active clasp arm in contact with the blue line, the proximal end will extend into the edentulous space. Estimate the angle of proximal bend required to reach the soldering spot. Remove the wire from the cast, and hold it with the Gordon contouring plier. The round beak of the plier must be away from the operator, so that the proximal bend will be made against the round surface. The beak of the plier is placed before the wax mark, that is, closer to the clasp tip by 1 to 2 mm (Fig. 9-11). The bending, again, is done with the thumb and forefinger to the approximate angle.

7. Return the wire to the master cast, and evaluate its position (Fig. 9-12). In most cases one additional bend will be needed for the wire to reach the soldering spot. If the wire is to be soldered to the minor connector, then this bend will not be necessary.

8. This additional bend may take the form of a sharp angle or a gentle curve, depending on the particular case. Since the wire at this bend will be covered with resin and at a distance removed from the active clasp arm, the three-pronged plier may be used. Place the middle beak on the spot where the bend is desired, and crimp (bend) the wire by closing the beaks. It may be possible to make this bend with the wire actually on the cast, or very close to it (Fig. 9-13).

9. With the basic bends completed, reposition the clasp on the master cast, and verify its contact and contour. Attaching the clasp to the framework some distance from the active arm allows a measure of adjustability before the final position is chosen.

10. As tooth contours become less ideal, additional bends may become necessary. In these instances, mark the wire with the wax pencil, hold it with the plier, and bend it with the hand. It is more important to maintain simple clasp contours than to introduce multiple bends in the hope of touching the designed blue line throughout every convolution. As long as the terminal third is in contact with the retentive area at the desired undercut, the clasp will function satisfactorily. When it is obvious that an undercut exists at the proximal line angle where the wire passes on its way to the retentive area, prepare the undercut with standard blockout techniques (Fig. 9-14). Adapt the wire to the wax in the undercut area (Fig. 9-15). Solder the clasp arm to the frame with this wax still in place. The wax will keep the proximal two thirds of the active arm from being placed into any amount of undercut. *This is critical* because a wire clasp arm that is forced to flex in the proximal third due to an undercut at that point will soon deform and stand away from the tooth.

11. It must be understood that these procedures

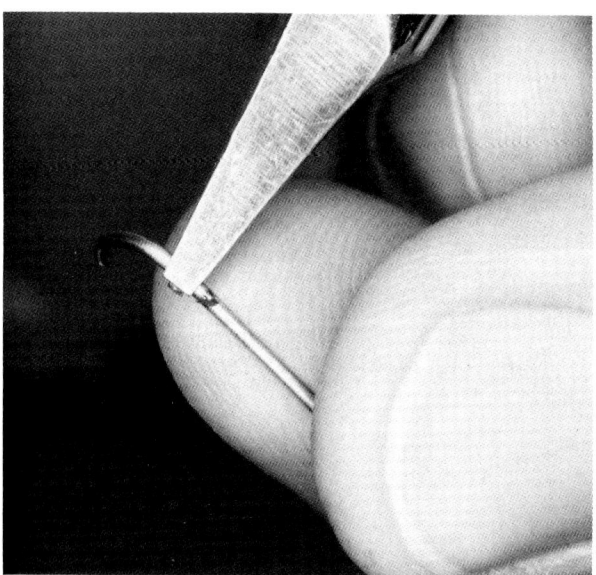

**Fig. 9-11.** Beaks of plier are placed before wax mark by 1 to 2 mm.

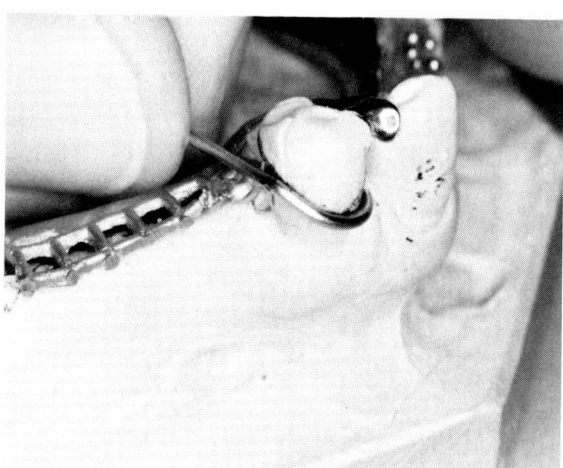

**Fig. 9-12.** Wire must be returned to master cast after each bend to evaluate its position.

are applicable for all wire circumferential retentive clasp arms be they buccal or lingual. The clasp tip is finished at this point by rounding the wire at the disk cut to remove any sharpness. This finishing is best done with a fine-pointed stone at relatively low speeds followed by a rubber point.

**Infrabulge clasps.** Although there are many possible forms that the infrabulge clasp can take, by far the most common shapes for wire clasp arms are the I bar and the L bar.

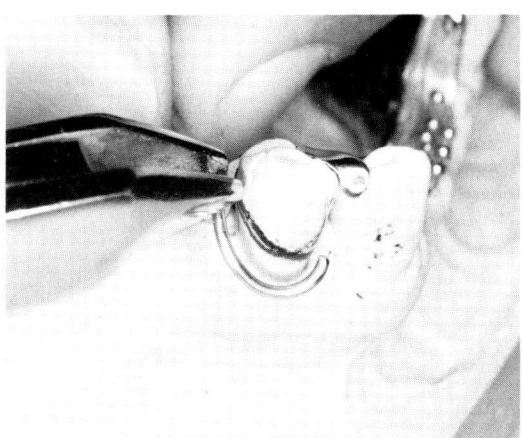

**Fig. 9-13.** Three-pronged plier can be used to make bends that will be within resin. This bend will bring wire to soldering spot.

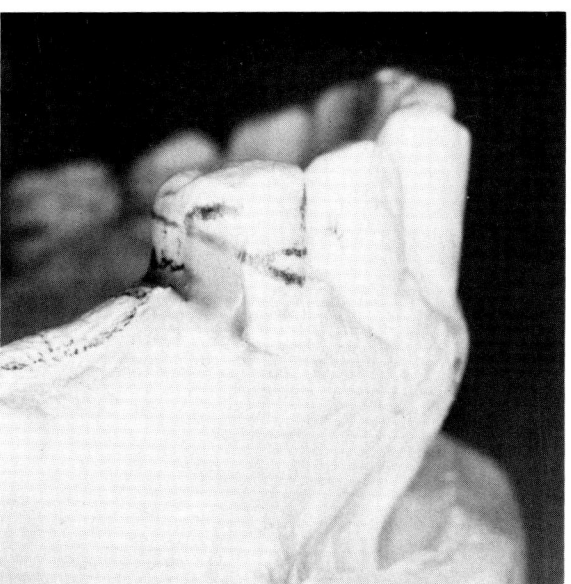

**Fig. 9-14.** Proximal undercuts are blocked out before wire can be adapted.

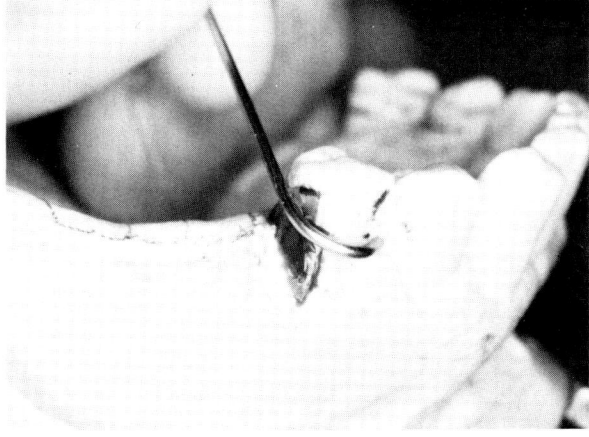

**Fig. 9-15.** Wire is adapted to wax to keep proximal two thirds from falling into undercut.

## I-BAR CLASP

1. The I-bar form is the easiest of all wire clasp arms to contour. Draw the clasp arm on the master cast in blue pencil (Fig. 9-16). Place the clasp tip into an undercut of 0.010 inch.

2. Decide on the contour of the tip with relation to the undercut area before the contouring can begin. If a round wire touches a round tooth, the contact area will invariably be only a point contact. It may be modified by bending the wire to allow a line contact vertically, or it can be modified by grinding or disking a contact area at the point where the wire will touch the tooth. If this modification is a flat disk cut, then the flat surface of the wire will still touch the rounded tooth surface in only a point. If the wire end is modified to a slightly concave surface (Fig. 9-17), then it may be possible to have a true surface contact with the undercut "spot" on the tooth. This surface area contact can be prepared with either a disk or pointed stones with slow speed.

3. With the shaping of the tip completed, the clasp contouring can begin. Use a boley gauge to measure the distance from the clasp tip drawn on the master cast to the first bend (Fig. 9-18). Transfer this length to the wire with a wax pencil. Hold the wire with the Gordon plier, and make a 90-degree bend against the round beak of the plier.

4. Place the wire on the master cast, and estimate the curvature of the second bend (Fig. 9-19). Hold the wire in the three-groove plier, and make the second bend to bring the proximal segment into the area of retentive mesh, minor connector, or metal retention.

5. It is often necessary to make a third bend to bring the wire over the ridge crest and down to the soldering spot away from the area to be occupied by the denture teeth. This third bend will be made at the ridge crest and can be accomplished with the three-pronged plier or any smaller beaked plier (Fig. 9-20).

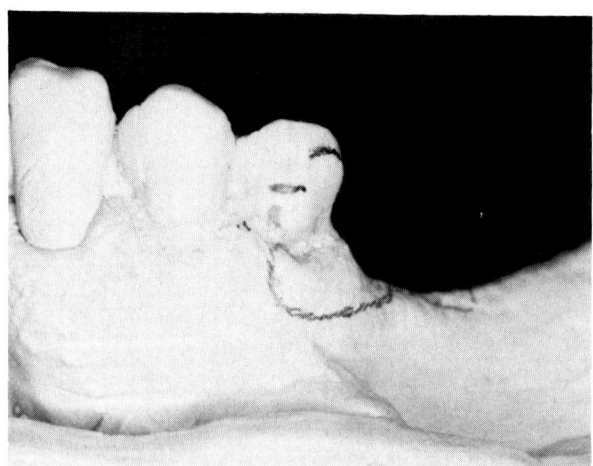

**Fig. 9-16.** I-bar clasp as designed on master cast. On distal extension situations, it is placed at or anterior to greatest convexity mesiodistally.

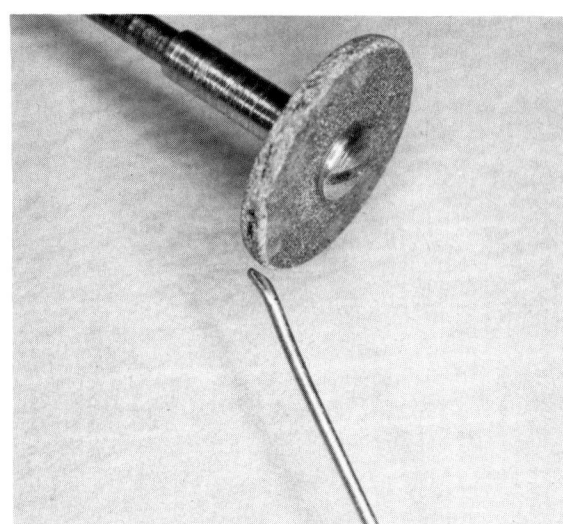

**Fig. 9-17.** Tip of I-bar clasp wire is modified with disk to provide concave surface that corresponds to curvature of tooth at retentive area.

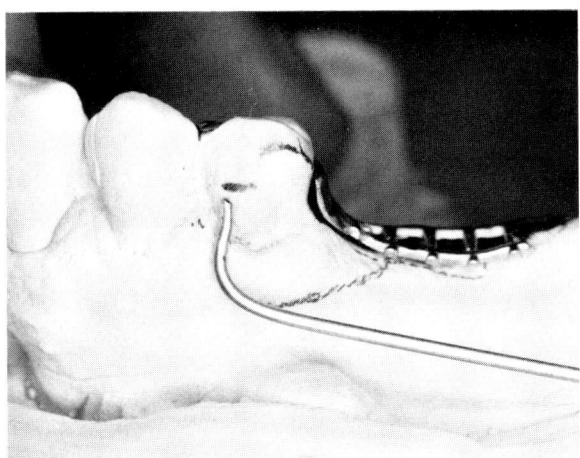

**Fig. 9-18.** First bend of I-bar clasp is usually made 2 to 3 mm past point where wire crosses gingival margin.

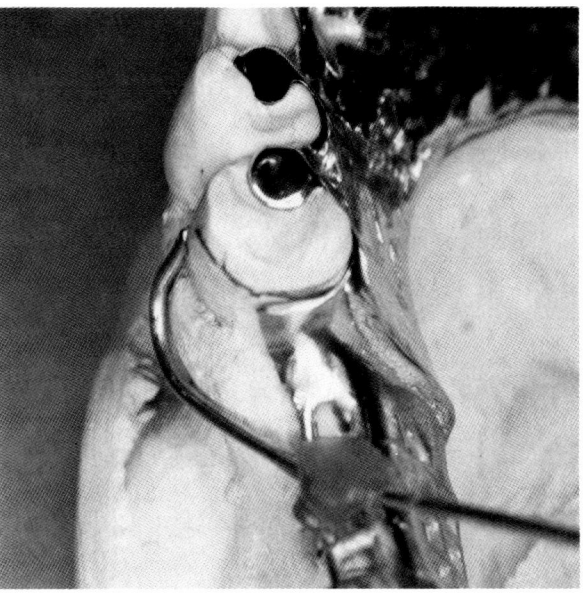

**Fig. 9-19.** Curvature of second bend of I-bar depends on curvature of soft tissue contour from first bend to point where wire will enter resin.

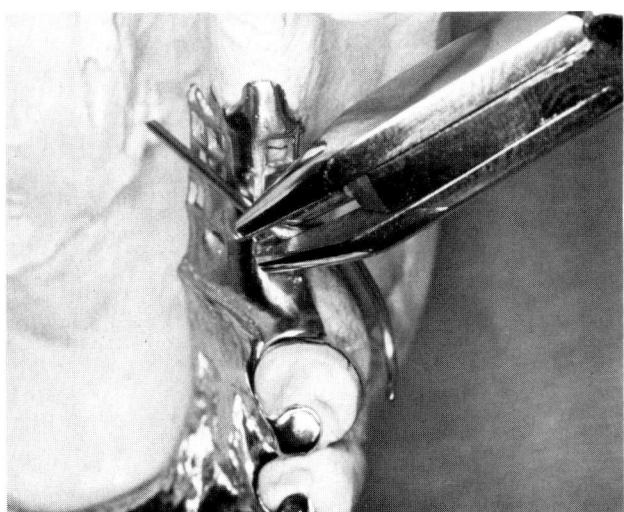

**Fig. 9-20.** Third and last bend of I-bar clasp. Since it will be within resin, it can be made with any wire-bending plier.

### L-BAR CLASP (MODIFIED T CLASP)

The other infrabulge clasp form in which wrought wire is desirable is the L bar. This clasp is a modification of the T-bar clasp, with the nonretentive tip of the clasp eliminated. The clasp normally employs a distofacial retentive area on an abutment anterior to an edentulous space (Fig. 9-21). The L-bar clasp is more difficult than the I bar in that it has one additional component. Other than this distal arm, all other parts of the clasp and its contouring are identical to the I bar previously described.

1. Draw the desired position of the clasp arm and body on the master cast.
2. The first bend is identical to that used on a circumferential clasp. In fact, the distal arm of the L-bar clasp may be viewed as the terminal third of a circumferential clasp (Fig. 9-22). The wire is contoured to a basic curve with the three-groove plier.
3. Move the curve of wire along the tooth until it corresponds to the curvature of the abutment tooth at the blue line.
4. Remove the excess wire at the tip with a disk after marking it with wax pencil.
5. Place the wire on the blue line, and make a wax mark at the point where the wire crosses the height of contour (Fig. 9-23). The second bend is made against the round beak of the Gordon plier and will usually be near 90 degrees.
6. Measure the distance from bend two to bend three, and transfer the measurement to the wire, since the wire can no longer be laid against the abutment tooth after bend two is complete (Fig. 9-24).
7. The wire from bend two to bend three is normally straight, but in those instances where gingival contours are somewhat horizontal, contour the wire to follow soft tissue curves (Fig. 9-25). This is a *difficult* step because it is not easy to maintain the previously established relation of the distal arm to the abutment tooth as the wire is bent. It is helpful if the contour of the plier beak approximates the contour of the desired curve in the wire. Attempting to use a small beak to create a large curve will usually result in an uneven contour and the possibility of nicking the wire.
8. Once bend three has been made successfully, estimate or measure the length of proximal wire needed to reach the soldering spot (or area), and cut the wire slightly beyond that length.
9. Bends four and five may take the form of a gradual curve (when the edentulous area is flat) or two distinct bends (when the ridge area is prominent). Since they will be within the denture base in the completed prosthesis, they can be made by finger pressure or with three-pronged pliers (Fig. 9-26).

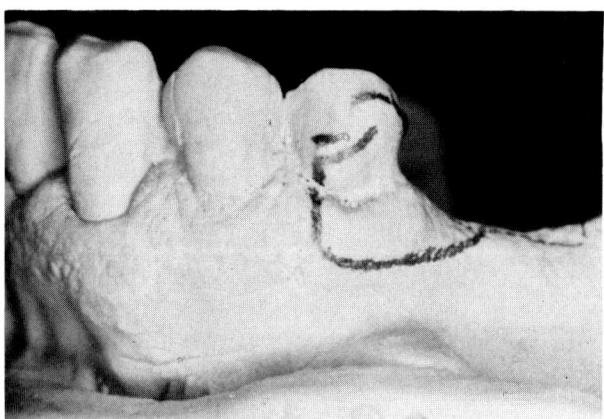

**Fig. 9-21.** L-bar clasp drawn on master cast in proper relation to survey line.

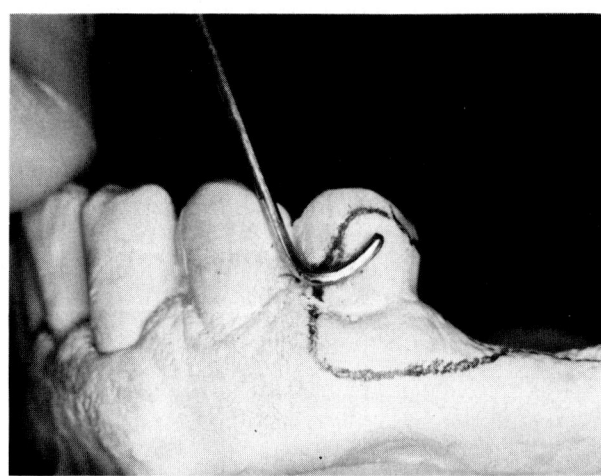

**Fig. 9-22.** Terminal portion of L-bar clasp after first bend.

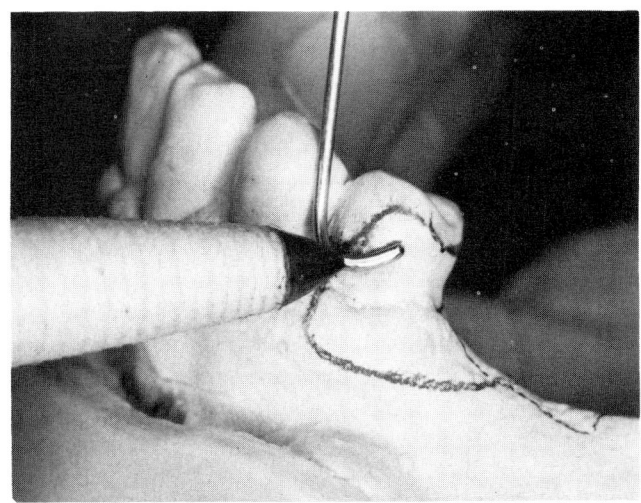

**Fig. 9-23.** In most situations, second bend will be made where terminal portion of L-bar clasp crosses height of contour.

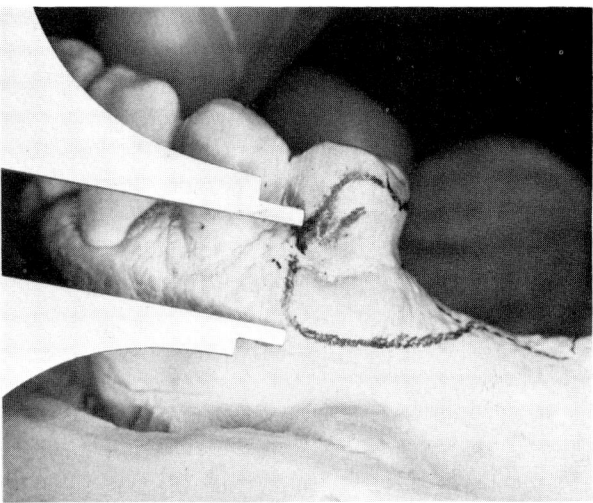

**Fig. 9-24.** Measurement taken for bend three.

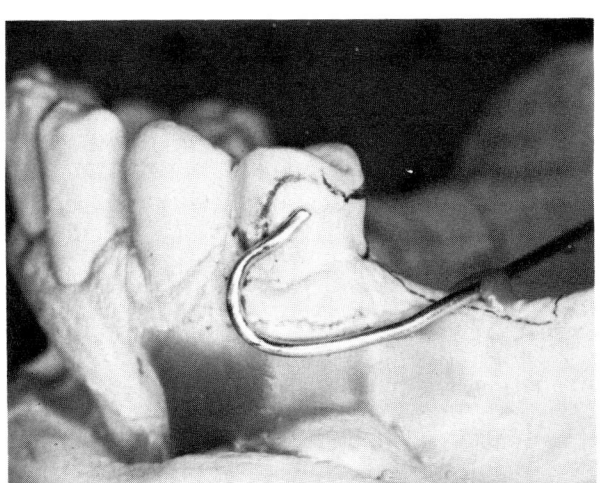

**Fig. 9-25.** Wire must follow contour of soft tissues and not impinge upon them. Wire should be contoured to lie passively 0.5 to 1 mm away from tissue where no undercuts are involved. Soft tissue undercuts in path of wire are treated in same manner as hard tissue undercuts in Fig. 9-14.

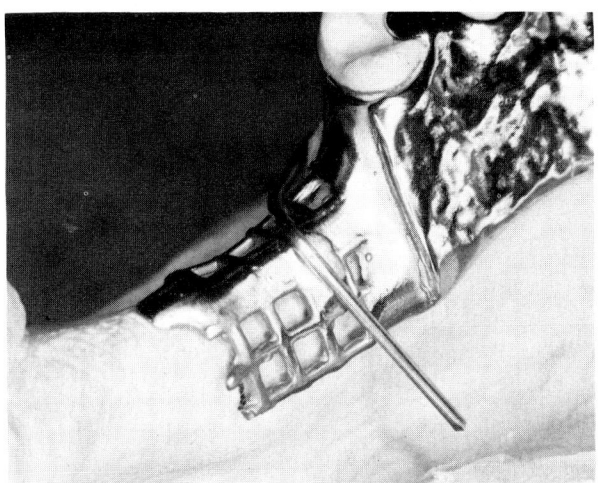

**Fig. 9-26.** Final bends bring proximal end of the L-bar clasp into contact with soldering spot.

**Embrasure clasps.** Although wrought wire can be used in the construction of embrasure clasps, it is not commonly used in this manner. The problems of attachment to the removable partial denture casting greatly complicate the contouring, and, even when successful, the resulting clasp is more rigid and more likely to distort or actually fracture than a routine circumferential clasp. This clasp requires more metal transocclusally than is normally present in even the most generous occlusal rest preparations. The wire will need to be surrounded by at least 1 mm of cast metal, or solder, where it passes transocclusally through the rest area so that it may have sufficient strength when completed. For an 18-gauge wire, this would require 2.4 mm of transocclusal space, not only in maximum interdigitation, but in excursive movements as well.

If the space exists, this clasp form can be constructed using an approach that differs slightly from those previously discussed.

1. Contour the clasp *during* the partial denture framework wax-up stage rather than after it, as in the case of the other clasps mentioned.

2. When the transocclusal portion of the framework is completed in wax, make the first bend in the same fashion as the routine circumferential clasp.

3. Begin the second bend at the proximal line angle and produce a section of wire that follows the contour of the marginal ridges as it passes lingually (Fig. 9-27). It must allow the active clasp arm to contact the blue line while the transocclusal portion passes 2 mm above the marginal ridges of the stone teeth.

4. As the wire reaches the lingual embrasure, mark it with the wax pencil at that point which will allow bend three to direct the wire lingually, staying approximately 1 mm from the stone cast for a distance of 3 to 4 mm (Fig. 9-28). Bends two and three must be done with finger pressure and small beaked pliers because they will normally be quite abrupt.

5. Cut the wire off 3 to 4 mm from bend three.

6. Bring the contoured clasp assembly to the waxed refractory cast, and warm the proximal portion over an open flame while the clasp is held by the terminal portion.

7. Seat the warmed clasp on the refractory cast, and hold it while it melts the transocclusal portion of the wax-up (Fig. 9-29).

8. Repeat step 7 a number of times so that the proximal wire will melt a "trenchlike" groove into the wax-up. If the wire is overheated the first time, it becomes difficult to hold, and the heat may destroy that portion of the wax-up.

9. In this manner the casting is made to fit the wire rather than attempting to contour the wire to fit an arbitrary recess. The recess is essential so that the wire can have a positive soldering area with a known amount of metal present. The 3- to 4-mm extension lingually is necessary so that the soldered connection is not limited to the occlusal aspect (Fig. 9-30). The solder joint may be compromised by occlusal equilibration, and without the lingual exten-

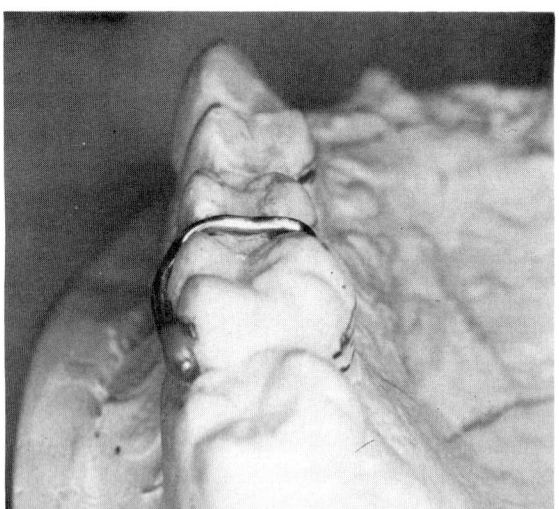

**Fig. 9-27.** Second bend must bring wire evenly into interproximal prepared area, but keep it approximately 1 mm above stone cast.

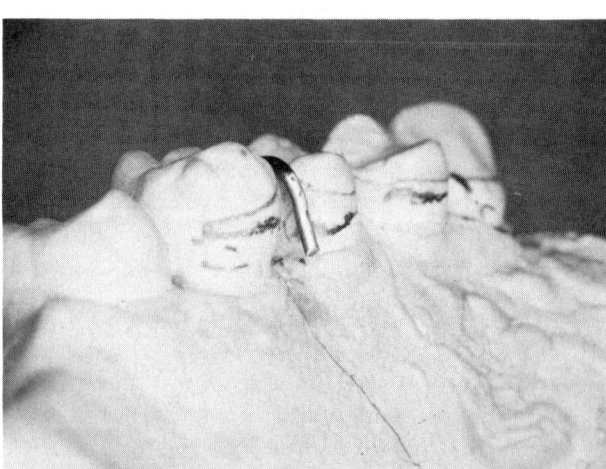

**Fig. 9-28.** Bend three on embrasure clasp brings proximal end to lingual side of embrasure and keeps it approximately 1 mm from soft tissue surface of stone cast.

sion the joint may be too weak and fracture or become distorted with use.

**Orthodontic clasps.** Certain preformed clasp forms may be used in temporary or transitional removable partial dentures. These clasps are routinely used in removable orthodontic appliances. The two forms that are applicable to prosthodontics are the ball clasp and the Adams clasp. Although it is possible to reconstruct and contour these clasps completely freehand, their availability in preformed sizes and gauges combined with their relatively low cost make this impractical.

**BALL CLASP**

1. Prepare the master cast to accept this clasp if in younger patients no usable undercut area is available gingival to the buccal contact points on the posterior teeth. Relieve the interdental papilla with a No. 11 scalpel blade to simulate the natural tooth contour beneath the gingival tissue (Fig. 9-31). This created undercut area need be only as large as the ball on the end of the ball clasp.

2. Measure the distance from the undercut area to the occlusal surface, and transfer it to the preformed ball clasp with the wax pencil. The first bend is made against the very tip of the round beak of the Gordon plier. The bend will be 90 degrees or slightly less (Fig. 9-32).

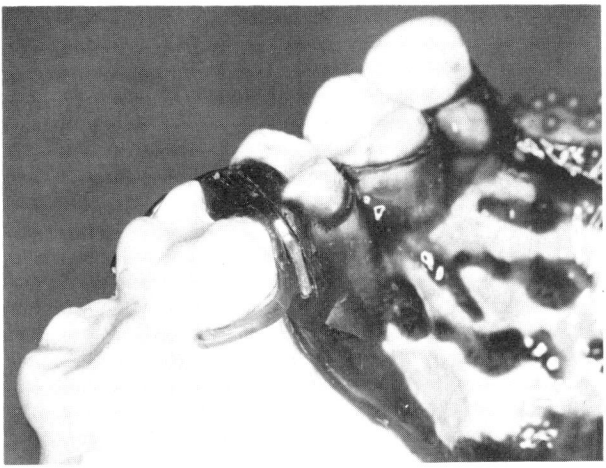

**Fig. 9-29.** Fully contoured clasp is warmed and seated into partial denture wax-up area.

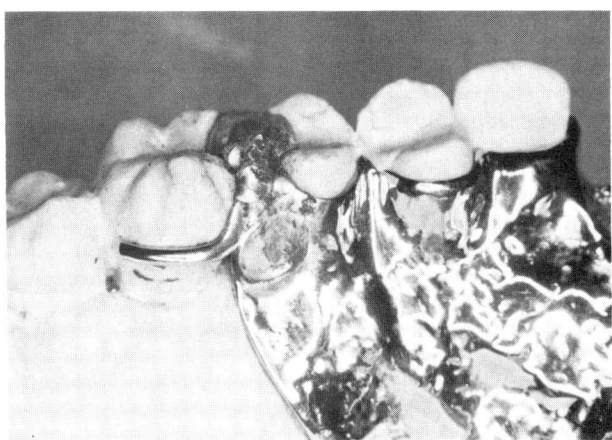

**Fig. 9-30.** Lingual view after soldering.

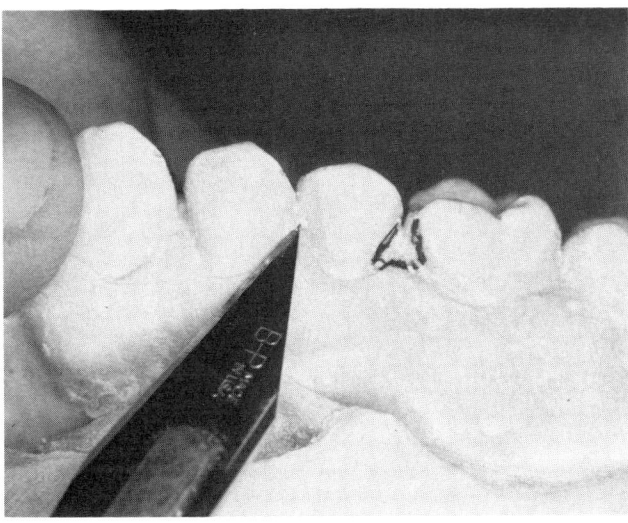

**Fig. 9-31.** Soft tissue contours are relieved for placement of ball clasp when there is no available retentive area interproximally.

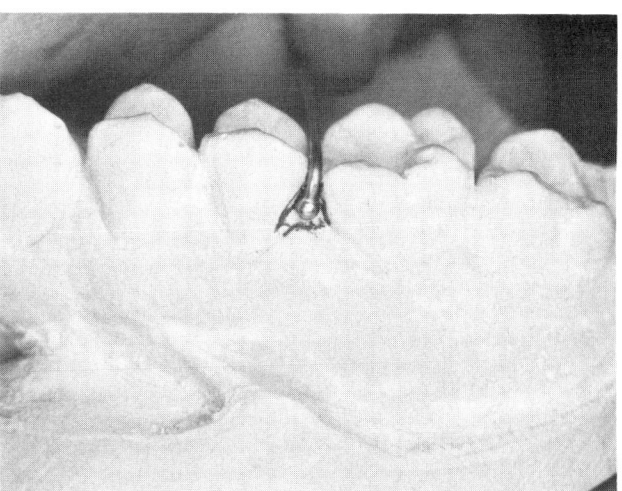

**Fig. 9-32.** First bend of ball clasp.

3. The second bend occurs at the point where the lingual occlusal embrasure begins. It is made at an obtuse angle that will correspond with the slope of the lingual soft tissues (Fig. 9-33).

4. Since this type of clasp is used exclusively on resin appliances, the proximal part of the clasp must be bent so that the clasp will have a retentive form within the resin. The clasp assembly is cut off ¾ inch (1.9 cm) from bend two.

5. The most common form of resin retention is a zigzag form bent out of the ¾-inch proximal segment. The bends can be done with any small-beaked plier, but the three-pronged plier is normally used. Three bends of ¼ inch (0.63 cm) will provide adequate retention and resistance against rotation within the resin (Fig. 9-34).

6. The proximal segment must not lay against the lingual soft tissue slope. This segment should be raised so that an adequate amount of resin can be processed beneath it. A *minimum* of 1 mm is *essential* for assuring adequate retention (Fig. 9-35). If the retentive bends result in the wire touching the cast, finger pressure on the proximal retentive area of the wire will normally bring about the proper relation.

## ADAMS CLASP

The preformed clasp also relies on the undercut that exists gingival to the buccal contact area of posterior teeth. If this area is not apparent on the master cast, the interproximal gingival area must be relieved on the master cast in the same manner as was used for the ball clasp.

1. Select the preformed clasp from available widths so that the "arrows" fall into the usual and distobuccal interproximal areas (Fig. 9-36).

2. If the preformed clasps do not fit exactly, select the one slightly longer mesiodistally than the one that is slightly too short in this dimension.

3. Correct the discrepancy in the clasp that is too long by placing a slight bend in the portion between the "arrows" (Fig. 9-37).

4. Once the "arrows" are properly related to the undercut areas, contour the proximal segments to bring the wire to the same relation to the master cast that was required for the ball clasp.

5. Place the bend required for the resin retention portion of the clasp at the beginning of the lingual embrasure.

6. Repeat the zigzag configurations used in the ball clasp for both arms of the Adams clasp (Fig. 9-38).

7. The Adams clasp gains its retention effect from the "arrows" dropping into the buccal proximal undercuts. It is most effective when it is employed on a tooth that has mesiodistal tooth contacts.

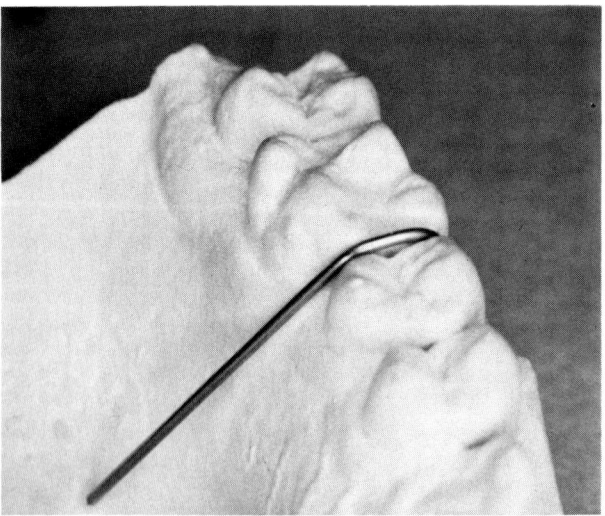

**Fig. 9-33.** Second bend begins at lingual embrasure and positions wire parallel to lingual soft tissue.

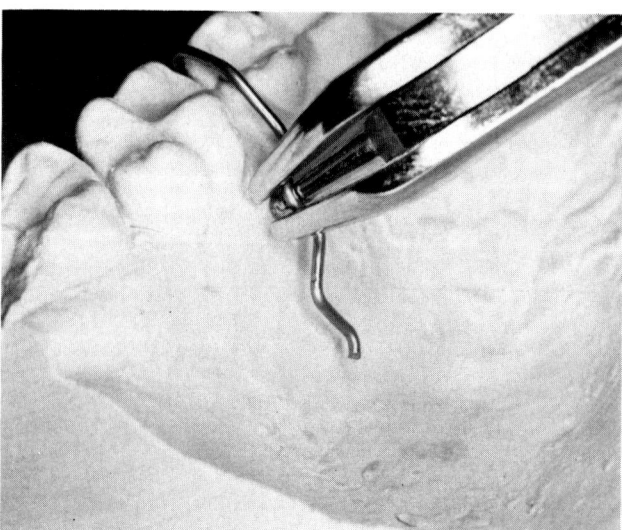

**Fig. 9-34.** Zigzag bends in wire for resin retention.

# Wrought wire clasps

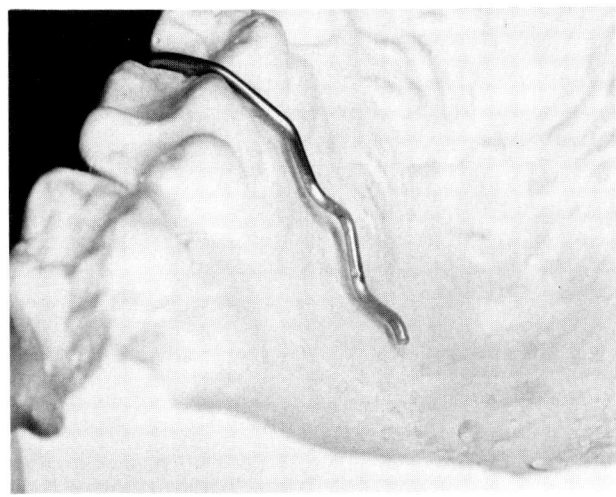

**Fig. 9-35.** Proper relation of resin retention portion of clasp to cast surface. This space should be about 1 mm.

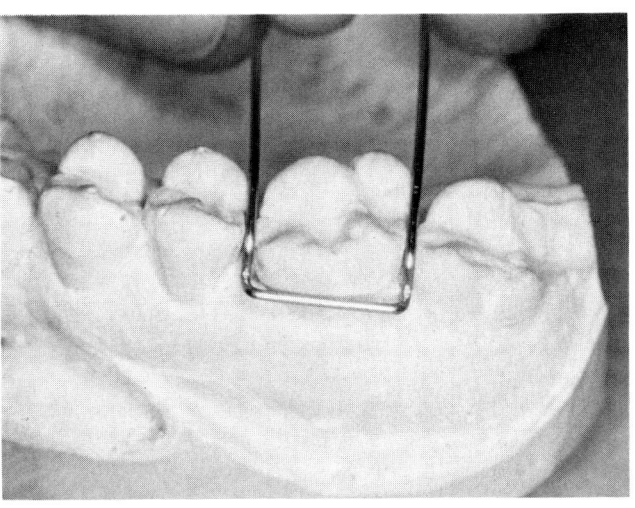

**Fig. 9-36.** Preformed Adams clasp in proper position on buccal surface of abutment tooth.

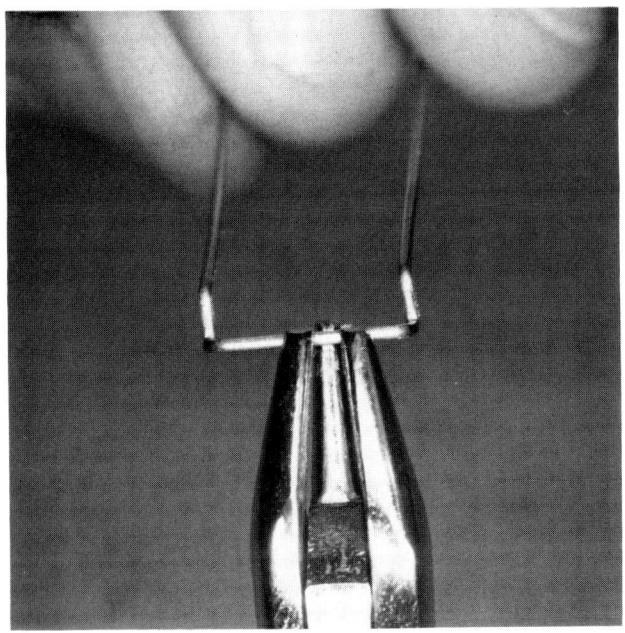

**Fig. 9-37.** Compensating bend made in buccal segment of Adams clasp to reduce its mesiodistal length.

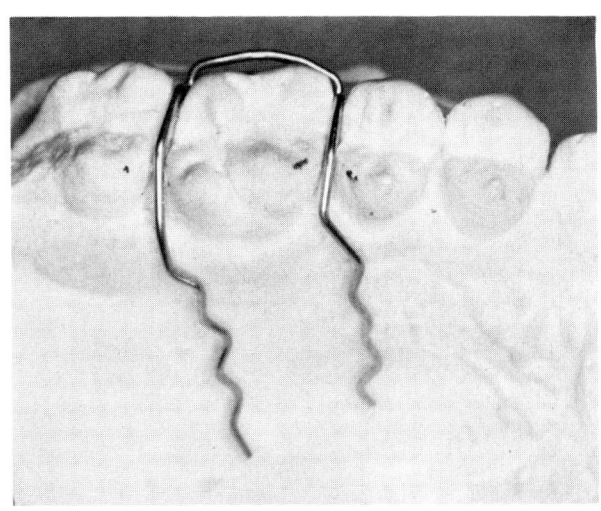

**Fig. 9-38.** Adams clasp properly contoured and ready for resin retention.

## Clasp attachment

The wrought wire clasp can be attached to the removable partial denture in three basic ways. Since the attachment is every bit as critical as the contouring, these attachment techniques must be practiced along with clasp contouring.

**Resin.** Wire clasps are joined to the partial denture with denture resin, primarily in temporary or transitional dentures or in clasp repairs.

1. If the temporary denture is to be made with autopolymerizing resin, then hold the contoured clasp with its proximal segment prepared for resin retention in its planned position while placing the sprinkle-on resin around it.

2. Position the clasp form (circumferential, infrabulge, ball, or Adams) on the abutment tooth, and verify its relation to the blue line. The proximal portion must clear the cast by at least 1 mm to have sufficient room for the resin.

3. Support the clasp in its designed position with a drop of sticky wax placed on the retentive tip while holding the clasp by its proximal end (Fig. 9-39).

4. After the resin has been added and cured, pick the sticky wax away carefully, and the clasp-tooth relation will not be altered.

5. If the resin partial denture is to be packed in a flask and cured, then support the proximal, resin retention end of the clasp before packing the resin.

6. Prepare and flask the partial denture in the standard manner.

7. After the investing gypsum material is fully set, immerse the flask in boiling water and separate it.

8. Eliminate the wax, and prepare the mold with a tinfoil substitute.

9. Support the proximal end of the clasp by adding a small amount of autopolymerizing resin under the wire (Fig. 9-40). This resin will support the wire during packing and will blend with the heat-cured resin.

**Cast to framework.** Circumferential and infrabulge bar clasps may be attached to the framework of a removable partial denture by incorporating the wire into the wax-up and casting the partial denture alloy to the preformed wire. This technique has been used for many years, but it produces a result that is inferior to a resin or soldered attachment. The molten metal appears to change the properties of the wire and results in a clasp that is much more rigid than one that had not experienced this thermal shock.

1. Contour the wire on the master cast as previously described.

2. Plan and position the proximal segment so that it will lie in a portion of the partial denture wax-up that will have adequate bulk to surround the wire. This area is most often found in the finishing lines for the resin (Fig. 9-41).

3. Transfer the wire from the master cast to the refractory cast with care to assure that it is in exactly the same position on both casts. This transfer may be made easier by forming a ledge at the blue line during the blockout stage so that the ledge will transfer to the refractory cast. Place the terminal portion of the wire on the ledge, and verify the position.

4. After casting, any finishing in the area of the wire must be done with extreme care so that the wire is not damaged. There is often a thin flashing of metal along the wire at the point where it exits

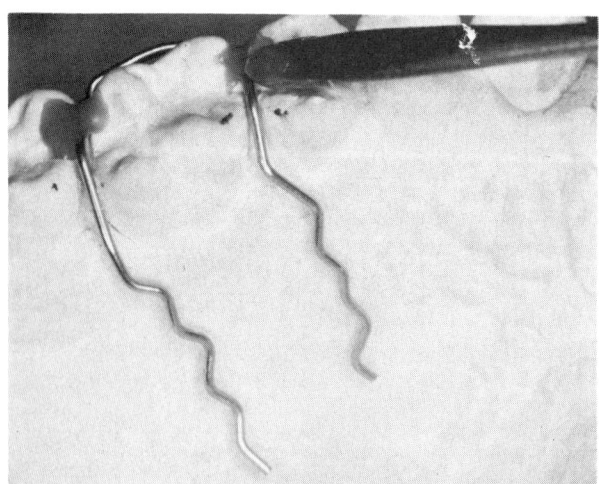

**Fig. 9-39.** Sticky wax added to clasp tip to maintain clasp-tooth relationship for addition of autopolymerizing resin.

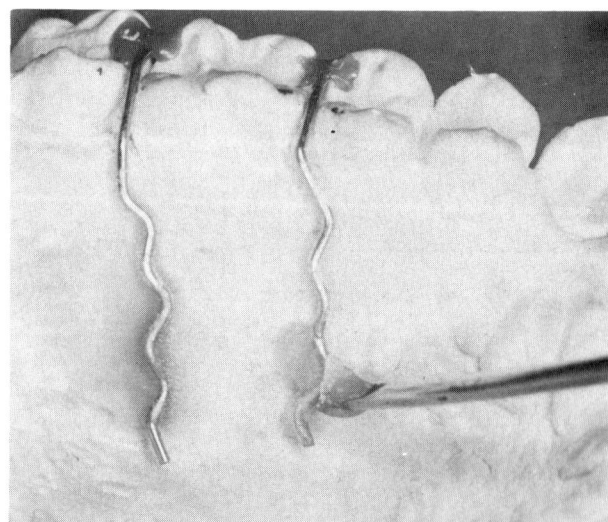

**Fig. 9-40.** Autopolymerizing resin is added to support proximal end of wire clasp.

from the casting. A No. 2 round bur in a high-speed, air-driven handpiece under magnification is the easiest way to remove the excess metal without touching the wire.

**Solder.** The simplest and surest way to join the wire clasp to the framework is by electrosoldering. This method also produces the most flexible clasp if the joint is placed in the retentive area some distance from the active clasp arm. The heat of the soldering operation affects the wire somewhat, reducing its flexibility. If this solder joint is within the denture resin area by at least ¼ inch (0.63 cm), the affected area does not have any measurable effect on the active clasp arm.

1. In designing the removable partial denture framework, consideration must be given to selecting the "soldering spot" for the attachment of the wire clasp arm later (Fig. 9-42). If the resin attachment is to be raised meshwork, then the mesh should be widened at the soldering spot (Fig. 9-43). If the resin attachment is to be through beads with ridge coverage in metal, then the plastic pattern stipple sheet should be beefed up by hand waxing a small area for soldering to give added bulk of metal in that area (Fig. 9-44). These critical areas should be identified on the master cast for reference in waxing the framework.

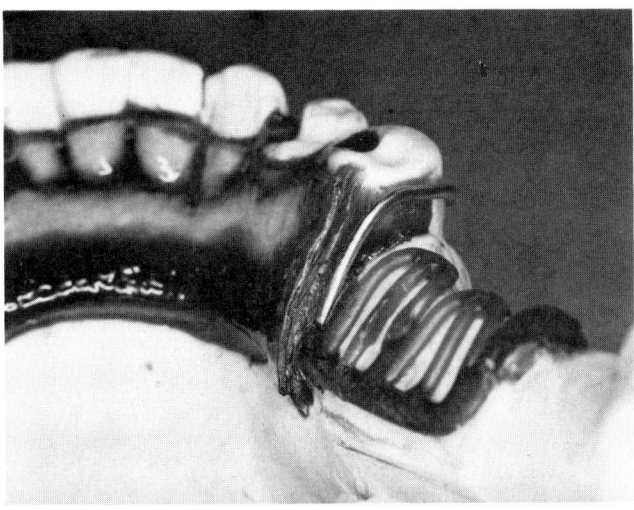

Fig. 9-41. Proximal end of wire is contoured to lie along external finishing line.

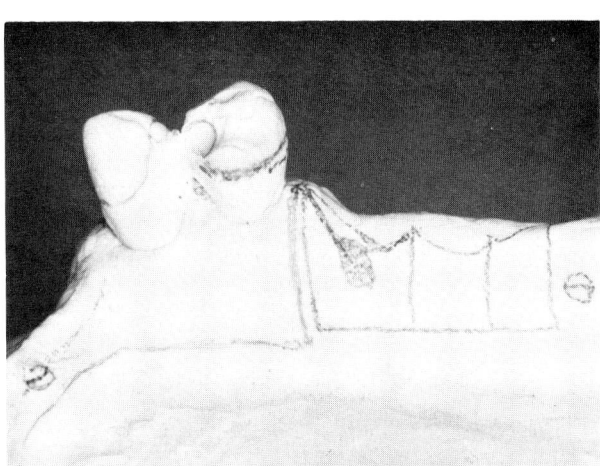

Fig. 9-42. Soldering spot indicated on master cast. It is placed lingual to crest of ridge and between first and second denture tooth.

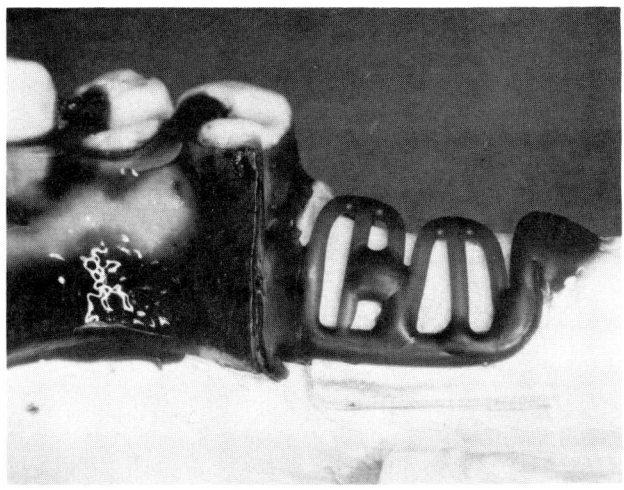

Fig. 9-43. Meshwork is prepared for soldering spot by widening mesh.

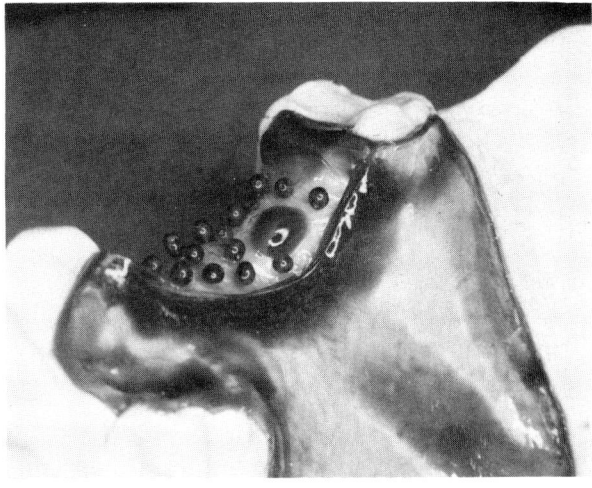

Fig. 9-44. Bulk of wax is added to metal retention in area of soldering spot.

2. When the casting has been fitted to the master cast and all finishing and polishing steps are completed, contour the wire clasps as described on pp. 269-280.

3. Position the wire clasp assembly so that the terminal portion (active clasp arm) is on the blue line. The proximal portion must at this point, lie passively across the soldering spot (Fig. 9-45). It is not necessary for the wire to terminate exactly on the spot. In fact, it is better to have the wire extend beyond the spot slightly. Cut the excess wire off after the soldering process. Hold the wire in position by the addition of a small amount of clay or rope-type window caulking material placed on the active clasp arm and the stone cast in that area (Fig. 9-46). Plaster or sticky wax can also be used, but both have disadvantages. The plaster takes time to set and is messy to remove. The wax may melt because the heat of soldering is conducted down the wire and the relationship may be lost.

4. The choice of solder used depends on the position of the soldering spot on the casting. If the solder joint will be exposed, then precious metal (800 fine) is indicated for the best long-term results. If the joint is back within the resin retention area, then a simple silver solder, or even a nonprecious solder, can be used because it will not be exposed to conditions that will cause it to tarnish. The joint is a physical one that combines the wire and the casting during the construction phases and will, in most cases, be covered and further retained with resin.

5. If an electrosoldering machine like the Torit Model 21A is used, it should be set on medium heat (Fig. 9-47). The electrodes consist of a carbon tip that can be contoured easily and will be placed passively on the solder joint and a copper tip. Place the copper tip on the framework a varying distance from the soldering spot and complete the electrical circuit through the casting. The copper tip must be clean to allow a good current contact.

6. Prepare the soldering spot and proximal segment with flux,* and lay a piece of strip solder that has been cut to approximately 3 mm and crimped slightly over the wire (Fig. 9-48).

7. Place the carbon tip on the solder without pressure, and place the copper tip on the casting. The exact distance separating these two contact areas is not critical but is normally a convenient relation determined by framework contour.

8. Hold the carbon tip in position without pressure until the solder flows (Fig. 9-49). Occasionally, no electrical circuit will be formed, and the copper tip will have to be moved slightly to complete the circuit.

9. An alternative method of placing the solder and completing the joint may prove easier to accomplish. Place the piece of solder on the workbench, and touch it with the carbon tip *very* briefly (Fig. 9-50). This action will complete the electrical cir-

*Drom-Flux, Canadian Refining Co., Ltd., Montreal, Canada.

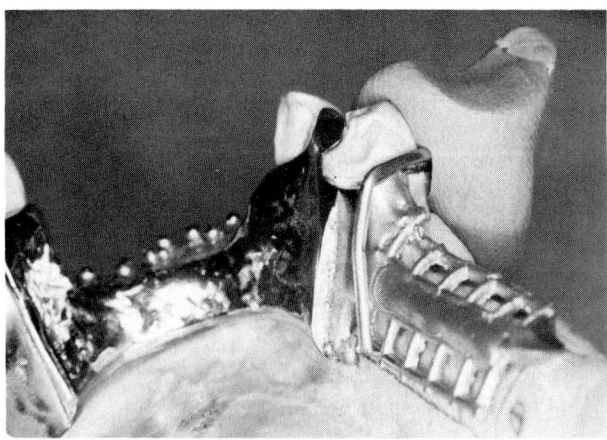

**Fig. 9-45.** Proximal wire lies across soldering spot.

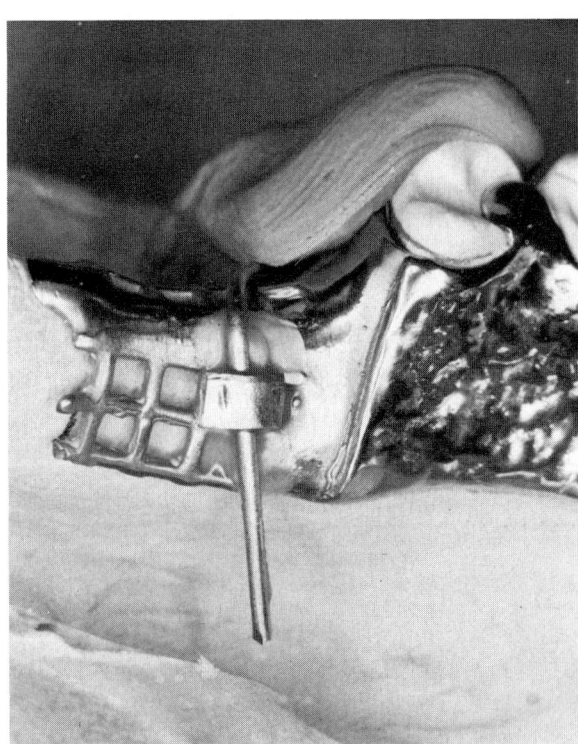

**Fig. 9-46.** Terminal wire is held in position with clay for soldering. Since no pressure is involved in soldering process, stabilization of wire need not be excessive.

Wrought wire clasps **285**

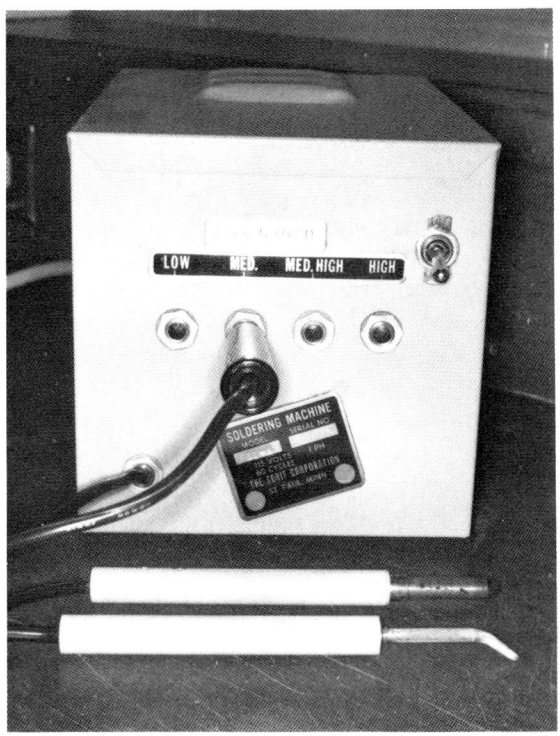

**Fig. 9-47.** Electrosoldering machine set on medium heat (Torit Model 21-A).

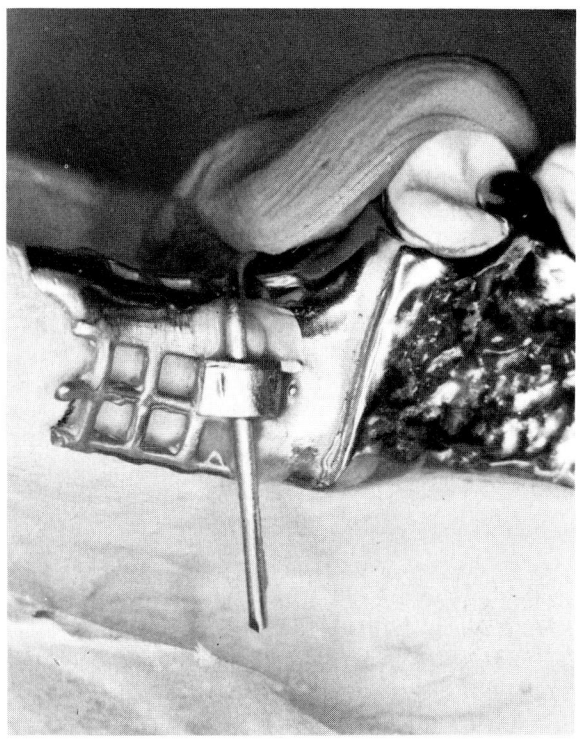

**Fig. 9-48.** Solder is laid over wire at soldering spot after flux has been added.

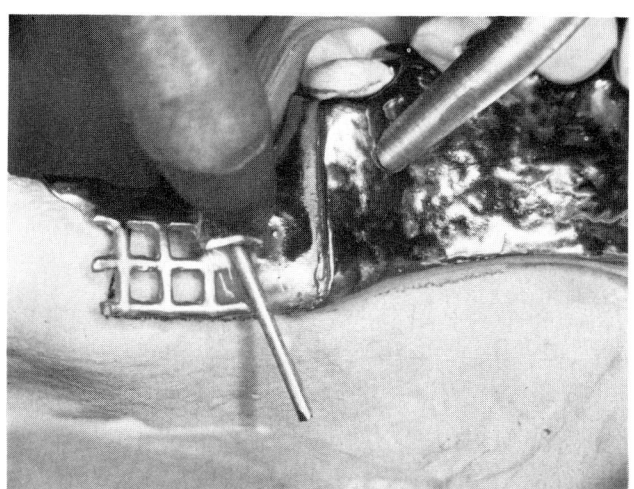

**Fig. 9-49.** Carbon tip properly placed on solder. This placement should always be without pressure.

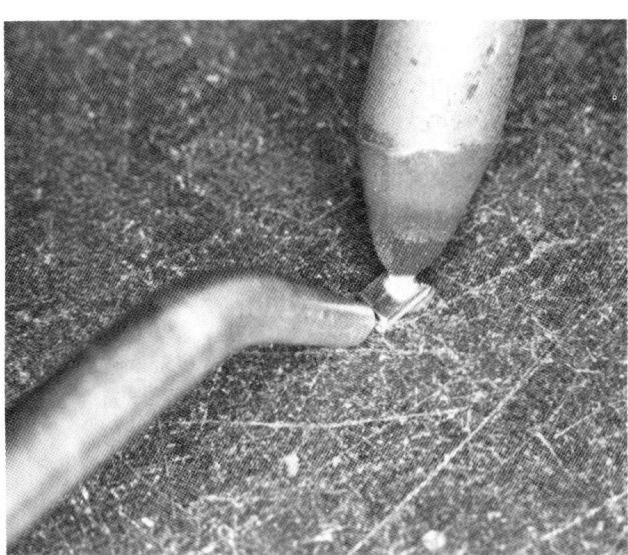

**Fig. 9-50.** Solder is attached to carbon tip by touching both tips to piece of solder *very* briefly.

cuit and make the solder adhere to the carbon tip. Transfer the solder to the already fluxed wire, and complete the joint. If the carbon tip is allowed to contact too long, the solder will melt completely and destory its effectiveness in forming the joint.

10. When the soldering joint is completed, remove any excess of wire past the joint with a disk. Remove any discoloration in the area quickly by sandblasting or liquid honing.

11. The soldering operation can also be completed with a torch, but the time involved and damage to the master cast that inevitably occurs make this technique inadequate by comparison.

12. If the soldering spot is to be outside the resin area (as in the case of an embrasure clasp or a circumferential clasp attached to a minor connector or rest area), more care and greater skill are required to complete a joint that will stand up in function. In most of these situations, more than one piece of solder will be necessary to complete the joint (Fig. 9-51). Move the carbon tip gently with a rolling motion from piece to piece. There must be *no pause* in this maneuver, since there is a good chance that oxides may form on the unheated solder particles which will prohibit the electrical circuit from forming. If this occurs, there is no recourse but to clean the area by sandblasting or honing and begin again. At no time should any force be exerted by the carbon tip because it can reposition the entire clasp assembly.

**Clasp adjustment.** When sufficient force is applied to a wire clasp, it will distort rather than break as a cast clasp will. It is therefore necessary to develop skill in re-adapting the wire clasp.

1. Evaluate the magnitude and direction of the distortion in relation to the retentive area before adjustments can be made.

2. The recontouring will almost always consist of repositioning the active clasp arm in two planes. The first bend should restore the vertical position of the arm, either gingivally or occusally until it is on the same horizontal plane with the desired undercut (Fig. 9-52).

3. The second bend will move the clasp horizontally until it again touches the tooth surface (Fig. 9-53). Ideally, in this position the clasp will be totally passive, but in practice total passivity is almost impossible to attain. The clasp will end up with some positive pressure against the tooth. If the clasp is well reciprocated, this slight pressure will cause no clinical problems, but if not, excessive tooth movement can occur. It will be necessary to try the partial denture back onto the arch and watch the clasp carefully to see if it is as passive as possible.

4. If it is not possible to achive the desired result in two bends, remove the clasp, and add a new one as a clasp repair.

**Clasp repair.** Wrought wire is most always employed in the replacement of a clasp arm that has been broken in use. The addition of the wire replacement requires that a cast be made with the partial denture in place in the mouth. Furthermore, the denture must remain in the impression on removal and have the dental stone poured against it in the impression.

1. Block out soft and hard tissue undercuts within the denture with clay or wax, so that the partial denture may be easily removed from the resulting cast without fear of breaking the stone teeth (Fig. 9-54).

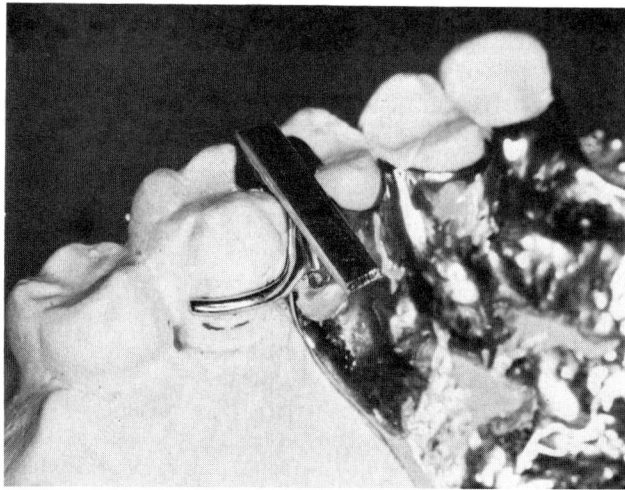

**Fig. 9-51.** Solder properly placed for wire attachment for wrought embrasure clasp.

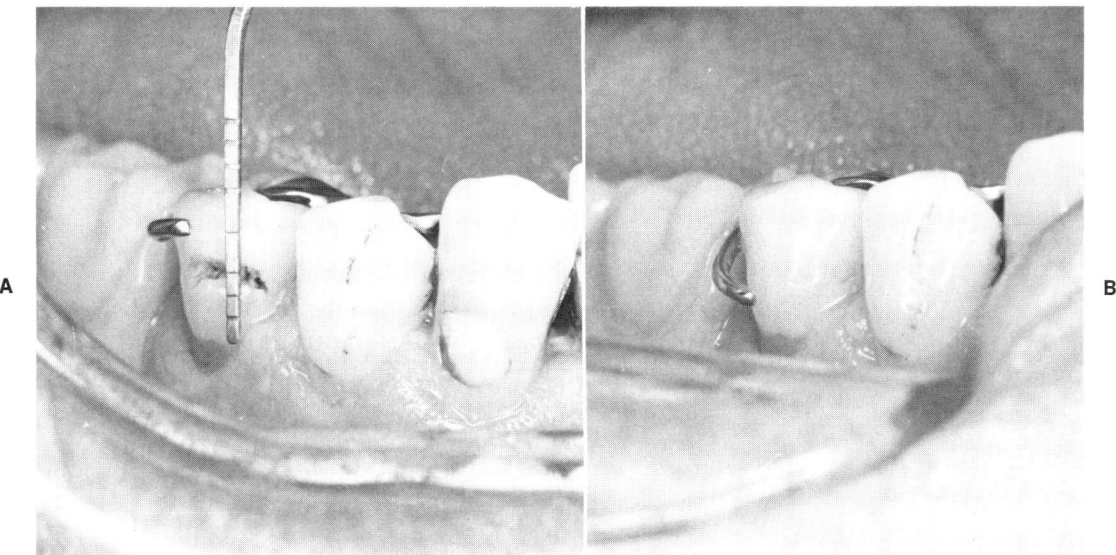

**Fig. 9-52. A,** Retentive area can be analyzed with periodontal probe and tooth marked with wax pencil before recontouring of distorted clasp is begun. **B,** First bend must restore vertical position of distorted clasp.

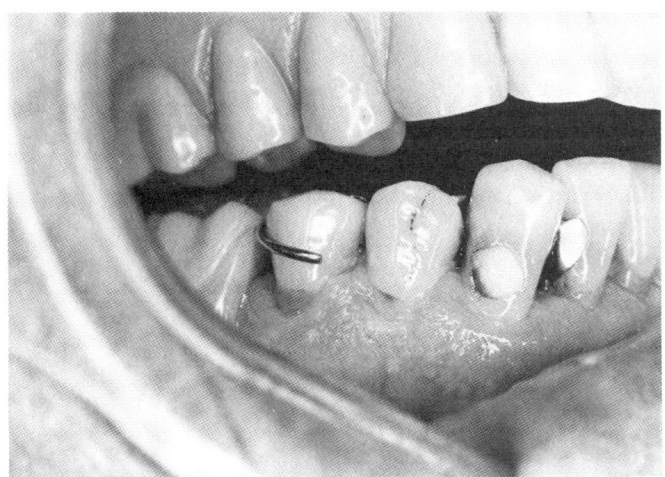

**Fig. 9-53.** Second bend brings wire back into contact with tooth. Wire should be passive when it touches tooth.

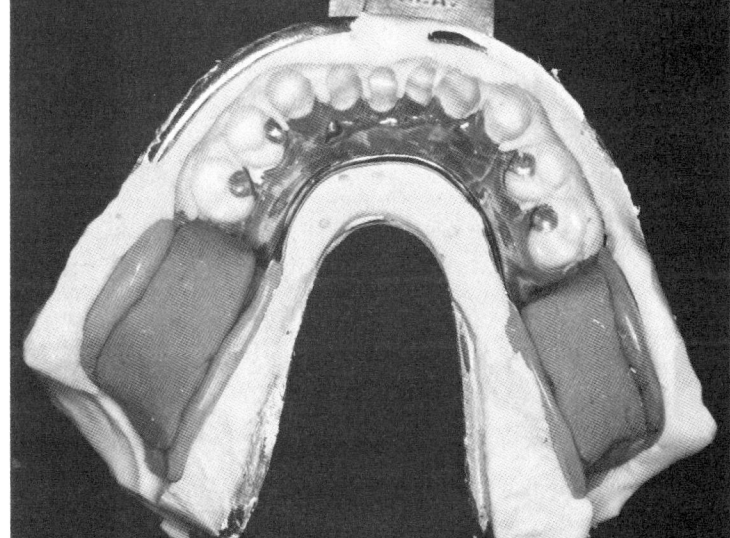

**Fig. 9-54.** Undercuts in denture are blocked out with clay or wax before dental stone is poured.

2. Analyze the stone tooth requiring the addition of the clasp with a surveyor in relation to the path of insertion so that its height of contour can be found. Find the most favorable position of the new clasp, and draw on the cast with the blue pencil (Fig. 9-55).

3. The new clasp may be circumferential or infrabulge, as the tooth contours and prescription indicate. The steps in contouring the replacement are identical to those described on pp. 269-280.

4. Before the contouring can begin, prepare the partial denture to accept the proximal end of the clasp assembly. The attachment can be completely within the resin on a combination of soldering and resin attachment.

5. Indicate a slot in the buccal flange of resin for the addition of the infrabulge clasp (Fig. 9-56). Cut the slot to half the depth of the available resin with a fissure bur. The slot should be ¼ inch (0.63 cm) occlusogingivally to accommodate the retentive zigzag on the proximal end of the wire. Contour the infrabulge wire clasp, and attach it to the tooth with sticky wax. Add autopolymerizing resin to fill in the prepared slot, completing the repair (Fig. 9-57).

6. Circumferential wires are best retained in the resin on the opposite side of the ridge from the active clasp arm. Prepare the slot in the same manner as in step 5, beginning at the minor connector and passing occlusally and then lingually. The occlusal portion of the slot need only be as wide as the wire itself. The lingual part of the slot should open immediately to ¼ inch (0.63 cm) for resin attachment (Fig. 9-58). Contour the clasp, and position it on the abutment tooth. Hold it in position with sticky wax while adding tooth-colored autopolymerizing resin to the slot where it passes over the occlusal surface of the denture tooth.

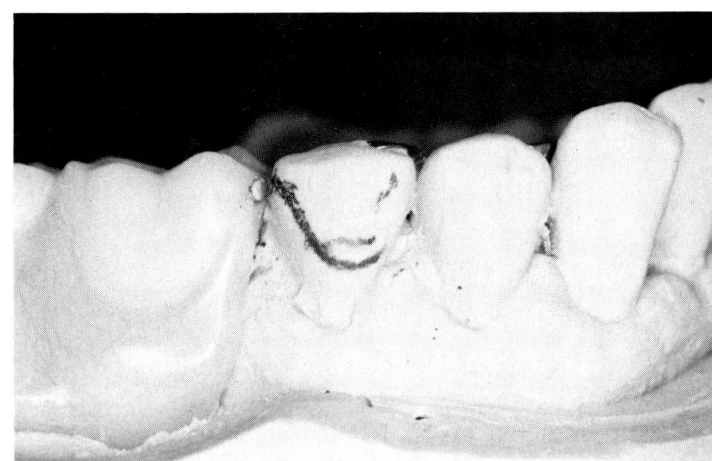

**Fig. 9-55.** Design for repair clasp is drawn on cast.

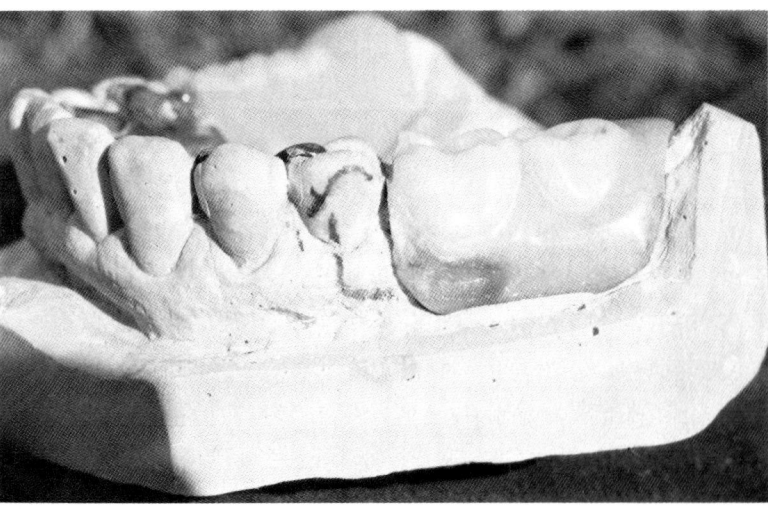

**Fig. 9-56.** Resin of partial denture is prepared for addition of repair clasp.

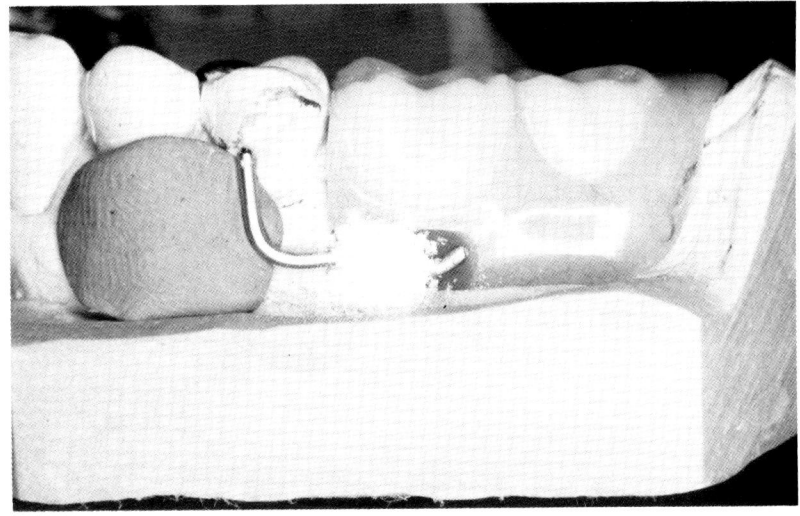

**Fig. 9-57.** Autopolymerizing resin is added to repair clasp to complete repair.

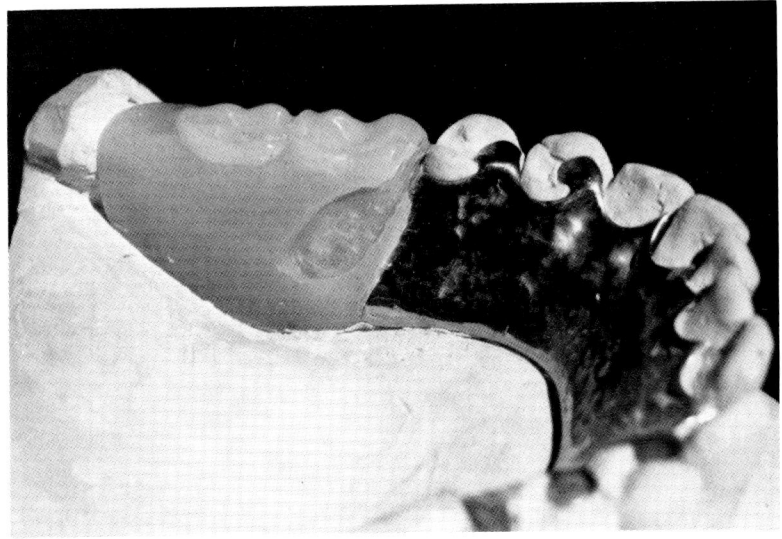

**Fig. 9-58.** Lingual preparation for addition of circumferential wire clasp.

**SOLDERED REPAIR ATTACHMENT**

If a clasp needs to be added to an area where no resin is available to retain it, the connection will be made by electrosoldering. Precious metal solder will be used to ensure that the joint will not tarnish.

1. Prepare the soldering spot by making a slot in the minor connector with a disk to recieve the proximal end of the wire (Fig. 9-59). Consideration must be given to selecting a soldering spot in an area where there is sufficient bulk of metal to support the soldered wire in function (a minimum of 1 mm of metal around the wire). If this amount of metal is not available (as in the case of some repairs of transocclusal clasps), the clasp repair cannot be expected to succeed.

2. Remove any resin immediately adjacent to the prepared slot to gain access for the soldering tip.

3. Contour the clasp arm as previously described, with special attention given to fitting the proximal segment into the slot formed in the minor connector.

4. Shape the carbon tip on a rough wheel to the contour that will allow the greatest contact at the soldering spot.

5. The soldering operation is completed as previously described (Fig. 9-60). Any resin that may

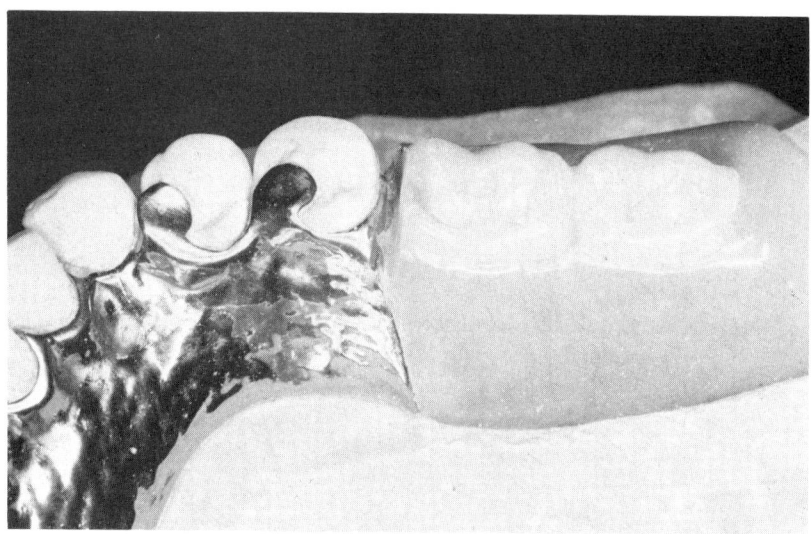

**Fig. 9-59.** Minor connector is prepared with disk cut to accept repair clasp.

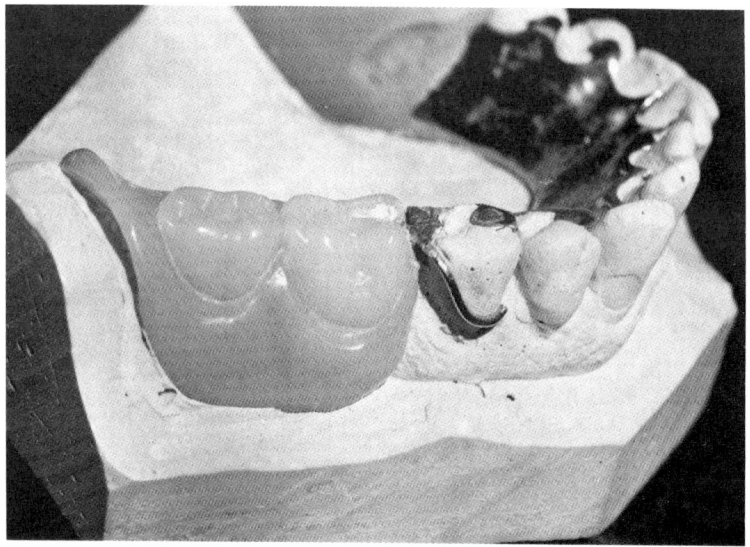

**Fig. 9-60.** Soldering operation completed for addition of repair clasp.

have been affected by the heat of soldering must be removed and replaced with autopolymerizing resin of the appropriate shade.

Soldered clasp repairs always result in more rigid clasp arms than those retained by resin. Special emphasis must be placed on the selection of the gauge of wire used and the depth of undercut in which they are placed.

## PROBLEM AREAS

Problem areas associated with the construction of wire clasp arms are (1) poor clasp adaptation, (2) faulty solder joints, and (3) breakage of the clasp arm in function (Table 9-1). These problems can be reduced by practicing each phase of wire construction. The tasks involved in constructing a quality wire clasp arm are not in themselves overly complex, but a reasonable level of experience is required before clasps can be made quickly with dependable results.

### Table 9-1. Wrought wire clasps

| Problem | Probable cause | Solution |
| --- | --- | --- |
| Wire not able to be adapted to tooth | Tooth contours too irregular | Reprepare abutment contours; change clasp design (example, circumferential to infrabulge bar if proximal tooth contours are sharp with high survey line); additional blockout of undesirable undercuts and irregularities |
| | Improper contouring sequence (resulting in multiple improper bends) | Begin again with new wire (multiple bends cannot be recontoured) |
| Wire does not contact tooth after soldering | Wire not passive on soldering spot | Cut or grind wire off and reposition for resoldering or begin again with new wire |
| | Excess pressure on carbon tip | Same as above |
| | Wire improperly held in place with sticky wax or clay | Same as above; if discrepancy is slight, it may be possible to adjust clasp arm (see procedure for clasp adjustment) |
| Unable to complete circuit for soldering | Carbon tip corroded or dirty | Recontour carbon tip with abrasive wheel or disk |
| | Film or debris on casting in contact area | Clean all polishing compound from casting in ultrasonic cleaner before soldering operation |
| Solder joint weak, wire breaks off or distorts with routine handling | Solder joint overheated (metal appears burned and grainy) | Cut or grind off wire, clean soldering spot, and begin again with new wire |
| | Solder joint cold | Clean joint with sandblasting or liquid honing and reflux before reapplication of heat (additional solder may be needed) |
| | Solder joint incomplete | Same as above |
| | Soldering spot too small | Unless another soldering area can be found, it may be necessary to remake casting |
| Wire breaks where it emerges from casting (when it has been incorporated into casting) | Wire has been nicked or sharply bent at or slightly within metal-wire junction | Smooth off junction, and contour new wire for soldering to minor connector or resin retention area |

**BIBLIOGRAPHY**

Brockhurst, P. J.: Comparison of the performance of materials for spring members in dental appliances, using the theory of simple bending, Aust. Dent. J. **15:**119, 1970.

Brockhurst, P. J.: Base metal wires for gold alloy soldering to cast cobalt-chromium alloy partial dentures, Aust. Dent. J. **15:**499, 1970.

Brudvik, J. S., Fisher, W. T., and Chandler, H. T.: Repairs of metal parts of removable partial dentures, J. Prosthet. Dent. **28:**205, 1972.

Brudvik, J. S., and Wormley, J. H.: Construction techniques for wrought wire retentive clasp arms as related to clasp flexibility, J. Prosthet. Dent. **30:**769, 1973.

Cecconi, B. T., Asgar, K., and Dootz, E.: The effect of partial denture clasp design on abutment tooth movement, J. Prosthet. Dent. **25:**44, 1971.

Clayton, J. A. and Jaslow, C.: A measurement of clasp forces on teeth, J. Prosthet. Dent. **25:**21, 1971.

Dykema, R. W., Cunningham, D. M., and Johnston, J. F.: Modern practice in removable partial prosthodontics, Philadelphia, 1969, W. B. Saunders Co.

Fenner, W., Gerber, A., and Muhlemann, H. R.: Tooth mobility change during treatment with partial denture prosthesis, J. Prosthet. Dent. **6:**520, 1956.

Frechette, A. R.: The influence of partial denture design on distribution of force to abutment teeth, J. Prosthet. Dent. **6:**195, 1956.

Henderson, D., and Steffel, V. L.: McCracken's removable partial prosthodontics, St. Louis, 1977, The C. V. Mosby Co.

Kaires, A.: Effect of partial denture design on bilateral force distribution, J. Prosthet. Dent. **6:**373, 1956.

Phillips, R. W.: Skinner's science of dental materials, ed. 7, Philadelphia, 1973, W. B. Saunders Co.

Scott, J. E., and Deary P.: The soldering of dental wires to a cast cobalt-chromium alloy, Dent. Pract. **19:**261, 1969.

Taylor, N. O., and Teamer, C. K.: Gold solders for dental use, J. Dent. Res. **28:**219, 1949.

# CHAPTER 10

# INVESTING, BURNOUT, AND CASTING

KENNETH D. RUDD, ROBERT M. MORROW, GEORGE KNIGHT, and ENNIS HOWARD

**investing** The process of covering or enveloping wholly or in part an object such as a trial denture tooth, wax pattern, or crown with an investment material before curing, soldering, or casting.
**casting investment** Refractory material from which the mold is made in fabrication of gold or cobalt-chromium castings.
**gypsum-bonded casting investment** Casting investment that can be bonded by alpha-hemihydrate, a derivate of gypsum, because the fusion temperatures of the metal alloys to be cast in it are relatively low.
**phosphate-bonded casting investment** Casting investment that is bonded by a phosphate and a metallic oxide that react to form a hard mass; generally used for high-fusing alloys.
**burnout** Elimination by heat of an invested pattern from a set investment to prepare the mold to receive casting metal.
**casting** To produce a casting in a mold.

In this chapter methods for investing a wax pattern for a removable partial denture, burning out the pattern, and casting metal into the mold will be described. The procedures will be for a low/gold content casting alloy.* Other alloys will require modification in the type of investment used and in the procedures used. Pattern thickness, type of investment, burnout temperatures, melting procedure, and postcasting mold treatment can vary significantly with other alloys. When other alloys/investment systems are used, it is imperative that the manufacturer's technical recommendations be closely followed.

---
*Alborium, J. F. Jelenko & Co., New Rochelle, N.Y.

## INVESTING THE SPRUED PATTERN

Investment for a removable partial denture wax-up consists of two parts. The first is the investment (refractory) cast on which the pattern is waxed, and the second is the outer investment that surrounds the cast and pattern.

The second, or outer, investment is applied in two separate steps. The first is a thin coat, sometimes called the paint-on investment, which is applied with a brush to ensure that air is not trapped adjacent to the pattern, and the second, sometimes called the outer investment, is poured or vibrated into the investment ring around the pattern and cast after the paint-on investment has set.

The purpose of the investment is as follows:
1. To provide strength necessary to resist the forces created by the stream of molten metal.
2. To make a smooth surface for the mold cavity so the casting will require as little finishing as possible.
3. To establish an avenue of escape for most of the gases created by the burnout and casting procedure.
4. To compensate for some of the dimensional changes of the metal when it goes from the molten to the solid state.

### PROCEDURE

1. Before mixing the investment material, line the investment ring with one layer of strip substi-

tute asbestos.* Leave the lining 7 mm short of the end of the ring toward the crucible former or sprue end of the flask (Fig. 10-1). This lining permits the gases to escape during burnout and also allows for mold expansion. The investment in contact with the ring at the crucible end prevents the investment from falling out when handling the ring. The liner must be wet after it is in place but should not be packed tightly against the ring (Fig. 10-2).

2. Even though the refractory cast was dipped in beeswax or sprayed with model spray, which prevent it from absorbing water, it is a good practice to soak the cast for 5 minutes in room-temperature water before applying the paint-on layer of investment (Fig. 10-3). This is a good procedure because sometimes it is necessary to trim the refractory cast some more after it has been dipped in wax or sprayed.

3. Mix 100 gm of investment with the same water-powder ratio, plus 1 ml of water that was used for the refractory cast. (If the investment for the refractory cast was 100 gm of powder to 29 ml of water, the mix for the paint-on investment will be 100 gm of powder to 30 ml of water.) NOTE: Always use distilled water. This slightly thinner mix allows better adaptation to the wax pattern and also permits easier escape of the gases formed during burnout (Fig. 10-4). Hand spatulation of the mix must be

---

*C & B Flask Liner, Buffalo Dental Manufacturing Co., Brooklyn, N.Y.

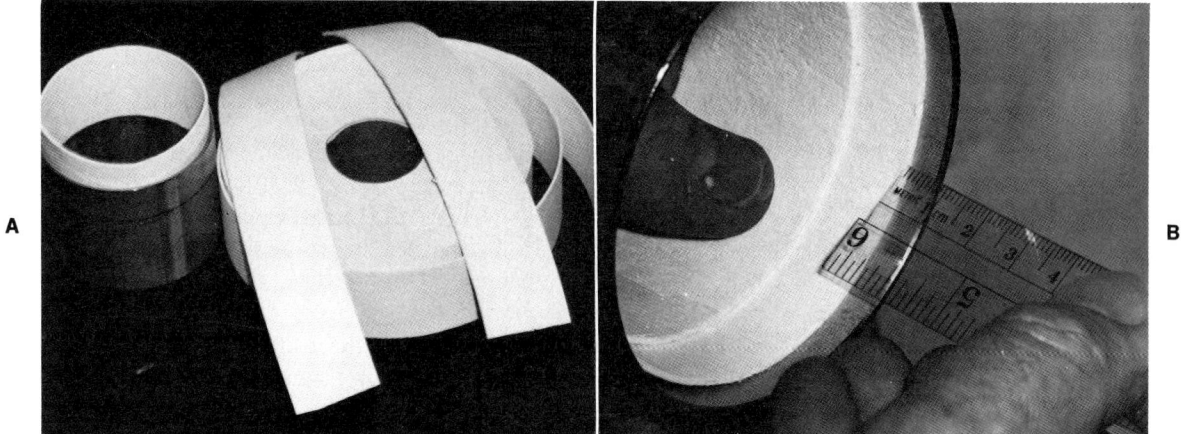

Fig. 10-1. A, Since asbestos is dangerous to health, this substitute lining material is used. It is much more difficult to use than asbestos but can be managed if handled adeptly. B, Strips of lining material in place in flask 7 mm short of sprue end.

*Investing, burnout, and casting* **295**

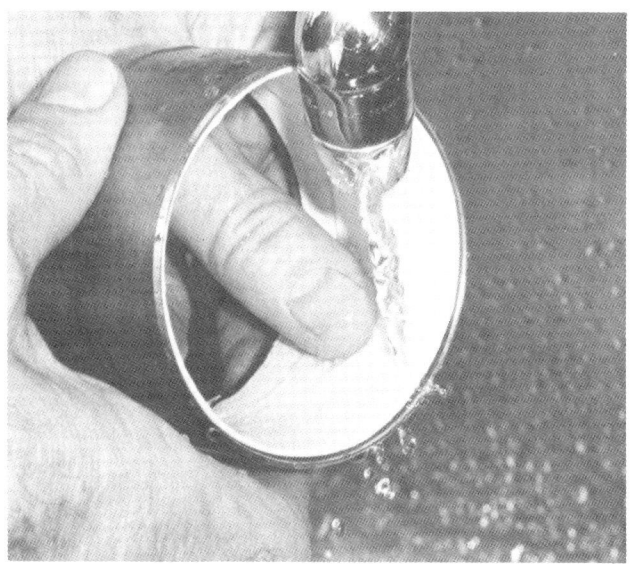

**Fig. 10-2.** Liner is saturated with water after it is in place in ring but is not packed tightly.

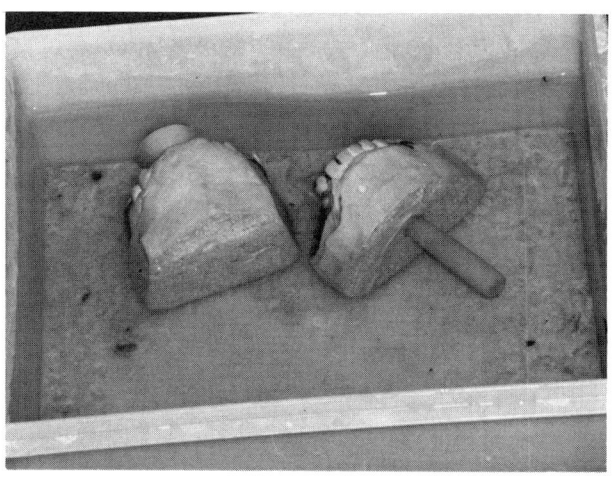

**Fig. 10-3.** Refractory cast is soaked for 5 minutes in room-temperature water before paint-on investment is applied.

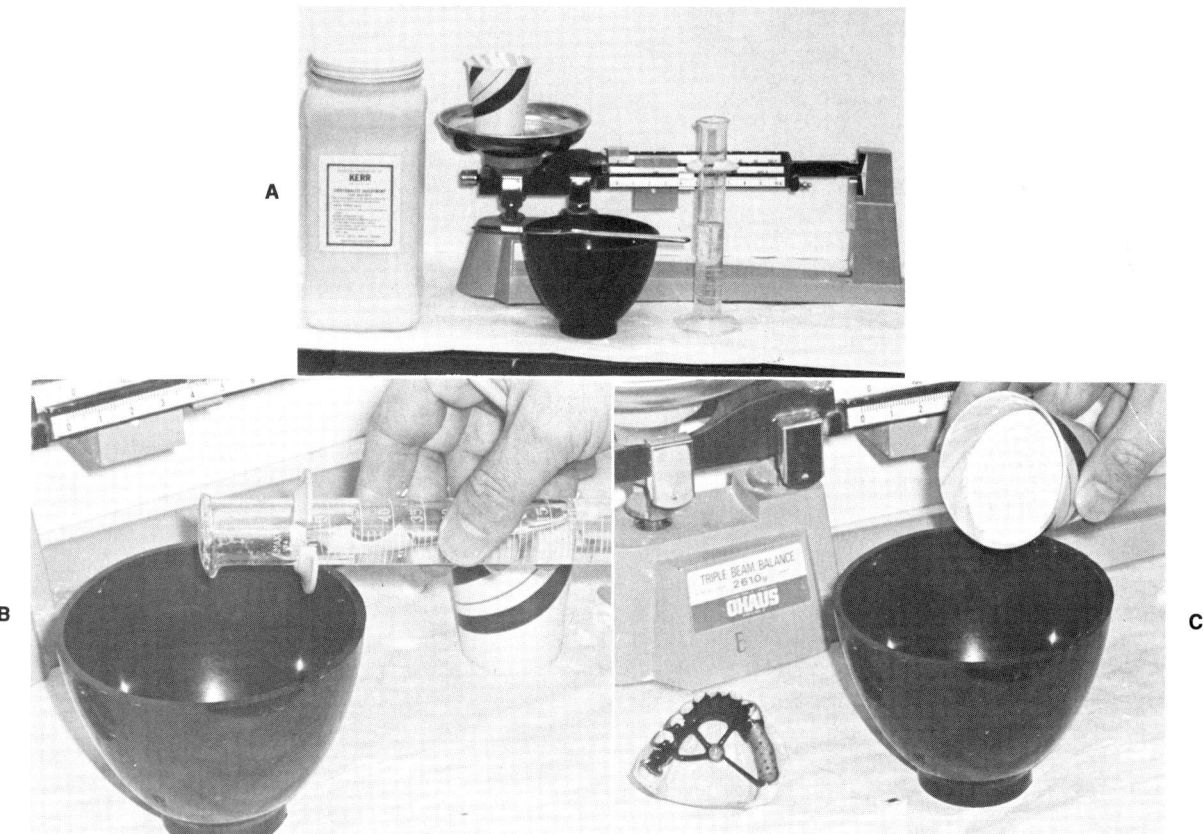

**Fig. 10-4. A,** Mix 100 gm of investment for paint-on layer. **B,** Always use distilled water. **C,** Always add powder to water.

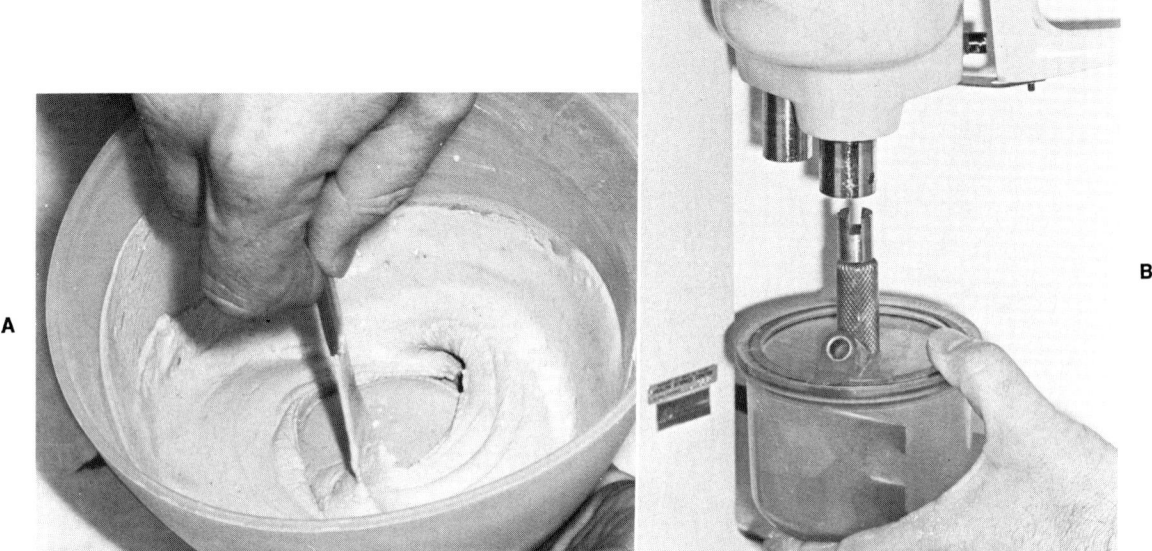

Fig. 10-5. **A,** Mix investment by hand for 60 seconds. **B,** If mechanical mixer is used, do not use vacuum.

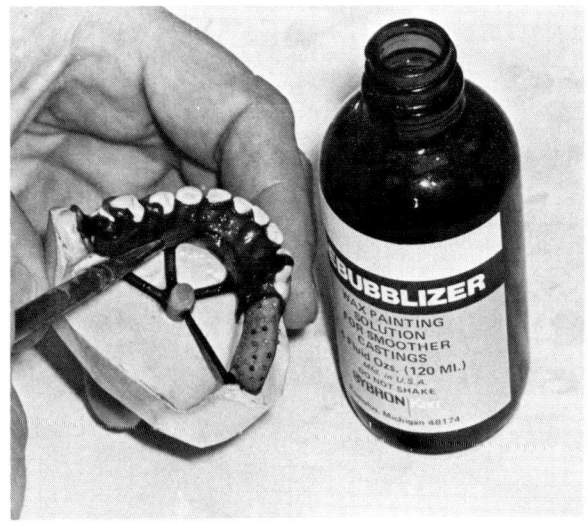

Fig. 10-6. Wax pattern and sprues are painted with surface tension reducer.

thorough and should continue for 60 seconds. If a mechanical mixer is used, do not use the vacuum (Fig. 10-5). Some air should be incorporated in the outer investment to make it more porous, which makes it easier for the gases to escape.

4. Paint the wax pattern and sprues with a wetting agent (debubblizer or surface tension reducer)* to reduce the surface tension of the wax so the outer investment will cover and adapt closely to the wax (Fig. 10-6).

5. Hold the investment cast by the end of the central sprue protruding from the base of the cast. If the wax-up is sprued from the top or the posterior side, hold the cast by the base. With a brush, pick up small portions of the investment, and work it under and around the sprues (Fig. 10-7). Continue to work the investment around the sprues and over the pattern moving from one side of the cast to the other. The entire pattern should be covered with 3 to 4 mm of investment. This layer should be as uniform in thickness as possible to ensure even expansion of the mold (Fig. 10-8).

During the paint-on procedure it may be helpful to use vibration to help the flow of the investment. This must be done indirectly to protect the pattern. The hand holding the brush can rest on the vibrator. The action of the vibrator will assist the flow of the investment over the pattern. Neither the hand holding the cast nor the cast should touch the vibrator (Fig. 10-9).

6. Set the invested pattern aside until this paint-on layer has reached its initial set. Support the cast during this time so the investment will not flow from the pattern (Fig. 10-10).

7. Attach the partially invested pattern to a crucible former, or, as an optional procedure, invest it directly in a ring, and carve the crucible in the investment. (Skip to step 15 for this optional procedure.) It is much more desirable to use a crucible

---

*Debubblizer—Wax Painting Solution, Kerr Manufacturing Co., Romulus, Mich.; Ti-Sol, Ticonium Co., Albany, N.Y.

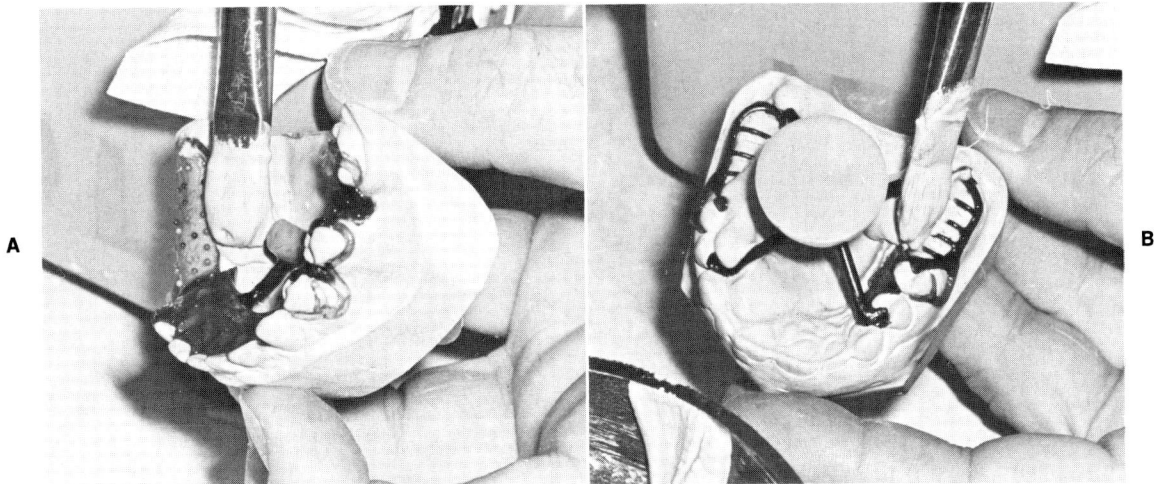

**Fig. 10-7. A,** Hold cast by end of central sprue protruding from base of cast or by base, and with brush paint investment over wax. **B,** When wax-up is sprued from top or distal side, hold cast by base, and paint on investment.

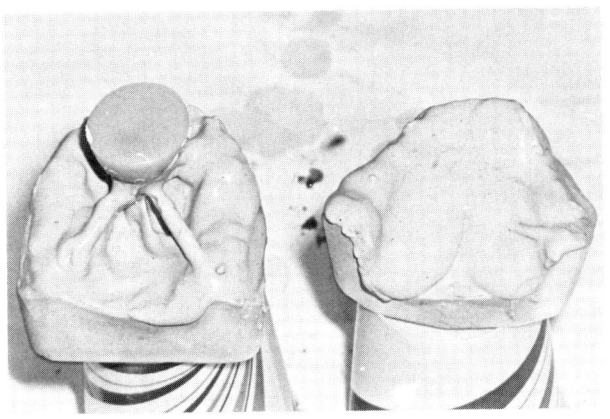

**Fig. 10-8.** Entire pattern is covered with uniform layer of paint-on investment between 3 and 4 mm thick. Mandibular pattern, right. Maxillary pattern, left.

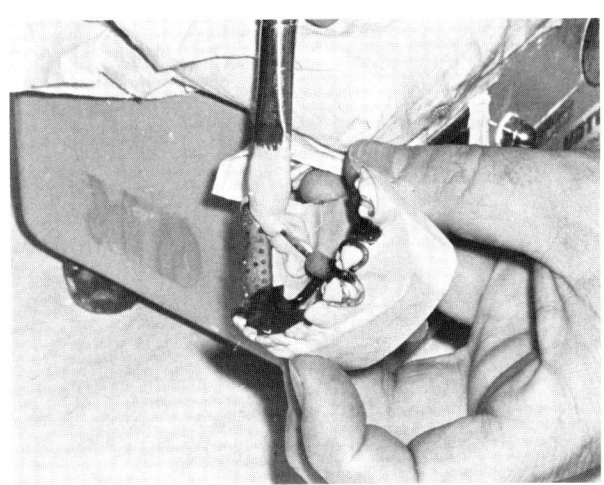

**Fig. 10-9.** Place hand holding paintbrush on vibrator. Action of vibrator will assist flow of investment.

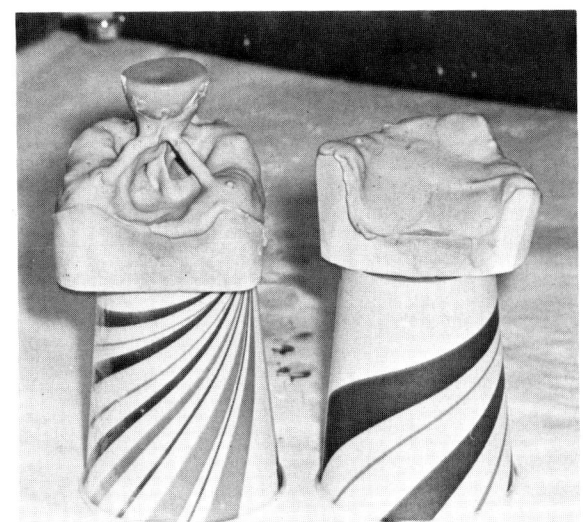

**Fig. 10-10.** Casts are supported while paint-on investment sets.

former than to carve the investment, but both methods will be shown.

Insert the wax central sprue through the hole in the crucible former. Place the casting ring over the cast, and seat it in the proper groove on the crucible former. Adjust the position of the cast in relation to the ring so that it is centered in the ring and the highest point of the wax pattern is 15 mm from the end of the ring (Fig. 10-11). This position is critical for complete escape of gases and for sufficient strength of investment to resist the force of the molten metal. Seal the central sprue to the crucible former with wax (Fig. 10-12). Cut the excess length of the sprue and be sure the wax is sealed well. If the reinforcing bur in the wax interferes, remove it, and fill the hole with wax (step 11). Do not overfill with wax because the crucible former must sit flat on the bench top (Fig. 10-13).

8. Seal the casting ring to the grooves in the crucible former with wax. A tacky wax such as round orthodontic wax or round beading wax used in boxing impressions is good for this purpose (Fig. 10-14). Fill the investment ring with water. This

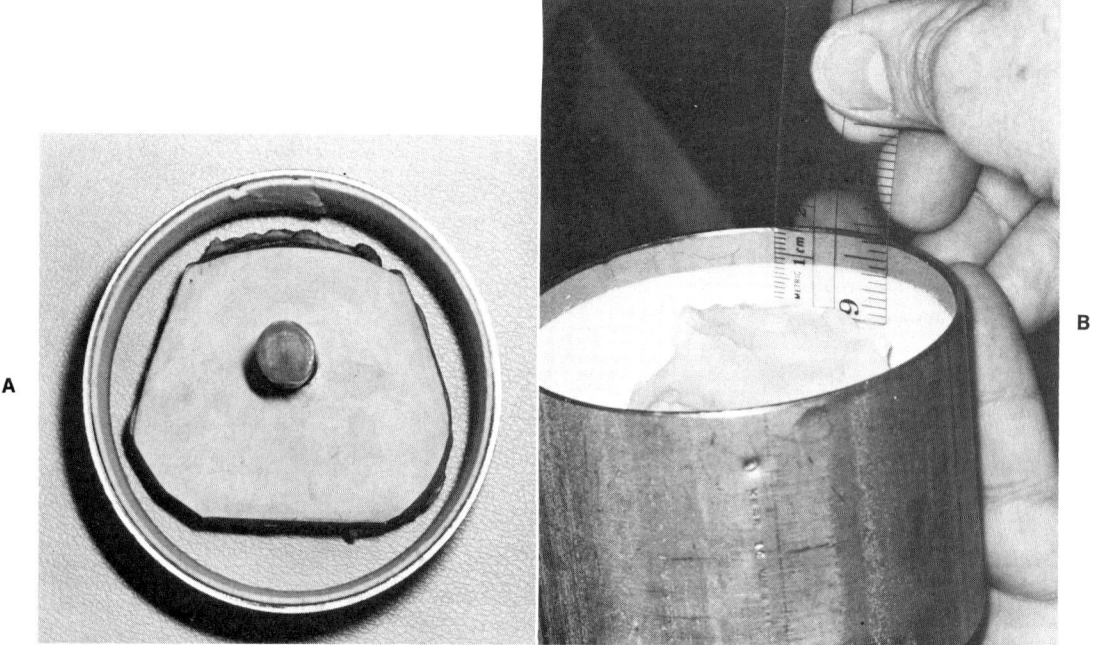

**Fig. 10-11. A,** Cast is centered in ring and must clear sides of ring by at least ¼ inch (0.63 cm). **B,** Highest point of wax pattern is 15 mm from bottom end of ring.

Investing, burnout, and casting **299**

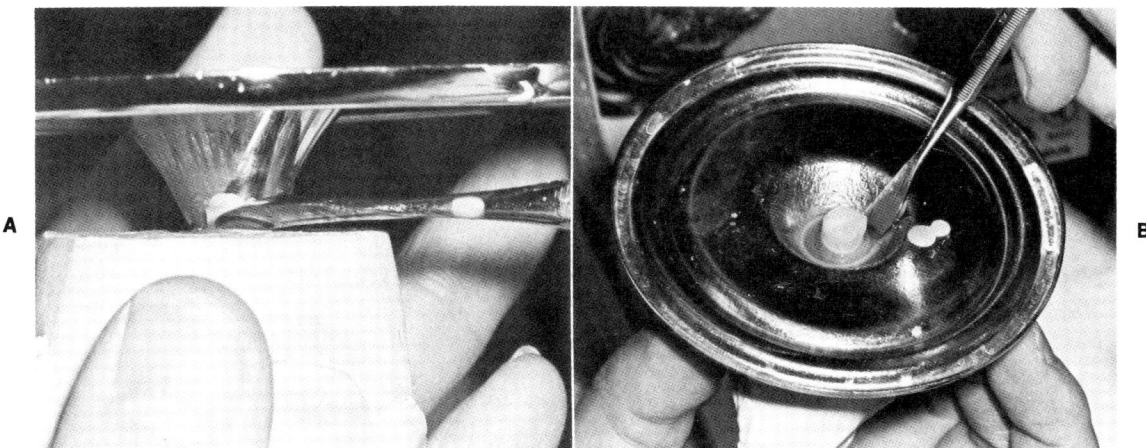

**Fig. 10-12.** Cast is held in this position while it is sealed with wax at top **(A)** and bottom of sprue former **(B)**.

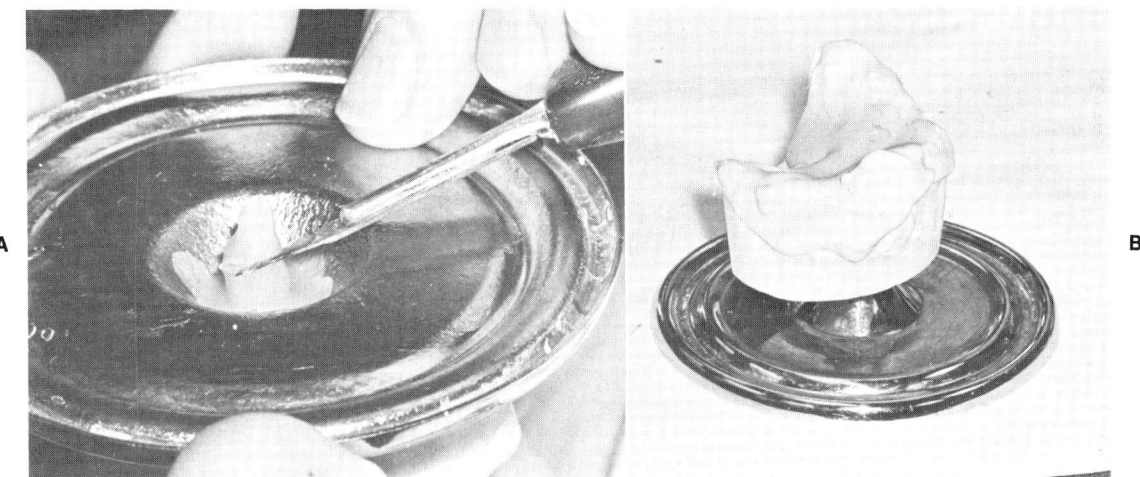

**Fig. 10-13. A,** Excess length of central sprue is cut off flush with bottom of sprue former. **B,** Crucible former must sit flat on bench.

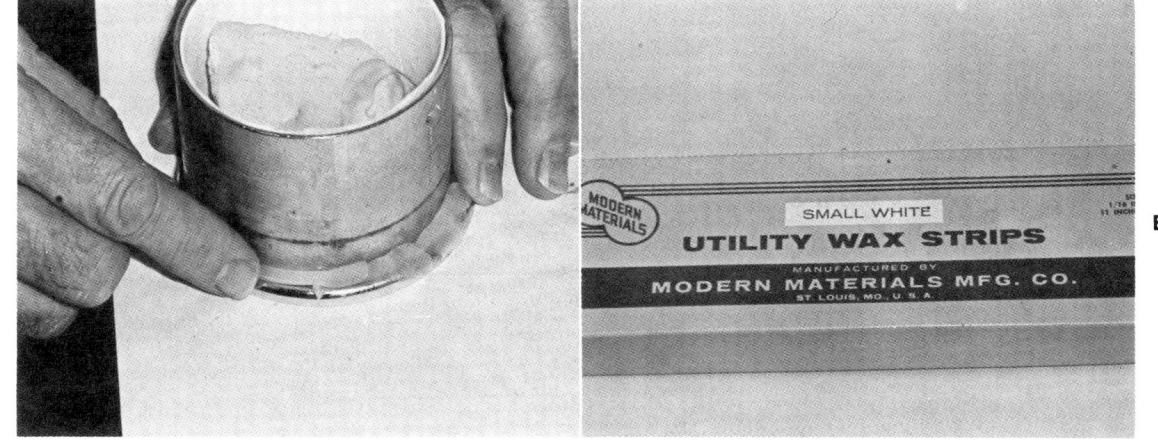

**Fig. 10-14. A,** Casting ring is sealed to sprue former with tacky wax. **B,** Good wax to use is utility wax strips or beading wax.

**300** *Dental laboratory procedures: removable partial dentures*

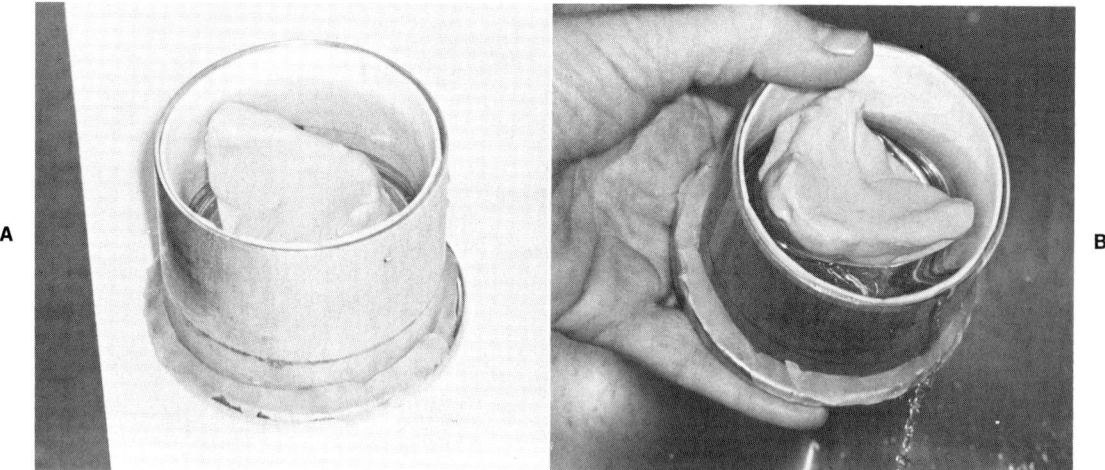

**Fig. 10-15. A,** Investment ring filled with water to soak investment and verify complete seal of ring. **B,** Empty water after 3 minutes and remove excess.

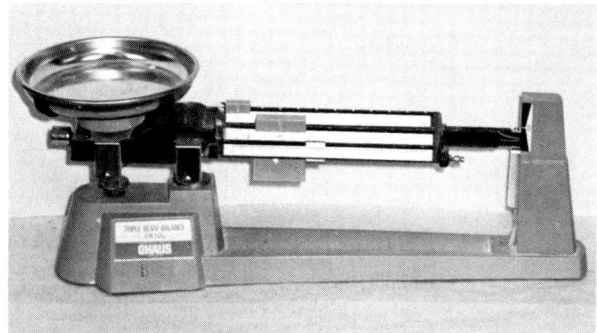

**Fig. 10-16.** Weigh accurately on good beam balance 450 gm of investment, enough to fill large casting ring, and measure water. Same water-powder ratio is used as for paint-on investment.

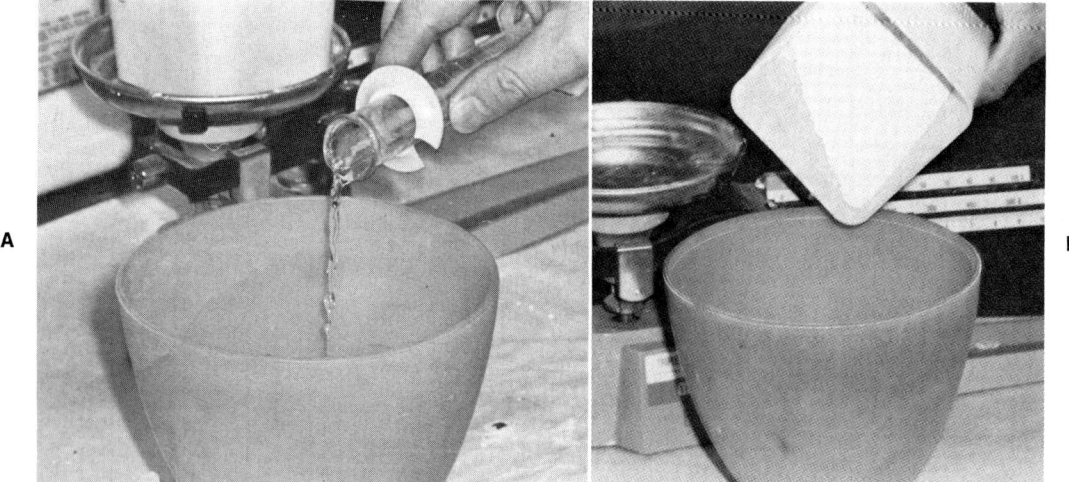

**Fig. 10-17. A,** Distilled water poured into bowl, **B,** Weighed investment added to distilled water. Mix is hand spatulated for 60 seconds.

will verify the complete seal of the ring and will soak the paint-on investment. Allow it to soak for 2 to 3 minutes, then empty the water. Be sure the excess water is all removed (Fig. 10-15).

9. Mix 450 gm of investment material for the large casting ring. Use the same water-powder ratio that was used for the paint-on investment (Fig. 10-16). Use distilled water, pour it into the mixing bowl, and then add the investment. Hand spatulate the mix for 60 seconds (Fig. 10-17). Vacuum mixing or mechanical spatulation is not desired because some air in this mix is necessary to aid in venting the gases that will occur during burnout and casting.

10. Place the crucible former ring on a vibrator, and use light vibrations to vibrate the investment slowly into the ring until it is completely filled. Take care to not trap air under the base of the investment cast (Fig. 10-18).

11. Allow the investment to set for at least 1 hour. Rotate the crucible former gently, and remove it from the casting ring (Fig. 10-19). If the reinforcing bur was not removed in step 7, grasp the end of it with pliers, and remove it with a pull in a straight line. If resistance is encountered, heat the sprue, and soften the wax before removing the bur (Fig. 10-20).

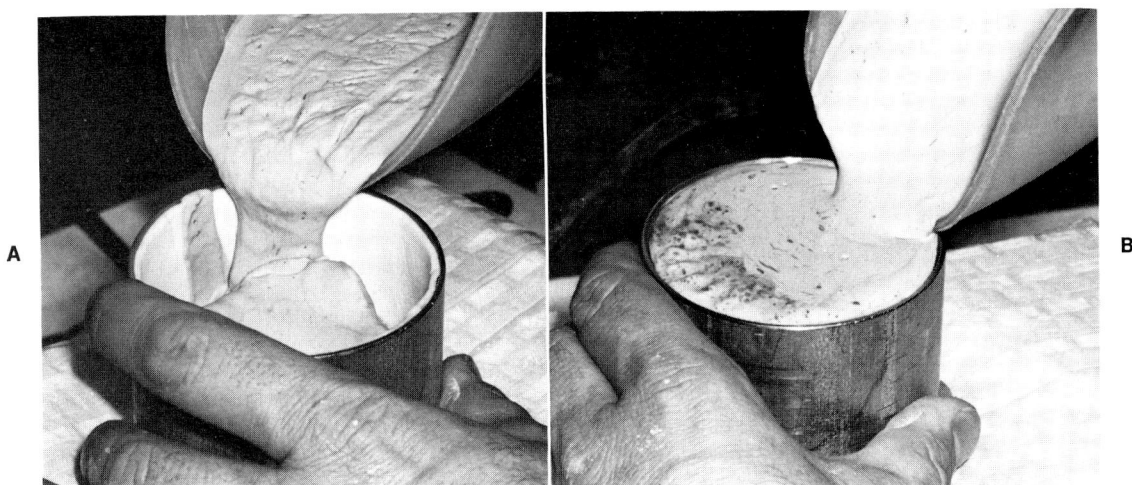

Fig. 10-18. A, With ring and crucible on vibrator, pour investment over cast. B, Light vibrations are used to slowly vibrate investment mix to fill ring. Allow investment to set.

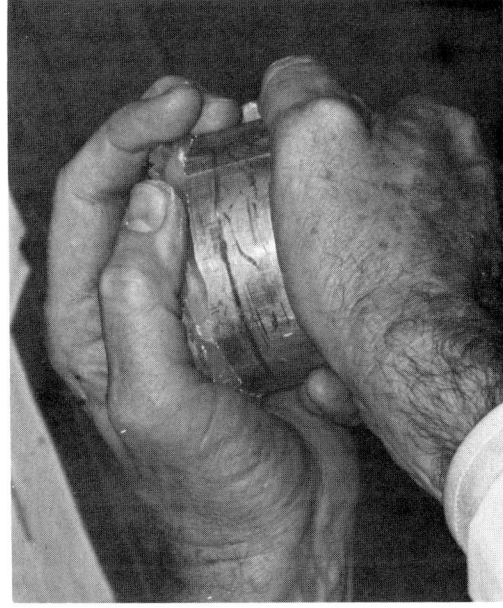

Fig. 10-19. One hand grips casting ring and other grips crucible former. Gently twist crucible former to remove it from casting ring.

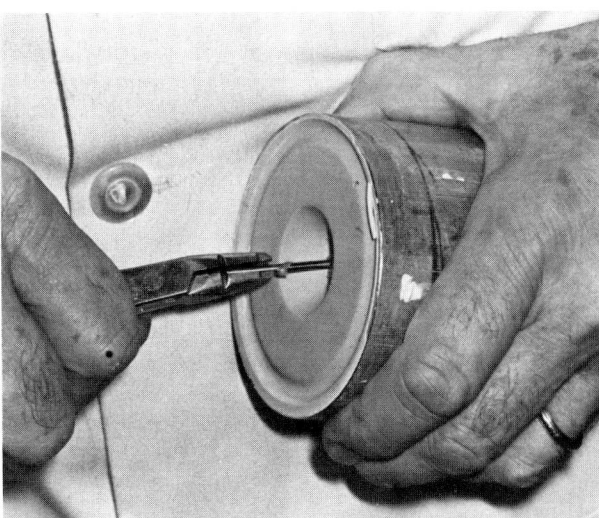

Fig. 10-20. Reinforcing bur is removed by pulling in straight line with pair of pliers.

12. Flatten the end of the investment opposite to the crucible with a knife. Make it level with the metal casting ring (Fig. 10-21). This is necessary so it will seat evenly in the casting machine.

13. Use jeweler's rouge to place some identification on the investment in the casting ring. This mark will stay on during the burnout and can be used to identify one casting from another if more than one ring is in the furnace at one time (Fig. 10-22).

14. The invested wax up is ready for burnout and casting (Fig. 10-23).

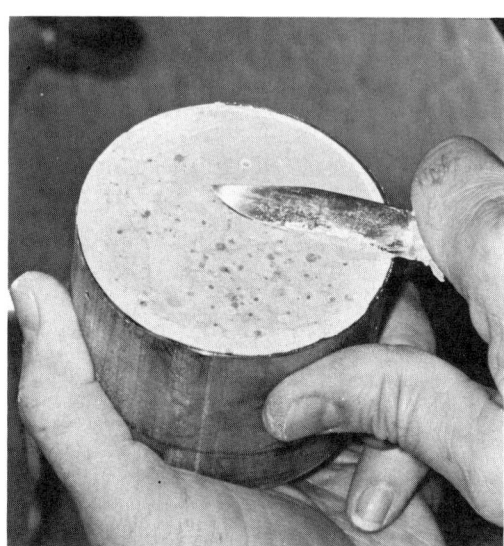

**Fig. 10-21.** Knife is used to trim investment level with metal casting ring.

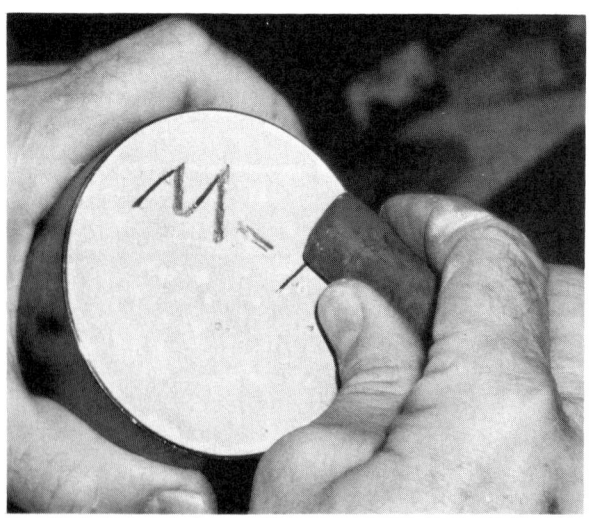

**Fig. 10-22.** Jeweler's rouge is used to identify casting. It will not be destroyed during burnout.

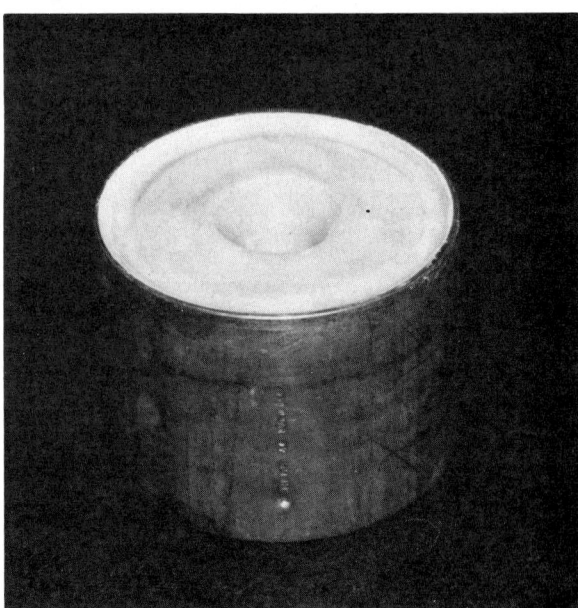

**Fig. 10-23.** Investing following recommended method is completed.

## OPTIONAL INVESTING PROCEDURE

This investing procedure is recommended for castings sprued in the preceding procedure that have their own preformed crucibles, as in the maxillary cast, which was sprued from above (Figs. 8-71 and 8-72). Some use this method for investing castings sprued through the cast as will be demonstrated by the mandibular cast. It is not recommended for through-the-cast spruing but has enough advocates to warrant description here.

1. The ring should be lined as described in step 1 of the procedure for investing the sprued pattern (Figs. 10-1 and 10-2). Hold the maxillary cast with the paint-on investment by the central sprue, and insert it into the prepared casting ring to determine if it still has the necessary clearance (Fig. 10-24). Place the mandibular cast in the casting ring until the cast with the paint-on investment is 15 mm from the end (Fig. 10-25). The central sprue will be sticking out the other end of the ring. Lay a spatula or straightedge, and make a mark on the wax sprue (Fig. 10-26). Remove the cast, and wrap a piece of half-round casting wax around the sprue at the level of the mark, and seal it in place (Fig. 10-27).

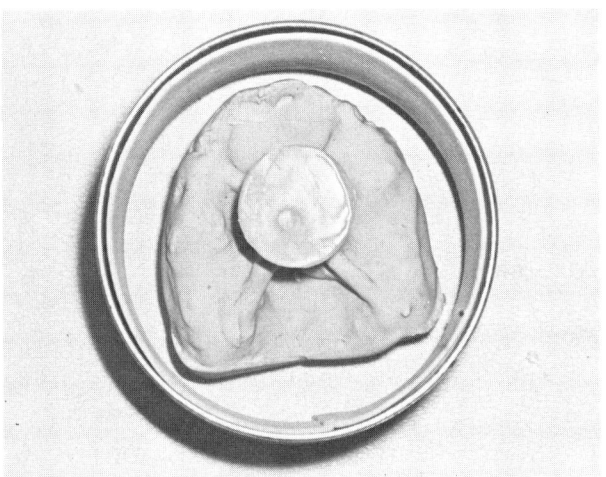

**Fig. 10-24.** In optional method, wax-up covered with paint-on investment is placed in lined casting ring to make sure there is sufficient clearance around sides. If not, it should be trimmed carefully.

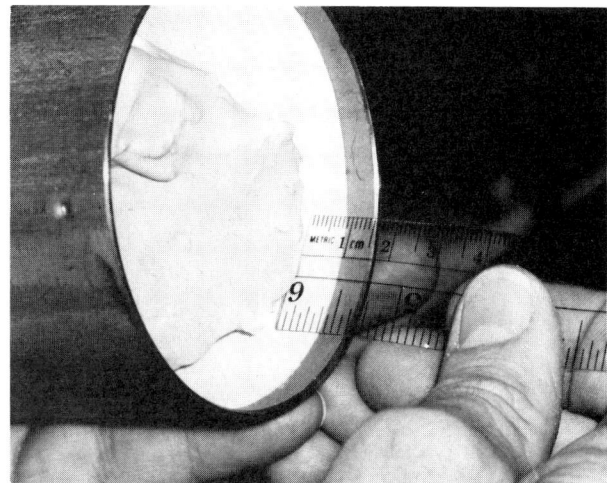

**Fig. 10-25.** Cast is positioned 15 mm from end of casting ring.

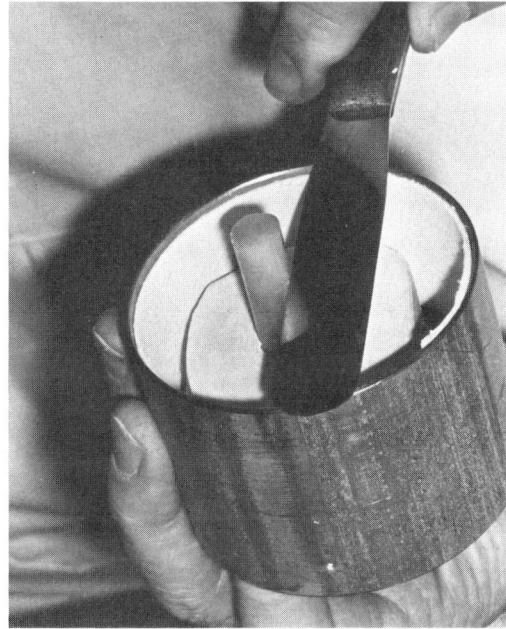

**Fig. 10-26.** Cast is held in position, and sprue is marked by laying spatula across casting ring.

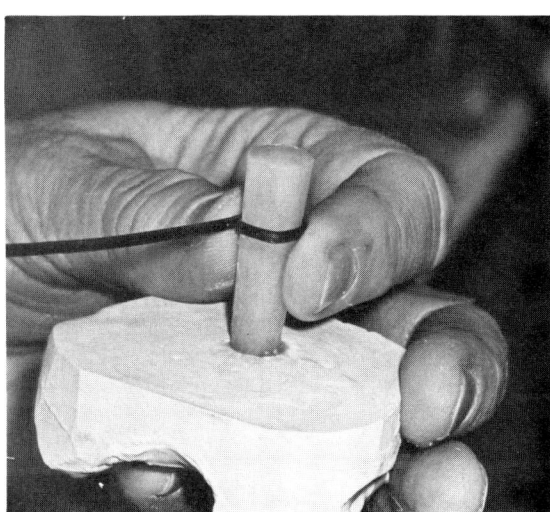

**Fig. 10-27.** Piece of half-round casting is wrapped around central sprue at level of mark made by spatula and sealed in place.

2. Place the investment casts in water for 2 or 3 minutes (Fig. 10-28).

3. While the casts are soaking, place the casting rings on a flat sheet of plastic or glass, and seal them in place with a rope of orthodontic wax or beading wax (Fig. 10-29).

4. Make a mix of investment for each casting ring as described in step 9 of the procedure for investing the sprued pattern.

5. Vibrate the mix of investment into each casting ring until it is about three-fourths full (Fig. 10-30).

6. Remove the investment casts from the water, and shake off the excess. Vibrate the sprued mandibular investment cast into one casting ring of investment to the level of the half-round wax shape wrapped around the central sprue (Fig. 10-31). This will position the refractory cast 15 mm from the bottom of the casting ring. Vibrate the maxillary cast into the other casting ring until the sprue former base is flush with the top rim of the casting ring (Fig. 10-

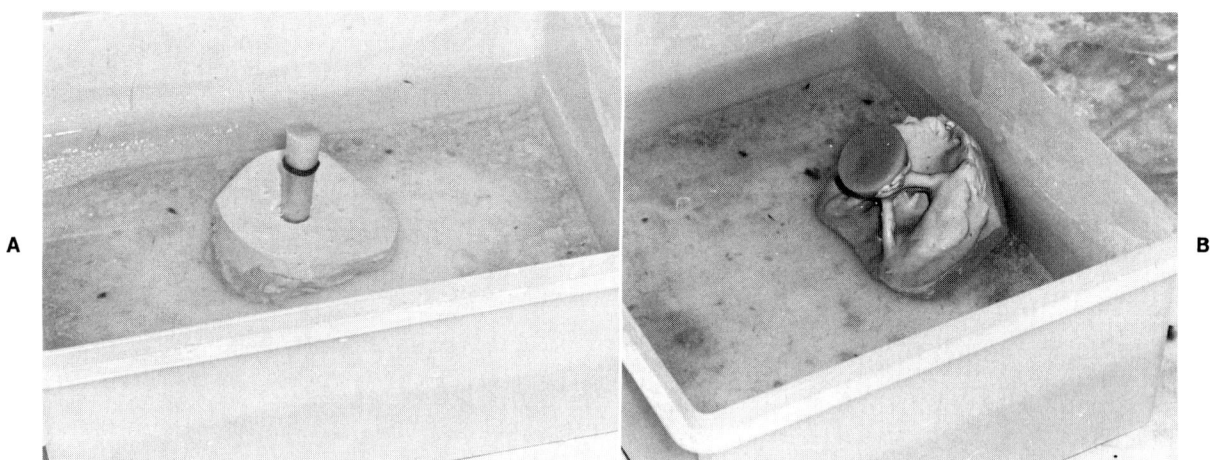

**Fig. 10-28.** Investment cast is immersed in water for 3 minutes. **A,** Pattern sprued through base. **B,** Pattern sprued from above.

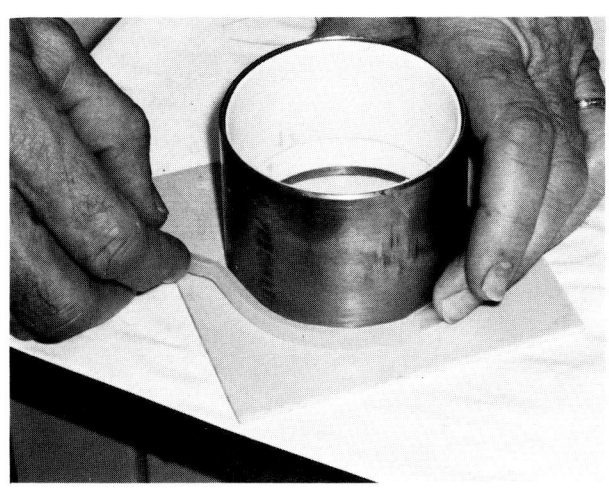

**Fig. 10-29.** Casting ring is sealed to plastic sheet with tacky wax.

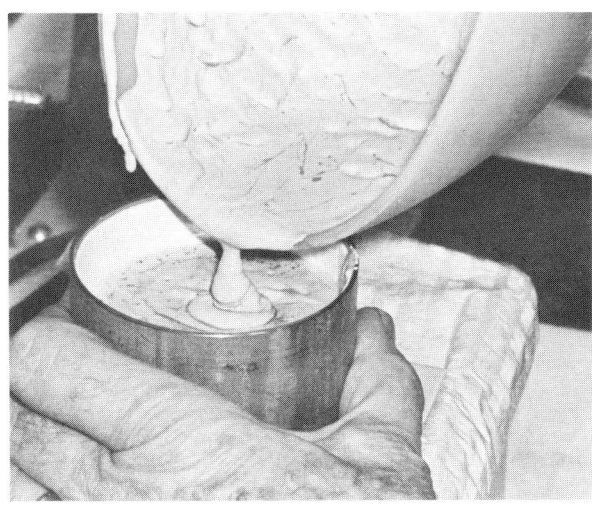

**Fig. 10-30.** Vibrate investment into casting ring until it is three-fourths full.

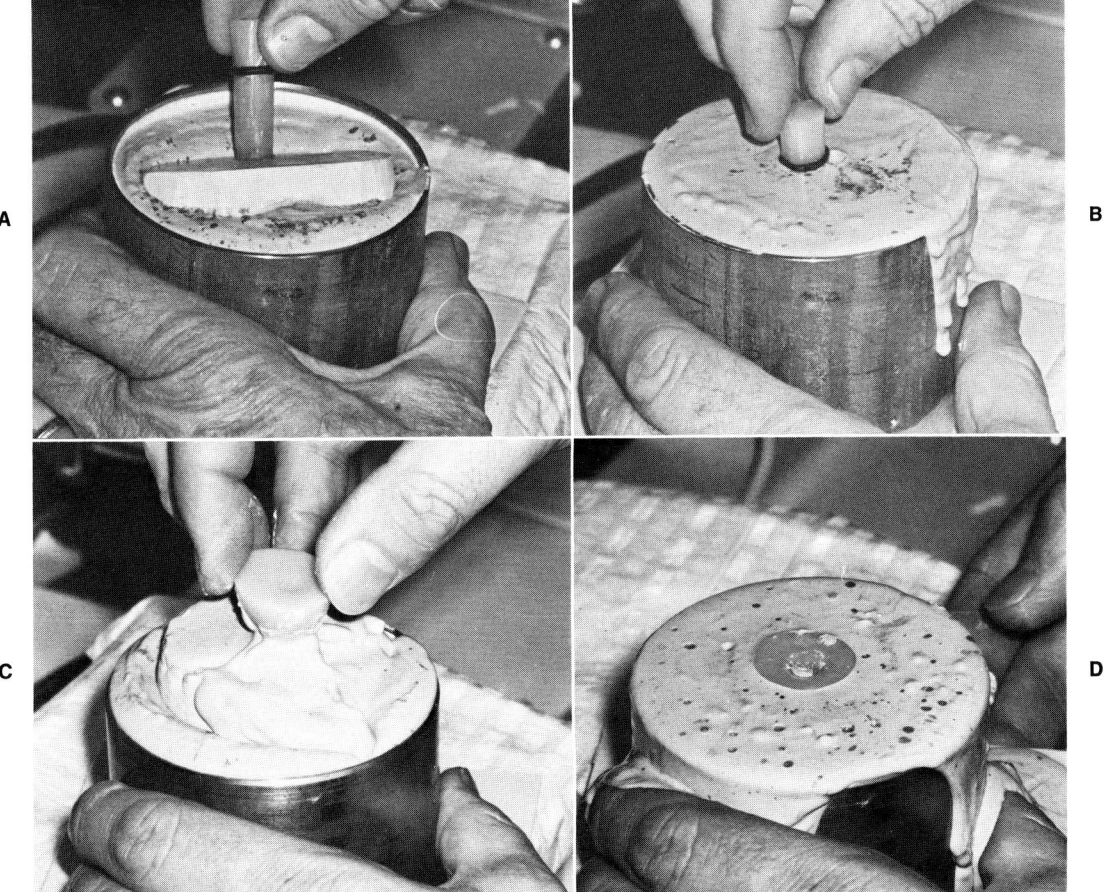

**Fig. 10-31. A,** Vibrate refractory cast into investment. **B,** Keep vibrating until half-round ring on central sprue is level with rim of flask. **C,** Pattern sprued from above is vibrated in same manner. **D,** Vibration is continued until sprue former is level with casting ring.

31). Be sure that as the casts are vibrated to place, they stay in the center of the casting ring (Fig. 10-32). Permit the investment to set for at least 1 hour.

7. After the investment has set, remove the central wax sprue to expose the reinforcing bur in the mandibular cast (Fig. 10-33). Heat the end of the bur, and remove it with pliers (Fig. 10-34).

8. With a knife, trim the central sprue and investment until it is flush with the rim of the casting ring (Fig. 10-35). The invested maxillary wax-up is ready for burnout and casting.

9. If necessary, enlarge the investment around the end of the central sprue with a knife to form a larger crucible (Fig. 10-36).

10. The invested mandibular wax-up is ready for burnout and casting (Fig. 10-37).

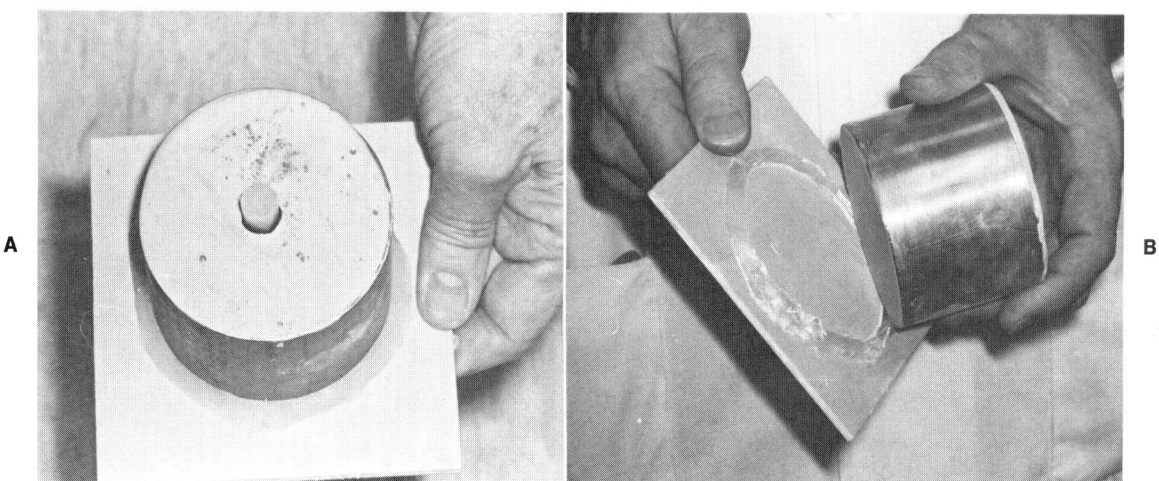

**Fig. 10-32. A,** Cast and sprue must be in center of casting ring. **B,** After investment sets, remove plastic sheet.

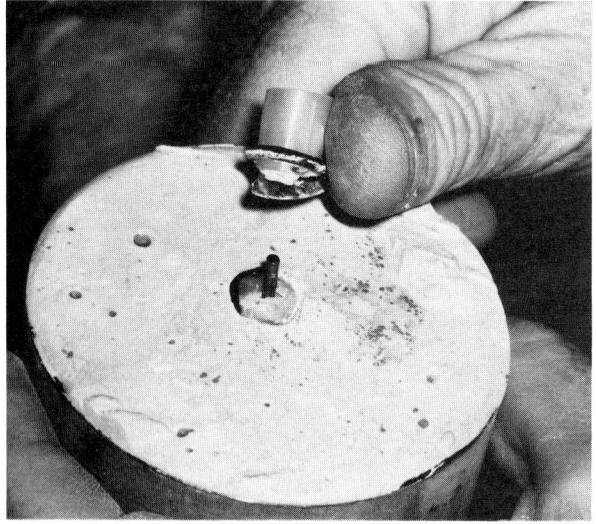

**Fig. 10-33.** Remove wax central sprue to expose reinforcing bur.

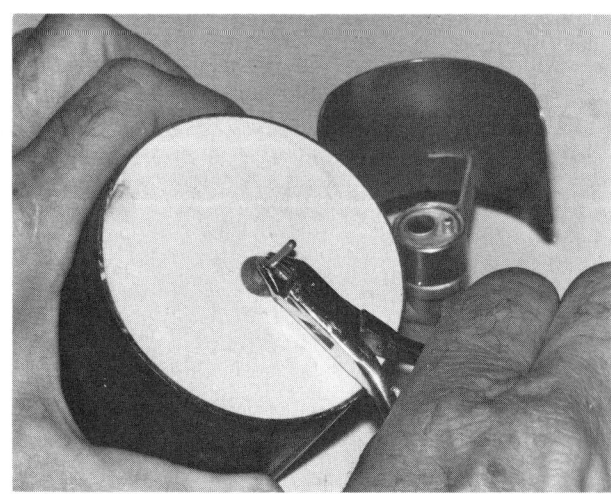

**Fig. 10-34.** End of bur is heated and removed with pliers.

*Investing, burnout, and casting* **307**

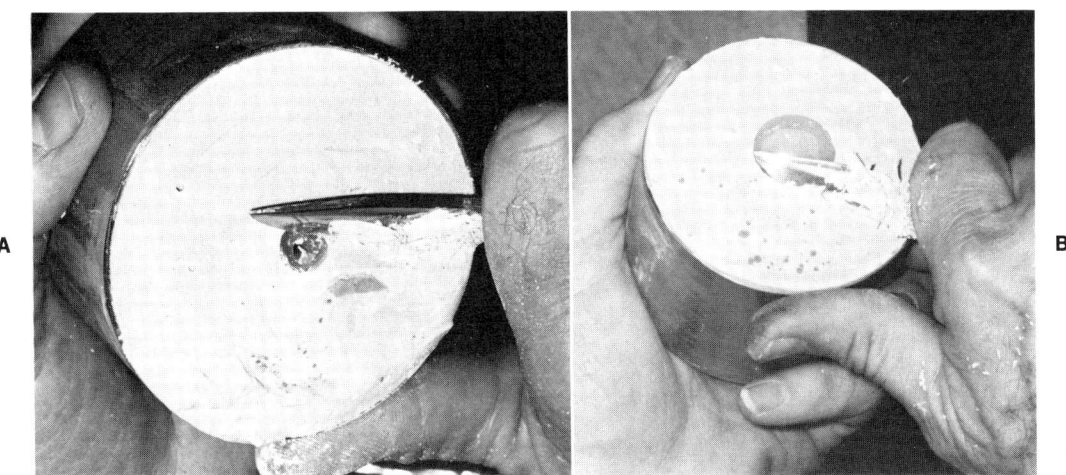

**Fig. 10-35.** Investment and sprue are trimmed flush with rim of casting flask. **A,** Pattern sprued through base. **B,** Pattern sprued from above.

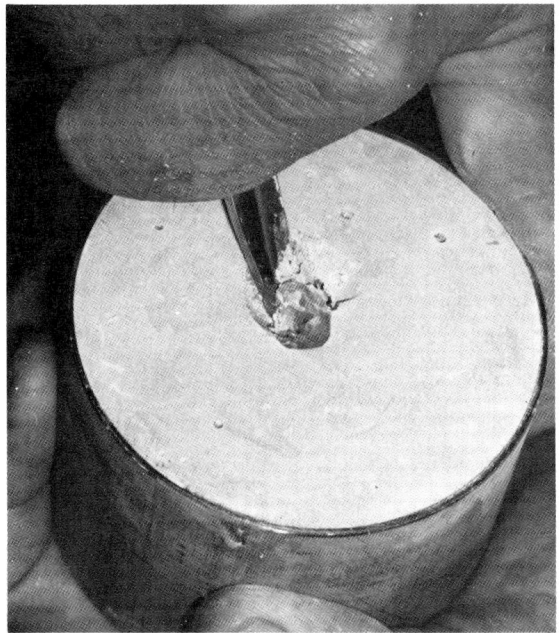

**Fig. 10-36.** Larger crucible may be carved into investment with sharp knife if necessary, but particles of roughened investment may be carried into mold by molten metal.

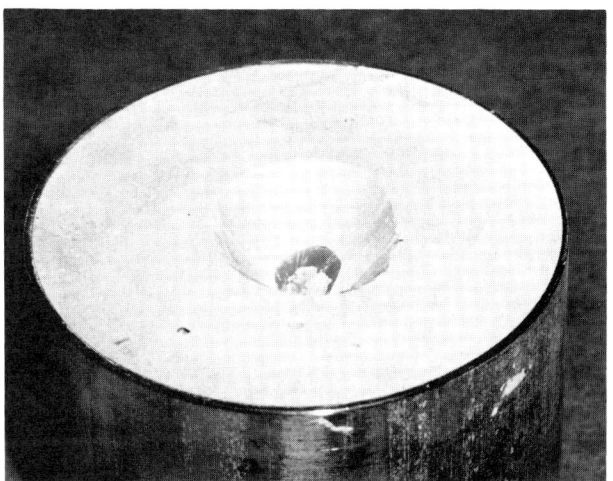

**Fig. 10-37.** Investing by optional method is completed.

**Table 10-1.** Investing a wax pattern

| Problem | Probable cause | Solution |
| --- | --- | --- |
| Casting will not seat on cast | Wrong water-powder ratio used for investment | Use manufacturer's recommended water-powder ratio for cast, paint-on, and outer investment |
| | Wrong type investment used | Select investment material that is compatible with alloy used |
| | Improper blockout procedure | Use surveyor to block out all undesirable undercuts |
| Miscast | Paint-on and outer investment vacuum spatulated | Do not vacuum spatulate paint-on and outer investment |
| Casting has numerous nodules and fins | Air trapped against pattern during paint-on of investment | Paint investment on carefully to minimize voids |
| | Surface tension reducer was not used on wax pattern | Paint wax pattern with surface tension–reducing agent (Ti-Sol) before adding investment |

### PROBLEM AREAS

The principal problems associated with the investing procedure are related to failure to use the proper water-powder ratio for the investment, using the wrong type of investment, vacuum spatulating the outer investments and trapping air when adding the paint-on investment (Table 10-1). Following the manufacturer's recommendations closely, selecting the proper investment material, and careful attention to technical procedures will significantly reduce problems.

### BURNOUT

The burnout operation dries the moisture out of the mold, eliminates the wax and plastic pattern by melting and vaporization, and expands the mold to compensate for the shrinkage of the metal. The time required for the burnout depends on the heat available, size of the furnace, and number of molds to be burned out at the same time. The temperature inside the mold is held down during the early stages of the burnout by the vaporization of the water in the mold, regardless of the temperature setting of the furnace. Water temperature will not rise above its boiling point so the internal temperature of the mold will remain at 212° F (100° C) until all of the water is vaporized.

The water is usually all driven off within an hour. The temperature inside the mold will then rise to the temperature of the furnace, but it may require another hour before the temperature within the mold is completely equalized. During this period, the furnace may be set at 1000° F (538° C). After this 2-hour period, the mold and the furnace should remain at a temperature between 1250° and 1300° F (675° and 710° C) for another 1½ to 2 hours. This time is necessary to complete the removal of the carbon residue resulting from the vaporization and oxidation of the wax and plastic pattern and to complete the removal of the moisture from the interstices of the investment.

The wax itself is eliminated early in the burnout,

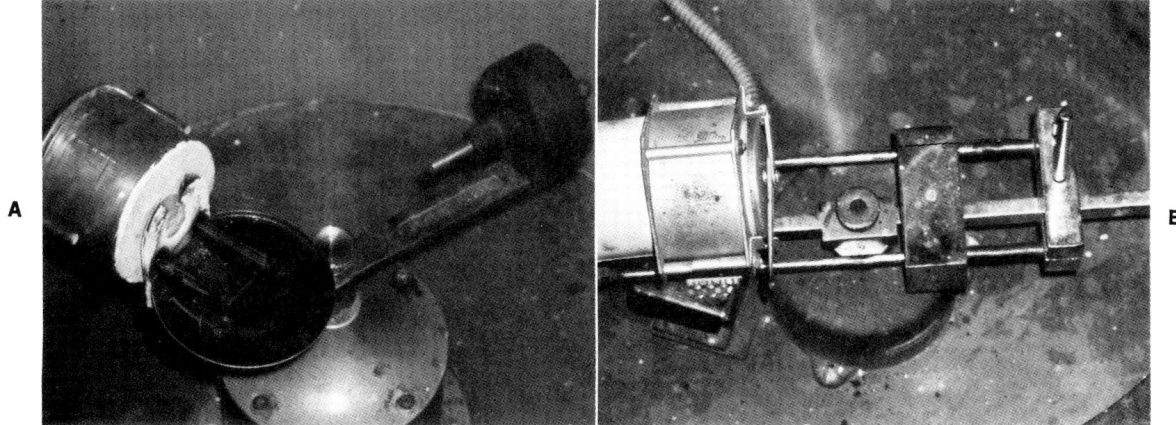

**Fig. 10-38.** Check casting machine by actually placing casting ring in it to see if it will hold ring properly. **A,** Spring-propelled broken arm casting machine with casting ring in place. **B,** Same procedure with straight-arm, electric-melt casting machine.

usually before the temperature has risen to 1000° F. The carbon residue takes much longer. The interstices or spaces between the particles of investment are the critical areas as far as complete elimination of moisture and carbon particles is concerned. These small spaces actually account for 50% of the total volume of the investment. The gases in the mold cavity must rapidly escape through these spaces when the stream of molten metal enters the cavity. If, because of insufficient burnout, all the moisture or carbon is not removed, an incomplete or porous casting will result because gases cannot escape.

To properly control the temperature inside the mold and make the heat more uniform, the investment should be moist when it is placed in the furnace. If the burnout is not done the same day the investment is poured, it should be soaked for several minutes before the burnout is begun.

**PROCEDURE**

1. Prepare and balance the casting machine before the casting ring is placed in the burnout oven. Be sure the casting machine will hold the casting ring (Fig. 10-38). If the machine is not an electric melt type, a fresh strip of substitute asbestos should be adapted to the large ceramic crucible. Cut the strip slightly longer than the crucible, and taper one end, wet the liner, make a funnel out of the tapered end and push it through the spout, adapt the main portion of the liner to the crucible, and with an instrument form the remainder around the spout opening to form a liner for it and lock the liner in position (Fig. 10-39). Balance the arm of the machine with the crucible, metal, and the flask in position (Fig. 10-40).

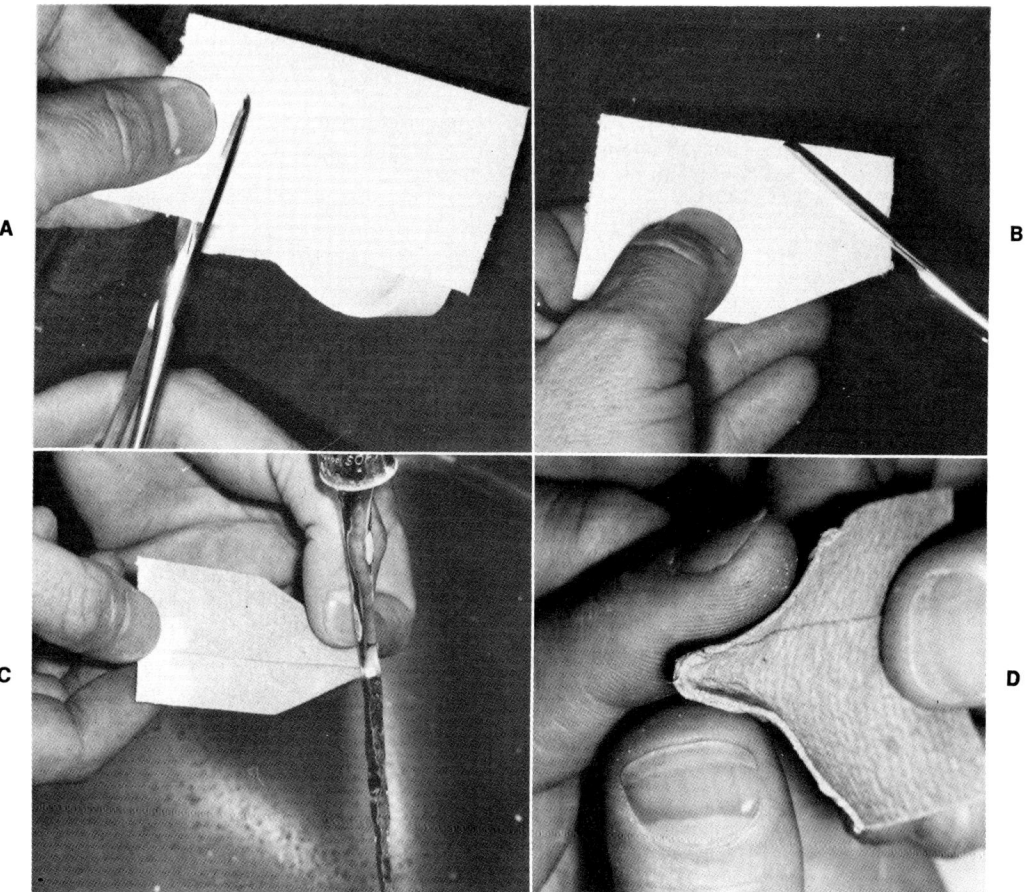

**Fig. 10-39.** Adapt strip of substitute asbestos to inside of large ceramic crucible. **A,** Double strip cut slightly longer than crucible. **B,** One end tapered by cutting with scissors. **C,** Liner is wet with water. **D,** Funnel is made at tapered end.

Investing, burnout, and casting **311**

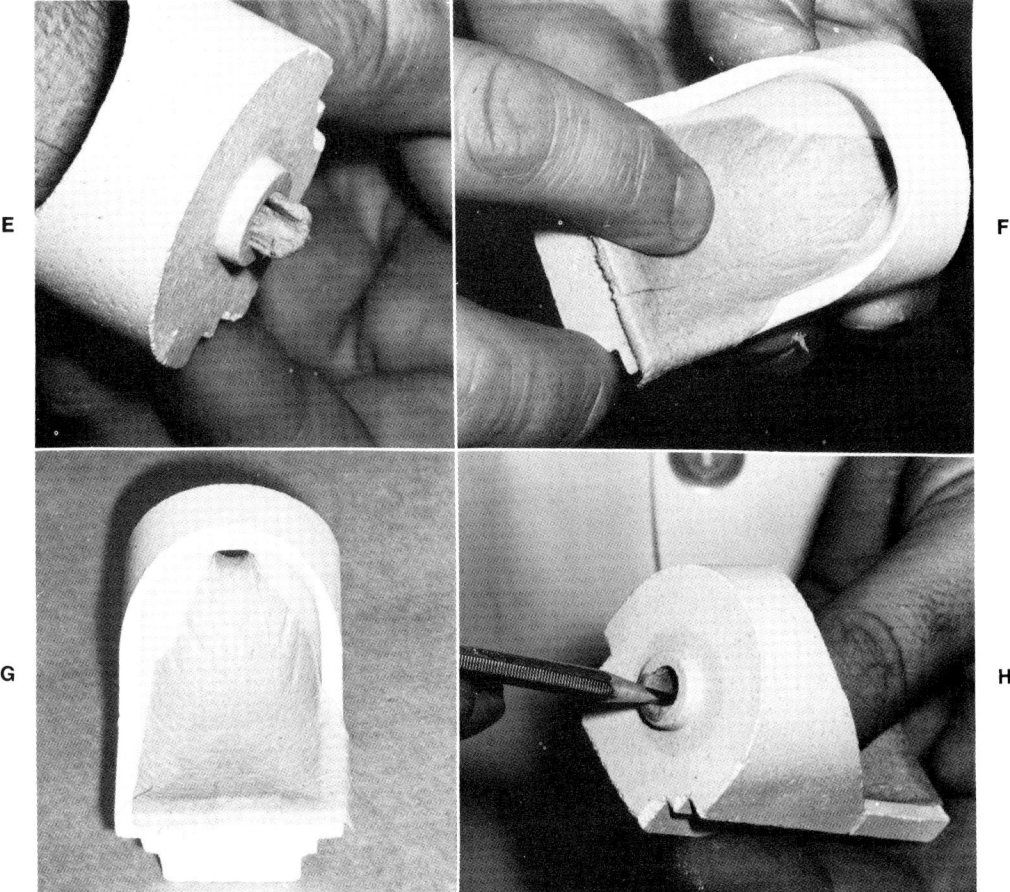

**Fig. 10-39, cont'd. E,** Funneled end is pushed through spout of crucible. **F,** Main portion of liner is adapted to inside of crucible. **G,** Funnel end is adapted to inside of spout with instrument to form liner for spout. **H,** Completed liner in crucible.

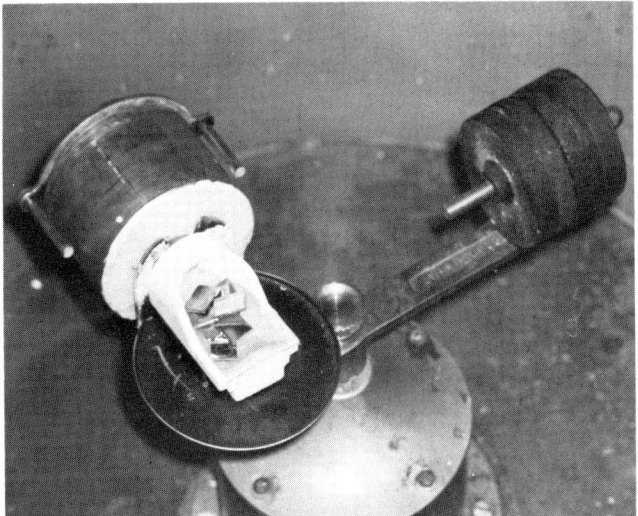

**Fig. 10-40.** Lined crucible, metal, and invested partial denture are placed in casting machine, and machine is balanced.

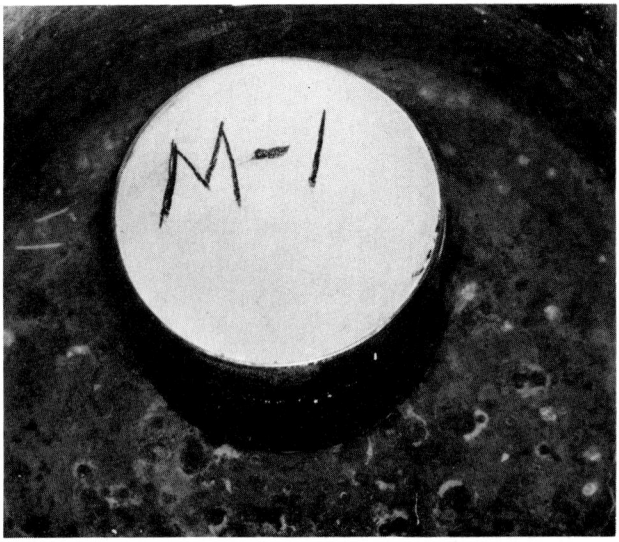

**Fig. 10-41.** Investment soaked in water for few minutes.

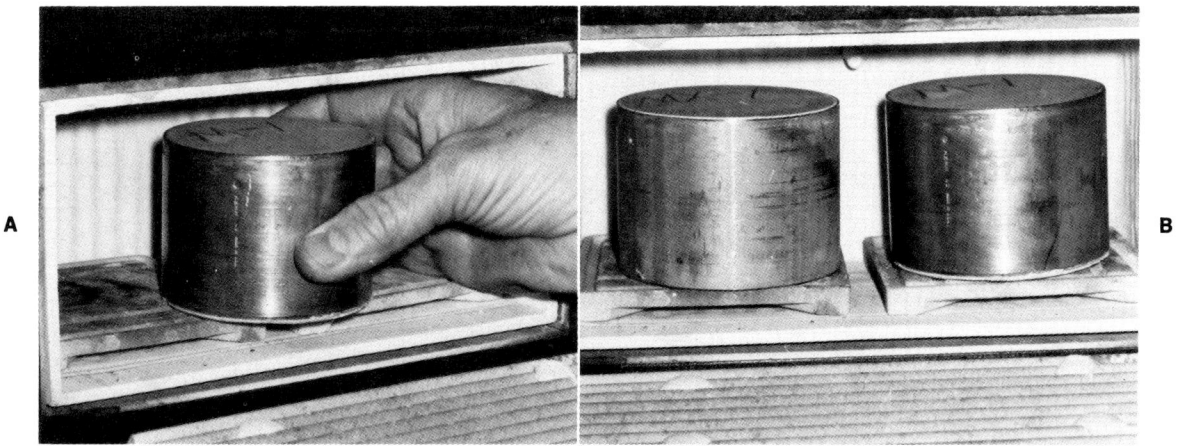

**Fig. 10-42. A,** Ring is placed in cool furnace, sprue hole down **B,** Ring does not touch side of furnace or another ring.

2. Soak the investment in water for several minutes (Fig. 10-41).

3. Place the ring in a cool furnace sprue side down. Do not let the ring touch the sides of the furnace or another ring (Fig. 10-42). If the side of the flask touches anything it will cause it to heat unevenly and distort.

4. Turn the burnout furnace on, and adjust it to reach 1000° F in about 1 hour.

5. Leave the furnace at the 1000° F setting for 2 hours. This is the period of greatest expansion. Then increase the temperature setting of the furnace so it will hold the temperature between 1250° and 1300° F (Fig. 10-43). NOTE: The temperature should not rise above 1300° F. Plaster-bound investment begins to contract at 1350° F, and breakdown of the binder occurs at 1450° F.

6. When the temperature of the furnace has reached 1250° F, the mold must heat soak at this temperature for at least 1½ hours.

7. The mold is ready to cast. If any doubt exists about the completion of the burnout, it is better to leave it for a longer time than to chance casting failure (Fig. 10-44).

*Investing, burnout, and casting* **313**

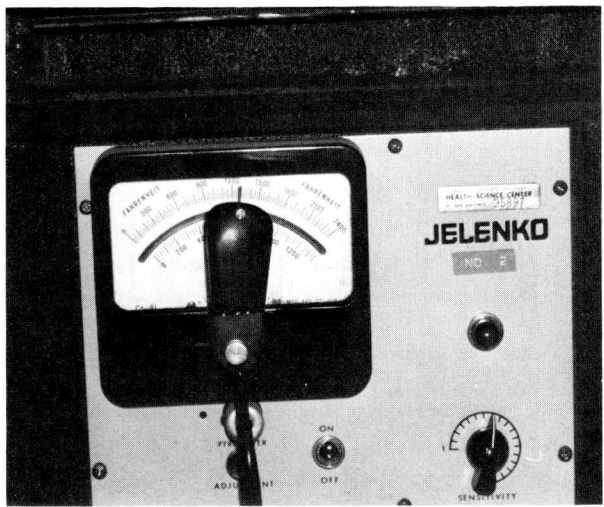

**Fig. 10-43.** Furnace turned on and set to reach 1000° F (538° C) in 1 hour. After 2 hours, set temperature control of furnace so it will maintain temperature between 1250° and 1300° F (675° and 710° C). Mold must heat soak at temperature between 1250° and 1300° F for at least 1½ hours.

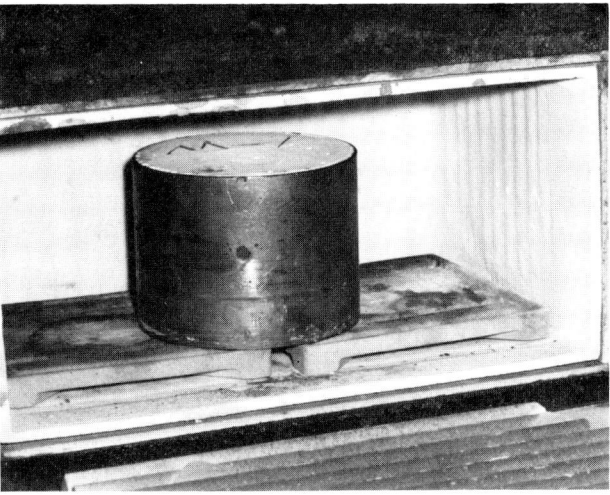

**Fig. 10-44.** Mold ready to cast.

## CASTING

The casting will be done in a centrifugal force casting machine. Failures can occur by having too much or too little force. Too little force may allow the metal to "freeze" before the mold is completely filled, and too much force may produce turbulence in the metal that can result in trapping gases in the casting. Three or four turns of the casting machine are correct for most castings.

The heat for melting the metal may be supplied by a blow torch using gas and air, gas and oxygen, acetylene, electrical conduction, or induction. It is much easier if the casting procedure is done with two persons when a blow torch is used. One person should control the blow torch and release the casting machine. The other person, at the proper time as determined by the melting of the metal, should remove the ring from the furnace and position it in the casting machine. In the interest of safety, it is best if no one but the person doing the casting is close to the machine when it is released.

### PROCEDURE

1. Examine the liner in the crucible to see if it is clean and continuous to and through the spout.
2. Wind the casting machine three or four turns, depending on the tightness of the spring, and lock it in position (Fig. 10-45).
3. Place the metal in the crucible on the asbestos liner (Fig. 10-46).

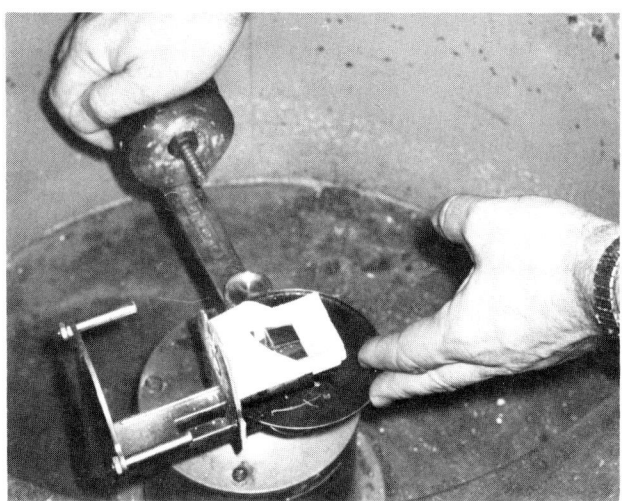

**Fig. 10-45.** Casting machine is wound and locked in position.

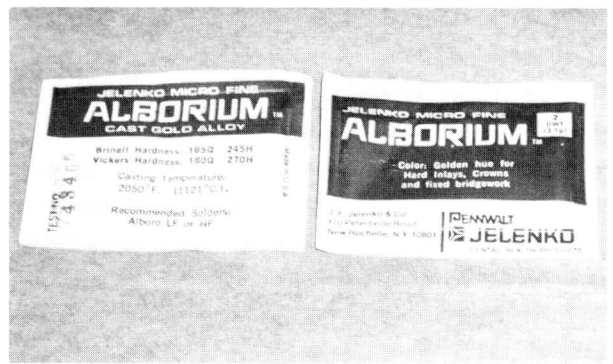

**Fig. 10-46.** Alborium metal is placed in crucible.

**314** *Dental laboratory procedures: removable partial dentures*

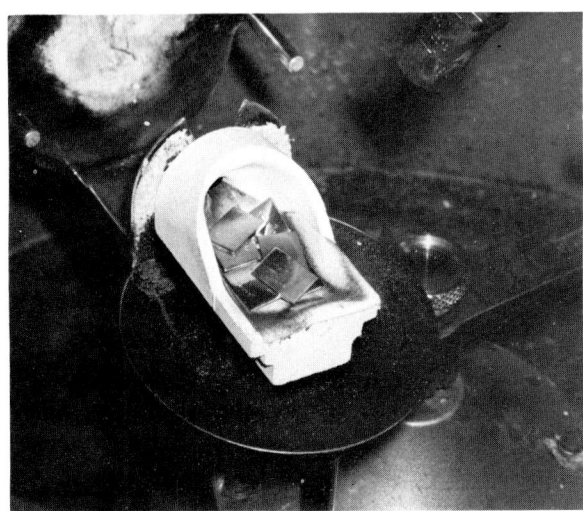

**Fig. 10-47.** Torch adjusted to produce reducing flame.

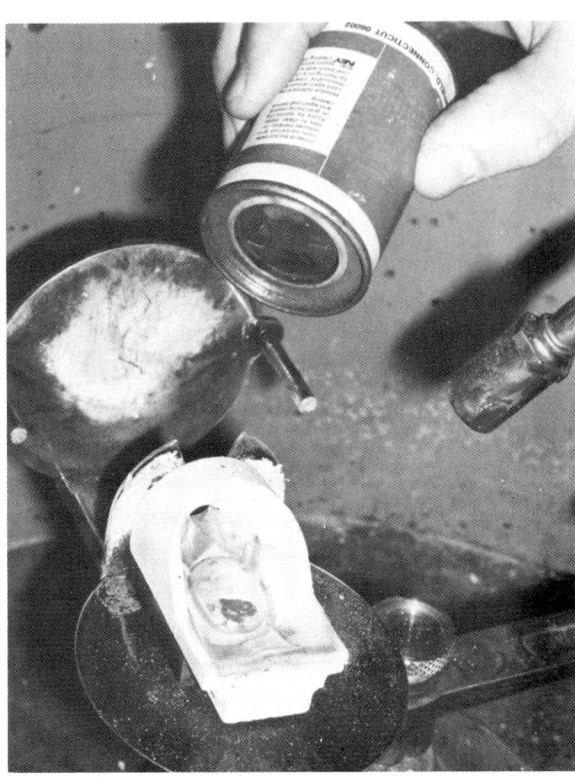

**Fig. 10-48.** Tip of blue flame cone is kept on metal. Powdered flux added when metal starts to ball up.

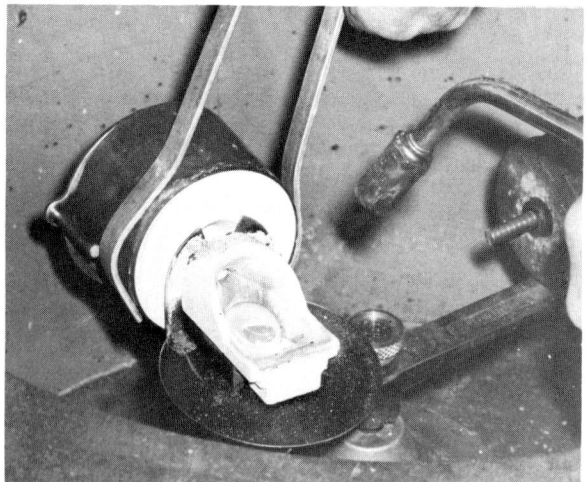

**Fig. 10-49.** Place casting ring in casting machine when metal is clean and fluid.

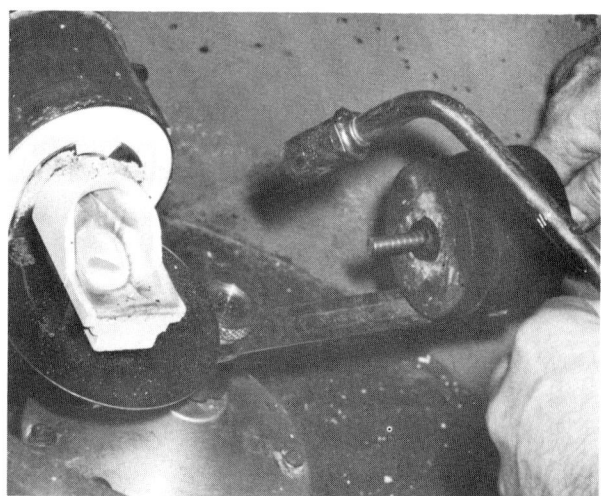

**Fig. 10-50.** Without moving flame, release casting machine.

*Investing, burnout, and casting* **315**

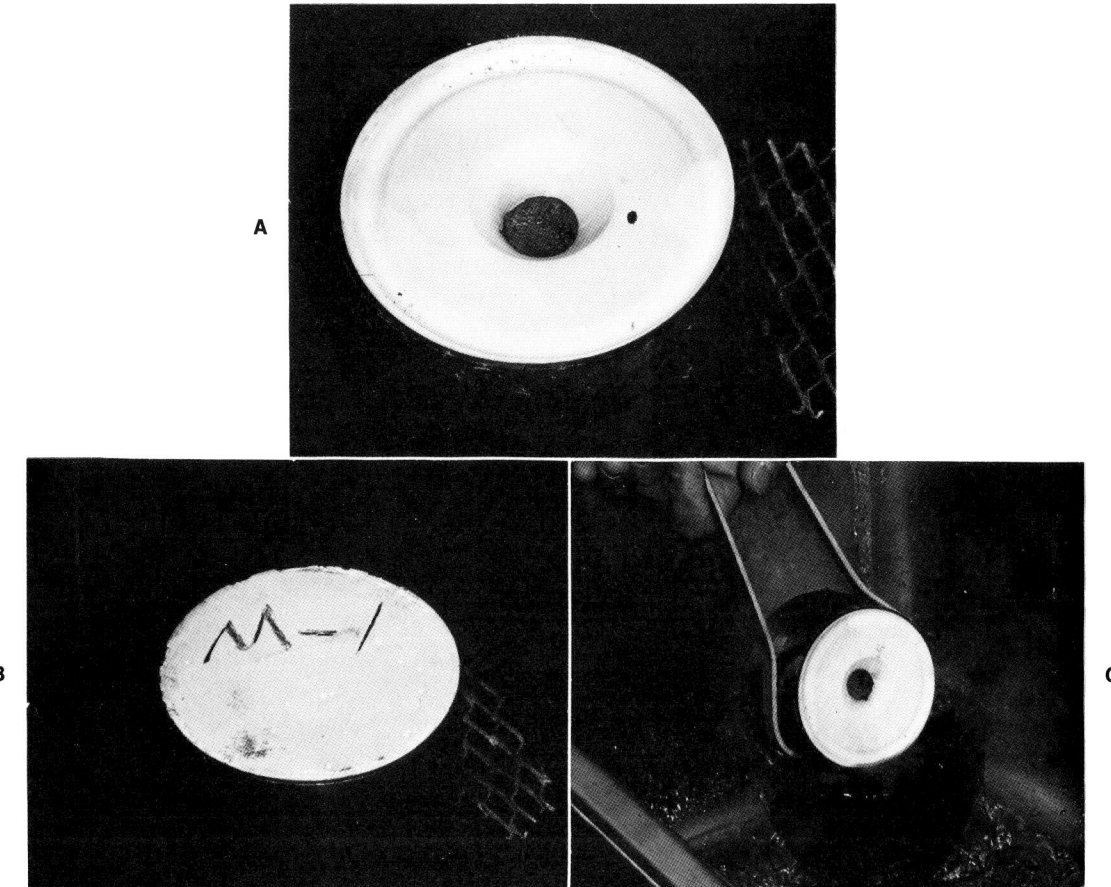

**Fig. 10-51. A,** Bench cool casting for 12 minutes after casting machine stops turning. **B,** Rouge marking is still on investment even though it has been in furnace at 1300° F for at least 2 hours. **C,** Then quench in water to soften casting, and cool investment.

4. Light the torch, and adjust it to form a reducing flame (Fig. 10-47).

5. Heat the metal, keeping the tip of the blue cone on the surface of the metal. A large bulk of metal takes several minutes to melt. When the metal begins to ball up, add powdered flux (Fig. 10-48).

6. When the surface of the metal is clean, and a swirling action can be seen, position the casting ring in the casting machine. Do not move the flame from the metal (Fig. 10-49).

7. If the metal surface is still clean and the metal is swirling, move the arm of the casting machine to drop the locking pin. Without moving the flame from the metal, release the casting machine (Fig. 10-50).

8. When the machine stops, remove the ring and allow it to bench cool for 12 minutes before quenching in water (Fig. 10-51).

### Recovering the casting

Quenching the casting in water after allowing the mold to bench cool for 12 minutes will produce the most ideal handling properties of gold alloy. The alloy will be in a fairly soft and ductile condition and will make the finishing much easier. This process of allowing the casting to cool slowly in the mold for a controlled time period and then quenching is known as heat softening the alloy.

After the metal has been finished, but before it is polished, the properties of the metal should be restored. This is known as heat hardening the metal. This process is done most simply by placing the framework in an oven that has been heated to 842° F (450° C) and permitting it to cool to 482° F (250° C) over a period of 30 minutes. At that time, it is removed from the furnace and bench cooled. It is now at its most hardened state. However, in the softening and hardening of any particular alloy, the recommendation of the manufacturer should be followed.

## Cleaning the casting

After the casting has been quenched, remove the casting and investment from the ring, and if necessary use a knife blade and run it around the ring (Fig. 10-52). Exercise care to avoid nicking the casting. Remove as much investment by hand as possible, then use a stiff brush and running water (Fig. 10-53). The casting should not be struck to dislodge the investment, and prying the material with a metallic instrument should be avoided. Most of the investment except for small particles in difficult to reach areas can be removed with the brush and water.

The remaining investment may be removed with a shellblaster* or sandblaster.† The shellblaster is usually used on gold and the sand blaster on cobalt-chromium (Fig. 10-54). A fine stream of air containing particles of walnut shell or fine particles of sand is blown from a nozzle under pressure. The casting should be rotated so that the airstream is directed toward those areas which contain the remaining particles of investment (Fig. 10-55).

*Shellblaster or sandblaster (cabinet type), Ruemelin Manufacturing Co., Inc., Milwaukee, Wis.
†Portable sandblaster, J. F. Jelenko & Co., New Rochelle, N. Y.

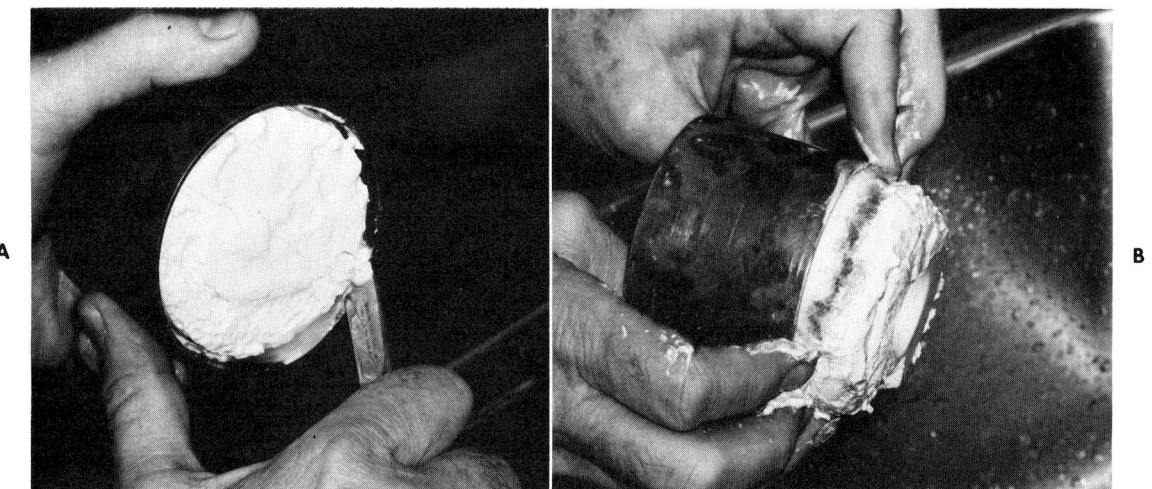

Fig. 10-52. **A,** Knife blade is used to loosen investment. **B,** Remaining investment is pushed from ring.

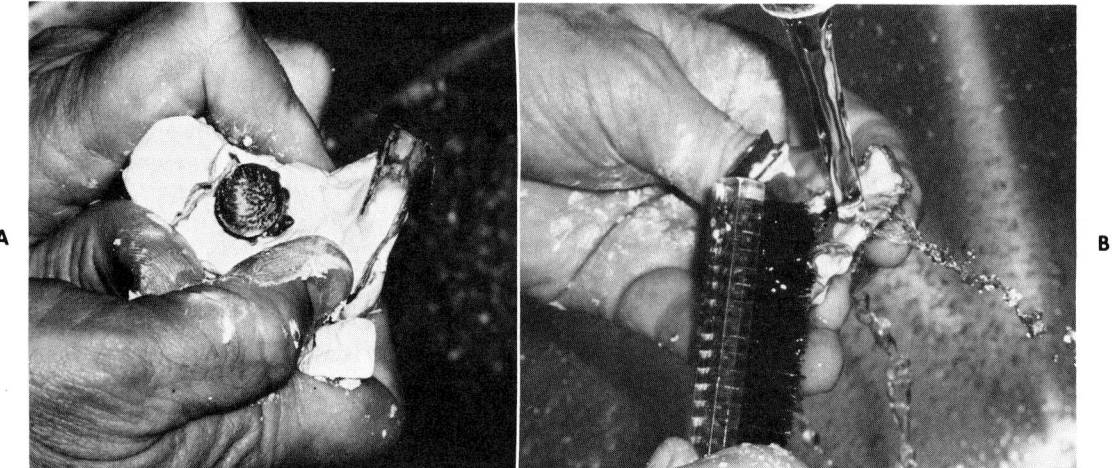

Fig. 10-53. **A,** Investment is removed by hand. **B,** Investment removed with stiff brush and running water.

*Investing, burnout, and casting* **317**

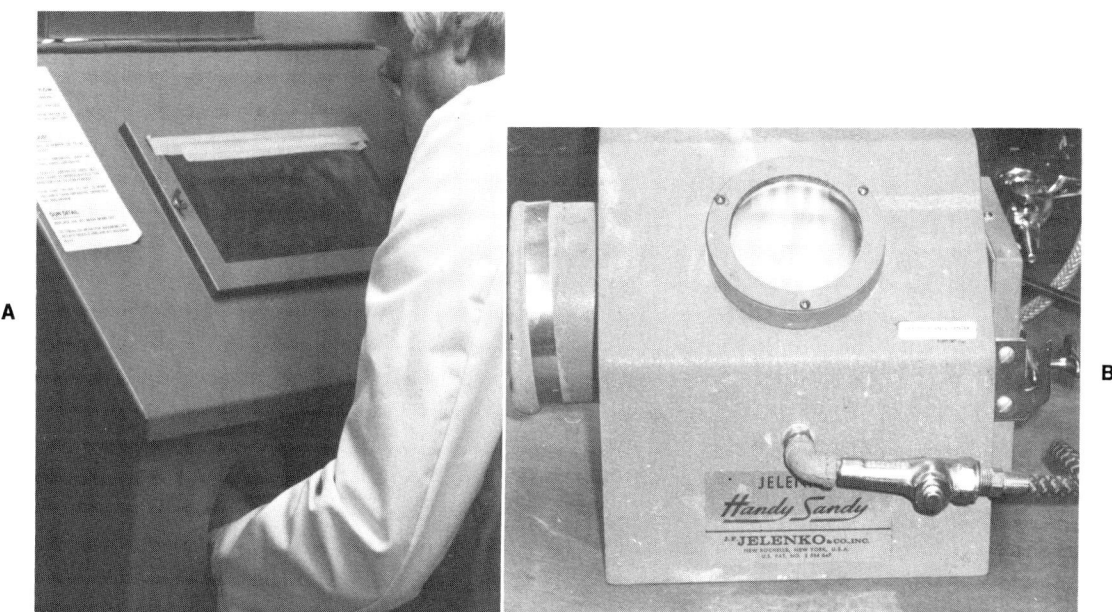

Fig. 10-54. **A,** Shellblast machine. **B,** Handy Sandy sandblast machine.

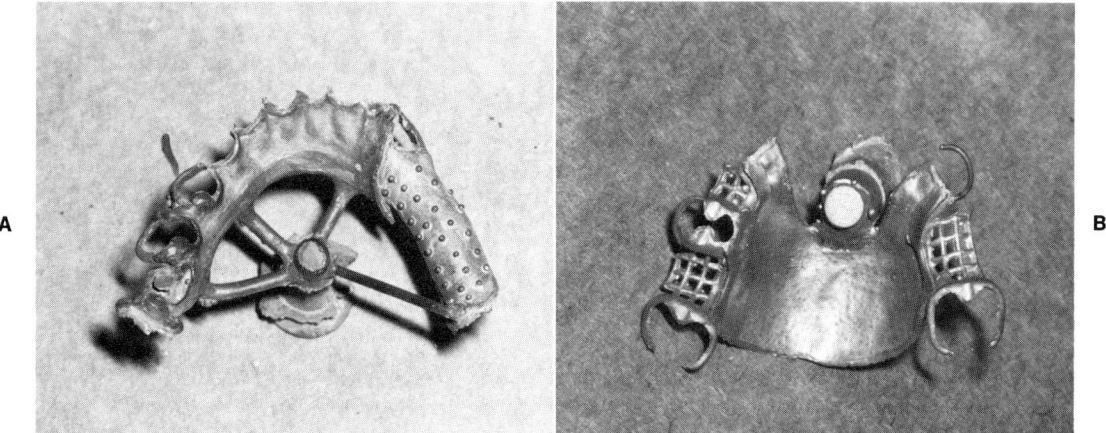

Fig. 10-55. **A,** Gold casting shellblasted. **B,** Cobalt-chromium casting sandblasted.

## Pickling the casting

Cobalt-chromium castings are not pickled. They are sandblasted only to remove the investment and oxide.

Gold alloy castings must always be pickled in an acid pickling solution.* This procedure removes base metal deposits, oxidation, and other contaminants from the surface of the gold alloy. If these contaminants are not removed, they will later lead to tarnishing and discoloration of the metal in the mouth.

Always use clean pickling solutions. Never heat a casting over a flame and plunge it into the solution. This is a sure way to warp the casting. Always place the casting into a cool pickling solution so it is completely covered, then heat the container over a flame until the surface of the metal brightens (Fig. 10-56). Remove the casting from the solution with plastic tongs, never metal, and rinse under water (Fig. 10-57). If bare metal tongs are used, the pickling solution and the casting will be contaminated with base metal, and the casting will tarnish in the mouth.

The casting is now ready for finishing and polishing (Fig. 10-58).

## PROBLEM AREAS

Problems associated with the burnout and casting procedures include failure to line the casting ring, permitting the investment to dry out prior to placing it in the oven, increasing the temperature too fast, overheating, casting the metal too cool or too hot, quenching the casting too soon, and contaminating the casting with other metals (Table 10-2). Each specific procedure should be executed with precision if casting problems are to be minimized.

---

*Jel-Pac, J. F. Jelenko & Co., New Rochelle, N.Y.

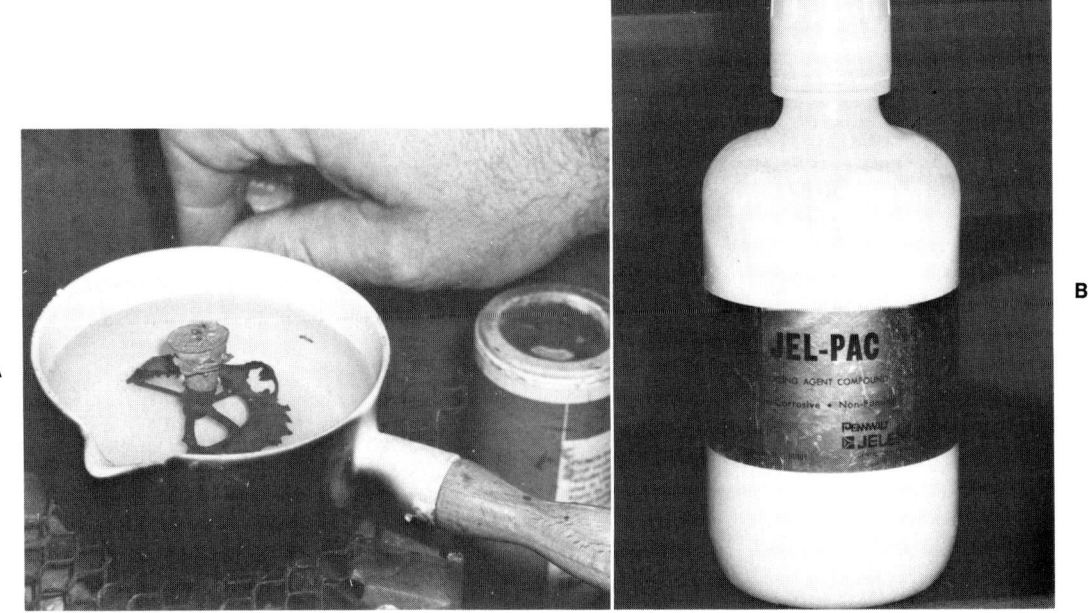

**Fig. 10-56. A,** Gold shellblasted casting placed in pickling solution. Solution is heated until gold brightens. **B,** Jel-Pac is noncorrosive pickling agent.

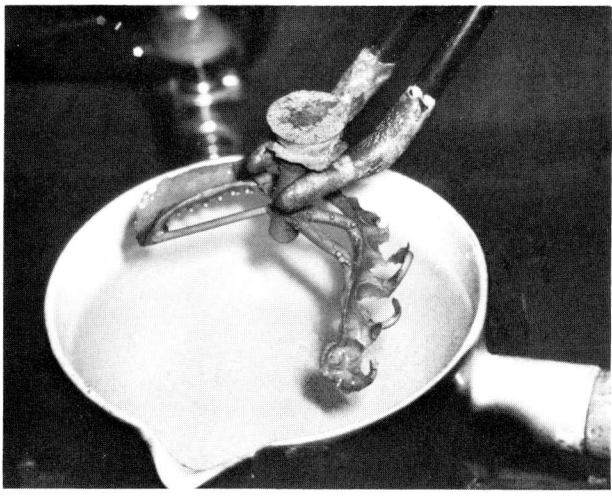

**Fig. 10-57.** Plastic tongs are used to remove casting from solution.

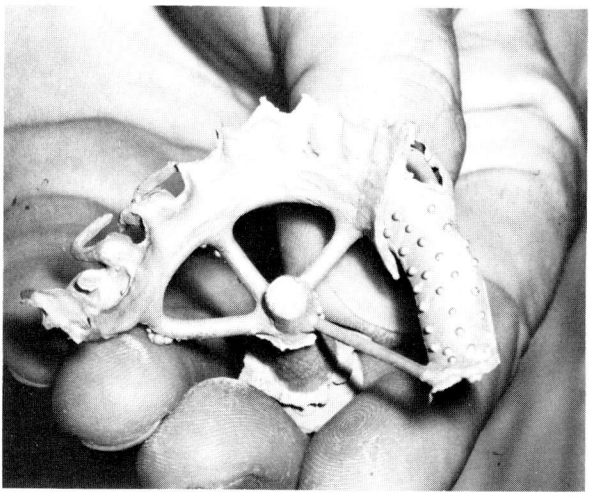

**Fig. 10-58.** Pickled casting ready for finishing and polishing.

**Table 10-2.** Burnout and casting

| Problem | Probable cause | Solution |
| --- | --- | --- |
| Excessive cracks in mold during burnout | Casting ring not lined | Line casting ring with substitute asbestos liner (C & B Flask Liner or equivalent) |
| | Investment too dry when placed in oven | Soak ring in water for few minutes before placing in oven; do not place in preheated oven |
| | Temperature raised too fast | Start burnout in cold oven and raise temperature gradually (reach 1000° F in 1 hour) |
| Pitted and discolored casting | Investment overheated | Do not overheat investment: start in cold oven and raise temperature gradually |
| Portions of framework did not cast | Metal too cold when cast | Have metal fluid and at proper temperature |
| | Improper spruing | Sprue framework to eliminate casting thick portions through thin portion |
| | Gas trapped in mold | Do not vacuum spatulate outer investments |
| Pattern failed to cast | Pattern separated from crucible former during investing | Reinforce main sprue with bur or wire; use proper diameter sprue; handle carefully during investing; do not vibrate too heavily |

## SUMMARY

Investing, burnout, and casting procedures for a low–gold content alloy were described in this chapter. Alhough significant variation in methods exists for other metal/investment systems, the one described is typical and was accomplished with equipment commonly available in a laboratory. As is the case for most technical procedures, experience is indeed the best teacher.

## BIBLIOGRAPHY

Air Force Manual 160-29: Dental laboratory technicians manual, United States Air Force, Washington, D.C., 1954, U.S. Government Printing Office.

Air Force Manual 162-6: Dental laboratory technology, United States Air Force, Washington, D.C., 1975, U.S. Government Printing Office.

Martinelli, N.: Dental laboratory technology, ed. 2, St. Louis, 1975, The C. V. Mosby Co.

Sowter, J. B.: Dental laboratory technology: prosthodontic techniques, Chapel Hill, N.C., 1968, The University of North Carolina Press.

3. Using a disk, barrel-shaped mounted stone, fine-tapered mounted stone, or carbide bur, depending on the access to the area, remove the flash from the clasp arms, minor connectors, rests, indirect retainers, and denture base retention areas (Fig. 11-6). Be very careful not to alter the shape of the clasp arms.

Mounted stones are made for grinding either gold or cobalt-chromium. They cannot be used interchangeably. The stones made for gold are too soft to use on cobalt-chromium, they disintegrate too rapidly. The mounted stones made for chromium castings are too hard for gold; they clog up with the softer metal and will not cut.

4. Use larger wheels or stones to smooth the contour of the major connectors and to remove small pits or defects. The stone should be kept moving forward and backward along the length of the major connector in strokes at least 15 mm long to avoid creating small depressions, waves, or uneven surfaces on the connector (Fig. 11-7).

5. Smooth the rest of the framework except for those areas which come in contact with the teeth, such as the undersurface of occlusal rests, the minor connectors, and the inner surface of clasp arms, with a fine tapered monted stone. Use this stone also to slightly round the sharp edge on the inferior border of the clasp arms (Fig. 11-8). This will permit the clasp to slide onto the abutment teeth easier. Do not decrease the width of the clasp in doing this.

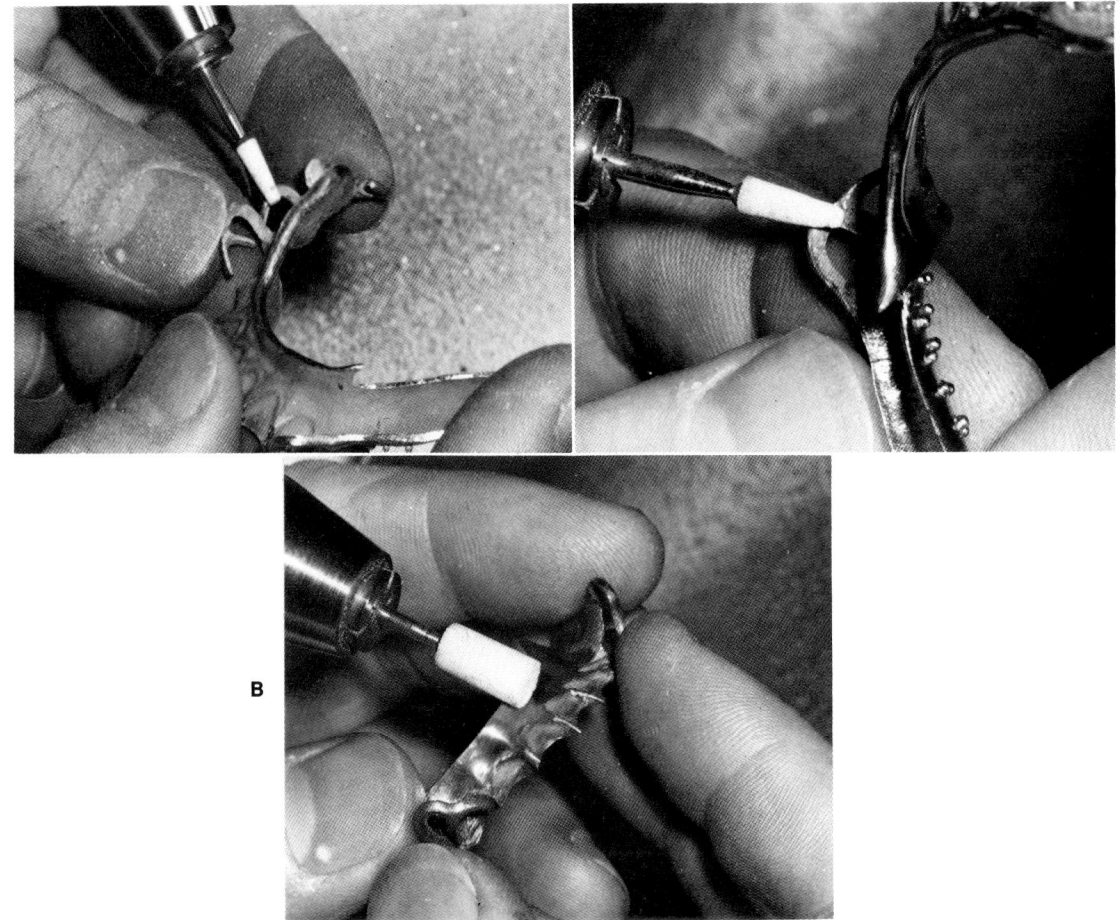

**Fig. 11-8. A,** Slightly round sharp inferior border of clasp arms or approach arms. **B,** Grind entire surface of casting with mounted stones except surfaces in contact with teeth and those areas to be left stippled or tissue side of maxillary major connectors.

6. Use an inverted cone stone or a separating disk to refine the undercut butt joint of the finish lines, both internally and externally (Fig. 11-9). The acrylic resin retention latticework need not be smooth or polished other than to remove nodules or flash that may be present. A wire brush is excellent for brightening nailhead or bead retention (Fig. 11-10).

7. Optionally a series of sandpaper disks of decreasing grit can be used to smooth all clasp arms and occlusal rests. The disk flexibility permits it to adapt itself to the contours of the clasp arms so that the shape is preserved as the surface is smoothed. Sandpaper disks cannot be used on cobalt-chromium castings (Fig. 11-11).

Rubber abrasive wheels, knife-edge wheels, disks, and points are preferred for fine finishing on the castings. The ones used for gold have fine pumice as an abrasive (Fig. 11-12). The ones with pumice will not polish cobalt-chromium, and the ones with carborundum may be too hard and cut the gold too fast.

8. Finish the metal surfaces that contact the teeth next. These are the inner surfaces of the clasp arms, occlusal rests, indirect retainers, and minor connectors. The important thing is to polish these but change the surfaces as little as possible, since they must fit the teeth accurately.

  a. Using magnification and a bright light, examine the surfaces that contact the teeth for nodules, small defects, and irregularities (Fig. 11-13). Remove these with small fine stones or burs. Grind only those areas where defects are visible (Fig. 11-14).

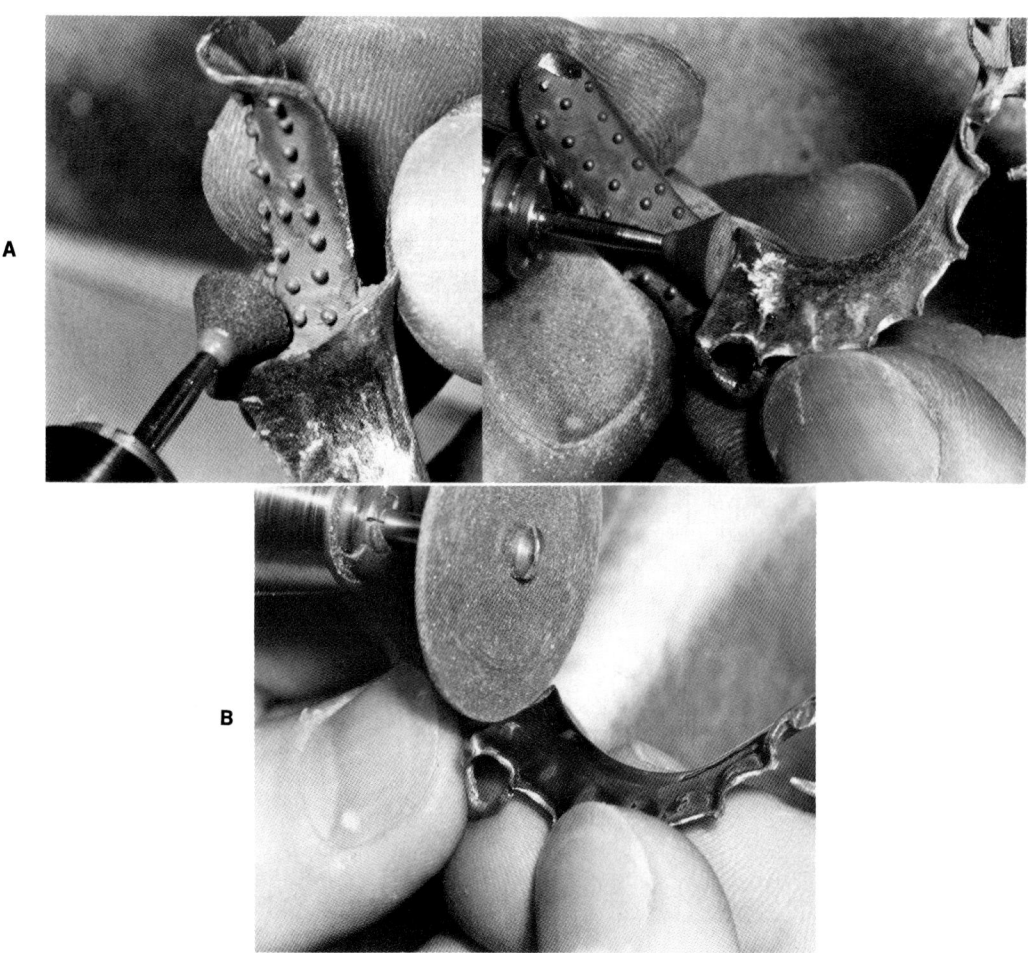

**Fig. 11-9. A,** Inverted cone stone used with sharp edge in undercut (left) or flat surface against finish line (right). **B,** Separating disk is used to finish and shape finish lines.

## Finishing and polishing the framework 327

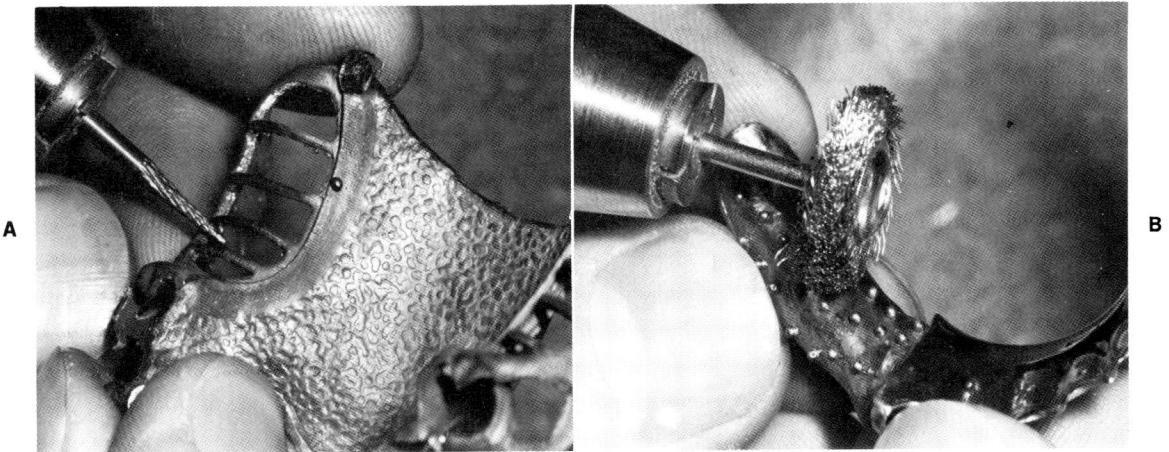

Fig. 11-10. **A,** Remove flash and nodules from acrylic retention latticework. They need not be polished. **B,** Wire brush works well to shine bead retention and nailheads.

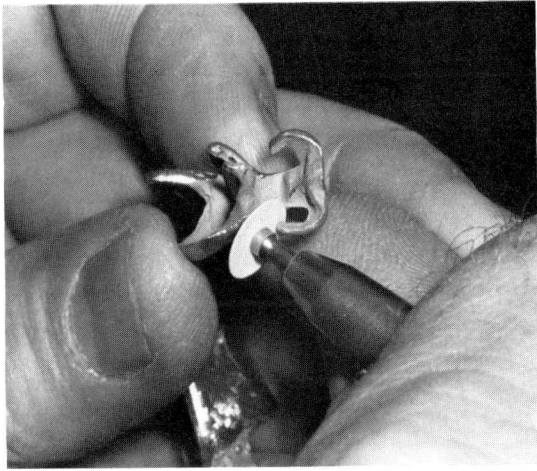

Fig. 11-11. Sandpaper disks may be used to finish accessible parts of castings made of gold. This is not recommended for cobalt-chromium.

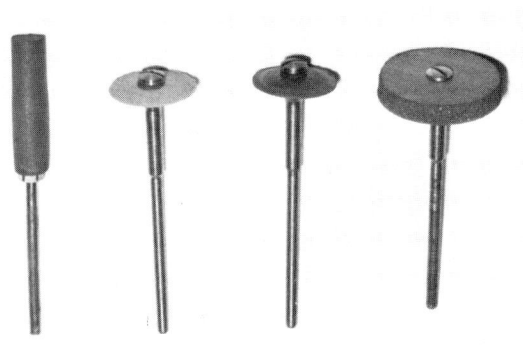

Fig. 11-12. Rubber abrasive wheels, knife-edge wheels, and points are used for gold and cobalt-chromium. Rubber wheels impregnated with pumice are used for gold and with Carborundum for cobalt-chromium.

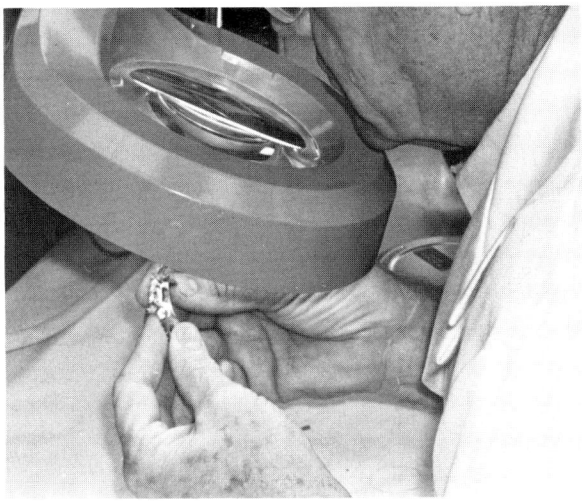

Fig. 11-13. Magnification and bright light used to examine casting and locate nodules and defects.

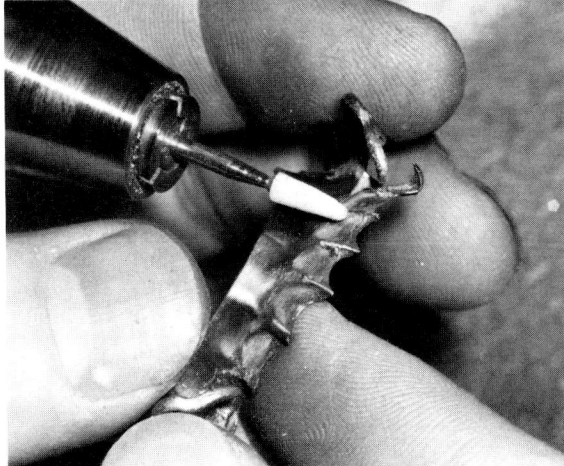

Fig. 11-14. Nodules are removed with fine stones or burs.

b. Shape a rubber abrasive point by running it against a truing stone or a heatless stone until it comes to a point (Fig. 11-15). Lightly smooth these surfaces with it.
c. Using a cylindrical felt cone with tripoli, produce a completely smooth surface (Fig. 11-16). Hollow out the end of the cone by holding a knife tip to the revolving cone; this depression is useful in polishing the underside of occlusal rests (Fig. 11-17). Remove the residue of tripoli with soap and water, a mixture of two thirds tincture of green soap and one third household ammonia, or ready-to-use Septisol solution* (Fig. 11-18).
d. Use another felt cylinder with jeweler's rouge to complete the finishing (Fig. 11-19).

---

*Septisol solution, Vestal Laboratories, Division of Chemed Corp., St. Louis, Mo.

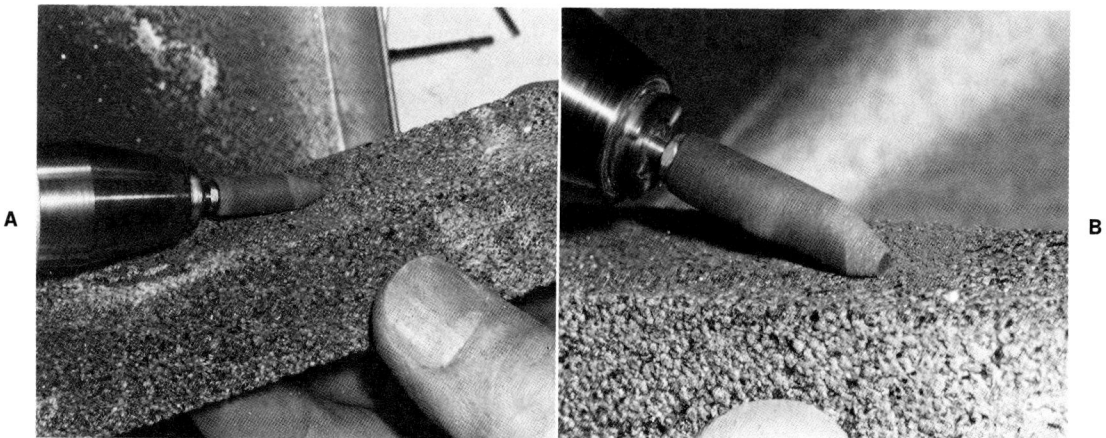

Fig. 11-15. **A,** Point is formed on rubber abrasive cylinder by running it against truing stone. **B,** NOTE: Mandrel is placed well into chuck.

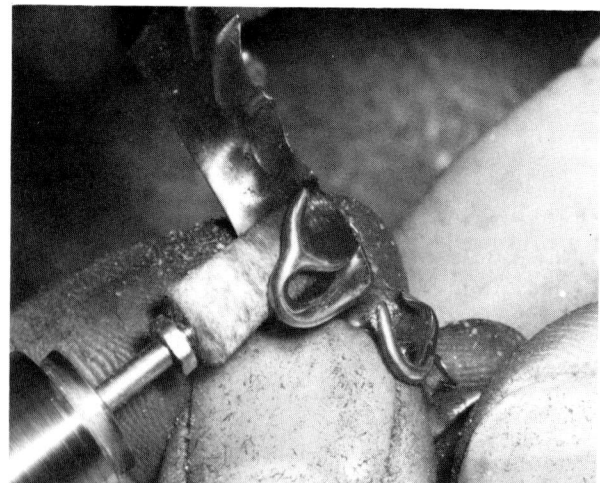

Fig. 11-16. Use tripoli on felt cylinder to smooth surfaces that contact teeth.

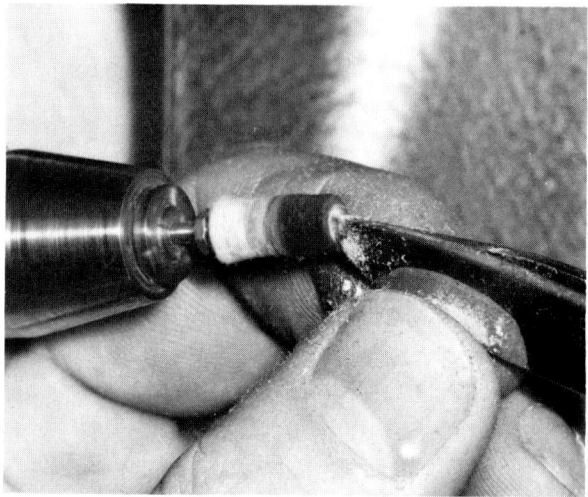

Fig. 11-17. Hollow end of felt cylinder by holding knife tip against it while it is turning. Use this with tripoli to polish under rests.

## Finishing and polishing the framework 329

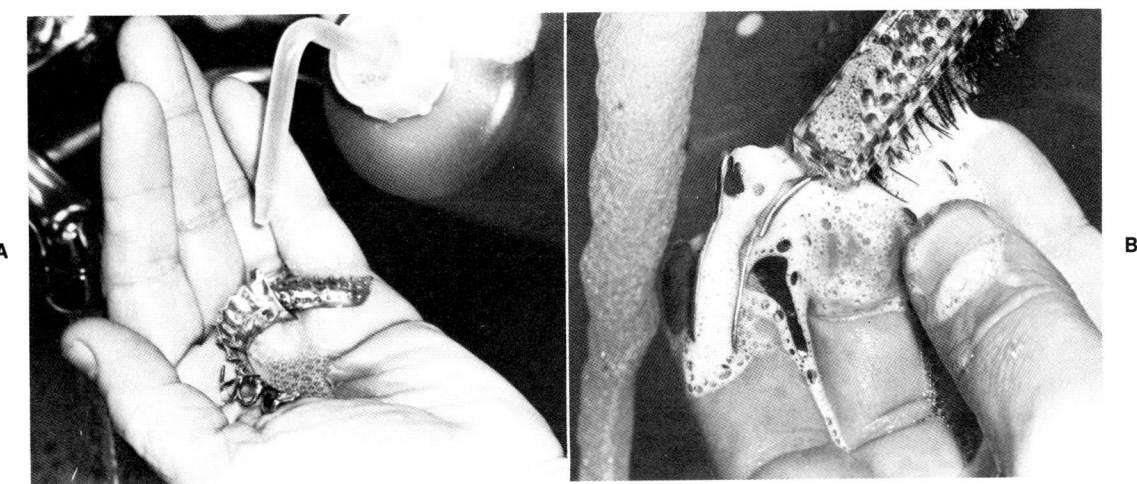

**Fig. 11-18.** Remove tripoli residue by washing with soap and water or liquid soap and ammonia. **A,** Use liquid soap generously. **B,** Scrub vigorously with small stiff brush.

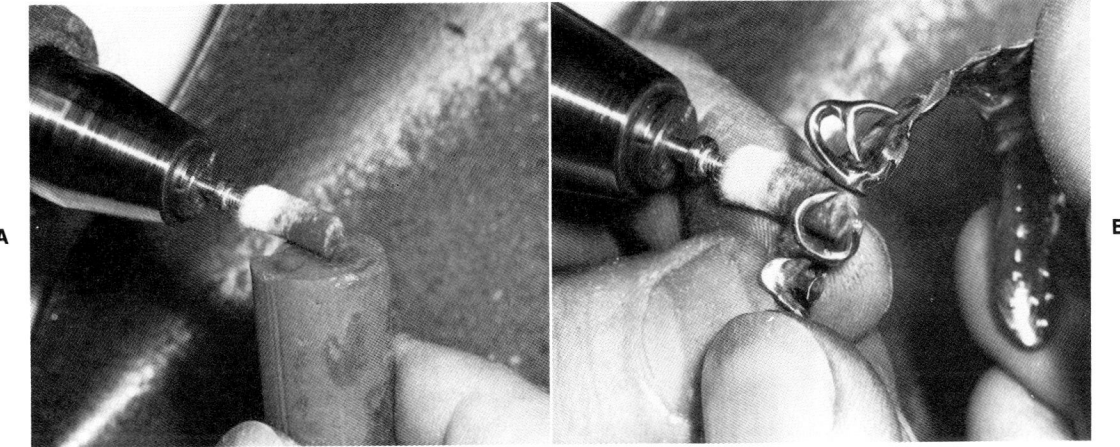

**Fig. 11-19.** Another felt cone is used with jeweler's rouge to complete polishing of surfaces. **A,** Applying rouge to felt cone. **B,** Polishing inside of clasps.

9. Smooth the entire remaining framework, except the clasp arms, using the rubber wheels and points (Fig. 11-20). When possible, use the rubber wheel by running it parallel to the length of the major connector, not across its width (Fig. 11-21). This will produce a smooth surface with less waves. The knife-edge wheels may be used to smooth finish lines (Fig. 11-22).

10. Use small felt wheels with tripoli next to remove traces of marks left by the rubber wheels and points on some of the more difficult to reach areas (Fig. 11-23).

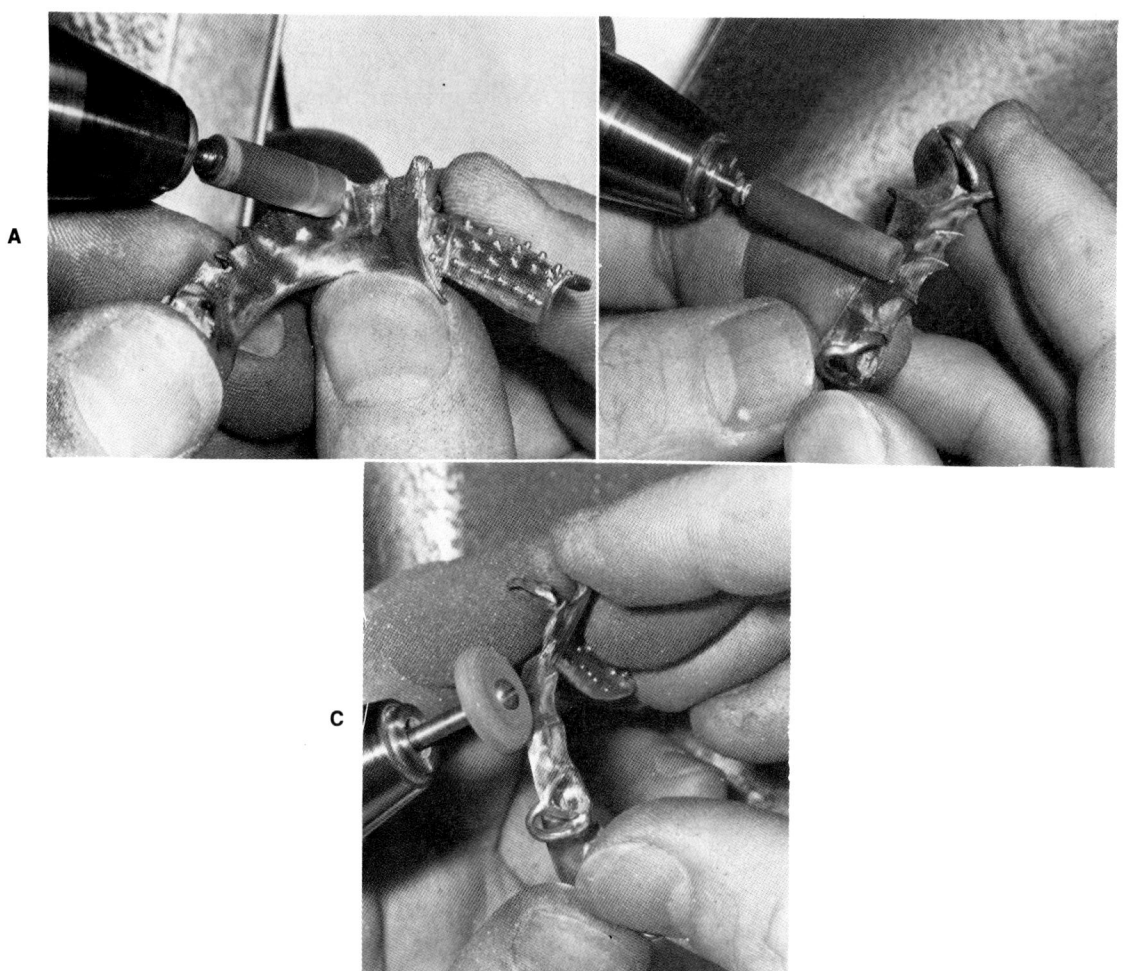

**Fig. 11-20.** Remaining portions of framework except clasp arms and part of metal that contact teeth are smoothed with rubber abrasive wheels and points. **A,** Points can be used in grooves. **B,** Points can be used on flat surfaces. **C,** Wheels can be used on major connectors.

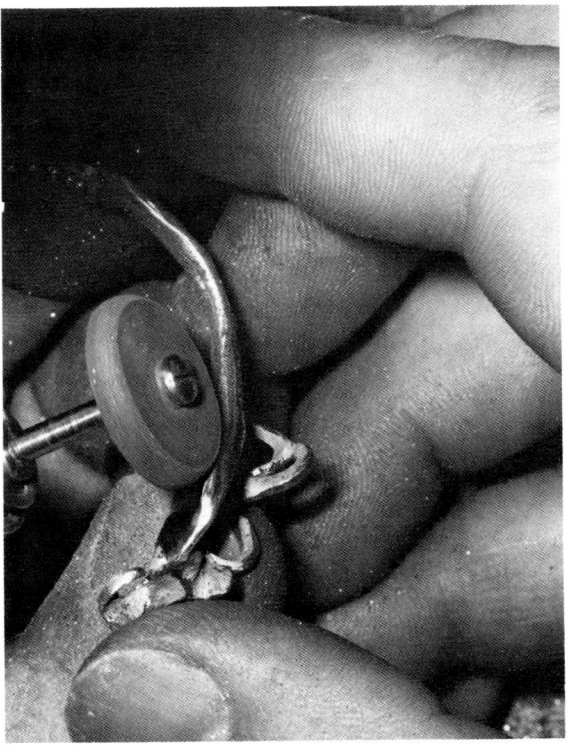

**Fig. 11-21.** Run rubber wheel the length of major connector as much as possible.

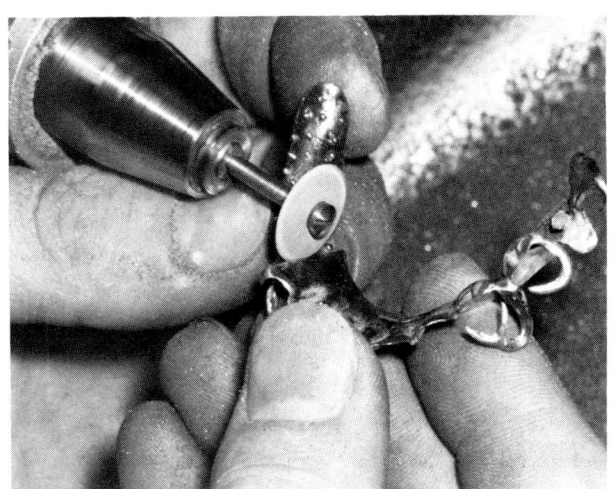

**Fig. 11-22.** Finish lines may be smoothed by knife-edge wheels.

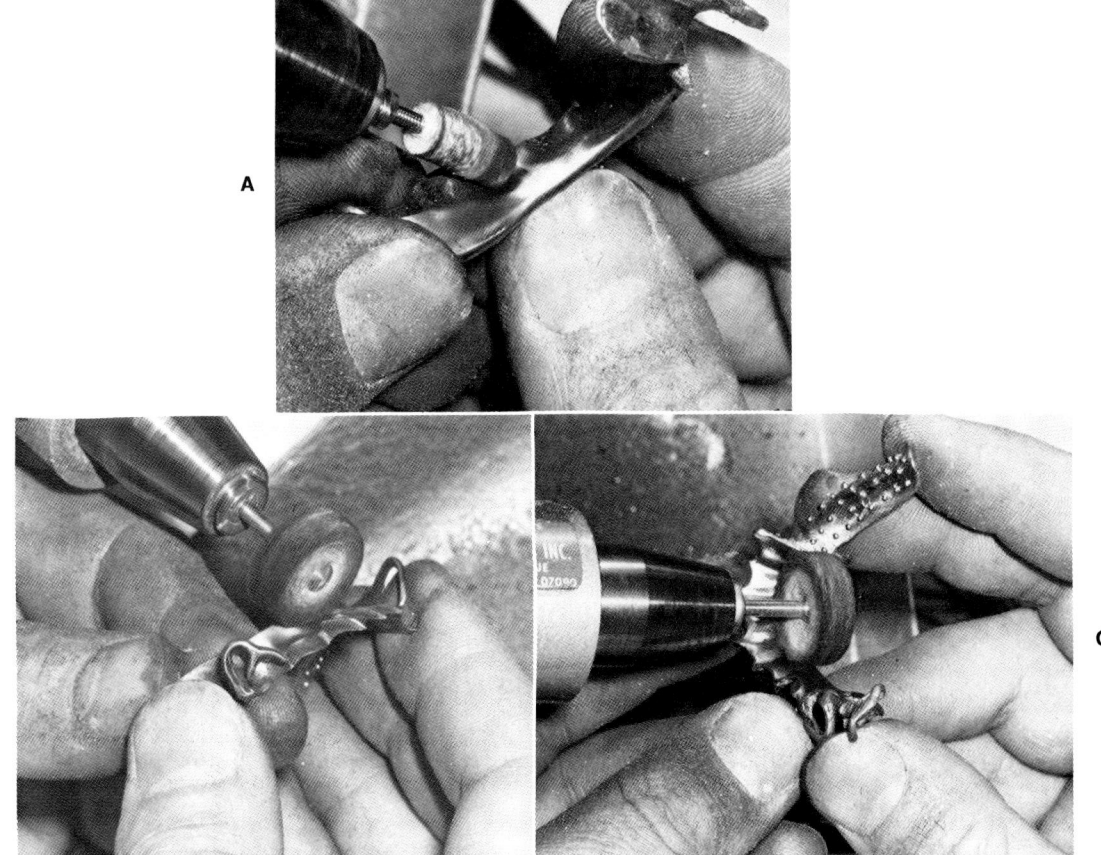

**Fig. 11-23.** Small felt wheels and points with tripoli can be used to get in difficult areas. Felt point and tripoli used to polish groove **(A)**. Tripoli on felt wheel used to polish tissue side **(B)** and tongue side **(C)** of major connector.

11. The entire framework, including the outer surfaces of the clasps, is polished with a small tripoli-impregnated cloth wheel (Fig. 11-24).
    a. Polish the clasp arms with he cloth wheel running parallel to the length of the clasp from shoulder to the tip (Fig. 11-25).
    b. Polish all other areas of the framework from several different directions to produce an even polished surface.

PREPARING A CLOTH OR RAG WHEEL FOR USE ON A LATHE. *Caution:* The use of a large rag or cloth wheel on a lathe for polishing a metal framework is very hazardous. It is easy to catch a clasp in the cloth and have the framework thrown with great force against the pan or anywhere in the room. A new cloth wheel should always be "broken in" before using it. This needs to be done to make it softer and fluffier and to remove the small strings that will be on the surface. If not removed these small strings can get tangled in the framework and result in damage.
    a. While the wheel is revolving on a lathe, press a dull edge of a stainless steel knife or spatula against the wheel with pressure. This will cause the surface of the wheel to fray, become more fluffy, and to produce more uneven strands of string (Fig. 11-26).
    b. Stop the wheel, and use a match to burn off these strands of string. Be careful to thoroughly extinguish the flame (Fig. 11-27).
    c. Repeat this procedure several times until no more string appears on the surface.
    d. A new wheel should be prepared exclusively for use with tripoli and one for rouge (Fig. 11-28). These should be kept for polishing gold restorations only.

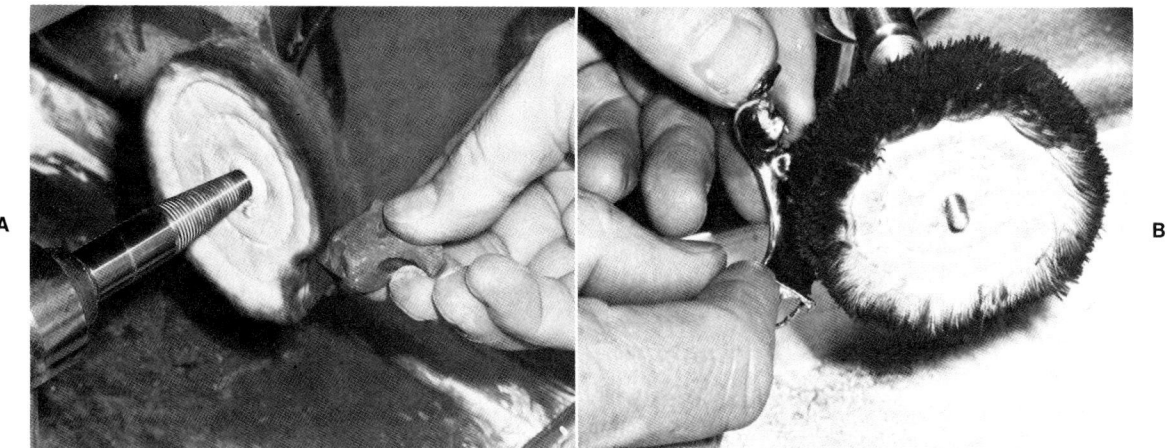

**Fig. 11-24.** Rag wheel and tripoli are used to polish rest of framework. **A**, Coating rag wheel with tripoli. **B**, Polishing major connector.

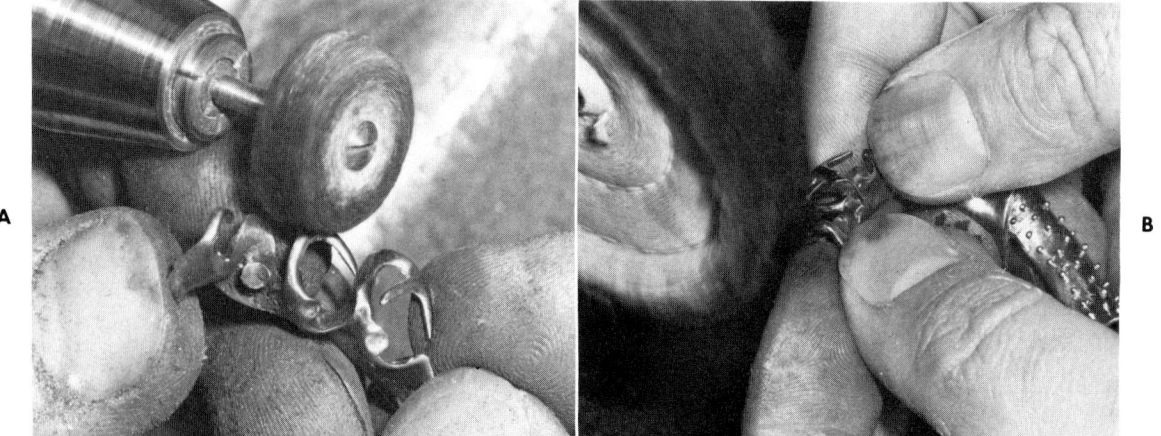

**Fig. 11-25. A**, Clasps may be polished from shoulder to tip with felt wheel and tripoli. **B**, Large rag wheel may be used for polishing if clasps are protected to prevent catching them in rag wheel.

### Finishing and polishing the framework 333

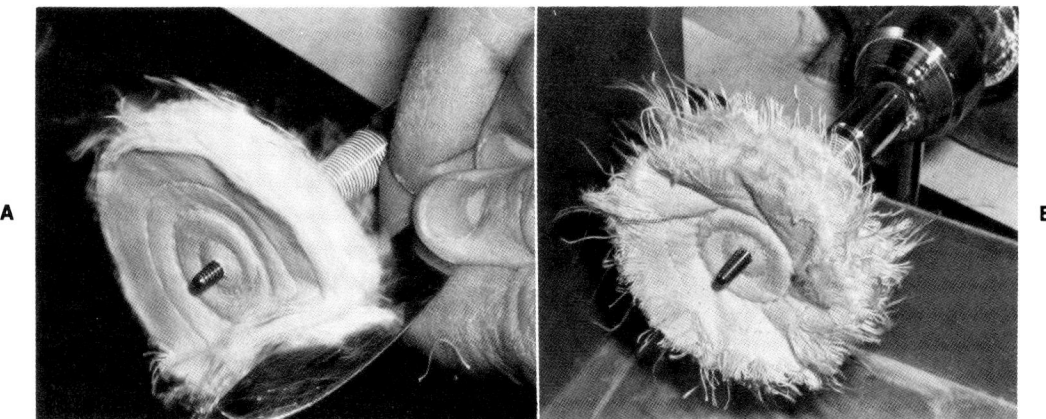

**Fig. 11-26. A,** New rag wheel on lathe being frayed by holding stainless steel blade against it while it is running. **B,** Frayed wheel.

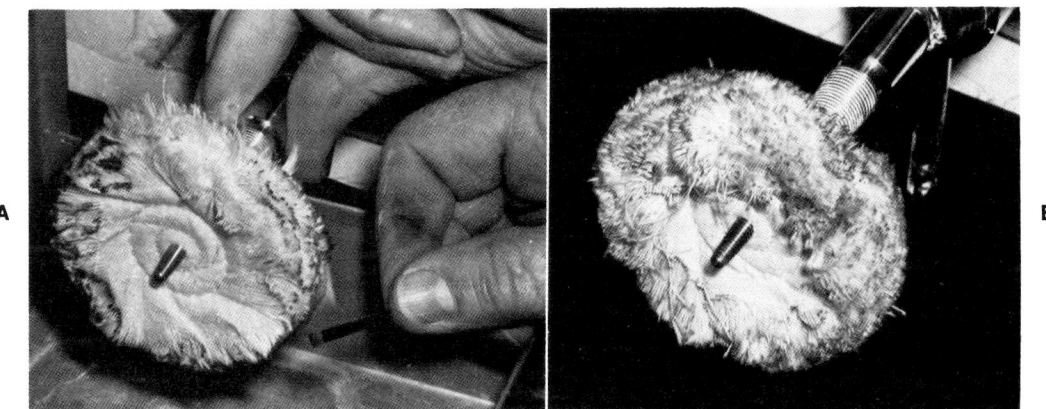

**Fig. 11-27. A,** Burn off strands with match, and extinguish flame by running rag wheel against stainless steel blade. **B,** New wheel broken in ready for polishing.

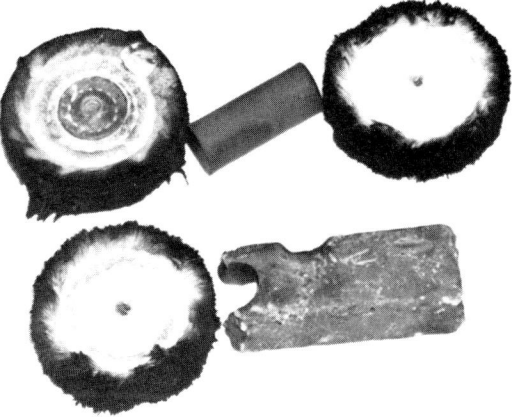

**Fig. 11-28.** One wheel for tripoli (bottom) and separate rag wheel or chamois wheel for jeweler's rouge (top).

12. After the casting has been thoroughly polished with tripoli, scrub the casting with soap, water, and a brush. Remove all traces of tripoli (Fig. 11-29). In some of the difficlt to reach areas, use chloroform on a pledget of cotton to remove traces of tripoli (Fig. 11-30).

13. Heat treat the casting, following the manufacturer's directions because different alloys are heat treated in various ways.

14. After heat treament, it will be necessary to pickle and repolish the casting with tripoli. Scrub it to remove the tripoli.

15. Polish the framework with a cloth wheel and rouge (Fig. 11-31).

16. Scrub the casting with soap and water or tincture of green soap and ammonia, and, if necessary, chloroform to remove all traces of the rouge (Fig. 11-32).

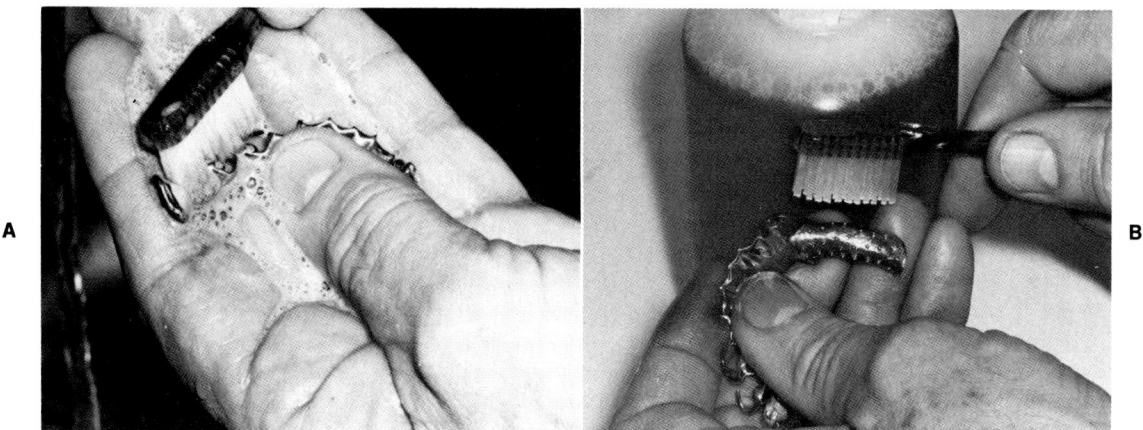

Fig. 11-29. **A,** Scrub casting to remove tripoli. **B,** Toothbrush with liquid soap and ammonia is good for this purpose.

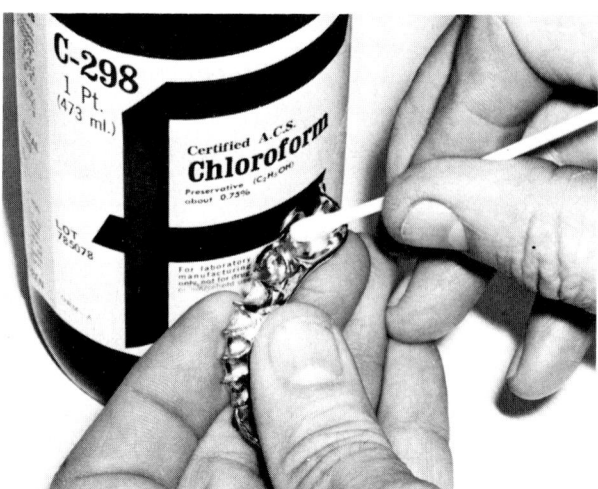

Fig. 11-30. Chloroform on cotton may be used to remove last traces of tripoli or rouge.

*Finishing and polishing the framework* **335**

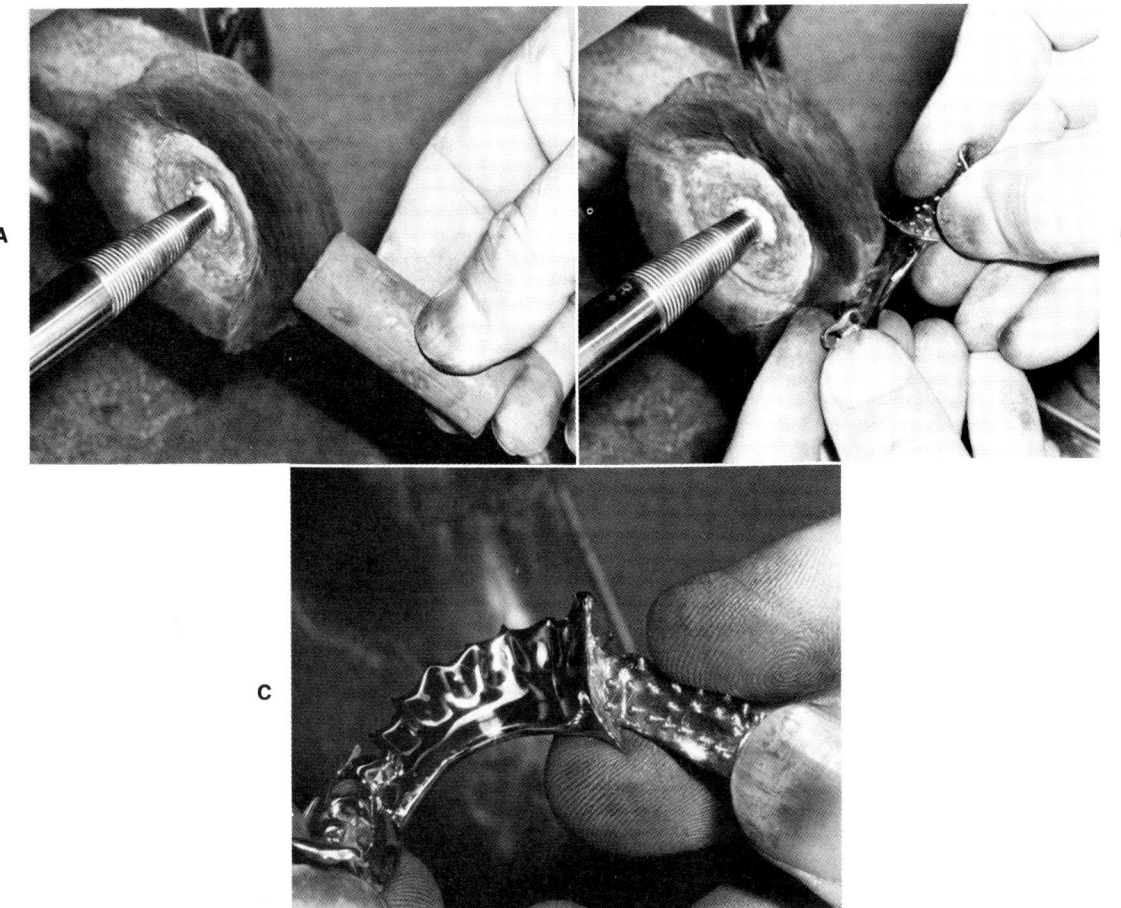

**Fig. 11-31. A,** Rag wheel or chamois wheel and jeweler's rouge used to polish casting. **B,** Rouge is used for final gloss polish. **C,** Final polish.

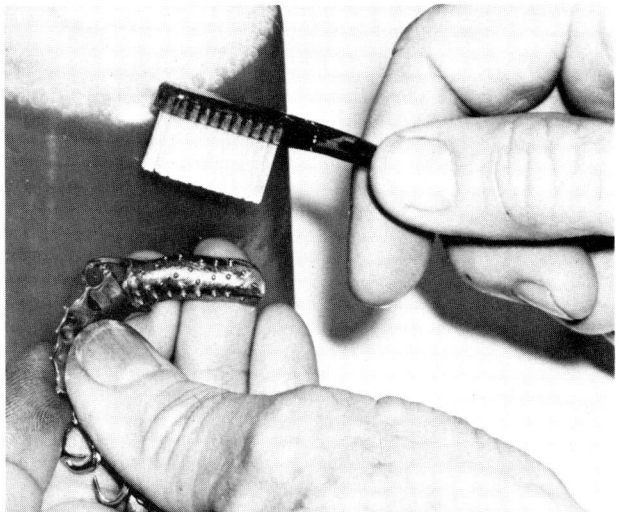

**Fig. 11-32.** Clean casting well to remove all traces of jeweler's rouge.

17. Dry the casting thoroughly with compressed air, and examine it carefully under a bright light and magnification for any scratches or defects. If any are present, the framework should be repolished in these areas (Fig. 11-33).

18. If the polish is satisfactory, the framework may now be tried on the master cast or duplicate master cast (Fig. 11-34).

19. If the blockout and relief wax is to be removed, it may be done by soaking the cast in warm (120° F; 49° C) slurry water for 5 minutes and then pouring hot (200° F; 95° C) slurry water over the cast to remove the wax (Fig. 11-35).

20. Check the fit of the framework on the master cast (Fig. 11-36).

## PROBLEM AREAS

The principal problems associated with finishing and polishing cast removable partial denture frameworks include failure to achieve the desired luster, overthinnng critical areas of the casting, notching or nicking clasps and minor connectors, and distorting the framework when polishing on a lathe (Table 11-1). A highly polished surface is achieved by completing each step in the sequence before going to the next step. In this manner, increasingly smooth and polished surfaces are developed. Obviously, it is important to use the correct instrument and polishing agent. Where imperfections exist in the casting, a soldering procedure may be indicated rather

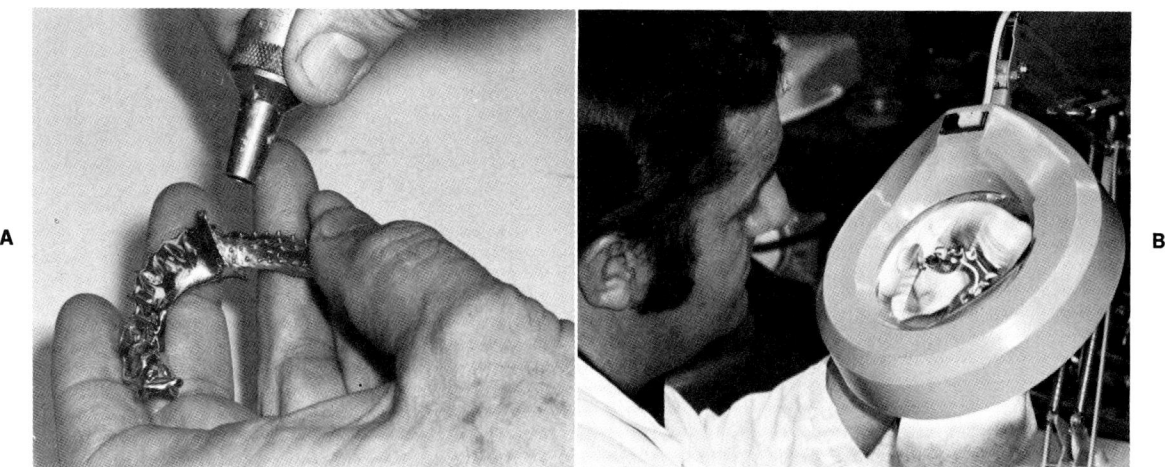

Fig. 11-33. **A,** Dry casting well with compressed air or cleansing tissue. **B,** Examine casting carefully under bright light and magnification. Repolish where necessary.

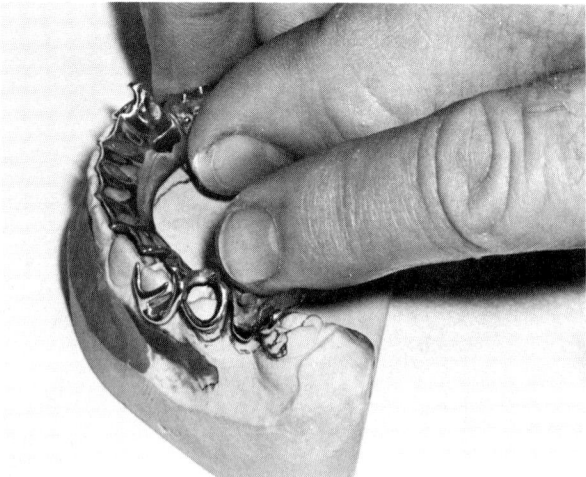

Fig. 11-34. If duplicate master casts are made, try casting on master cast or duplicate master cast.

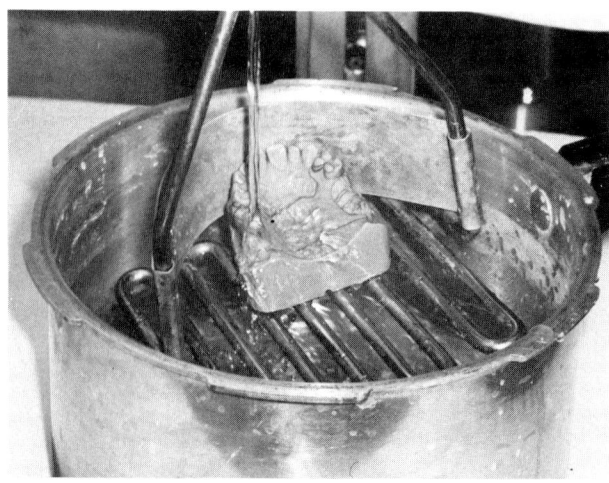

Fig. 11-35. If desired, remove relief wax and blockout from master cast by soaking cast in slurry water (120° F; 49° C) for 5 minutes. Flush with hot slurry water (200° F; 95° C).

*Finishing and polishing the framework* **337**

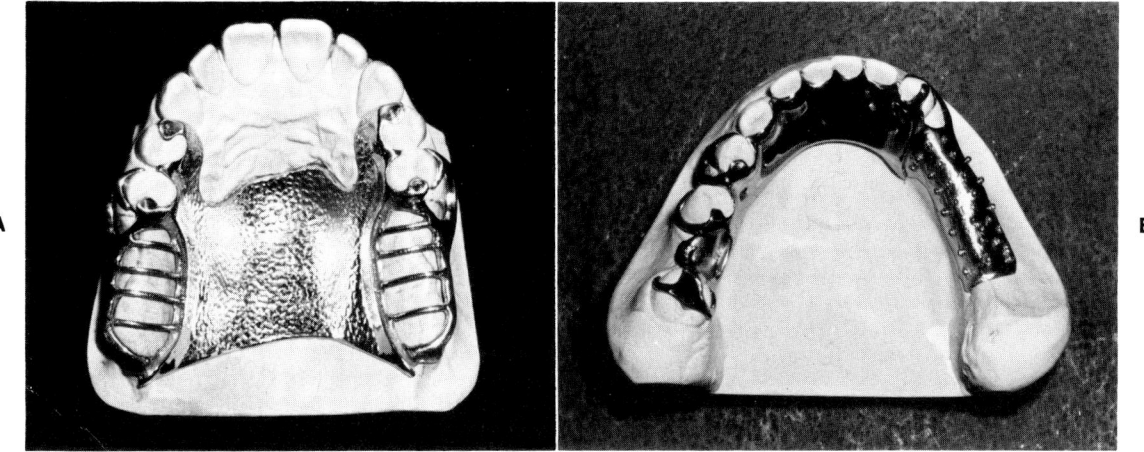

**Fig. 11-36.** Examine fit of casting on master cast. **A**, Maxillary cast. **B**, Mandibular cast. If it fits well, casting is ready for framework try-in in mouth. If it does not fit, perhaps it can be adjusted by fitting it to cast. If this cannot be done, framework should be remade.

**Table 11-1.** Finishing and polishing

| Problem | Probable cause | Solution |
|---|---|---|
| Polished surface is dull with fine scratches | Sequence of finishing steps not followed | Follow steps as outlined; do not "jump" steps |
| | Steps not carried to completion before proceeding to next step | Complete each step before proceeding to next one |
| Major or minor connector overthinned and flexible | Casting too thin as a result of incorrect wax-up | Use correct gauge of wax during wax-up; do not flame with alcohol torch |
| | Framework overthinned with abrasive stones during finishing | Use care when finishing connectors to avoid overthinning; check frequently during finishing |
| Clasp is nicked or notched | Clasp was miscast | Use correct wax thickness on pattern |
| | Clasp was nicked with stone or bur during finishing | Take care to avoid nicking framework with bur or wheel |
| Framework distorted | Framework caught in lathe during finishing | Take care when using lathe to prevent framework from being caught in polishing wheel |

than eliminating it by grinding. The latter may produce a thinned area in a critical portion of the framework and can reduce rigidity significantly. Care should also be taken when smoothing clasp arms to prevent notching that can result in stress concentration and early failure of the clasp due to breakage. It is obviously important to not "catch" the framework when polishing on a lathe, otherwise the casting may be ruined.

## SUMMARY

In this chapter the procedures for finishing and polishing a cast metal framework were discussed. Procedure sequence and materials will vary with the particular alloy used; however, the principles are basically the same. Achieving a correcly finished and highly polished framework requires knowledge and skill, which are best obtained through experience.

## BIBLIOGRAPHY

Air Force Manual 160-29: Dental laboratory technicians manual, United States Air Force, Washington, D.C., 1959, U.S. Government Printing Office.

Air Force Manual 162-6: Dental laboratory technology, United States Air Force, Washington, D.C., 1975, U.S. Government Printing Office.

Martinelli, N.: Dental laboratory technology, ed. 2, St. Louis, 1975, The C. V. Mosby Co.

Sowter, J. B.: Dental laboratory technology: prosthodontic techniques, Chapel Hill, N.C., 1968, The University of North Carolina Press.

CHAPTER 12

# SELECTING AND ARRANGING TEETH

WADE D. SMITH, WILLIAM A. KUEBKER, and JAMES A. FOWLER, Jr.

Although similarities exist between the arrangement and articulation of artificial teeth for complete dentures and for removable partial dentures, the variations must be explored. The remaining natural dentition dictates many decisions regarding type and size of artificial teeth to be selected and arranged. The functional and esthetic excellence of the prosthesis is critically dependent on proper selection and positioning of the teeth on the framework.

## SELECTING THE ARTIFICIAL TEETH

With few exceptions, acrylic is the material of choice for denture teeth incorporated into removable partial dentures. Over time, opposing porcelain teeth will severely abrade gold and amalgam restorations, as well as the natural dentition. Because artificial teeth incorporated into a removable partial denture require a great deal of adjustment for fit and occlusion, the necessary mechanical retention of porcelain teeth may need to be sacrificed to fit the tooth in place. Also, porcelain teeth require more laborious efforts to reduce them to appropriate size and to contour the occlusal and incisal surfaces to harmonize with the patient's existing dentition.

A variety of artificial teeth are available for replacements. Generally, the dentist will specify the types of replacement teeth desirable, and the retention for the artificial teeth will have been incorporated into the wax-up of the removable partial denture framework. The esthetic success of artificial tooth replacement on a removable partial denture begins with proper design of the underlying framework. Positioning the teeth for maximum esthetics requires that the underlying acrylic retentive devices do not interfere with the desired tooth position. *Therefore esthetic considerations must be planned at the time of framework design and framework wax-up.* (See Table 12-1.) Otherwise, tooth positioning for maximum esthetic results is not possible. For example, it is often better to select bead retention for anterior replacement teeth, especially if the residual ridge is large. The retentive latticework is considerably thicker, making esthetic positioning of the artificial replacement teeth difficult (Fig. 12-1). If a latticework is used, its design and position should not interfere with the esthetic placement of the necks of the anterior artificial teeth (Fig. 12-2).

Similarly, framework design can enhance the natural appearance of posterior teeth on a removable partial denture. When the retentive latticework distal to natural maxillary canines or first premolars is not carefully planned, positioning artificial replacements distal to the natural teeth is difficult. Often, the replacement teeth require excessive reduction at the gingival margin to avoid the improperly located latticework. This results in a disharmony of the gingival crest heights of the natural and denture

### Table 12-1. Selecting and arranging teeth

| Problem | Probable cause | Solution |
|---|---|---|
| Inability to interdigitate artificial teeth with opposing natural dentition mesiodistally | Incorrect size of posterior tooth replacements selected | Select posterior artificial teeth as close to size of remaining natural teeth as possible |
| Inability to interdigitate with opposing natural dentition occlusogingivally | Pin not raised 1 mm to accomplish occlusion harmonious with remaining dentition | Raise pin 1 mm before setting teeth and grind in occlusion |
| Maxillary posterior tooth replacements do not appear to harmonize esthetically with adjacent natural teeth | Incorrect size of posterior tooth replacements selected | Select posterior artificial teeth as close to size of remaining natural teeth as possible |
| Maxillary posterior teeth must be adjusted too short occlusogingivally to create harmonious appearance with adjacent natural teeth | Incorrect position of retentive latticework on ridge, making esthetic grind in impossible | Retentive latticework must be stepped back to permit esthetic placement of replacement teeth, especially maxillary first and second premolars |
| | Incorrect retentive element selected for replacement teeth | On tooth-supported partial dentures with well-healed ridge, bead retention on metal base allows more space for setting teeth esthetically |
| Insufficient space to set posterior tooth replacement | Latticework too bulky or struts positioned in improper location to position teeth properly | Latticework should be proper diameter and struts located buccal to crest of ridge |
| Anterior replacement teeth too short for satisfactory esthetics | Improper location of latticework | Grind replacement teeth and position prior to waxing framework; fabricate stone matrix to assist stabilization of replacement teeth during framework wax-up |
| | Latticework selected rather than bead retention on metal base | If ridge is well healed, metal base with bead retention will provide more space for esthetic placement of teeth |

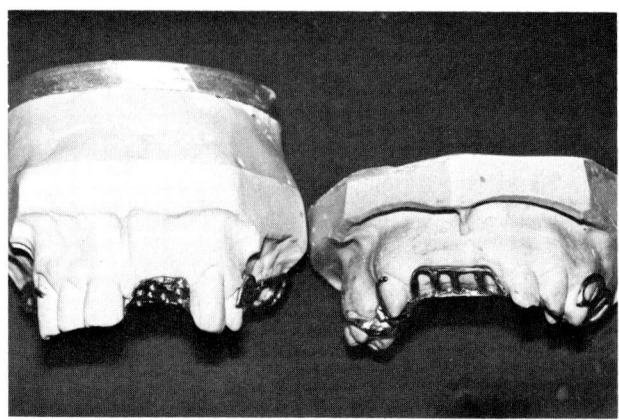

**Fig. 12-1.** Bead retention on left provides greater space for anterior replacement teeth than latticework on right. NOTE: Labial major strut on right coincides with position that necks of replacement teeth should assume. Esthetic positioning of teeth becomes very difficult.

teeth, which gives an artificial appearance (Figs. 12-3 and 12-4).

To cope with the problem of framework design for maximum esthetics, it is often advisable to select and grind in anterior replacement teeth prior to the wax-up of the framework. Or, the dentist may wish to have a try-in of the denture teeth to be placed on the partial denture to ensure that the shade, mold, and position of the teeth are satisfactory to the patient. An index may be fabricated to maintain the teeth in the desired position while the framework is waxed. Because the denture teeth are often butted to the tissue for maximum esthetic results, it is important that the index be cut short at the gingival margin to reveal the necks of the denture teeth in proper relationship with the tissue (Fig. 12-5). The framework may then be waxed to provide a strong and esthetically pleasing result (Fig. 12-6).

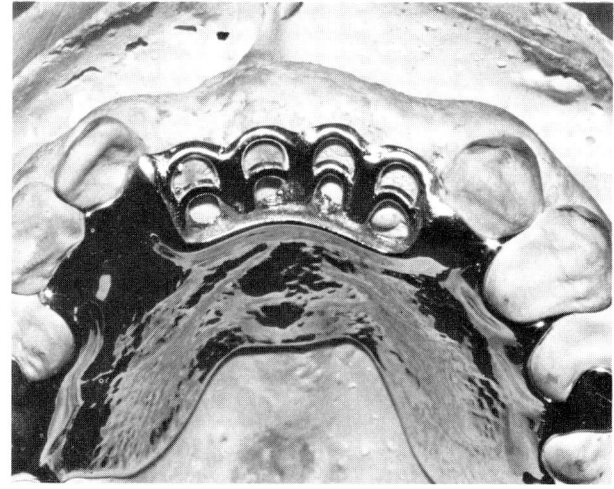

**Fig. 12-2.** Retentive latticework is located to allow maximum esthetic positioning of replacement teeth.

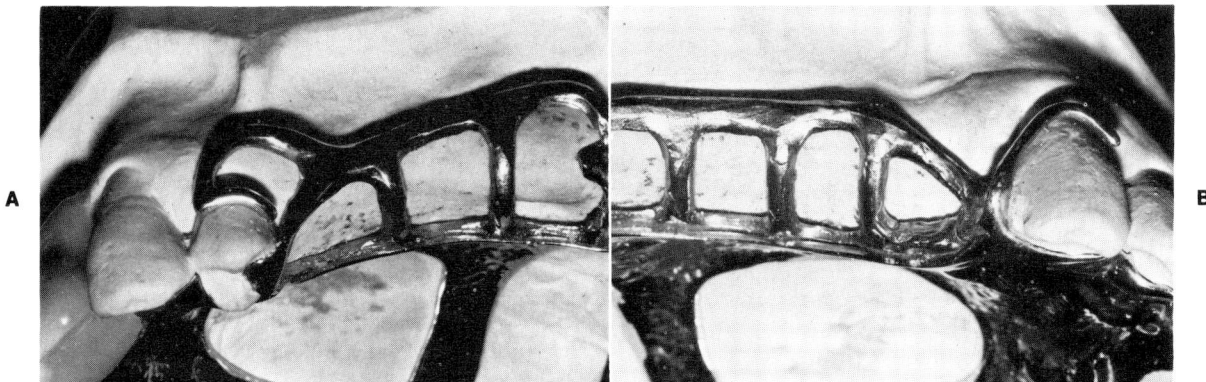

**Fig. 12-3. A,** Retentive strut is positioned to interfere with proper positioning of artificial second premolar. **B,** Retentive strut has been designed to allow esthetic positioning of neck of artificial first premolar and provides space necessary to retain maximum length of replacement.

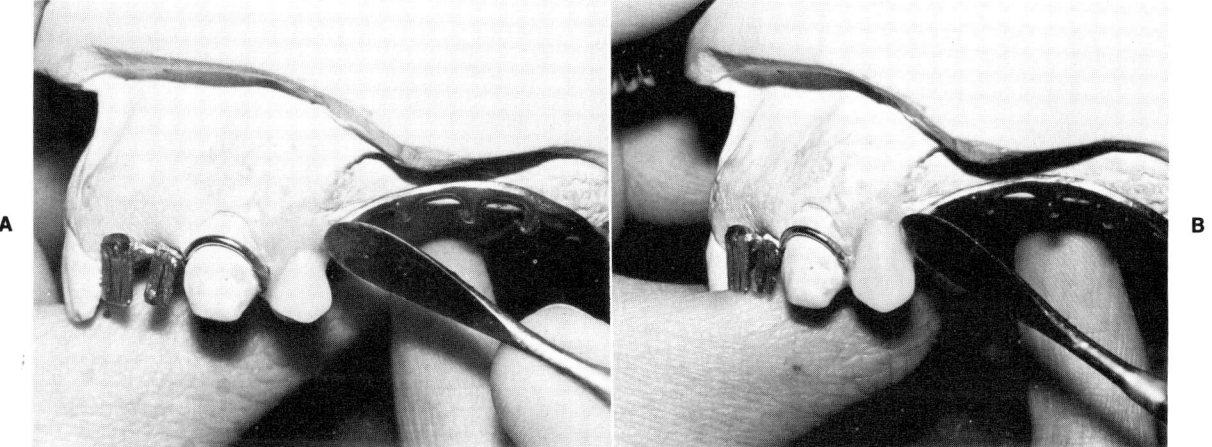

**Fig. 12-4. A,** Neck of denture tooth required excessive shortening to clear improperly positioned retentive strut. Result is unnatural appearance due to disparity in height of gingival margin of canine and first premolar. **B,** Properly designed latticework results in longer replacement tooth and more natural and harmonious length of natural canine and artificial first premolar.

**342** *Dental laboratory procedures: removable partial dentures*

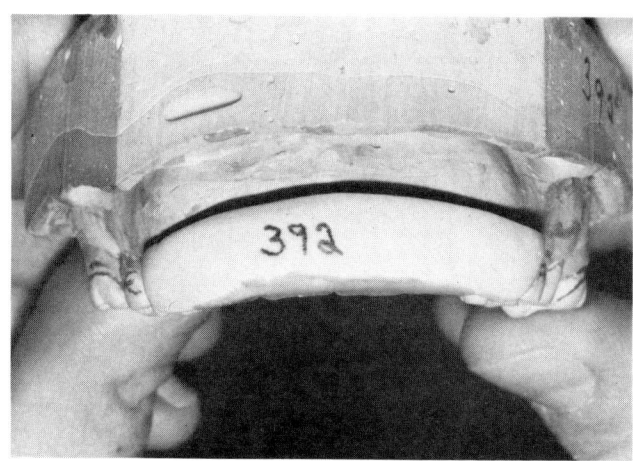

**Fig. 12-5.** Index is trimmed to reveal necks of denture teeth (in shadow).

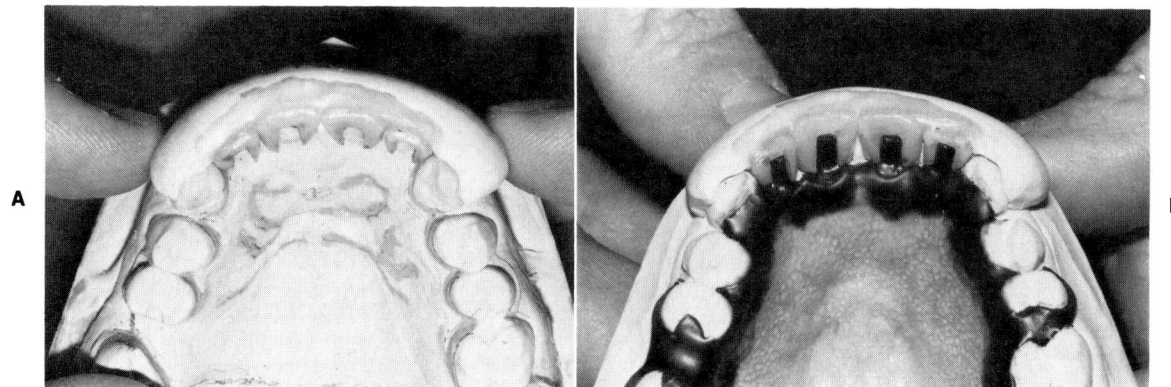

**Fig. 12-6. A,** Teeth are positioned in index with spaces prepared on lingual surface to wax retentive devices. **B,** Wax-up of framework on refractory cast is determined by prearranged tooth position. Maximum esthetics and strength may be achieved.

*Selecting and arranging teeth* **343**

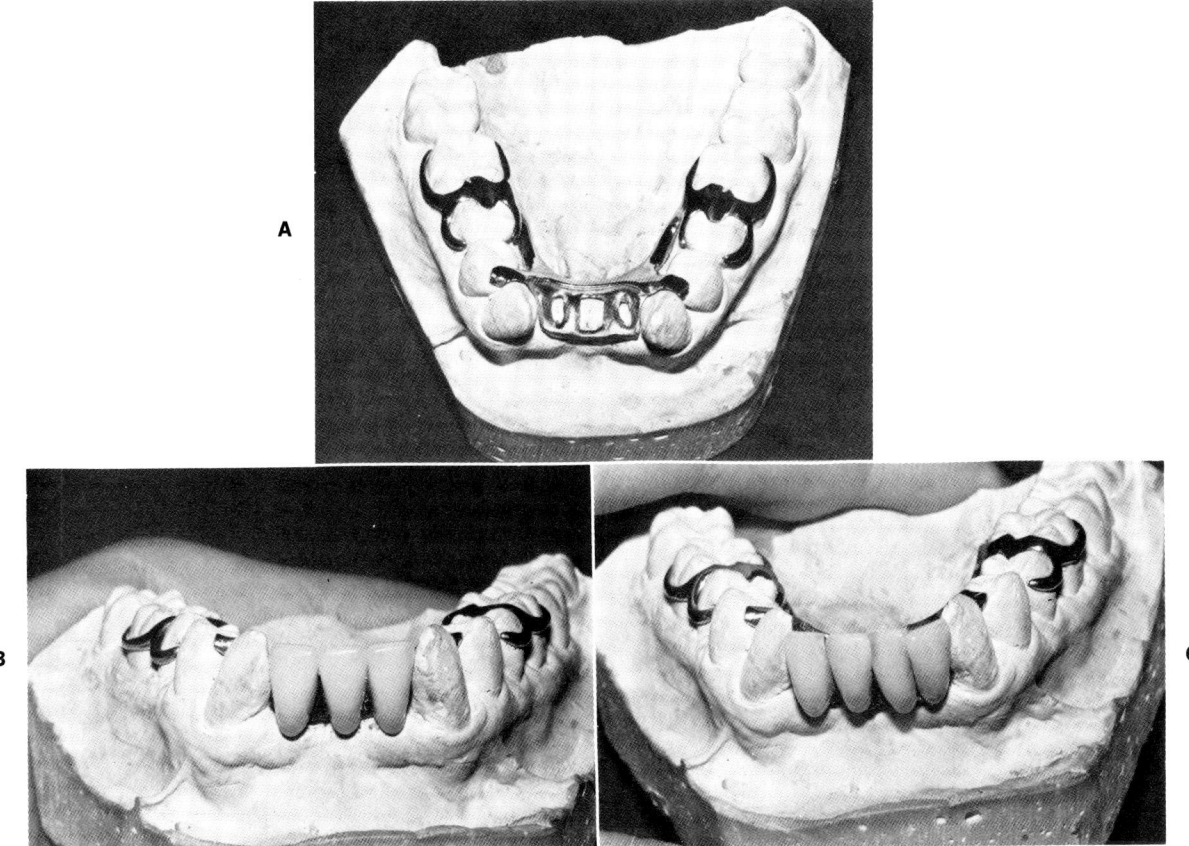

**Fig. 12-7. A,** Minimum space is available to replace mandibular incisors on removable partial denture framework. **B,** Three incisors of proper size appear artificial when set without horizontal overlapping. **C,** Four properly sized incisors may be adjusted to fit reduced space and create more lifelike appearance.

A major problem with removable partial dentures is accomplishing an esthetic blend with the patient's remaining natural dentition. Shade and mold selection becomes critical to a realistic appearance. Both anterior and posterior teeth must be selected to appear as if they belong with the natural dentition. Often, crowding properly sized maxillary or mandibular anterior teeth is far more satisfactory than selecting a smaller mold or eliminating one tooth because of reduced space. Nothing appears more artificial than placing three mandibular incisor teeth into the space where four natural teeth were removed. Therefore crowding four teeth into the space is far more cosmetically pleasing than placing three teeth uniformly (Fig. 12-7).

Selection of a posterior mold is also critical to the esthetic results, especially if maxillary first or second premolars are being replaced on the removable partial denture. Generally, the technique suggested for selecting a posterior mold is to measure the space available distal to the most distal abutment and select a mold that will fill this space. However, in removable partial prosthodontics, the artificial replacement teeth must appear to compliment the patient's natural dentition. Therefore it is better to select a posterior mold that is similar in size with existing posterior teeth adjacent to or opposing the artificial teeth to be selected. Remember, that most natural posterior teeth are larger buccolingually than are denture teeth, and the dimension to consider is the mesiodistal and the occlusogingival dimension of the facial surface of the teeth for size comparison. In the absence of posterior teeth, a mold should be selected to harmonize with the size of the remaining anterior teeth.

## ARRANGING THE ARTIFICIAL TEETH
### Anterior teeth

Although missing anterior teeth are ideally replaced with a fixed prosthesis, often, the removable partial denture will incorporate anterior replacements into the design. Primary considerations for anterior tooth replacements are esthetics and strength. For the patient, a natural esthetic appearance is an important consideration. However, the removable partial denture must not interfere with the patient's remaining natural dentition in either centric or eccentric positions.

### PROCEDURE

1. With the casts mounted on a semiadjustable articulator, set the incisal guide table to allow the remaining stone teeth to dictate the lateral and protrusive excursions without abrading the master casts (Fig. 12-8).

2. If the removable partial denture is scheduled for an esthetic try-in, paint tinfoil substitute onto all edentulous areas of the cast to the peripheral roll. Alternatively, the framework may be removed from the cast, and a small piece of tinfoil burnished to the edentulous ridge using a pencil eraser. The tinfoil will then adhere to the baseplate wax and may be trimmed to the peripheral roll, and carried with the framework to the try-in. The advantage of using tinfoil is to be able to recognize when wax gets onto the tissue side of the edentulous area, preventing the framework from reseating completely onto the master cast.

3. Generally, replacement teeth for removable partial dentures must be adjusted on the ridge lap in order to position them properly. However, it is important to remember that the replacement teeth must appear to belong with the remaining natural dentition. Therefore, when adjusting the denture teeth, do not shorten them incisogingivally any shorter than the natural teeth adjacent to the edentulous space. With a soft lead pencil, heavily mark the retentive components in the area where the first tooth is to be placed (Fig. 12-9).

4. Rub the ridge-lap area against the retentive components for acrylic resin to mark the area of the tooth to adjust. Alternatively, a piece of articulating paper may be interposed between the tooth and the framework, marking the tooth where it should be adjusted. With an acrylic bur or heatless stone, reduce the area marked on the tooth without sacrificing the facial esthetics of the tooth being ground in. Re-mark the retentive area, and again rub the ridge-lap surface against the latticework. When marking and adjusting the denture tooth results in an esthetic and functional positioning of the tooth, lightly wax the tooth into position with baseplate wax.

5. Continue to position the remaining anterior

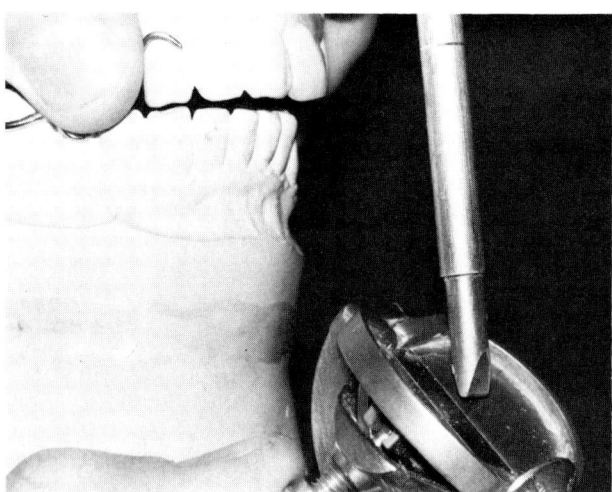

**Fig. 12-8.** Incisal guide table is adjusted to allow natural teeth to dictate functional movements without abrading stone surface.

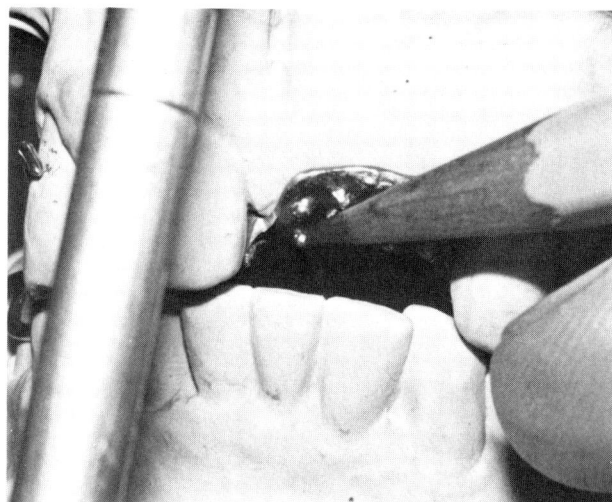

**Fig. 12-9.** Soft lead pencil is used to mark acrylic retentive areas and cast guiding planes prior to positioning first tooth.

Selecting and arranging teeth

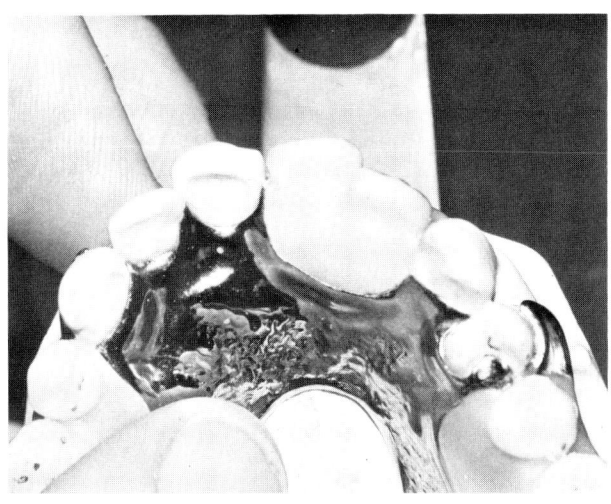

Fig. 12-10. Observing arch form from incisal edges provides information for esthetic positioning of replacement teeth. Note relative positions of distal surfaces of central incisors with mesial surfaces of lateral incisors.

replacement teeth until a pleasing esthetic and functional result develops. Care must be exercised to ensure that proper faciolingual positioning of the anterior teeth has resulted. Often looking down on the incisal edges of the anterior teeth provides information to ensure correct positioning of the teeth (Fig. 12-10). Observe proper arch form and symmetry, and combine them with subtle techniques to improve the natural esthetic results. Some of these include (1) setting one central incisor slightly facial to the other; (2) varying the long axes of the anterior teeth slightly; (3) overlapping centrals with laterals, or tucking laterals slightly behind centrals; or (4) reshaping the facial and incisal surfaces of the teeth for a more natural appearance (Fig. 12-11). Remember, it is often necessary to remove a considerable amount of acrylic from the lingual and ridge-lap areas of anterior replacements. If a shade has been selected to harmonize with the existing natural dentition, and if the tooth must be reduced considerably, be sure to check that the shade has not been lightened with the thinning procedure. Sometimes a darker shade must be selected to compensate for the reduction in thickness of the denture tooth. Often, to create a natural appearance, different shades or different molds must be selected to create the desired appearance (Fig. 12-12).

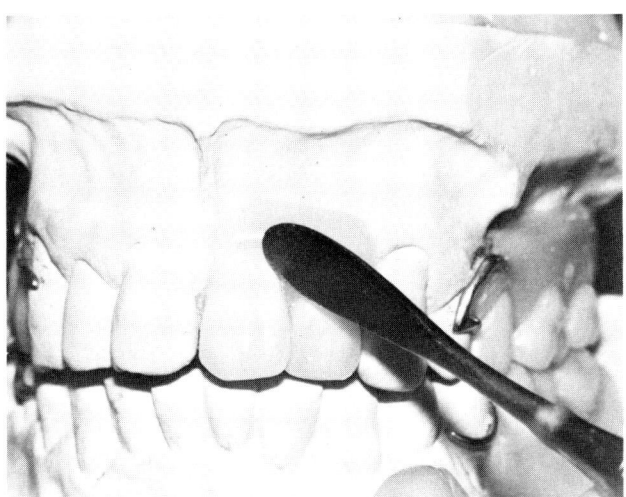

Fig. 12-11. Incisal edges and facial surfaces of denture teeth have been reshaped to provide appearance closely resembling natural counterparts.

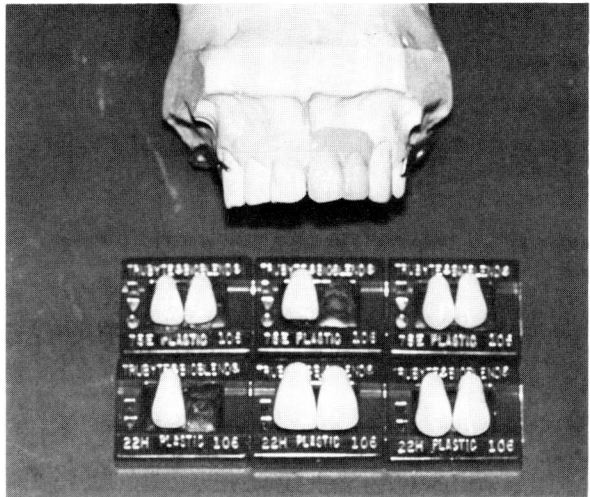

Fig. 12-12. To more nearly match shape and size of natural central and lateral incisor, two different molds were selected.

## Posterior teeth

A number of different factors must be considered when selecting and arranging posterior artifical denture teeth for a removable partial denture. First, the teeth must have the proper mesiodistal width to occlude most nearly with the opposing natural dentition. Also, the tooth must be long enough occlusogingivally to create a natural appearance when compared with the remaining natural teeth (Table 12-1). If all posterior teeth are being replaced with artificial denture teeth, they must be selected to harmonize in shade and size with the remaining natural teeth. The teeth selected for the removable partial denture should not extend onto the ascending portion of the mandibular residual ridge or beyond the anterior extent of the maxillary tuberosity, to prevent unfavorable leverage forces from being transferred to the natural abutment teeth (Fig. 12-13). If, however, a natural second or third molar remains in the opposing area, an artificial denture tooth should be articulated with it to prevent its extrusion.

Often, the space remaining to arrange artificial denture teeth does not allow replacement of those teeth lost by the patient. For example, a patient might be missing only a first molar on one side of the arch. But because of drifting of the second molar, only a small space remains. In this case, it is sometimes necessary to position another second premolar for a total of three premolars and one natural second molar on one side of the arch (Fig. 12-14). Or, a premolar and a molar may be indicated for a distal extension removable partial denture replacing two molar teeth.

It is important to recognize that *commercially available posterior teeth are not designed to articulate accurately with the natural human dentition.* Indeed, they are designed to properly articulate only with their opposing artificial teeth. Therefore it *must* be borne in mind that artificial posterior teeth opposing a natural dentition should be considered as blocks of acrylic to be modified to harmonize with the opposing natural dentition. Only then will the artificial teeth be shaped to articulate properly with the natural dentition. This concept is essential if a functional and esthetic result is to be expected from a removable partial denture. The positioning and modification of the occlusal surfaces are properly done tooth by tooth to achieve maximum function from the arrangement.

### PROCEDURE

1. Remove the acrylic resin denture base with which the jaw relation records were made to mount the master casts. Flame the tissue side of the acrylic until it has softened, and then remove it with an instrument (Fig. 12-15). Heating should be done over a bowl of water to quench the acrylic should it ignite. Clean any residue from the removable partial denture framework, and position it on the master cast. If a corrected cast impression has been accomplished, the tissue stop incorporated into the framework of a distal extension removable partial denture no longer contacts the tissue of the cast. Paint tinfoil

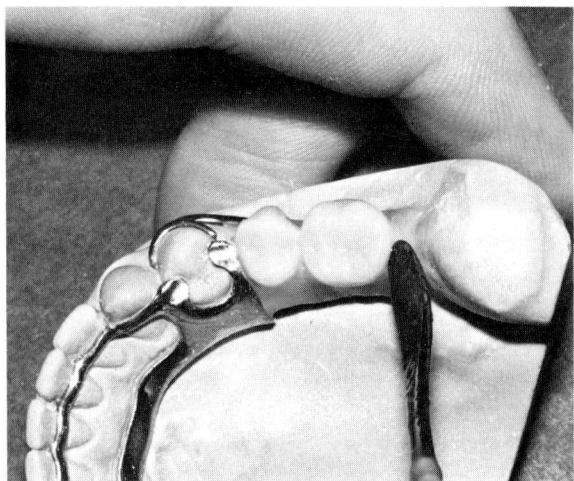

**Fig. 12-13.** Premolar and molar are selected for this edentulous space because extending denture teeth further distally would create unfavorable leverages on remaining natural dentition.

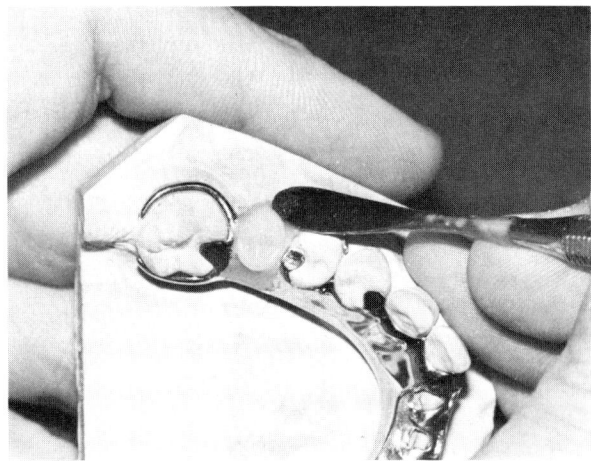

**Fig. 12-14.** Space remaining where natural first molar was lost is greatly reduced due to tipping of second molar. Second premolar denture tooth is used to fill space.

substitute on the residual ridge beneath the tissue stop. Moisten the tip of a sable brush with the monomer supplied with pink autopolymerizing resin. Pick up a small ball of the powder with the brush tip, and place it under the tissue stop to reestablish contact with the stone cast below (Fig. 12-16). This will prevent distortion of the framework during the trial packing procedure. Allow the acrylic to polymerize.

2. If the removable partial denture is to be tried in the patient's mouth after the setup, paint tinfoil substitute onto the ridge before reseating the framework into place, as with a removable partial denture replacing anterior teeth (Fig. 12-17). Often a piece

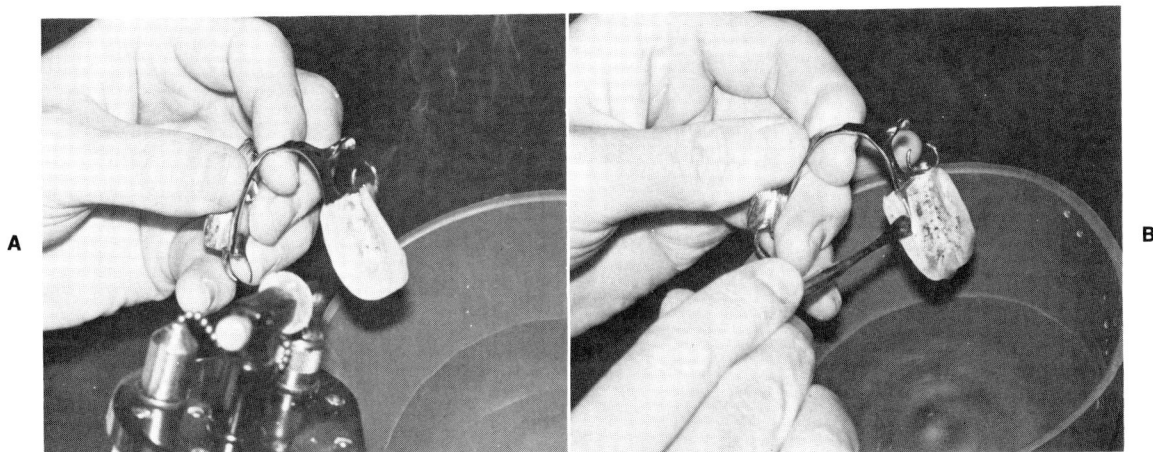

**Fig. 12-15. A,** Tissue side of acrylic resin base is flamed with torch to soften acrylic. With careful heating, acrylic will not ignite and will result in framework free of carbon residue. NOTE: Heating is accomplished over water for safety should acrylic ignite. **B,** Softened acrylic is removed with instrument and drops into water.

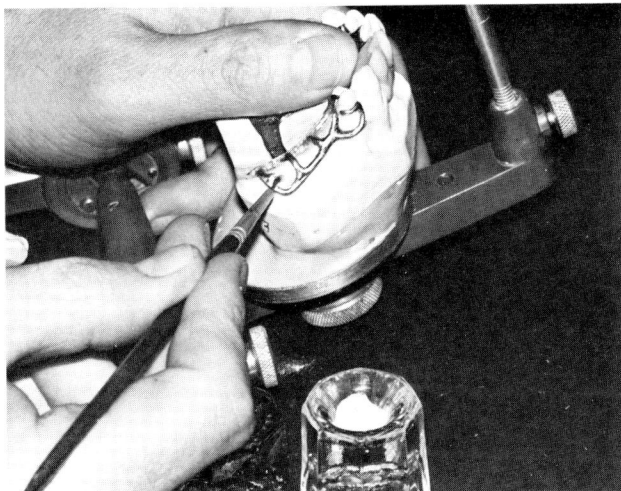

**Fig. 12-16.** Small amount of pink autopolymerizing resin is placed beneath tissue stop using sable brush moistened with monomer.

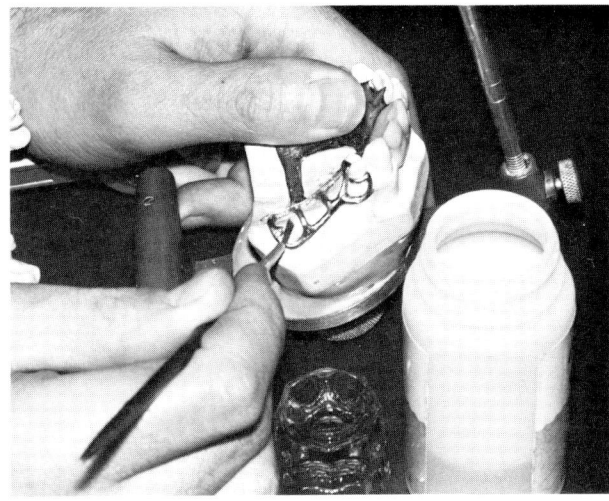

**Fig. 12-17.** Tinfoil substitute is dispensed into separate container, diluted slightly, and painted onto ridge.

of tinfoil may be burnished to the ridge rather than using tinfoil substitute (Fig. 12-18). By using tinfoil, wax that may become lodged on the tissue surface of the distal extension base may be located and removed. If wax is incorporated on the tissue surface during the try-in appointment and is undetected, it may prevent the framework from seating accurately back on the master cast for the final wax-up. Remove the tinfoil after the try-in and before the partial denture wax-up. After the separating medium is placed on the cast, flow baseplate wax around the retentive latticework to stabilize the framework to the cast.

3. Adjust the incisal guide table and wings so that the remaining stone natural teeth dictate the lateral and protrusive excursions of the articulator without abrading the stone casts (Fig. 12-19).

4. Open the incisal guide pin 1 mm. This, of course, will bring the remaining natural (stone) teeth out of occlusion by a corresponding distance (Fig. 12-20).

5. Position the first tooth distal to the remaining natural teeth. Depending on the opposing occlusion, it is usually necessary to adjust the mesial and ridge-lap areas of the denture tooth to bring it into intimate contact with the adjacent natural tooth. The tooth must be marked to determine where reduction is to take place. Either of two techniques may be used. The first is to mark the retentive latticework and the minor connector with a soft lead pencil and transfer the lead to the tooth by rubbing it against the marked framework (Fig. 12-21). The second technique is to place articulating ribbon between the tooth and the framework and rub the tooth against the articulating ribbon (Fig. 12-22). The tooth will thus be marked and may be reduced until excellent proximal and gingival adaptation occurs with the natural tooth adjacent to it and the latticework of the framework (Fig. 12-23). It is important to recognize that where esthetics is a factor on maxillary partial dentures, extreme care must be exercised when adjusting the teeth for fit to the frame-

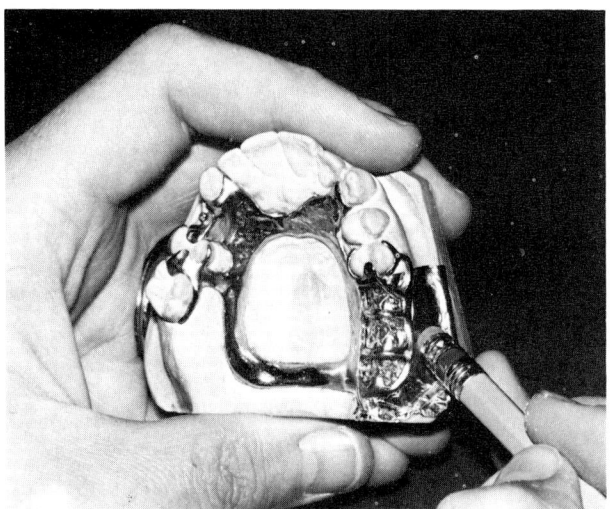

**Fig. 12-18.** Tinfoil may be burnished to ridge, using pencil eraser.

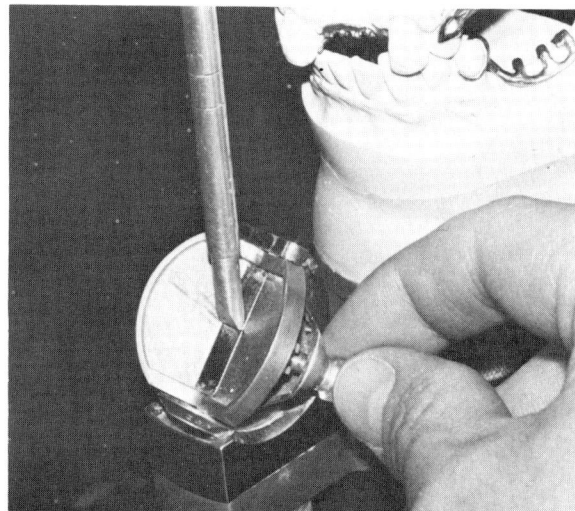

**Fig. 12-19.** Incisal guide table and wings are adjusted so that lateral and protrusive excursions of articulator are dictated by natural teeth without abrading stone casts.

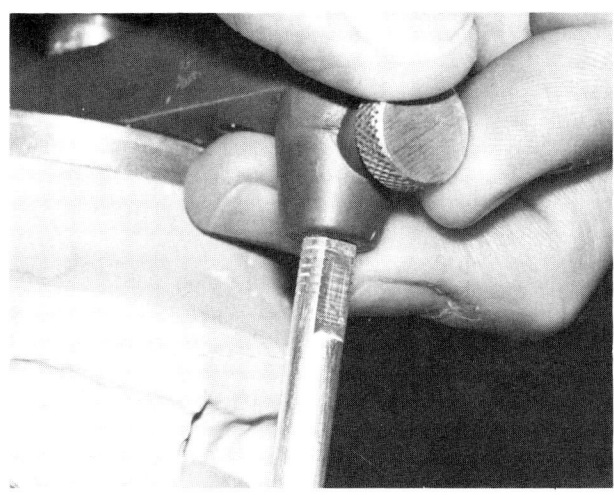

**Fig. 12-20.** Incisal guide pin is opened 1 mm, bringing remaining natural teeth out of occlusion.

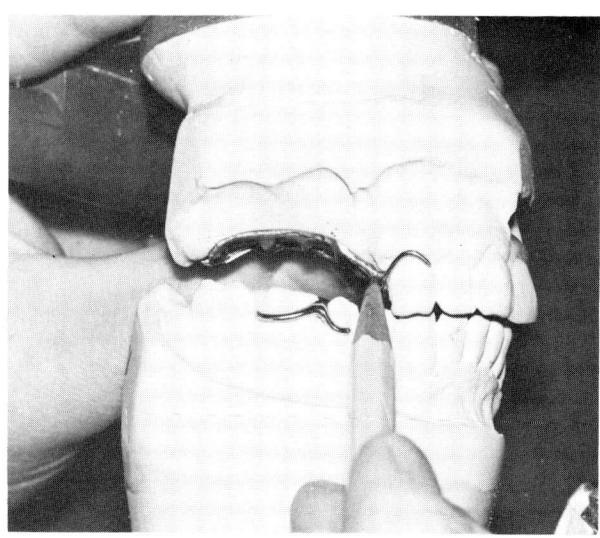

**Fig. 12-21.** Latticework, cast metal guiding plate, and clasp are marked with soft lead pencil.

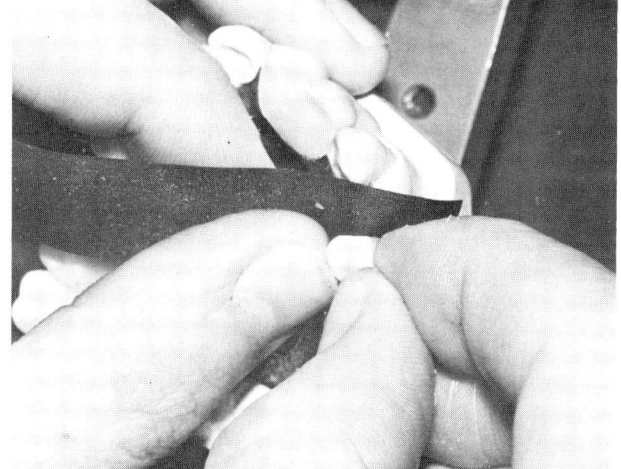

**Fig. 12-22.** Articulating ribbon is placed on latticework and cast guiding plane, and replacement tooth is rubbed against it.

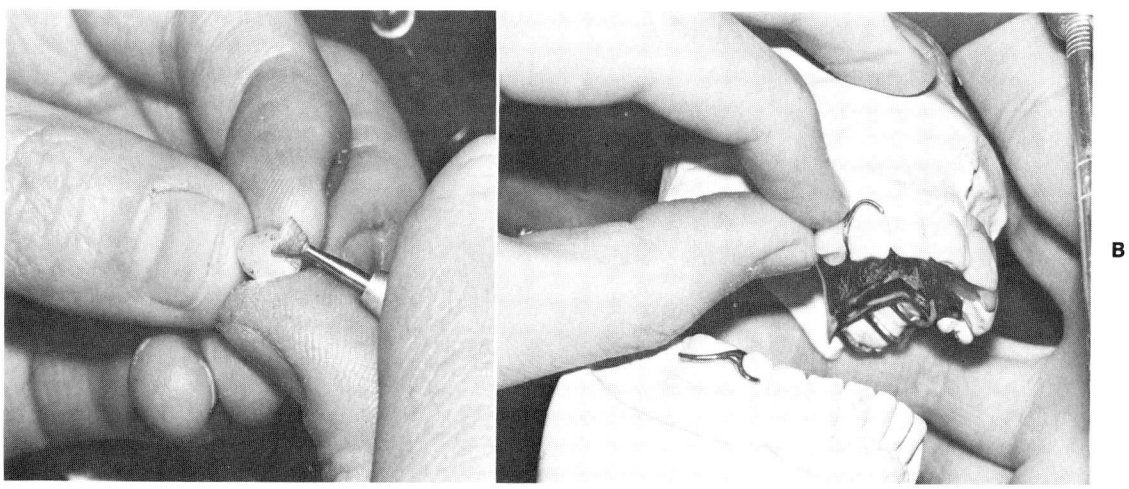

**Fig. 12-23. A,** Marking is transferred to proximal and ridge-lap areas of denture tooth, and these areas may be reduced with a stone. **B,** Repeated marking and careful adjusting allow denture tooth to be brought into intimate contact with natural tooth, creating more esthetic appearance.

work. If the teeth are not carefully and precisely adjusted, an unsightly space develops between the natural tooth and the artificial replacement (Fig. 12-24). Be sure that the maximum occlusogingival length of the denture tooth is preserved at this phase, so that the artificial tooth appears as long, or nearly as long at the gingival margin as the adjacent natural tooth (Fig. 12-25). To accomplish this, the gingival portion of the denture tooth must often be reduced to near paper thinness, without shortening the tooth appreciably.

6. Lute the tooth to the framework with baseplate wax, and check the occlusion for contact. If contact is slightly high, adjust it until even contact is made with the pin contacting the incisal guide table. (Remember, the incisal guide pin remains 1 mm open.)

7. If the tooth opposes a natural dentition, check to see if the intercuspation that is developing mesiodistally appears to be proper (Fig. 12-25, *B*). Are the cusp tips of the tooth set in the proper relationship with the opposing teeth? Does it appear that the remaining teeth to be set will continue an ac-

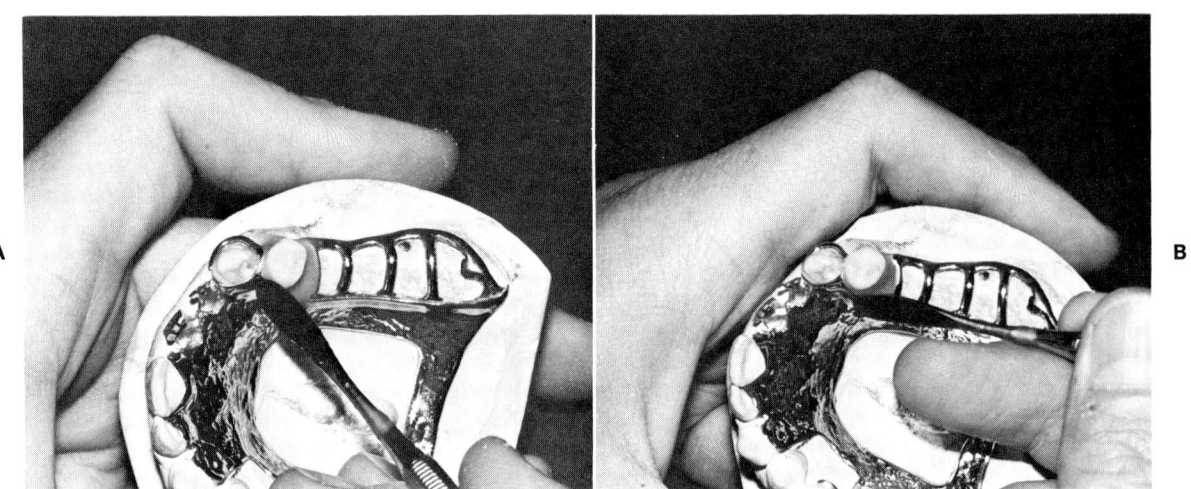

**Fig. 12-24. A,** Denture tooth has not been adjusted sufficiently, leaving space between it and natural abutment tooth. **B,** With careful alteration of ridge-lap contours, denture tooth may be positioned immediately adjacent to abutment tooth.

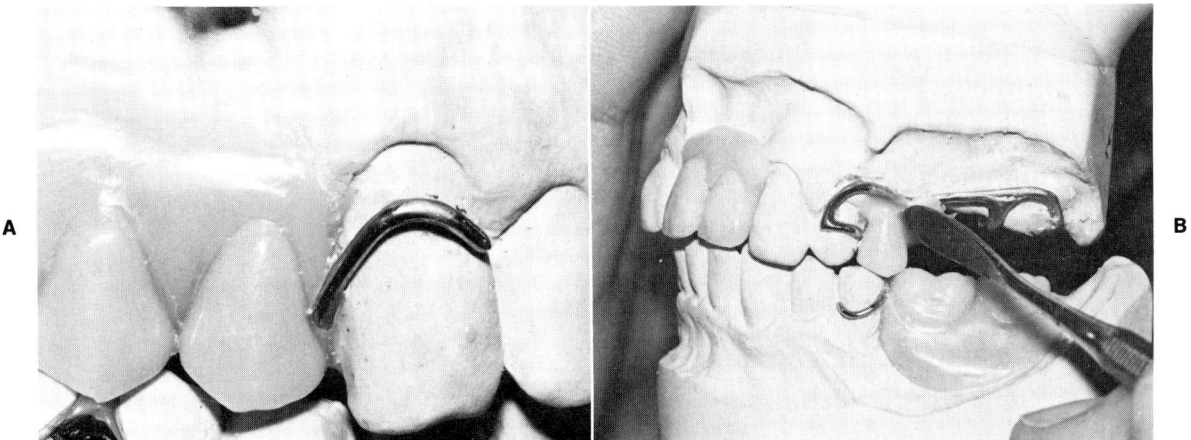

**Fig. 12-25. A,** Although first premolar has been nicely positioned mesially to contact adjacent canine abutment, tooth is too short at gingival margin when compared to canine abutment. Longer first and second premolars would have created more natural appearance. **B,** Second premolar denture tooth has been properly adapted at gingival margin, preserving length of artificial tooth closely matching that of its adjacent abutment. Note properly developing cusp-fossa relationship with opposing natural and artificial teeth.

ceptable interdigitation? Be sure proper cusp-fossa relationships are developing.

8. Select the next tooth distal, and mark the latticework and the tooth with a lead pencil or articulating paper. Adjust it until its mesiodistal, buccolingual, and occlusogingival position appears correct, and adjust the occlusion to refine its position (Fig. 12-26). Check the working relationship to be certain that the maxillary buccal cusp tips are relating properly with the mandibular teeth (Fig. 12-27). Inspect the teeth from the lingual aspect to ensure development of tight cusp-fossa relationships (Fig. 12-28).

9. Continue to mark and position the remaining posterior teeth until an acceptable arrangement has been created (Fig. 12-29).

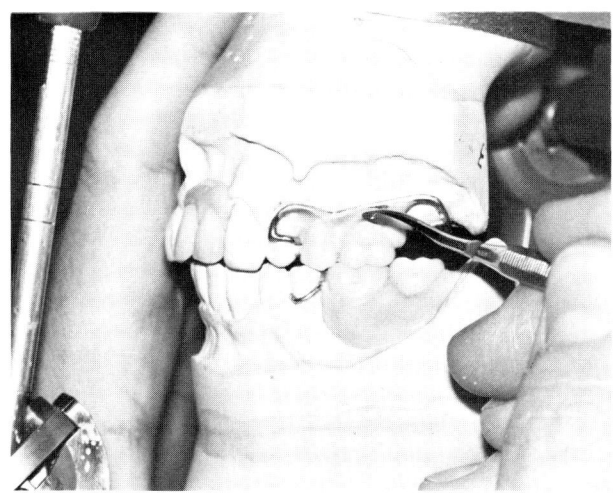

**Fig. 12-26.** Ridge-lap area of next tooth is adjusted, and tooth is positioned for proper mesiodistal and buccolingual relationships with opposing teeth.

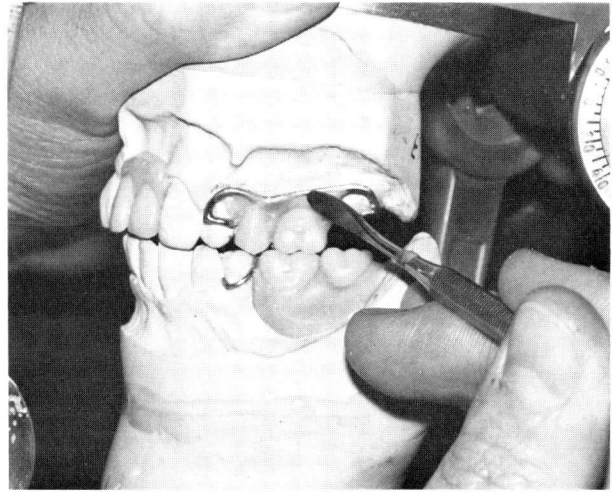

**Fig. 12-27.** Articulator is moved to working relationship, and tooth is adjusted to provide proper relationships of buccal cusps without interferences.

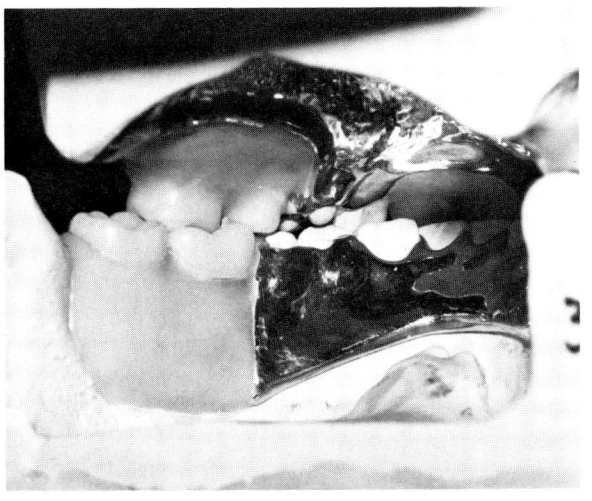

**Fig. 12-28.** Cusp-fossa relationship is inspected from lingual aspect to verify tight contacts.

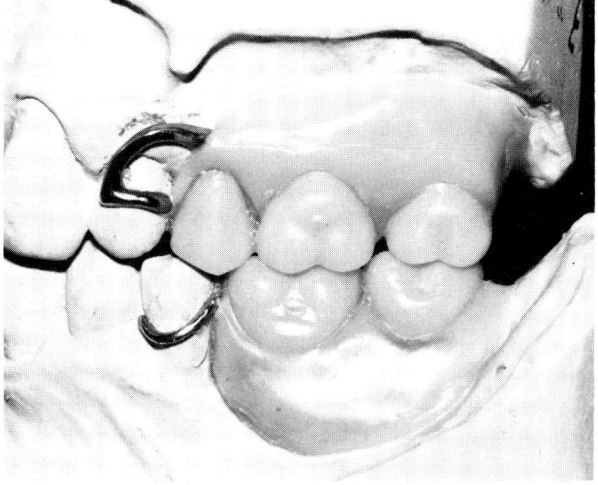

**Fig. 12-29.** Completed set-up is inspected for proper tooth position.

10. Reposition the incisal guide pin to the neutral position (Fig. 12-30). It should now be 1 mm from contacting the incisal guide table. Mark the occlusal contacts with articulating ribbon (Fig. 12-31). (Articulating paper should not be used because the heavy inking will build up on the opposing stone teeth and create inaccurate markings.) Adjust the occlusion using a small green stone until contact is uniform and *the incisal guide pin once again contacts the guide table* (Fig. 12-32). Mark the final occlusal contacts with the articulating ribbon (Fig. 12-33).

11. Next, unlock the condylar elements, and check the lateral and protrusive excursions. Remember that the artificial teeth on the removable partial denture should not dictate lateral or protrusive excursions. With another color articulating ribbon, mark any interferences in lateral excursions *without* eliminating the centric contacts previously established and marked (Fig. 12-34).

As a final check for adequate occlusion, a shim stock may be used to check all teeth, both natural and artificial, for adequate contact. The incisal guide pin should be contacting the guide table (Fig. 12-35).

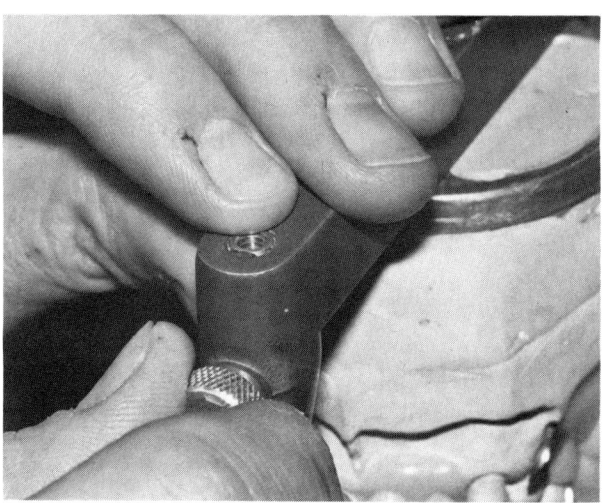

**Fig. 12-30.** Incisal guide pin is repositioned to neutral position.

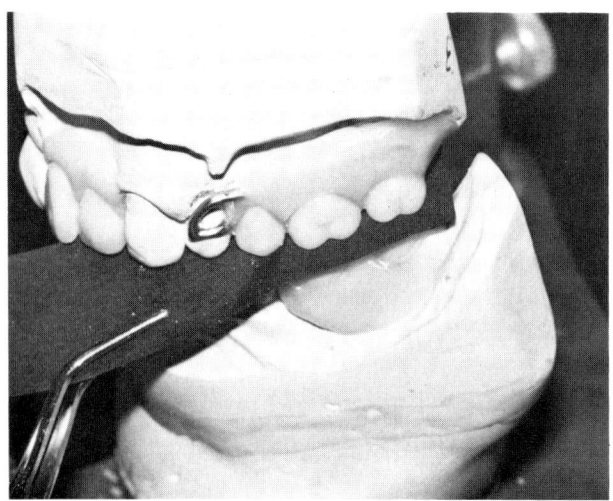

**Fig. 12-31.** Articulating ribbon is used to mark occlusal contacts.

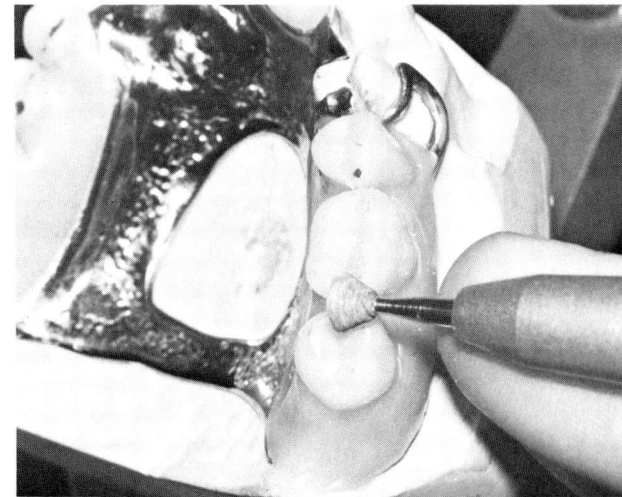

**Fig. 12-32.** Small green stone is used to reduce contacts until occlusion is uniform and *incisal guide pin once again contacts guide table.*

## Selecting and arranging teeth 353

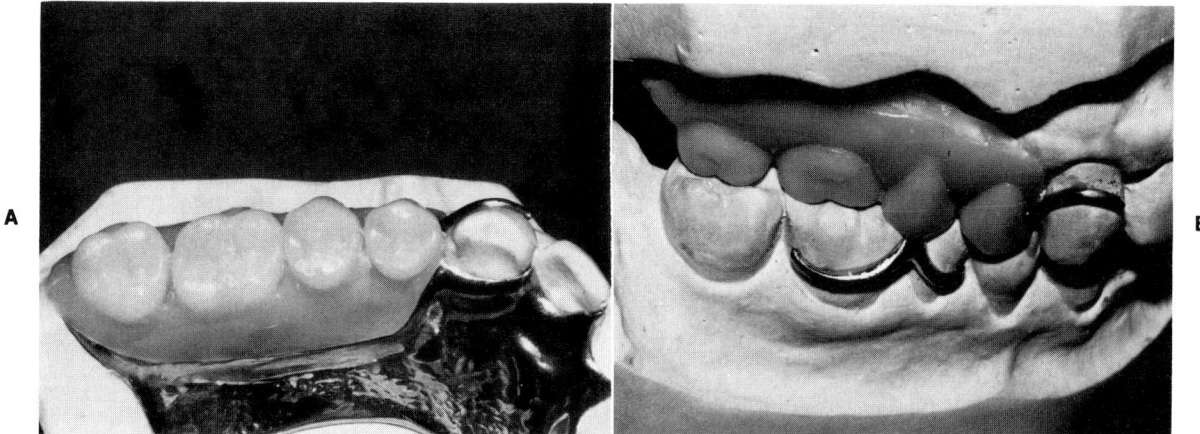

**Fig. 12-33. A,** Occlusal anatomy of denture teeth has been modified to harmonize with opposing natural dentition. **B,** In this way, harmonious occlusion is possible despite variations in opposing dentition.

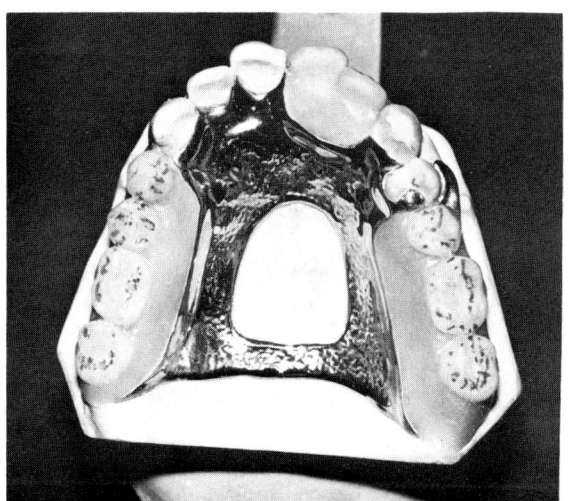

**Fig. 12-34.** Final occlusal contacts are marked with articulating ribbon.

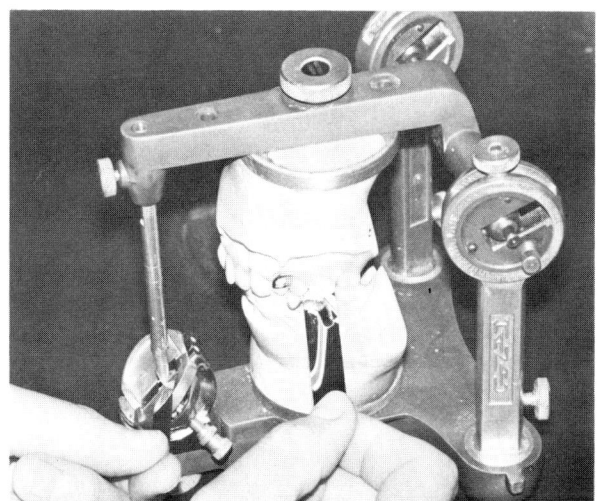

**Fig. 12-35.** Occlusion is checked for adequate contacts and to ensure that incisal guide pin once again contacts guide table.

## SETTING ARTIFICIAL POSTERIOR TEETH TO A FUNCTIONALLY GENERATED PATH TEMPLATE

Occasionally, a dentist will wish to set the posterior teeth on a removable partial denture to a functionally generated path. With this technique, the patient actually "chews in" the occlusal relationships of the teeth to be replaced by the removable partial denture. In this way, the possibility of establishing an occlusal interference in the removable partial denture is reduced to nearly zero.

After the framework has been properly fitted and the corrected cast impression procedure has been completed, an acrylic record base is attached to the retentive latticework of the removable partial denture framework. When the dentist establishes that neither the framework nor the acrylic record base interferes with the patient's normal occlusion, an occlusion rim is fabricated. This occlusion rim is constructed from a type of wax easily altered by the patient's functional movements. The occlusal surface of the wax occlusion rim must be wide enough to record completely the lateral and protrusive excursions of the mandible. The occlusion rim is constructed slightly high so that, by functional movements of the mandible, the patient wears away the wax and "grinds" a functional anatomy using the teeth opposing the removable partial denture. The dentist may have the patient wear the partial denture for a variable length of time, up to a few days, to establish the proper occlusion. Sometimes, the dentist uses a softer wax and guides the patient into excursive movements, rapidly wearing away the wax until a functional record is achieved. This record is then used to set the artificial teeth.

The master cast is received with the wax functionally generated path on the framework (Fig. 12-36). A template must be constructed from the functionally generated path to be used to set the teeth for the removable partial denture.

### PROCEDURE

1. Seat the framework carefully onto the master cast to ensure that it is completely seated and properly positioned. Lute the framework to the master cast with modeling plastic or sticky wax (Fig. 12-37).

2. The generated path must be beaded and boxed so that the stone template may be poured. Carefully enclose the functionally generated path wax with beading wax (Fig. 12-38). Be careful not to distort the wax record by heating. Include the stone abutment teeth as positive stops in the beading procedure. Follow the same procedure on the functionally generated path on the other side of the partial denture. If the path is recorded only on one side, bead the occlusal surfaces of the natural teeth on

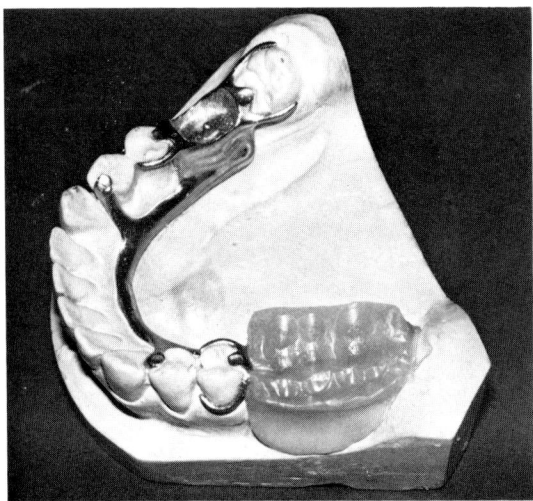

**Fig. 12-36.** Functionally generated path record is received from dentist on framework. Notice that record is considerably wider buccolingually than teeth that will replace record.

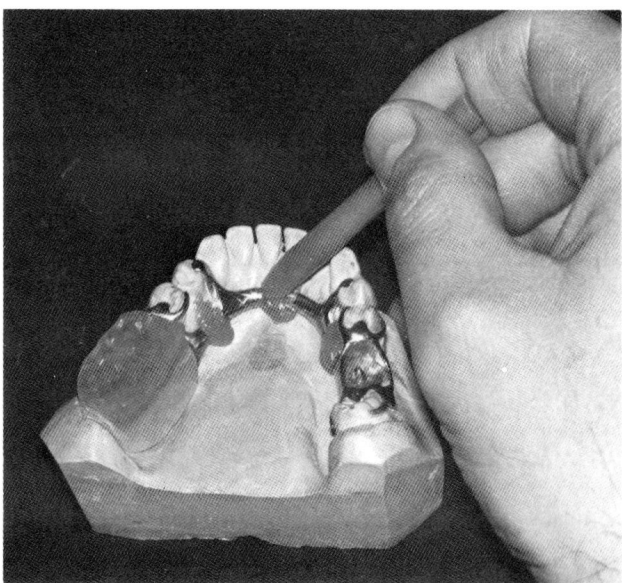

**Fig. 12-37.** Framework is checked for complete seating on master cast. It is then luted to position using modeling plastic or sticky wax.

the other side of the arch to create positive stops (Fig. 12-39).

3. Warm a piece of boxing wax, and trim it to fill in the space between the right and left beaded areas. Lute the wax into position (Fig. 12-40).

4. Enclose the beaded areas by trimming and fitting boxing wax to the beaded areas until an enclosure is formed around the functionally generated path or paths, abutment teeth, and beaded natural teeth (Fig. 12-41).

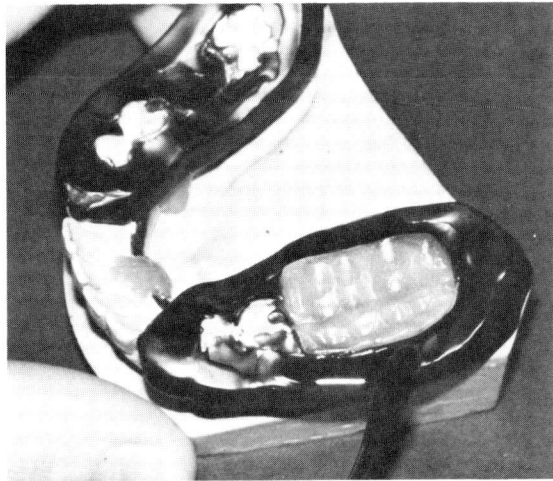

**Fig. 12-38.** Functionally generated path wax is enclosed with soft beading wax. Caution must be exercised to prevent distortion of wax record by heating. Notice that posterior abutment teeth on this side are enclosed to serve as positive occlusal stop.

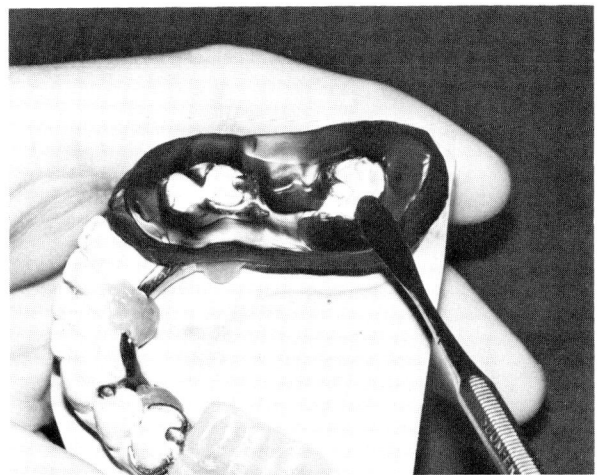

**Fig. 12-39.** If functionally generated path is on only one side of partial denture framework, occlusal surfaces of natural teeth on other side of arch must also be enclosed with beading wax.

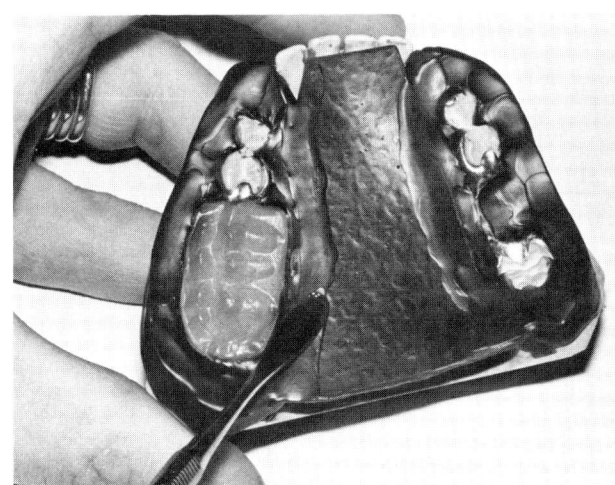

**Fig. 12-40.** Boxing wax is trimmed to fill space between right and left sides of arch. It is then luted into position.

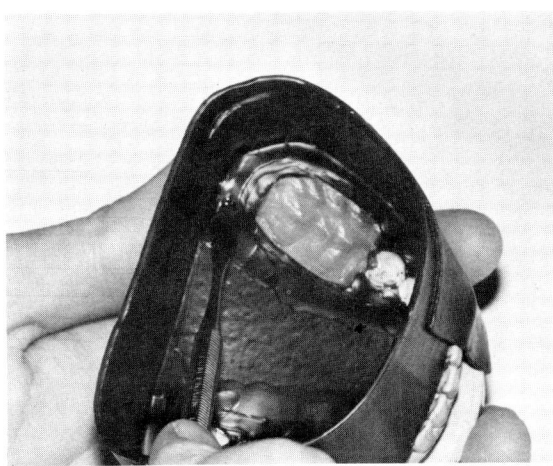

**Fig. 12-41.** Boxing wax is trimmed to enclose all areas previously beaded.

5. Paint a coating of separating medium* onto the exposed and boxed stone occlusal surfaces of the teeth (Fig. 12-42). Do not use a separating medium that occupies space, such as petroleum jelly.

6. Pour clear slurry water into the boxed cast, and seal any leaks evident (Fig. 12-43).

7. Vacuum mix 150 mg of improved dental stone† with the correct amount of water, and vibrate the stone carefully into the boxed generated path (Fig. 12-44). Remove the cast from the vibrator, and build a thickness of approximately 15 mm of stone covering all exposed and boxed areas.

8. After the stone has set, carefully remove the boxing wax, leaving the template affixed to the master cast and generated path (Fig. 12-45).

---

*Super-Sep, Kerr Manufacturing Co., Romulus, Mich., or equivalent.
†Vel Mix, Kerr Manufacturing Co., Romulus, Mich., or equivalent.

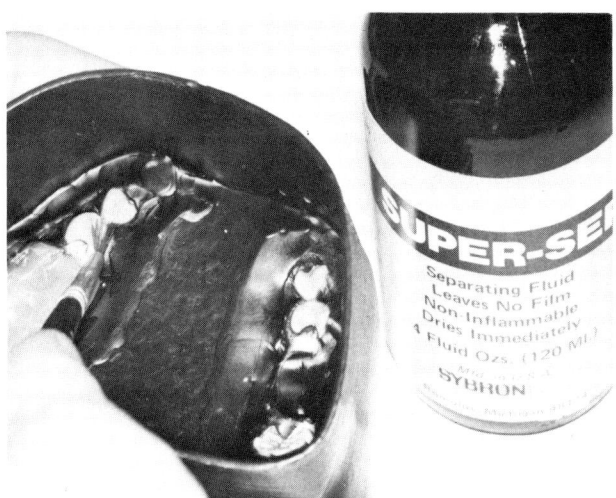

Fig. 12-42. Separating medium is painted onto all exposed stone occlusal surfaces.

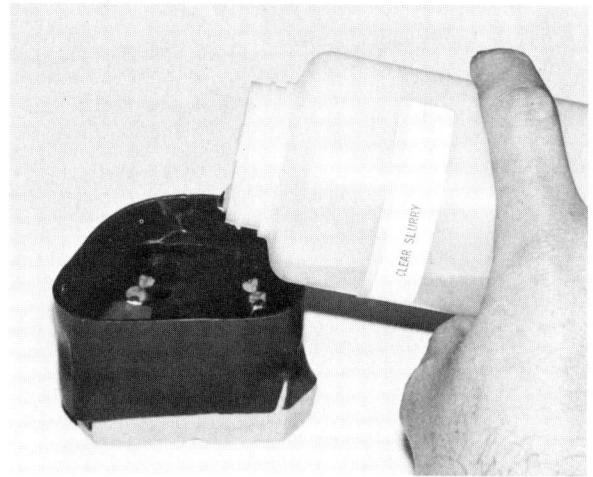

Fig. 12-43. Clear slurry is poured into boxed cast to check for leaks.

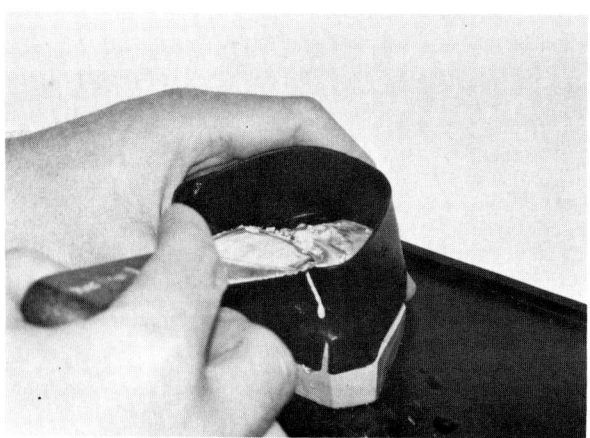

Fig. 12-44. Improved dental stone is vacuum mixed and vibrated carefully into boxed functionally generated path.

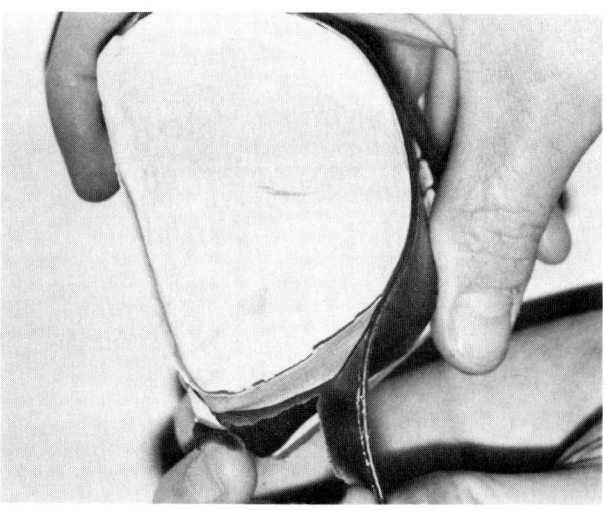

Fig. 12-45. Boxing wax is removed, leaving master cast sealed to template.

## Mounting the template

The template and master cast should now be mounted on a hinge or semiadjustable articulator. It is important to preserve the relationship of the template to the master cast and functionally generated path by not separating the two prior to mounting on the articulator.

**PROCEDURE**

1. Index the bases of both the template and the master cast, and add a separating medium to the index grooves. Soak the bases of both casts in clear slurry water.
2. With a mix of dental stone, lute the lower half of the cast-template complex to the articulator. Place stone on the upper half, and close it to lute the master cast and template to the articulator (Fig. 12-46). Although a semiadjustable articulator may be used to orient the cast and template, it will be used strictly as a hinge when positioning the replacement teeth.
3. After mounting the casts in the proper relationship on the articulator, the master cast and template may be separated from one another (Fig. 12-47). Critically examine the master cast and the template to be sure no voids appear in the template and that no damage was done to the master cast (Fig. 12-48).

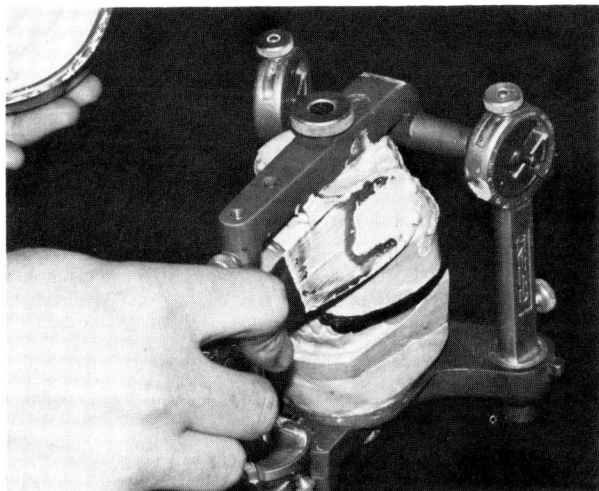

**Fig. 12-46.** Master cast and template are oriented to articulator using dental stone.

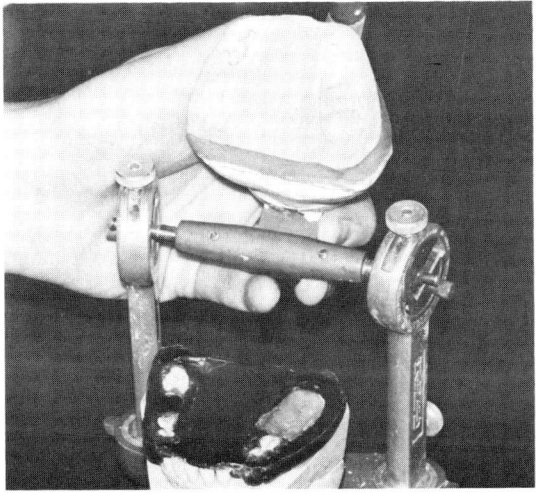

**Fig. 12-47.** After casts have been mounted on articulator, template is separated from master cast.

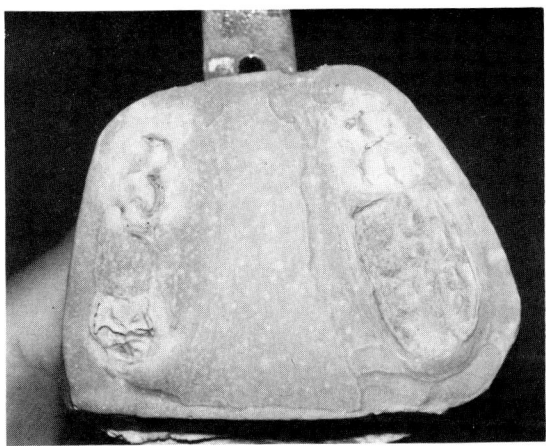

**Fig. 12-48.** Template is critically examined to be sure that no voids are present.

## Arranging the artificial teeth and adjusting the occlusion to a functionally generated path occlusion

Once the master cast is mounted on the articulator opposing the occlusal template, the mounting should be examined carefully to ensure its accuracy (Fig. 12-49). After verifying its accuracy, the removable partial denture may be removed from the master cast and the wax occlusal record removed from the baseplate.

The acrylic resin baseplate may be removed by carefully heating the acrylic with a torch over a bowl of water. Soften the acrylic with heat, without igniting the acrylic. When the acrylic surrounding the latticework has softened, pull the acrylic resin off the latticework and allow it to drop into the water. If a carbon residue was formed on the framework, it should be removed prior to reseating the framework on the master cast. Check to be sure that the framework is accurately positioned on the master cast (Fig. 12-50).

### PROCEDURE

1. If a corrected cast impression has been accomplished, the contact of the tissue stop of the framework must be reestablished with the master cast using autopolymerizing acrylic resin.

2. Flow baseplate wax around the retentive latticework to stabilize the framework to the cast. Once again, if the removable partial denture is scheduled for a try-in after the setup, paint tinfoil substitute on the residual ridge prior to the addition of wax to the latticework, to allow removal of the framework with the teeth in place.

3. Adjust the incisal guide pin or centric holding device on a hinge articulator to open a space of approximately 1 mm between the teeth of the master cast and the positive tooth stops on the occlusal template (Fig. 12-51).

4. Position the first tooth distal to the remaining natural teeth. The mesial and ridge-lap areas of the denture tooth generally require considerable adjustment to bring them into intimate contact with the natural (stone) abutment tooth. Mark the latticework with a soft lead pencil or use articulating paper, and rub the denture tooth against the latticework (Fig. 12-52). The markings noted on the proximal and ridge-lap areas of the denture tooth may now be adjusted until intimate proximal contact results with the adjacent tooth (Fig. 12-53). The tooth may now be waxed into its proper position (Fig. 12-54). The template will guide proper buccolingual positioning. The occlusal surface of the denture tooth should be somewhat higher than the adjacent stone abutment tooth (Fig. 12-55).

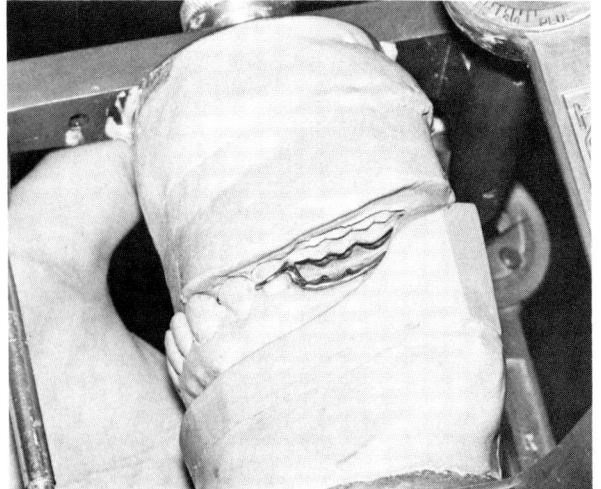

**Fig. 12-49.** Carefully examine mounting to ensure its accuracy.

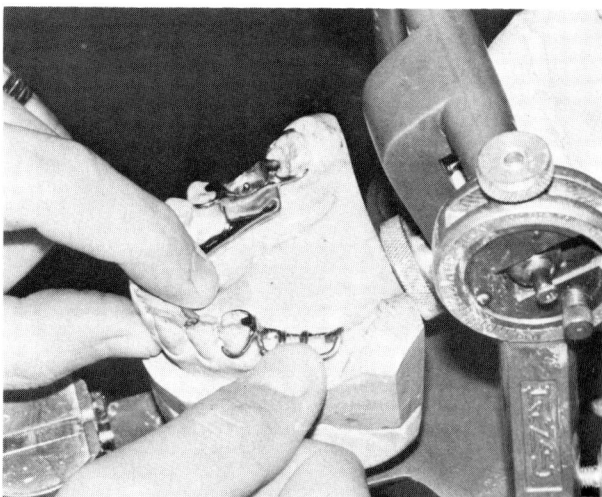

**Fig. 12-50.** Framework is reseated onto master cast and checked for accurate positioning.

## Selecting and arranging teeth

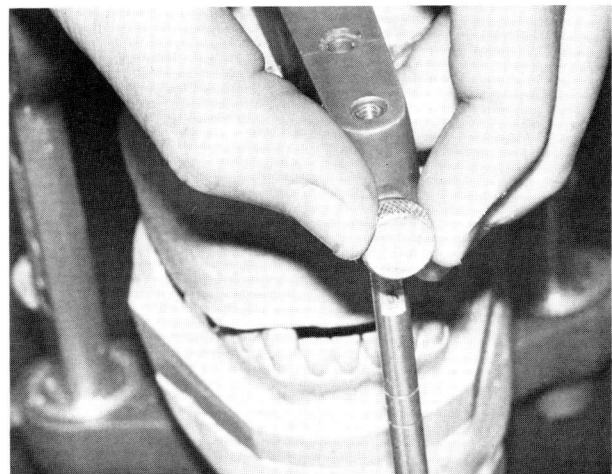

**Fig. 12-51.** Incisal guide pin is adjusted open 1 mm to provide space between master cast and template.

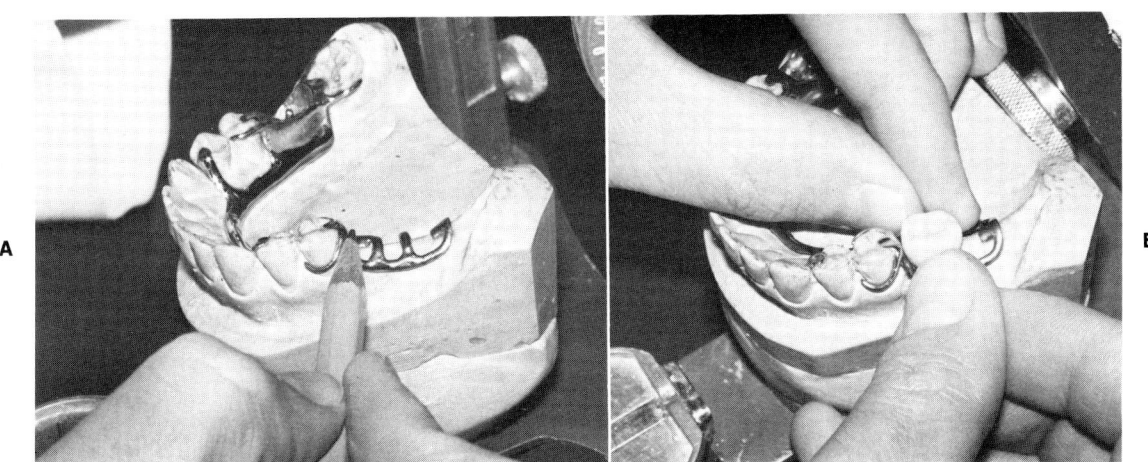

**Fig. 12-52. A,** Latticework is marked with soft lead pencil. **B,** Denture tooth is positioned and rubbed against latticework to mark areas needing adjustment.

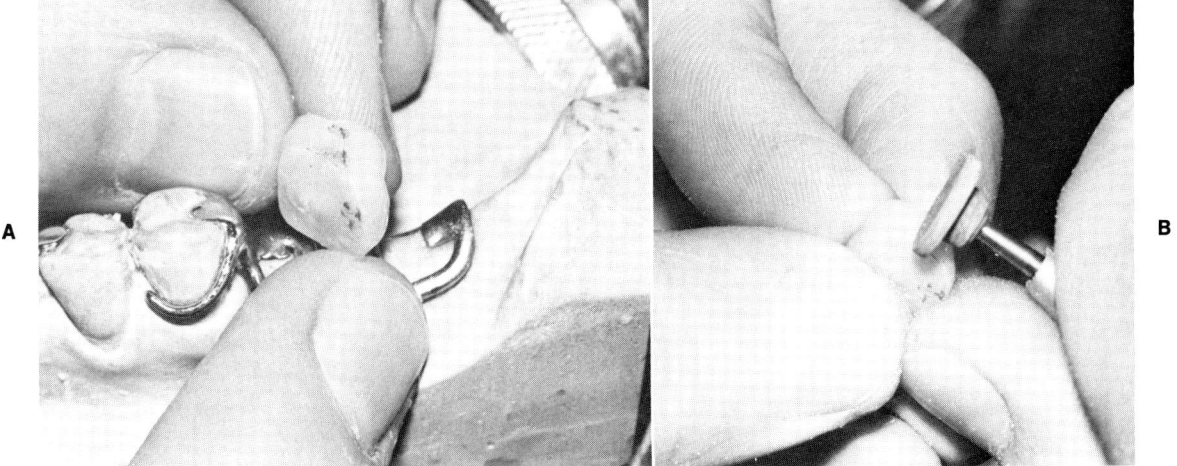

**Fig. 12-53. A,** Areas requiring adjustment are transferred from latticework to denture tooth. **B,** Denture tooth is adjusted only in areas indicated.

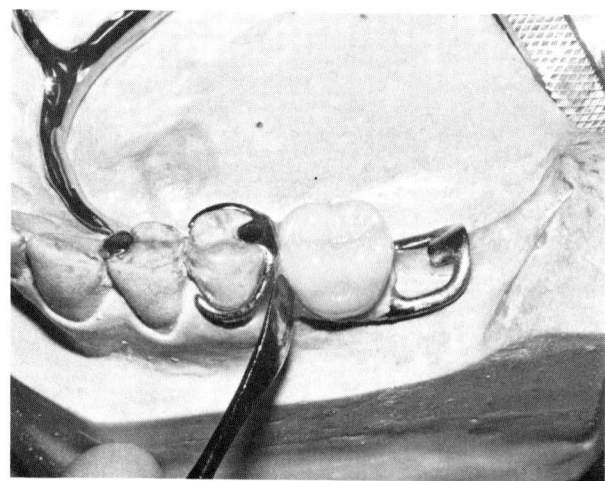

**Fig. 12-54.** Denture tooth is waxed to its proper position.

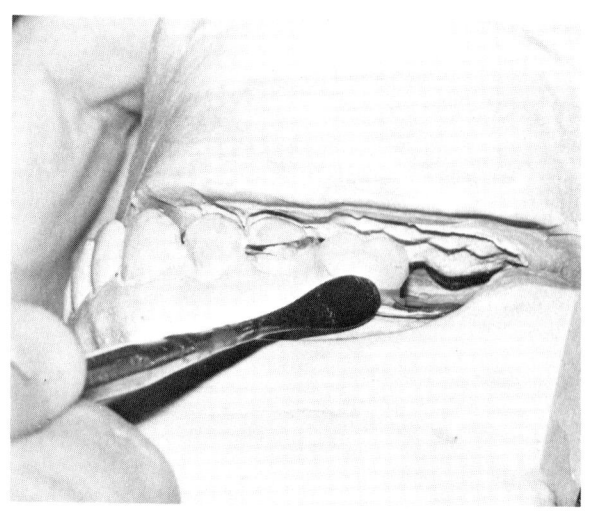

**Fig. 12-55.** Occlusal surface of denture tooth will be somewhat higher than adjacent stone abutment tooth.

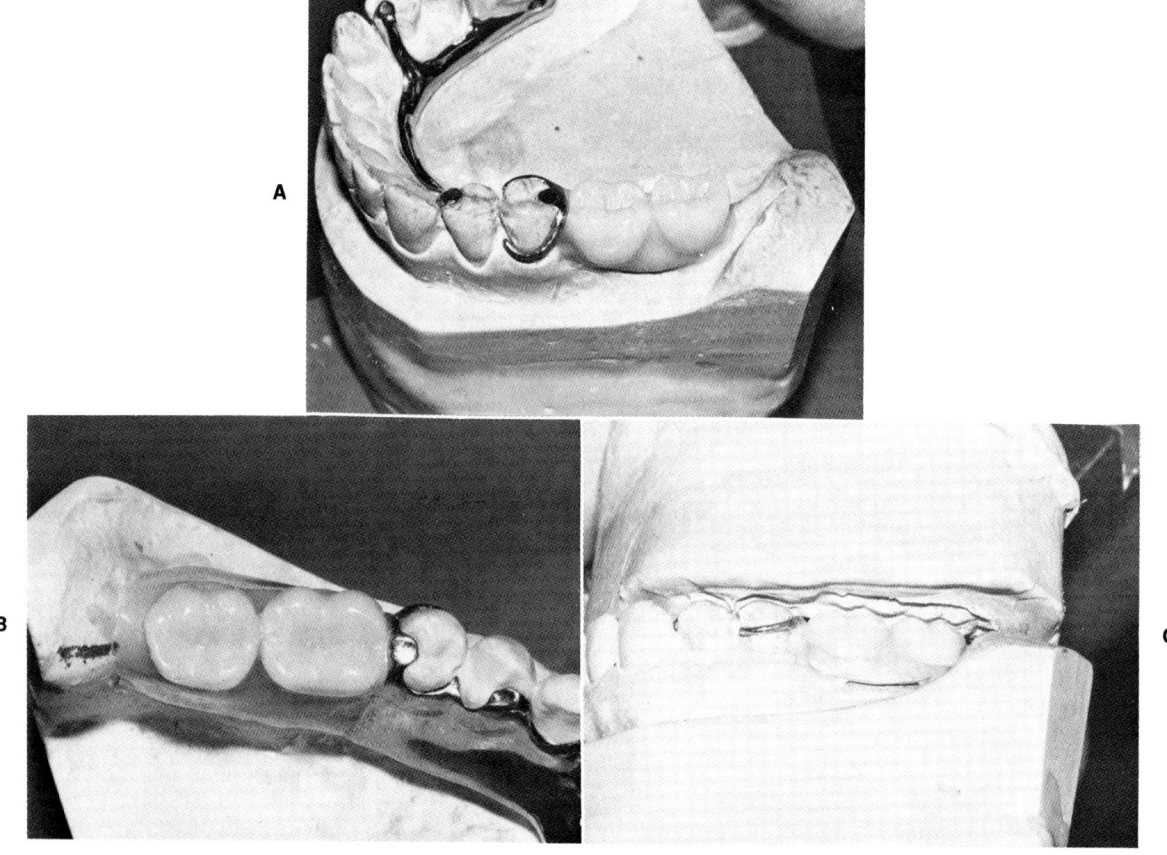

**Fig. 12-56. A,** Remaining teeth in arch are positioned and waxed to place. **B,** Correct buccolingual orientation is dictated by occlusal template. **C,** Denture teeth have been set in high occlusion. Note space between stone abutment teeth and template. Denture teeth are contacting template.

*Selecting and arranging teeth* **361**

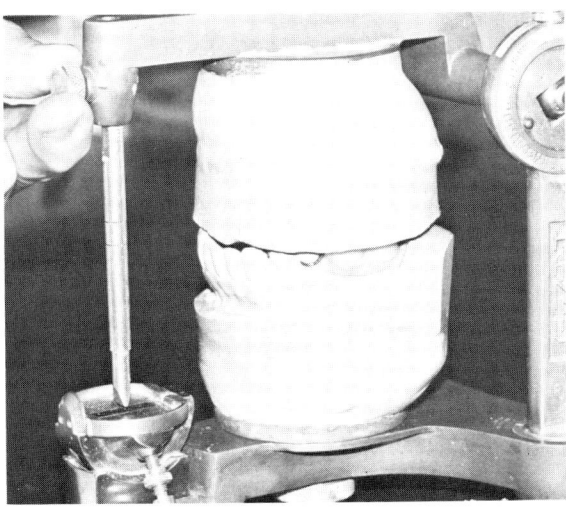

Fig. 12-57. Incisal guide pin is repositioned to neutral position. Note space between incisal guide pin and incisal guide table.

5. When proper positioning of the first tooth has been achieved, mark the ridge lap of the next tooth distally, and position it in its correct relationship.

6. Position the remaining teeth in the arch in the same manner (Fig. 12-56).

7. Reposition the pin on the articulator to the neutral position. There should now be 1 mm of space between the incisal pin and the incisal guide table (Fig. 12-57). Using articulating ribbon, rather than articulating paper, mark the areas of contact, and adjust the denture teeth until the pin contacts the table and the stone abutment teeth contact the occlusal template (Fig. 12-58). If articulating paper is used, there is a tendency for the material to build up on the template and provide inaccurate markings.

Fully balanced occlusion of the denture teeth is created on a hinge articulator by adjusting the artificial denture teeth for uniform contact with the occlusal template (Fig. 12-59). Because the template

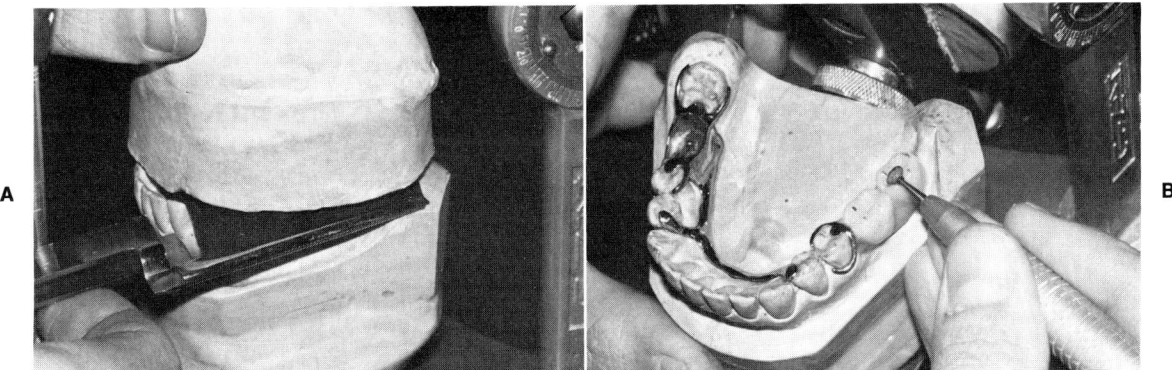

Fig. 12-58. **A,** Contact areas between denture teeth and template are marked with articulating ribbon. **B,** Denture teeth are adjusted until pin contacts table and stone abutment teeth contact template.

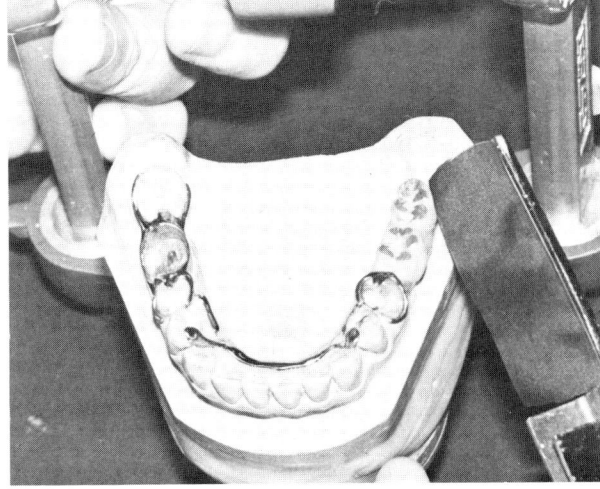

Fig. 12-59. Fully balanced occlusion is created when denture teeth have been adjusted for uniform contact with occlusal template. Notice large surface area of denture teeth in contact with occlusal template when denture teeth have been properly adjusted.

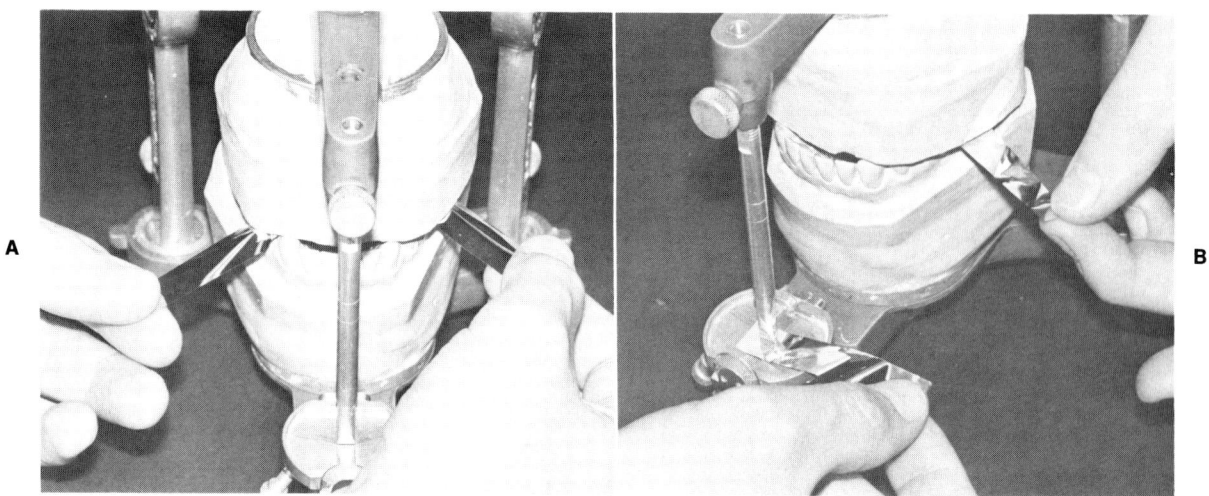

**Fig. 12-60. A,** After processing, occlusion is once again reestablished so that even occlusal contact exists between template and denture teeth and template with stone abutment teeth. **B,** At this time, incisal guide pin should also be in tight contact with incisal guide table.

was fabricated from a functionally generated path on the removable partial denture in the patient's mouth, this path represents all occlusal contacts in every position that the mandible achieves during function. The beauty of the functionally generated path concept of balancing occlusion is that the resultant denture teeth set to the template balance perfectly when placed in the patient's mouth because the contacts were dictated by the patient and not by a semiadjustable articulator, which *approximates* the patient's jaw motion.

8. After processing the removable partial denture, the master cast may be oriented to the mounting. The processing error may be corrected by once again adjusting the occlusion until contact of the template reaches the stone natural teeth of the master cast and the incisal guide pin contacts the incisal guide table (Fig. 12-60). When this has been accomplished, the removable partial denture will be in harmonious balance with the patient's natural dentition.

CHAPTER 13

# FLASKING, PROCESSING, DEFLASKING, AND FINISHING

KENNETH D. RUDD, ROBERT M. MORROW, and GEORGE KNIGHT

**deflasking** The procedures involved when retrieving the cured prosthesis from the investment and flask.
**finishing** Smoothing, contouring, and polishing procedures incident to completing the prosthesis.
**flasking** The act of investing a pattern in a flask. The process of investing the cast and a wax denture in a flask preparatory to molding the denture base material into the form of the denture.
**process** A series of operations that convert a wax pattern such as that of a denture base into a solid denture base of another material.

After the teeth have been set in the removable partial dentures, they may or may not be tried in the mouth. In either instance, the occlusion and arrangement of the teeth should be examined critically and adjusted if necessary (Fig. 13-1).

Usually in setting the teeth, especially if they are to be tried in the mouth, the wax in the denture base area is not extended to the peripheral roll on the cast in all areas. It is convenient if at sometime during the procedure, the outline of the denture base area is drawn on the cast. This will serve as a guide when the denture base areas are being waxed for flasking (Fig. 13-2).

Some prefer to mark the outline by beading it. A sharp instrument may be used to scrape the cast over the outline of the denture base. This bead will be transferred to the acrylic resin when it is processed and can be used as a guide when trimming the acrylic resin (Fig. 13-3).

Special attention should be given to the anatomy of the wax-up before the partial dentures are flasked. A great amount of finishing time can be saved if the contours and extensions are waxed exactly the way the denture base should look when finished. The exception to this is at the finish lines on the partial denture. They should be slightly overwaxed to permit finishing precisely to the finish line and not have the metal more prominent than the plastic. The joint should have a smooth transition from the plastic to the metal (Fig. 13-4).

When the partial dentures are ready to invest, give them another thorough examination to determine if all defects in the wax have been corrected and the contours are proper (Fig. 13-5). Reexamine the occlusion, and make any necessary adjustments before the casts are removed from the articulator (Fig. 13-6). If the mounting procedure was accomplished accurately and carefully, the casts will separate cleanly from the mounting, and the grooves will be smooth and uniform (Fig. 13-7).

If dirt or carbon paper marks are on the denture teeth, they may be removed by wiping them with cotton saturated with chloroform (Fig. 13-8). *Caution:* Use the liquid sparingly, especially on plastic teeth.

Even though the bases of the casts were painted with a separating medium* when they were mounted on the articulator, they should be given another uniform coating so they will separate read-

---
*Super-Sep, Kerr Manufacturing Co., Romulus, Mich.

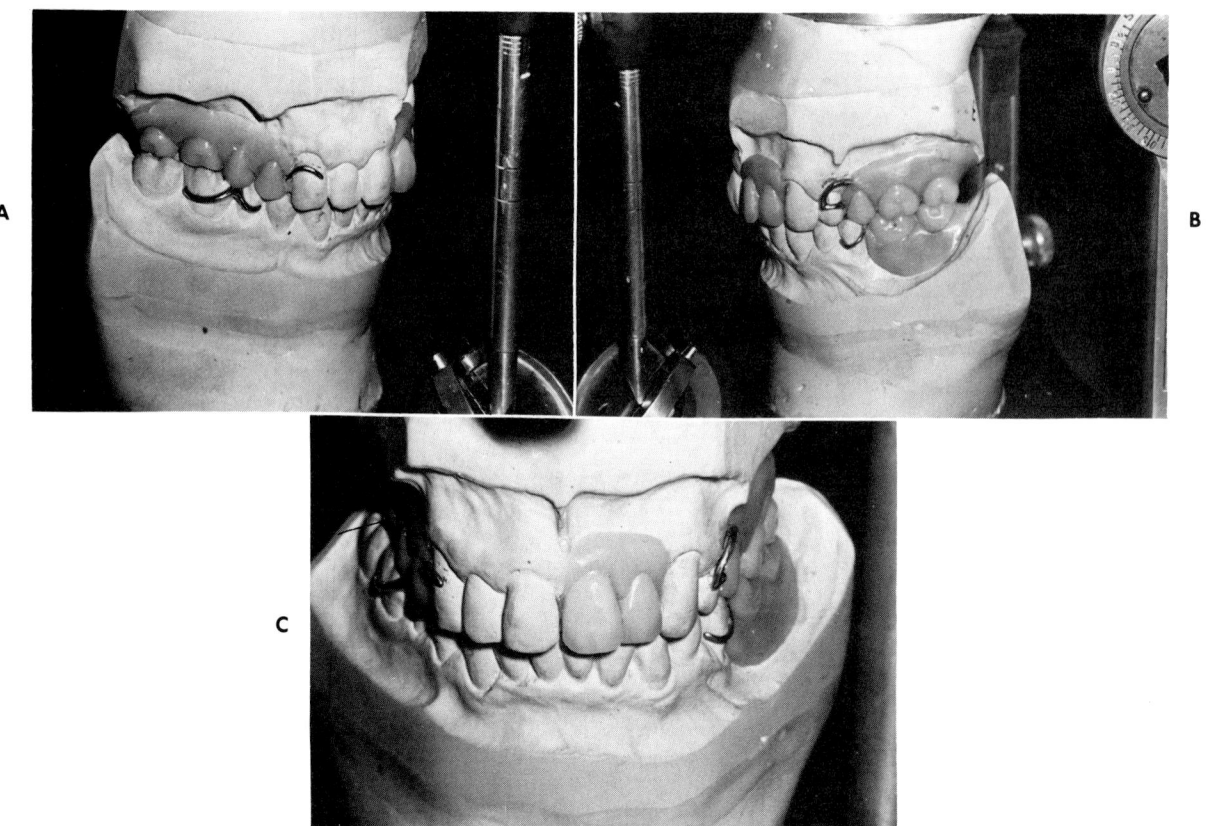

**Fig. 13-1.** When teeth have been set, partial dentures may or may not be tried in mouth. Either way, occlusion should be examined carefully and readjusted if necessary. **A,** Right side. **B,** Left side. **C,** Anterior view.

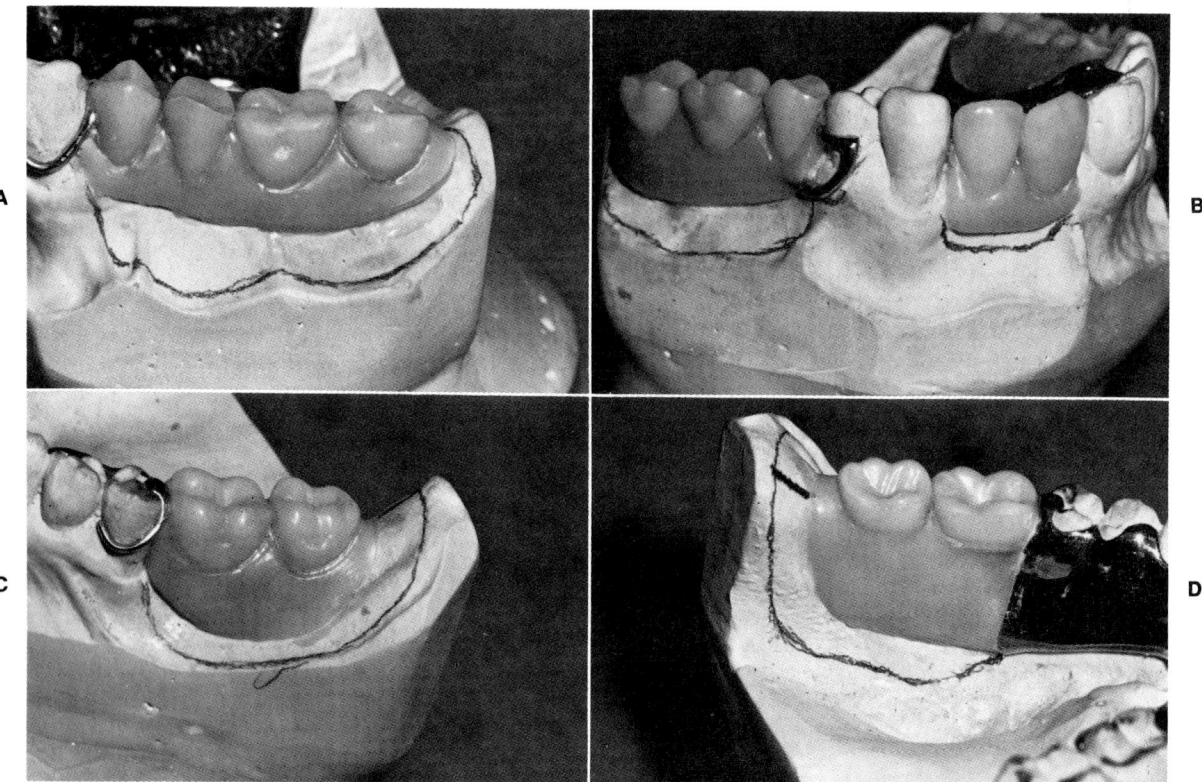

**Fig. 13-2.** Outline of extent of denture base makes it more convenient to wax to proper outline. **A,** Maxillary right side. **B,** Maxillary left side. **C,** Mandibular facial side. **D,** Mandibular lingual side.

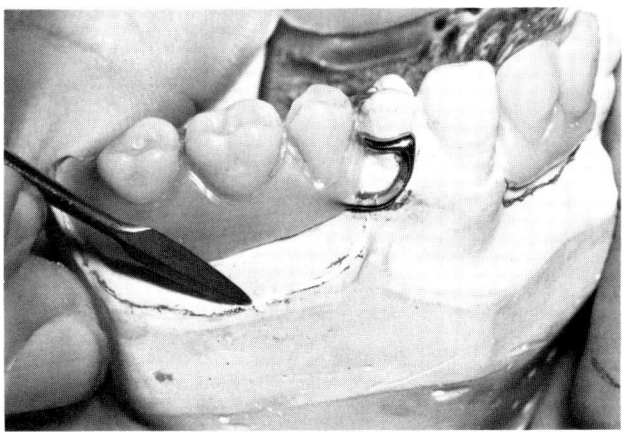

**Fig. 13-3.** Some prefer to bead cast at outlined border. This beading will be transferred to acrylic to act as guide in trimming.

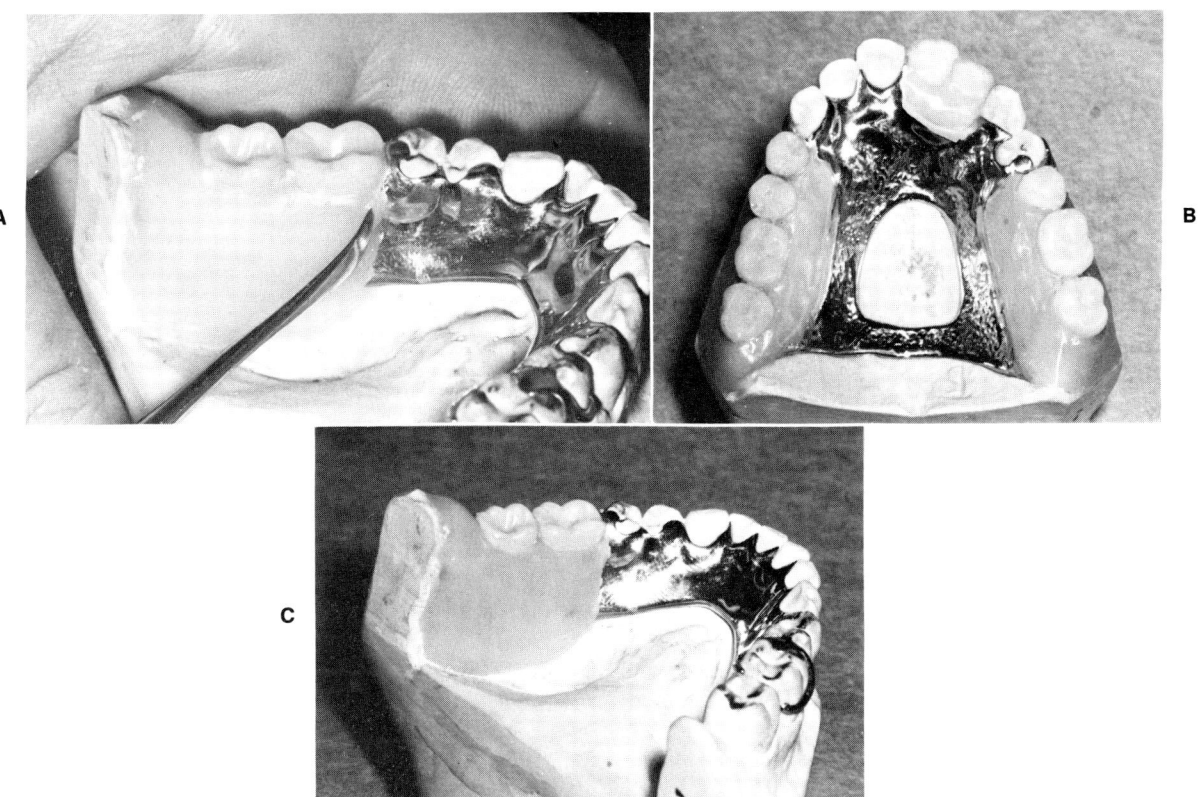

**Fig. 13-4. A,** Overwax denture base slightly at finish lines to allow for finishing and polishing acrylic resin. **B,** Finish lines on maxillary partial denture. **C,** Finish lines on mandibular partial denture.

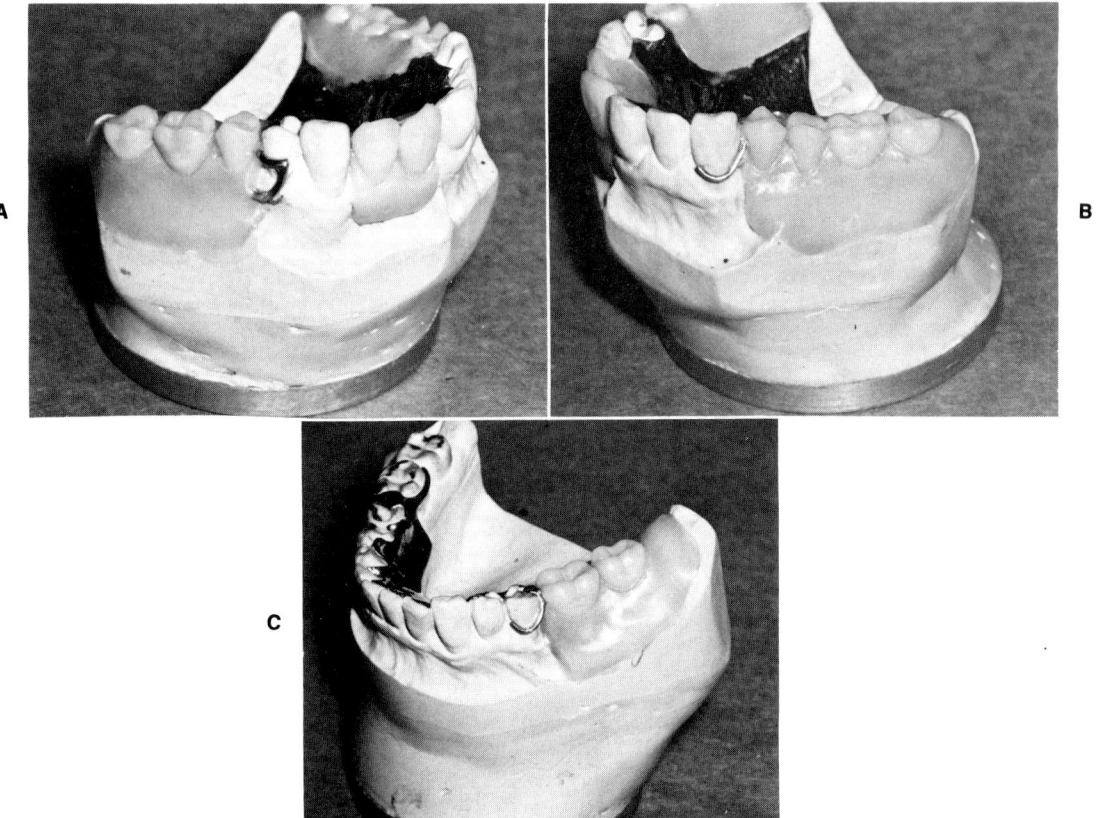

**Fig. 13-5.** Maxillary partial denture ready to invest. **A,** Left side. **B,** Right side. **C,** Mandibular partial denture ready to invest.

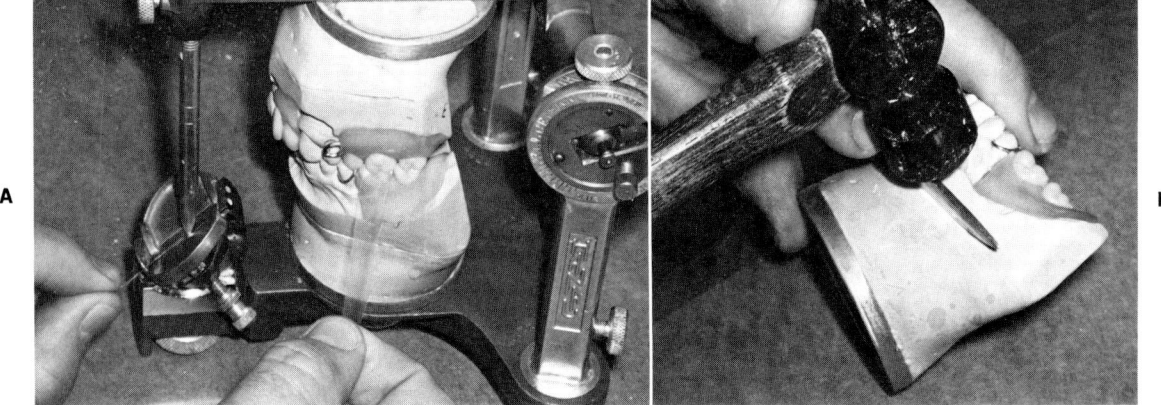

**Fig. 13-6. A,** Carefully reexamine occlusion and make any necessary adjustments. **B,** Remove cast from its mounting.

*Flasking, processing, deflasking, and finishing* **367**

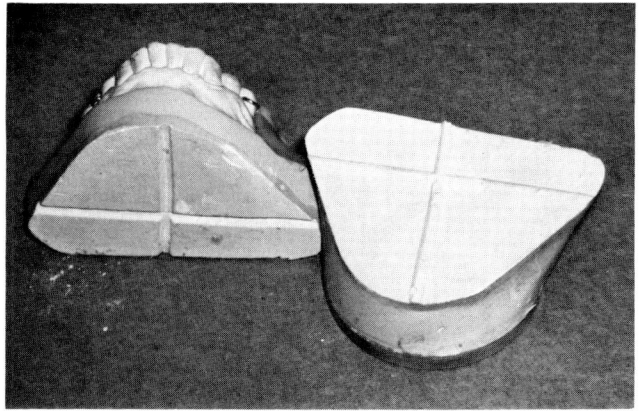

**Fig. 13-7.** If cast was carefully indexed and mounted, its base will be smooth, and grooves will be uniform when separated.

ily from the investing stone. The bases should be soaked in slurry water for a few minutes to prevent the cast from dehydrating the investing stone and leaving a soft area adjacent to the cast that will be easily compressed during packing (Fig. 13-9).

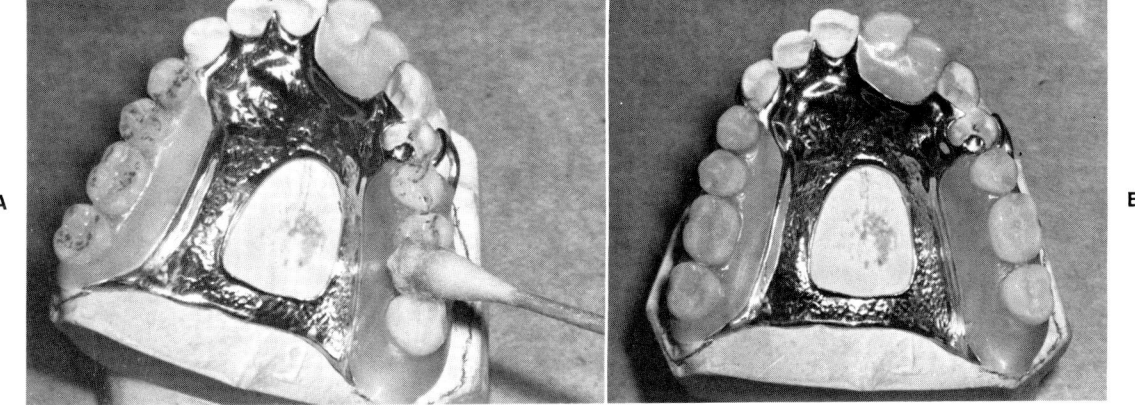

**Fig. 13-8. A,** If carbon paper marks are on denture teeth, they may be removed with cotton-tipped applicator dipped in chloroform. **B,** Teeth are easily cleaned.

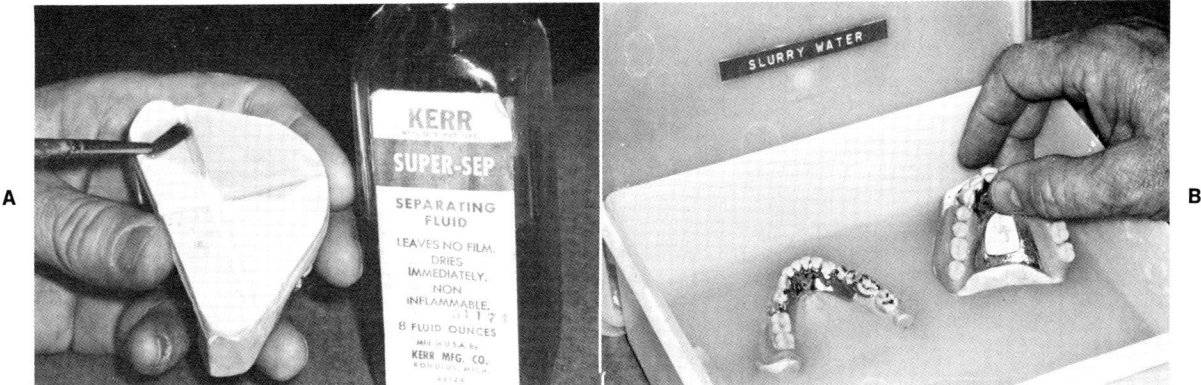

**Fig. 13-9. A,** Base of cast is painted with Super-Sep. **B,** Bases are soaked in slurry water.

## FLASKING

Flasking is investing the removable partial denture in dental stone for processing a resin denture base on it. It is done as follows in four steps:

1. Half flasked in lower half
2. Framework covered to eliminate undercuts
3. Upper half flasked
4. Stone cap

The first step is the same as for flasking a complete denture (Morrow et al., 1980). The base is painted with a gypsum separating medium, and the cast with the partial denture on it is seated in the lower half of the flask with the investing stone level with the land area of the cast (Fig. 13-10) (150 gm of Hydrocal is usually sufficient). It is important that there be at least 15 mm clearance between the occlusal surfaces of the teeth on the cast and the top of the upper half of the flask. This is another reason why it is important to control the thickness of the cast at the time it is poured. If the cast is so thick that it must be thinned in order to flask it properly, the indices on the base of the cast will be lost and the cast cannot be remounted for correction of occlusal errors after processing.

When the first investment has set, the surface of the stone and the entire surface of the master cast, except for the wax and artificial teeth, are painted with the gypsum separating medium (Fig. 13-11). NOTE: It is critical not to allow the separating medium to contact the wax or artificial teeth because the color will be transferred to the acrylic resin.

The flask should be soaked in slurry water for a few minutes before the second investing coating of dental stone is added (Fig. 13-12). The second mix of Hydrocal should be the same as the first mix, 150 gm of powder. Follow the manufacturer's directions for the water-power ratio. Form it over the master cast and metal framework, covering everything but

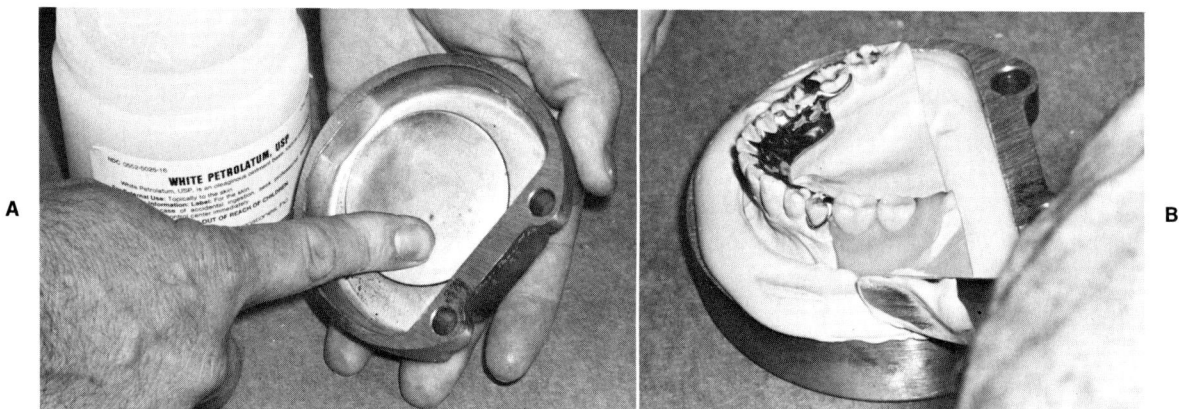

Fig. 13-10. **A,** Lubricate flasks lightly with petroleum jelly. **B,** Cast seated in stone in lower half of flask.

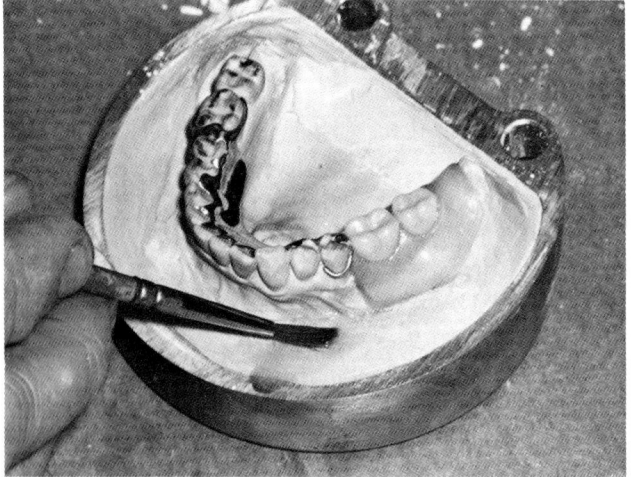

Fig. 13-11. After stone has set, trim it level with rim of flask, taper it to land of cast, and paint all exposed stone surfaces in this portion of flask with Super-Sep.

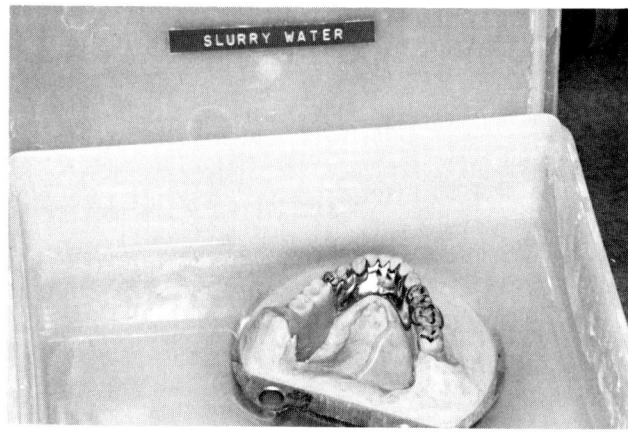

Fig. 13-12. Soak half-flasked partial denture in slurry water for a few minutes.

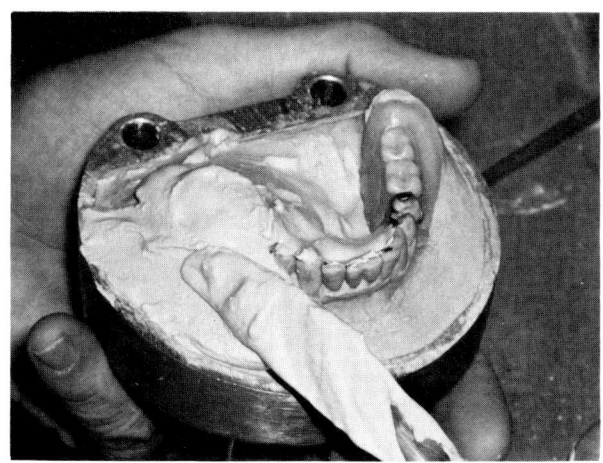

Fig. 13-13. Apply stone mix to cover cast and metal framework. Do not cover wax or artificial denture teeth.

the waxed denture base and artificial teeth (Fig. 13-13). It is essential that this second mix be contoured so that no undercuts are created in a vertical direction (Fig. 13-14). Sharp angles should be avoided. When the third pour or cope is made, there should be no thin projections of stone that may fracture during the boilout or packing procedure. There should be at least 7 mm clearance between the top of the second mix and the top of the upper half of the flask. The edges of the second mix should end even with the rim of the lower half of the flask.

After the second pour sets, trim it with a knife to accentuate the taper. If there are still slight undercuts or the taper is too steep, a thin layer of wax may be flowed into and over them (Fig. 13-15). Paint the stone with a separating medium, and soak it in slurry water a few minutes (Fig. 13-16). *Caution:* Do not permit the separating medium to touch the wax or artificial teeth.

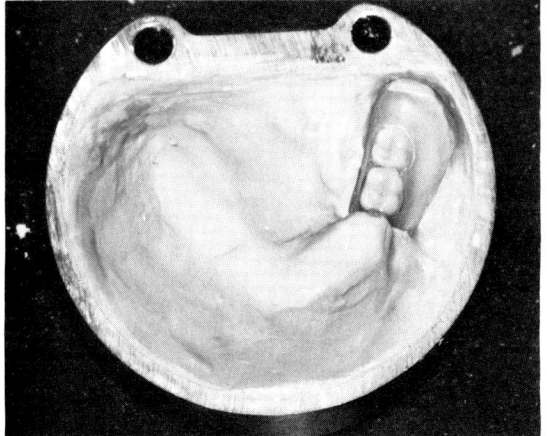

Fig. 13-14. Edges of second pour should taper to inner edge of flask.

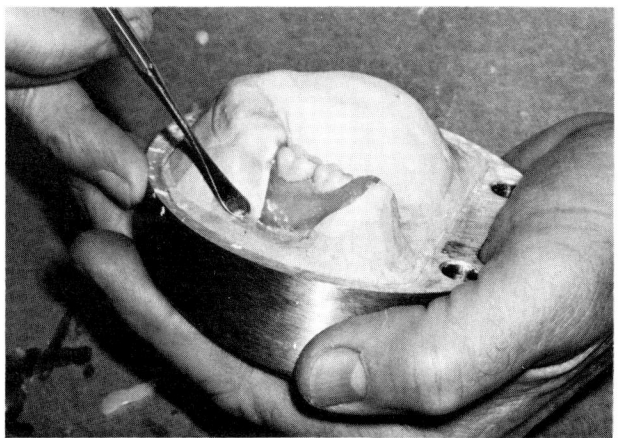

Fig. 13-15. When second pour sets, trim it to accentuate and smooth the taper. If undercuts remain or angle is too steep, thin layer of baseplate wax is flowed over them.

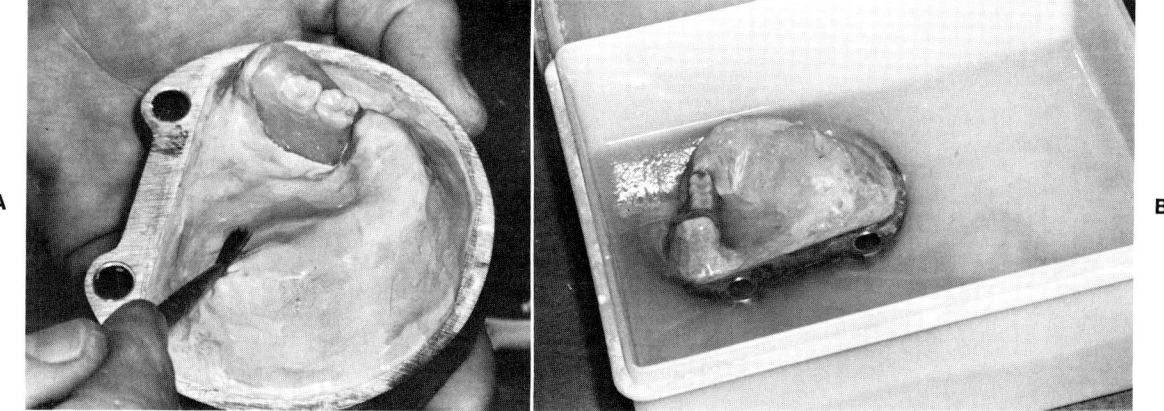

Fig. 13-16. **A,** Paint stone with Super-Sep. **B,** Soak it in slurry water for a few minutes.

Paint surface tension reducer* on the surface of the wax and teeth to permit the next layer of stone to adapt more closely to them (Fig. 13-17). The third investment of stone (150 gm of powder) is accomplished in the same way as the second layer in complete denture flasking (Morrow et al., 1980). The upper half of the flask is positioned. Make sure that it is completely seated. The stone mix is vibrated into the flask and filled just short of the top rim (Fig. 13-18). The occlusal surfaces of the plastic teeth are uncovered, and the soft stone is shaped to form a concavity (Fig. 13-19). The fourth or final mix will be poured into this. The surface of the concavity should be left slightly roughened and/or small undercuts may be cut into the surface after the third pour has set (Fig. 13-20). This is necessary to prevent the lid from accidentally coming off during the packing procedure.

Gypsum separating medium is painted on the set surface of the third mix, avoiding contact with the exposed surfaces of the artificial teeth (Fig. 13-21). Slurry water is added to the concavity (Fig. 13-22). After soaking for several minutes, the slurry water is poured off, and the fourth mix of stone (100 gm of powder) is vibrated into the flask until filled (Fig. 13-23). Press the top of the flask into position (Fig.

---

*Debubblizer, Kerr Manufacturing Co., Romulus, Mich., or equivalent.

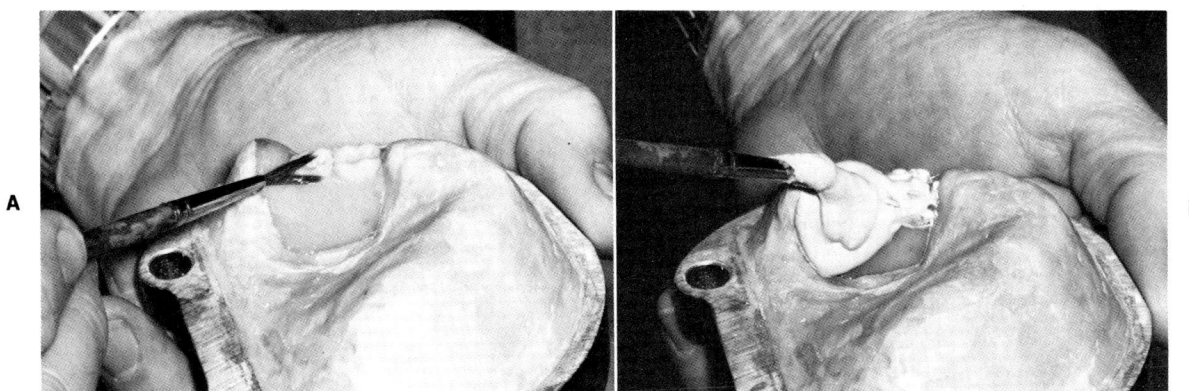

**Fig. 13-17. A,** Paint artificial teeth and wax with surface tension reducer. **B,** Apply layer of stone over wax and denture teeth with brush.

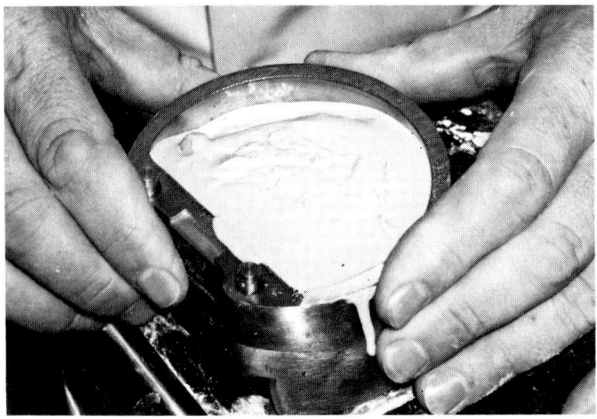

**Fig. 13-18.** Vibrate stone mix into flask and fill it just short of top rim.

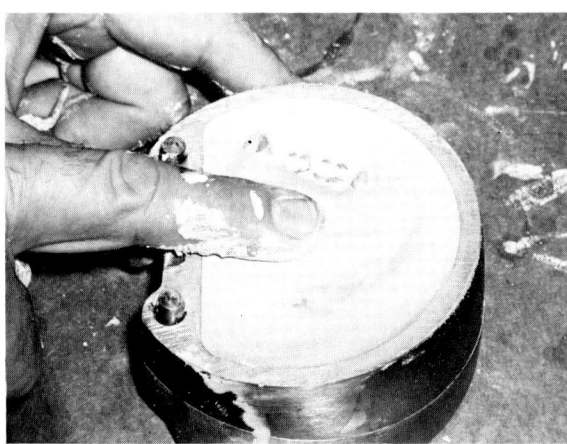

**Fig. 13-19.** Uncover occlusal surfaces of artificial teeth and second investment. Soft stone is shaped to form concavity.

## Flasking, processing, deflasking, and finishing 371

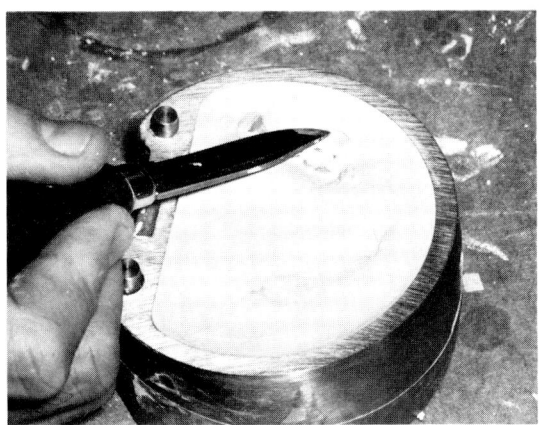

**Fig. 13-20.** Surface is left slightly roughened, and small undercuts are cut into third pour when it sets.

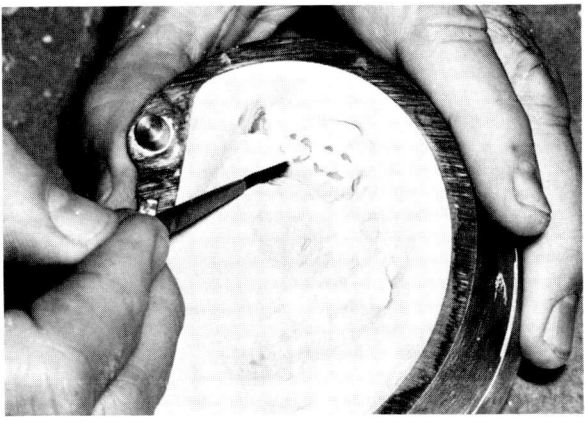

**Fig. 13-21.** Paint surface with Super-Sep. Avoid getting it on artificial teeth.

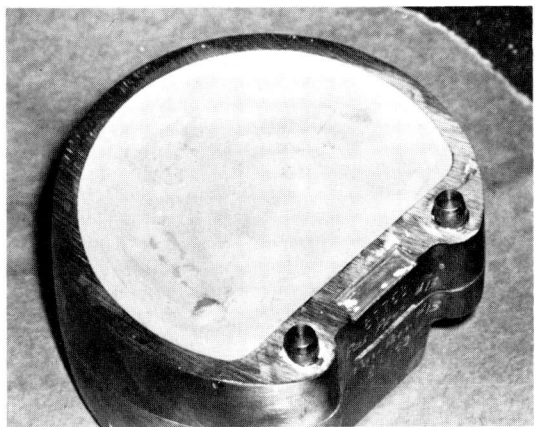

**Fig. 13-22.** Add slurry water to concavity and soak for several minutes.

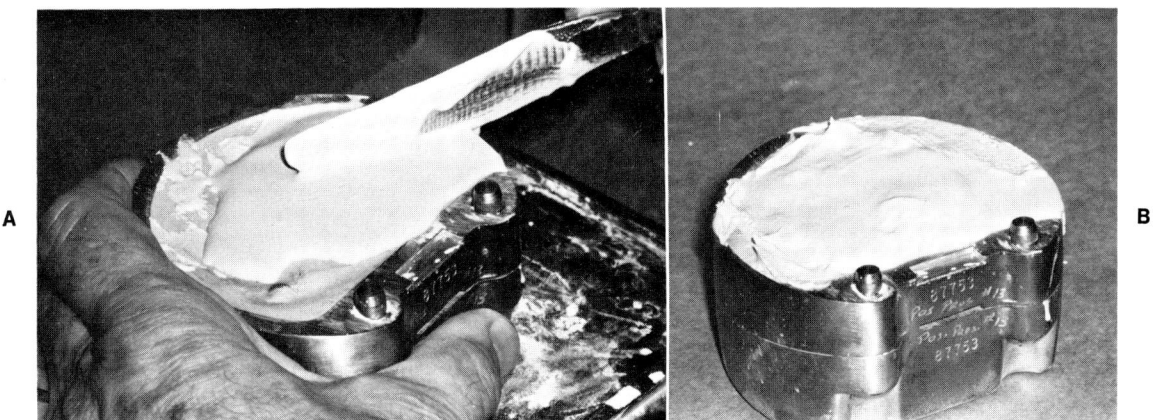

**Fig. 13-23. A,** Pour slurry water off, and vibrate stone mix in top. **B,** Overfill flask slightly.

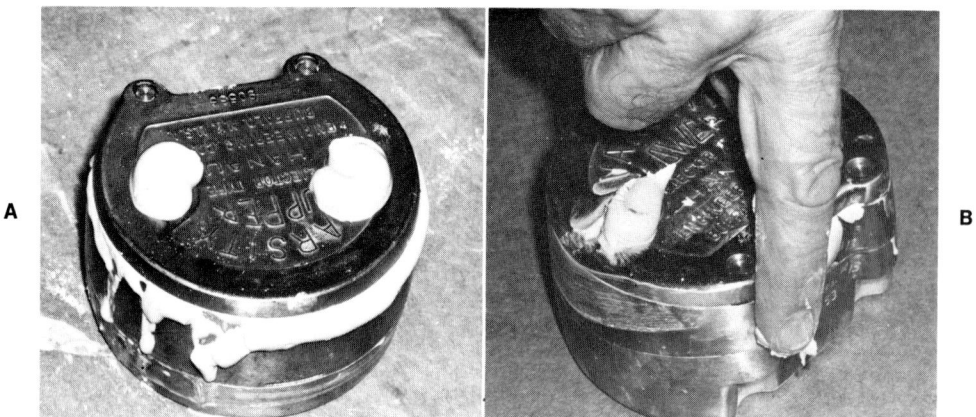

**Fig. 13-24. A,** Press top of flask in position. **B,** Remove excess stone around sides with fingers.

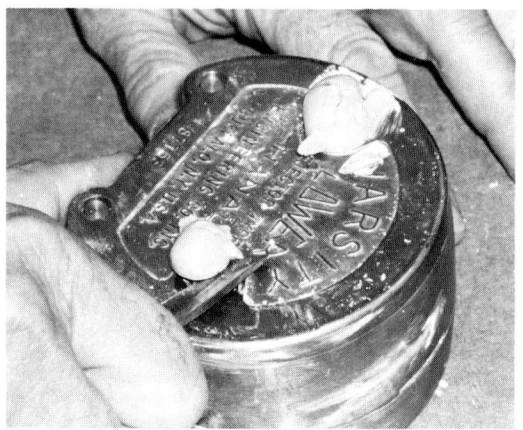

**Fig. 13-25.** Remove any remaining excess from flask after mix has set.

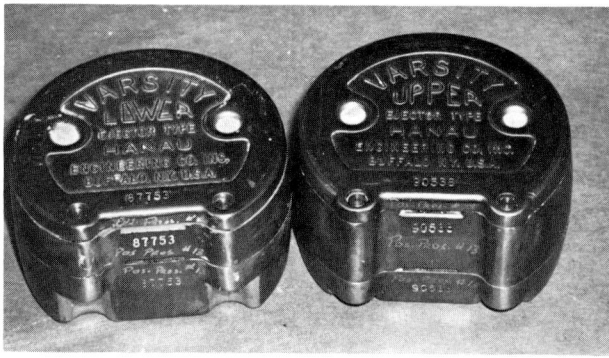

**Fig. 13-26.** Cleaned flasks. Do not start wax elimination procedure until at least 1 hour has elapsed from time of fourth pour.

13-24). After the stone has set, remove any remaining excess with a knife (Fig. 13-25). Permit the flask to set for a minimum of 1 hour before wax elimination is begun (Fig. 13-26).

### PROBLEM AREAS

The principal problems associated with flasking include failure to properly trim the cast to assure proper thickness, not eliminating undercuts in flasking stone, and forgetting to paint the stone with separating medium before adding the next mix (Table 13-1).

### Wax elimination

If the wax elimination procedure is delayed beyond the hour or so required for the stone to set, the flask should be soaked in room-temperature water at least 1 hour before the boilout procedure is started (Fig. 13-27). The procedure for wax elimination is exactly the same as for complete dentures (Morrow et al., 1980). The flask is placed in boiling water for 5 minutes (Fig. 13-28). The flask is pried open carefully and separated in a vertical direction to prevent breaking the stone investment (Fig. 13-29). Remove as much wax as possible with a knife or spatula (Fig. 13-30). The remaining wax is

## Table 13-1. Flasking

| Problem | Probable cause | Solution |
| --- | --- | --- |
| Cast too high when placed in flask | Cast base is too thick | Trim base to provide 15 mm clearance between occlusal surfaces of teeth and top of upper flask (cope) |
| Flask halves cannot be separated after boilout | Stone undercuts present preventing separation<br>Separating medium not applied | Contour investing stone to eliminate undercuts<br>Paint stone surfaces with separating medium before pouring |
| Investing stone fractures on separating flasks | See above | See above; after boilout separate flask halves in straight upward direction using prying instrument in each slot |

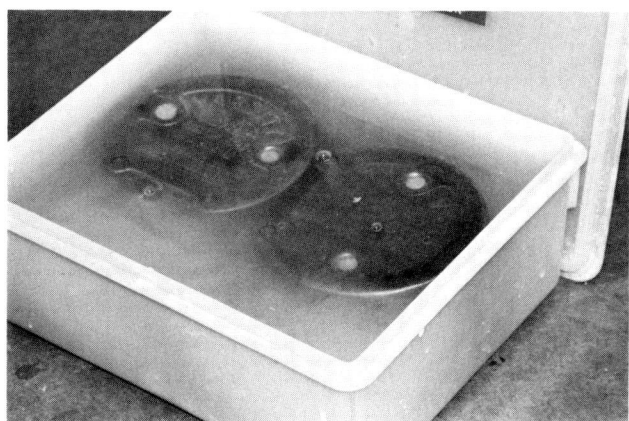

Fig. 13-27. Soak flask in water for at least 1 hour if wax elimination procedure has been delayed.

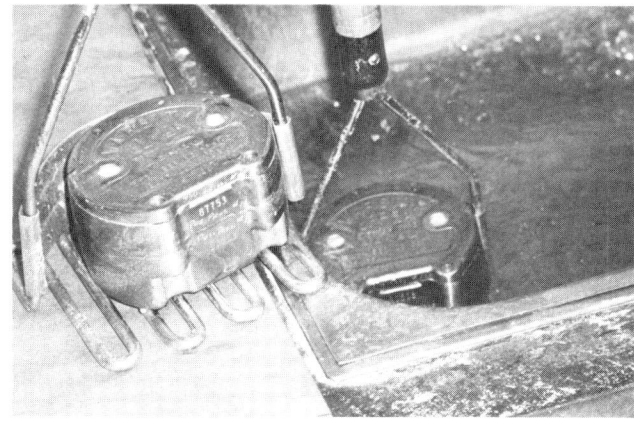

Fig. 13-28. Flask is placed in boiling water for 5 minutes.

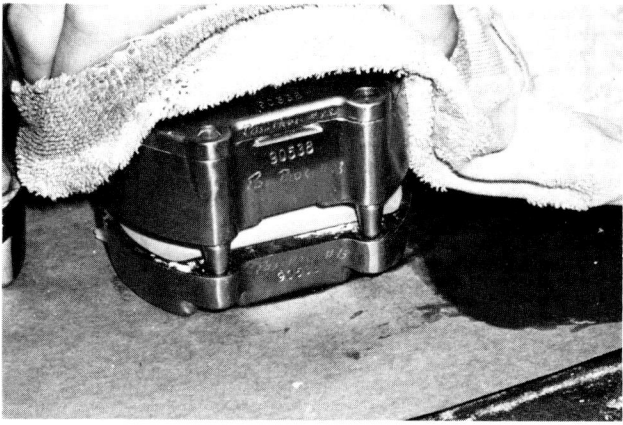

Fig. 13-29. Flask is pried open carefully and removed in vertical direction.

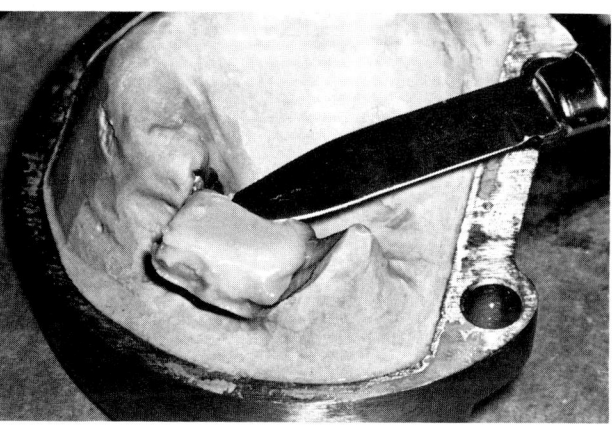

Fig. 13-30. Remove bulk of wax with knife or spatula.

flushed out with boiling water (Fig. 13-31). Use a soft brush and detergent to clean thoroughly both halves of the flask (Fig. 13-32). Clean under the acrylic resin retention struts thoroughly. Finally, flush the molds well with clean boiling water. Place both halves of the flask on end for several minutes to allow the water to drain completely (Fig. 13-33). Trim thin stone investment edges with a sharp blade to prevent the stone from breaking during packing and mixing with the acrylic resin (Fig. 13-34). When the flasks stop steaming but are still quite warm, grind diatorics in plastic denture teeth, remove the debris, and apply a coating of tinfoil substitute.*

A good method of ensuring that plastic artificial denture teeth are locked firmly to the denture base is to provide mechanical retention in the base of the tooth. This is done by cutting a small undercut hole in the tooth using a No. 6 round bur. The hole should not be too deep because the pink denture base resin may show through the denture tooth (Fig. 13-35). Permit the flasks to cool until they can be handled comfortably, then a second coating of tinfoil substitute may be added. It is essential that a smooth and solid coating of tinfoil substitute be applied to prevent the stone from adhering to the resin during processing. The ridge-lap areas of the artificial teeth should not be painted, since this could prevent the acrylic resin denture base material from attaching securely to the teeth. Make sure that the area under the acrylic resin retention of the denture base is coated with tinfoil substitute (Fig. 13-36). When the flask is completely cool, it is ready for packing with acrylic resin.

*Al-Cote, The L. D. Caulk Co., Milford, Del., or equivalent.

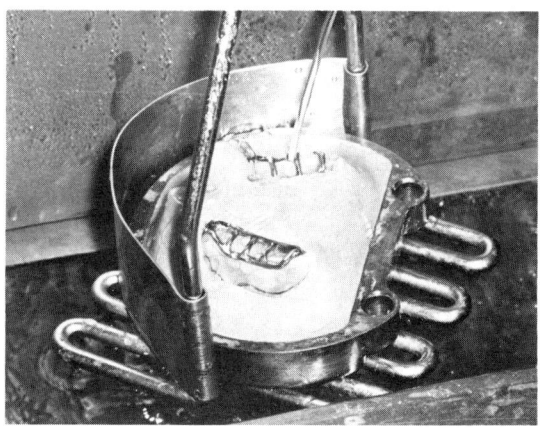

**Fig. 13-31.** Flush out remaining wax with boiling water.

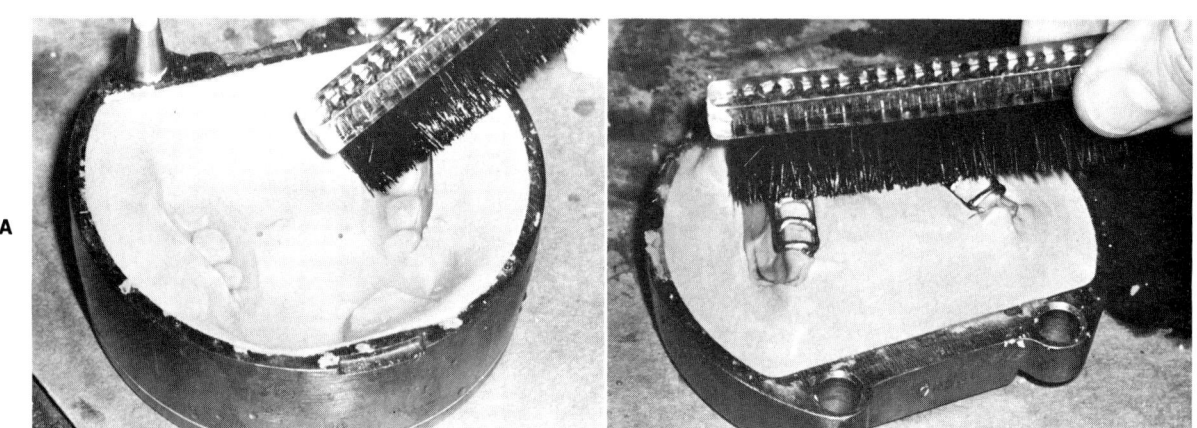

**Fig. 13-32.** Clean two halves of flask with soft brush and detergent. **A,** Top half. **B,** Bottom half.

## Flasking, processing, deflasking, and finishing 375

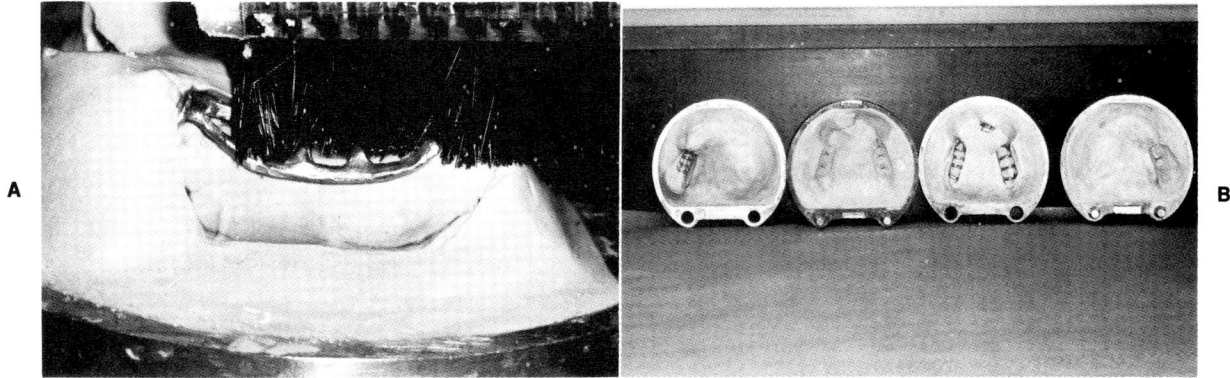

**Fig. 13-33. A,** Clean under resin retention lattice very thoroughly. **B,** Flasks on end to permit water to drain.

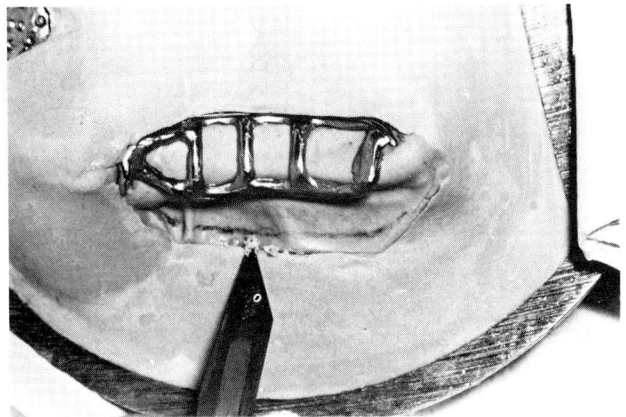

**Fig. 13-34.** Trim sharp stone edges with sharp blade.

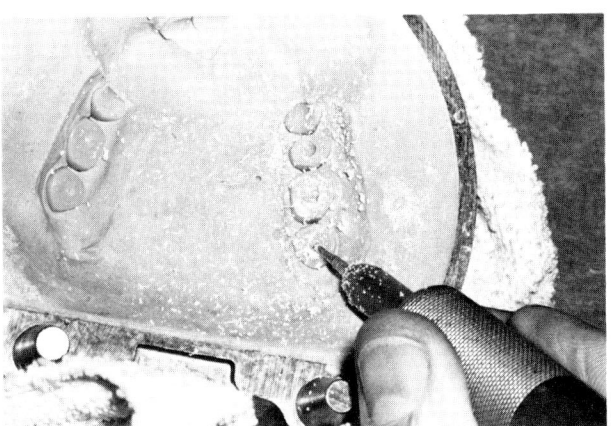

**Fig. 13-35.** Grind diatorics in plastic teeth.

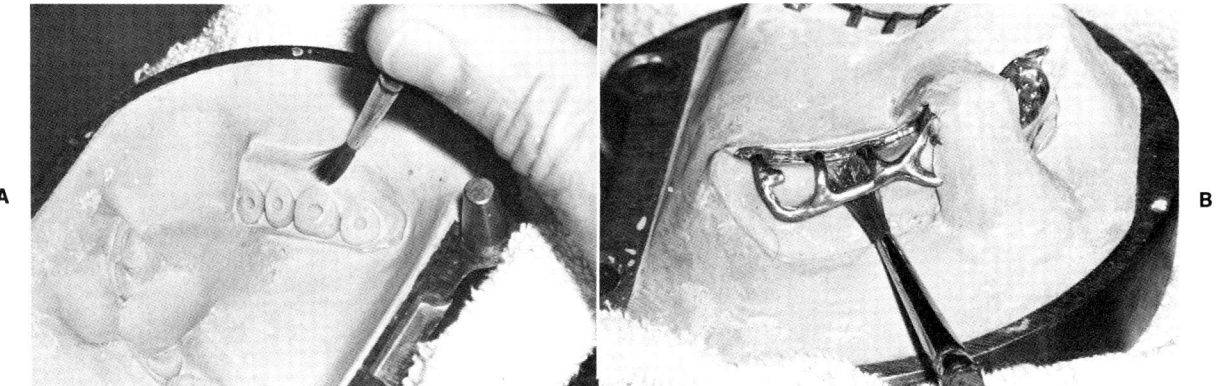

**Fig. 13-36.** Coat all of stone in both halves of flask with tinfoil substitute. **A,** Paint carefully around teeth to avoid excess puddling. **B,** Make sure that stone under retention framework is coated.

## Packing

If it is desired to characterize or stain the denture base, the procedure is the same as for complete dentures (Morrow et al., 1980). This is indicated usually when anterior teeth are being replaced by denture teeth on a denture base.

NOTE: When the master cast for a distal extension partial denture has been repaired or altered from a corrected cast impression, the tissue stop at the end of the retentive latticework usually will not be in contact with the underlying edentulous ridge. The closing pressure of the packing procedures may distort or depress the unsupported extension of the framework. To prevent this from happening during the flask closure, a small amount of self-curing resin should be sprinkled on or painted under the distal end of the latticework and allowed to set before the denture resin is packed.

Use a good acrylic resin such as Lucitone,* and add the powder to the liquid and stir for 30 seconds or until the powder is thoroughly wet (Fig. 13-37). Close the jar and allow it to set until the mix reaches a doughy stage, separates cleanly from the sides of the jar, and does not stick to the spatula. The mix should be checked periodically to test its progress. The time will vary depending on the brand of acrylic resin and the temperature of the room. The resin should not be handled with bare fingers either during the mixing or packing. If plastic gloves are not available, the material should be handled between plastic sheets that will be used during the trial packing procedure (Fig. 13-38). The oils from the hands contaminate the acrylic resin, and many people are allergic to the monomer, which may cause a contact dermatitis.

When the resin has reached the proper consistency, packing should be accomplished as quickly as possible. The main difference between packing a partial denture and a complete denture is that a "split-packing" technique is used for the partial denture. The framework is retained in the lower half of the flask and the teeth in the upper. If the conventional packing technique is used, when the flask is opened during the trial packing procedure, either the framework or the teeth could be dislodged. To prevent this from happening, split packing is done.

A small amount of acrylic resin dough is finger pressed through and around the latticework of the framework in the lower half of the flask and another portion of the mix is pressed against the teeth in the upper half of the flask (Fig. 13-39). A plastic sheet is placed over one half of the flask, and the flask is closed (Fig. 13-40). Place the flask in a press, and

---

*Lucitone denture base resin, The L. D. Caulk Co., Milford, Del.

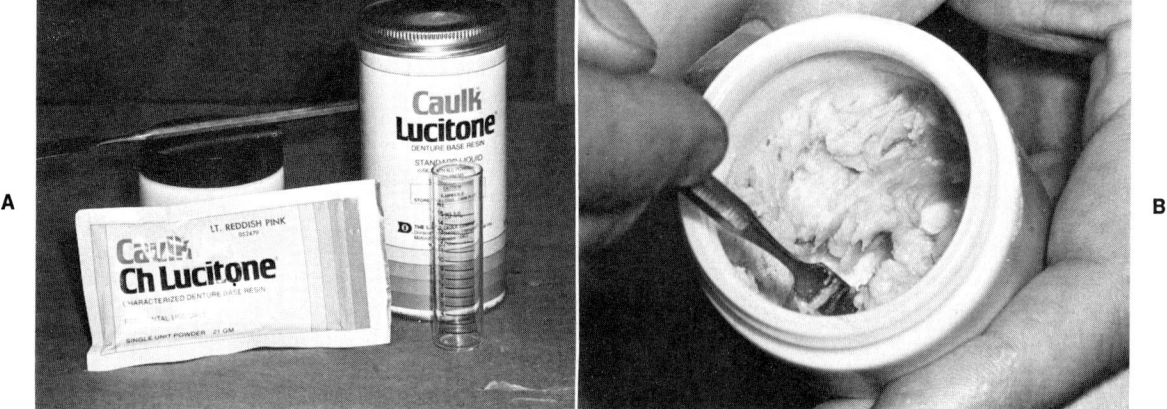

Fig. 13-37. **A,** Use good quality acrylic resin, and mix it in jar that can be sealed. **B,** Add powder to liquid and mix thoroughly.

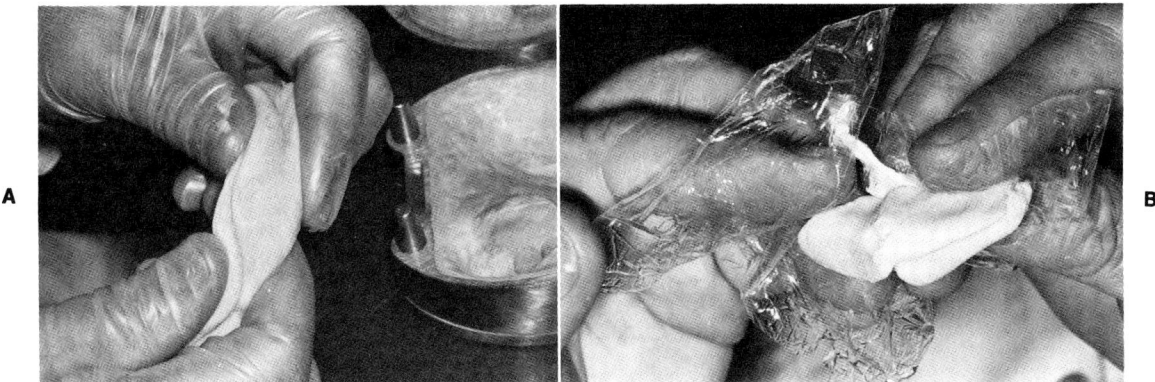

**Fig. 13-38.** Handle acrylic resin with plastic gloves **(A)** or plastic squares **(B)**. Do not touch it with bare fingers.

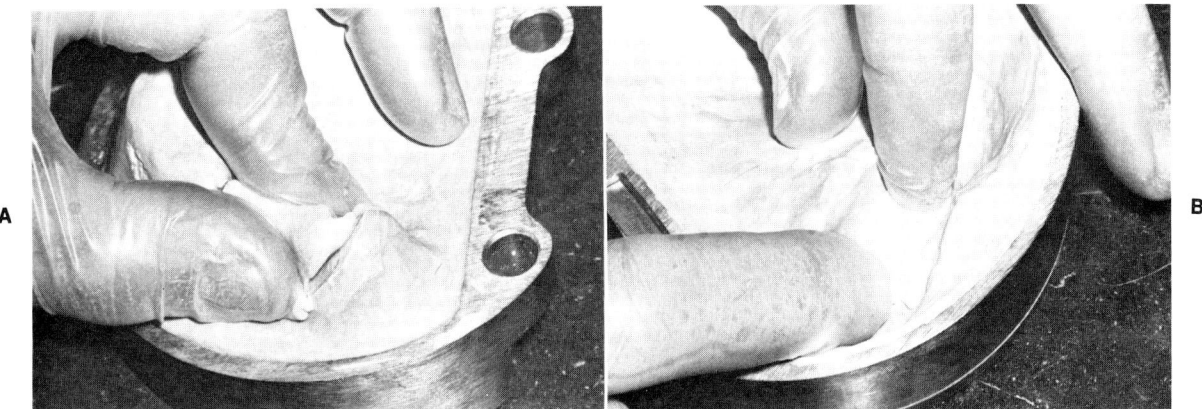

**Fig. 13-39. A,** Using finger pressure, pack dough around and under metal for acrylic retention. **B,** Force some around denture teeth in upper half of flask.

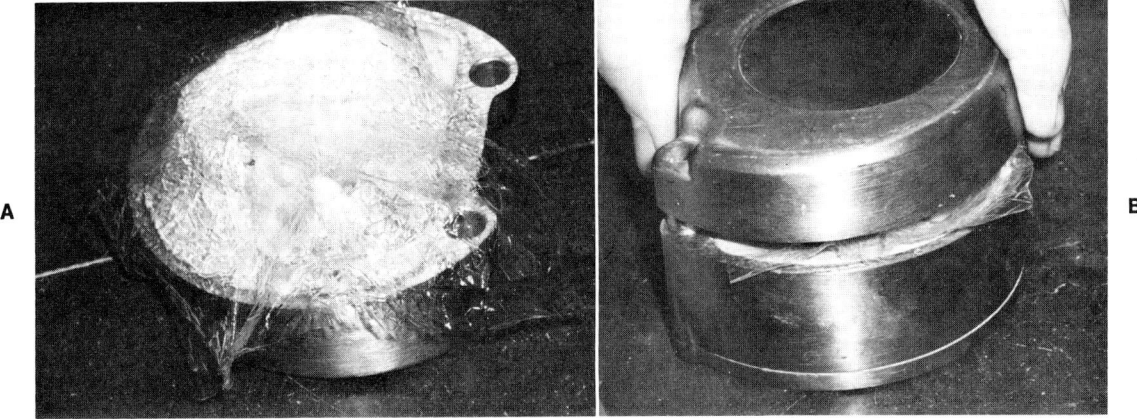

**Fig. 13-40. A,** Place plastic sheet between two halves of flask. **B,** Close flask.

**378** *Dental laboratory procedures: removable partial dentures*

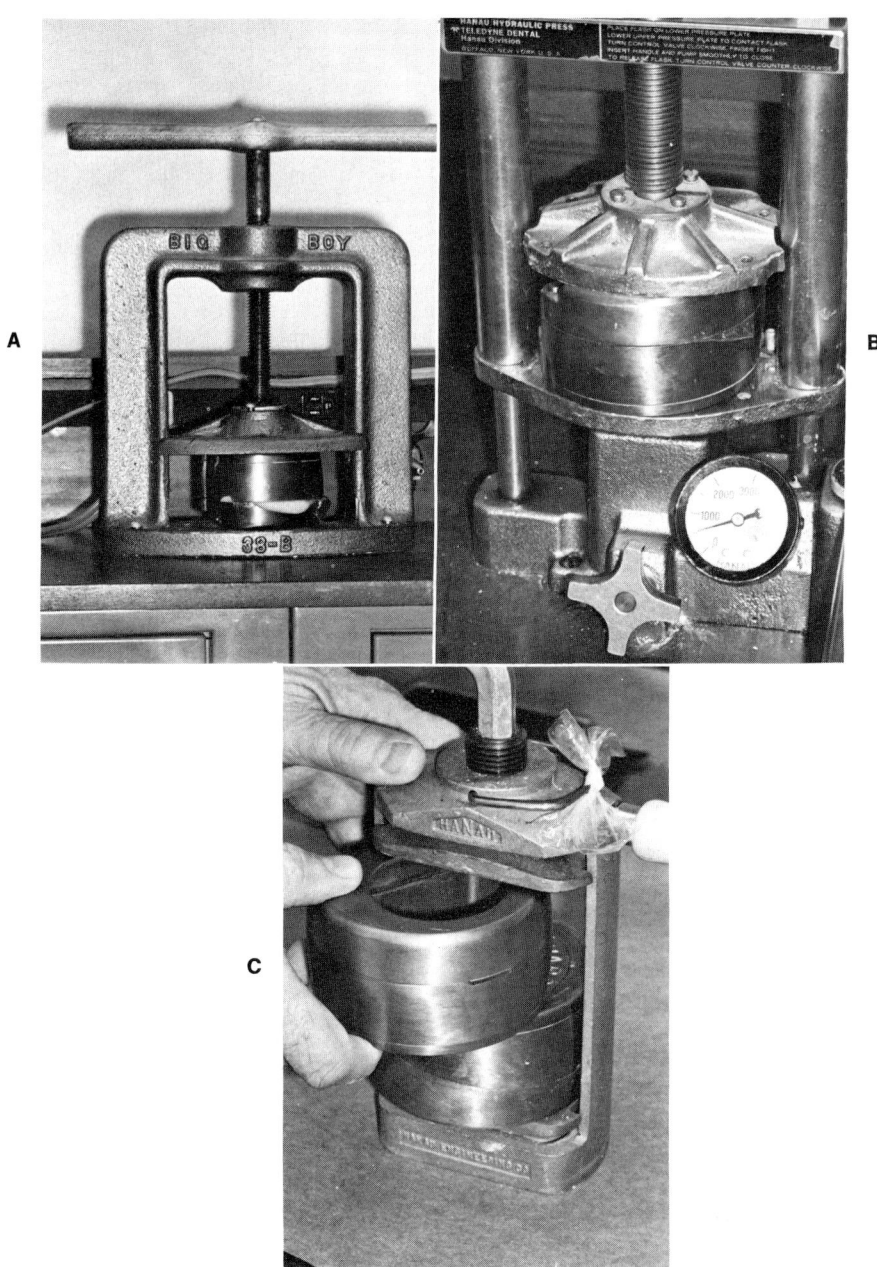

**Fig. 13-41.** Flask is placed in press and pressure applied slowly. **A,** Bench press. **B,** Pneumatic press. **C,** Empty flask may be used as spacer in flask press.

*Flasking, processing, deflasking, and finishing* **379**

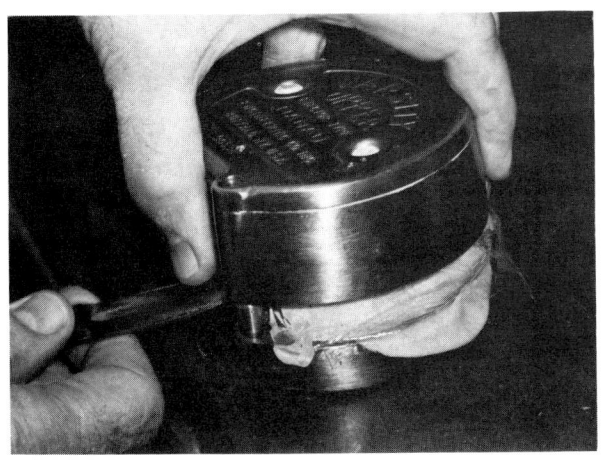

**Fig. 13-42.** When considerable resistance is felt in closing flask, remove it from press and open it.

apply pressure slowly to permit the resin to flow. An empty flask may be used as a spacer in the flask press (Fig. 13-41). When considerable resistance to closing the flask is encountered, release the press, and remove and open the flask (Fig. 13-42). If sufficient resin was used in each half of the flask, there will be a flash of acrylic resin around all margins of the denture base. Trim the flash with an instrument, replace the plastic sheet between the halves of the flask, and repeat the trial closure (Fig. 13-43). If flash was not present around all of the margins, add a small portion of resin to the deficient area. Repeat the trial packing until a minimal amount of flash is present. Remove the plastic sheet, wet the two surfaces of acrylic resin with monomer, and close the flask (Fig. 13-44). Tighten the flask press com-

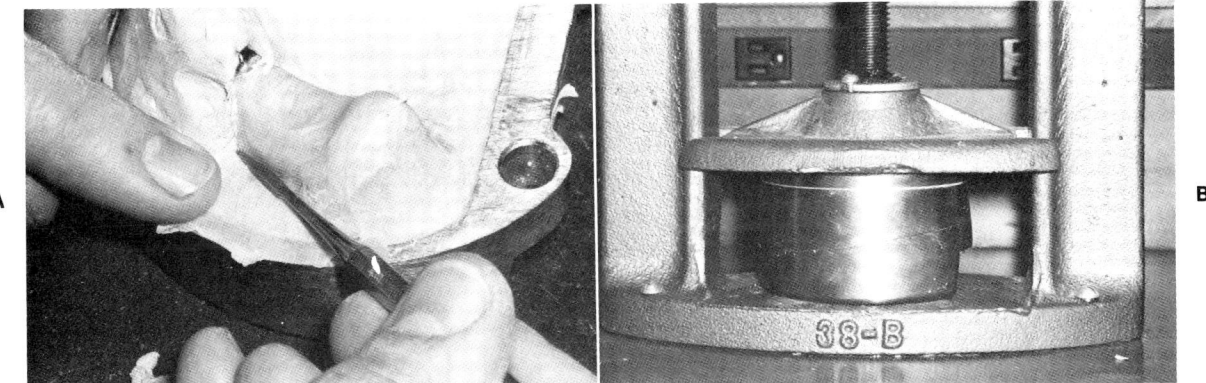

**Fig. 13-43. A,** Remove flash with dull instrument. Replace plastic sheet between flask halves, and press it again. **B,** Repeat until no flash is seen.

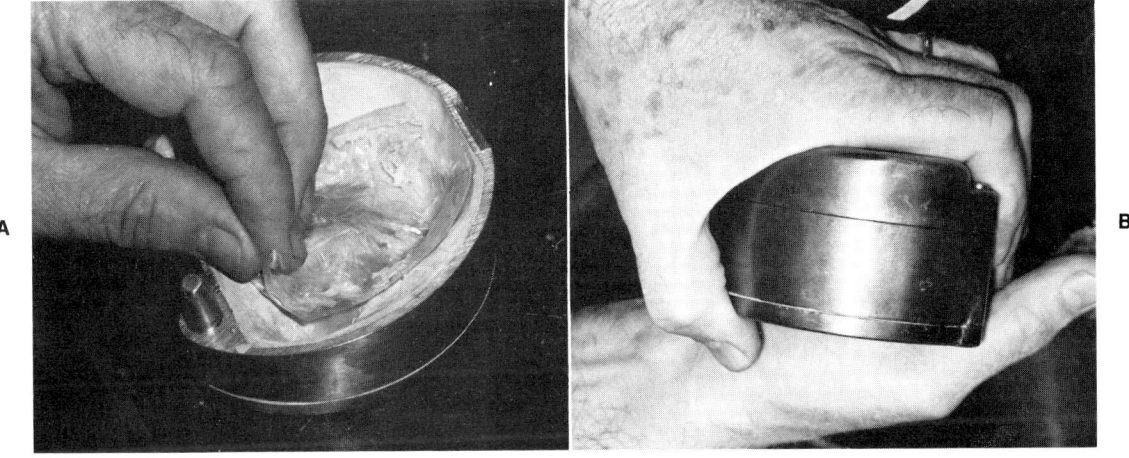

**Fig. 13-44. A,** Plastic sheet is removed. **B,** Both surfaces are wet slightly with acrylic liquid, and flask is closed without plastic sheet and placed in two-flask hand press.

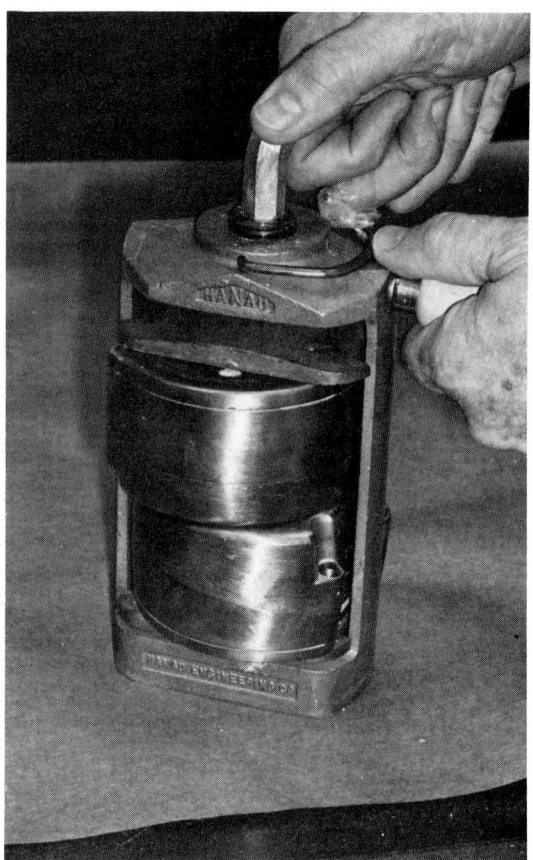

**Fig. 13-45.** Tighten press as much as possible, then unscrew press one turn. Partial denture is ready to process after it has bench cured for 1 hour.

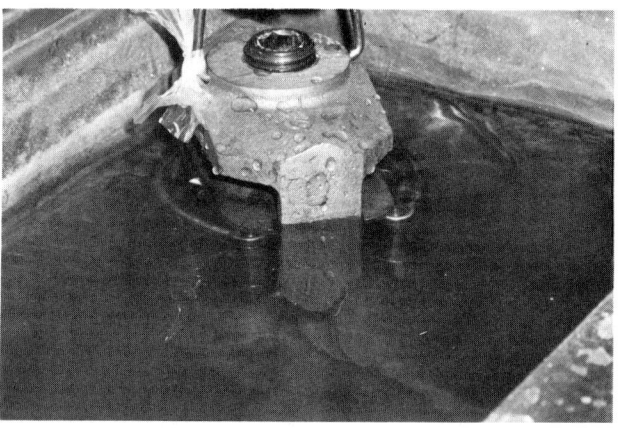

**Fig. 13-46.** Curing unit should be at room temperature, and water must cover flask with partial denture.

pletely, and then back off the press one-quarter turn. The flask should be permitted to bench cure for 1 hour before processing is started (Fig. 13-45).

## PROCESSING

When the 1-hour bench-curing time is over, place the press in a curing unit. The unit should be at room temperature, and the water should completely cover the flask containing the partial denture (Fig. 13-46). As a general rule the long cure is used for both complete and partial dentures. This is usually done overnight, and the denture will be ready to recover and complete the following morning. A two- or three-stage curing unit is recommended. To set the Hanau curing unit* for the long cure, set the time dial on station one at 8 hours, and set the corresponding temperature control below the time dial at 160° F (71° C). Set the time dial on station two at 9 hours, and set its temperature control at 212° F (100° C) (Fig. 13-47). This setting of the curing unit means that the water temperature will be raised to 160° F rapidly and will be held at that level for 8 hours. Then the temperature will automatically be raised to and maintained at boiling for 1 hour.

There may be instances when not enough time is available for the long cure. In these cases it is possible to use the short cure, which consists of holding the temperature at 130° F (54° C) for 1½ hours and then boiling for ½ hour. Needless to say, there is a certain element of risk involved in this procedure. If deflasking cannot be done immediately after processing and cooling, the investment should not be allowed to dry. Keep the flask covered with room-temperature water until deflasking is accomplished. Do not deflask until the flask and its contents are at room temperature (Fig. 13-48).

### PROBLEM AREAS

The principal problems associated with the boil-out and packing procedures include incorrect time and temperature for wax elimination, failure to coat the mold with uncontaminated tinfoil substitute, improper trial packing, and incorrect curing cycle selection (Table 13-2).

---

*Hanau Curing Unit, Hanau Division, Teledyne Dental Products Co., Buffalo, N.Y.

*Flasking, processing, deflasking, and finishing* 381

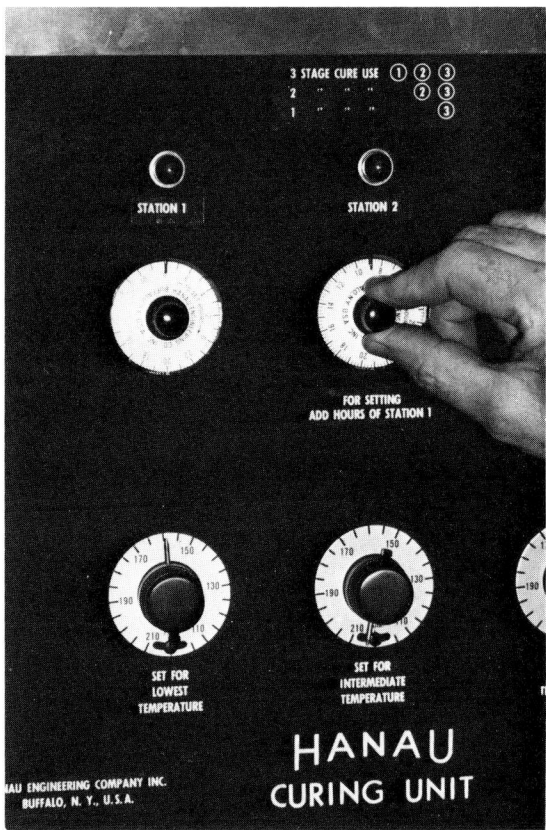

**Fig. 13-47.** Hanau two- or three-stage curing unit. For long cure, set top dial in stage one for 8 hours and temperature for 160° F (71° C). Set top dial on stage two for 9 hours, and set temperature dial for 212° F (100° C).

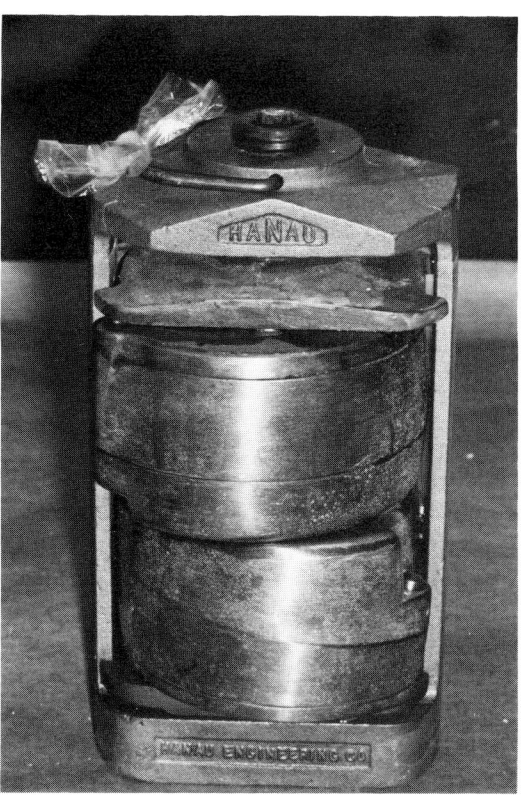

**Fig. 13-48.** Partial denture is ready for deflasking when it has cooled to room temperature.

**Table 13-2.** Boilout and packing

| Problem | Probable cause | Solution |
|---|---|---|
| Wax too firm on flask separation, causing teeth to be retained in wax | Flask not immersed in boiling water for 5 minutes | Permit flask to remain in boiling water for 5 minutes |
| Wax liquefied and penetrates stone and cast | Time of boilout too long | Permit flask to remain in boiling water for only 5 minutes |
| Cured resin adhered to flasking stone, making removal difficult | Tinfoil substitute not applied | Apply tinfoil substitute before packing |
|  | Tinfoil substitute contaminated | Use care to not contaminate tinfoil substitute |
| Cured denture base has porosity | Denture base was underpacked | Trial pack several times to be assured that mold is not underpacked |
|  | Denture base cured at too high temperature initially | Bench cure for 1 hour after packing, place in room-temperature water, and use long-cycle cure |
| Framework of cured distal extension partial denture is warped | Distal extension for resin retention was not supported by unit and was distorted during compression molding | Make certain that cast stop is in contact with cast before trial packing; use autopolymerizing resin to achieve stop if required |

**382** *Dental laboratory procedures: removable partial dentures*

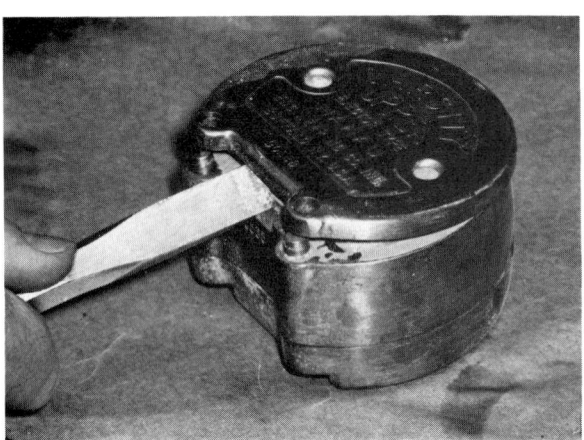

Fig. 13-49. Remove top of flask.

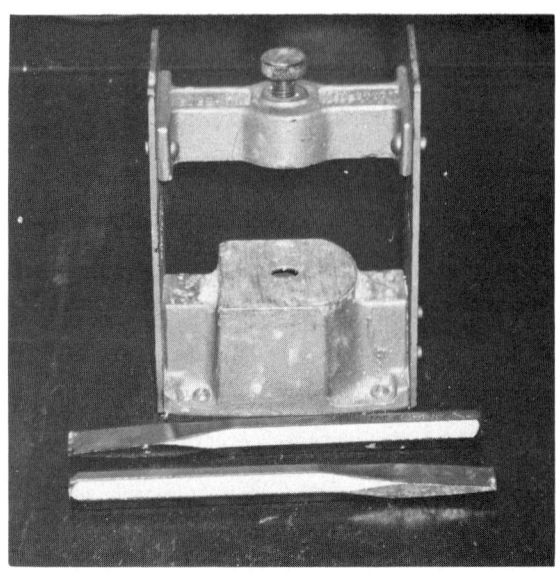

Fig. 13-50. Hanau flask ejector complete with chisels.

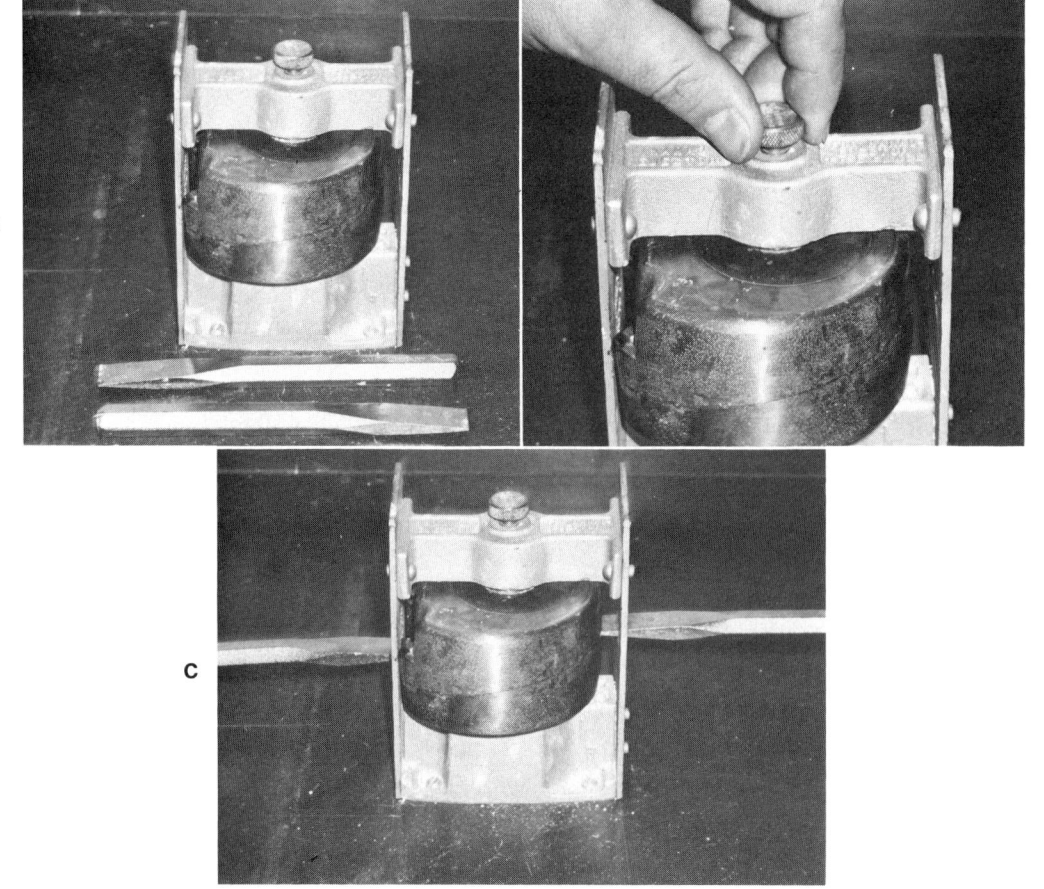

Fig. 13-51. **A,** Flask in ejector upside down. **B,** Tighten screw in top of ejector against knockout plate. **C,** Place chisels into slots of flask.

## DEFLASKING

The basic procedure for deflasking the removable partial denture is the same as that for the complete denture. The first step is to remove the top of the flask by prying gently with a laboratory knife (Fig. 13-49). A Hanau flask ejector* is used to remove the stone from the flask in one piece without damage to the flask (Fig. 13-50).

Place the flask in the ejector with the bottom up. Tighten the screw in the top of the ejector against the round knockout plug in the bottom of the flask. Use the chisels to engage the slots of the flask, one on each side (Fig. 13-51). Use an upward and then a downward motion. Both halves of the flask will come loose and can be removed from the ejector (Fig. 13-52). Hold the edge of the laboratory knife against the cap (fourth pour) of the stone invest-

---
*Hanau Flask Ejector, Hanau Division, Teledyne Dental Products Co., Buffalo, N.Y.

ment, and, with a light tapping force, the lid will separate (Fig. 13-53). Make a saw cut on the upper half of the stone investment between the central incisors (Fig. 13-54). Care must be taken not to overcut and damage the teeth on the stone cast. Next, two cuts are made, one on each side of the stone investment at the posterior ends (Fig. 13-55). The cuts should be made deeply enough to reach the master cast, but not to damage it. The blade of the laboratory knife can be inserted into the anterior cut, and, with a twisting motion, the labial and buccal portions of the investment should come loose (Fig. 13-56).

Clear the lingual surfaces of the artificial teeth that are now exposed, and, with the blade of the knife, pry gently from the rear to remove this portion of the stone investment (Fig. 13-57). Two layers of investment remain. Make three saw cuts, one between the central incisors and the other two at each posterior end of the first and second stone invest-

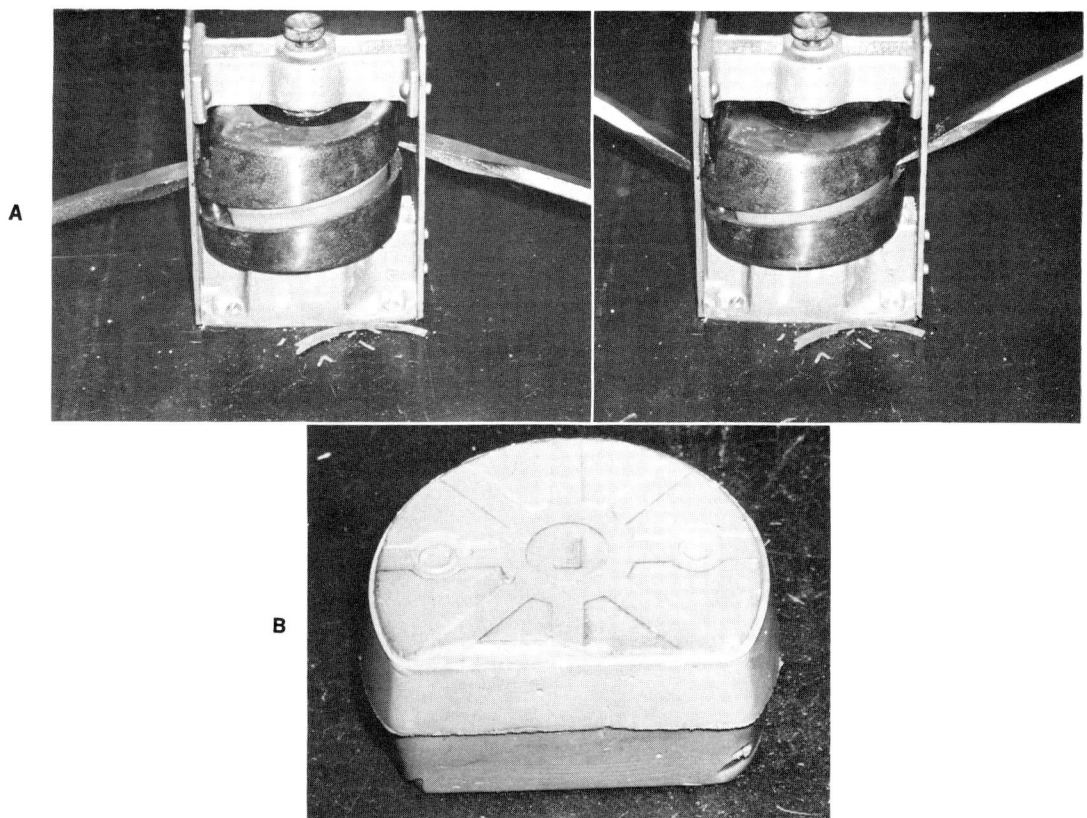

Fig. 13-52. **A,** Pry upward (right), then downward (left), and flask is loosened from stone. **B,** Remove from ejector. Flask can be separated, leaving stone in one piece.

**384** *Dental laboratory procedures: removable partial dentures*

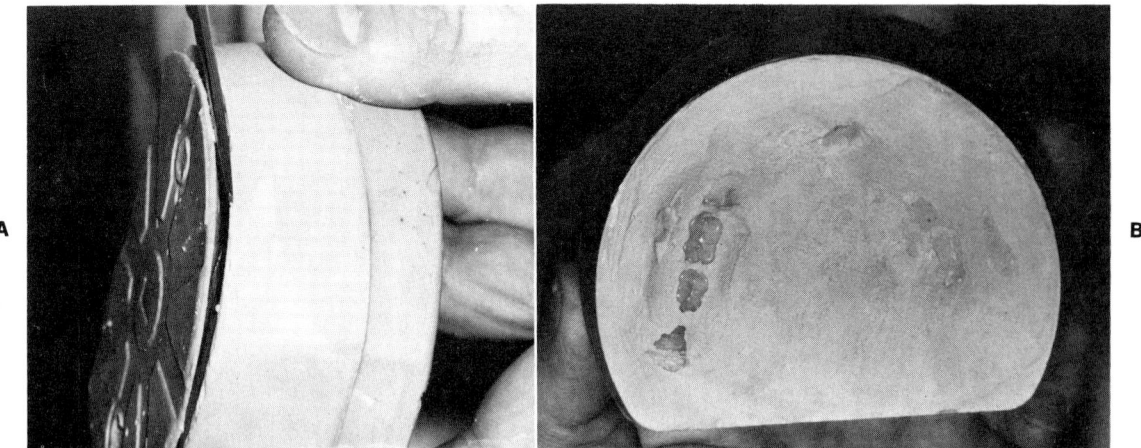

**Fig. 13-53. A,** Hold edge of knife against stone cap, and tap lightly to remove it. **B,** Cap removed to expose occlusals of teeth.

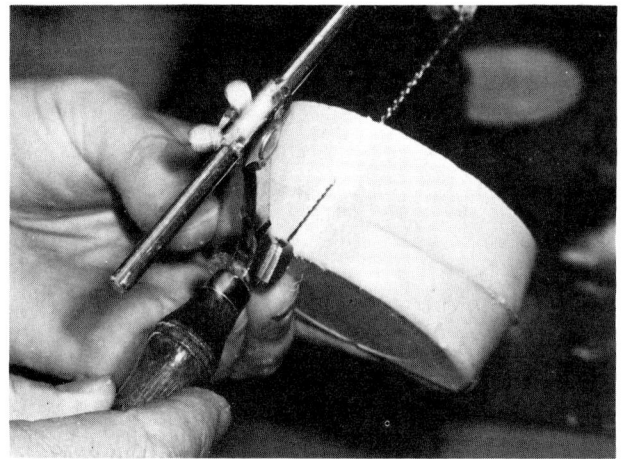

**Fig. 13-54.** Use saw to cut stone between central incisors.

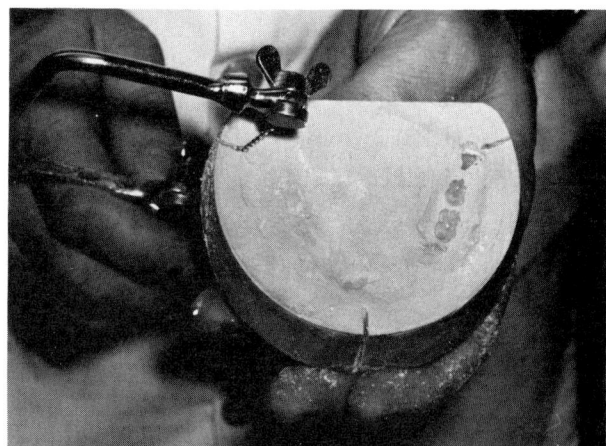

**Fig. 13-55.** Cut is made on each side at posterior portion of investment of stone.

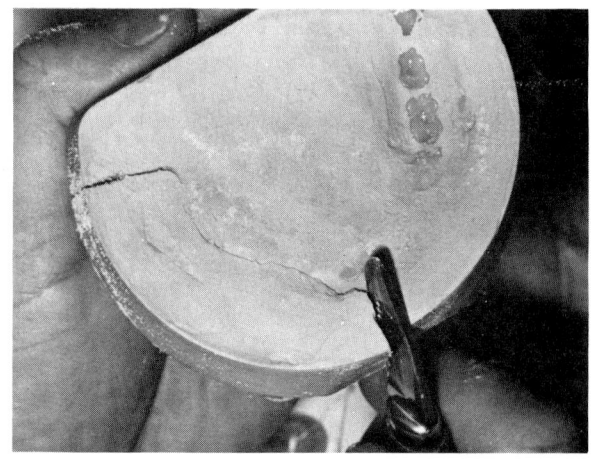

**Fig. 13-56.** Insert knife blade in anterior saw cut, and twist it to loosen stone.

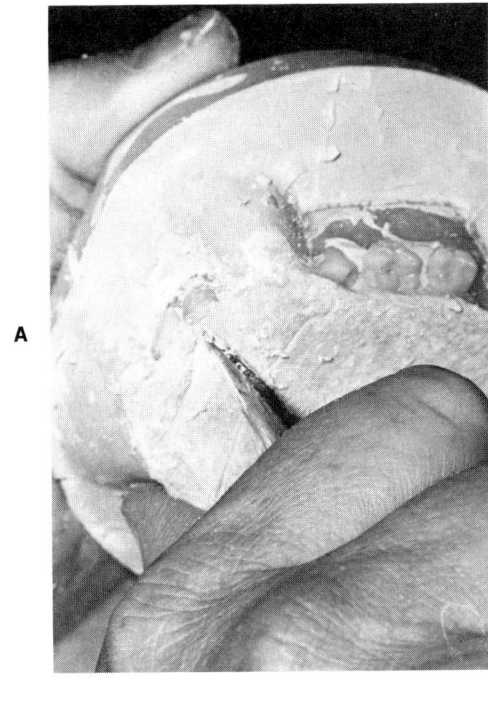
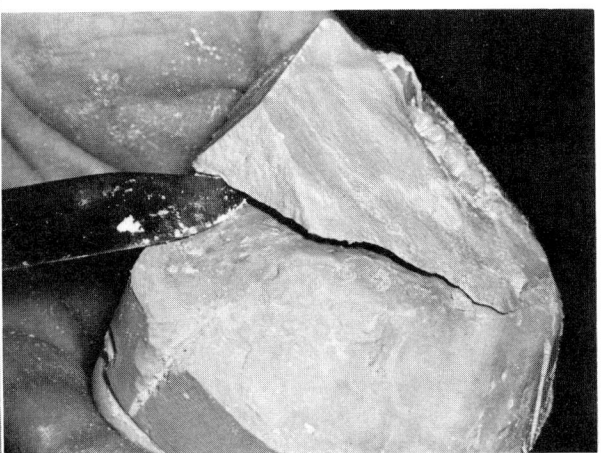

Fig. 13-57. **A,** Free lingual surfaces of teeth with knife. **B,** Pry lingual portion loose with knife blade.

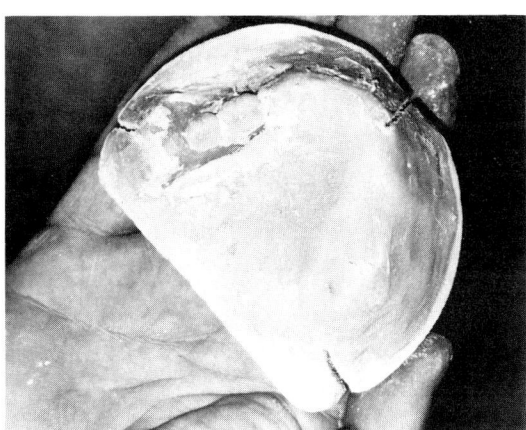

Fig. 13-58. Make three saw cuts in stone investment in positions shown.

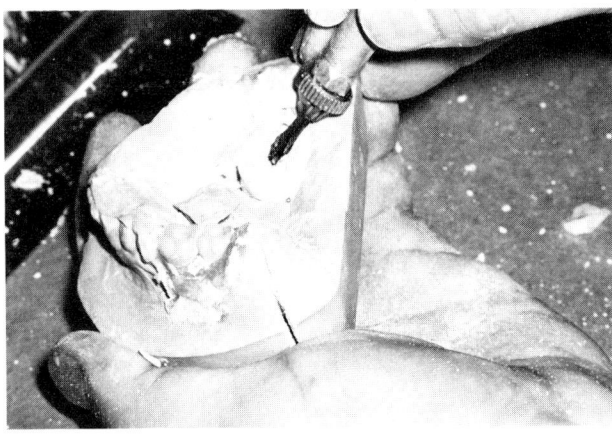

Fig. 13-59. Pry labial and buccal portions of stone loose. Remove any lingual stone that is left. Pneumatic chisel is helpful.

ment layers (Fig. 13-58). The blade of the laboratory knife may now be used to pry the labial and buccal portions of the stone investment free and a knife or pneumatic chisel used to remove the remaining lingual portion (Fig. 13-59). Be careful not to distort or damage the lingual bar or the reciprocal clasp arms of the partial denture. When this portion is completely removed, the final stone investment layer can be removed (Fig. 13-60). Hold the master cast and the first stone investment layer with one hand, and, using the handle of the laboratory knife,

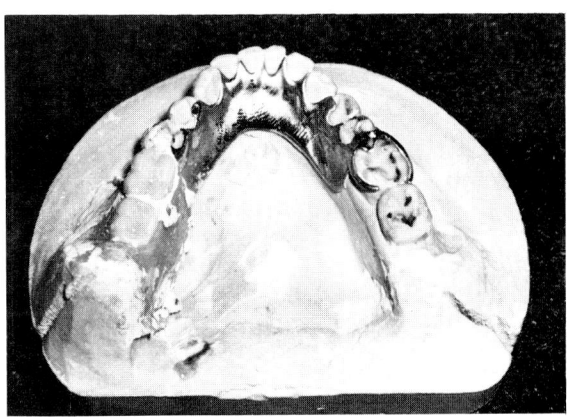

Fig. 13-60. Cast ready for removal of final layer.

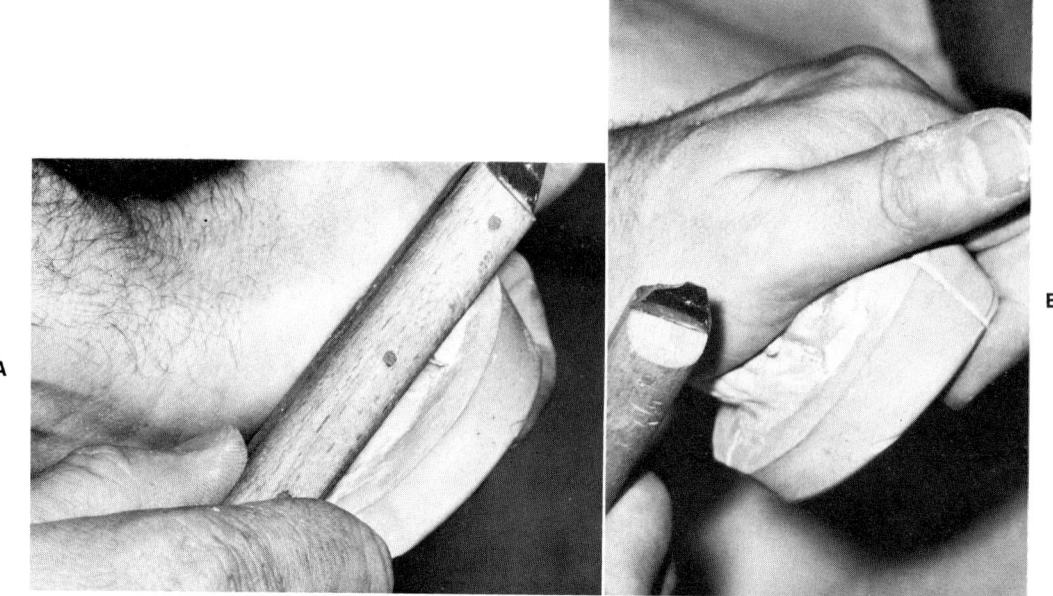

**Fig. 13-61. A,** Hold cast in one hand. Note grip. **B,** Strike stone investment with handle of laboratory knife to remove it.

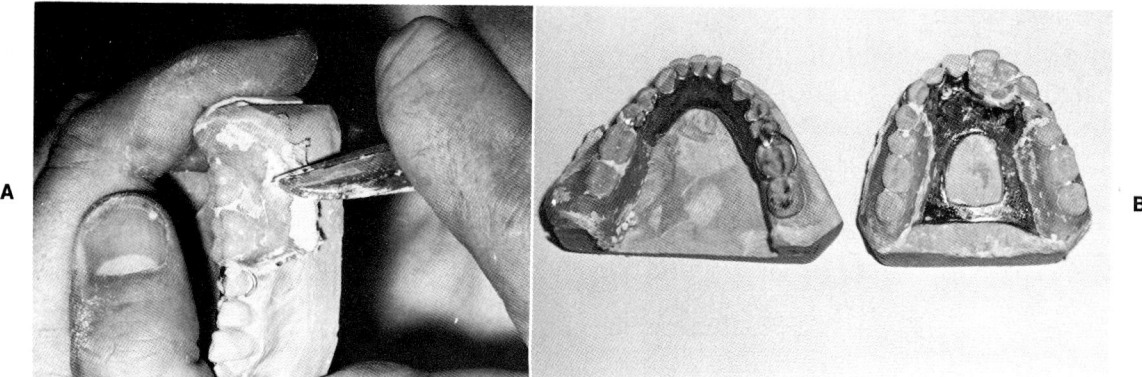

**Fig. 13-62. A,** Remove any remaining large pieces of investing stone with knife blade. **B,** Casts with partial dentures recovered from stone investment.

**Fig. 13-63.** Clean base of cast with brush.

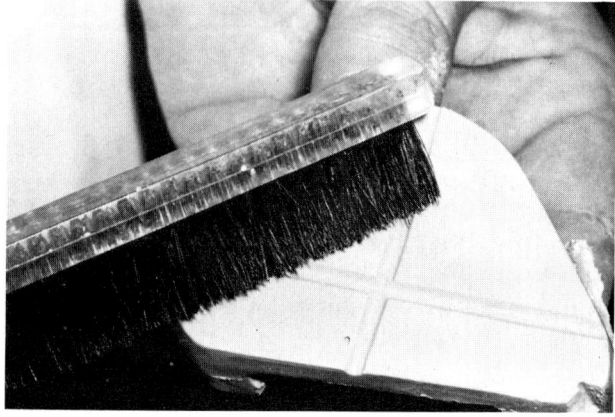

tap against the top of the first layer. It should separate from the master cast. Note the grip used to hold the cast (Fig. 13-61). Use the blade of the laboratory knife to remove any investment that may stay on the base of the master cast (Fig. 13-62). With a brush, remove all small particles of investment layer that may cling to the indices on the base of the master cast (Fig. 13-63).

## REMOUNTING AND CORRECTING PROCESSING ERRORS

Place the cast on the mounting stone in the articulator, and verify that the fit is extremely accurate. No space should be visible between the stone mounting and the base of the cast (Fig. 13-64). Seal the master cast to the stone mounting using baseplate wax or sticky wax. Apply enough wax so that the cast will not be loosened while the occlusal adjustment is being accomplished (Fig. 13-65). Close the articulator, and observe the amount of pin opening (Fig. 13-66). If there is 1 mm or less of pin opening, the technique used in investing and processing was acceptable. If there is more than 1 mm of pin opening, some errors occurred during the investing procedure. If an excessive amount of pin opening occurs, the anatomy of the teeth may be destroyed in reestablishing the proper occlusal relationship, thereby reducing the efficiency of the removable partial denture by having the opposing teeth articulate against a wide flattened surface.

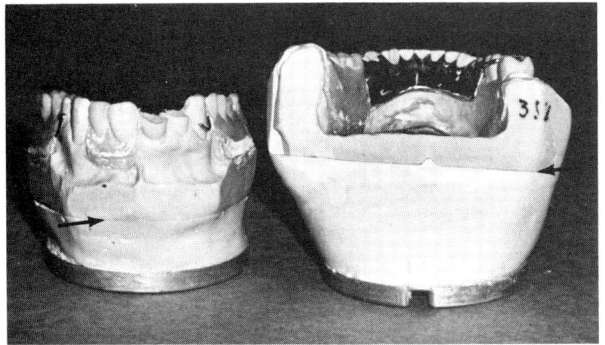

**Fig. 13-64.** Replace casts on mounting stone of articulator. There should be no visible space.

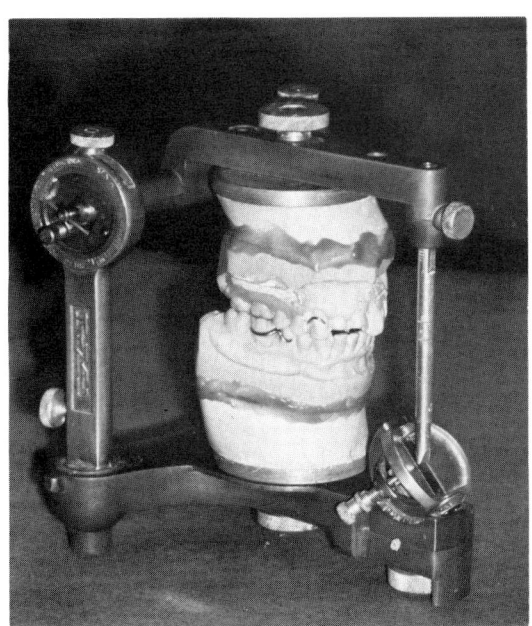

**Fig. 13-65.** Seal casts in place with sticky wax or baseplate wax.

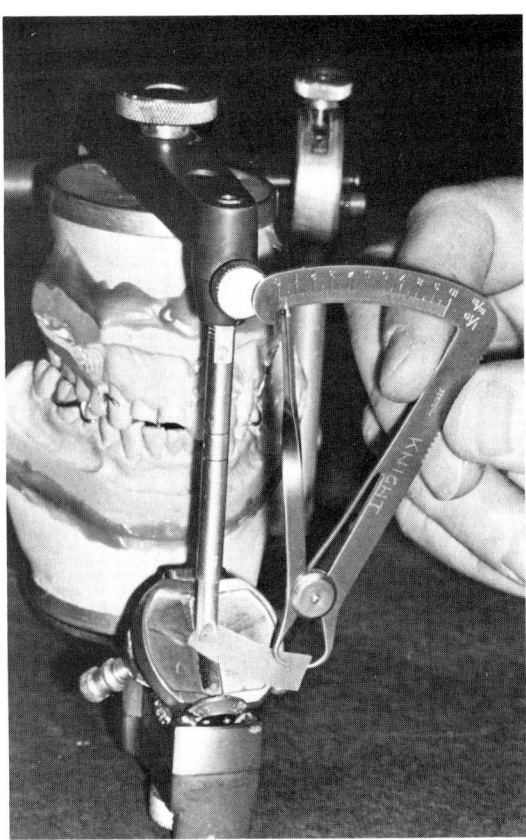

**Fig. 13-66.** Close articulator and look at pin opening. Opening 1 mm or less is good; opening shown is 0.5 mm.

The condyles of the articulator should be locked in the centric relation position (Fig. 13-67). The errors that occurred during processing can be located with articulating paper (Fig. 13-68). Adjust plastic teeth by grinding with a bur, and porcelain teeth are ground with a mounted stone (Fig. 13-69). Grind the occlusion so that the opposing stone teeth are returned to equal contact. In correcting the pin opening, do not remove the cusp tips but deepen the fossae and adjust the inclined planes. Reshape the occlusal surface to provide inclines, grooves, and escape ways. Use very thin tissue paper or 0.0005-inch plastic shim stock* to test the contacts between opposing teeth (Fig. 13-70). When the vertical dimension of occlusion has been restored, check the relationship of the teeth in working and balancing occlusion on both sides. Never let the artificial teeth keep the natural, or stone teeth, from contacting in any of the eccentric positions (Fig. 13-71). Be sure to check for any balancing contacts that may have been created, and eliminate them by grinding the artificial teeth.

---

*The Artus Corp., Englewood, N.J.

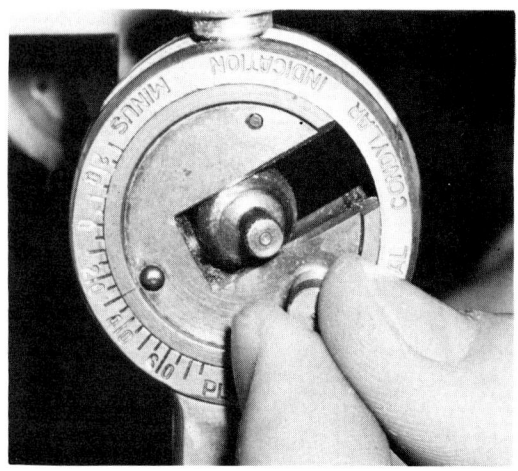

Fig. 13-67. Lock condyles of articulator in centric position.

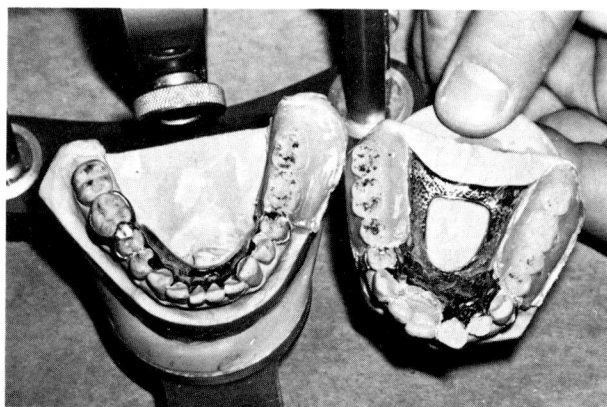

Fig. 13-68. Mark occlusal surfaces with articulating paper to find high spots.

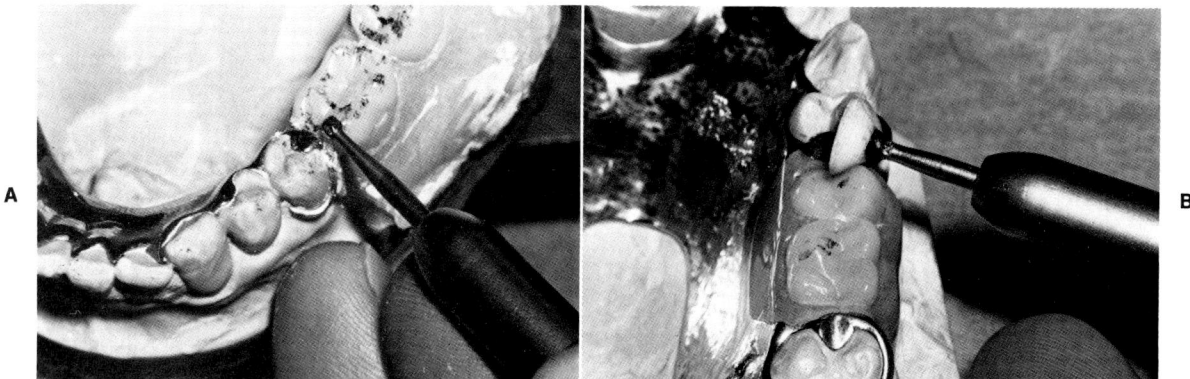

Fig. 13-69. A, Grind plastic teeth with bur. B, Grind porcelain teeth with mounted stone.

*Flasking, processing, deflasking, and finishing* **389**

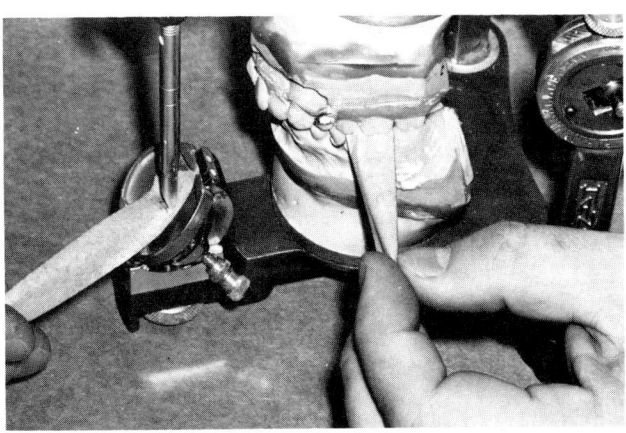

**Fig. 13-70.** Contacts between all of opposing posterior artificial and stone teeth should hold very thin tissue paper or 0.0005-inch shim stock.

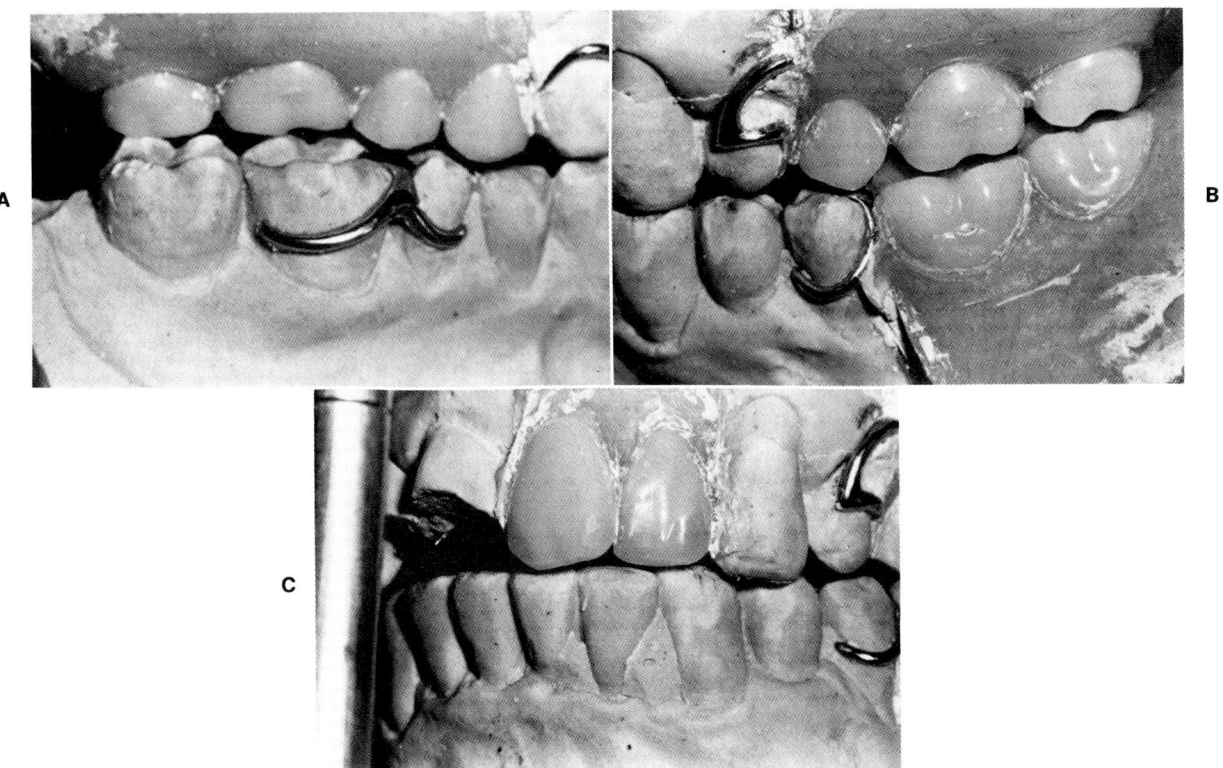

**Fig. 13-71.** Examine teeth in right lateral **(A)**, left lateral **(B)**, and protrusive **(C)** positions. Artificial teeth should not keep natural teeth or stone teeth from contacting in any eccentric position.

## FINISHING AND POLISHING

Cut the abutment from the master cast by using a bur, laboratory knife, or plaster saw (Fig. 13-72). Generally, when this is done, the removable partial denture can be teased off the master cast (Fig. 13-73). If resistance is encountered in removing the partial denture, the master cast must be sectioned and removed piece by piece as is done with complete dentures. The sectioning is described in Chapter 9 of volume 1 (Morrow et al., 1980). When the partial denture has been removed, stone particles should be removed from around the teeth and from the resin-metal joints using a small instrument, explorer tip, stiff brush, or shellblaster (Fig. 13-74). Care must be taken in using these instruments to avoid damaging the plastic or metal. Remove the

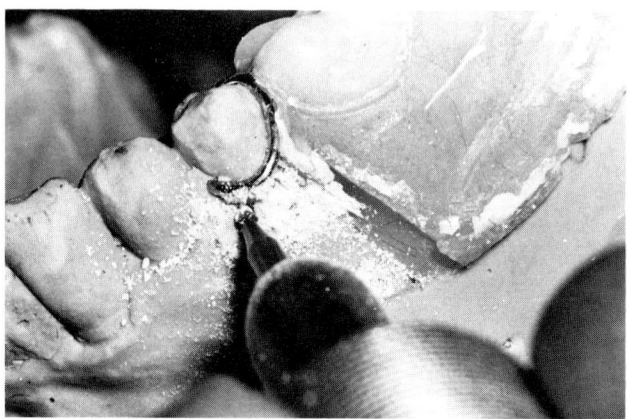

**Fig. 13-72.** Bur is used to cut abutment teeth from master cast.

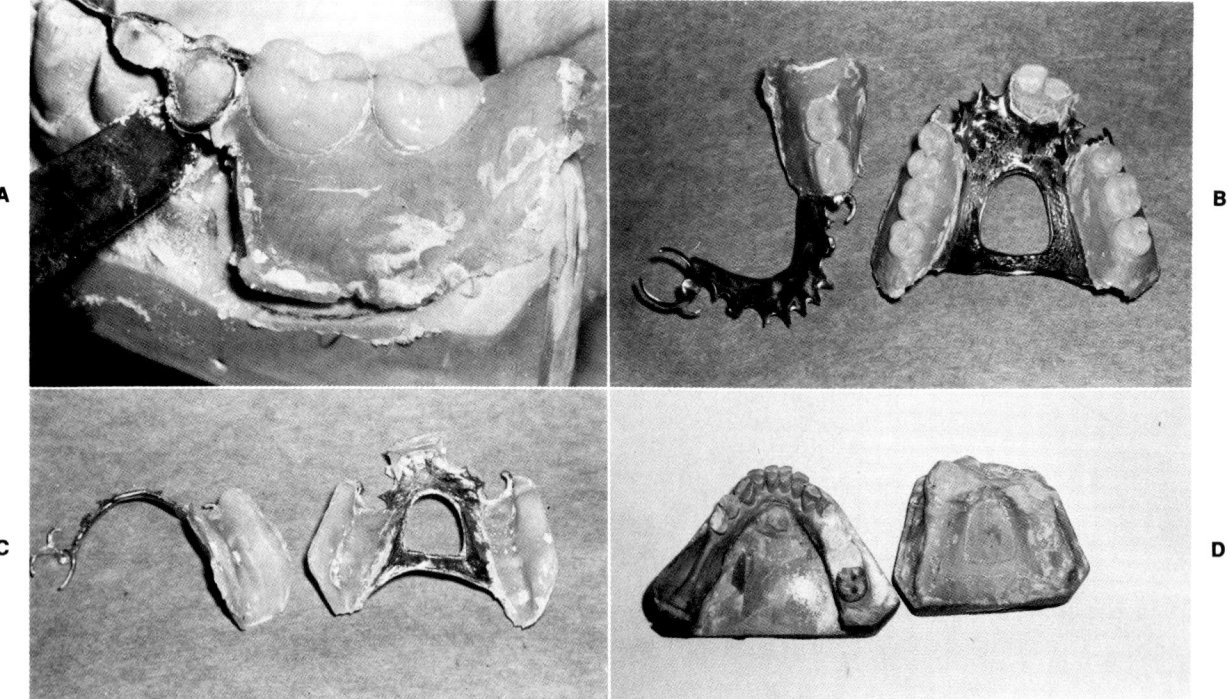

**Fig. 13-73. A,** Gently pry partial denture from cast. **B,** Occlusal view. **C,** Tissue side. **D,** Casts are destroyed.

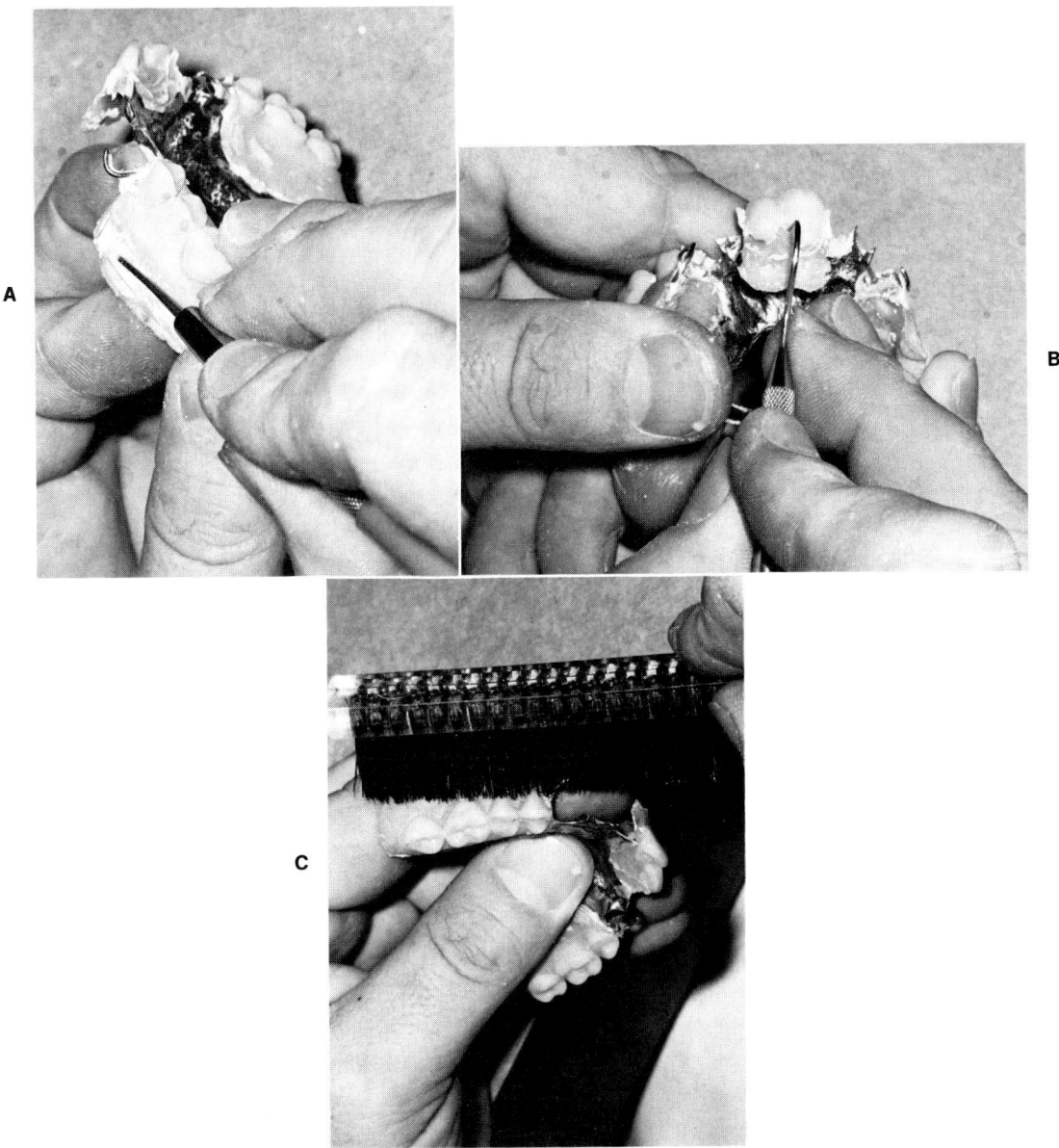

**Fig. 13-74.** Remove stone particles around partial denture with small instrument **(A)**, explorer tip **(B)**, or stiff brush **(C)**. Shellblaster may also be used.

peripheral flash with vulcanite burs, mounted stones, or an arbor band (Fig. 13-75). Keep the peripheries smooth and rounded. They should be a minimum of 2 mm thick. The joint between the metal and the resin at the external and internal finish lines should be trimmed, using a rubber abrasive wheel, vulcanite bur, or small mounted stone (Fig. 13-76). Avoid scratching or damaging the metal. Small fissure burs should be used to remove any flash that has occurred around the clasp assembly (Fig. 13-77). The distal extension base is shaped next. On the buccal surface, a slight concavity should be developed just above the peripheral roll (Fig. 13-78); on the lingual surface, a gentle concavity should be produced from the gingival crest of the teeth to the peripheral roll (Fig. 11-79). The distolingual extension of the mandibular distal extension denture bases should be thinned to approximately 2 to 2.5 mm (Fig. 13-80). This is one of the areas on the denture that is trimmed arbitrarily to provide room for the tongue.

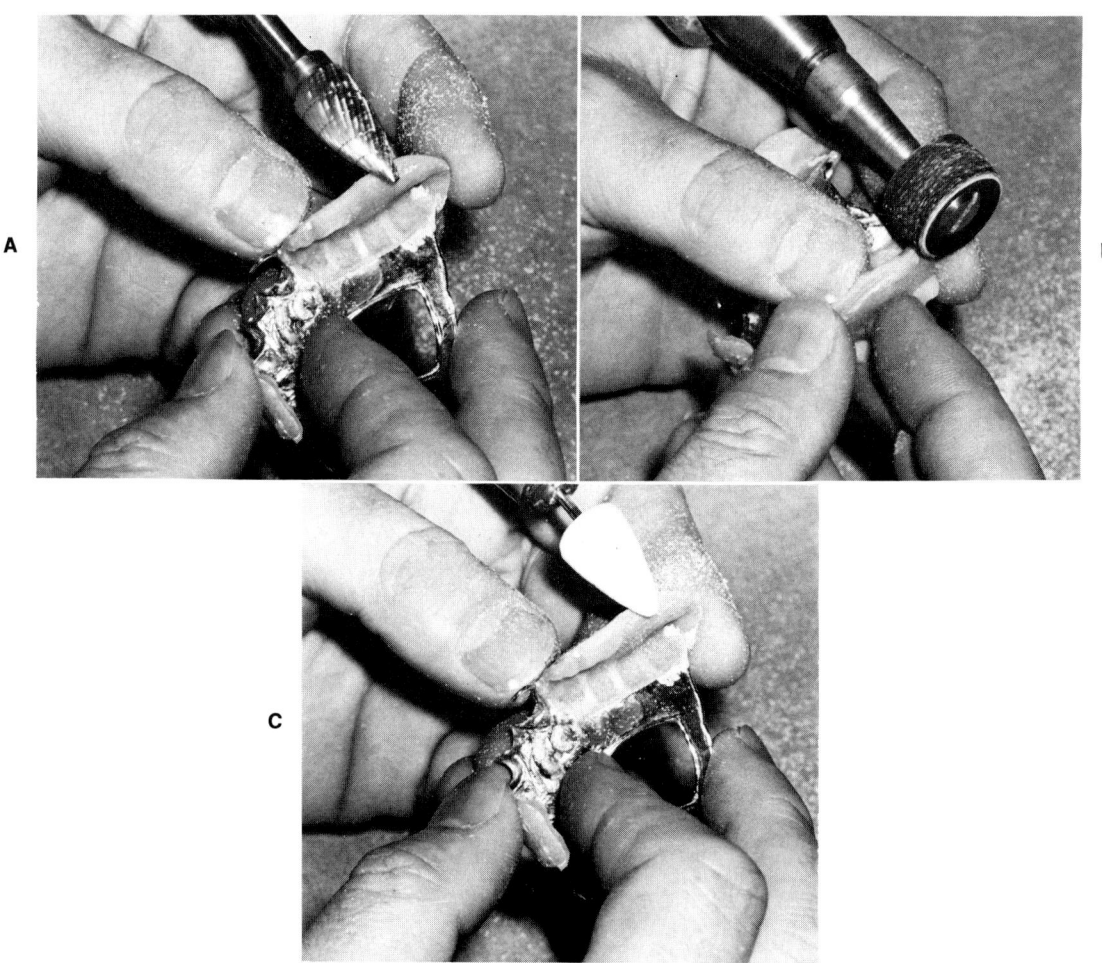

**Fig. 13-75.** Grind peripheral flash with vulcanite bur **(A)**, arbor band **(B)**, or mounted stone made for cutting acrylic resin **(C)**.

*Flasking, processing, deflasking, and finishing* **393**

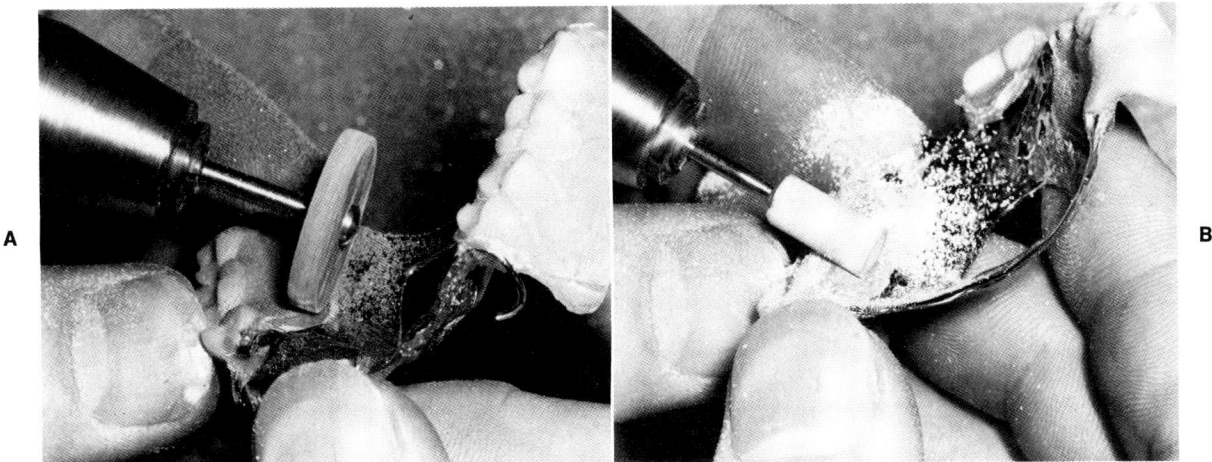

**Fig. 13-76.** Trim acrylic resin at finish line with rubber abrasive wheel **(A)**, or vulcanite bur **(B)**, or small mounted stone. Be particularly careful not to mar metal.

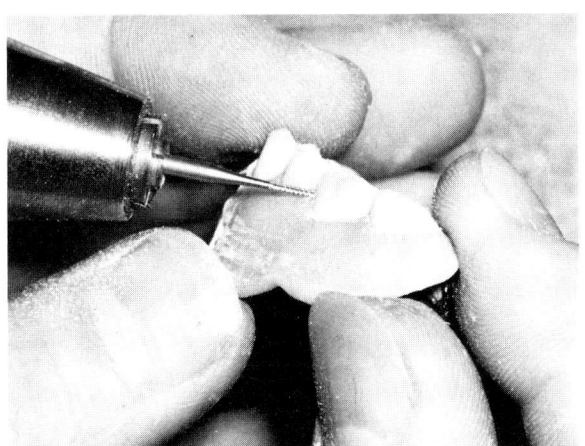

**Fig. 13-77.** Remove flash around teeth with small fissure bur.

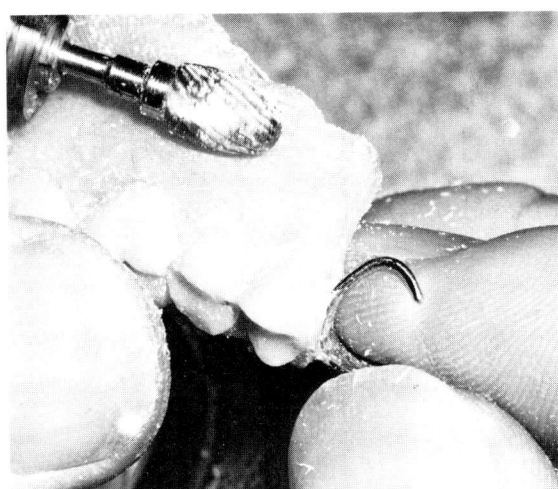

**Fig. 13-78.** Develop slight concavity on facial surface.

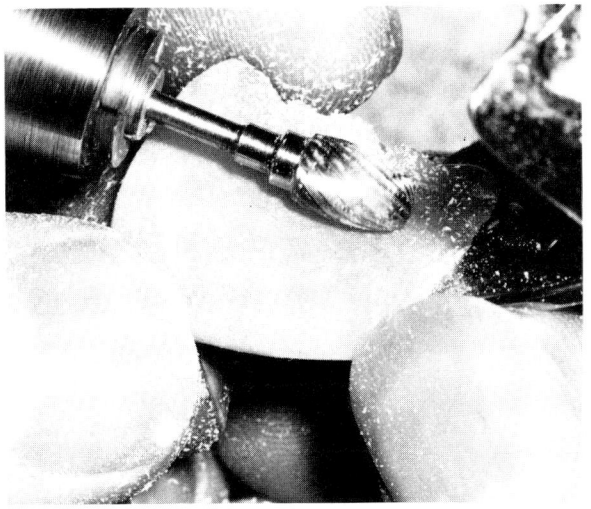

**Fig. 13-79.** On lingual surface develop slight concavity just below gingival crest.

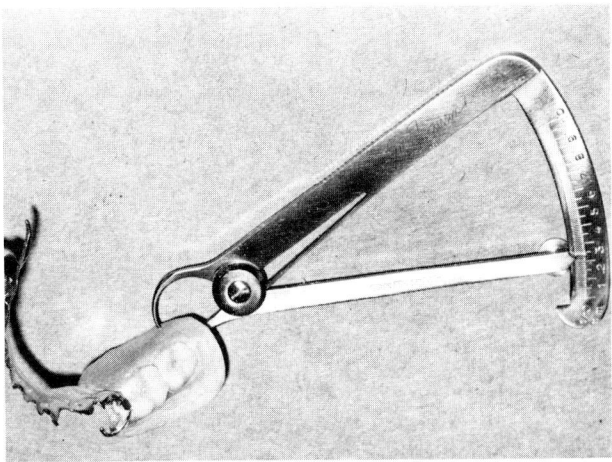

**Fig. 13-80.** Thin distolingual side of denture base to about 2 to 2.5 mm.

The acrylic resin at the external finish lines should be trimmed smooth, but slightly elevated above the height of the metal (Fig. 13-81). This slight elevation will be removed during the final polishing and will ensure a smooth flowing surface from metal to plastic (Fig. 13-82). The gingival margins around the teeth are cleaned of acrylic resin flash and nodules with an explorer point, small chisel, or bur. Often, a tip of a bar-type T or modified T clasp will be embedded in the acrylic resin. It can be freed by cutting or sanding the bulk of the resin away and then working a metal lightning abrasive strip between the resin and clasp. Move the strip up and down until sufficient clearance is obtained. If a bur is used to gain this clearance, invariably too much acrylic resin will be removed (Fig. 13-83). This cleaning operation will emphasize the value of a good wax-up. The better the wax-up, the fewer the problems encountered in finishing.

The first stage of polishing should now be accomplished. Flour of pumice or fine pumice on a wet cloth wheel should be used to remove all the scratches on the external surface of the acrylic resin (Fig. 13-84). Do not overpumice around plastic teeth. It is possible to destroy the shapes of the teeth by overzealous use of pumice. The juncture of

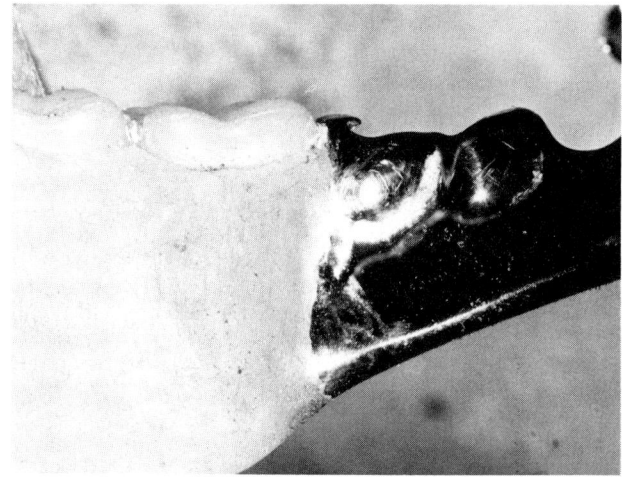

**Fig. 13-81.** Acrylic is smoothed but not finished flush with finish line.

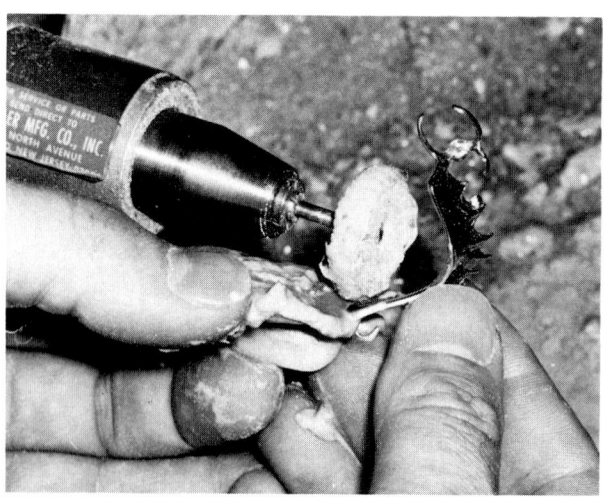

**Fig. 13-82.** Smooth surface at finish line is developed with pumice on rag wheel or small felt wheel.

*Flasking, processing, deflasking, and finishing* **395**

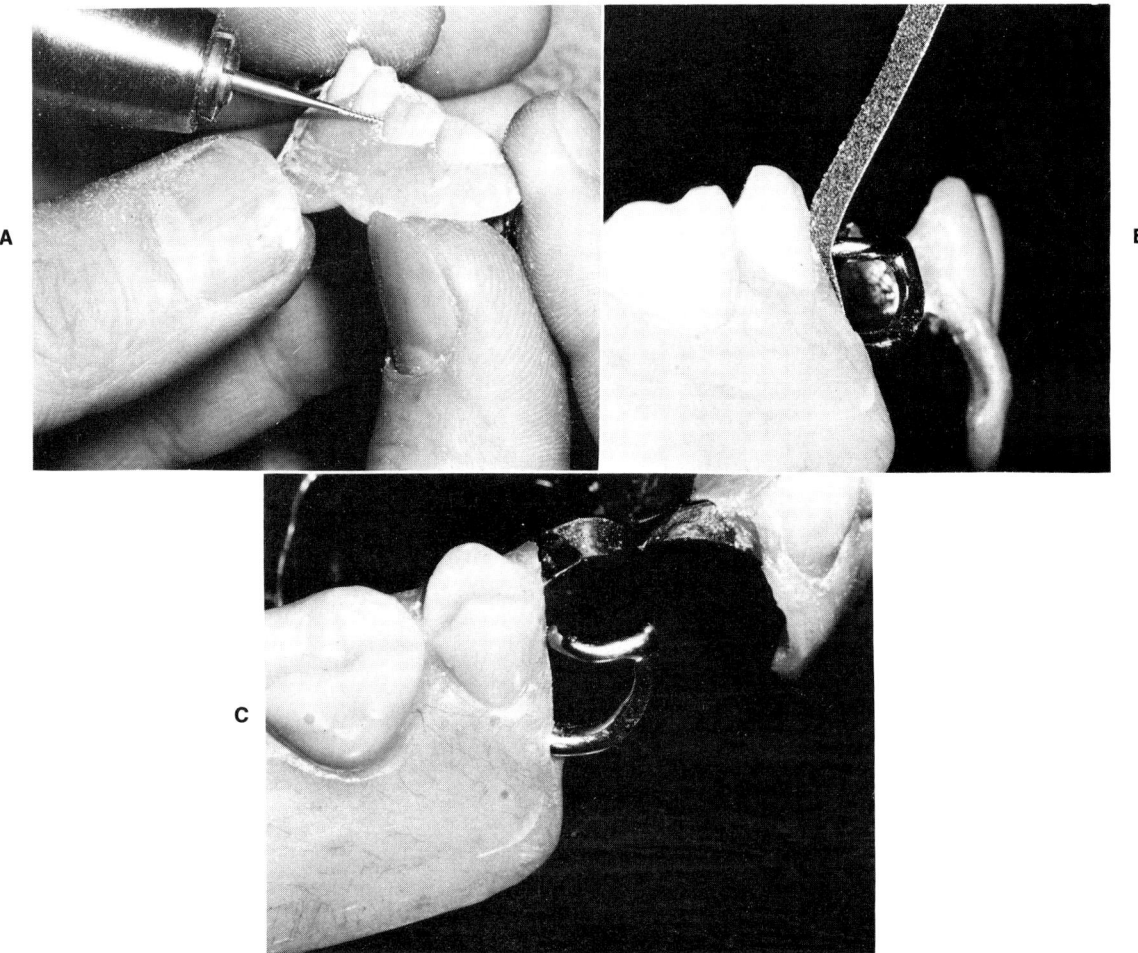

**Fig. 13-83. A,** Clean flash and sharpen acrylic around gingival margins of teeth. **B,** Bar-type clasp may be freed from acrylic resin by using lightning abrasive strip. **C,** Freed bar clasp.

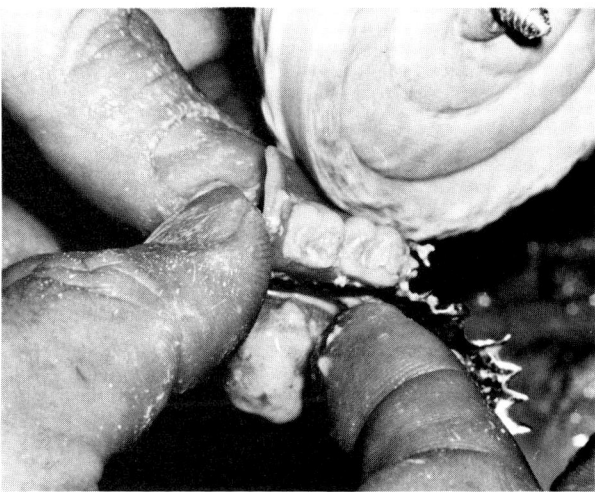

**Fig. 13-84.** Polish external surface of acrylic resin with flour of pumice on rag wheel.

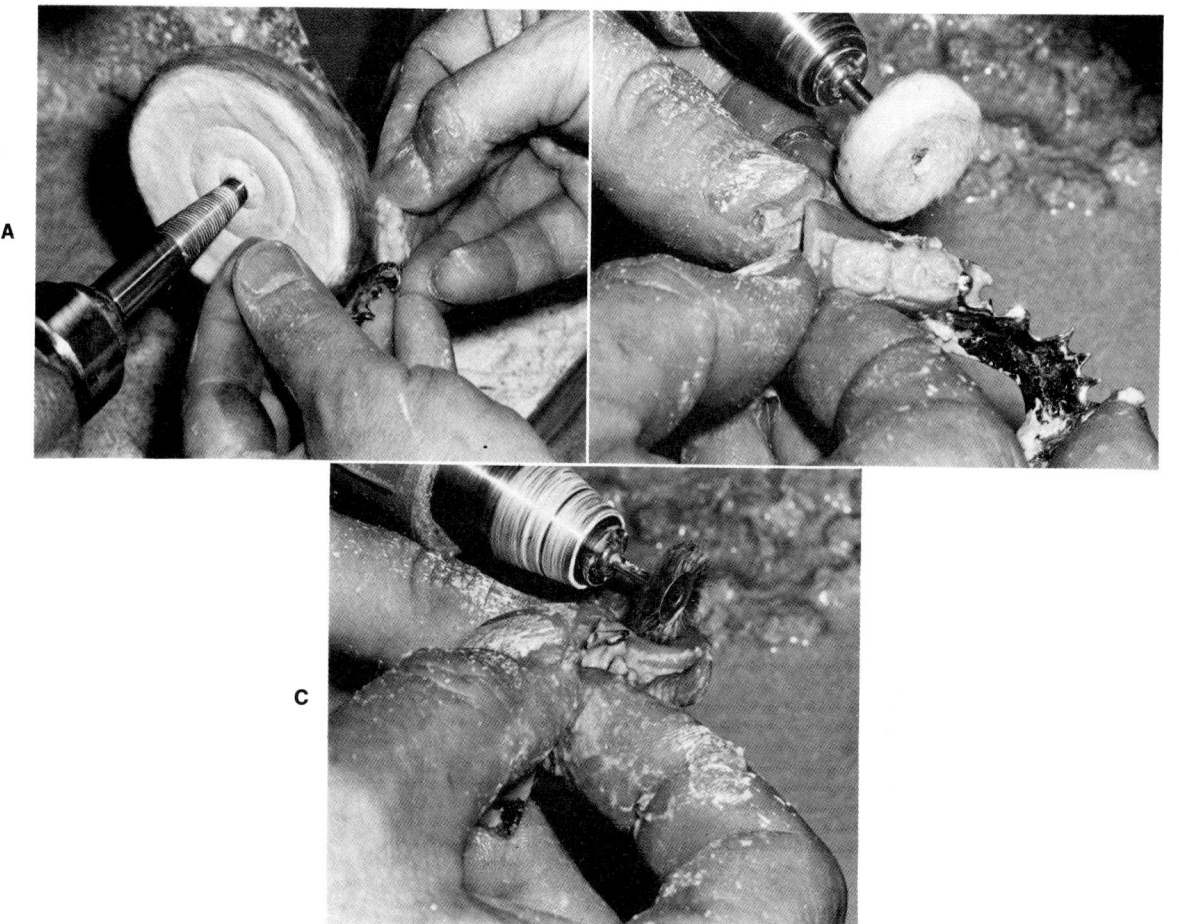

**Fig. 13-85. A,** Do not reduce acrylic below surface of metal at finish line. **B,** Use small felt wheel to reach areas inaccessible to large rag wheel. **C,** Soft bristle brush is good for pumicing around teeth.

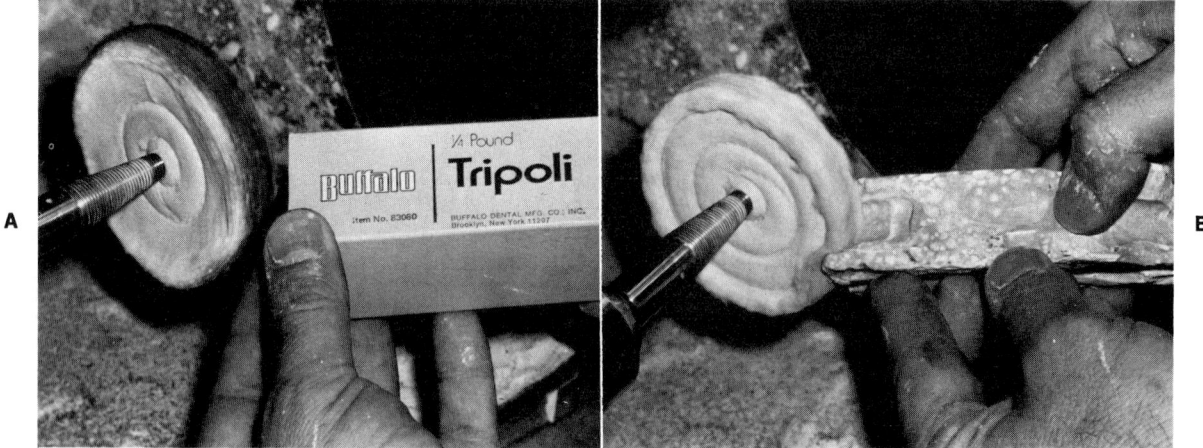

**Fig. 13-86.** Apply final polish with dry, clean cloth rag wheel. Tripoli is applied first **(A)**, then White Diamond for a high shine **(B)**.

the external and internal finish line may be pumiced lightly, but again, care must be taken not to reduce the height of the resin below that of the metal (Fig. 13-85). If the pumicing is done thoroughly, the final polish will take a very short time. For the final polish, dry, clean cloth wheels with resin polishing compounds such as Tripoli* for a smooth finish and White Diamond† for a high shine should be used (Fig. 13-86). Restore a high gloss to all the resin surfaces and to the occlusal surfaces of the teeth. It may be necessary to repolish the metal with rouge or high shine again. Do not let the rag or felt wheel or cone touch the acrylic resin because it burns very easily (Fig. 13-87).

Wash the removable partial denture with soap and water and a soft brush. Tincture of green soap and ammonia is also very good for this (Fig. 13-88). Finally, inspect all surfaces, preferably with magnification, to be certain that all scratches and other minor defects have been removed (Fig. 13-89). The partial dentures are ready for delivery (Fig. 13-90).

---

*Tripoli, Buffalo Dental Manufacturing Co., Inc., Brooklyn, N.Y.
†White Diamond, William Dixon Co., Carlstadt, N.J.

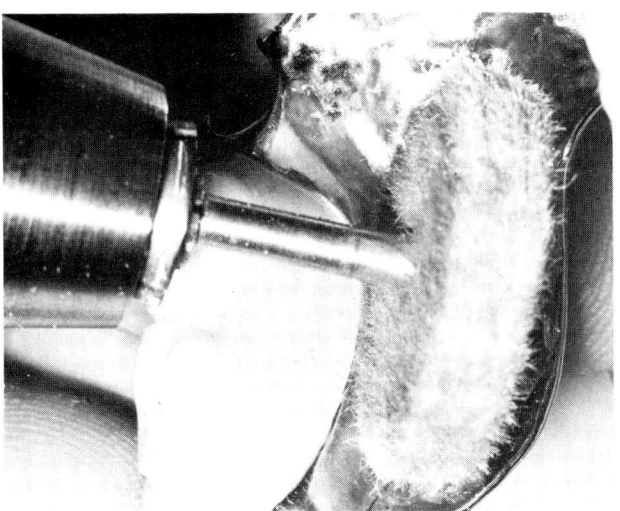

**Fig. 13-87.** Repolish metal. Do not touch acrylic.

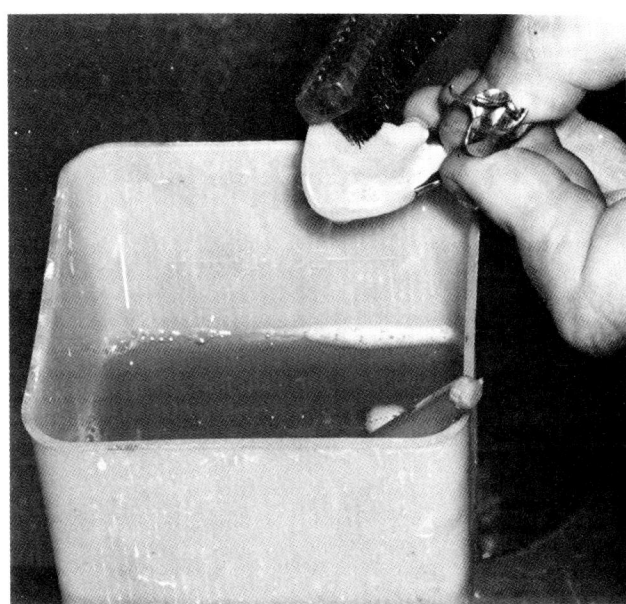

**Fig. 13-88.** Clean with tincture of green soap, hot water, and brush.

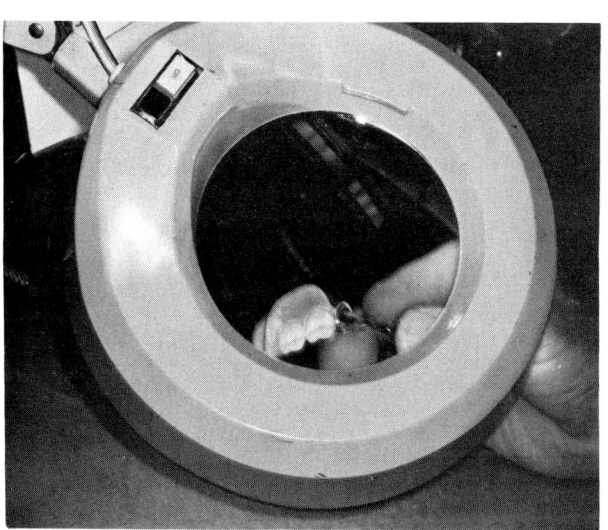

**Fig. 13-89.** Inspect finish with magnification.

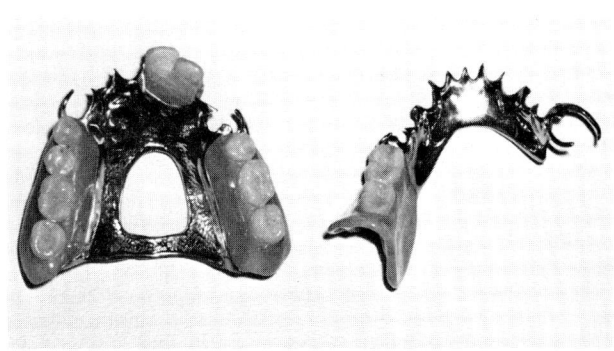

**Fig. 13-90.** Completed partial dentures ready for delivery.

## DUPLICATE MASTER CASTS

If partial dentures were processed on the master casts, the only thing available to send back to the dental office is the two partial dentures and the diagnostic casts. The partial dentures will not fit the diagnostic casts (Fig. 13-91). When adjustment is required, it must be done in the mouth. Duplicate master casts can be very valuable.

Duplicate master casts are made at the time the refractory casts are made. After the cast has been removed from the duplicating medium for the refractory cast, remove any blockout or relief on the soft tissue areas of the denture base. If none are present, they may be used without further preparation. Put the casts in duplicating flasks and pour hydrocolloid around them as described in Chapter 7. Cool the hydrocolloid, and recover the cast from the duplicating material. Vibrate a mix of dental stone into the mold to make a duplicate master cast. This duplicate master cast can be used for fitting the metal framework when polishing. Since it can be mounted in an articulator, the teeth can be set up

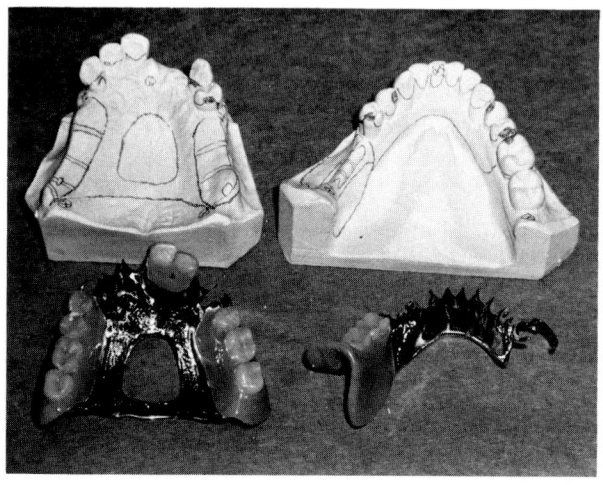

**Fig. 13-91.** Completed partial dentures and diagnostic casts ready to be returned to the dental office. NOTE: Master casts are destroyed if partial dentures are processed on them.

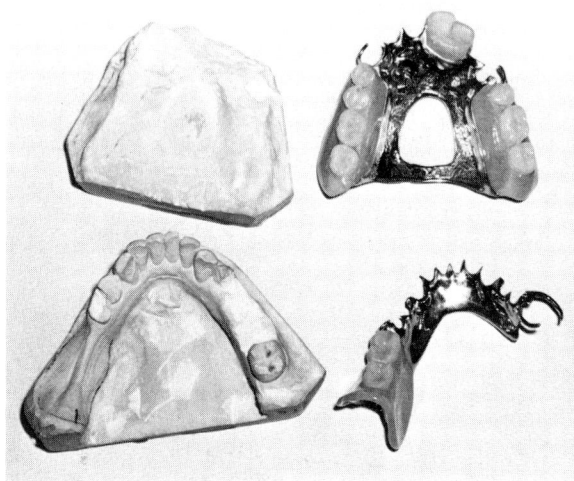

**Fig. 13-92.** Alternatively, partial dentures can be processed on duplicate master casts that will be destroyed during procedure, leaving master casts intact.

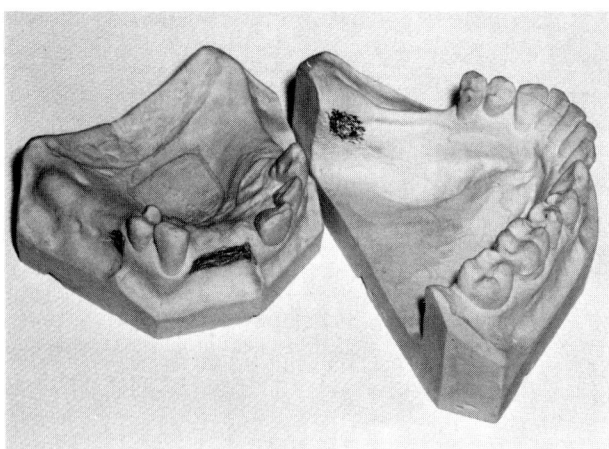

**Fig. 13-93.** Master casts will be preserved, and partial dentures can be fitted to them by removing undercuts, indicated by dark marks, in denture base area to permit seating completed partial dentures on them.

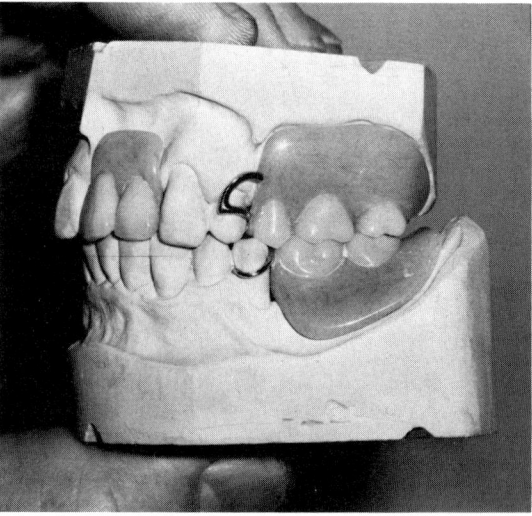

**Fig. 13-94.** Completed partial dentures can be returned to dental office on master cast.

on the duplicate master cast rather than on the master cast. Partial dentures can be processed on the duplicate master cast, remounted on the articulator, and the occlusion corrected. Remove it from the cast as just described, and finish and polish it. The duplicate master casts will be destroyed but the master casts are intact (Fig. 13-92). Fit the finished partial denture to the master cast. It will be necessary to remove some undercuts in the denture base area on the cast (Fig. 13-93). The partial dentures are placed on the master casts ready to be returned to the office (Fig. 13-94).

Fitting and processing on the duplicate master cast has the following advantages:

1. Arbitrary blockout wax and blockout wax need not be removed from the master cast unless it is in a denture base area.

2. The master cast is not scarred and damaged if the framework is not fitted to it in the laboratory.

3. By mounting the master casts and the duplicate master casts, the jaw relation record is double-checked.

4. The master cast is not destroyed when recovering the partial denture after processing.

5. Finished partial dentures can be sent back to the office on the master cast.

6. Completed partial dentures can be mounted easily on the articulator, when they are returned on the master cast. The occlusal adjustments may be done on the articulator rather than in the mouth.

7. If the framework or a clasp has been bent or sprung, it is easier to adapt it to the cast than to the mouth.

8. It will help to identify whoever is at fault if the completed partial denture does not fit. If the framework fits the mouth at the time of the try-in, but does not fit after the partial denture is completed, it is easy to place it on the master cast to see if it still fits the cast as it did before the plastic was finished. If the cast is not available, it is one person's word against another's.

## SUMMARY

In this chapter flasking, processing, deflasking, and finishing procedures have been described and potential problem areas identified. The methods presented are those which have proven to be effective and have stood the test of time. Since it is possible to ruin an acceptable framework through careless flasking, processing, deflasking, and finishing, it is particularly important to develop a thorough understanding of the methods.

### REFERENCES

Morrow, R. M., Rudd, K. D., and Eissmann, H. F.: Dental laboratory procedures: complete dentures, vol. 1, St. Louis, 1980, The C. V. Mosby Co.

### BIBLIOGRAPHY

Air Force Manual 160-29: Dental laboratory technicians' manual, United States Air Force, Washington, D.C., 1959, U.S. Government Printing Office.

Air Force Manual 162-6: Dental laboratory technology, United States Air Force, Washington, D.C., 1975, U.S. Government Printing Office.

Sowter, J. B.: Dental laboratory technology: prosthodontic techniques, Chapel Hill, N.C., 1968, The University of North Carolina Press.

Stewart, K. L.: Removable partial denture laboratory manual, San Antonio, 1979, The University of Texas Health Science Center.

# CHAPTER 14

# RELINING AND REBASING

WILLIAM A. KUEBKER, JAMES A. FOWLER, Jr., and AMBROCIO V. ESPINOZA

**rebase** A process of refitting a denture by the replacement of the denture base material without changing the occlusal relations of the teeth. (All the denture base resin is replaced; the metal framework and the denture teeth are unchanged.)

**reline** To resurface the tissue side of a denture with new denture base material to make it fit more accurately. (The metal framework, artificial teeth, and external denture bases are not changed.)

## RELINING

Removable partial dentures are relined to improve the fit of the denture base to the residual ridge. This procedure is indicated when the prosthesis fulfills the following criteria: (1) the framework is in good condition and fits well; (2) the occlusion can be corrected with simple equilibration; (3) the denture base material is in good condition, and its appearance is acceptable to the patient; (4) the artificial teeth are in good condition, and their appearance is acceptable to the patient; and (5) the denture base borders are reasonably accurate.

The denture base to be relined may be of the distal extension type or may be entirely tooth supported. Or the prosthesis may have both types of bases. The reline impression may be made with one of several different materials such as mouth-temperature wax, metallic paste, rubber base, or silicone impression material. The laboratory procedures for relining the removable partial denture are essentially the same regardless of the type of edentulous area or type of impression material used in making the impression.

The laboratory procedure of flasking and processing a removable partial denture *reline* is definitely *contraindicated.* Incomplete flask closure of even the smallest degree will result in severe clinical problems. The framework may not seat completely, resulting in continuous stress being placed on the abutment teeth by the retentive clasps as well as the rests not being completely seated into the rest seats. There may be excessive pressure over the residual ridge, resulting in considerable soreness for the patient. The use of one of the reline jigs is the safest way to process a removable partial denture reline.

The laboratory may receive the reline impression in one of two forms. The dentist may make the reline impression of the denture base areas and send the prosthesis to the laboratory in this condition. Or an alginate impression may be made over the prosthesis after the reline impression has been made of the denture bases. The laboratory will then receive an alginate impression with the prosthesis embedded in the alginate. Different procedures will have to be followed in making the reline master cast, depending on the form in which the prosthesis is received. Once the reline master cast has been made, the reline procedures are the same for both types of reline impressions.

### Reline master cast
#### *Framework and bases with reline impression*
**PROCEDURE**

1. Pour artificial stone into the relined bases using the two-stage pour technique (Fig. 14-1).
2. After the reline master cast has completely set, it is shaped on a model trimmer, and its base is indexed (Fig. 14-2).

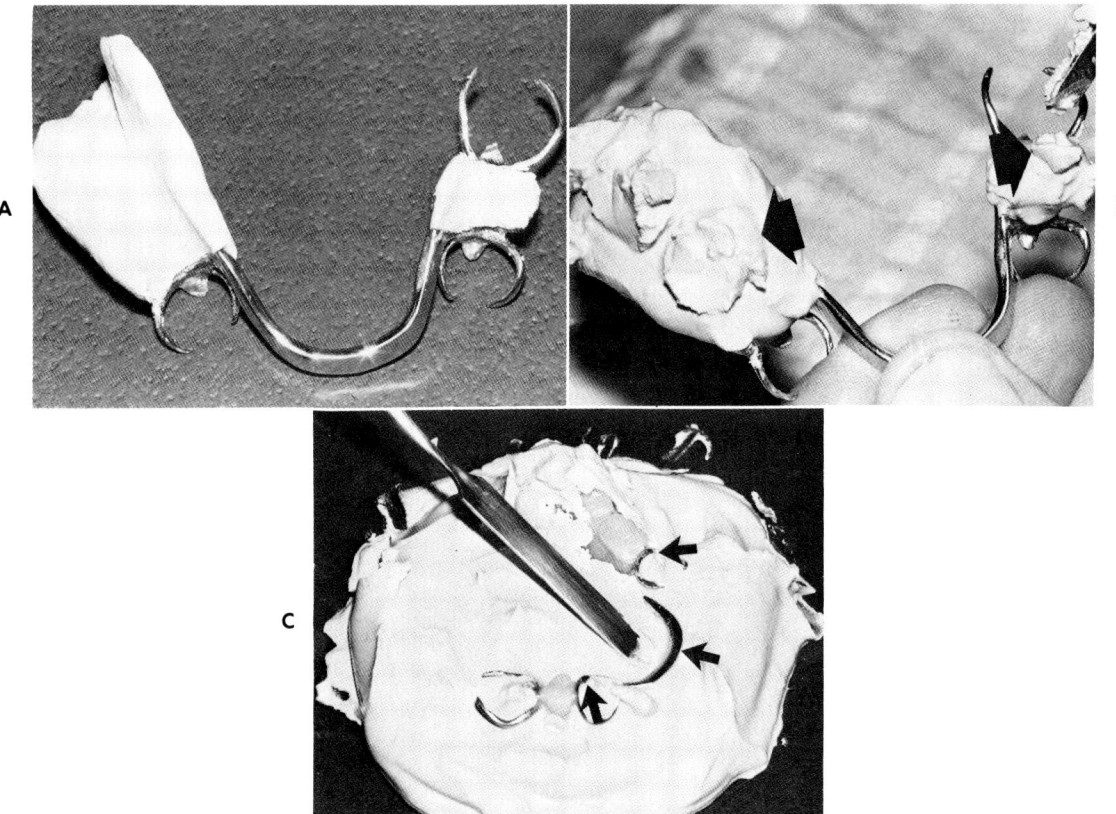

**Fig. 14-1. A,** Impression is made in denture bases of removable partial denture that is to be relined. **B,** Artificial stone is poured into denture base impression areas, making certain borders are covered. Small irregular mounds of artificial stone (arrows) are added to assist in retention of second stage of pour. **C,** After first pour has reached its initial set, it is soaked in clear slurry water and then inverted into second mix of stone. Soft artificial stone is shaped so that it contacts undersurface of major connector and occlusal rests (arrows). Care is taken to avoid locking framework into stone cast.

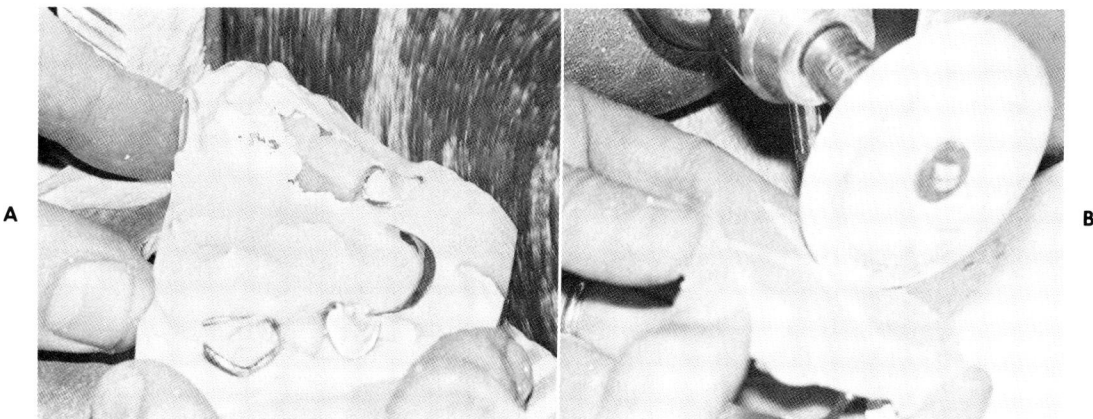

**Fig. 14-2. A,** After soaking cast in clear slurry water for 3 to 4 minutes, it is trimmed on cast trimmer. **B,** Base of cast is indexed with tapered cutting wheel.

**402** *Dental laboratory procedures: removable partial dentures*

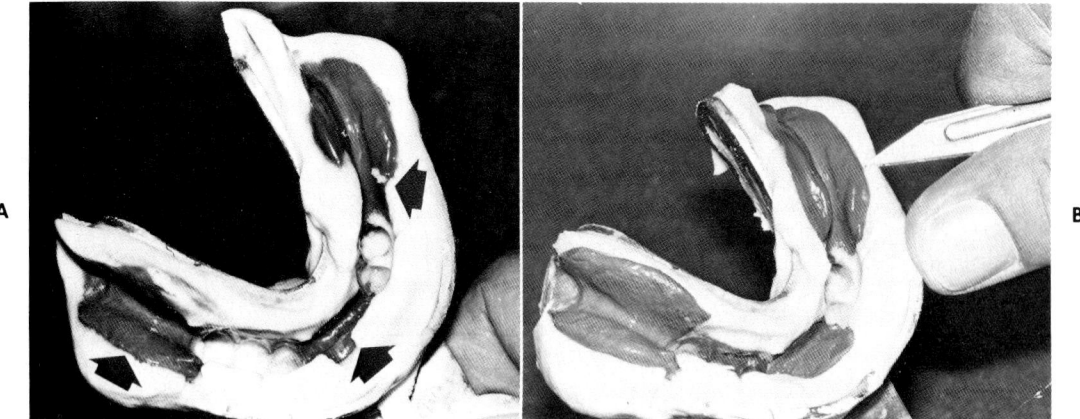

**Fig. 14-3. A,** Bases have been relined with rubber base impression material, and alginate impression was made over removable partial denture while it was seated in mouth. Note that alginate impression material covers borders (arrows) of relined denture bases. **B,** Sharp knife is used to trim alginate to expose all border roll areas of relined bases.

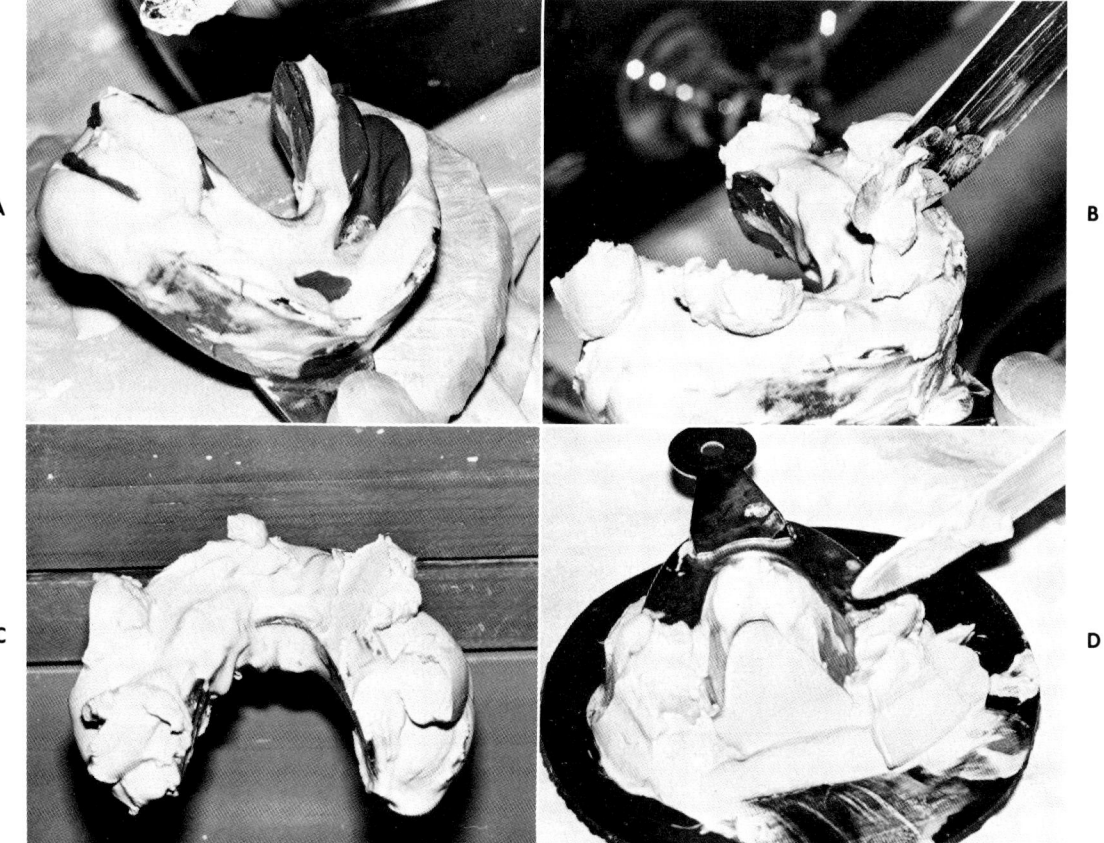

**Fig. 14-4. A,** Mix of artificial stone is vibrated into impression. Entire impression is filled, and all borders are covered. **B,** Small irregular mounds of artificial stone are placed to provide retention for second stage of pouring cast. **C,** Impression tray is suspended by its handle, and Hydrocal is allowed to complete its initial set (10 to 15 minutes). **D,** After soaking first stage of pour in clear slurry water for 5 minutes, tray is seated into patty of Hydrocal. Stone is shaped around borders of first pour to provide support for heels of cast and to create good union between first and second stages of pour.

## Alginate impression over framework and relined bases

**PROCEDURE**

1. Prepare the alginate impression with its picked up removable partial denture for pouring the reline cast (Fig. 14-3).
2. Pour the master reline cast in Hydrocal using the two-stage pour technique (Fig. 14-4).
3. Remove the alginate impression from the set cast, shape the cast on a model trimmer, and index the cast (Fig. 14-5).

## Reline using a reline jig*

The same procedures may be followed using a Hooper Duplicator† or any other suitable reline jig.

**PROCEDURE**

1. Make an index of the occlusal and incisal surfaces of the teeth of the cast and removable partial denture. Attach this index to the lower half of the jig (Fig. 14-6). NOTE: The removable partial denture *must not be removed* from its cast until indicated later in the reline procedure.

---

*Reline Jig, Howmedica, Inc., Chicago, Ill.
†Hooper Duplicator, Hanau Division, Teledyne Dental Products Co., Buffalo, N.Y.

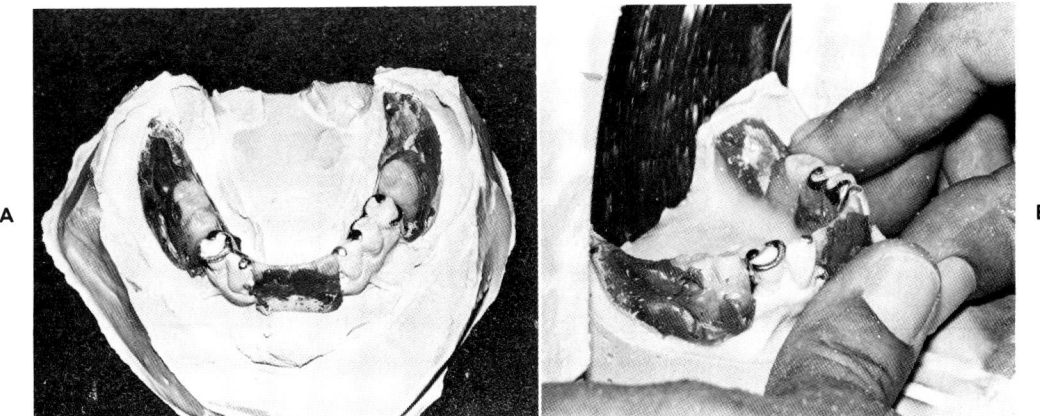

**Fig. 14-5. A,** Alginate impression is removed from cast 45 to 60 minutes after first stage of pour. Note that relined partial denture remains on cast. **B,** After thoroughly soaking cast in clear slurry water, cast is shaped on model trimmer, and its base is indexed with tapered index wheel.

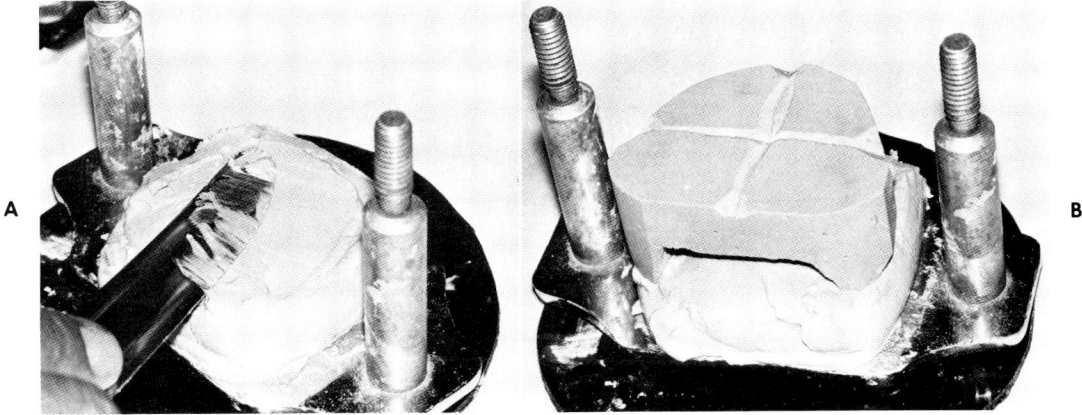

**Fig. 14-6. A,** Artificial stone is mixed and placed in retention area of lower half of reline jig. Additional Hydrocal is placed and shaped into flat patty of larger dimensions than reline cast. **B,** Reline cast is seated into soft patty of Hydrocal so that occlusal third of teeth are embedded into stone. Hydrocal is allowed to set.

2. While the cast is still seated in the occlusal index, attach it to the upper member of the reline jig with Hydrocal. Take care to ensure that the upper member is in complete metal-to-metal contact with the cylindrical shafts of the lower half of the reline jig and that the wing nuts are completely tightened (Fig. 14-7).

3. After the Hydrocal has completely set, separate the two halves of the reline jig. Verify the adequacy of the occlusal index before separating the removable partial denture from its reline cast (Fig. 14-8).

4. Carefully remove the removable partial denture from the reline cast (Fig. 14-9).

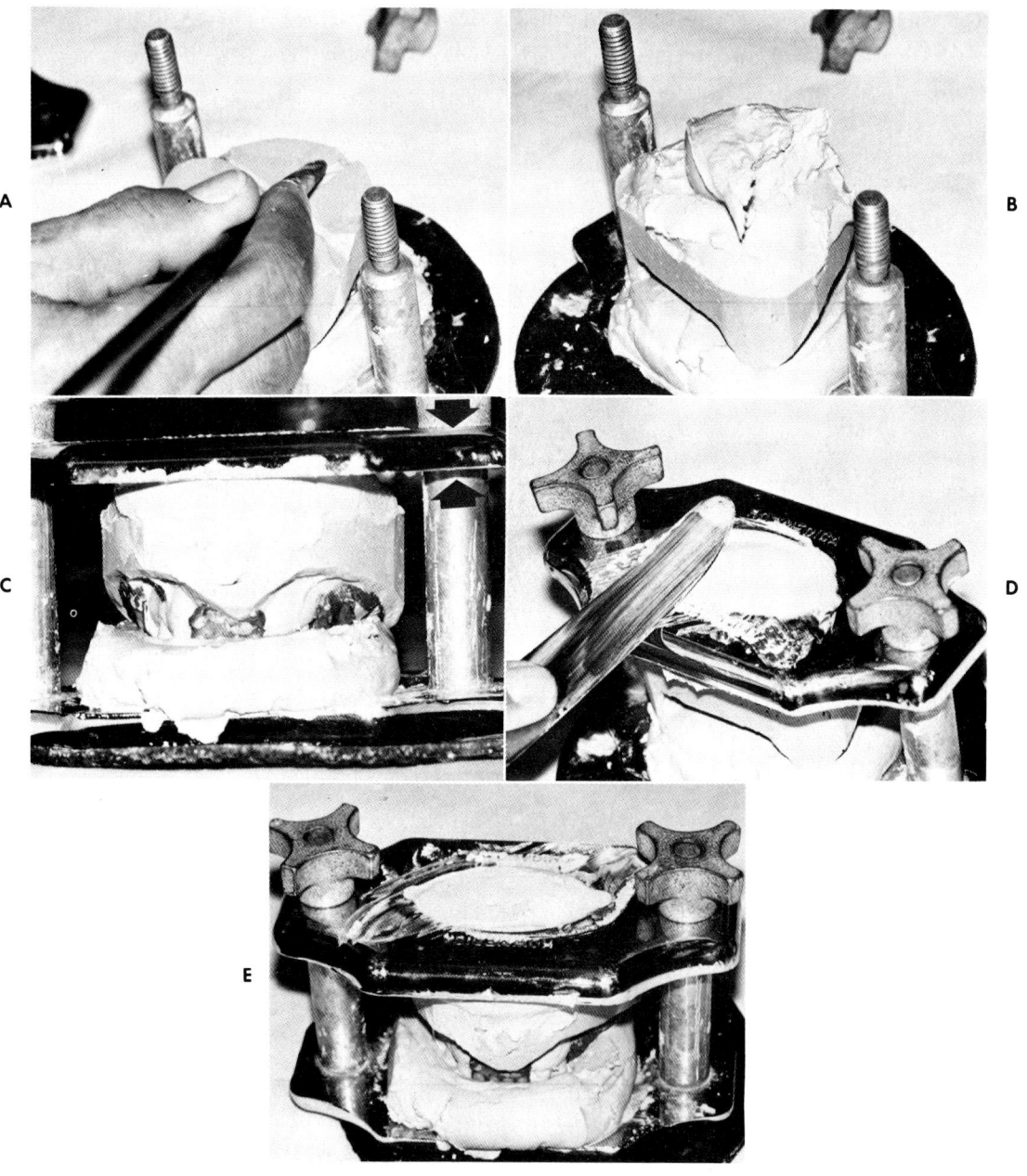

Fig. 14-7. **A,** While reline cast is still seated in its occlusal index, base of cast is painted with separating medium. **B,** Mix of Hydrocal is built up on base of reline cast. **C,** Upper half of reline jig is positioned over cylindrical shafts (arrows) of lower member. Wing nuts are closed down until complete metal-to-metal contact is present between beveled shoulders of cylindrical shafts and beveled seats of upper member of reline jig. **D,** Additional Hydrocal is added and smoothed to completely fill retention area of upper half of reline jig. **E,** Hydrocal is allowed to reach its final set.

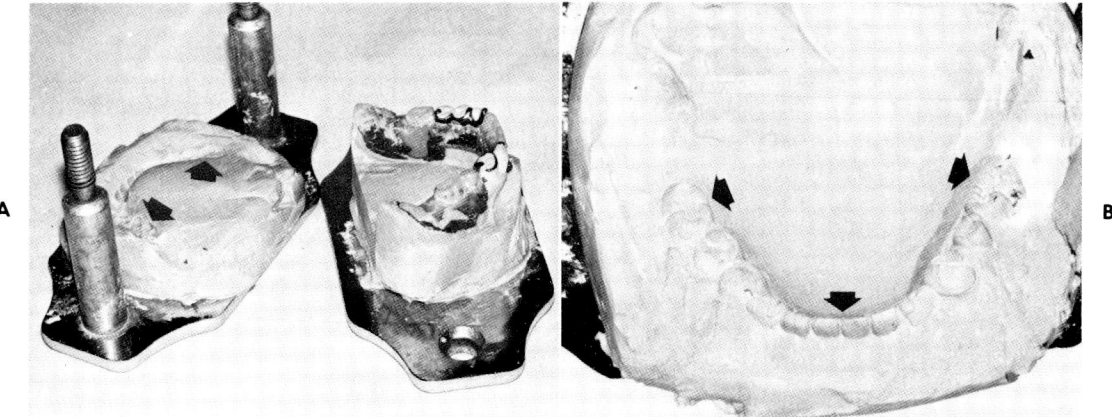

**Fig. 14-8. A,** After Hydrocal has completely set, wing nuts are removed, and two halves of reline jig are separated, exposing occlusal index (arrows). **B,** Before removing partial denture from reline cast, occlusal index is carefully examined to ascertain that clear, definite indices are present (arrows) so that prosthesis can be accurately repositioned into index.

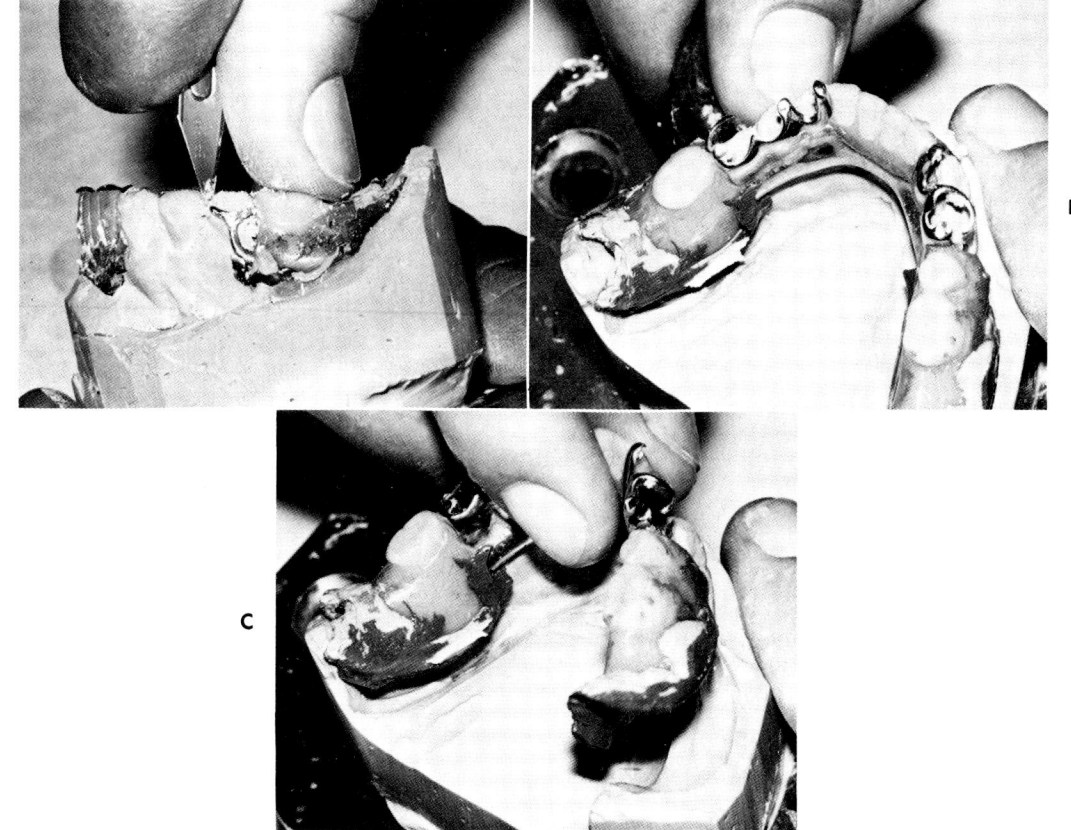

**Fig. 14-9. A,** Sharp knife is used to trim abutment teeth and any other areas of reline cast that may be locking partial denture into cast. **B,** After soaking the cast in 140° F (60° C) water for 3 to 4 minutes, instrument is used to carefully tease removable partial denture from cast. If resistance is met, cast should be inspected for areas where prosthesis is locking, and cast is then resoaked in warm water. **C,** Partial denture is removed when removal can be accomplished without danger of distorting clasps or other components of prosthesis.

5. Apply two layers of tinfoil substitute to the reline cast and the occlusal index (Fig. 14-10).

6. Remove the impression material from the denture base areas (Fig. 14-11).

7. Remove all traces of impression material from the tissue surfaces of the denture bases. A fresh clean surface of resin should be exposed (Fig. 14-12).

8. Freshen the borders of the denture bases, and prepare them for a butt joint of new resin (Fig. 14-13).

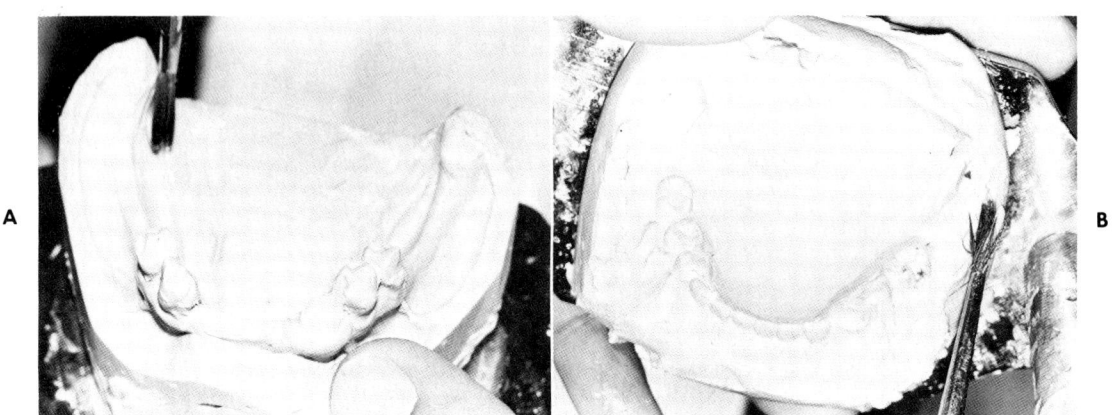

**Fig. 14-10. A,** Brush is used to flow tinfoil substitute onto reline cast. When first layer has dried, second layer is applied. **B,** Two layers of tinfoil substitute are applied to all areas of occlusal index that may be contacted by acrylic resin during reline procedure.

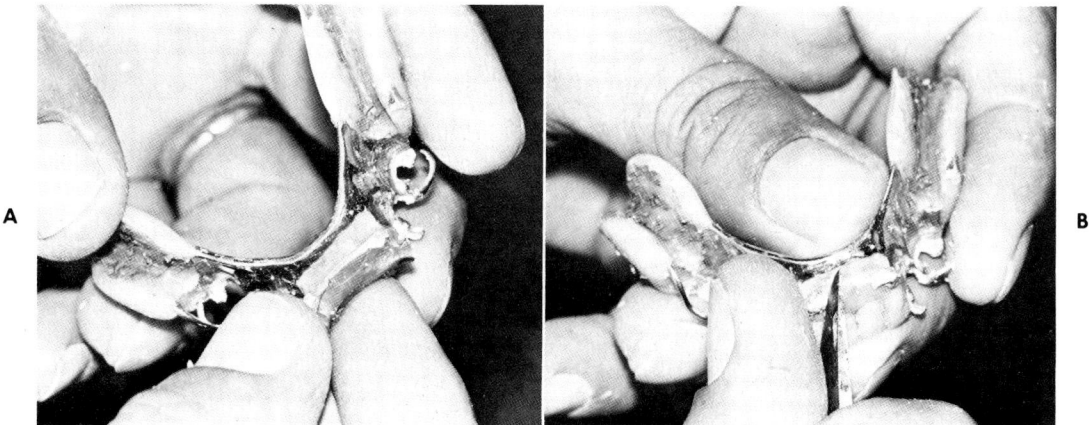

**Fig 14-11. A,** Rubber base impression material is removed from denture base areas. **B,** Sharp knife is used to scrape off modeling plastic used in border molding and any other impression material adhering to denture bases.

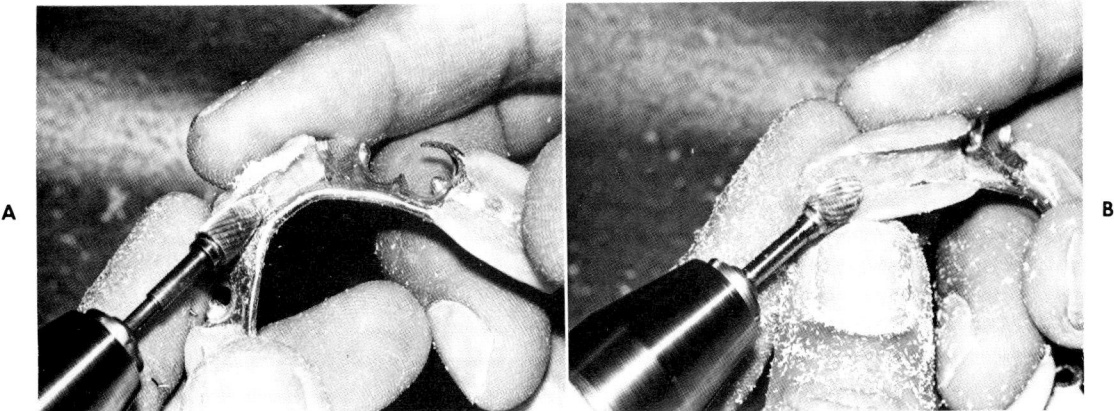

**Fig. 14-12. A,** Vulcanite bur is used to remove impression material that remains on anterior denture base. Acrylic resin is relieved to expose acrylic resin minor connector of framework. **B,** Posterior bases are relieved to clean and freshen resin and to remove any undercuts.

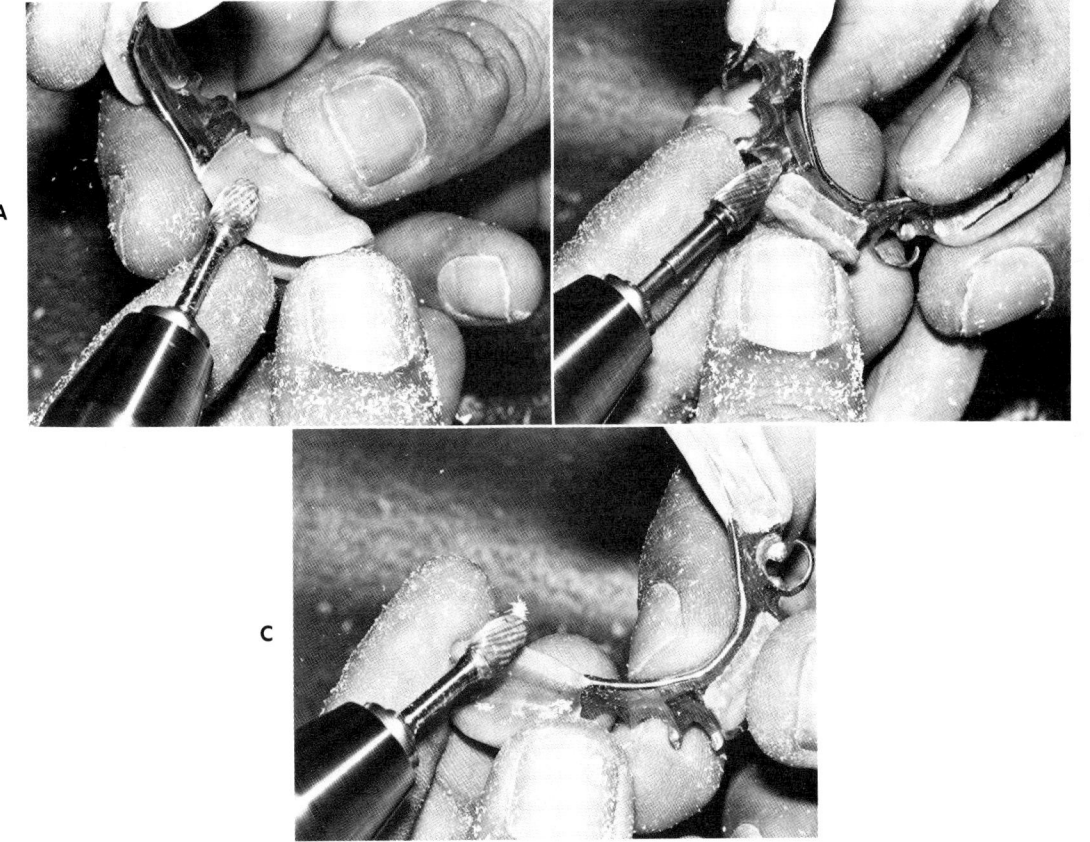

**Fig. 14-13. A,** Vulcanite bur is used to prepare clean fresh surface extending several millimeters onto polished surfaces of borders of denture bases. **B** and **C,** All borders are shortened approximately 1 mm and are cut flat to provide for butt joint of new acrylic resin.

9. Seat the removable partial denture into the index, and lute it in position with wax (Fig. 14-14).

10. Mix autopolymerizing acrylic resin according to the manufacturer's instructions (Fig. 14-15).

11. Place the soft acrylic resin on the denture bases and on the tissue areas of the cast, and assemble the two halves of the reline jig. Screw the wing nuts down to ensure that the two halves of the jig are in metal-to-metal contact (Fig. 14-16).

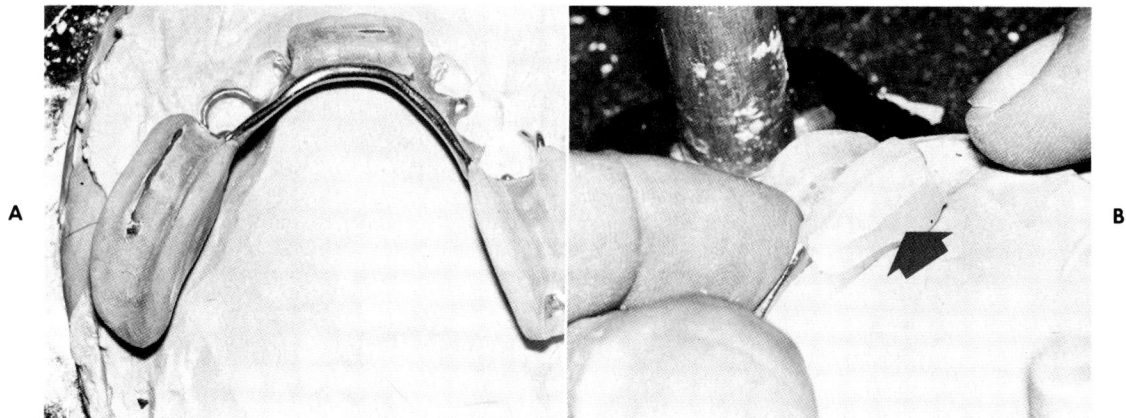

**Fig. 14-14. A,** Prosthesis is seated into occlusal index and inspected to make certain it seats accurately. **B,** Wax is used to lute prosthesis to cast (arrow) to prevent movement during placement of new acrylic resin.

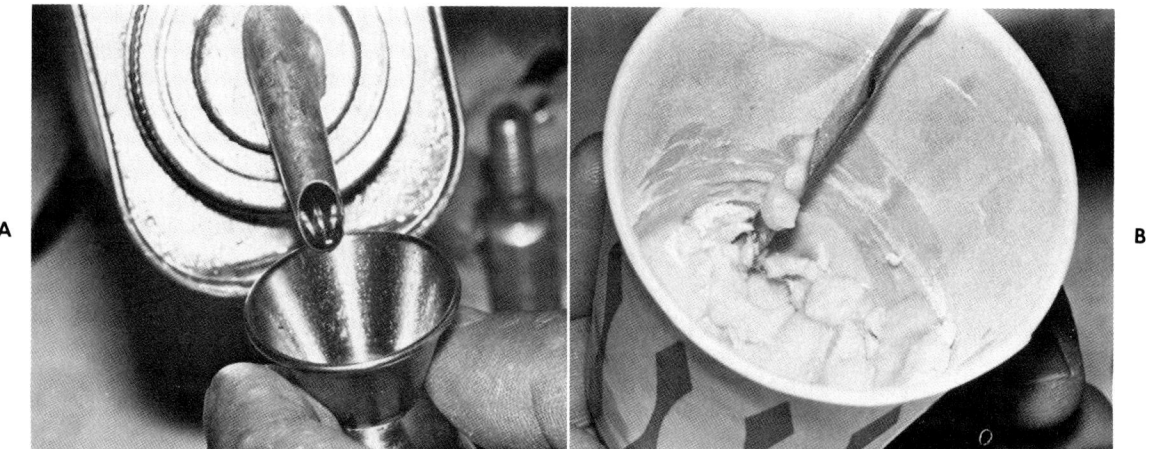

**Fig. 14-15. A,** Autopolymerizing acrylic resin that is suitable for relines is measured according to manufacturer's instructions. **B,** Resin is mixed to make certain that all of polymer is wetted by monomer.

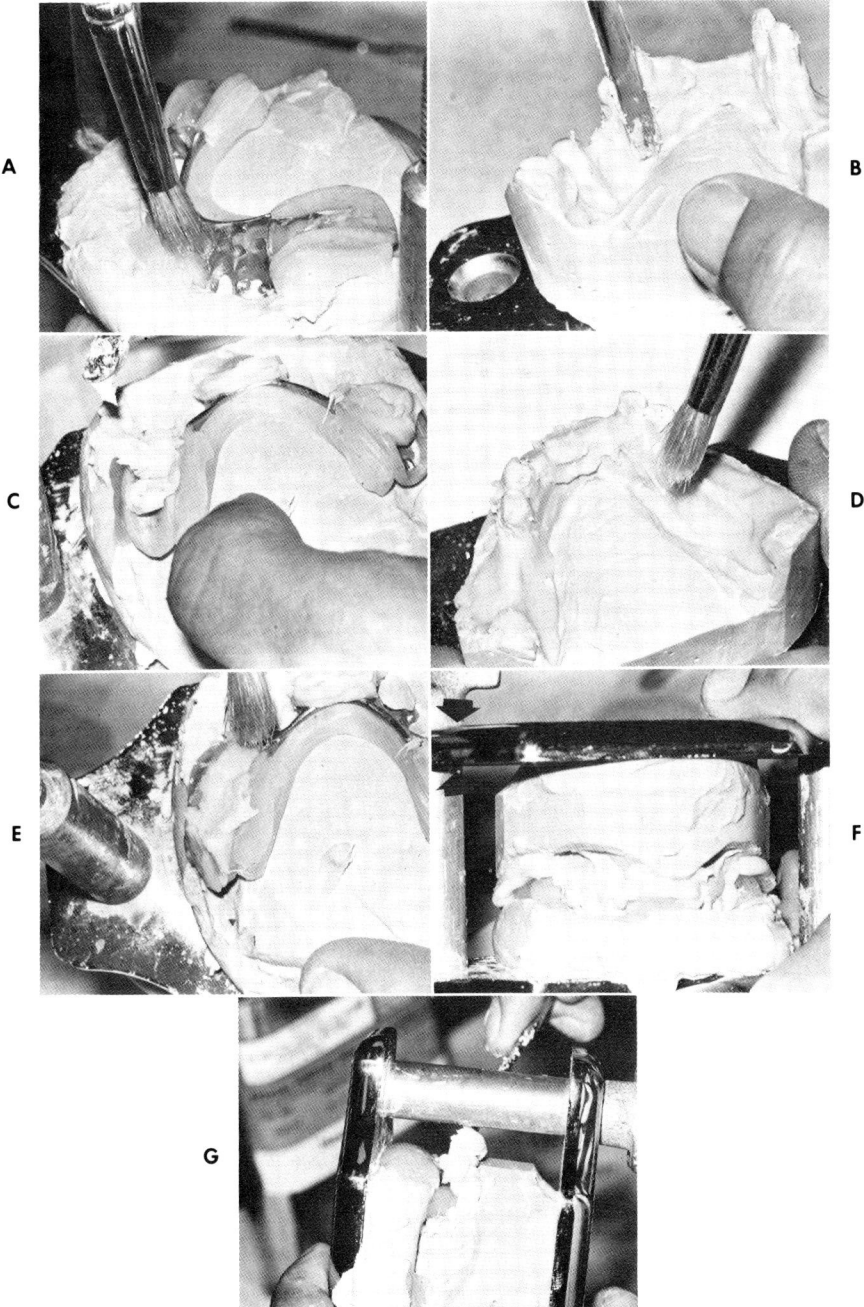

**Fig. 14-16. A,** Resin bases are painted with same type of autopolymerizing resin monomer as was used in making mix of resin. **B,** Spatula is used to flow soft resin onto ridge areas of reline cast in attempt to avoid trapping air. **C,** Soft resin is also placed onto tissue surfaces of denture bases. **D,** Monomer is painted to dampen surface of resin that was placed on reline cast. **E,** Monomer is also painted on resin placed in denture bases. **F,** Two halves of reline jig are assembled, and wing nuts are tightened down until there is metal-to-metal contact between beveled recesses of upper member and beveled cylindrical shafts of lower member of reline jig. **G,** Spatula is used to remove excess soft acrylic resin and to compress resin into border areas of reline cast to prevent air entrapment or incomplete filling of border areas.

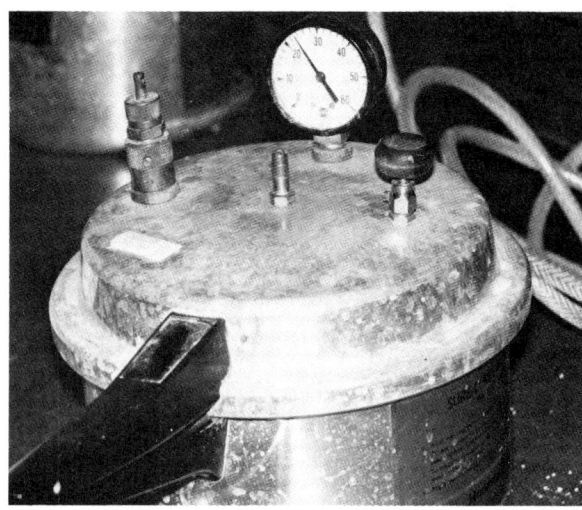

**Fig. 14-17.** Reline jig is placed in pressure container that contains water at 100° F (39° C). Reline is cured for 30 minutes under pressure of 15 to 25 psi.

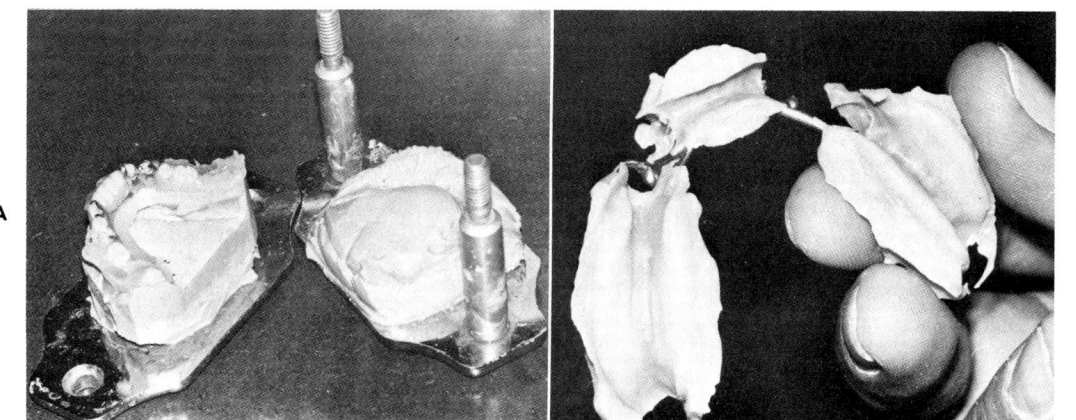

**Fig. 14-18. A,** After processing, wing nuts are removed, and two halves of reline jig are separated. **B,** Relined prosthesis is recovered from reline cast.

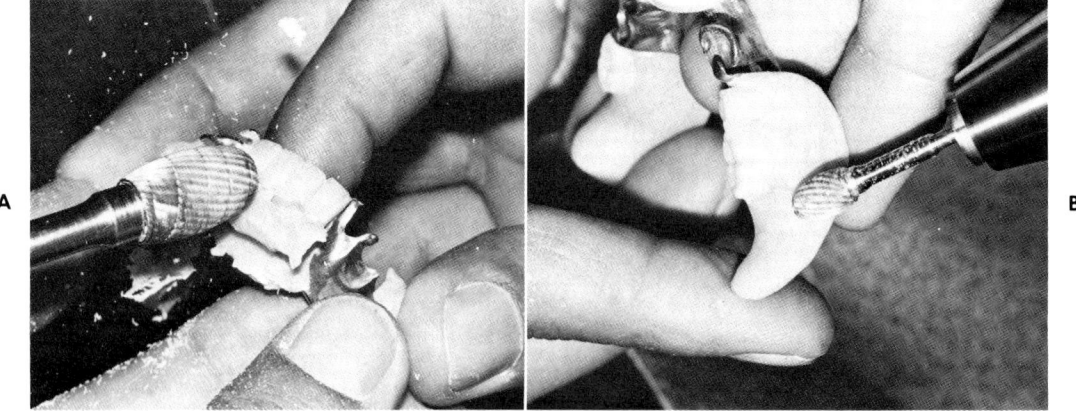

**Fig. 14-19. A,** Vulcanite bur is used to remove flash from processed reline. **B,** External contours of prosthesis are refined with vulcanite bur.

# Relining and rebasing 411

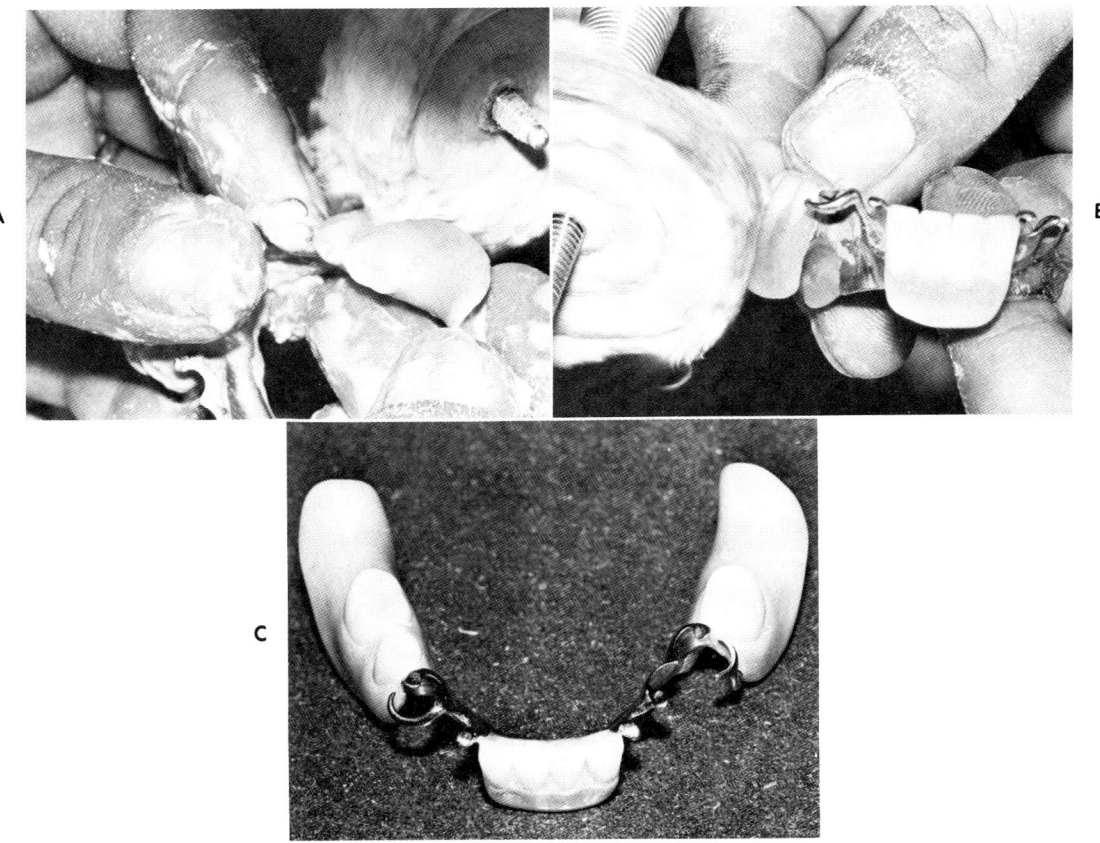

**Fig. 14-20. A,** Wet rag wheel and wet flour of pumice are used to polish external surfaces and borders of prosthesis. **B,** Clean dry rag wheel and fine polishing compound are used to produce final polish. **C,** Relined removable partial denture.

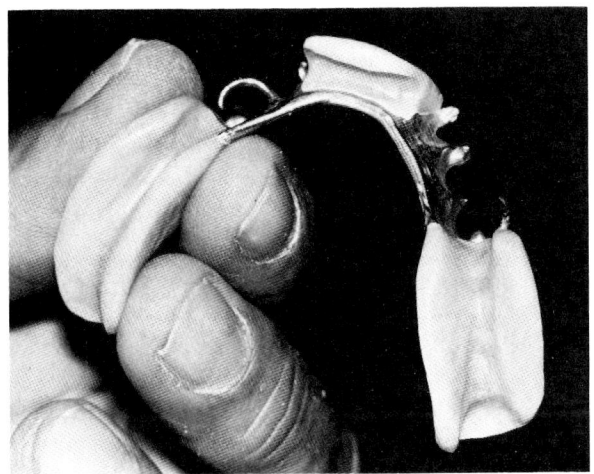

**Fig. 14-21.** Both tissue side and polished surfaces are carefully inspected for presence of voids, nodules, porosity, or any other defects.

12. Process the reline for 30 minutes in a pressure container (Fig. 14-17).

13. After processing, remove the relined removable partial denture from the reline cast (Fig. 14-18).

14. Remove the flash, and refine the contours of the removable partial denture (Fig. 14-19).

15. Polish the borders and external surfaces (Fig. 14-20).

16. Carefully inspect the relined removable partial denture for voids, nodules, or any other defects (Fig. 14-21).

## PROBLEM AREAS

The major problems associated with relining removable partial dentures can be eliminated by using the reline jig method rather than flasking the prosthesis for processing. Problems associated with

**Table 14-1.** Removable partial denture reline procedures

| Problem | Probable cause | Solution |
|---|---|---|
| Voids in resin of relined prosthesis | Insufficient autopolymerizing acrylic resin used | Use adequate volume of resin |
| | Air trapped over ridge areas | Carefully place resin over tissue areas of reline cast and onto tissue surfaces of denture bases |
| Voids in border areas | Insufficient resin used | Use adequate volume of resin |
| | Resin not compressed into border areas of cast | Use cement spatula to compress resin into all border areas after closure of reline jig |
| Demarcation lines or wrinkle on tissue surface of relined prosthesis | Surfaces of resin placed on cast and in denture bases become too dry before closure of reline jig | Place resin on cast and bases when it is at proper stage, and paint surfaces with monomer before closing reline jig |
| Unsightly line between new and original resin on denture border areas | Original denture resin not thoroughly cleaned and freshened prior to addition of new autopolymerizing resin | Thoroughly remove all traces of impression material; freshen all surfaces to be contacted by new resin by grinding with vulcanite bur |
| | Aerosol of oil in compressed air supply coated denture resin | Avoid using air to remove resin grindings if air source is contaminated with water or oil |
| | Resin too dry when placed in denture | Use correct liquid-powder ratio; place on denture and cast at proper stage |
| | Resin too dry when reline jig is closed | Paint surfaces of original resin with monomer before adding new resin |
| Relined denture is porous | Reline not cured in pressure container | Cure reline in pressure container for 30 minutes at 15 to 25 psi |
| Removable partial denture cannot be removed to clean off impression material without breaking reline cast | Undercuts were not removed from denture bases before making reline impression | Remove undercuts from denture bases before making impression |
| Rests of relined prosthesis will not seat completely into rest seats of abutment teeth | Reline processed in flask with incomplete flask closure | Use reline jig method rather than flasking |
| | Rests were not seated when impression was made | Open mouth impression should be used with finger pressure over rests only |
| | Reline jig not completely closed | Make certain thumbscrews of reline jig are completely tightened when processing reline |
| Relined partial denture rocks in mouth | Reline impression made with teeth in occlusion | Make open mouth impression |
| | Reline impression made with finger pressure over denture base areas | Hold prosthesis in place with finger pressure over rests only |
| | Framework not designed with three points of metal-to-tooth contact for correct orientation of framework when making impression | Avoid attempting to reline prosthesis that is not designed with three points of contact |
| | Prosthesis not accurately seated into occlusal index, or it moved during packing and processing | Inspect carefully to ensure that prosthesis is accurately seated in occlusal index; lute prosthesis in place with wax |
| Removable partial denture will not go completely into place in mouth | Resin left on guide plane areas or under rests | Carefully inspect completed reline for resin left on rests and guide planes |
| | Resin base interferes with flexing of clasp | Contour resin bases so they will not interfere with flexing of clasps |
| | Framework distorted when removing prosthesis from cast | Avoid use of force when removing prosthesis from cast |

the reline jig method, probable causes, and solutions to the problems are described in Table 14-1.

## REBASING

Removable partial dentures are rebased to improve the fit of the denture base to the residual ridge and to replace all of the denture base material. Rebasing is usually done because the denture base material has discolored or deteriorated. A new partial denture is sometimes rebased if the base developed porosity during the processing of the acrylic resin. Rebasing is indicated when the prosthesis fulfills the following criteria: (1) the framework is in good condition and fits well, (2) the artificial teeth are in good condition and the patient approves of their appearance, (3) the occlusion can be corrected with simple equilibration, (4) the denture base borders are reasonably accurate or can be extended to proper length in the impression making procedure.

The removable partial denture to be rebased may be of the distal extension type or may be entirely tooth supported or may have a combination of the two types of bases. The rebase impression may be made with the same materials and may be made by the same procedures as those described for the reline impression. The laboratory procedures for rebasing the removable partial denture are the same regardless of the type of edentulous area or the type of impression material used in making the impression.

The laboratory may receive the rebase impression in either of the two forms described for the reline impression. The laboratory procedures for making the rebase master cast are the same as for making a reline master cast.

### PROCEDURE

1. The rebase impression is received in the laboratory, and a rebase master cast is made using the two-stage pour technique (Fig. 14-22).

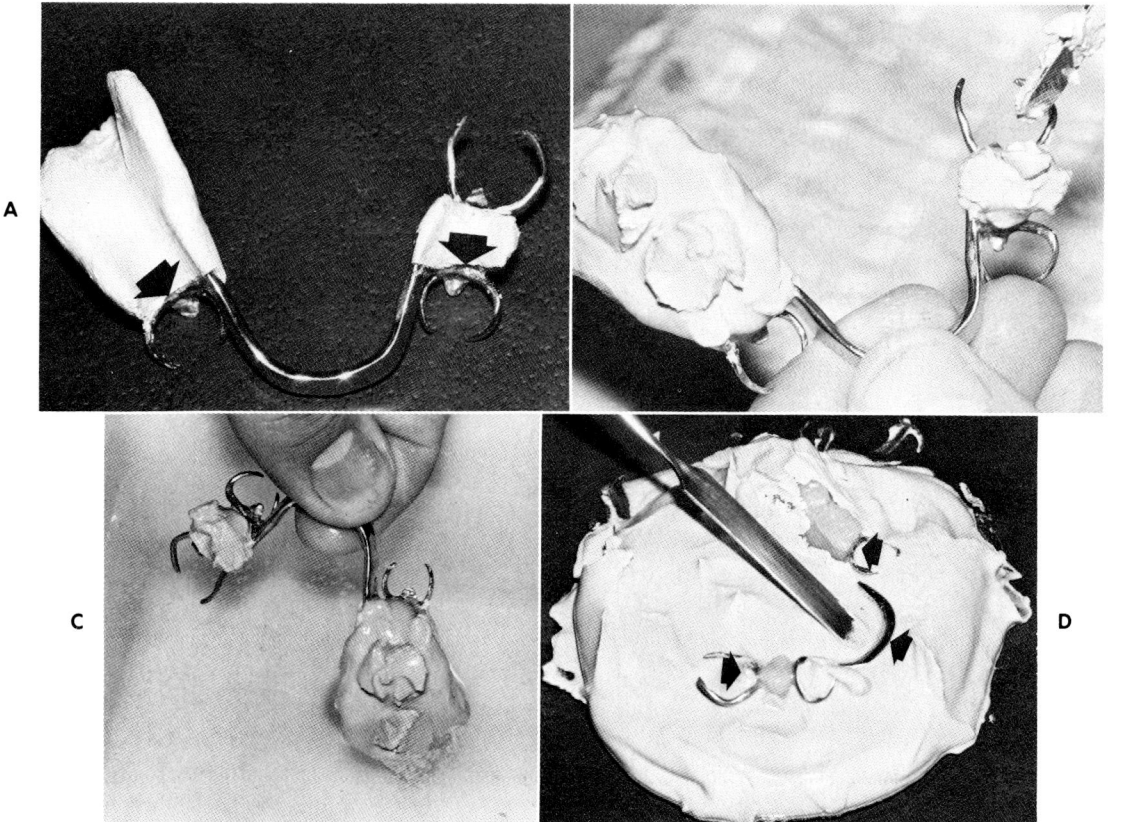

**Fig. 14-22. A,** Rebase impression has been made with zinc oxide–eugenol impression paste. Impression material is trimmed from minor connector areas (arrows). **B,** First stage is poured into denture base areas being certain to cover all borders. Small undercut mounds of stone are added for retention of second pour. **C,** After first pour has reached its initial set, it is soaked in clear slurry water for 2 to 3 minutes to wet first pour. **D,** First pour is inverted into patty of stone. Stone is shaped to contact undersurface of major connector and rest seats (arrows), but care must be taken to avoid locking framework into stone.

**414** *Dental laboratory procedures: removable partial dentures*

2. After the stone cast has set, shape it on a cast trimmer, and index the base (Fig. 14-23).

3. Paint the base of the cast with a stone separating medium,* and mount the cast on the lower half of a hinge-type articulator (Fig. 14-24).

4. Clean the artificial teeth of any impression material that is present, and lute the master rebase cast to its stone mounting on the articulator (Fig. 14-25).

---

*Super-Sep, Kerr Manufacturing Co., Romulus, Mich.

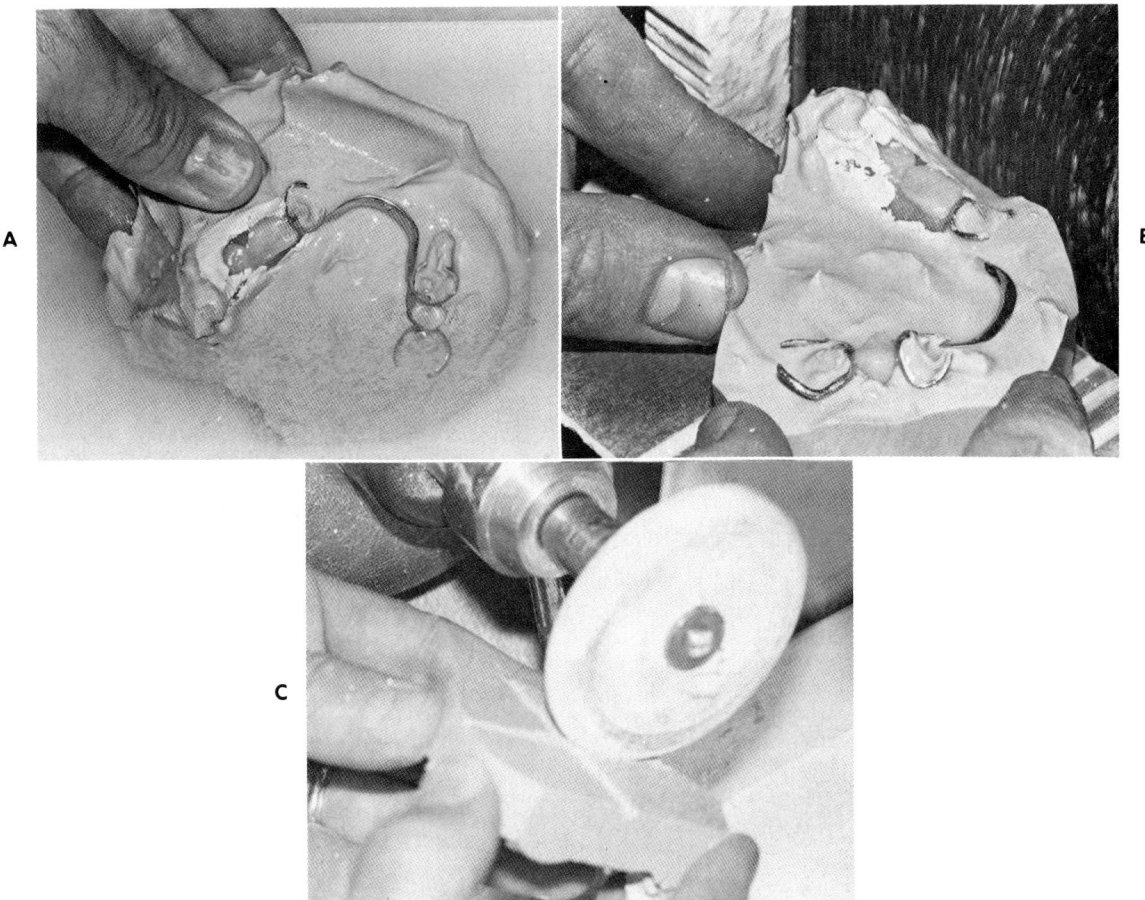

Fig. 14-23. A, After dental stone has reached its final set, cast is placed in clear slurry water for 2 to 3 minutes to thoroughly wet its surface. B, Cast is shaped on model trimmer using good flow of water. C, Base of cast is indexed with intersecting V-shaped grooves.

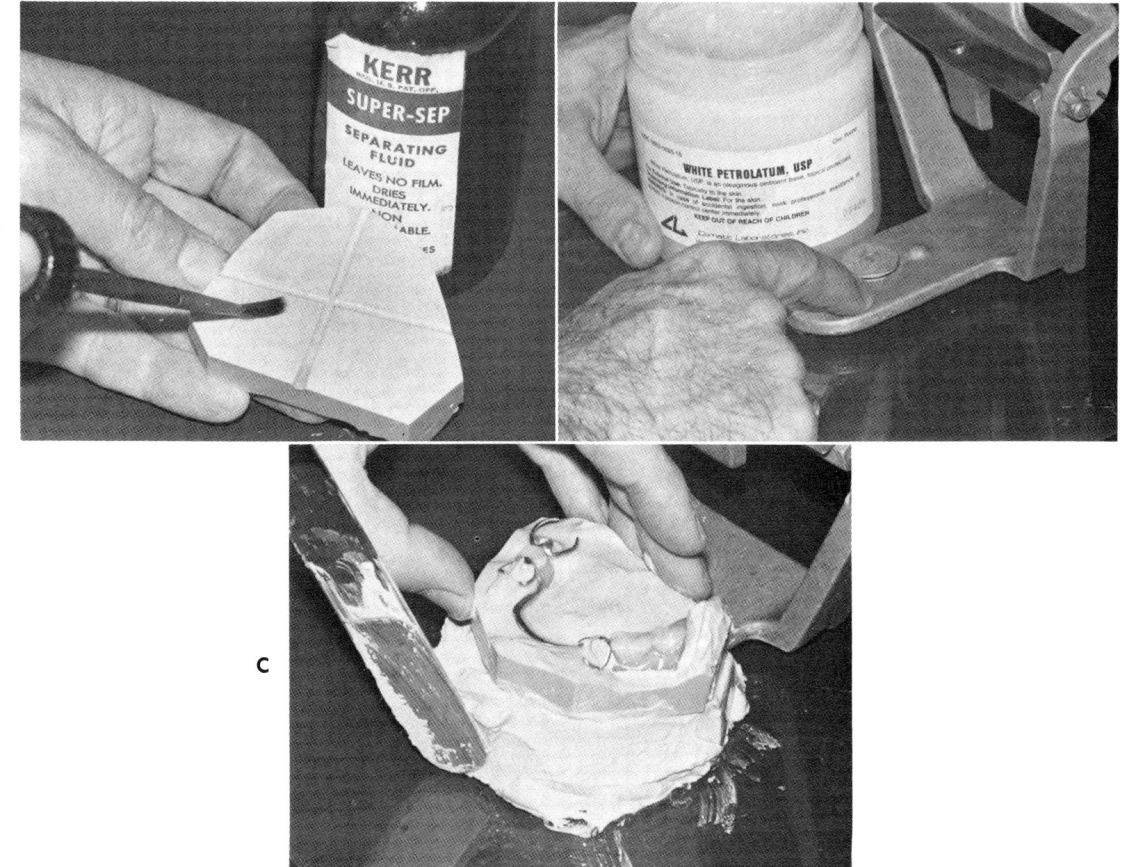

**Fig. 14-24. A,** Base of cast is painted with artificial stone separating medium and placed in clear slurry water for 2 to 3 minutes. **B,** Bottom half of articulator is lubricated with petroleum jelly. **C,** Mix of dental stone is used to mount rebase master cast. Occlusal plane is parallel with base of articulator.

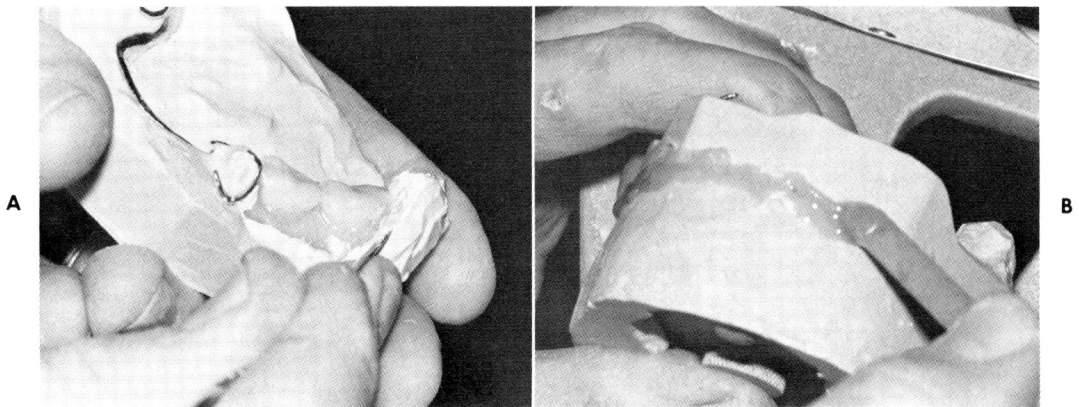

**Fig. 14-25. A,** Master rebase cast is removed from its mounting. Impression material that flowed onto polished surface and artificial teeth of prosthesis is cleaned off with instrument. **B,** Modeling plastic (or sticky wax) is used to lute cast onto its stone mounting.

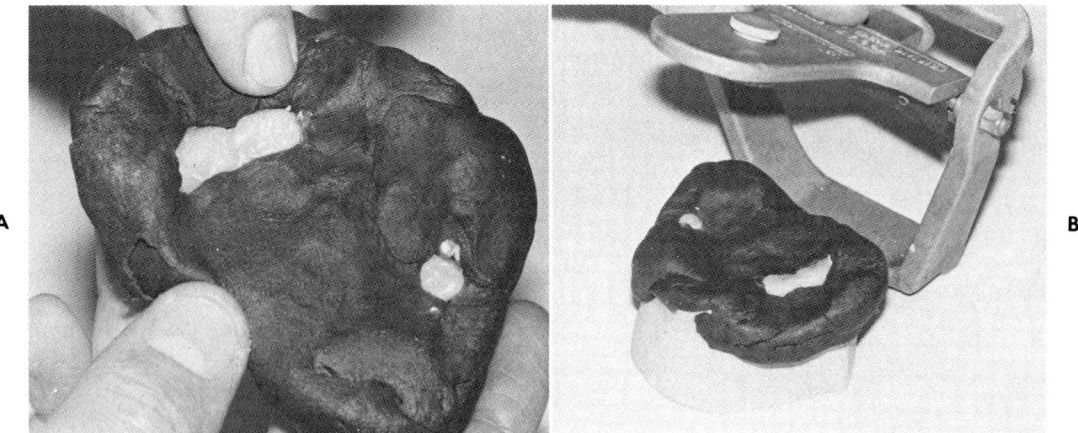

**Fig. 14-26. A,** Matrix for pouring of occlusal index is made by shaping blockout material so that only artificial teeth are exposed. Sufficient amount of tooth must be exposed to ensure that teeth can be accurately placed into index after they have been cut out of denture base. **B,** Completed matrix on articulator. Top half of articulator is lubricated with petroleum jelly in preparation for attachment of stone occlusal index. Estimate is made of amount of artificial stone required to fill space between matrix and upper half of articulator.

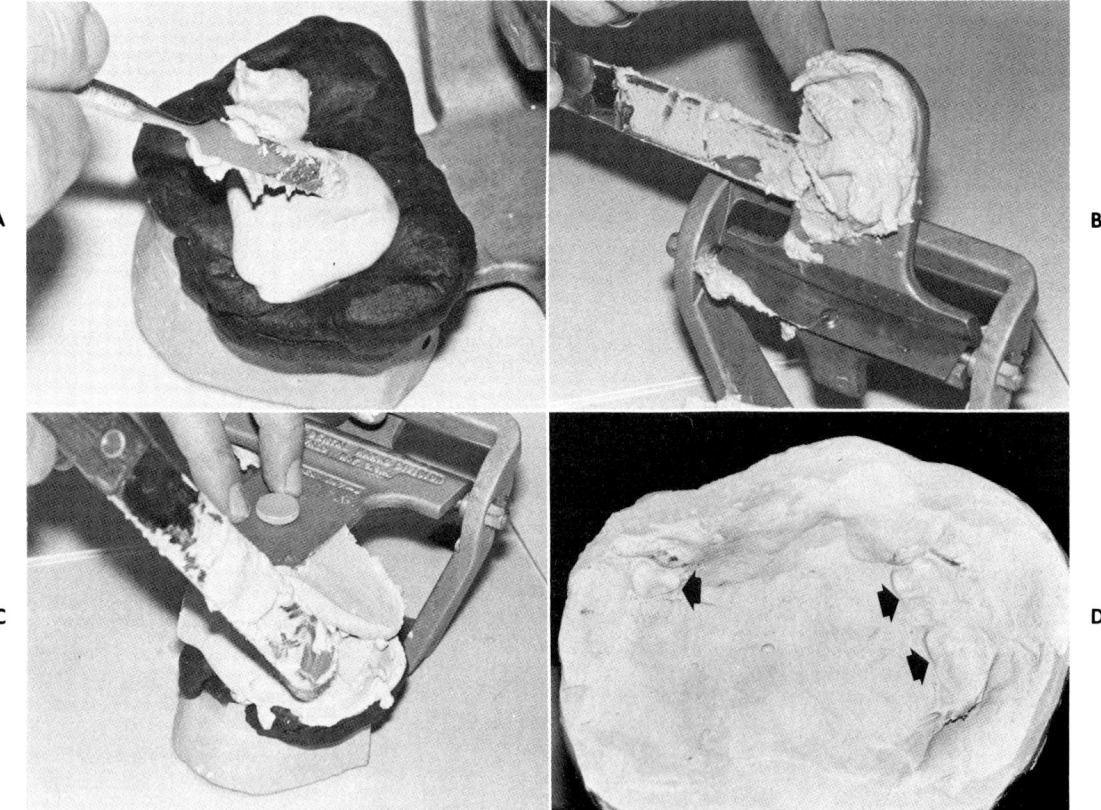

**Fig. 14-27. A,** Using correct water-powder ratio, mix of stone is made that is large enough to pour occlusal index and attach it to upper half of articulator. Entire matrix is filled with stone. **B,** Stone is added to retention area of upper member of articulator. **C,** Additional stone is added to complete pouring of occlusal index. **D,** After dental stone has reached its final set, articulator is opened to expose completed occlusal index. Note indentations for placement of artificial teeth (arrows).

5. Use blockout material to make a matrix for pouring an occlusal index (Fig. 14-26).

6. Use a single mix of stone to pour the occlusal index and to attach the index to the upper half of the articulator (Fig. 14-27).

7. Remove the removable partial denture from the rebase master cast (Fig. 14-28).

8. Remove the impression material from the cast and denture base areas. Cut the artificial teeth off the denture bases (Fig. 14-29).

9. Trim the artificial teeth, place them into the occlusal index, and lute them into position (Fig. 14-30).

10. Burn the resin bases off of the framework, and seat the framework on the rebase master cast to see if the tissue stop contacts the cast (Fig. 14-31).

11. Use autopolymerizing acrylic resin to establish contact between the tissue stop area of the framework and the ridge area of the rebase master cast (Fig. 14-32).

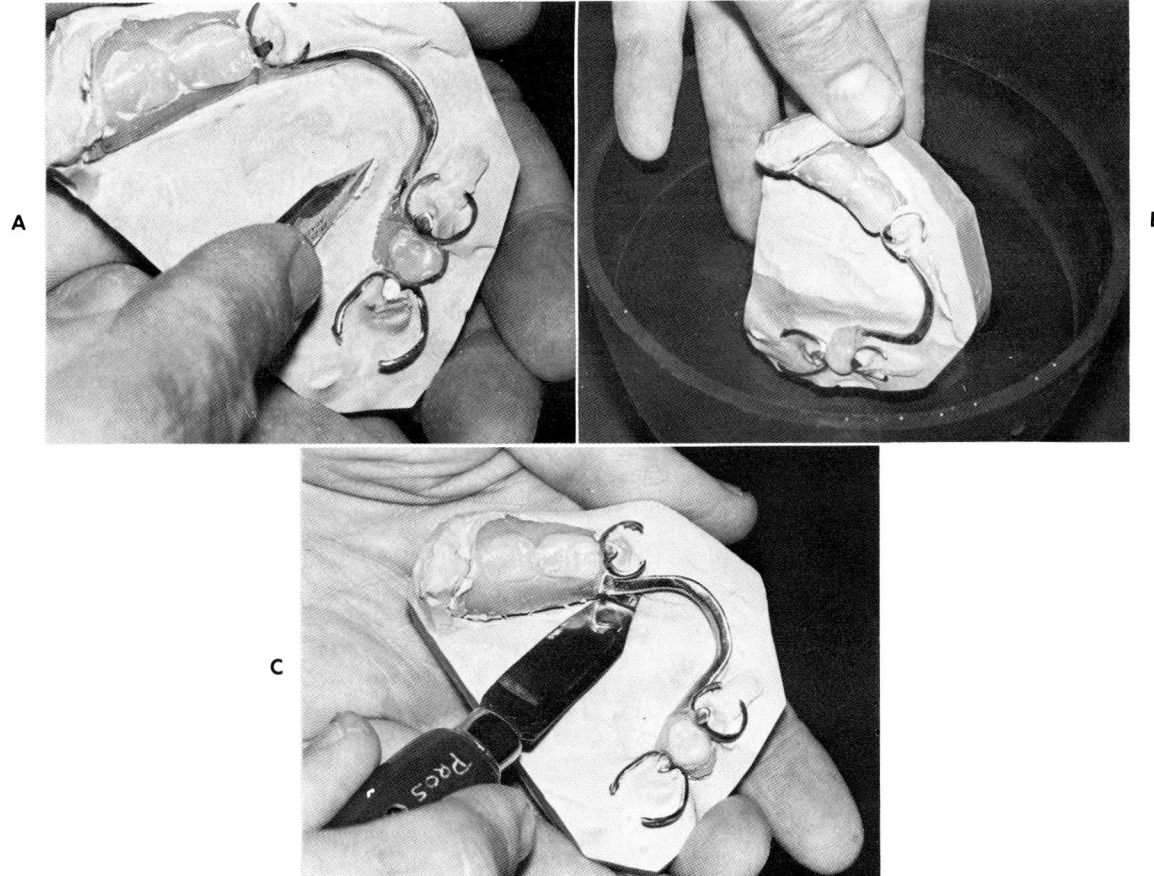

**Fig. 14-28. A,** Sharp laboratory knife is used to remove stone that may be locking framework or denture base areas of removable partial denture onto cast. **B,** Rebase cast is placed into bowl of 130° to 140° F (54.5° to 60° C) water for 3 to 4 minutes to soften impression material. **C,** Knife is used to tease prosthesis off rebase master cast. Excessive force must be avoided, or damage may be done to framework.

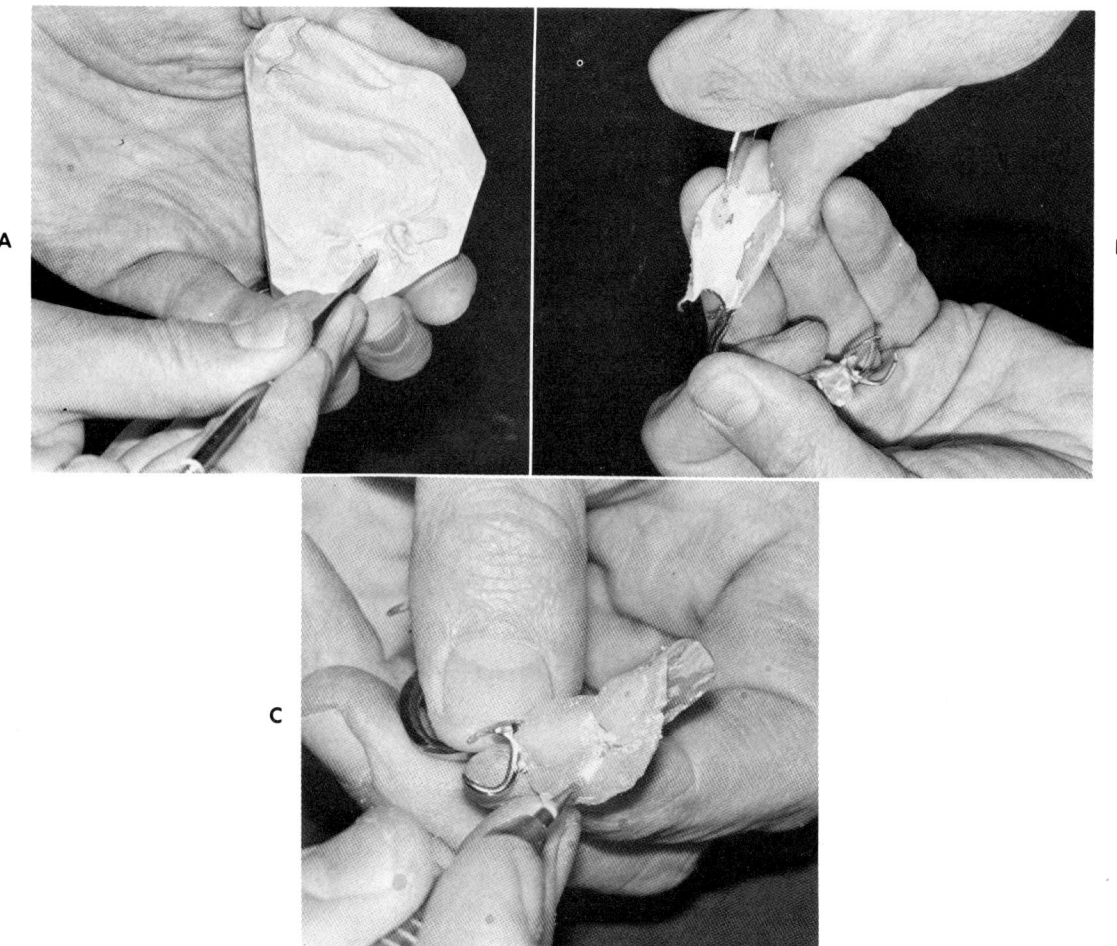

**Fig. 14-29. A,** Instrument is used to remove impression material that has adhered to cast. **B,** Laboratory knife is used to remove impression material from denture bases. **C,** No. 557 or 558 straight fissure bur in straight laboratory handpiece is used to remove artificial teeth from denture base.

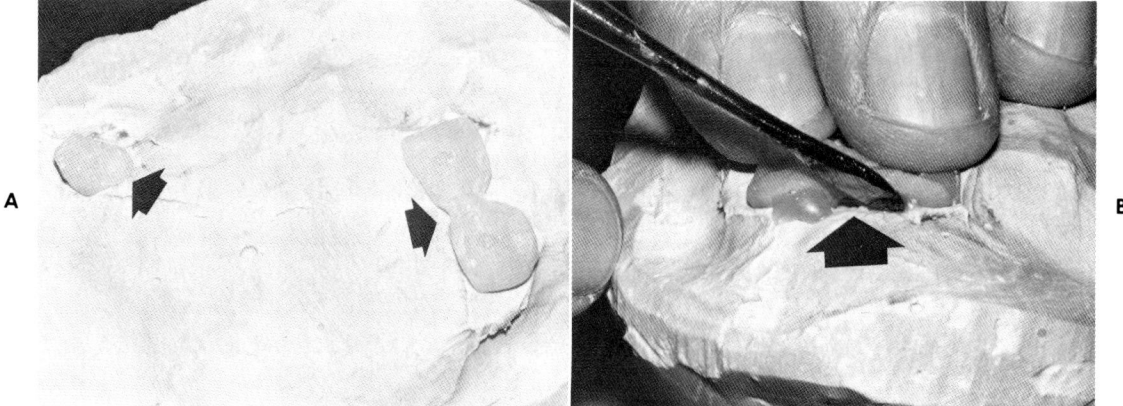

**Fig. 14-30. A,** After trimming all excess resin from artificial teeth and preparing diatoric hole in base of each tooth with round bur, teeth are placed into their respective indentation (arrows) in occlusal index. **B,** No. 7 wax spatula and baseplate wax are used to lute each tooth firmly to occlusal index (arrow).

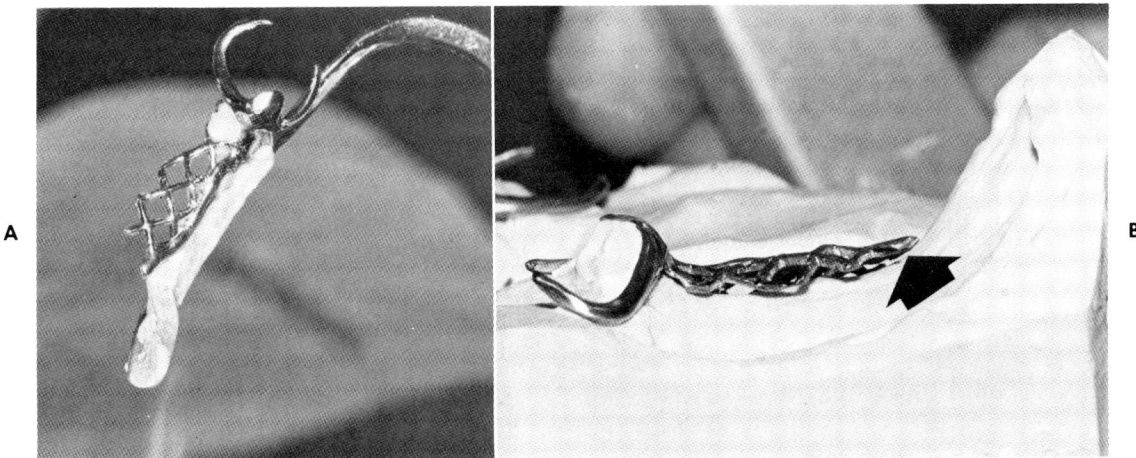

**Fig. 14-31. A,** Resin bases are burned off framework by placing base area over flame. When resin has softened sufficiently, instrument is used to pull resin from framework. **B,** Framework is seated on cast to verify fit of tissue stop. Usually space will be present (arrow). Failure to establish contact can result in movement or distortion of framework during packing of acrylic resin for processing.

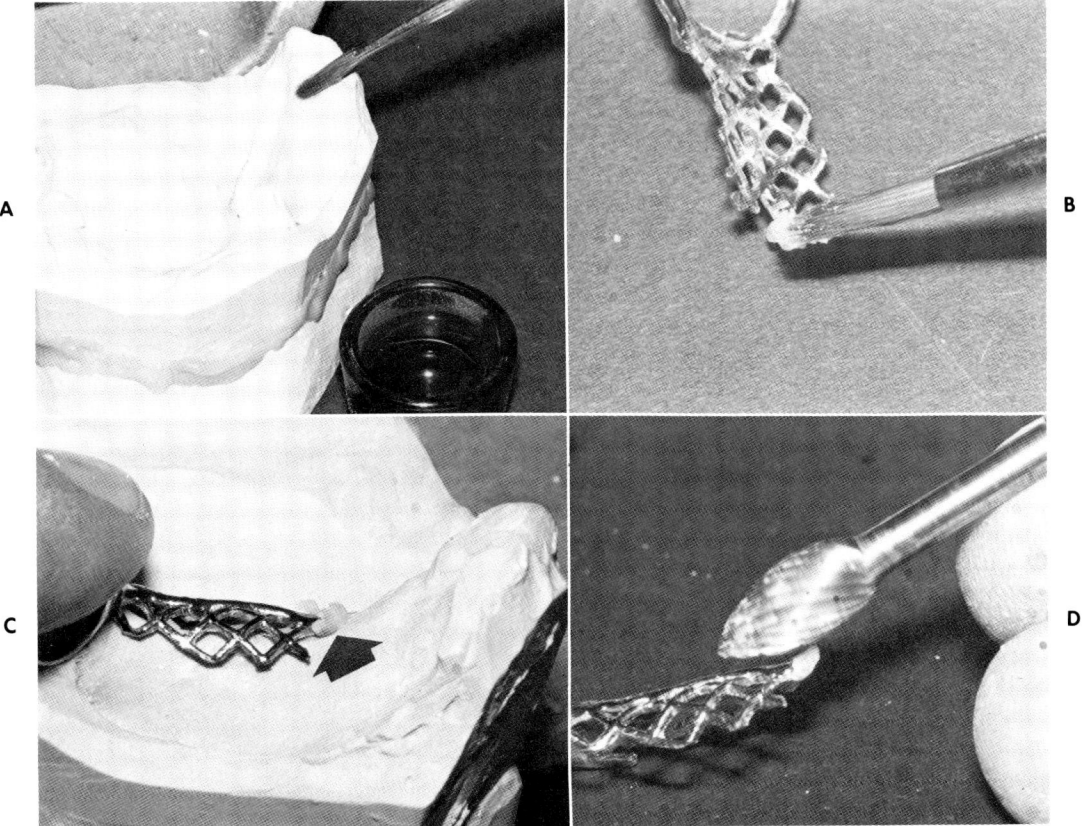

**Fig. 14-32.** Establishment of tissue stop. **A,** Small amount of tinfoil substitute is poured into small glass dish, and brush is used to flow material onto tissue stop area of cast. **B,** Small amount of autopolymerizing acrylic resin is placed on tissue stop of framework. **C,** Framework is seated on rebase cast making certain rests are accurately seated and sufficient resin is present to establish contact with cast (arrow). **D,** After resin has polymerized, excess resin is removed with vulcanite bur, leaving area of resin contact with cast of 2 to 3 mm in diameter.

**420** *Dental laboratory procedures: removable partial dentures*

12. Place softened baseplate wax on the denture base areas of the framework, and close the articulator to pick up the artificial teeth from the occlusal index (Fig. 14-33).

13. Wax up the denture bases, and polish the wax (Fig. 14-34).

14. Paint the rebase master cast with stone separating medium in preparation for flasking (Fig. 14-35).

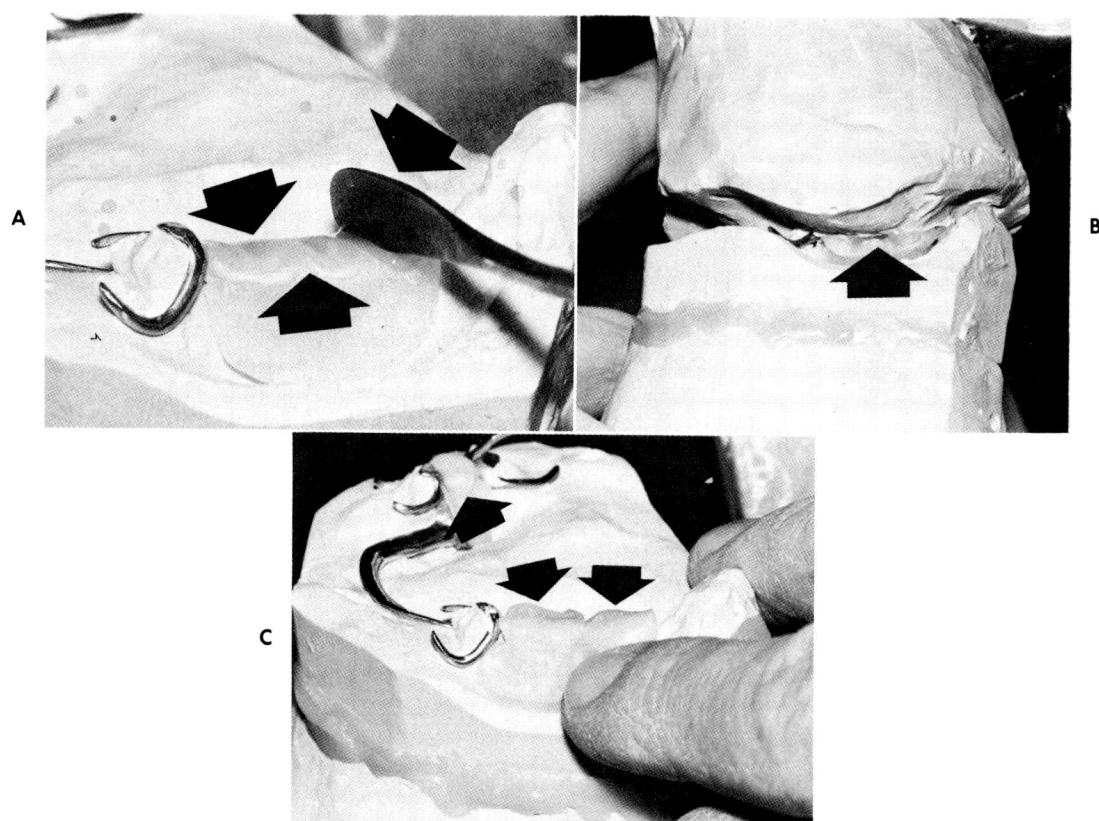

**Fig. 14-33. A,** Strip of baseplate wax is softened over flame and is adapted over denture base areas of framework. Hot No. 7 wax spatula is used to pool wax overlying crest of ridge (arrows). **B,** Articulator closed, and wax is allowed to harden around necks of teeth (arrow). **C,** Articulator is opened with teeth remaining in correct relationship to framework (arrows).

*Relining and rebasing* **421**

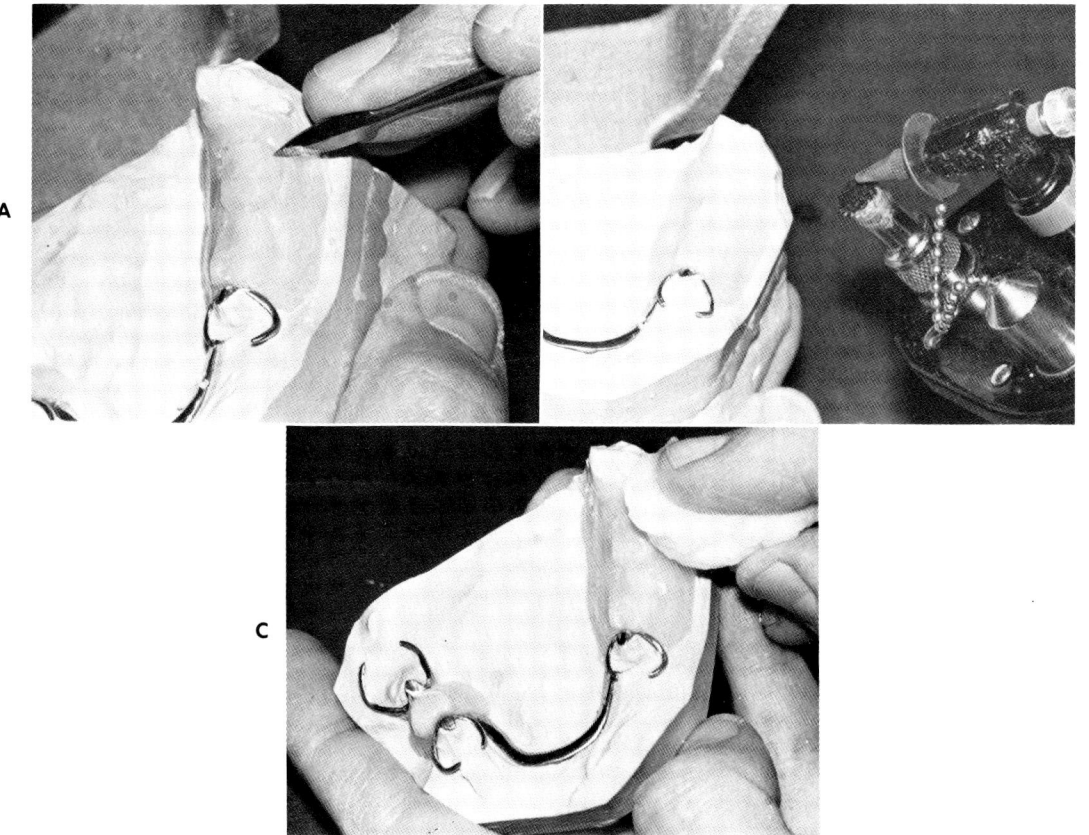

**Fig. 14-34. A,** Wax is added to complete denture bases and is carved to anatomic contours. **B,** Wax is lightly flamed with brush flame from alcohol torch. **C,** Surfaces of wax are polished with dampened cotton and cool water.

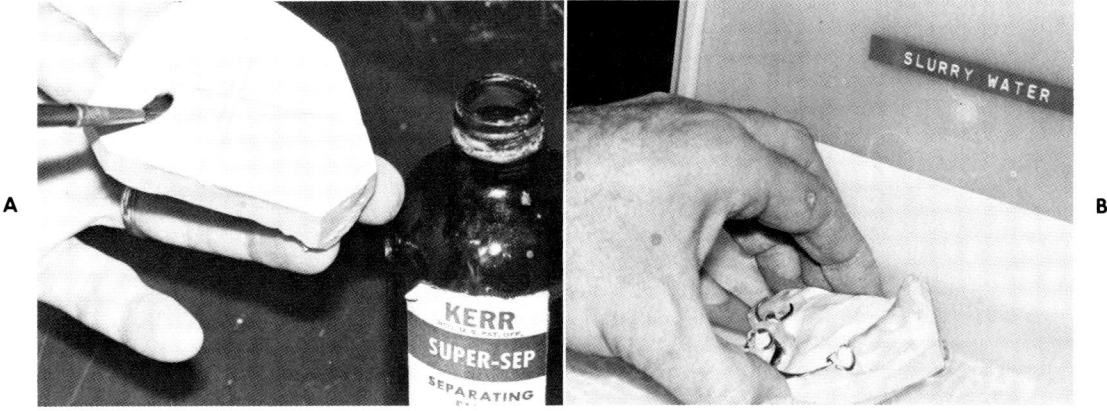

**Fig. 14-35. A,** Brush is used to paint stone separating medium on entire rebase cast. Care must be taken to avoid placement of separating medium on wax because this could result in discoloration of denture base resin. **B,** Painted rebase cast is soaked in clear slurry water for 4 to 5 minutes before flasking.

15. Half flask the rebase master cast in a lower complete denture flask using artificial stone (Fig. 14-36).

16. Boil out the flask, and paint both halves with tinfoil substitute (Fig. 14-37).

17. Pack the flask with heat-curing acrylic resin (Fig. 14-38).

18. After processing, recover the rebased removable partial denture, and remove excess resin with arbor bands and vulcanite burs (Fig. 14-39).

19. Polish and carefully inspect the rebased removable partial denture in preparation for delivery to the dentist (Fig. 14-40).

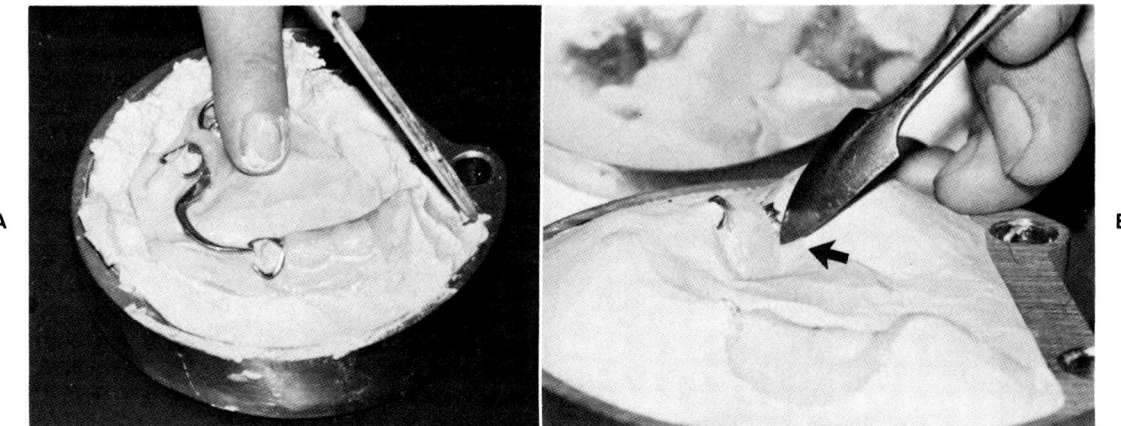

**Fig. 14-36. A,** Mix of artificial stone is placed in bottom half of lower complete denture flask. Rebase cast is placed into flask, and additional stone is used to cover entire rebase cast, exposing only denture base areas and artificial teeth. **B,** Baseplate wax is flowed into any undercut or irregular areas (arrow) of flasking stone that could interfere with opening of flask at boilout. Entire surface of flasking stone is painted with stone separating medium, and flasking is completed in usual manner.

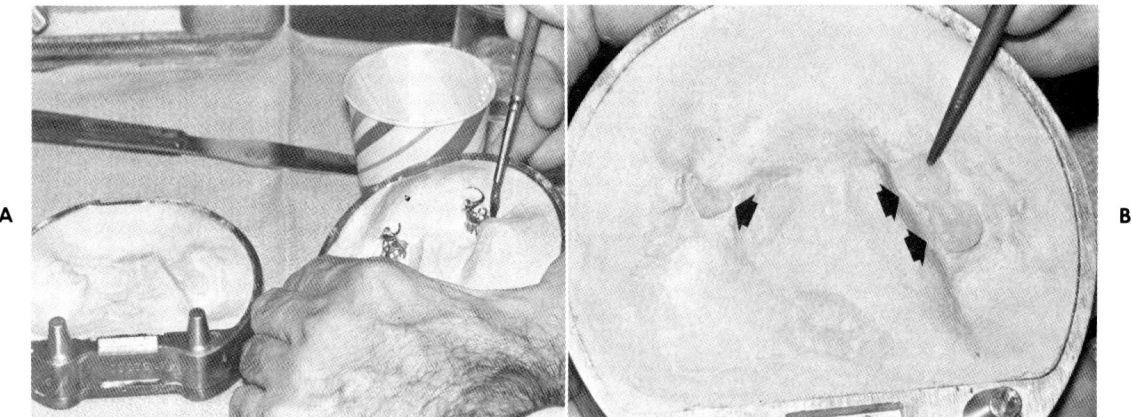

**Fig. 14-37. A,** After flask has been boiled out and all traces of wax have been carefully removed, hot flasks are painted with two coats of alginate tinfoil substitute. Foil substitute should always be placed in small container, and any excess should be discarded. Care must be taken to cover all denture base areas under acrylic resin retention components of framework. **B,** Artificial teeth are inspected to make certain that they are firmly and completely seated in the cope half of flasking stone (arrows). Diatoric holes are prepared in base of artificial teeth if this was not accomplished previously.

*Relining and rebasing* **423**

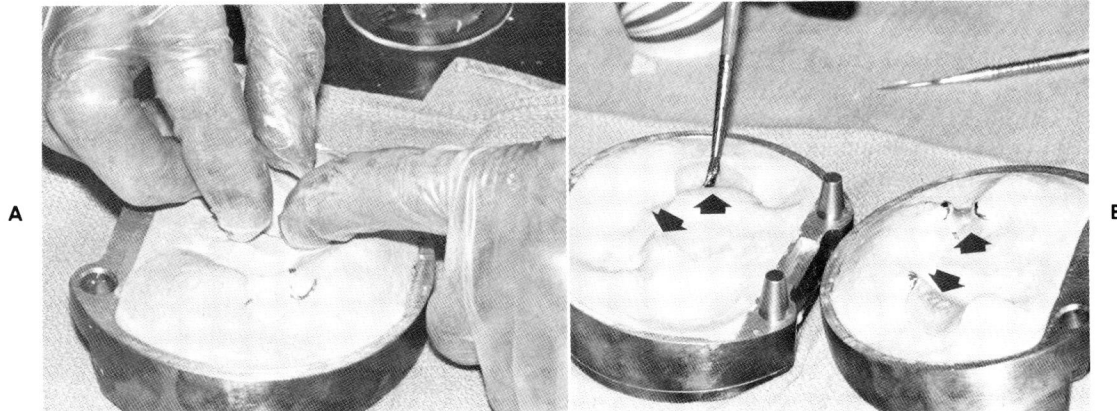

**Fig. 14-38. A,** Acrylic resin polymer and monomer are measured, mixed, and packed at dough stage using split-pack method. **B,** After two or three trial packs and removal of excess resin, resin surfaces of both halves of split pack are painted with monomer (arrows). Flask is closed and processed in usual manner.

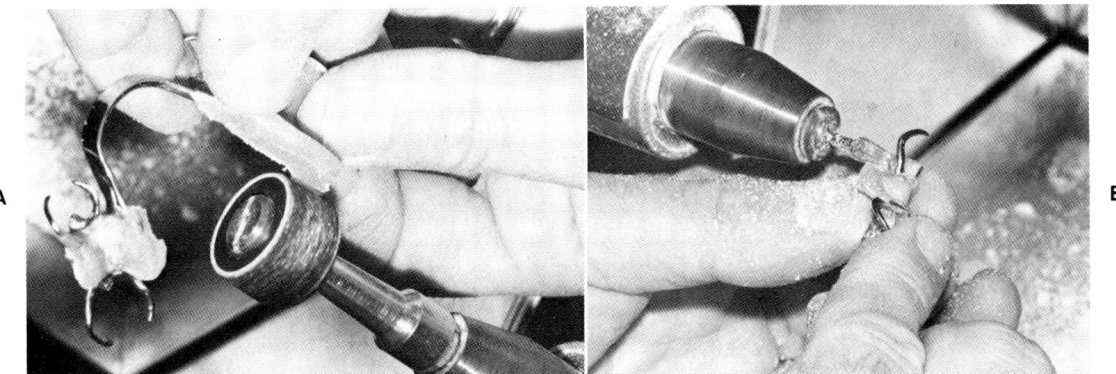

**Fig. 14-39. A,** After rebased removable partial denture is recovered from flask following processing, arbor band is used to remove resin flash. **B,** Vulcanite bur is used to complete fine finishing of denture bases.

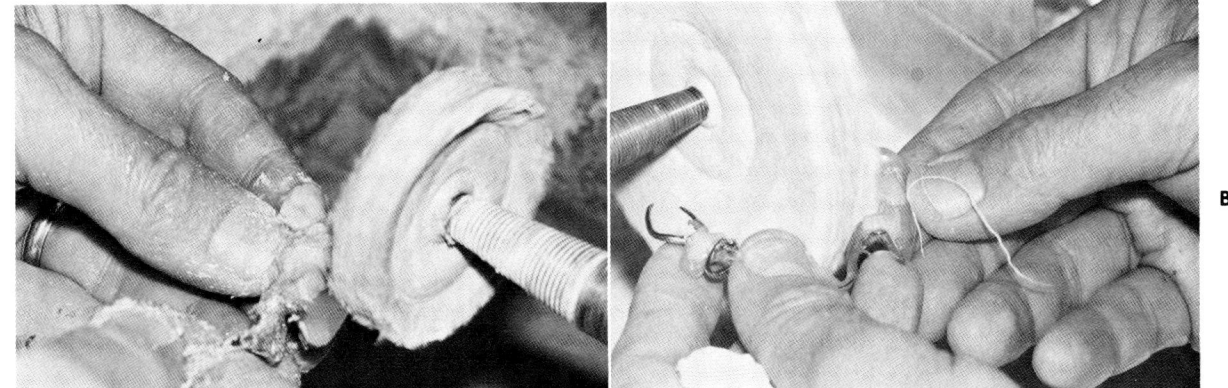

**Fig. 14-40. A,** Denture base areas are polished with fine pumice and wet rag wheel. **B,** High shine compound on clean rag wheel is used to place final polish on prosthesis. Tissue side, border, and polished surfaces are inspected with magnification for presence of nodules, scratches, voids, or other defects in rebased denture bases.

**Table 14-2.** Removable partial denture rebase procedure

| Problem | Probable cause | Solution |
|---|---|---|
| Difficulty removing removable partial denture from rebase master cast | Undercuts not removed from denture bases before making rebase impression | Use vulcanite bur to remove all undercut areas from tissue surfaces of denture bases |
| | Prosthesis locked into stone cast during pouring of rebase cast | Take care when pouring remount cast to contact tissue side of major connector only and to avoid carrying stone too far onto polished surface areas of resin bases |
| Cannot separate two halves of flask at time of boilout | Undercuts created when flasking lower half | Carefully shape dental stone covering framework and rebase cast to avoid creating undercuts; flow baseplate wax into stone undercuts or irregular areas |
| | Failure to paint lower half of flasking stone with separating medium before pouring rest of flask | Paint all stone surfaces with separating medium, avoiding contact with wax |
| Demarcation lines in resin bases | Resin in two halves of split-packed resin dried out before final closure of flask | After final trial pack, paint surfaces of both halves of split-packed resin with monomer before final closure |
| Orange discoloration of resin bases or artificial teeth | Stone separating medium flowed on artificial teeth or waxed up denture bases | Take care when painting stone separating medium to avoid contact with wax or teeth; when painting around teeth or wax, hold flask so excess medium will flow away from area to be protected |
| Dental stone adheres to resin after processing | Contaminated tinfoil substitute | Never apply tinfoil substitute directly from storage container; always pour amount to be used into another container and discard unused material |
| | Failure to flow tinfoil substitute under acrylic resin retention component of framework | Apply generous amounts of tinfoil substitute, forcing it under acrylic resin retention with fine brush |
| Porosity in denture base | Insufficient amount of resin used in packing denture bases | Trial pack using split-pack method, making sure that excess resin is present on both halves of split pack; trim and repeat trial packs to complete flask closure |
| | Too much monomer in resin when processed | Use manufacturer's recommended liquid-powder ratio; do not pack until resin reaches dough stage; bench cure for 30 minutes before placing flask in processing tank |
| Rebased removable partial denture will not seat completely into rest seats in mouth | Impression not completely seated when rebase impression was made | Maintain prosthesis in place with finger pressure over rests and not denture bases; make open mouth impression; do not allow patient to close while impression is being made |
| | Framework moved or distorted during packing of resin | Establish tissue stop with autopolymerizing acrylic resin if tissue stop is out of contact with cast |

**Table 14-2.** Removable partial denture rebase procedure—cont'd

| Problem | Probable cause | Solution |
|---|---|---|
| | Resin on guide plane areas of framework | Carefully check finished rebase, and remove any resin that flowed onto guide planes or under rests |
| | Denture base resin prevents clasp from flexing | Trim denture base resin away from terminal areas of retentive clasp arms to allow clasp to flex during insertion and removal of prosthesis |
| | Framework distorted when recovering prosthesis from flask | Use separating medium between various stages of flasking prosthesis; section dental stone rather than forcing framework during recovery from flasking stone |
| Artificial tooth covered with resin or displaced in rebased resin bases | Tooth moved out of index in cope half of flasking stone | Check position of each artificial tooth in its index in cope half of flasking stone; when waxing up prosthesis, uncover sufficient amount of tooth so that definite index will be formed that is capable of retaining artificial tooth in its proper position during boilout and packing |

### PROBLEM AREAS

The principal problems associated with rebasing removable partial dentures are described in Table 14-2. Probable causes and the solutions to these problems are also described in this table.

## RECONSTRUCTION OF REMOVABLE PARTIAL DENTURES

Reconstruction of a removable partial denture is a process of remaking a prosthesis in which only the framework is retained. Both the denture base material and the teeth are changed. This procedure is indicated when the partial denture framework fits well but the condition of the teeth or the occlusal relationships are so poor that the teeth would be unsatisfactory when the proper occlusal relationships were reestablished.

### PROCEDURE

Basically, the procedures involved in reconstruction are the same as those for constructing a new removable partial denture from the point of completion of the framework. The important consideration in reconstruction is the production of a cast on which the framework fits accurately. To achieve this, it is necessary to make an impression with the prosthesis in the mouth.

### Making a reconstruction cast

The dentist can make a corrected cast impression on the existing denture bases and make an alginate impression over the prosthesis. The laboratory can then make the reconstruction cast in the same manner as that used for making a reline cast (Figs. 14-3 to 14-5). The resin bases are then burned off as for a rebase (Fig. 14-31). Clinical and laboratory procedures then follow the same sequence as for a new removable partial denture.

The dentist may go one step farther at the time of making the reconstruction impression. After constructing the corrected cast impression on the denture bases, the teeth and, if necessary, part of the denture base are ground to create clearance with the opposing occlusion. This step allows a jaw relation record to be made before the dentist makes the alginate impression over the prosthesis. After pouring the cast and careful removal of the alginate impression, the reconstruction cast is ready for mounting against an opposing cast. The next step is the arrangement of teeth, which is accomplished as for a new removable partial denture.

### PROBLEM AREAS

The main problems involve making a cast on which the framework fits accurately. Movement of

**Table 14-3.** Removable partial denture reconstruction

| Problem | Probable cause | Solution |
|---|---|---|
| Framework not completely seated on reconstruction cast | Impression tray contacted distal extension bases while making alginate impression, causing displacement of framework | Use tray that has 5 to 7 mm clearance around both prosthesis and remaining teeth; do not use excessive force in seating tray |
| | Body of alginate too heavy or begins to set when seating tray, causing displacement of framework | Use correct water-powder ratio; use cool water to prolong working time |
| | Corrected cast impression made with finger pressure over ridge areas, displacing framework from teeth | Maintain prosthesis in position with finger pressure over rest areas only |
| | Prosthesis lifts slightly out of alginate impression during removal of impression from mouth | Allow alginate to set additional 2 minutes before removal to increase strength of alginate; add retention to denture base areas such as bent paper clip attached with sticky wax; inspect carefully to make certain prosthesis is completely seated in impression |
| | Prosthesis displaced during pouring of cast | Avoid overvibration during pouring of stone |

the prosthesis from its correct position while making the impression or pouring the reconstruction cast are the most common causes of problems (Table 14-3).

## SUMMARY

Indications and methods of relining and rebasing a removable partial denture were described in this chapter. The most satisfactory method of relining a removable partial denture is with the use of a reline jig and autopolymerizing resin. The rebase procedure replaces all the denture base resin and uses conventional flasking and processing techniques. The open mouth impressions are made the same way for both reline and rebase procedures; consequently, the occlusion is usually high and must be corrected in the mouth.

Care must be taken in every laboratory step of reline and rebase procedures to achieve a successful result. Complete success also depends on the quality of the prerequisite clinical procedures and the final fitting procedures.

## BIBLIOGRAPHY

Blatterfein, L.: Rebasing procedures for removable partial dentures, J. Prosthet. Dent. 8:441-467, 1958.

Henderson, D., and Steffel, V. L.: McCracken's removable partial prosthodontics, ed. 5, St. Louis, 1977, The C. V. Mosby Co.

Miller, E. L.: Removable partial prosthodontics, Baltimore, 1978, The Williams & Wilkins Co.

Morrow, R. M., Rudd, K. D., and Eissmann, H. F.: Dental laboratory procedures: complete dentures, vol. 1, St. Louis, 1980, The C. V. Mosby Co.

Smith, D. E., Lord, J. L., and Bolender, C. L.: Complete denture relines with autopolymerizing resin processed in $H_2O$ under air pressure, J. Prosthet. Dent. 18:103-115, 1967.

Sowter, J. B.: Dental laboratory technology: prosthodontic techniques, Chapel Hill, N. C., 1968, The University of North Carolina Press.

Steffel, V. L.: Relining of removable partial dentures for fit and function, J. Prosthet. Dent. 4:496-509, 1954.

# CHAPTER 15

# REPAIRS

JAMES S. BRUDVIK

The need to repair the removable partial denture can be separated into two basic areas that often overlap: repairs that are required before the partial denture is returned to the prescribing dentist and those which occur after delivery when the dentist must either repair it himself or return the denture to the laboratory.

The construction of a removable partial denture is complex with many opportunities for error. Clasps can be cast short, rests are often overlooked and omitted, and voids can be found in major connectors. These problems do not necessarily mean that the entire partial denture must be remade. A thorough knowledge of repair techniques, coupled with well-defined standards of acceptance, will allow the technician to deal ethically with the partial denture repair.

Those repairs generated by the patient or occasionally by the dentist make up the bulk of removable partial denture repairs. The technician needs to apply the same standards of acceptance he uses in house and inform the dentist when he cannot perform an acceptable repair on the submitted denture. In a more practical sense, repairs can be divided into (1) metal repairs and (2) resin and denture tooth repairs.

## METAL REPAIRS

Repairs of major connectors, minor connectors, rests, clasps, and resin and tooth retention make up the bulk of metal repairs. The majority of these involve the use of dental solder. Both precious and nonprecious solders can be used in these situations. Historically, the precious solders have been indicated when the repair was to be exposed to the oral fluids. The less expensive nonprecious solders were indicated when the repair was to be covered with resin, when the possibility of tarnish was eliminated.

### Precious metal solders

Dental solders are classified as "hard solders," in contrast with the soft solders (lower melting temperatures) used in industry. Generally, hard solders are stronger, more resistant to tarnish, and have a higher fusing temperature. Those solders associated with fixed partial dentures and crowns are composed primarily of precious metals. Tarnish resistance is directly related to gold and platinum metal content with a fineness of .760 required to prevent discoloration. When the restoration can be readily removed from the mouth and repolished, as in the case of the removable partial denture, precious solders of a lower fineness can be used. Since the strength of the solder is inversely proportional to its gold content, this reduction in the required fineness results in a stronger repair.

Precious metal solders are usually composed of gold, silver, copper, zinc, tin, and, occasionally, phosphorus. Silver increases the fluidity and narrows the melting range, making high silver content solders ideal for use with electrosoldering devices.

Solder joints of precious metal should always be quenched immediately after the soldering is completed so that solution heat treatment can occur. This treatment increases ductility and reduces the chance of joint fracture in function.

The strength of soldered repairs in removable partial denture alloys is estimated to be in the range of 50,000 psi (ultimate tensile strength). Although this figure is about one third of that found for the alloys themselves, it is more than enough to resist the stresses of normal wear on the properly designed repair.

Silver, copper, and zinc can be alloyed to make excellent solders that are far less expensive than those containing gold. These "silver solders," although not completely resistant to tarnish, are often used as a substitute when the joint will not be exposed to oral fluids.

**Nonprecious metal solders**

Repairs of dental prostheses have historically been made using precious metal solders. However, nonprecious solders can be used successfully; they are best used with electric soldering devices because they melt at high temperatures. The great majority of these are industrial brazing alloys (typical composition is 70% nickel, 25% chromium, and 5% trace elements). The trace elements are usually silicon, boron, and manganese.

Electric solder,* is a good example of this alloy. It is quite similar in content to the Ticonium 100 alloy,† with a flow temperature of 1950° F (1065.5° C). This soldering alloy is almost impossible to control with a torch but responds well to electric soldering. Soldering alloys of this type provide a stronger repair joint and do not tarnish in the mouth. They can be used with confidence in removable partial denture repairs at a great reduction in cost compared to precious metal solders.

**Soldering techniques**

Removable partial dentures can be soldered using the gas-oxygen flame commonly associated with precious metal soldering in fixed restorations. Over the last few decades, the use of electric soldering devices for removable repairs has become so commonplace that they are used almost exclusively in modern dentistry. Because the gas-oxygen flame heats an area rather than a specific point, it has a tendency to destroy the dental cast if the repair is made on it.

Electric soldering can be expected to cause less microstructural change and reduce decay corrosion in the joint. There are a number of these units on the market, the best known perhaps being the one manufactured for many years by Torit* (Fig. 15-1). They are simple electronically, consisting of a transformer that can be varied in its output (usually in four stages: low, medium, medium high, and high heat) and that has two electrodes. One electrode is made of a copper rod with an insulated handle; the other is a carbon rod within a copper casing with an identical handle. The carbon tip is placed on the solder and the electrical circuit completed through the copper rod when it contacts the framework (Fig. 15-2). The position of the copper rod in relation to the solder and the carbon tip alters the electrical circuit theoretically, but practically, the distance between them is not critical.

The carbon tip is constantly being eroded from the heat of the soldering operation and needs to be reshaped to provide a pointed tip rather than a blunt end. The tips can be replaced when they become worn. With properly contoured carbon tips the soldering operation can be carried out very close (3 to 5 mm) to areas of resin without destroying the resin. This fact alone makes electric soldering the technique of choice for removable partial dentures.

Areas to be joined with solder must be clean and free from oxides. Fluxes are required and are most commonly those which contain fluoride (usually a potassium fluoride). The fluoride is necessary to dissolve the passivating film associated with alloys containing chromium that are used for removable partial denture frameworks. The flux is available as either a paste or a powder and is diluted for use to a watery consistency. It is applied liberally to the joint area.

The easiest way to handle the small pieces of solder is to join them to the carbon tip by placing the carbon tip on the piece of solder and then only one *very briefly* touching the solder with the carbon tip (Fig. 15-3). This action melts the surface of the solder and lightly joins it to the carbon tip. The solder can now be carried exactly to place over the fluxed joint, and, with the copper tip already in place, the soldering operation is completed as soon as the solder and carbon tip touch the framework and complete the circuit.

Every attempt should be made to complete the joint with one application of heat. Oxides form quickly, and, should the first try not be satisfactory, the joint may have to be freshened by stoning before a second attempt is made. A longer joint can be

---

*J. F. Jelenko & Co., New Rochelle, N.Y.
†Ticonium Co., Albany, N.Y.

*The Torit Corp., St. Paul, Minn.

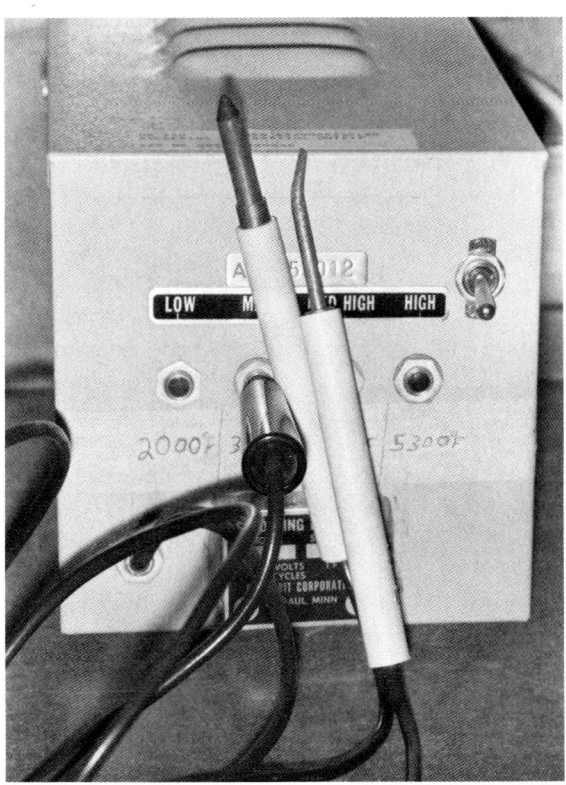

Fig. 15-1. Torit Soldering Unit.

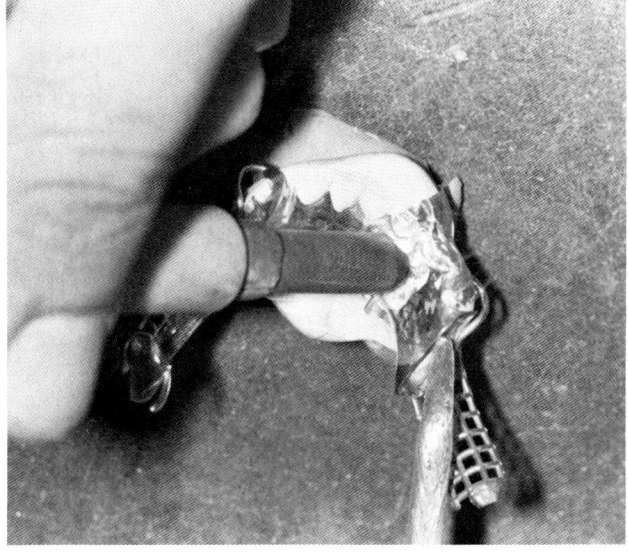

Fig. 15-2. Carbon tip on solder while copper tip completes circuit.

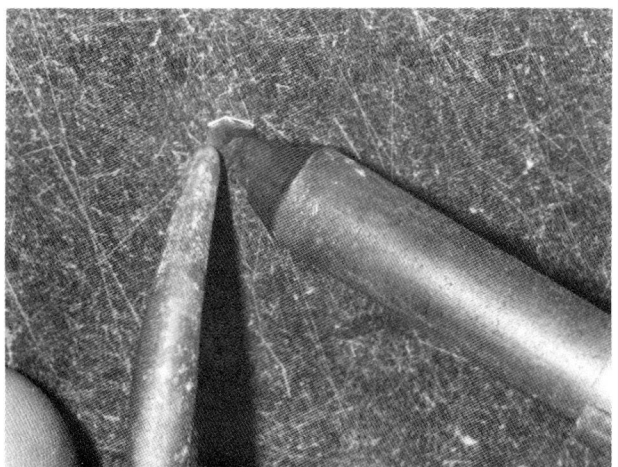

Fig. 15-3. Carbon tip placed on solder and briefly contacted with copper tip to superficially melt solder and attach it to carbon tip.

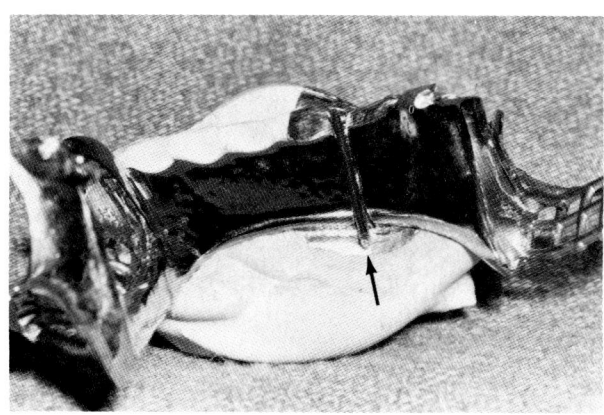

Fig. 15-4. Eighteen-gauge nickel-chromium wire used as filler with solder to bridge wide gap (arrow).

made by carrying a long piece of solder by one end and then slowly moving the carbon tip along the solder as it melts without removing the tip.

The gap to be bridged by the solder plays a role in the success of the repair as well. If the gap is greater than the diameter of an 18-gauge wire, then the gap should be filled with either a platinum-gold-palladium wire, chromium-nickel-cobalt wire, or a piece of the same partial denture alloy. The use of a filler metal will give a stronger joint than a wide joint filled only with solder (Fig. 15-4).

The settings on the electric soldering transformer

are influenced by the alloys involved in the repair as well as the techniques employed. The medium range is satisfactory for most partial denture repairs using precious metal solders. There is no advantage in overheating the solder joint, so some practice repairs are indicated when alloys or techniques change. Incomplete cold joints are also less than desirable, so the technician must watch the solder carefully through colored (dark blue) lenses to be certain that the solder completely melts and flows. The light from the carbon tip is intense when the circuit is completed, making the colored lenses an essential safety requirement.

### Major connector repair

Major connectors can be sectioned and rejoined in a new relationship with solders and exhibit sufficient strength to function clinically. Distortions that occur in the casting and finishing process, causing the frame *not* to fit passively on the master cast or in the mouth, are indications for major connector repair.

**PROCEDURE**

1. Section the casting with a thin Carborundum disk* at the point where the distortion appears to be (Fig. 15-5). (Some experience in fitting and finishing removable partial denture frameworks is usually necessary to make this appraisal.) If the two independent sections fit satisfactorily on the master

---

*Dedeco 1¼-inch Koolies, Dental Development and Manufacturing Corp., Brooklyn, N.Y.

cast, a major connector repair is indicated. It is usually not practical to attempt more than one sectioning and repair on a connector even though it is technically possible to make and repair a series of these cuts. Major connectors that are broad and thin do not lend themselves as well to this approach. The greatest success can be expected on lingual and palatal bars.

2. If the contour of the master cast in the area of the repair is not critical (as in the case of the lingual bar), then the soldering operation can be completed on that cast. When the integrity of the cast surface is essential to the completion of the partial denture, then make the repair on a duplicate cast or on a countercast. A great potential for error exists in both of these situations. The fabrication of the duplicate cast requires zero-degree expansion stone and a careful blockout of gross undercuts that might distort the duplicating media. A matrix normally relates the sectioned partial framework using either plaster or autopolymerizing resin (Fig. 15-6). It is in this manner that the repair would be received from the dentist. In either case, pour a countercast against the matrix and framework (Fig. 15-7). Again use zero-degree expansion stone should be used to assure accuracy. Apply a separating media, liquid soap or tinfoil substitute, to the matrix to ease separation.

3. When the countercast is completely set, remove the impression matrix, and separate and prepare the partial denture sections for soldering by freshening the metal joint with a fine stone or disk.

4. To obtain a relatively smooth tissue surface at

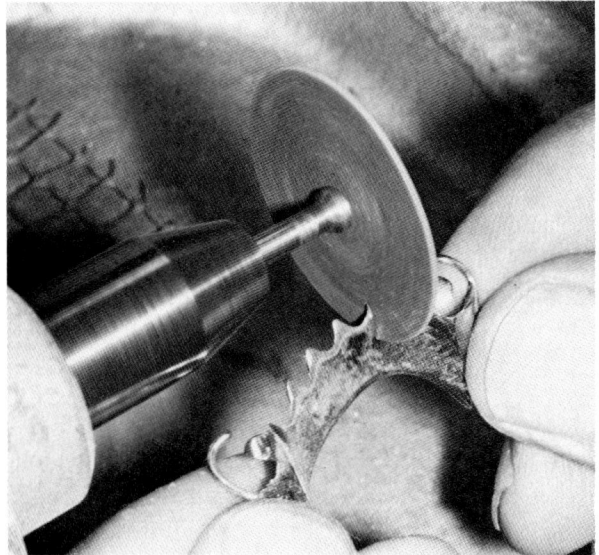

**Fig. 15-5.** Sectioning of casting with thin Carborundum disk.

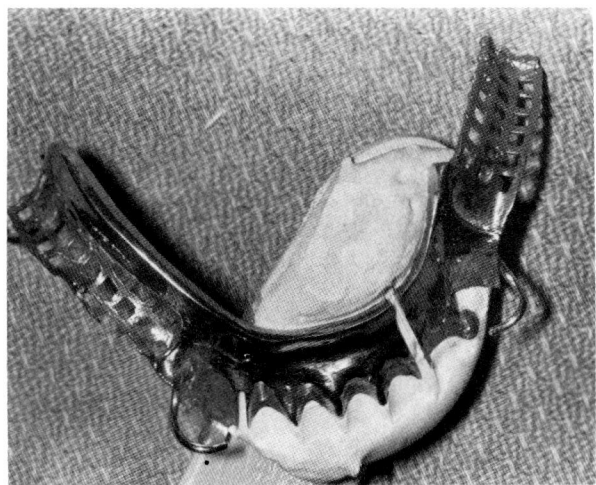

**Fig. 15-6.** Plaster matrix relating sectioned parts in new relationships from master cast.

the repair site, adapt high-heat metal foil of 0.001 inch or thinner to the countercast or soldering cast, and extend it 3 to 5 mm beyond the soldering space (Fig. 15-8). Flux the joint area, and carry solder to the site on the carbon tip (Fig. 15-9). The solder piece should be of sufficient size to complete the joint in a single operation.

### Rest and minor connector repair

Minor connectors can be sectioned and soldered with the same technique. When a rest does not seat completely, the minor connector should be sectioned some distance from the rest itself. In this approach the solder joint will *not* be on the occlusal surface.

Attempts to add a complete rest to the framework with solder are usually not satisfactory. When a rest has been omitted during the wax-up or broken from an existing frame, a quality repair requires the casting of the rest and adjacent minor connector and the soldering of the cast portion to the framework.

#### PROCEDURE

1. Make a shallow V cut or box cut in the minor connector to allow for a positive positioning of the repair (Fig. 15-10). Lubricate the model used for the

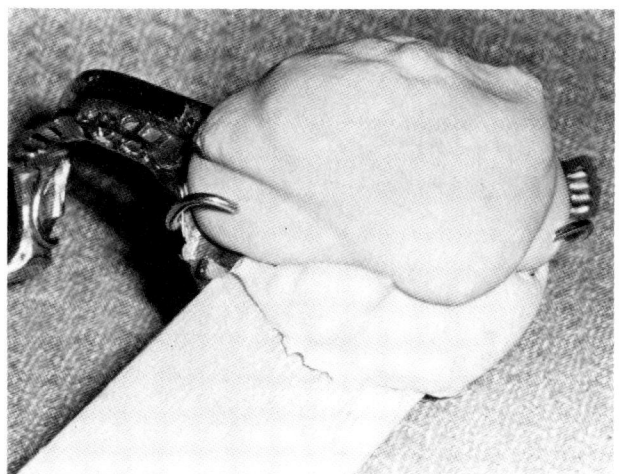

**Fig. 15-7.** Dental stone poured against sectioned casting and matrix.

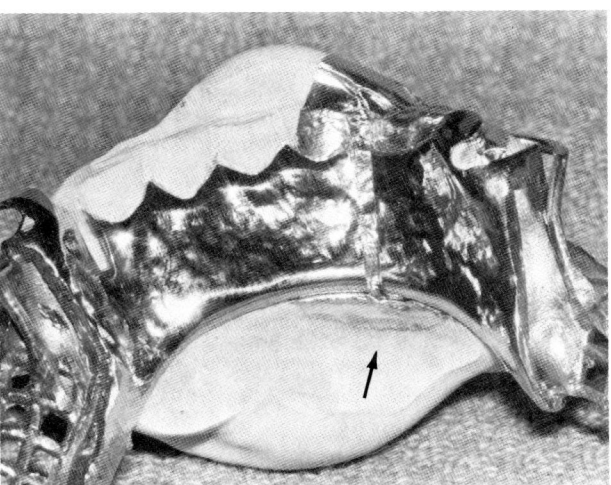

**Fig. 15-8.** Thin foil is adapted on countercast to protect area of soldering (arrow).

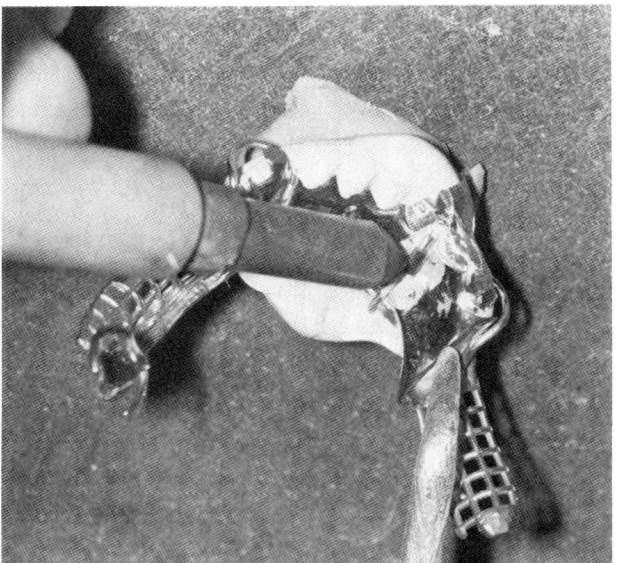

**Fig. 15-9.** Solder joint covered with flux. Solder is carried to place on carbon tip.

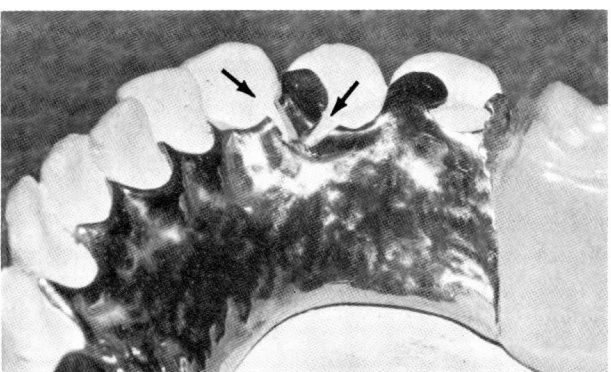

**Fig. 15-10.** Shallow V cut made in minor connector to accept repair addition (arrow).

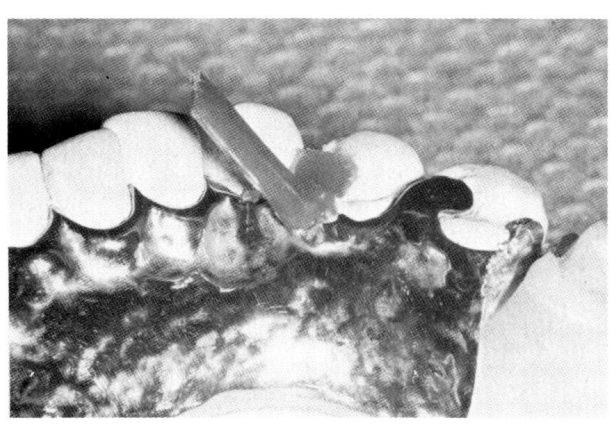

Fig. 15-11. Waxed repair addition sprued and ready for removal.

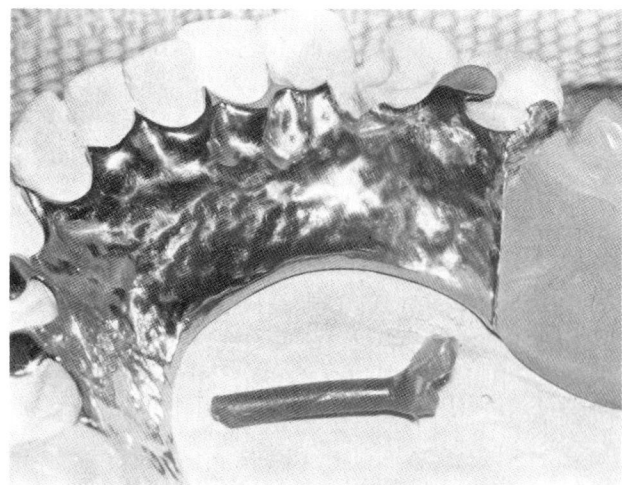

Fig. 15-12. Sprued repair addition.

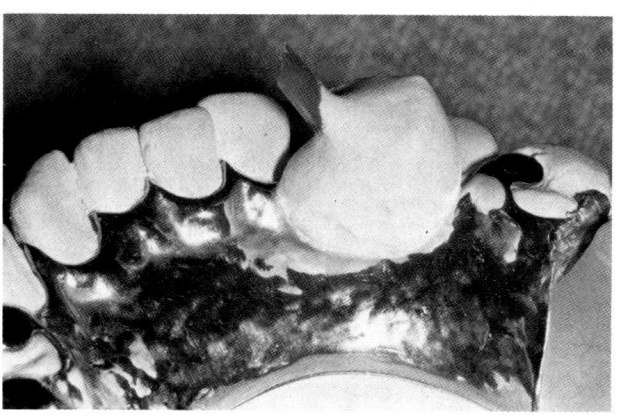

Fig. 15-13. Refractory material painted on wax repair addition.

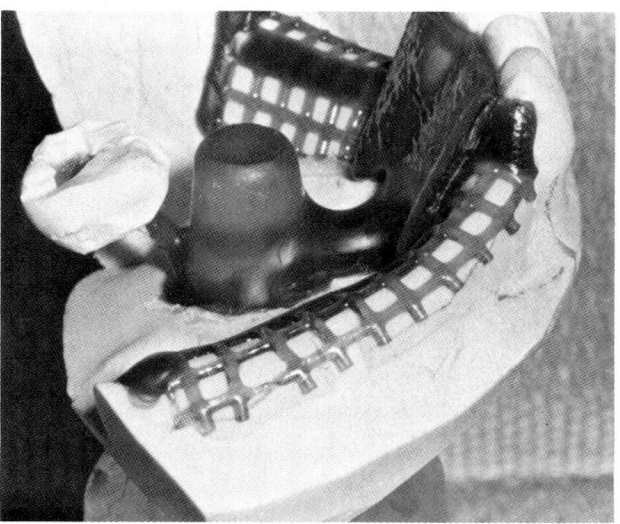

Fig. 15-14. Sprue lead attached to complete removable partial denture wax-up as "rider."

repair with die separator, and wax the repair parts directly on the master repair cast. The technician *must* evaluate the height of contour before a direct wax-up and make certain that there are no infrabulge areas in the tooth structure over which the wax-up still can be made. Should an undercut exist, it must be either blocked out or relieved from the casting. Carefully place and lubricate blockout wax to prevent the adherence of wax from the construction.

2. Sprue the waxed repair addition, and remove it from the repair cast (Figs. 15-11 and 15-12). If obvious distortion is observed on removal, then replace and recontour the waxed addition. To prevent distortion, paint a small amount of refractory material around the wax-up, and, when it is set, free the entire segment from the repair cast (Fig. 15-13). Use the sprue lead to manipulate the wax-up. Once freed, join the repair by the sprue lead to a sprue base, and invest and cast it. These small additions are normally added to another partial denture wax-up as a "rider" and cast in a normal fashion (Fig. 15-14).

3. Recover the repair segment after casting, fit it to the repair cast, and then solder it as previously described (Fig. 15-15). Since the repair is made in the minor connector area and well away from the rest itself, no interference with occlusal contact will occur.

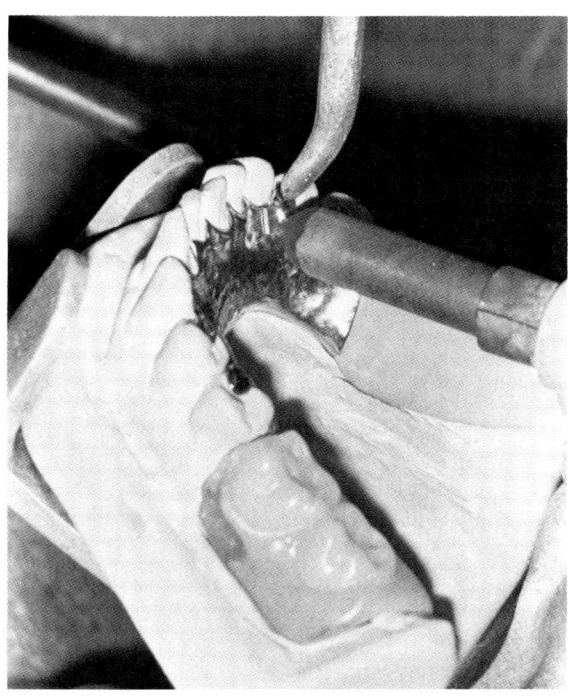

Fig. 15-15. Repair addition fitted and prepared for soldering.

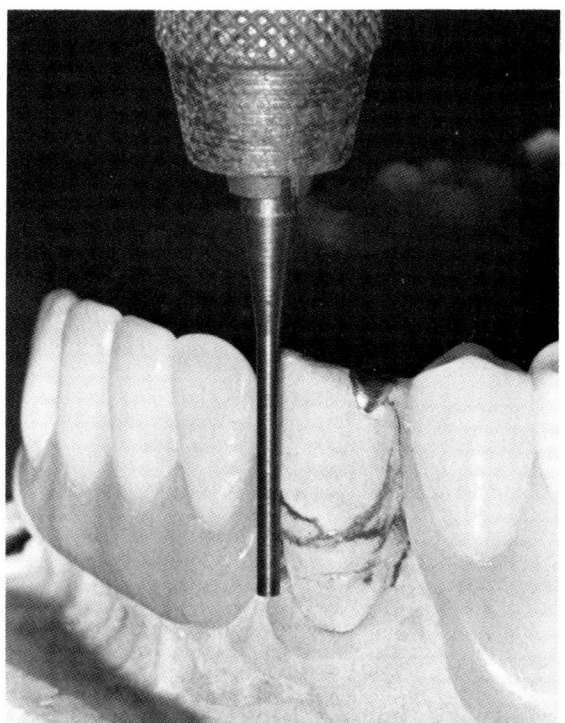

Fig. 15-16. Clasp repair tooth analyzed on surveyor.

## Clasp repair

The most common removable partial denture repair is the replacement of the retentive clasp arm. The constant stressing of metal inevitably results in work hardening, even if the clasp is constructed from a wrought alloy. Attempts at adjustment by the technician, dentist, and, unfortunately, the patient can easily result in clasp failure and fracture. The fractured clasp arm can be replaced with either a cast or wrought substitute. An analysis of the possible causes of the failure is essential before the repair is begun so that the contributing factors can be eliminated.

## Repair with wrought alloys

The great majority of clasp arm repairs are made with wire, because in most situations, it is far simpler to replace the broken clasp arm in this manner. Both circumferential and infrabulge clasps adjacent to resin denture bases are easily replaced with wire. Wire replacements become technically difficult only when associated with embrasure clasps or when adjacent to metal denture bases.

The wire clasp can be either added to the resin denture base with autopolymerizing resin or soldered to the rest/minor connector using the same techniques discussed earlier in this chapter and in Chapter 9.

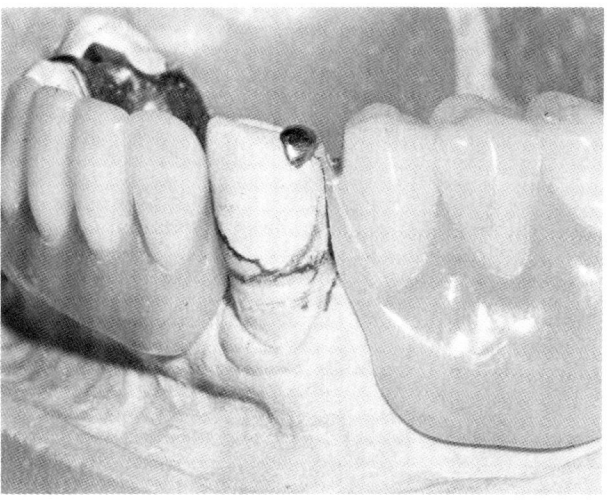

Fig. 15-17. Pencil line drawn on cast for wire placement.

### PROCEDURE

1. The abutment tooth requiring the addition or replacement of a circumferential retentive clasp arm adjacent to a resin denture base is ideally suited for a wire clasp.

2. Analyze the abutment of the repair cast on the dental surveyor to determine the height of contour, and mark it on the tooth (Fig. 15-16).

3. Draw a single pencil line on the cast to indicate the desired placement on the repair cast and aid in the positioning of the wire clasp (Fig. 15-17).

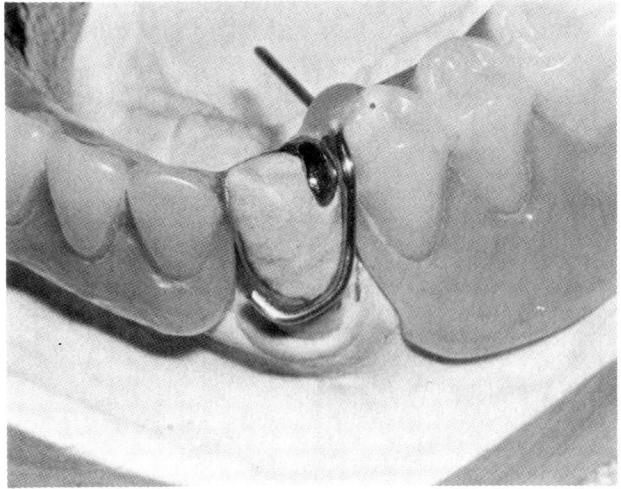

**Fig. 15-18.** Wire clasp adapted to line.

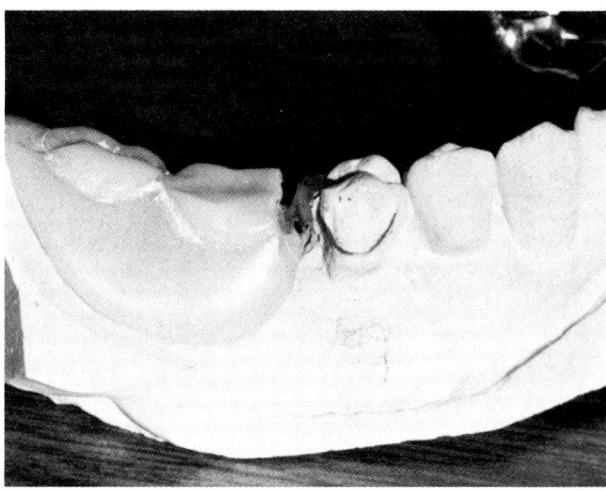

**Fig. 15-19.** Disk cut through resin to gain access to minor connector for soldering.

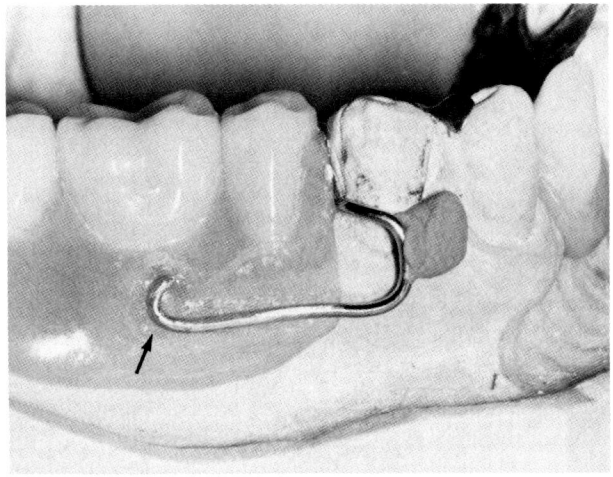

**Fig. 15-20.** Resin retentive contour in infrabulge clasp (arrow).

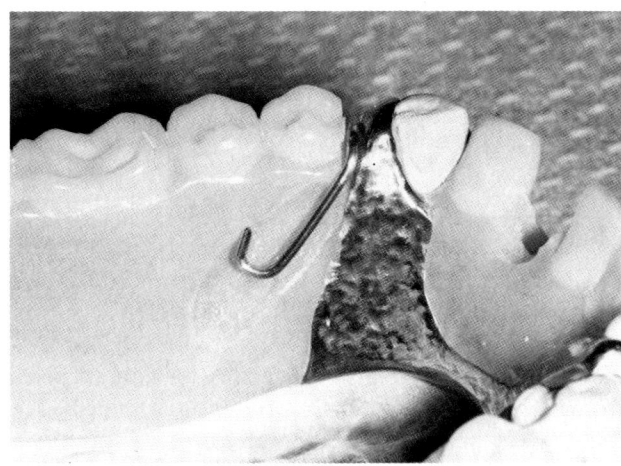

**Fig. 15-21.** Circumferential clasp contoured to pass to lingual flange area for resin retention.

4. Adapt wire of the prescribed gauge and alloy to be along the design line (Fig. 15-18).

5. When the clasp is to be soldered into the minor connector area, remove the resin with a disk cut to gain access to the metal (Fig. 15-19).

6. Always retain infrabulge clasps in the resin in wire repairs. Cut a trough in the buccolabial flange to accept the base of the wire. Bend the wire so that some physical retention to rotation exists within the resin (Fig. 15-20).

7. Solder circumferential clasps at the minor connector, or contour them to pass over the minor connector and attach them on the lingual flange area with resin (Fig. 15-21). Wire is the repair clasp of choice when only the retentive clasp arm is to be replaced. When the entire clasp assembly is required, then it is more practical to wax and cast it as a unit.

## Repair with cast clasps

The embrasure clasp and those clasps associated with single-tooth replacements are best repaired with cast alloys. There is seldom enough bulk of metal available in the area where a wire addition would need to be soldered for a dependable repair. Cast clasp repairs, involving more than the actual clasp arm, can be constructed and then attached to the metal of the framework by soldering them in an area not subject to flexion or the restrictions of occlusion.

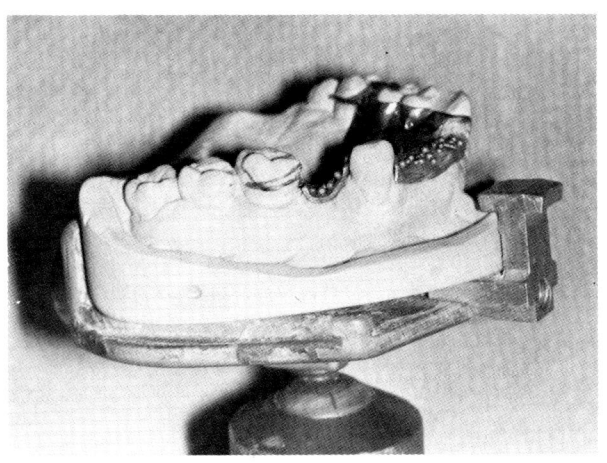

Fig. 15-22. Clasp designed on stone tooth for cast clasp repair.

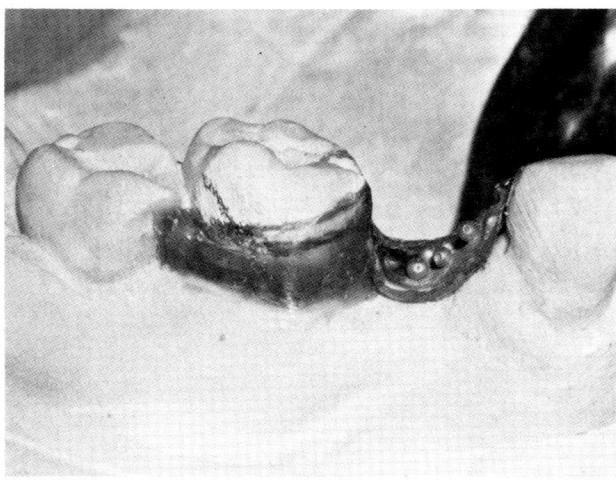

Fig. 15-23. Cast clasp repair, blocked out.

**PROCEDURE**

1. The clinician submits a repair cast poured into an impression made over the denture. The denture must have been completely seated on the abutment teeth in the mouth during the impression procedure and must be removed from the mouth in the impression. The impression need not be made of the complete arch. In many instances a sectional impression of the repair area may be the technique of choice because it allows the clinician to maintain and verify the frame-tooth relation while the impression is being made.

2. Remove the denture from the repair model, and evaluate the denture for the addition of the clasp assembly.

3. It may be necessary to remove some areas of denture resin to gain access (usually when veneered, single tooth replacements are involved).

4. Section the clasp assembly in the minor connector area with shallow V-shaped disk cuts. Use a boxlike cut to give positive placement of the repair section when fitting and finishing the metal.

5. Analyze the tooth or teeth that are involved with the repair for existing undercuts to determine usable retentive areas. Place the repair cast on the survey table, and attempt to find the original path of insertion. By examining the proximal guiding planes of the other abutments, this path can be identified and related to the abutment to be repaired. The tolerances are such that this repositioning is not absolutely critical. Since most removable partial dentures have a path of insertion roughly parallel to the long axis of the abutment teeth, any repair planned at this path should be successful with a minimum of adjustment at insertion. Draw the desired clasp design on the repair cast (Fig. 15-22).

6. Treat the cast with model spray and seat the denture. Add blockout wax, and shape it in the conventional manner (Fig. 15-23). Due to the uncertainties of the repair situation, the retentive clasp arm should be as long as possible with no more than the terminal third in a retentive undercut. The most desirable retentive depth will be 0.010 inch. Ledge the blockout wax to conform to the clasp retention area.

7. Arbitrarily block out gross undercuts on the denture and the repair cast with clay or wax. Duplicate the cast, with the denture still in place, according to standard techniques and materials recommended by the manufacturer of the alloy to be used.

8. Recover the refractory cast, trim it just short of the repair area, and dip it in beeswax. Model spray can also be used to seal the cast. (These steps will be identical to those described in Chapters 7 and 8.)

9. When the refractory cast has cooled and dried, wax the repair components to the cast with techniques identical to those used in normal framework construction (Fig. 15-24). If commercial plastic clasp patterns are to be used for the clasp arms, use a pattern with a width-thickness ratio approaching 2:1 to gain maximum flexibility for the repaired retentive clasp arm. Select the reciprocal clasp arm from those patterns having a width-thickness ratio closer to 1:1 to assure sufficient rigidity to stabilize the tooth.

**436** *Dental laboratory procedures: removable partial dentures*

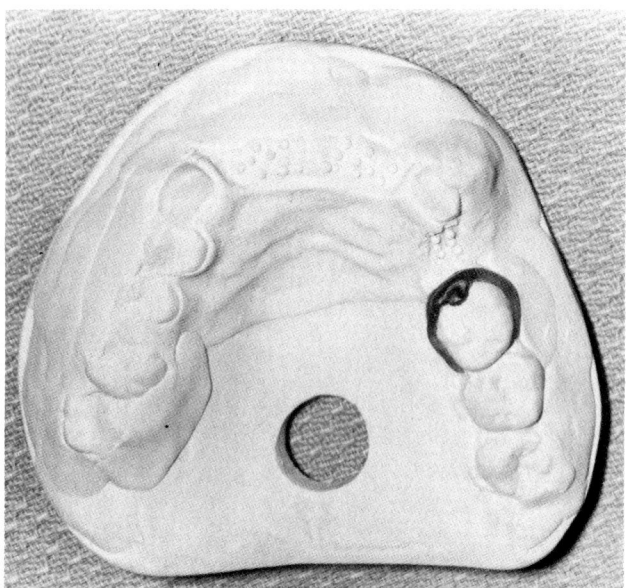

Fig. 15-24. Clasp assembly waxed on refractory cast.

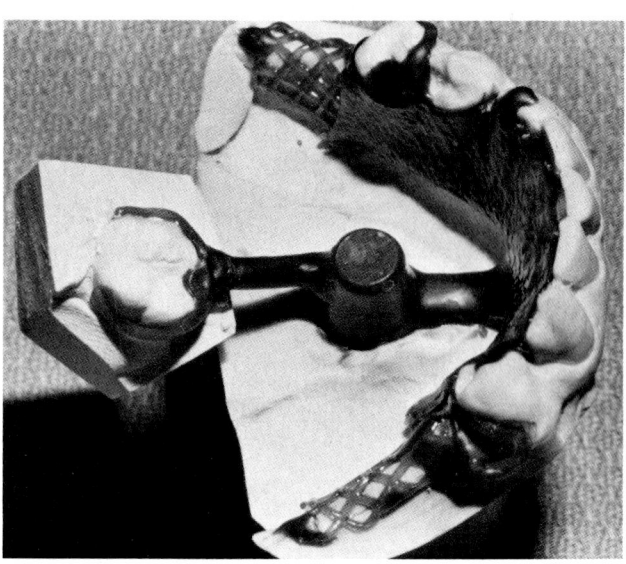

Fig. 15-25. Completed wax-up of cast clasp assembly added to routine framework for casting.

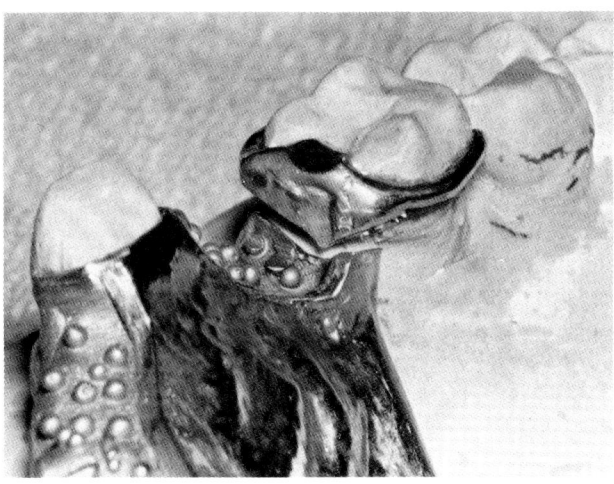

Fig. 15-26. Cast clasp assembly fitted to partial denture.

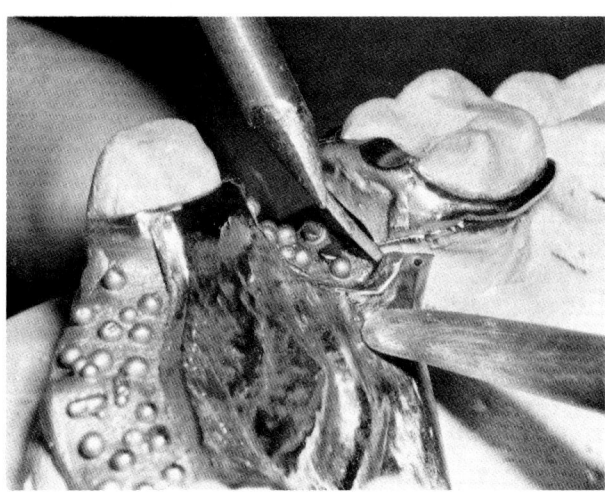

Fig. 15-27. Cast clasp assembly being soldered.

10. Sprue the completed wax-up in a nonfunctioning area, and add it to a routine framework casting as a "rider" (Fig. 15-25). If the repair addition is too large to be added safely to another casting (more than a simple clasp assembly), the technician may elect to invest the repair by itself.

11. The burnout and casting procedures are a factor of the alloy to be used and should pose no problem at all to the technician.

12. Recover the casting and fit it to the denture and the repair cast as required (Fig. 15-26). Once the repair components are fully seated, open the solder joint area slightly (no more than 1 mm) by disking the casting.

13. Protect the soldering area with foil, seat the components completely, and complete the repair with the electric soldering techniques described earlier (Fig. 15-27).

14. The resulting cast alloy repair can be expected to function as well as the original denture. If

**Fig. 15-28.** Cross section of finishing lines, showing offset.

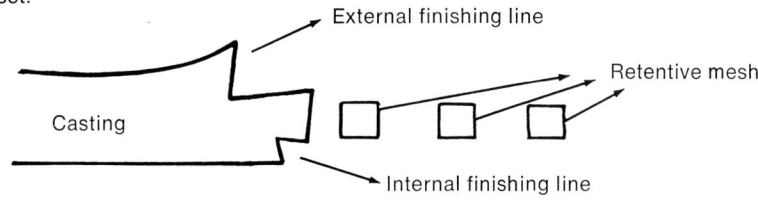

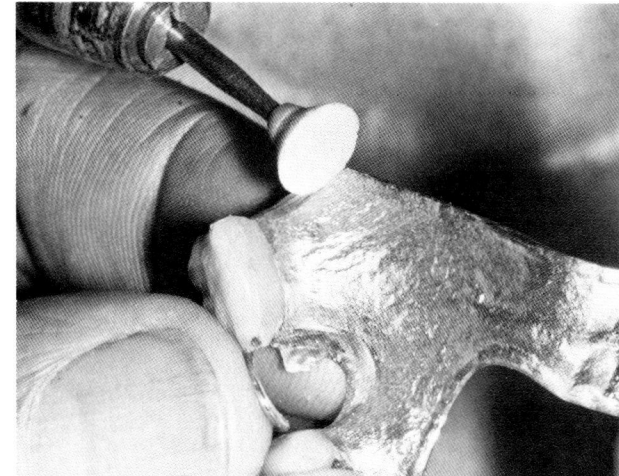

**Fig. 15-29.** Internal finishing line cut into tissue surface of casting.

the factors that caused the fracture have been reduced or eliminated, the repair may well be an improvement.

## Resin retention repairs

When abutment teeth are lost, many removable partial dentures can be salvaged by a combination of clasp, tooth, and denture base additions. Most additions can be attached through the resin of the adjoining denture base. Some situations require the addition of denture base retention to hold the resin repairs.

Resin retention, no matter what form it takes, requires the establishment of finishing lines for a quality repair. Wherever resin contacts metal in the partial denture, a definite finishing line allowing a minimum of 1 mm of resin bulk must be created. Resin not confined by the internal and external finishing lines will tend to percolate with oral fluids, trap and hold debris, and serve as a vehicle for the growth of microorganisms. Since the finishing line is normally adjacent to the abutment tooth, the septic condition created by unbutted resin furthers soft and hard tissue destruction. Finishing lines are usually offset so that no weak spot is created in the framework (Fig. 15-28). Finishing lines created in the repair situation must likewise be offset.

Since the great majority of these repairs involve a recent extraction, provision must be made for the inevitable resin reline. The internal finishing line must be placed as far from the extraction site as possible so that resorption of the alveolar process will occur primarily in the area of the resin addition.

There will seldom be sufficient thickness in the major connector of the partial denture to allow both internal and external finishing lines to be cut in. The external finishing line may have to be created with wire and/or solder to assure sufficient bulk. The actual resin retention addition associated with these finishing lines is the easiest part of the repair to construct. Loops of wrought wire or mesh fragments from scrapped partial denture frameworks are simple to fabricate and solder to the denture. Regardless of where the resin retention addition is required, the technical steps involved are basically the same.

### PROCEDURE

1. A repair cast with the denture in place must be received from the dentist. The cast should be accurate and free from blebs or voids in the area of the repair.

2. Remove the partial denture from the cast, and plan the placement of the internal finishing line and the desired resin retention as previously mentioned.

3. Mark the internal finishing line on the tissue surface of the casting with a wax pencil, and cut to a depth of at least 1 mm. With an inverted cone-shaped bur or stone, using high speed, form the resin-metal junction to 90 degrees or greater to achieve sufficient bulk of resin (Fig. 15-29).

4. Using a Boley gauge (or similar measuring caliper), measure the thickness of the casting at the finishing line. If more than 3 mm of metal remains, cut the external finishing line into the major connector in the same manner.

5. When insufficient metal remains, that is, when the rigidity of the casting has been compromised, *add* the entire external finishing line to the framework. The addition may be made of solder alone by laying a long strip of solder along the proposed line and blending it into the framework with the carbon tip of the electric soldering unit (Fig. 15-30).

6. Cut the external finishing line in the solder addition.

7. In an alternative approach, a 17- or 18-gauge nickel-cobalt-chromium wire* forms the core for the soldering operation. Cut the wire ½ inch (1.3 cm) longer than required for the line adapted, and then position it with ¼ inch (0.6 cm) excess at both ends, and hold it in place with clay or plaster.

8. Add solder to the junction of wire and framework to blend the two together (Fig. 15-31).

9. Cut the external finishing line at the expense of half of the wire, leaving an ample area for resin bulk (Fig. 15-32).

10. Position the required resin retention, and join it to the framework with solder (Fig. 15-33).

When the major connector is a lingual plate or in some way blankets the lingual surface of the remaining teeth, the construction of resin retention for the addition of one or more teeth that are not adjacent to the existing denture resin is as follows:

1. Design the internal finishing line, and cut into the framework as previously described (Fig. 15-34).

2. Cut a piece of wire (18-gauge nickel-cobalt-chromium), and adapt it to the contours of the lingual plate at the repair site, so that it will form a retention loop or post for the denture tooth to be added (Fig. 15-35).

---

*Ti-Wire, Ticonium Co., Albany, N.Y.

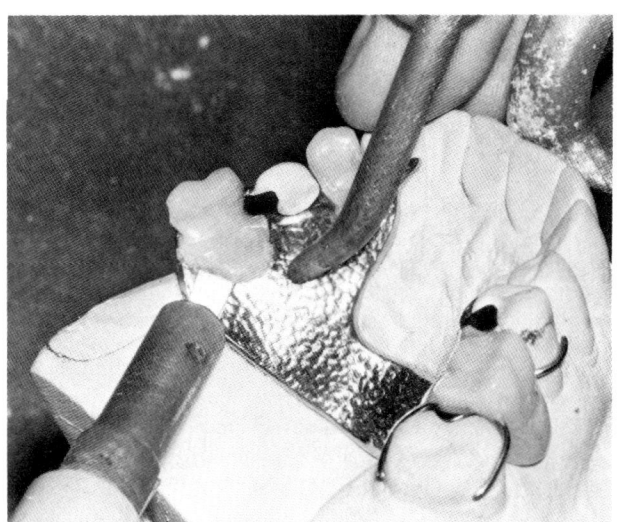

Fig. 15-30. Long strip of solder fused to frame to form finishing line.

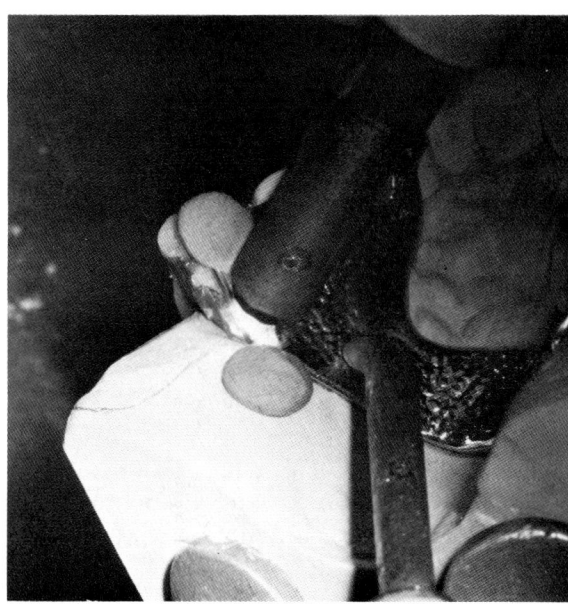

Fig. 15-31. Solder added to frame and wire junction.

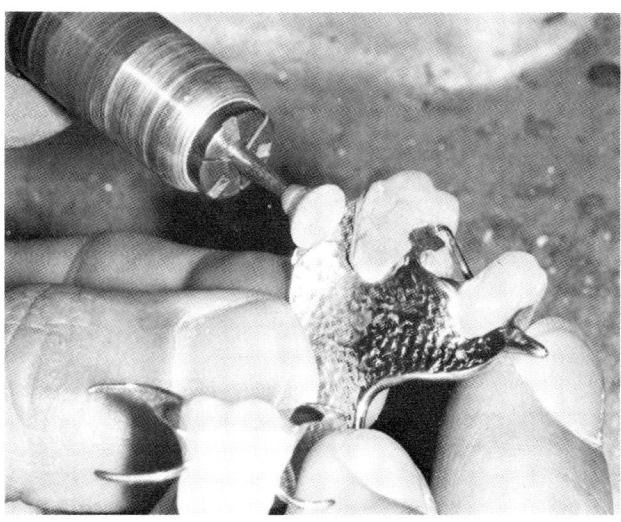

**Fig. 15-32.** External finishing line cut into wire-frame junction.

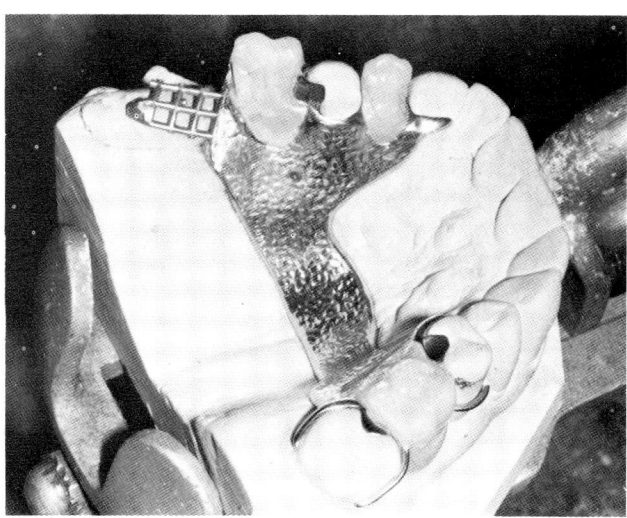

**Fig. 15-33.** Resin retention in place prior to soldering.

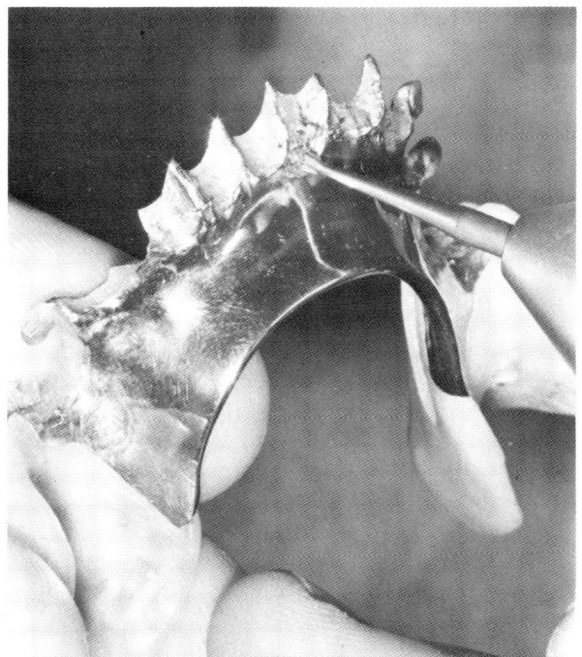

**Fig. 15-34.** Internal finishing line cut into lingual plate.

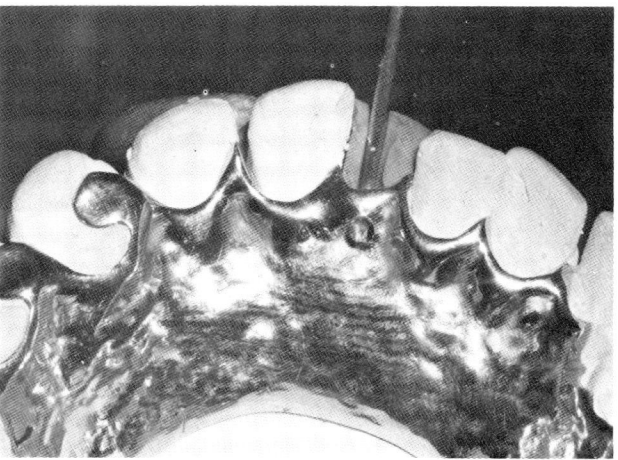

**Fig. 15-35.** Wire post adapted for single tooth resin retention through lingual perforation.

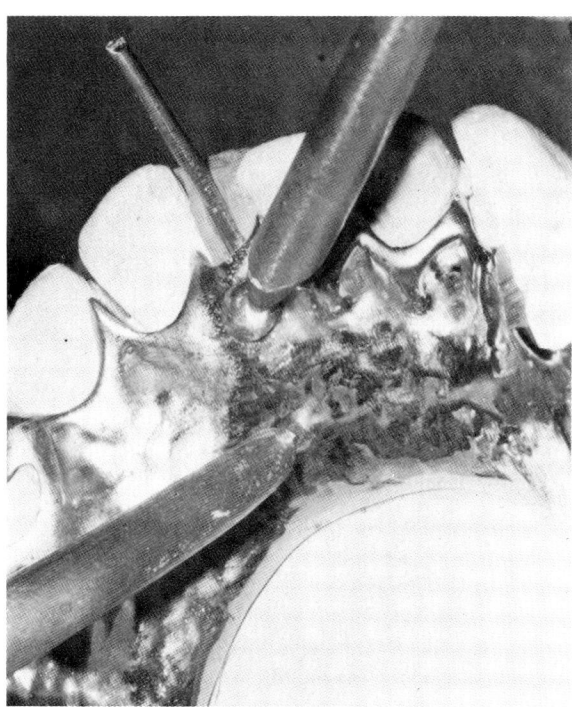

**Fig. 15-36.** Wire post soldered through perforation.

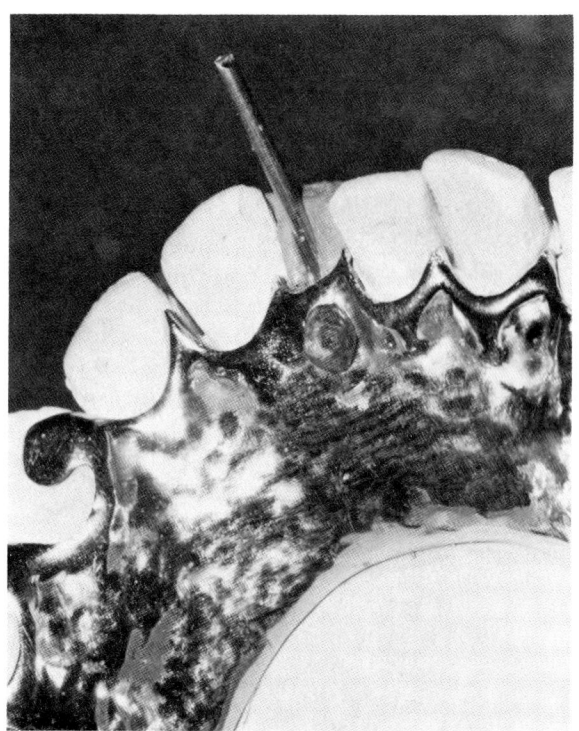

**Fig. 15-37.** Soldered post before finishing.

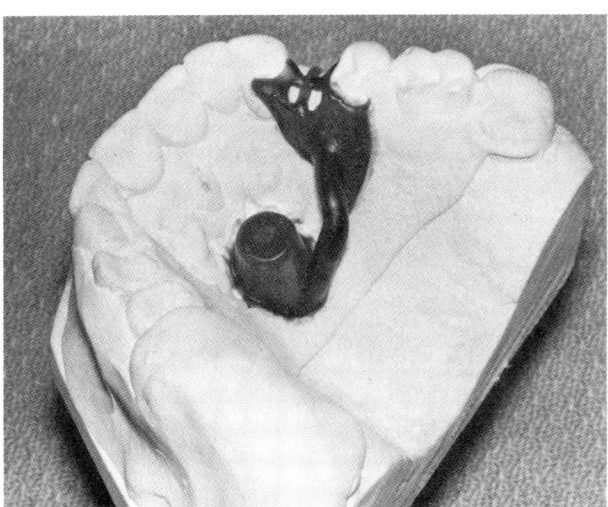

**Fig. 15-38.** Single tooth replacement waxed on refractory cast.

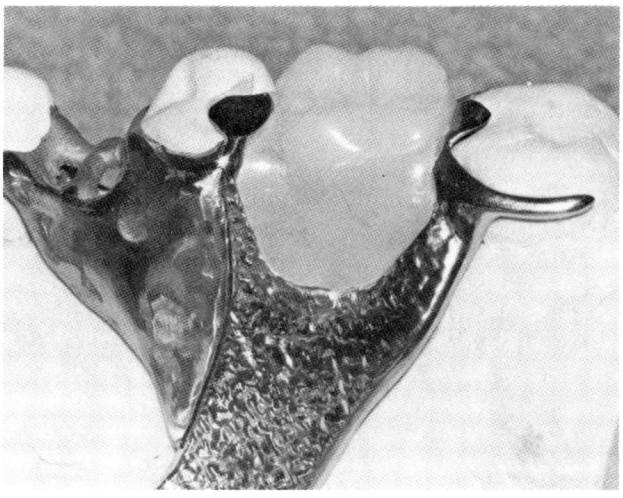

**Fig. 15-39.** Single tooth replacement fitted for soldering.

3. Since the smallest carbon tip of the electrosoldering unit has a diameter of 3.5 mm, it may not always be possible to reach the wire from the tissue side. In that case the lingual plate should be notched or perforated (Fig. 15-36). The wire loop is extended through the perforation and soldered on the outer surface of the casting where access for the soldering element presents no problem (Fig. 15-37).

When the major connector does not plate the tooth to be added, the repair becomes much more complex. A loop or strut of wire can be soldered to the major connector and extended to the now edentulous space. The addition is seldom rigid and results in repair that is only temporary or transitional. To add a single tooth replacement to a lingual bar or maxillary major connector that is some distance

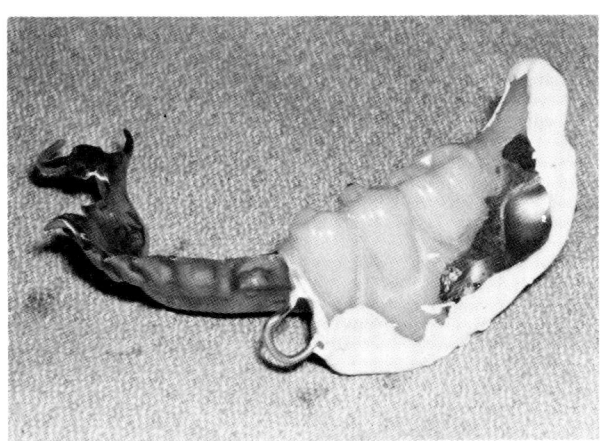

Fig. 15-46. Missing segments developed in modeling plastic, and reline impression made.

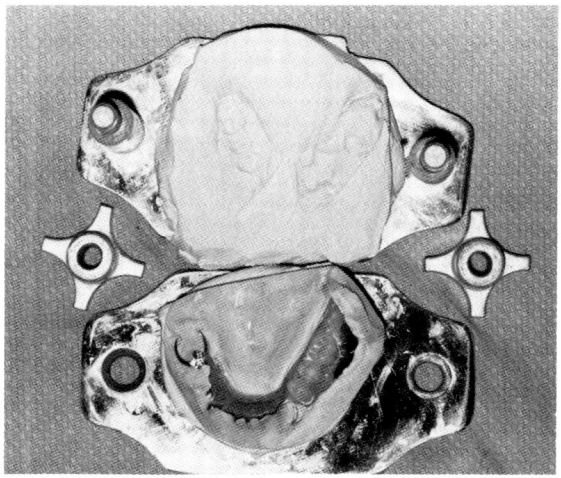

Fig. 15-47. Repair placed in remount jig.

removable partial denture as part of the repair. Missing segments of the resin base may have been reshaped in the patient's mouth with modeling plastic and a wash impression made as for a rebase or reline (Fig. 15-46). The following procedure produces the best possible repair results but obviously requires a longer chairside procedure:

1. Treat the reconstructed denture as a rebase. Flask in a denture flask, or place it in a reline jig.

2. If the missing parts are extensive, the repair is best handled in the denture flask. When the missing part(s) involves only the periphery and is not extensive, complete the rebase in the reline jig (Fig. 15-47).

### FRACTURED AND MISSING TEETH

The replacement of denture teeth may well be considered the easiest of all partial denture repairs. Given the necessary countermodel the technician can be expected to add the new denture teeth quickly and return a denture that requires little or no equilibration.

The denture base must be prepared to accept the replacement tooth. Fractured porcelain teeth may be removed by prying with a hot spatula from the lingual surface. Resin teeth must be ground out of the denture base with a resin bur.

#### PROCEDURE

1. Remove the fractured tooth or teeth from the resin base. Access for removal must always be made on the lingual surface to protect the faciogingival contours (Fig. 15-48).

2. Estimate the mold and shade for the replacement teeth, and fit the teeth to the existing tooth

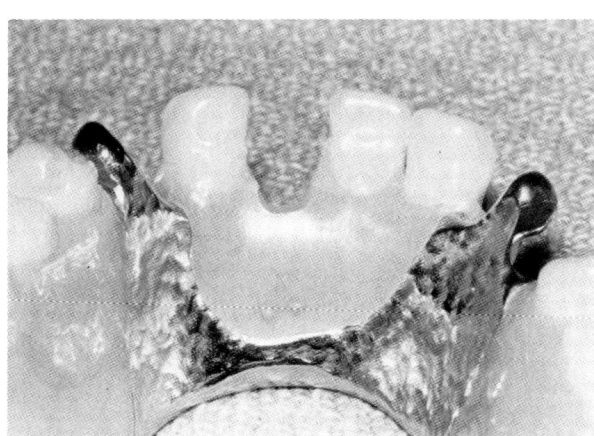

Fig. 15-48. Access for replacement of missing teeth cut lingually.

space. In the great majority of repairs, resin teeth will be selected as the replacement. Since they will bond to the denture base, a stronger repair can be expected. Porcelain teeth depend on diatoric recesses or pins and are more difficult to adapt by grinding.

3. Make every effort to fit the replacement tooth to the faciogingival contours, since a misfit in this area will result in repair resin extruding onto the denture tooth. Recontouring and finishing this resin is difficult, and esthetic compromises often result.

4. Fit the replacement tooth into a position that is in acceptable alignment by grinding both the tooth and denture base.

5. Tack the tooth in position with sticky wax applied to the lingual surface.

6. Evaluate occlusal relationships by placing the denture against the countercast. It is easier to ad-

base repair on the countermodel, and hold it in place with sticky wax.

8. Sprinkle autopolymerizing repair resin polymer into the repair area to just cover the countermodel and add monomer with an eyedropper to completely wet the polymer (Fig. 15-43). Polymer that is not wetted will result in a granular porous layer adjacent to the soft tissue and will greatly compromise the repair.

9. Fill the repair void to excess by adding monomer and polymer in succession, and then place it in a pressure pot at 28 psi with a small amount of warm water (100° F; 39° C), and allow it to complete polymerization according to the manufacturer's instructions.

10. Finish and polish to complete the resin repair.

### Simple fractures involving teeth

When the fracture area involves one or more teeth, the use of a second countercast can reduce finishing time by keeping the repair resin from the facial and occlusal surfaces of the denture teeth.

#### PROCEDURE

1. After the basic repair countercast has been poured and is set, vibrate a facial core of plaster onto the denture (Fig. 15-44). The core should cover the facial and occlusal surface of the associated denture teeth and extend onto the gingival surface of the denture base 2 to 3 mm.

2. Treat this facial core with tinfoil substitute, and sticky wax it into position before adding the repair resin (Fig. 15-45).

3. The core will prevent the repair resin from flowing into the gingival contours that may be difficult to finish. The small (2 to 3 mm) lip will not hinder the addition of the repair resin.

### Complex fractures

The primary differences between the complex repair situation and the simple one already described are those of multiple fractures and missing pieces. The clinician must submit these repairs to the laboratory on a repair cast that has been made with the partial denture completely seated in the mouth. Without the repair cast any attempt to repair this type of situation must be considered only temporary and may require a good deal of adjustment at insertion.

#### PROCEDURE

1. Remove the segments of the partial denture from the repair cast, and make any slight correc-

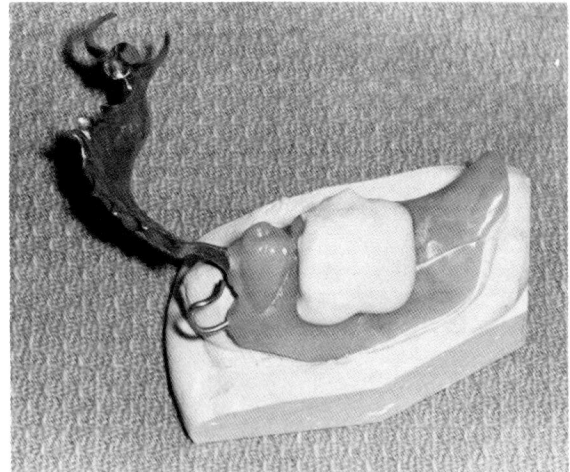

**Fig. 15-44.** Facial core placed on teeth of repair.

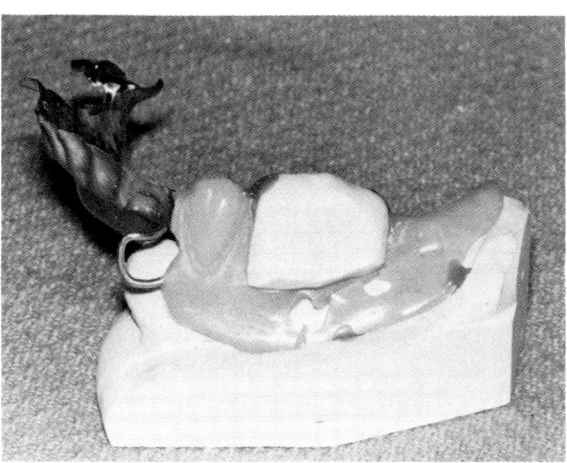

**Fig. 15-45.** Facial core sticky waxed into position.

tion by shaping the dental stone that might have been vibrated into cracks and voids.

2. Trim the segments as previously described, and replace them on the repair cast. Shape all missing and defective areas to normal contours with baseplate wax.

3. Now a decision must be made whether to flask the repair and replace most or all of the denture resin or to proceed as in the simple repair. If the areas now composed of wax are extensive, then the repair must be flasked.

4. Flask the repair cast in the conventional manner, boil it out, and pack it in autopolymerizing resin. Measure, mix, and pack the resin according to the manufacturer's directions; casual manipulation results in a repair of poor quality.

The clinician may have elected to reconstruct the

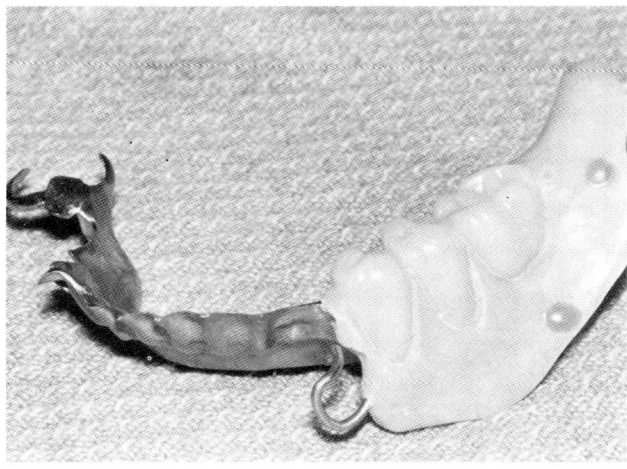

Fig. 15-40. Resin segments are related with sticky wax.

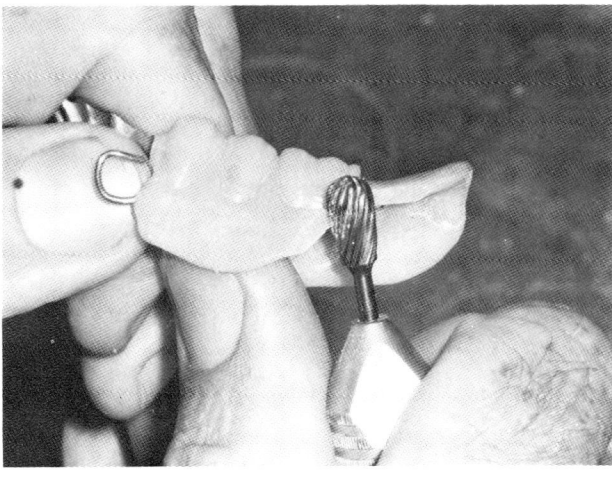

Fig. 15-41. Butt joint being prepared in resin.

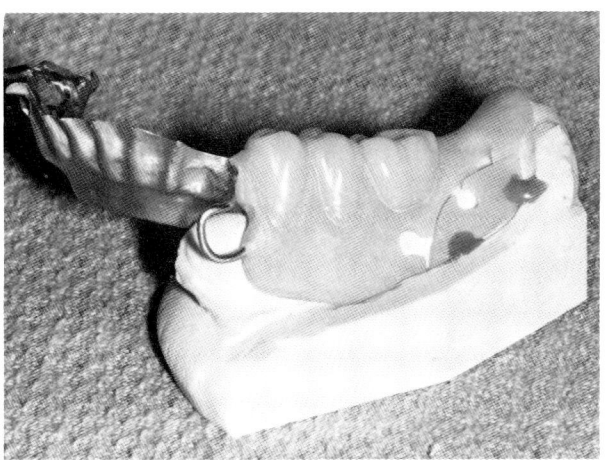

Fig. 15-42. Dovetailed slots cut in resin for repair.

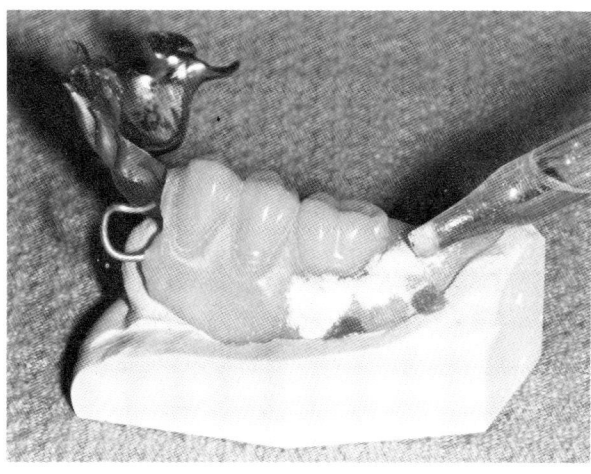

Fig. 15-43. Monomer added to resin in repair area.

must be cut back to a more bulky area. The dimensions of the repair site are critical only if they are minimal. When occlusal interference is suspected (over retromolar pad or tuberosity) and the resin is too thin, remove the entire area and replace it with an adequate (4 mm or greater) amount of repair resin. The clinician must now be informed that some equilibration will be required. Attempting to repair the very thin section of resin without increasing its thickness results in a poor quality of autopolymerized resin.

4. Trim the borders of the fractures site with a resin bur to provide for adequate bulk of resin (4 to 5 mm). Hold the bur 90 degrees to the outer surface of the denture base segments so that a right angle "butt joint" will be formed between the new resin and the old (Fig. 15-41). The right angle interface reduces the resin interface to the minimum, which is a disadvantage in thin sections, but this approach greatly reduces the chances of a noticeable junction line. Thin sections of repair resin overlaid on old resin will result in a visible line that may be objectionable. The butt joint is inherently weaker than a rounded joint because of stress concentrations at the right angles. Where the joint cannot be seen the edges should be rounded.

5. To increase the contact area of the denture repair, cut dovetailed slots along both sides of the fracture line (Fig. 15-42). This is particularly indicated in longitudinal fractures of the single maxillary denture opposed by natural teeth.

6. Paint the countermodel with tinfoil substitute, and allow it to dry.

7. Reposition the prepared section of the denture

from the extraction site, the following steps are indicated:

1. The laboratory receives a repair cast with the denture in place from the clinician. Tooth modification to include guiding planes and rest preparation will have been completed before the repair impression was made. A shallow notch is cut in the connector to receive the repair segment.
2. Spray the cast, and block it out with the denture in place in the conventional manner.
3. Duplicate the cast, and pour it in refractory material.
4. Form retention for the single tooth replacement on the refractory model, and wax a minor connector to connect it to the notch in the major connector (Fig. 15-38).
5. Sprue, invest, and cast the repair segment.
6. Recover, finish, and polish the casting and seat it on the repair cast. Some adjustment of the notch is necessary to create space for the solder. A solder gap of 1 mm is adequate for a successful solder repair.
7. Solder the single tooth replacement to the major connector as previously described (Fig. 15-39).

Multiple tooth replacement segments to distant major connectors are constructed as described here for a single tooth.

## RESIN REPAIR

The vast majority of resin repairs for removable partial dentures are made with autopolymerizing methyl methacrylate. The advantages of not having to process in the conventional denture flask are obvious, primarily speed and safety. Safety is especially important because flasking and recovery of an existing removable partial denture are frought with possibilities for error and damage to the denture.

### Autopolymerizing repair resins

The basis of methyl methacrylate polymerization is the decomposition of benzoyl peroxide. This breakdown forms free radicals (that is, compounds with an unpaired electron that are very reactive). The radicals serve as the links that join the long chain polymers together. In the standard heat-curing denture resin, the breakdown of the peroxide is caused by the heat of processing (above 140° F; 60° C). The autopolymerizing resin is activated by some form of a tertiary amine (such as *N,N*-dimethyl-*p*-toluidine) that is added to the monomer. After mixing with the polymer, the amine-peroxide reaction releases the free radicals, and polymerization takes place. In any case the size of the particles of polymer affects the rate of polymerization. The smaller the particle, the faster the reaction.

Because the reaction is chemically activated, once it begins it is difficult to stop. Working time with these resins is definitely limited, which can have both a positive and negative effect, depending on the particular need.

On the positive side, initial hardening occurs in 20 to 30 minutes for most resins of this type. Many technicians treat the resin as completely polymerized at this point, but greater end strength will occur if the resin is undisturbed for 2 to 3 hours. When major additions to the partial denture base are made, it is important to keep the flasked repair under pressure for the entire polymerization time. To not do so may result in warpage of the denture resin.

It can be expected that the autopolymerizing resins will have a greater dimensional stability than the heat-cured resins.

Autopolymerizing resins have a much greater tendency to be porous and lack color stability. The advantages of autopolymerization outweigh these deficiencies, and heat-cured resin is seldom used in removable partial denture repairs.

As with any dental material, the best results will occur from strict adherance to the manufacturer's directions. Unfortunately, repair resin is often abused by the technician. It is only in the long-term evaluation of the resin repair that proper handling becomes apparent.

### Denture base fractures

Resin fractures range from the very simple, where a clean break and the presence of all the pieces make the repair easy, to the complex, multiple fracture with missing segments.

#### Simple fractures

The simple fracture is usually received from the clinician as is. When the pieces can be *positively* related, no repair impression is necessary.

##### PROCEDURE

1. Reposition the segments and hold them with sticky wax while a countercast is poured (Fig. 15-40). Plaster may be used because no load will be placed on the cast. The countercast must extend well beyond the fracture line so that the segments will have a stable seat during the repair.
2. Remove the denture base segments as soon as the final set of the countercast is reached.
3. Remove the sticky wax, and prepare the fracture site for the addition of resin repair. Evaluate the fracture site as to its possible contribution to the denture base fracture. When the thickness of the resin is minimal (2 mm or less), the denture base

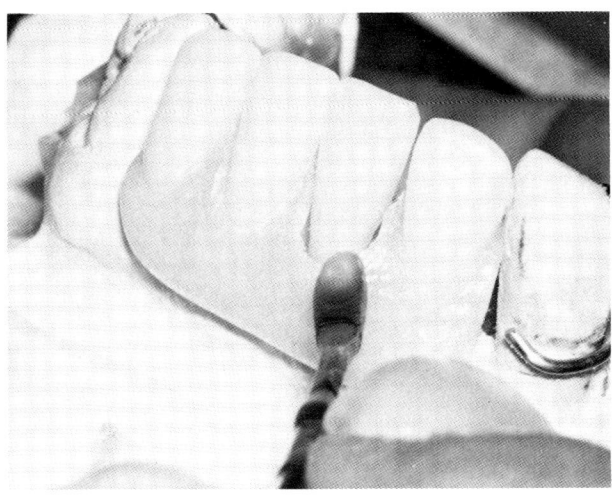

Fig. 15-49. Defects in labial contours are waxed in.

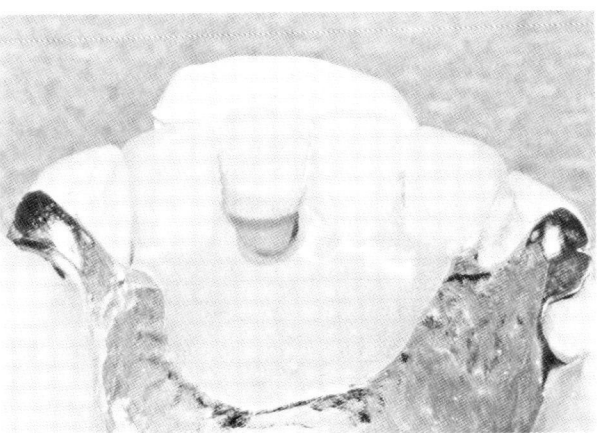

Fig. 15-50. Facio-occlusal matrix vibrated on repair denture.

just occlusal contacts after the denture teeth are attached with resin as long as alignment is satisfactory. Should the tooth be grossly in hyperocclusion, a decision to alter the alignment may be in order.

7. With the replacement tooth in position, fill in any labial defects in the gingival resin contours with wax, and festoon as in routine denture construction (Fig. 15-49).

8. Vibrate a plaster matrix onto the replacement tooth and a portion of adjacent teeth or denture base. The matrix must cover all the facial surface to include the denture base well beyond the waxed areas. It must also cover most of the occlusal or incisal surface (Fig. 15-50). By mixing the plaster with slurry water, the time to set can be greatly reduced.

9. Remove the wax from the denture with boiling water, and paint the plaster with tinfoil substitute.

10. Attach the denture tooth or teeth to the matrix with a small amount of sticky wax on the linguo-occlusal area.

11. Moisten the denture base with monomer, add a predetermined amount of autopolymerizing repair resin to the denture base, and seat the matrix with the denture teeth. The most satisfactory repair occurs when just the right amount of resin is added. Experience alone will allow neither too little resin, causing voids, nor too much, causing incomplete seating and a flash of excess resin.

12. Excess repair resin will extrude from the lingual aspect, where it can be shaped with a spatula to approximate the desired lingual contour, and the repair is placed in a pressure pot (Fig. 15-51).

13. When the repair resin is fully polymerized according to the manufacturer's instructions, finish

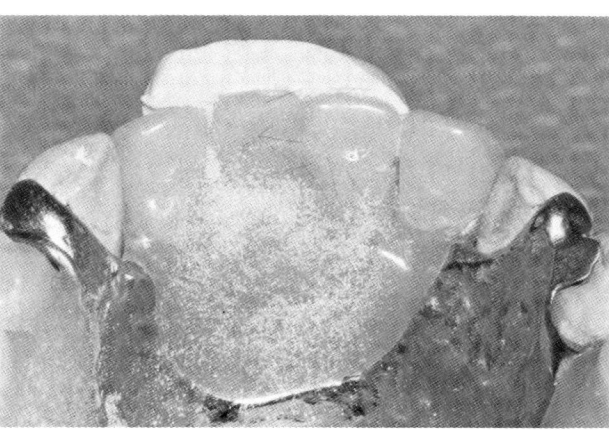

Fig. 15-51. Excess repair resin extruding from tooth repair area.

and polish the repair. If care has been taken in the previous steps, no resin will be present on the facial or occlusal surfaces. Remove the excess on the lingual surface with a finishing bur.

## TOOTH AND DENTURE BASE ADDITIONS

Additions of this sort are usually associated with the loss of terminal abutments where the tooth-borne denture is converted into a tooth-and-tissue-borne denture. The laboratory must receive a repair cast with the denture in place. The area to be added must be an accurate reproduction of the mouth. An opposing cast must also be included.

### PROCEDURE

1. If necessary, add the metal components of denture base retention as described earlier to the

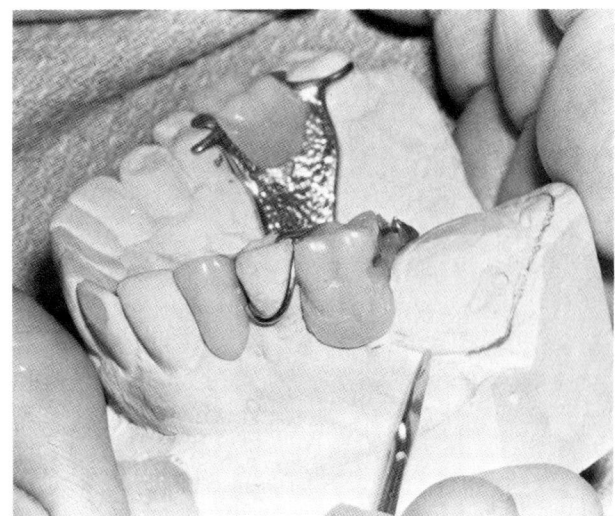

Fig. 15-52. Scribing peripheral extent onto repair cast.

denture before the teeth and denture base material are added.

2. Articulate the cast with the opposing cast on a simple articulator, grind and position teeth, and wax the new denture base to the estimated periphery. The clinician should indicate the desired extent of the denture base with a pencil line on the repair cast. The technician can scribe the line with a sharp instrument to create a witness mark that will aid in finishing the denture base to the desired extension (Fig. 15-52).

3. Flask the fully waxed repair as described before, and complete the repair with autopolymerizing resin in the flask.

4. It may be necessary to include a clasp change in this type of addition if the existing terminal abutment clasping is not suitable for the distal extension removable partial denture. Wrought circumferential or bar clasps may replace cast clasp arms to minimize loading the terminal abutment. In some cases it may be necessary to add a rest and minor connector as well as the clasp arm. When repairs of this complexity are encountered, the final result must merit the expense of the repair. The denture, with its new components, must function as well as a new removable partial denture.

### PROBLEM AREAS

Problems most commonly associated with the repair of the removable partial denture are primarily related to soldering operations: (1) solder joint separation, (2) inadequate metal surface for soldering, (3) reluctance to prepare repair surfaces and cast new repair elements, and (4) unfamiliarity with basic soldering techniques. In addition, inadequate bulk of repair resin also contributes to the problems encountered with removable partial denture repairs (Table 15-1). A logical analysis of the repair situation by both the clinician and the technician is required to determine if a quality repair is possible. The careful adherence to a sequential approach with predetermined standards of quality control is the most dependable way to reduce repair problems.

**Table 15-1.** Metal and plastic repairs

| Problem | Probable cause | Solution |
|---|---|---|
| Solder joint separates | Improper fluxing | Use only fluoride fluxes that have been mixed to thin consistency; only very watery surface of flux can be used; when surface begins to thicken, add more water and stir vigorously |
| | Metal surfaces not clean | Before soldering any metals (frameworks or clasps) freshen surfaces to be soldered with fine stone to remove oxides and debris |
| | Improper solder | Check with alloy manufacturer for recommended solders |
| | Soldering machine not operating properly | Verify heat setting with manufacturer's directions; keep both copper and carbon tip clean for current conduction |
| Solder balls up and will not complete soldering | Metal surfaces not clean or properly fluxed | See above |
| | Heat inadequate to complete soldering | Keep carbon tip on solder, and keep current flowing until solder flows; do not remove carbon tip from solder until solder flows |
| | Improper solder and/or flux | Check alloy manufacturer's recommendations |
| | Soldering machine not giving sufficient heat | Check heat setting |
| Electrosoldering terminals will not complete circuit, and no heat is generated | Oxide layer on metal | Lightly stone both surface area to be soldered *and* area where copper tip will be placed to complete circuit |
| | Either copper tip or carbon tip or both are not clean | Clean both tips with abrasive stone or disk before soldering |
| | Flux too thick | Thin fluoride flux to watery consistency and then use only surface material |
| | Malfunction of machine | Check circuit with ohmmeter to detect shorts or open circuit |
| Resin repair fractures immediately | Separating material on repair surfaces | Let separating material set completely before attempting repair |
| | Inadequate bulk of resin | Thicken repair site, and verify overall resin thickness (this may require occlusal adjustment) |
| Resin repair porous | Improper monomer-polymer ratio | Make repair resin as thick as possible when sprinkling on polymer but be sure to wet *all* polymer |
| | Neglecting pressure pot | Place resin repair in pressure pot as soon as possible; use 100° F (38° C) water at 28 psi pressure |

# CHAPTER 16

# FRICTIONAL WALL PRECISION ATTACHMENT PARTIAL PROSTHESIS

JACK H. SWEPSTON

**precision attachment (parallel attachment, frictional attachment, internal attachment, key and keyway attachment, slotted attachment)** A retainer, used in fixed and removable partial denture construction, consisting of a metal receptacle and a closely fitting part; the former is usually contained within the normal or expanded contours of the crown of the abutment tooth, and the latter is attached to a pontic or to the denture framework.

Precision attachments are basically classified as follows (Goodkind and Baker, 1976):
1. Intracoronal
    a. Resilient
    b. Nonresilient
2. Extracoronal
    a. Resilient
    b. Nonresilient

Additional terminology is used to identify specific types of attachments for specific uses. These include pawl connectors, screw units, stabilizers, studs, telescopic studs, and the custom-made channel-shoulder-pin (CSP) system. This chapter will be oriented specifically to the intracoronal nonresilient attachment.

A thorough knowledge in the technical procedures of fabrication of one of the more detailed demanding attachments can, with very little modification and ingenuity, be adapted to any of the other types. Attachments of different classifications are described in Chapters 11 and 19 of *Dental Laboratory Procedures: Fixed Partial Dentures*.

The objective of this chapter is to help the novice dentist and/or technician gain proficiency in attachment procedures. However, the experienced dentist and/or technician may also benefit from the procedures described.

Technical laboratory procedures described in the literature vary in completeness. Although many of the steps may be modified as the individual operator gains experience, it is essential that fundamental principles be adhered to in the fabrication of this or any other type of restoration.

## GOALS

The goals for fabrication of frictional wall precision attachment partial denture are as follows:

1. To provide an efficient masticating replacement of lost dental organs.
2. To be removable and replaceable without stress or strain on the abutment teeth.
3. To allow normal anatomic form to the abutment teeth.
4. To be capable of being tissue supported in a controlled manner.
5. To allow for various occlusal prescriptions.
6. To provide many years of comfortable service.

7. To be made of materials that are compatible with the oral tissues.
8. To be esthetically acceptable.
9. To have a minimal amount of tooth structure removed.
10. To avoid endodontic procedures.
11. To be hygienically clean.
12. To place minimum amount of strain on the abutment teeth.

These goals parallel the classical objectives of restorative dentistry, that is, to restore function, esthetics, comfort, and be nondestructive.

## INDICATIONS

Frictional wall precision attachment partial dentures (precision bridges) are indicated in most partial denture situations. In mouths with missing teeth, the first idea should be: Is a fixed partial denture indicated? If a removable partial denture is indicated, then consideration should be given to the precision partial denture over the clasp-type partial denture. The precision partial denture is indicated in the following situations:

1. Long-span replacements
2. Free-end saddles
3. Periodontal involvement that has contraindicated fixed partial dentures
4. For maximum esthetics

## CONTRAINDICATIONS

Frictional wall precision attachment partial dentures are contraindicated in the following situations:

1. Teeth with short clinical crowns (this can be overcome with periodontal surgery).
2. Teeth that are narrow faciolingually.
3. Teeth that have extremely large pulps (young people).
4. Any patient who has a contraindication for a fixed partial denture (health, noncooperative, small mouth).
5. Patient's lack of dexterity or ability to use the hands.

## ADVANTAGES

Frictional wall precision attachment partial dentures direct the forces on the abutment with the long axis of the tooth. The fulcra are reduced in height, closer to the crestal bone level. This improves the longevity prognosis of the abutment teeth and increases patient satisfaction.

Disadvantages are minimal, but must be considered. The abutment teeth must be restored and there may be an economic limitation for some patients.

## TECHNICAL PROCEDURES

To illustrate many of the fundamental principles used in the fabrication of a frictional wall precision attachment partial prothesis, a technique typodont will be used (Fig. 16-1). The maxillary second premolar, and first, second, and third molars are missing on one side. The maxillary second premolar and first molar are missing on the opposite side. This presents a combination type of restoration in that one side is a free-end denture base, and the other side is tooth supported. The spacing of the teeth on this typodont in a clinical situation would more than likely indicate a fixed prosthesis on the right side and a removable prosthesis on the left side with cross arch stabilization.

The fabrication of this particular type of prosthesis would be facilitated by a previous background in machine shop work, although it is not essential. The time, effort, and attention to details exerted for any phase of dentistry will suffice to adequately fabricate a successful precision attachment partial denture.

Few true frictional wall precision attachments are available on the market today. The type that will be described here is the Stern No. 7 frictional wall precision attachment* (Fig. 16-2). It comes with a standard metal or iridium-platinum female that can be used in conjunction with high-fusing metal designed for accepting porcelain. It has a slot buccally and lingually down the longitudinal axis of the male attachment that will be used in subsequent years for tightening the prosthesis as wear takes place.

---

*Stern Division, Sterndent Corp., Mt. Vernon, N.Y.

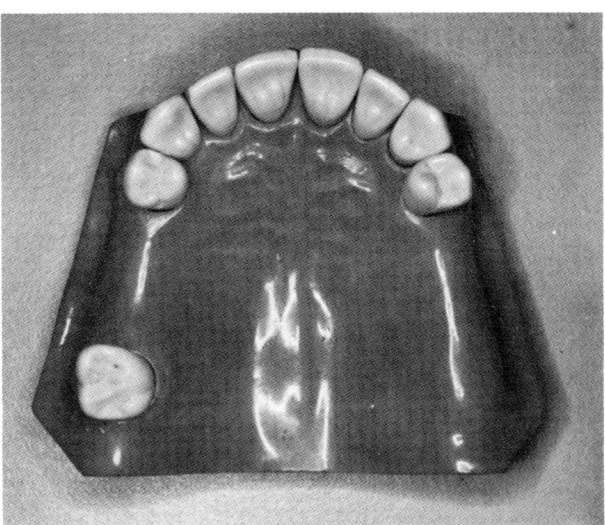

**Fig. 16-1.** Sample technique case.

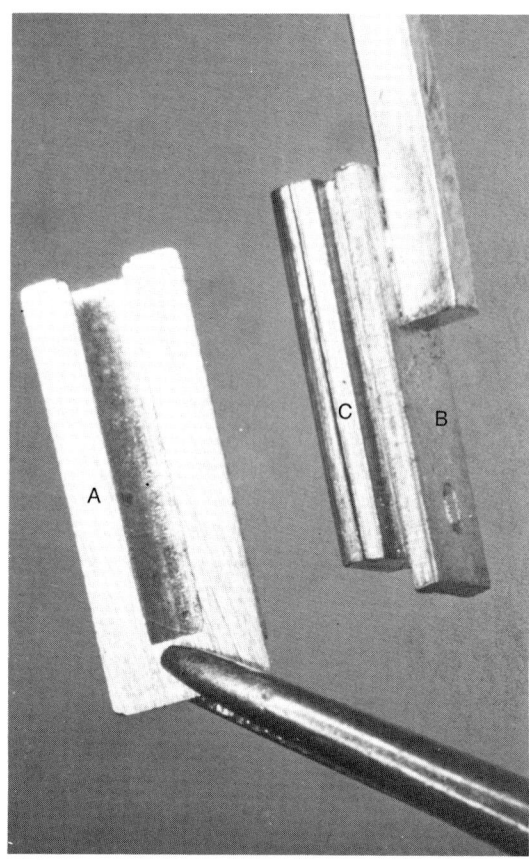

Fig. 16-2. Stern No. 7, .096 frictional wall precision attachment. *A,* Proximal contact plate of female attachment. *B,* Surface plate of male attachment. *C,* Slot for spreading leaves to tighten attachment.

## TREATMENT PLANNING

Diagnostic casts are made of the patient's mouth along with adequate face-bow transfer and interocclusal records. The casts are mounted in an articulator,* preferably of the arcon type. The articulator will have a point that indicates the axis of opening and closing of the jaws. A compass is used to scribe the arc of opening and closing in the midpoint of the replacement area (Fig. 16-3). This arc of opening and closing will be useful at a subsequent time in the diagnostic procedures.

The diagnostic cast is now oriented in an adjustable survey table.† The platform of the surveyor is sprinkled with acrylic resin powder, which allows the survey table to slide smoothly. The analyzing rod is placed in the vertical shaft of the surveyor (Fig. 16-4). The survey table is tilted to eliminate all of the undercut on one of the abutment teeth (Fig. 16-5). The survey table is now positioned so that the analyzing rod can be brought in close approximation with the art portion of the cast. A line is scribed parallel to this analyzing rod (Fig. 16-6). Similarly, the analyzing rod is brought against a second abutment tooth (Fig. 16-7), and the survey table is tilted

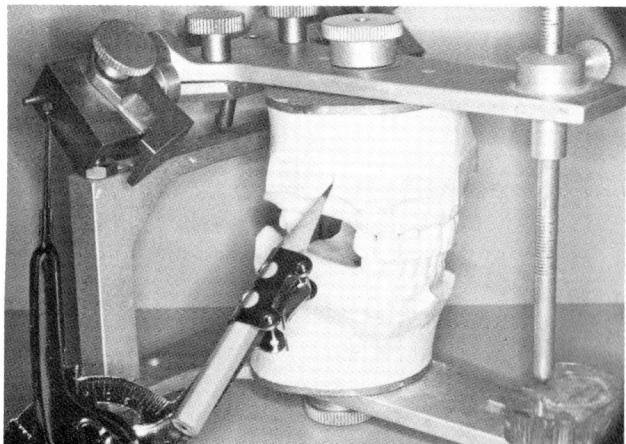

Fig. 16-3. Arc of opening of jaws scribed on land portion of cast.

*Whip-Mix Corp., Louisville, Ky.
†The J. M. Ney Co., Bloomfield, Conn.

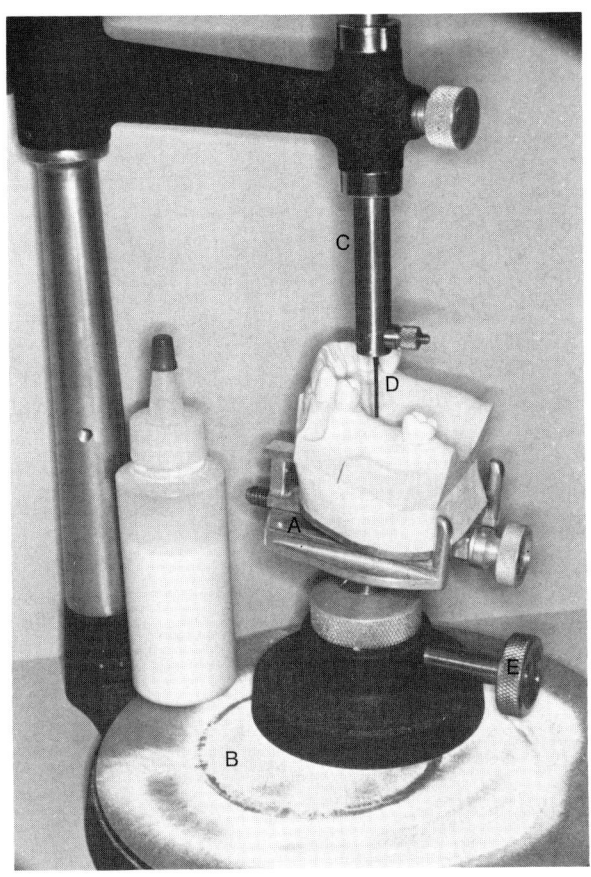

**Fig. 16-4.** Surveyor. *A*, Adjustable cast holder. *B*, Survey platform (sprinkled with acrylic powder for lubrication). *C*, Vertical shaft. *D*, Analyzing rod. *E*, Locking nut.

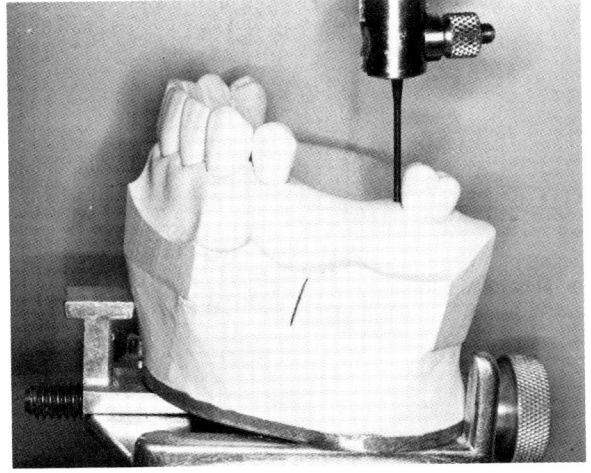

**Fig. 16-5.** Undercut eliminated.

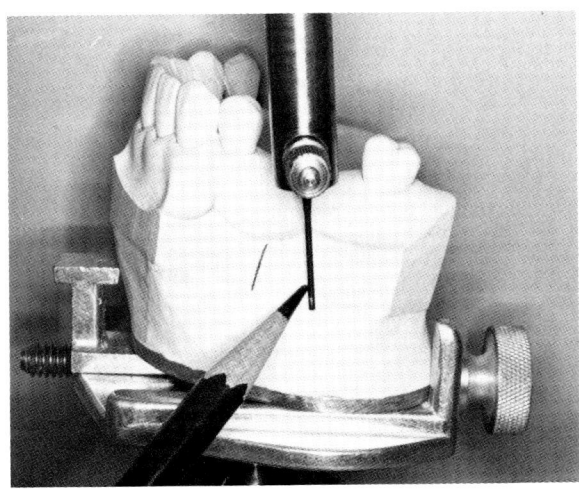

**Fig. 16-6.** Line drawn on art portion of cast parallel to analyzing rod.

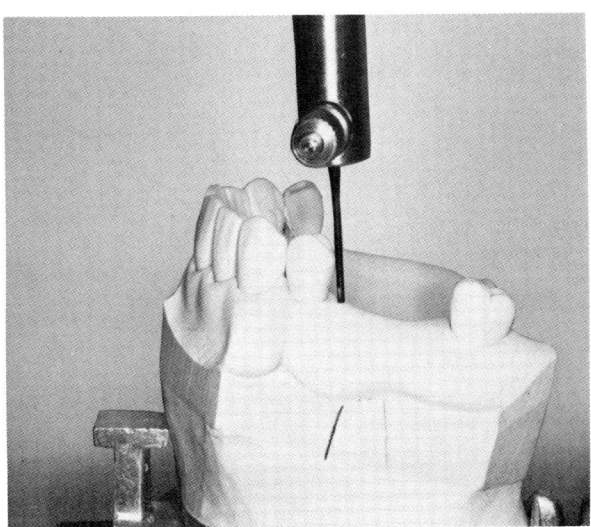

**Fig. 16-7.** Analyzing rod placed against second abutment tooth.

to make the analyzing rod parallel to the proximal surface, leaving no undercut (Fig. 16-8). Again, the survey table is shifted to the side, the analyzing rod is placed adjacent to the art portion of the cast, and a line is scribed parallel to the analyzing rod (Fig. 16-9). Each subsequent abutment tooth, however many there may be, is surveyed in the same way to eliminate all of the undercut, and a line parallel to that line is drawn on the art portion of the cast.

A bisecting line is then drawn between the most divergent of these lines (Fig. 16-10). This is the most common path of insertion with a minimal average undercut among all abutments. This line should be 5 degrees off of the arc of opening and closing scribed earlier on the art portion of the cast.

In a mediolateral configuration, the same type of analysis takes place. Each abutment tooth in turn (Fig. 16-11) is analyzed to allow the greatest length for attachment. The line for each abutment tooth is then scribed on the posterior aspect of the art portion of the cast. All abutment teeth are analyzed in the same manner. Subsequent to all abutment teeth being analyzed in the mediolateral direction, a bisecting line is drawn on the art portion of the cast that will bisect the most divergent abutment teeth (Fig. 16-12). This bisecting line will give the greatest attachment length among all of the combined abutment teeth. Each tooth should be measured to determine the available length. This length must permit use of at least two thirds of the attachment. Retention of a prosthesis is inversely proportional to the manufactured length, and consequently crown lengthening procedures may be indicated from this analysis. It is desirable but not essential that all attachments be of approximately the same length.

It now becomes necessary to parallel the bisecting lines in both the anteroposterior position and the mediolateral position (Fig. 16-13). These two lines are paralleled to the analyzing rod and by mathematics they are parallel to each other. This is the common path of insertion and withdrawal of the prosthesis.

During the treatment planning stages, adequate full-mouth radiographs, as well as the patient's medical and dental history and clinical examination, are vital aids in determining if this type of prosthesis is indicated.

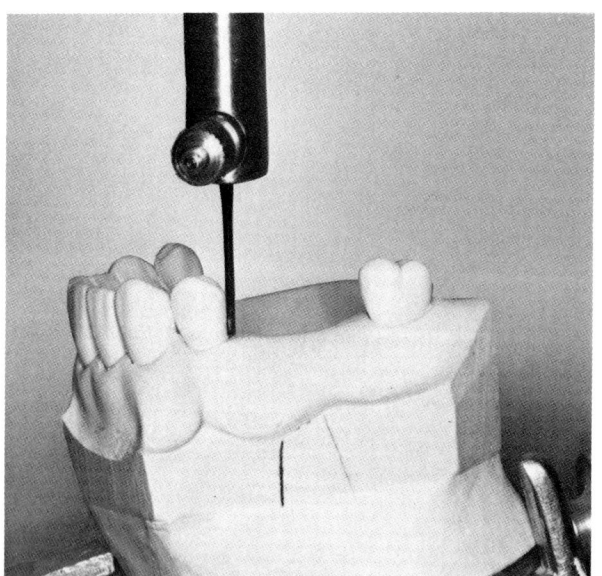

**Fig. 16-8.** Undercut eliminated on second abutment tooth by tilting cast.

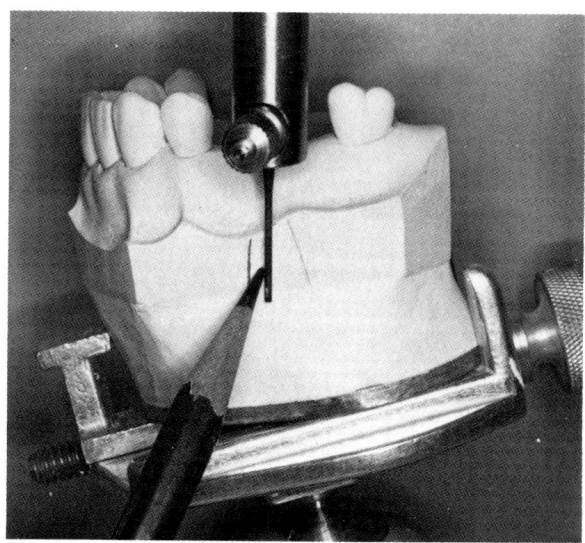

**Fig. 16-9.** Line scribed on land portion of cast parallel to analyzing rod for second abutment tooth.

## Frictional wall precision attachment partial prosthesis 453

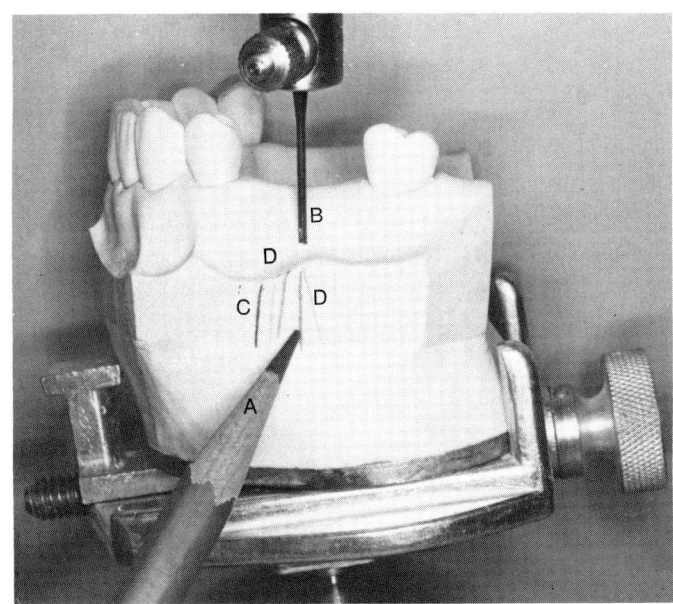

Fig. 16-10. Most divergent lines are bisected. *A,* Bisecting line. *B,* Analyzing rod. *C,* Arc of opening. *D,* Lines representing minimized undercut for each abutment tooth.

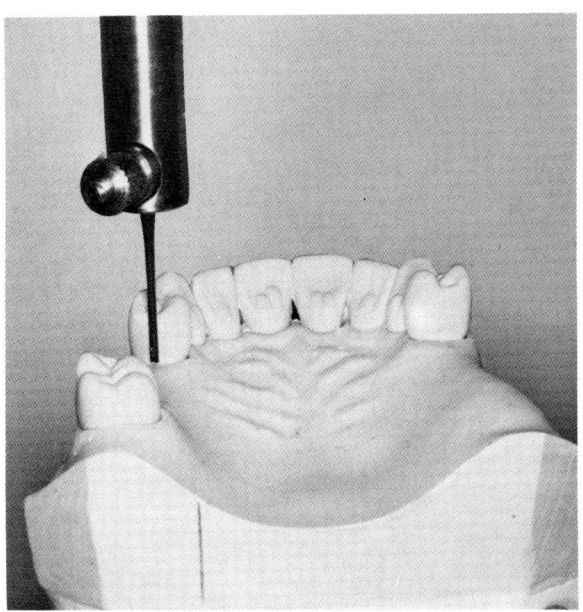

Fig. 16-11. Analysis in mediolateral dimension.

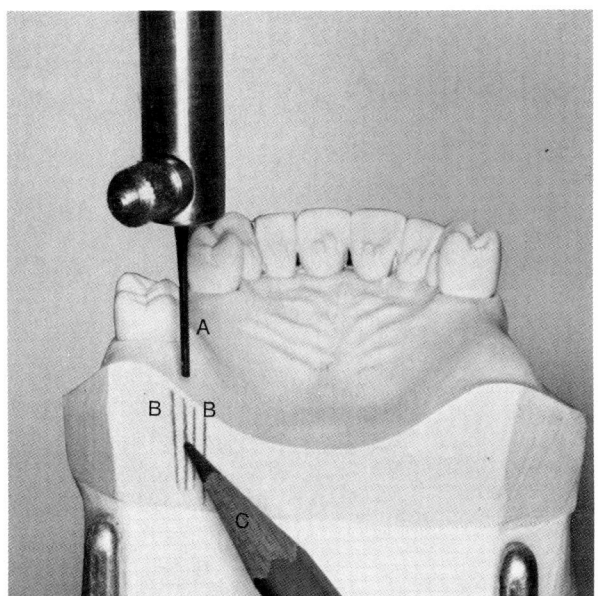

Fig. 16-12. Optimum path of insertion for maximum length in mediolateral dimension. *A,* Analyzing rod. *B,* Lines representing maximum length of each abutment tooth. *C,* Bisector for optimum length (mediolateral).

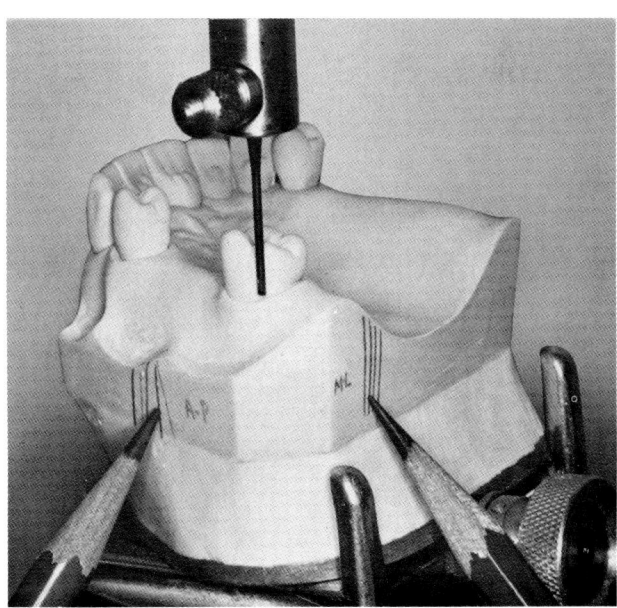

Fig. 16-13. Parallel bisector for minimal undercut (anteroposterior) and maximum length (mediolateral).

## PREOPERATIVE PROCEDURES

The common path of insertion must be transferred to the preparations on the teeth in the mouth. The receptacles that will receive the female precision attachment will also be transferred to the mouth. To accomplish this, some preoperative procedures are required on the diagnostic cast. A line is drawn down the center of the crest of the ridge in each abutment tooth area. The female portion of the attachment is placed on the mandrel, which is locked in the vertical shaft of the surveyor. The female is aligned on the proximal surface of the abutment and over the crest of the ridge (Fig. 16-14). Using a jig,* a handpiece may be assembled to the vertical shaft of the surveyor. This handpiece will carry a No. 558 fissure bur that will be used to cut the recess in the abutment teeth on the diagnostic cast and will be in the common path of insertion and removal of the prosthesis (Fig. 16-15). The female attachment is carried to the proximal surface of the abutment tooth in which it will lay. Lines are scribed on this proximal surface of the tooth to reflect the dimensions buccolingually of the female attachment in its innermost and outermost aspects. A line is also scribed at the gingival extent of the female attachment as it is planned for this particular abutment tooth (Fig. 16-16). By use of the handpiece and the jig assembled to the vertical shaft of the surveyor, a recess is prepared in the abutment tooth of the diagnostic cast so that the female attachment will be confined within the normal contours of the abutment tooth (Figs. 16-17 and 16-18).

These recesses, or slots, that will receive the female attachment in all abutment teeth are then lubricated with a separating medium that accompanies DuraLay autopolymerizing acrylic* (Fig. 16-19). The acrylic is then painted on the occlusal surface and into the recesses prepared on the diagnostic cast (Fig. 16-20). Before the acrylic sets, a short handle such as a contra-angle bur is embedded in the occlusal surface (Fig. 16-21). These become the

*The J.M. Ney Co., Bloomfield, Conn.

*Reliance Dental Manufacturing Co., Chicago, Ill.

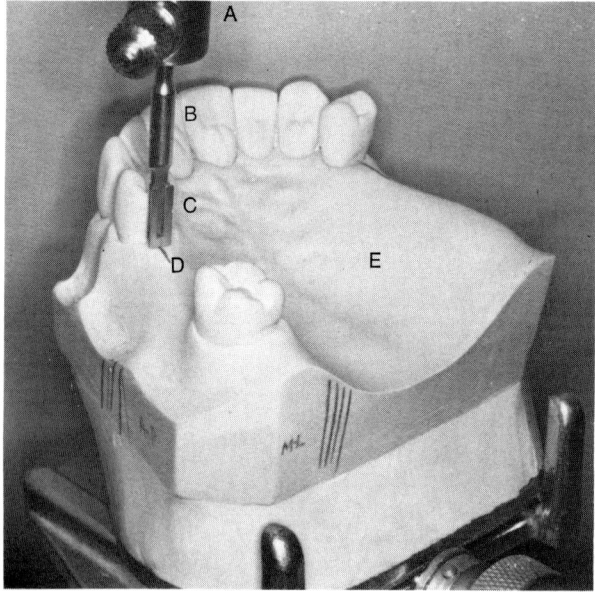

**Fig. 16-14.** Design for recess preparation. *A,* Vertical shaft of surveyor. *B,* Mandrel. *C,* Female attachment. *D,* Crest of ridge. *E,* Analyzed cast.

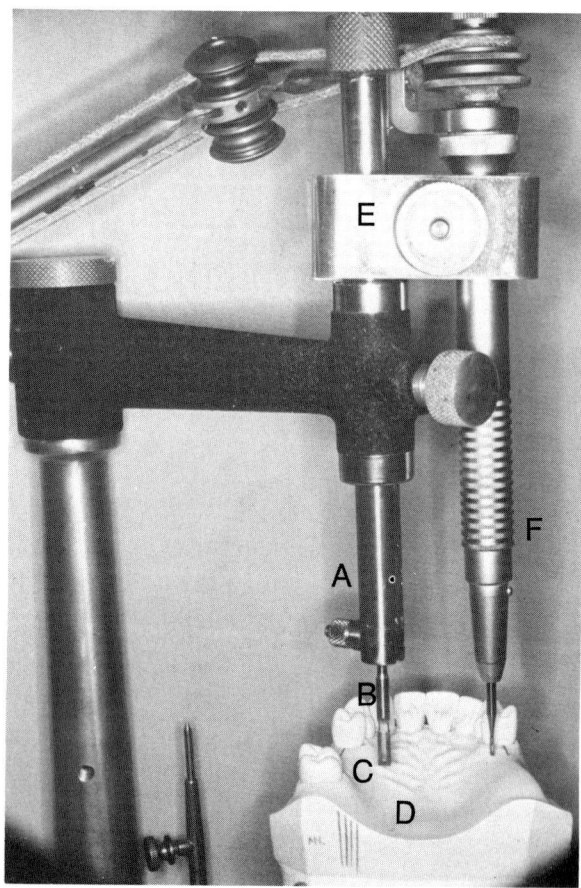

**Fig. 16-15.** Recess preparation setup. *A,* Vertical shaft of surveyor. *B,* Mandrel. *C,* Female attachment. *D,* Analyzed cast. *E,* Jig for holding handpiece. *F,* Handpiece with fissure bur.

*Frictional wall precision attachment partial prosthesis* **455**

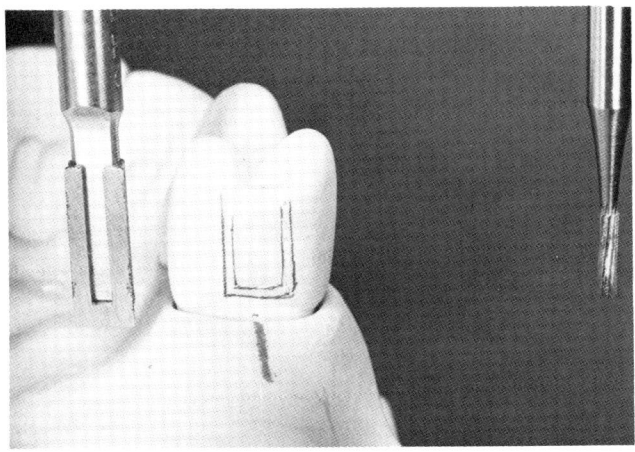

**Fig. 16-16.** Outline for recess preparation.

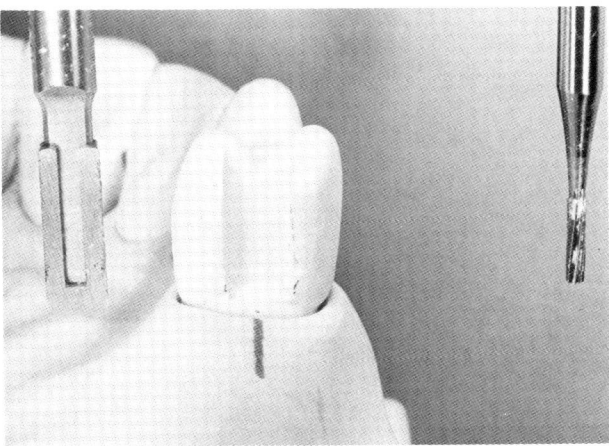

**Fig. 16-17.** Recess preparation completed.

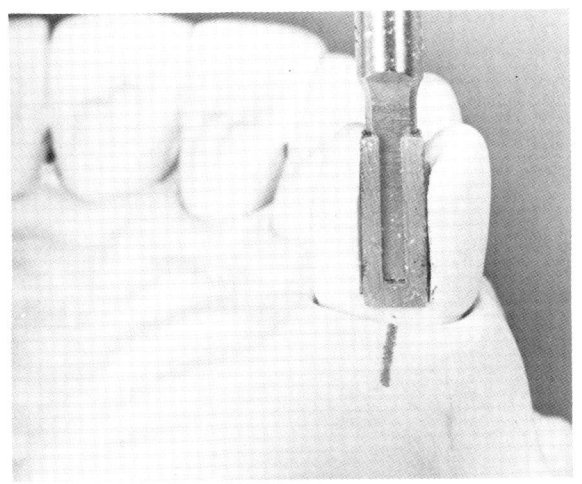

**Fig. 16-18.** Female attachment fits within normal contour of tooth.

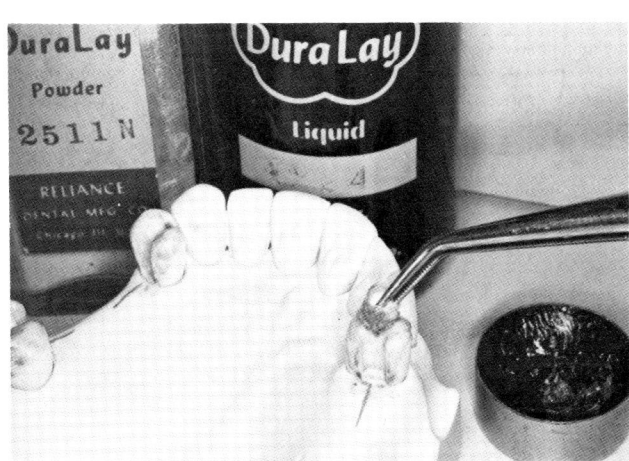

**Fig. 16-19.** DuraLay lubricant painted on occlusal and recess surfaces.

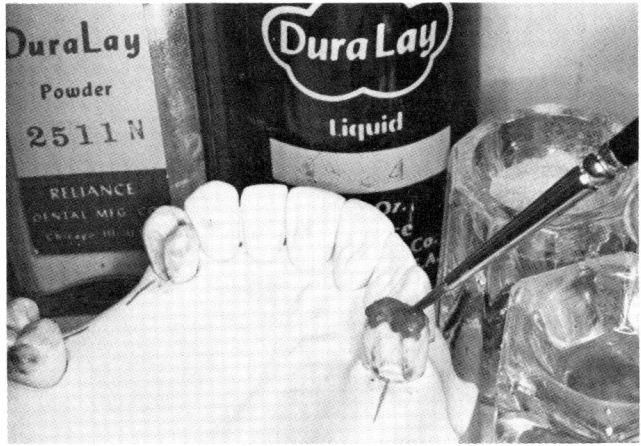

**Fig. 16-20.** DuraLay painted on occlusal surface.

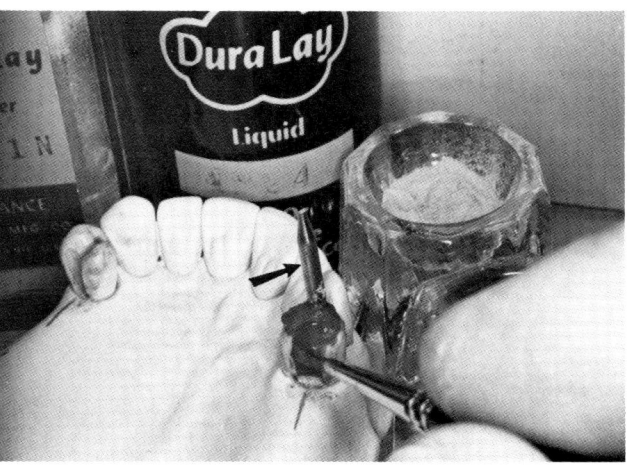

**Fig. 16-21.** Retention handle embedded in occlusal surface of DuraLay (arrow).

recess grinding guides (Fig. 16-22). The excess flash is trimmed from the buccal and lingual aspects of the recess (Fig. 16-23). These recess preparation guides are used in the mouth as aids in determining the exact location and depth of the recesses in the abutment teeth. The dentist marks the internal aspects of acrylic recess preparation guide with a soft lead pencil and completes the recess preparation in the abutment in its entirety before continuing with any other tooth preparation. The preparation that is indicated is completed.

Impressions are made along with face-bow transfer and interocclusal records. Solid casts are mounted in the articulator for fabrication of the wax patterns. The casts should incorporate the use of Artic-U-Locs* to facilitate the placement of the casts on the surveyor and subsequent accurate return to the articulator mounting. Individual or quadrant impressions for the gingival margins or the finishing lines of the preparations are separate (Fig. 16-24).

The articulated casts are now used to create the wax patterns to the occlusion requested in the prescription (Fig. 16-25). Completion of the occlusal four fifths of the wax pattern is followed by a preparation of the recess for the female attachment in the wax pattern itself.

The wax patterns are removed from the master cast. The cast is removed from the articulator and placed in the adjustable surveyor table. A mandrel is locked in the vertical shaft of the surveyor. The cast is moved adjacent to the mandrel and tilted until parallelism is reestablished. The wax patterns are replaced on the cast.

The female attachment held on the mandrel in the vertical shaft of the surveyor is placed adjacent to the wax pattern on the abutment tooth in the center of the crest of the ridge. An outline is scribed for the innermost and outermost dimensions of the female attachment (Fig. 16-26). The bulk of wax is then carved away with a mandrel that has been shaped in the form of a knife or chisel. This is held in the vertical shaft of the surveyor and moved up and down and sideways to carve the bulk of wax away (Fig. 16-27). The female will not fit within the confines of the pattern at this time.

To accurately reproduce the recess in the wax pattern for the female attachment, the attachment is placed on its mandrel, which in turn is placed in the vertical shaft of the surveyor. An alcohol torch is used to gently warm the female attachment (Fig. 16-28). The female attachment is then placed adjacent to the wax pattern and used as a molding instrument. Small increments of wax are removed in this fashion. Each subsequent removal should be very small, and the heat should be kept to a minimum to prevent distortion of the wax pattern (Fig. 16-29). At this time an excess amount of wax will appear along the contact plates or the surface plates of the female attachment. The chisel previously

---

*The J. M. Ney Co., Bloomfield, Conn.

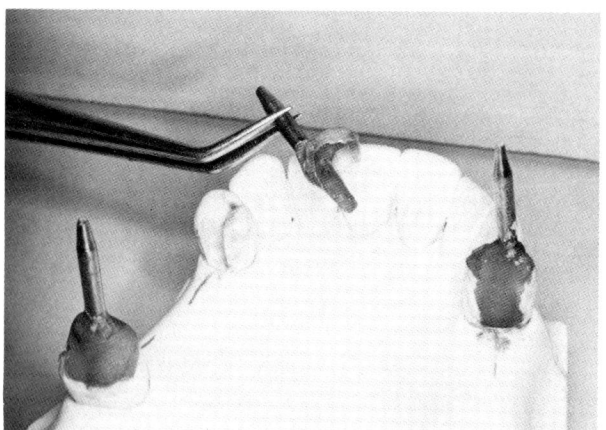

Fig. 16-22. Recess grinding guides made on diagnostic casts.

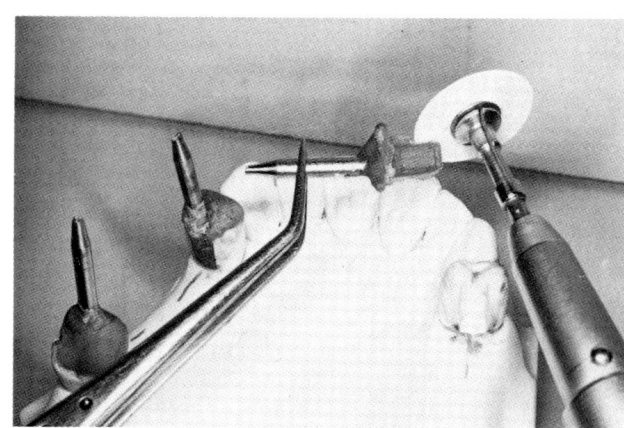

Fig. 16-23. Excess flash removed from recess grinding guide.

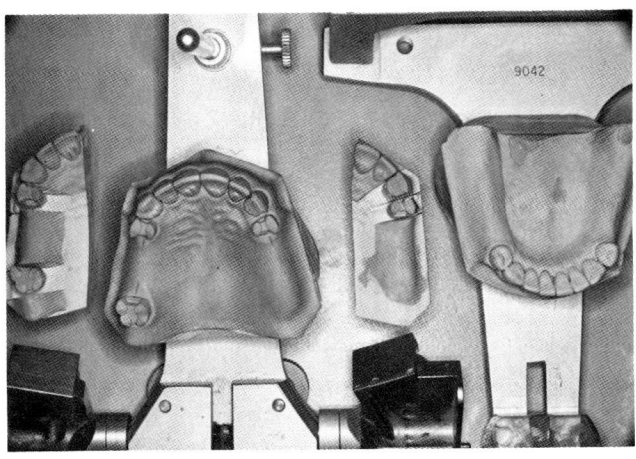

**Fig. 16-24.** Solid master cast mounted in articulator. Quadrant impressions are used for dies.

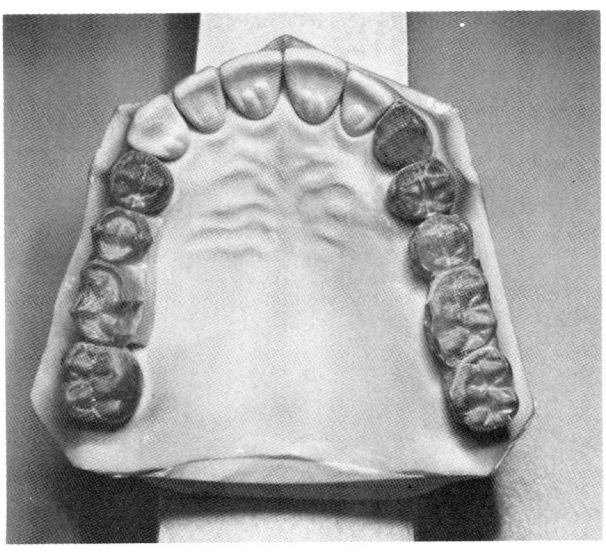

**Fig. 16-25.** Wax patterns created to dentist's prescription.

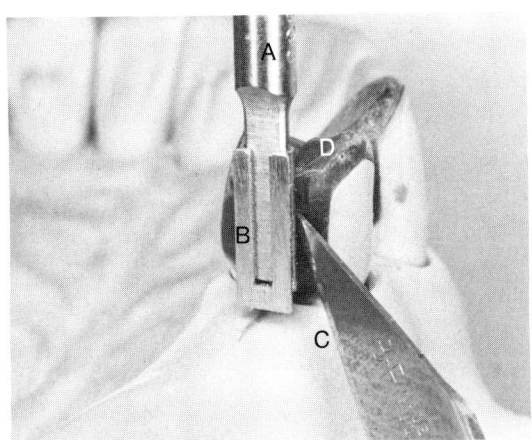

**Fig. 16-26.** Scribing of outline for female attachment on wax pattern. *A,* Mandrel. *B,* Female attachment. *C,* Bard-Parker blade No. 25. *D,* Wax pattern.

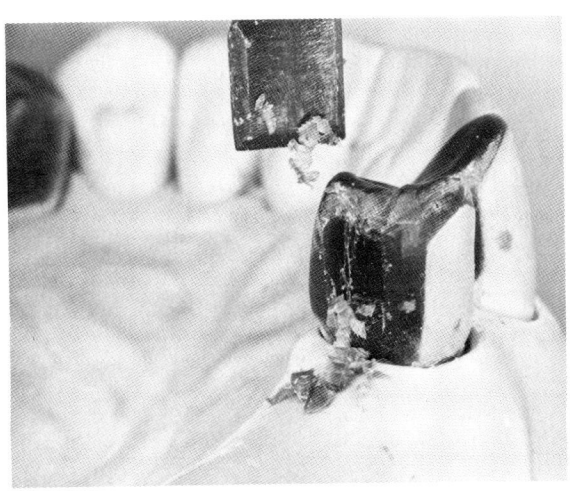

**Fig. 16-27.** Bulk of wax carved away with chisel.

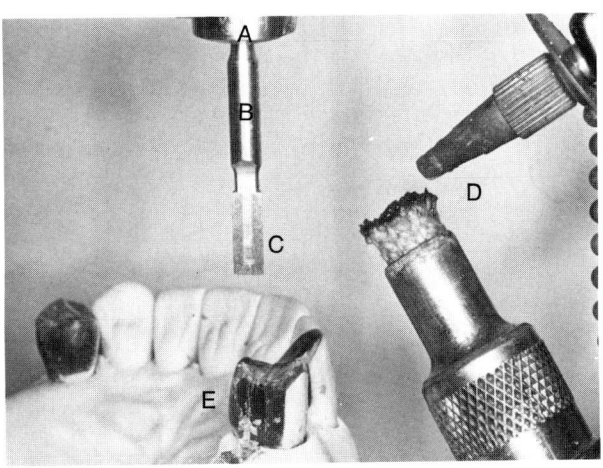

**Fig. 16-28.** Female attachment used as molding instrument. *A,* Vertical shaft of surveyor. *B,* Mandrel. *C,* Female attachment. *D,* Alcohol torch. *E,* Wax pattern.

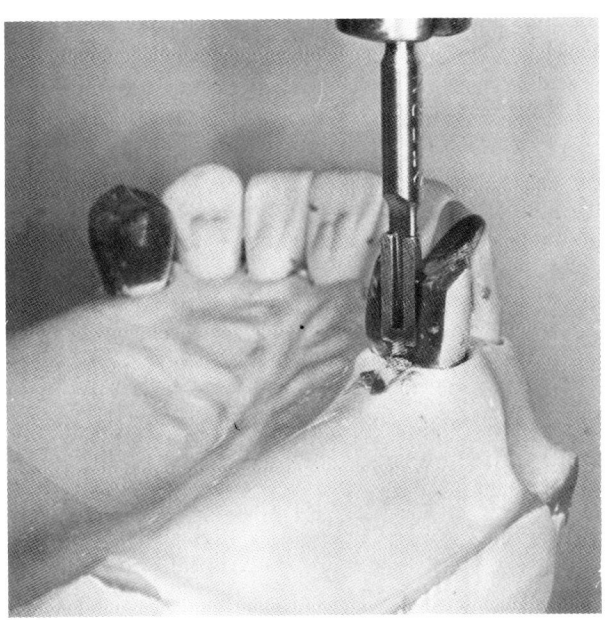

**Fig. 16-29.** Small increments of wax removed at a time.

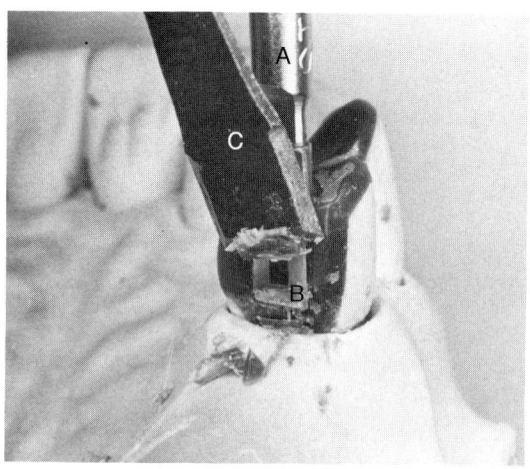

**Fig. 16-30.** Excess wax on contact plate of female attachment removed parallel to contact plate. *A,* Mandrel. *B,* Precision attachment. *C,* Wax chisel.

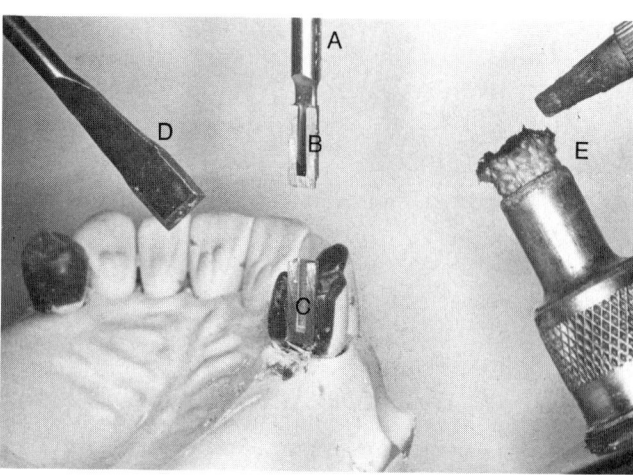

**Fig. 16-31.** Female attachment in wax pattern. *A,* Vertical shaft of surveyor holds mandrel. *B,* Female attachment. *C,* Female attachment seated in wax pattern. *D,* Wax carving chisel. *E,* Alcohol torch.

used for carving out the bulk of wax is used to shave the wax from the contact plate (Fig. 16-30). (A spare female attachment can be silver-plated to an oversize thickness of approximately 0.003 inches. This will make it easier to fit the female attachment within the casting at a later time.)* Fig. 16-31 shows the two methods of placing the female attachments within the wax patterns.

The wax patterns are then removed from the solid cast and transferred to the individual dies. The margins of the wax patterns are then completed, and the patterns are sprued, invested, cast (without the female attachments), and fitted to the dies as accurately as possible.

It is possible to cast gold to a female attachment and get an unbreakable union. However, no more than one female should be cast in a retainer, since parallelism will be lost when the castings are accurately fitted to the teeth.

A rigid impression tray that will cover the tissue-bearing areas is made (Fig. 16-32). This tray may be made of cast aluminum (the first choice) or a heavy vinyl or thick acrylic. It should not impinge on any of the castings themselves. A spare diagnostic cast may be used to fabricate this impression tray. The castings are ready to be returned to the mouth for the final fitting of the castings on the teeth at this time.

*Van Kirk, R. W.: Personal communication, 1976.

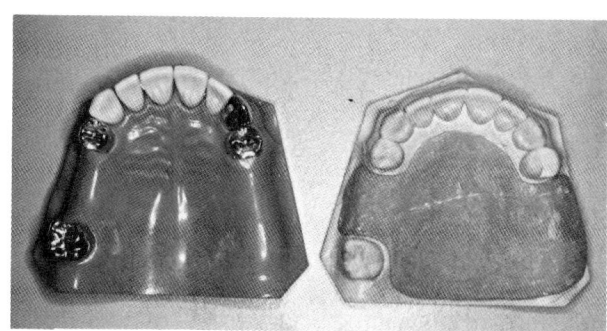

**Fig. 16-32.** Rigid tray for tissue coverage area of cast aluminum, vinyl, or acrylic.

## TRANSFER PROCEDURE

The dentist may select a transfer procedure that uses a combination of mucostatics and plaster. The tray made in the laboratory is fitted to the mouth and all impingements removed. A mucostatic impression of the tissue surface in the mouth (Fig. 16-33) is made using an accurate zinc oxide–eugenol cement.* An overall plaster impression† is

*Impression cement, Ackerman Dental Manufacturing, Chandler, Ariz.
†Snow White Impression Plaster No. 2, Kerr Manufacturing Co., Romulus, Mich.

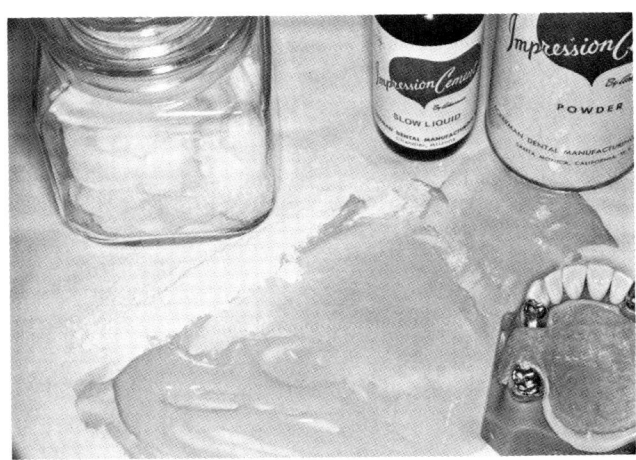

Fig. 16-33. Mucostatic impression of tissue-bearing areas.

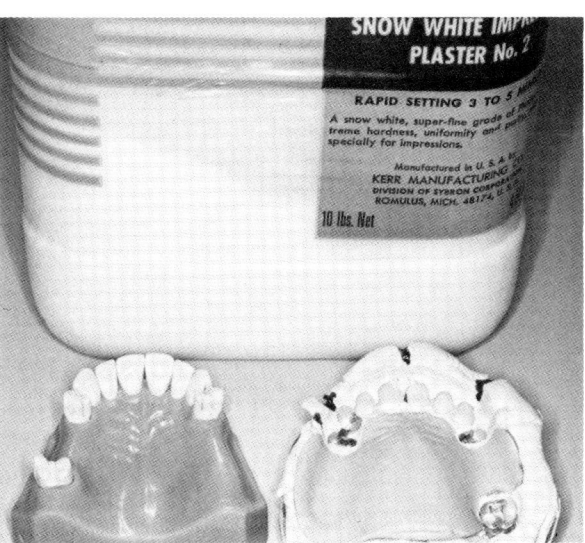

Fig. 16-34. Overall plaster impression.

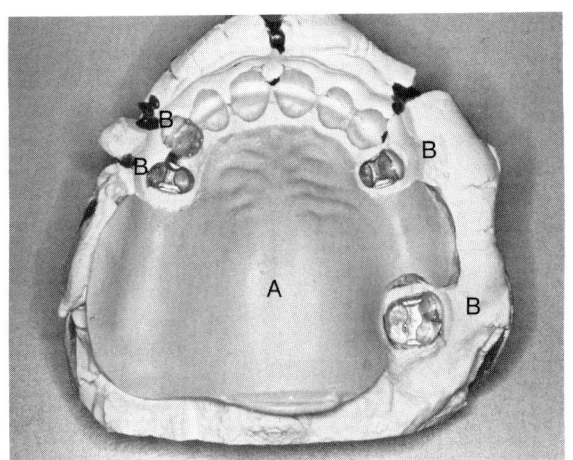

Fig. 16-35. Transfer impression as received in laboratory. *A*, Mucostatic impression of tissue-coverage area. *B*, Retainer castings.

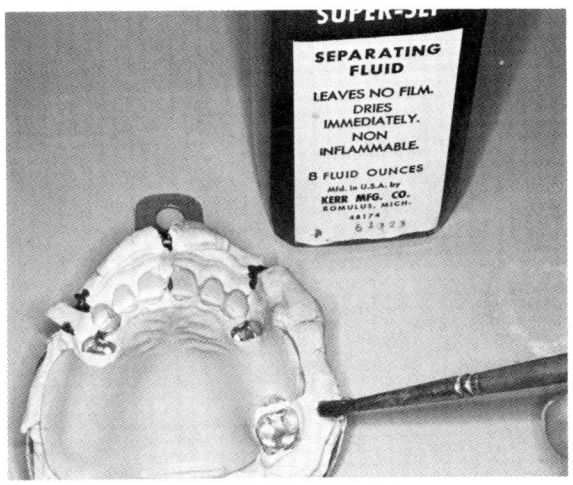

Fig. 16-36. Super-Sep painted on exposed plaster.

then made that will include not only the mucostatic tissue impression but also the remaining teeth including the abutment teeth (Fig. 16-34). The castings may or may not come out in the plaster impression. This transfer impression is returned to the laboratory for fabrication of a transfer cast (Fig. 16-35).

The exposed portions of plaster are treated with a plaster separating solution such as Super-Sep* (Fig. 16-36). The castings are then protected by a separating medium such as (1) Steel's antiflux† mixed with lighter fluid; (2) Ney's antiflux,‡ or an art store yellow ocher mixed with turpentine; and

---

*Kerr Manufacturing Co., Romulus, Mich.
†Columbus Dental, Columbus, Ohio.
‡The J. M. Ney Co., Bloomfield, Conn.

(3) Kiwi* white liquid shoe polish, some of which has been allowed to remain open and become thickened (Fig. 16-37). The difference between using a thick or thin separating medium will depend on the type and size of the casting to be protected. The thin material should be used for short, onlay-type restorations. The thicker material should be used for long, full-coverage restorations. One reason for using the separating medium is to protect the castings from contamination by low-fusing metal that will be poured into the castings at a later time. The other reason is to allow the castings to be removed and replaced accurately back on the cast, after the cast has been fabricated.

Hydrocolloid is injected directly over the margins of the casting to protect the margins against damage when removing the castings from the low-fusing metal and to prevent their contamination by the low-fusing metal (Fig. 16-38). This hydrocolloid will stand up nicely right on the edge of the margins of the castings. The areas to be poured in low-fusing metal are then dammed off with damp cotton (Fig. 16-39). Low-fusing metal† is then poured into the castings themselves (Fig. 16-40). The melting point of the metal should be about 160° F (71° C). Baker's B metal works well for this procedure. The low-fusing metal supporting the castings must be retained in the stone to be poured at a later time. Sufficient retention can be obtained by heating machine screws of a 2-56 size, ⅜ inch (0.9 cm) long and embedding them in the low-fusing metal (Fig. 16-41). Washers have been used, and wood screws also are suitable. Paper clips are not strong enough to resist the subsequent forces used on this cast. The cotton dam that prevented the excessive flow of the low-fusing metal is removed (Fig. 16-42). The entire impression is boxed with Mortite,* a weather-stripping compound that is commercially available in any hardware store (Fig. 16-43). The armamentarium needed for fabricating a transfer cast includes Ney antiflux, shoe polish, Steele's antiflux, a brush, Super-Sep, cotton, Mortite, Baker's B metal, and retention screws (Fig. 16-44).

*Mortite-Mortell Co., Kankakee, Ill.

*Kiwi Polish Co., Pottstown, Penn.
†Baker Dental Division, Engelhard Industries, Carteret, N.J.

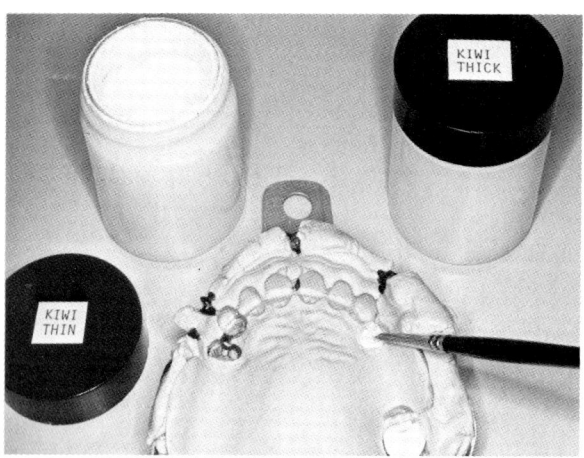

Fig. 16-37. Separating and protecting medium painted in retainer castings.

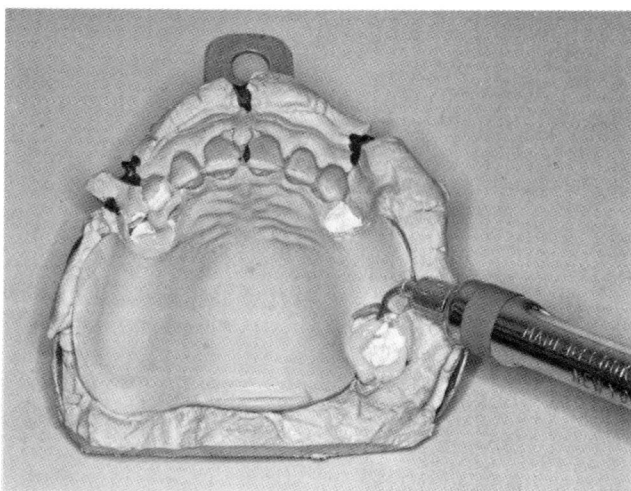

Fig. 16-38. Hydrocolloid injected on margins of abutment castings.

# Frictional wall precision attachment partial prosthesis

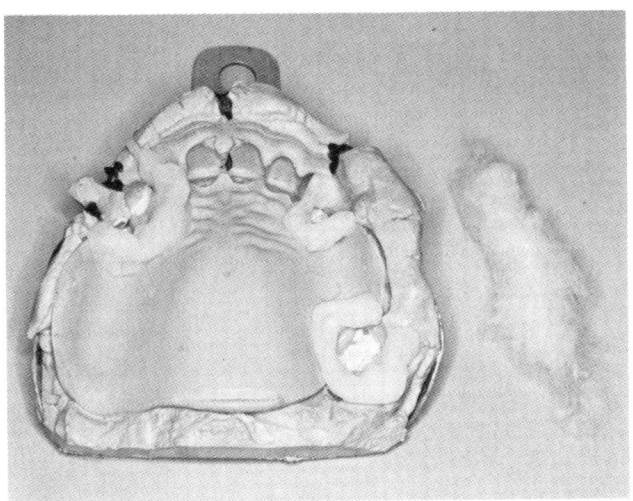

Fig. 16-39. Area around abutment castings dammed off with damp cotton.

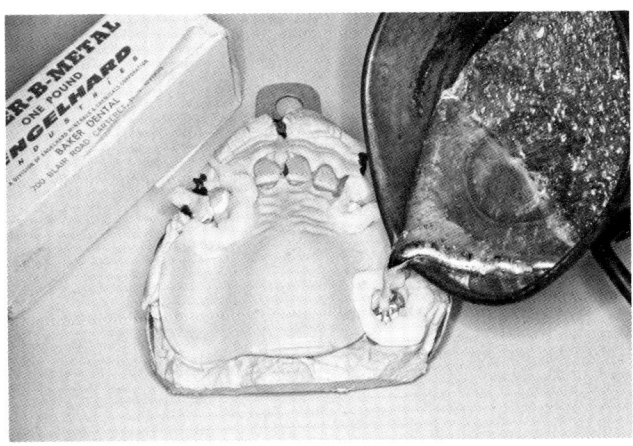

Fig. 16-40. Low-fusing metal poured in abutment castings.

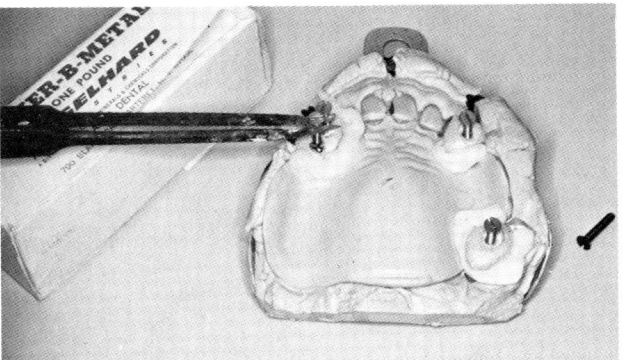

Fig. 16-41. Retention screws heated and embedded in low-fusing metal.

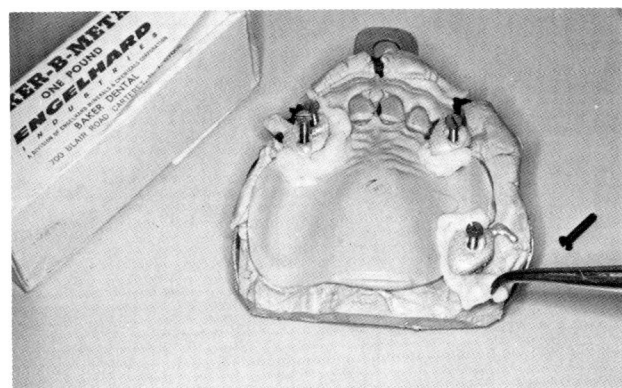

Fig. 16-42. Cotton dam removed.

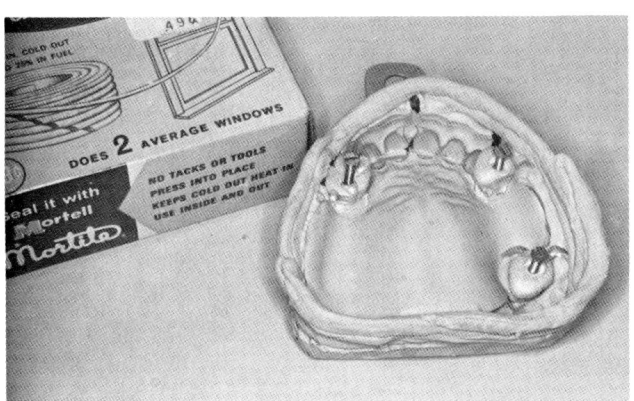

Fig. 16-43. Impression boxed with Mortite.

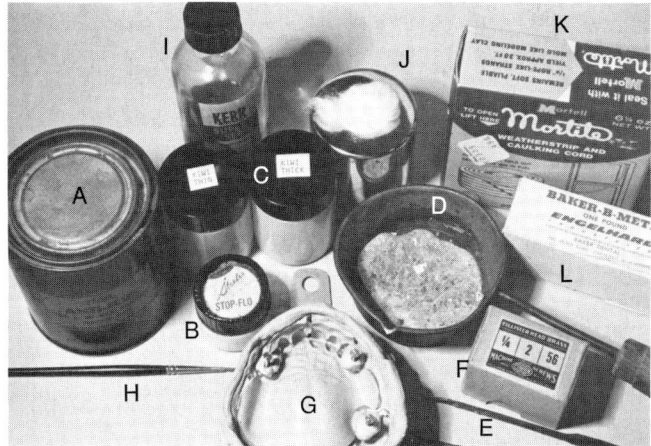

Fig. 16-44. Armamentarium for making transfer cast. *A,* Ney's antiflux. *B,* Steele's antiflux. *C,* Kiwi shoe polish (thick and thin). *D,* Ladle for metal. *E,* Cotton pliers. *F,* Retention screws. *G,* Transfer impression. *H,* No. zero sable brush. *I,* Super-Sep. *J,* Cotton. *K,* Mortite. *L,* Low-fusing metal.

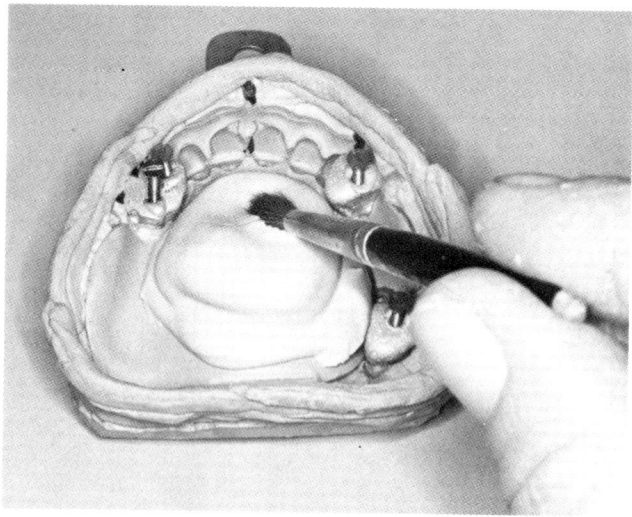

Fig. 16-45. Die stone painted in impression. Do not vibrate.

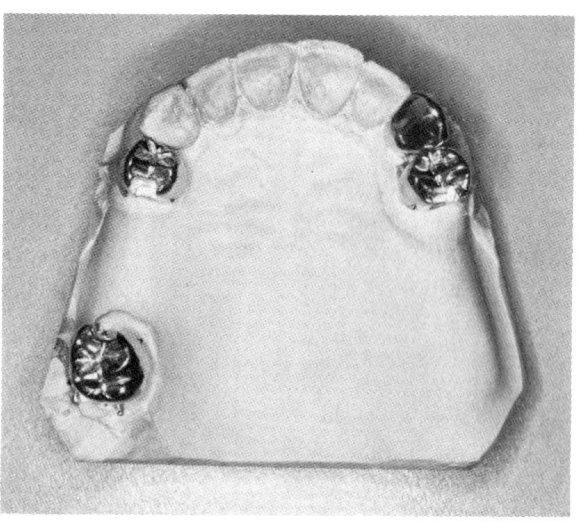

Fig. 16-46. Transfer cast.

The impression is now ready to be poured in a good grade of die stone (Fig. 16-45). This impression should not be vibrated. Vibration may cause some of the low-fusing metal dies and castings to come out of the impression, creating an inaccuracy. The die stone should be carefully painted into the impression. The resulting cast will show good detail in the tissue coverage area, but the residual unprepared teeth will probably not show as good a detail (Fig. 16-46). This detail depends on the accuracy and the ability of the dentist to make a plaster impression.

## ALTERNATE PROCEDURE

This alternate procedure can be used to make a transfer cast that will give more accurate detail of the remaining unprepared teeth. Prior to the time of fitting the castings directly in the mouth, the individual cast restorations are covered with a thickness of 0.003 inch of tinfoil (Fig. 16-47). This tinfoil is not burnished tightly to the gold restorations. Autopolymerizing acrylic is placed over the tinfoil and down on the buccal and lingual surfaces for 1 to 1.5 mm. Coat hanger wire is used to join opposite sides of the mouth. The transfer tray fits the castings quite loosely in the laboratory, as well as in the mouth, and therefore will not influence the spatial relation of the teeth. This transfer tray is used by the dentist to take an accurate index of the castings after they have been fitted on the teeth. The impression or index of these castings is made with a hard zinc oxide–eugenol cement* (Fig. 16-48). Next, the dentist will take an overall alginate impression that will reproduce the tissue areas and capture in great detail the transfer tray containing the castings, as well as the unprepared teeth. When the impression is received in the laboratory, the technician should be prepared to move quickly to make the transfer cast.

First, excess alginate, particularly in interproximal areas, is removed with iris scissors (Fig. 16-49) to allow the castings to be positively seated in the transfer tray index. At this point the procedure is the same as for the plaster-mucostatic impression, except that there is a time limitation of 12 minutes before the alginate begins to distort.† The castings are painted with a separating medium (Fig. 16-50). The margins are protected by injecting hydrocolloid over them (Fig. 16-51). The areas to be poured with low-fusing metal are blocked off with damp cotton. Low-fusing metal is poured into the castings. Retention screws are heated and embedded into the low-fusing metal (Fig. 16-52). The resulting transfer cast looks much neater, particularly in the areas of unprepared teeth. The accuracy of this procedure,

---

*Ackerman Dental Manufacturing Co., Chandler, Ariz.
†Rudd, K. D.: Personal communication, 1966.

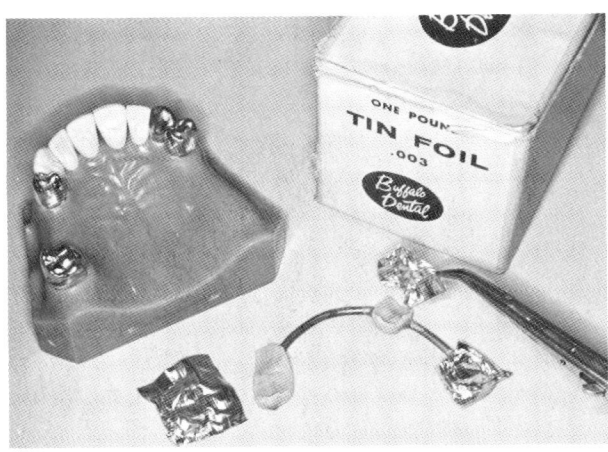

Fig. 16-47. Transfer tray for alternate transfer cast procedure.

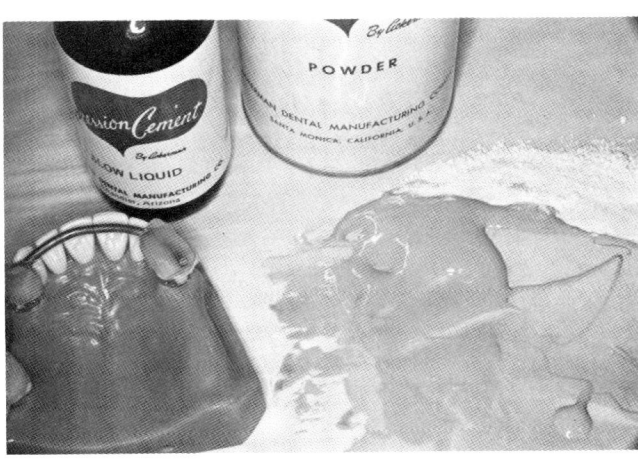

Fig. 16-48. Impression or index of castings in transfer tray.

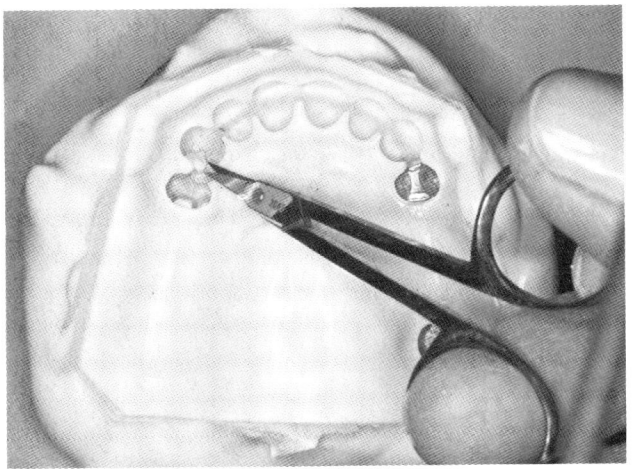

Fig. 16-49. Alginate removed interproximally with iris scissors.

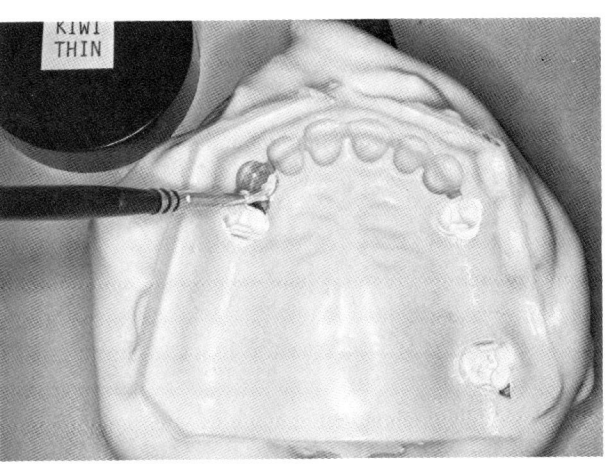

Fig. 16-50. Castings painted with separating medium.

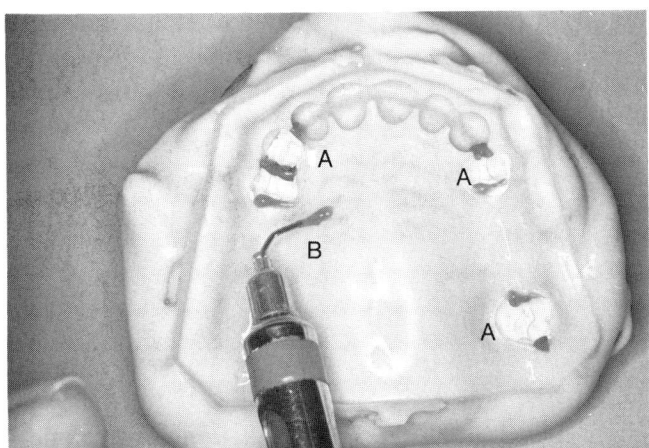

Fig. 16-51. *A*, Margins protected by ejected hydrocolloid. *B*, Demonstration of hydrocolloid ejection.

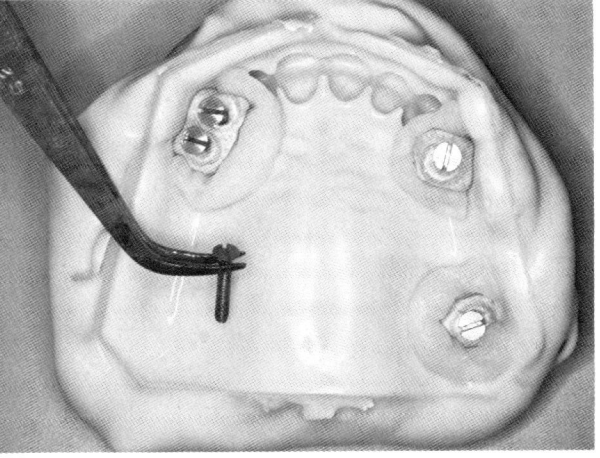

Fig. 16-52. Heated retention screws embedded in low-fusing metal.

as far as retainer castings are concerned, is equal to the plaster type of impression (Fig. 16-53). The detail of the unprepared teeth is superior to that made with a mucostatic impression; however, the tissue-bearing areas may not be quite as accurate.

The transfer cast is now mounted in the articulator by use of the face-bow transfer and the interocclusal records supplied by the dentist. The occlusion is refined to the tolerance and to the concept desired by the dentist.

At this time, the transfer cast is removed from the articulator and remounted in the surveyor table for refinement of the castings to receive the female attachment (Fig. 16-54). An analyzing rod is placed in the vertical shaft of the surveyor and brought into contact with the recesses (Fig. 16-55, A). The cast is tipped until the maximum amount of parallelism can be obtained between all the retainer castings (Fig. 16-55, B and C).

A small amount of machining may be necessary to encompass the female attachment without any impingement. Using a jig attached to the vertical shaft of the surveyor, a straight handpiece is mounted. The vertical shaft of the surveyor will carry the analyzing rod (Fig. 16-56). Alternately move the analyzing rod up to the recess in the retainer casting and refine it with the fissure bur. Replace the analyzing rod with the mandrel holding the female attachment and repeat the process. To facilitate the milling process, coat the recess with machinist's pattern ink (Dykem).* Shiny spots will appear where the binding occurs and can be milled accurately. The milling continues until the female attach-

---

*Dykem Co., St. Louis, Mo.

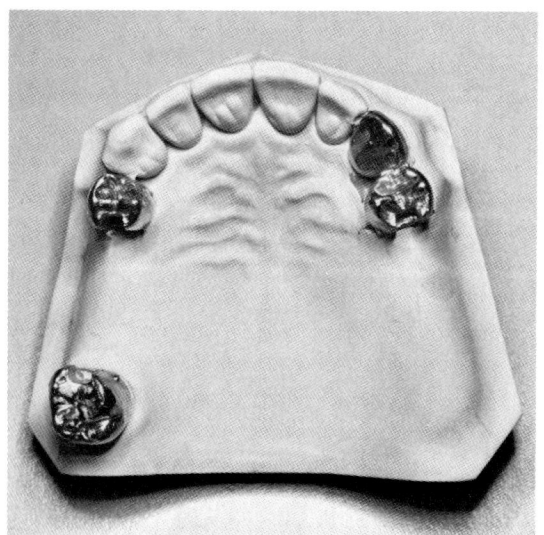

**Fig. 16-53.** Transfer cast made by alternate method.

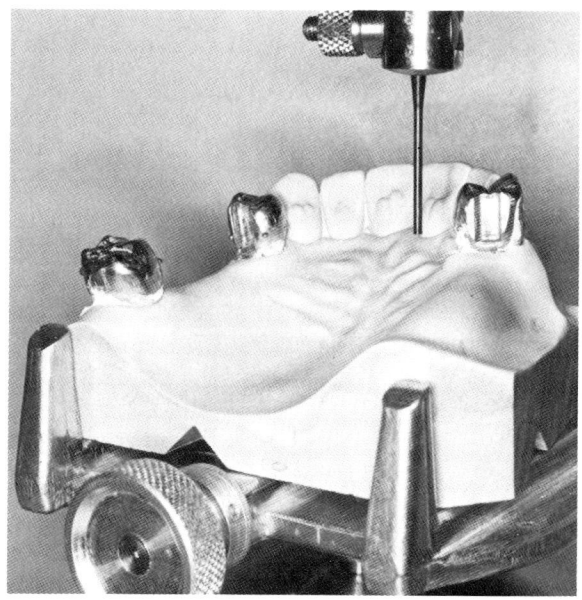

**Fig. 16-54.** Transfer cast mounted in surveyor table for realignment.

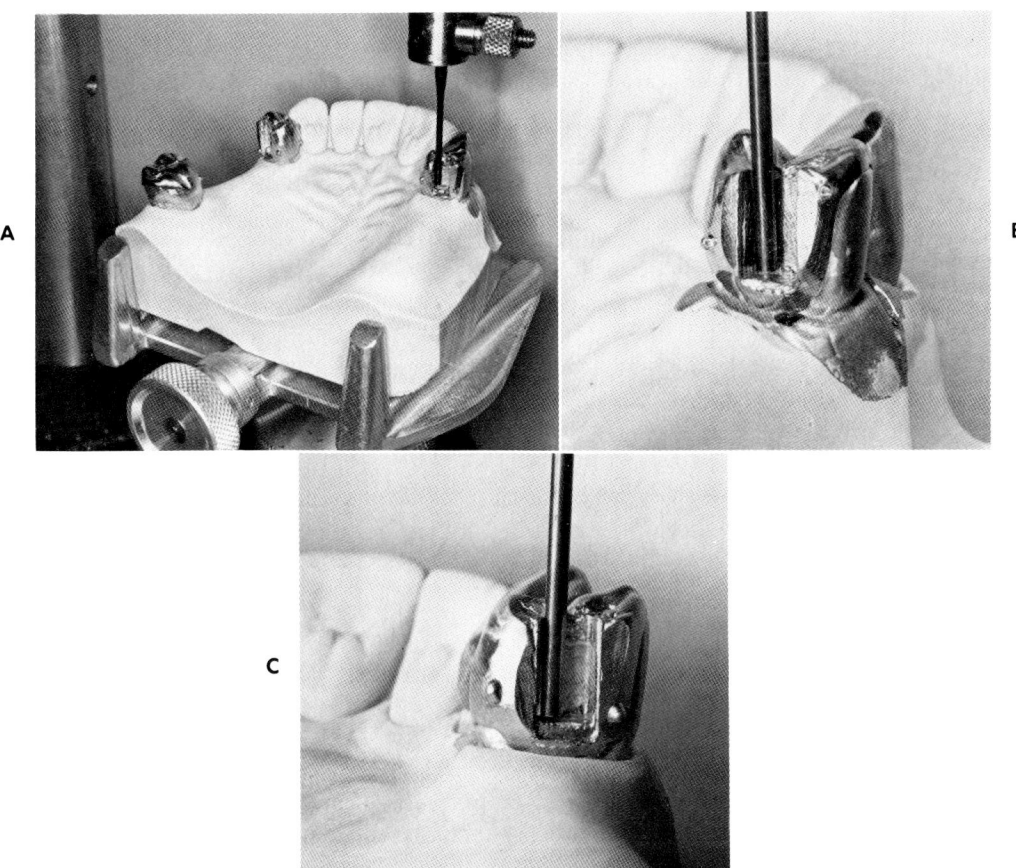

**Fig. 16-55. A,** Analyzing rod used to approximate parallelism between retainer castings. **B,** Lack of parallelism. **C,** Parallelism reestablished.

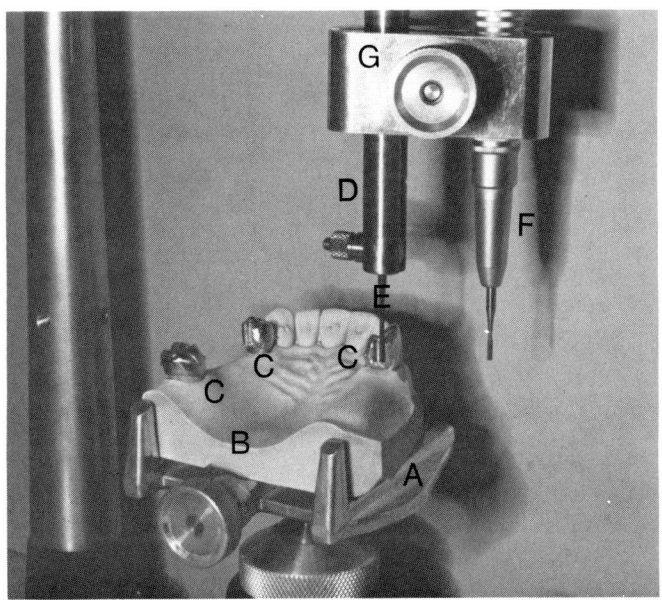

**Fig. 16-56.** Setup for milling recesses. *A,* Survey table. *B,* Transfer cast. *C,* Abutment castings. *D,* Vertical shaft of surveyor. *E,* Analyzing rod. *F,* Straight handpiece with plain fissure bur. *G,* Jig.

ment is completely retained within the normal contours of the abutment casting (Figs. 16-57 and 16-58). Notice that there is a minimum amount of space around the female attachment. This will result in the most accurate and the strongest solder joint. With proper attention to the soldering procedure, solder will be sucked around the female attachment by way of capillary attraction. The minimal space will allow a minimal amount of solder, which in turn, on congealing, will create the least amount of shrinkage and will reduce the amount of distortion. The female attachment on the mandrel is located in the recess in the casting with no binding in any way on the retainer casting. *This is a very delicate operation, requiring an ultimate sense of touch.* The long, vertical shaft of the surveyor held against a cast on a surveyor table may be flexed and thereby creates nonparallelism between female attachments.

Sticky wax is placed around the entire periphery of the female attachment (Fig. 16-59). The sticky wax serves two purposes: to prevent investment from getting into the area where solder is desired and to retain the female attachment in position until it is invested in correct relationship to the retainer castings. The mandrel is now removed from the female attachment. A carbon rod supplied with the precision attachment is checked for fit within the female attachment (Fig. 16-60). This carbon rod should fit quite loosely. A thin mix of cristobalite investment is then painted in the female attachment and the wetted carbon rod inserted into the female attachment (Fig. 16-61). This is allowed to set completely. The castings with the sticky-waxed female attachment and the embedded carbon rod are then immersed in a thick mix of soldering investment of the technician's choice (Fig. 16-62). Prior to the complete set of the soldering investment, trimming is initiated. The resulting refractory cast will

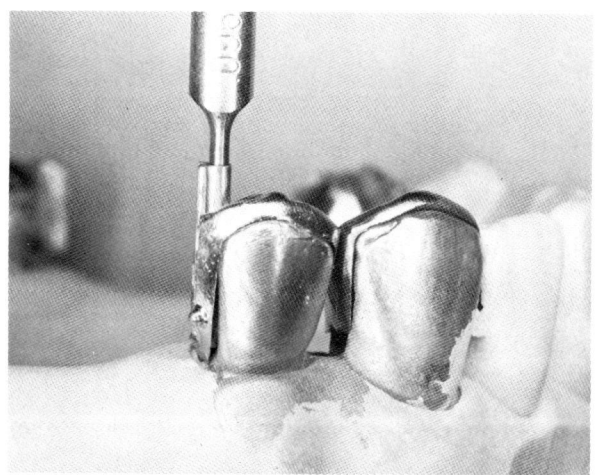

**Fig. 16-57.** Facial view of female attachment in abutment casting.

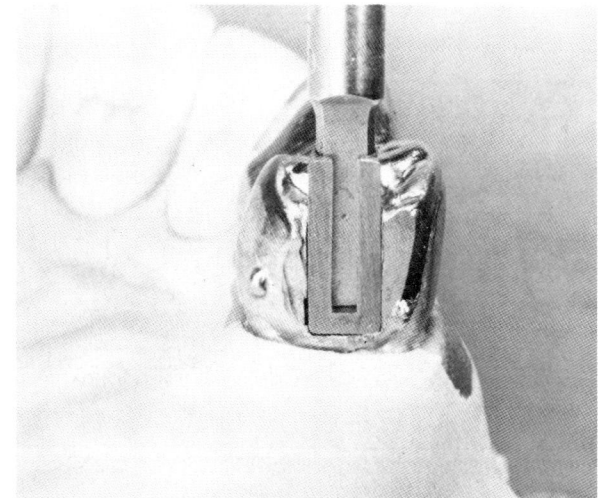

**Fig. 16-58.** Proximal view of female attachment in abutment casting. NOTE: Minimal space is present between female attachment and casting.

### Frictional wall precision attachment partial prosthesis 467

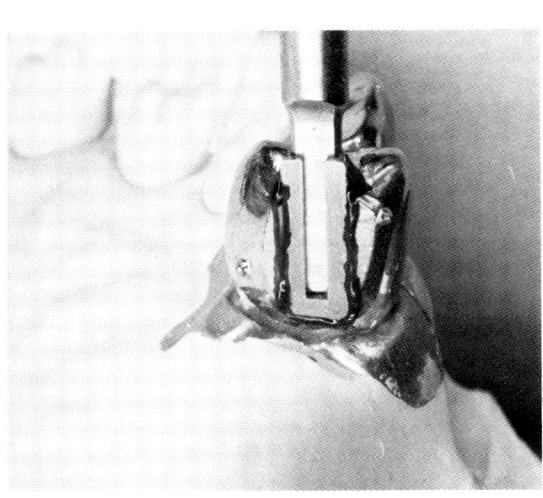

**Fig. 16-59.** Female on mandrel in vertical shaft of surveyor is sticky waxed to abutment castings.

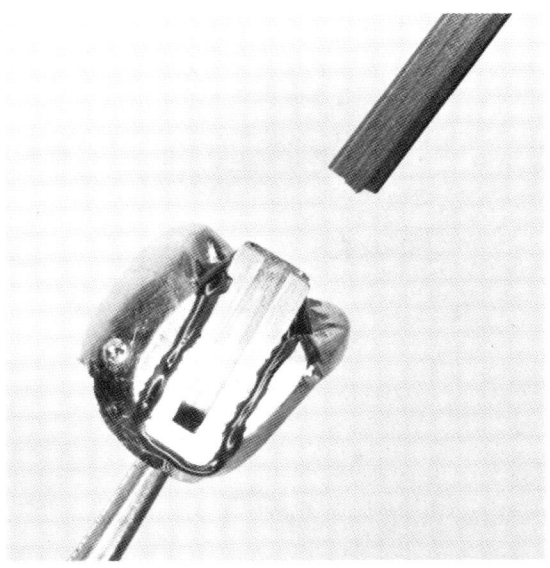

**Fig. 16-60.** Carbon rod (supplied by manufacturer) is checked for loose fit.

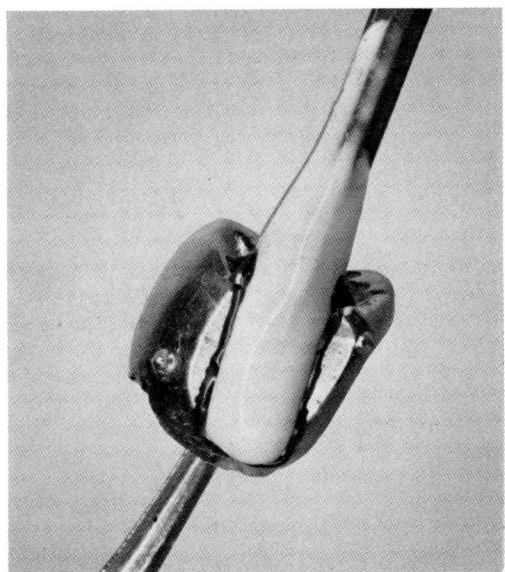

**Fig. 16-61.** Carbon rod held in female attachment with thin mix of cristobalite inlay investment.

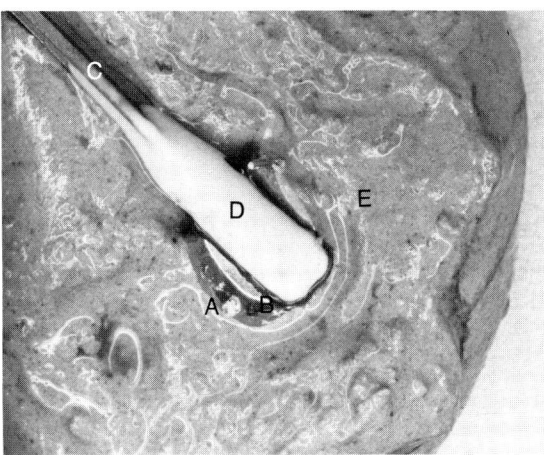

**Fig. 16-62.** Retainer castings with sticky waxed female attachment containing invested carbon rod embedded in soldering investment. *A,* Retainer casting. *B,* Sticky wax. *C,* Carbon rod. *D,* Cristobalite. *E,* Soldering investment.

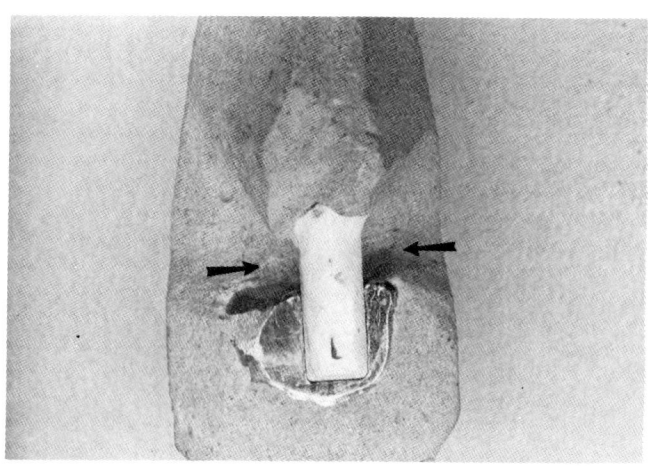

Fig. 16-63. Refractory investment prepared for soldering. Note open sluiceways (arrows).

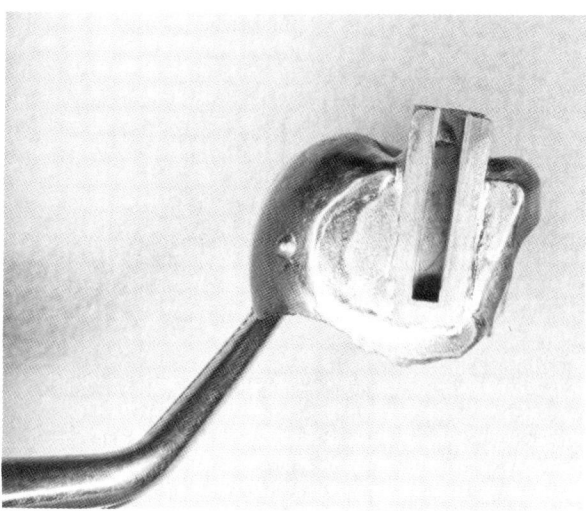

Fig. 16-64. Female soldered to abutment casting.

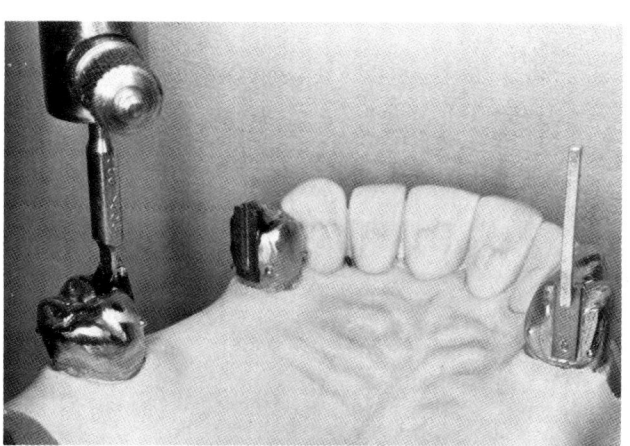

Fig. 16-65. Parallel and sticky wax female attachments to remaining abutments.

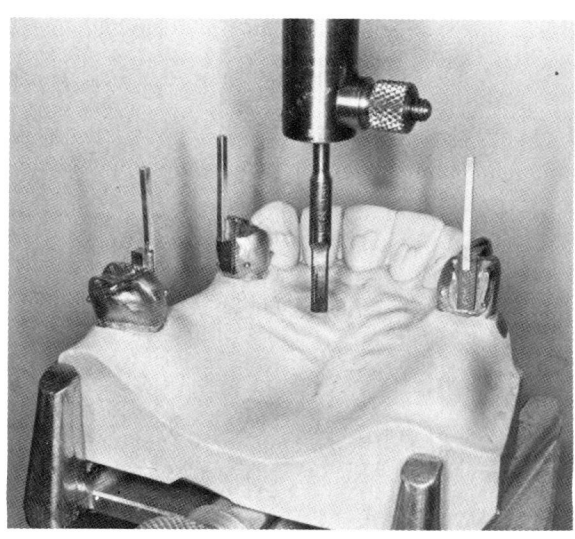

Fig. 16-66. All female attachments soldered to abutments. Male portion of attachments in place.

resemble Fig. 16-63. Notice that the sluiceways have been created to give aerodynamic access for heat from the soldering torch. The wax has been boiled out and a soldering flux added. Solder may be added at this time, or it may be added at the time the heated casting is ready to receive the solder. Using the generally accepted principles of soldering operation: (1) the parts should be clean, (2) the parts should be hot, (3) the parts should be close together, (4) gravity should be used wherever possible, and (5) the area should be accessible. The resulting soldering operation is illustrated in Fig. 16-64. For the novice it is wise to solder one retainer female attachment at a time.

The male attachment should be tested in the female. The fit should be with the same degree of smoothness as it was prior to the soldering operation. Occasionally, a tightness will be encountered. Fine powdered graphite as a dry metal lubricant will usually be sufficient. With excessive tightness it may be necessary to disassemble and repeat the soldering procedure.

Check the soldering procedure for parallelism, and align the remaining female attachments with sticky wax at this time (Fig. 16-65). All of the male attachments (Fig. 16-66) must be verified for fit after soldering.

## VERIFYING PARALLELISM

There are several methods of verifying parallelism of the female attachments. One is to sight the mandrel in the female to a nearby tall building if available or to the vertical shaft of the surveyor (Fig. 16-67). A second method is to sight across mandrels in each attachment in turn to see if superimposition exists, indicating parallelism (Fig. 16-68). Each pair of attachments must be checked in turn for all combinations. These methods are the most accurate. A third method to check the parallelism of the female attachments is to insert mandrels into each one of the female attachments and, using a jig, attach them to the vertical shaft of the surveyor (Fig. 16-69). The vertical shaft of the surveyor can be removed so that each one of the mandrels will come out without breaking the sticky wax if all female attachments are parallel (Fig. 16-70). This method is not as reliable as the sight method.

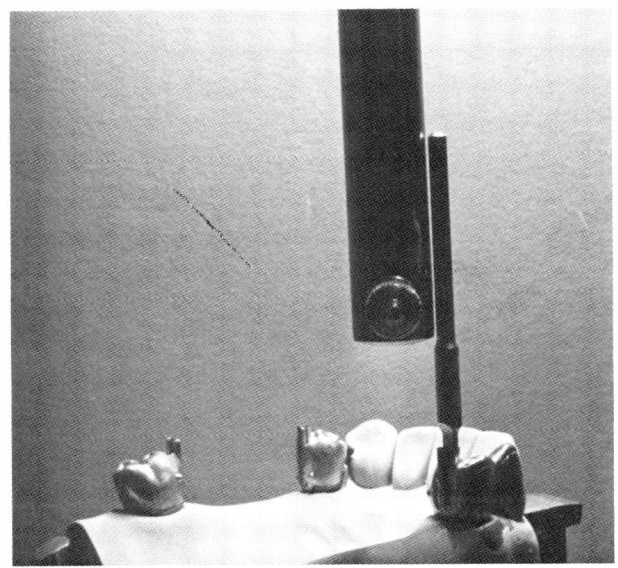

**Fig. 16-67.** Mandrel in female attachment sighted against vertical shaft of surveyor.

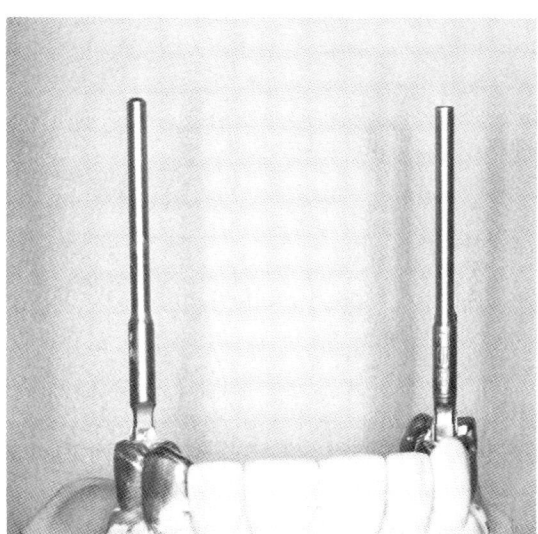

**Fig. 16-68.** Superimposition of mandrels in female attachments in right premolar and molar prove parallelism.

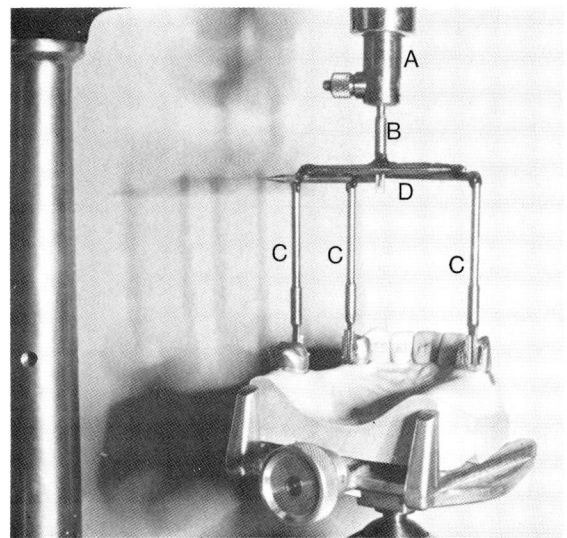

**Fig. 16-69.** Jig used in alternate method of proving parallelism. *A,* Vertical shaft of surveyor. *B,* Mandrel. *C,* Mandrels in female attachments. *D,* Metal rods sticky waxed to mandrels in female attachments and mandrel in vertical shaft of surveyor.

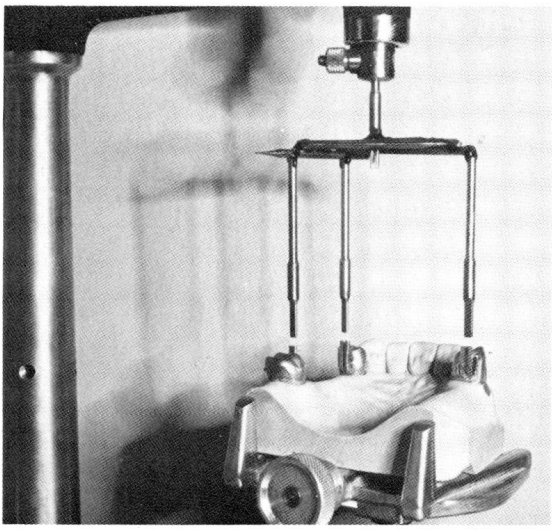

**Fig. 16-70.** Vertical shaft of surveyor is raised, lifting mandrels from female attachments without breaking sticky wax.

The retainer castings are then polished with the male attachment in place to prevent any destruction of the proximal contact plate of the female attachment (Fig. 16-71).

Rods of silver or nickel-silver come soldered to the proximal surface of the male attachment and can be removed by softening the solder in a flame (Fig. 16-72). These rods should be retained because they will be used at a subsequent time in assembling the male attachments to the partial denture framework.

The master cast is blocked out to eliminate all undercuts. Wax is added to give greater bulk over the occlusal surfaces behind or in front of the male attachment to give additional rigidity in the refractory cast material (Fig. 16-73). Great care must be taken to eliminate all possible undercuts. This will prevent the possibility of tearing the duplicating colloid. The blockout along the side of the male attachment toward the lingual surface and down the proximal surface or the surface plate of the male attachment should be parallel with the surfaces of the male attachment. At the gingival extent of the male attachment, the wax should be carried all the way to the ridge parallel with the male attachment. A line is lightly scribed in the wax to indicate the gingival extent of the male attachment (Fig. 16-74). The blocked out master cast on the duplicating flask base is partially immersed in slurry water so that only a portion of the master cast is under water. Duplication should not proceed until the cast has become saturated with the slurry water (Fig. 16-75). This eliminates air bubbles from coming to the surface while the duplicating colloid is congealing. Slurry water prevents dissolution of the master cast itself.

The duplicating colloid is best made from reversible hydrocolloid that is used in the operatory and ground up into fine particles with a food chopper.

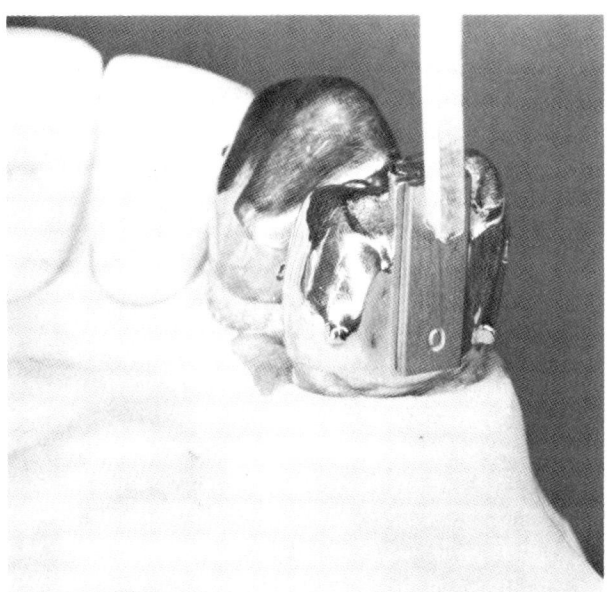

Fig. 16-71. Retainer castings polished with male attachments in place.

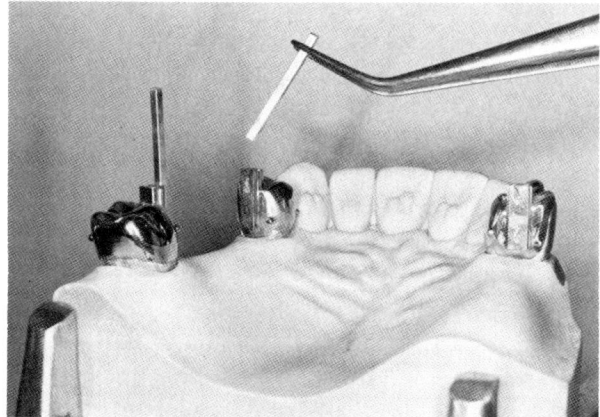

Fig. 16-72. Silver rods removed from male portion of attachments.

Duplicating colloid, as purchased, is not as accurate as the impression material used in the operatory. The duplicating colloid should be liquefied and the temperature reduced slowly to 138° F (53.5° C). The reduction in temperature can be accelerated by adding finely ground additional hydrocolloid from the operatory. This is contrary to what has been taught in the past in that it was believed that the duplicating colloid should always be smooth with no lumps in it. The extra hydrocolloid added before pouring reduces the temperature as well as reduces the bulk that will have to undergo congealing. This in turn reduces the amount of possible distortion that could take place during congealing.

As the duplicating colloid escapes through the vent holes in the top half of the flask, they are closed with small pieces of clay. The reservoir is completely filled. The duplicating flask is placed in ice water (circulating if possible) that just barely covers the base of the flask. Duplicating colloid then shrinks down toward the cast, providing greater accuracy.

The refractory cast material is poured into the duplicating colloid that is damp but does not contain free moisture. (Free moisture may be removed by using a pointed facial tissue to absorb it, eliminating the need for a blast of air that might break or tear the fragile portions of hydrocolloid.) Consistent records should be maintained of the water-powder ratio used in each one of the pours of the refractory investment material. Cristobalite model investment is a satisfactory material, and the ratio for the cast should be 31 ml of water to 100 gm of powder, vacuum mixed. Subsequent mixes will be of different ratios. The refractory cast is allowed to set in the duplicating colloid for 30 minutes. The cast is then elevated by the art portion on the sides uniformly with a snap.

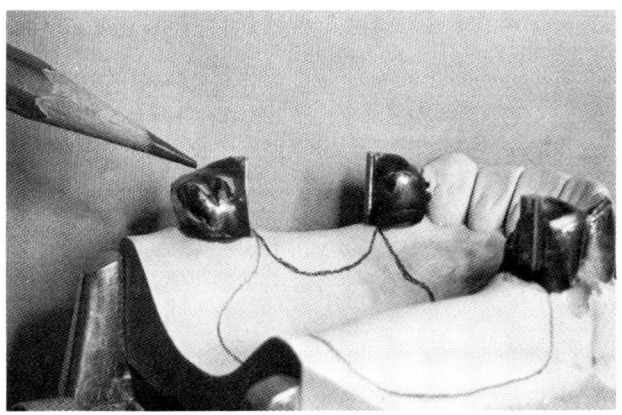

**Fig. 16-73.** Wax added adjacent to male attachment to give strength to subsequent refractory cast.

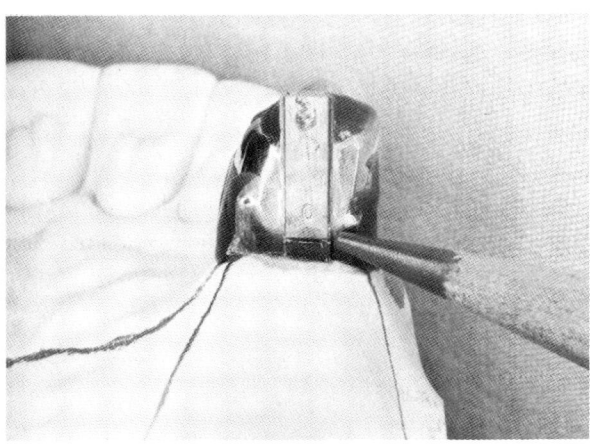

**Fig. 16-74.** Blockout gingival to male attachment. Shallow line is scribed at gingival extent of male attachment.

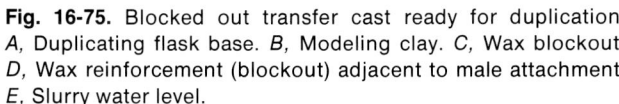

**Fig. 16-75.** Blocked out transfer cast ready for duplication. *A*, Duplicating flask base. *B*, Modeling clay. *C*, Wax blockout. *D*, Wax reinforcement (blockout) adjacent to male attachment. *E*, Slurry water level.

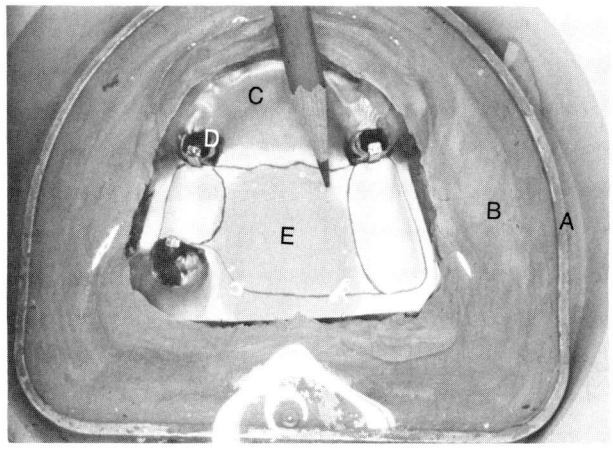

## CARE OF REFRACTORY CAST

The cast should not be handled for 24 hours. At the end of 24 hours, a coat of model spray* is sprayed on the cast. The cast is trimmed very carefully—preferably on a dry cast trimmer so that slurry does not accumulate on the working surfaces of the cast. The cast should always be handled by the base. It never should be touched in the areas where there will be a wax pattern and subsequently gold. The cast is then dried out in a circulating oven at 280° F (138° C) for 1 hour. The cast is removed from the oven and allowed to cool until it can be held comfortably in the hand. Two coats of model spray are applied to the working surface of the cast.

## FRAMEWORK WAX-UP

The scribe line at the gingival end of the male attachment that was created in the wax pattern prior to duplication will be evident. This area gingival to the male attachment should be carved back carefully to the approximate thickness of the male contact plate and carried to the gingival tissue surface (Fig. 16-76). In this fashion, wax and, subsequently, gold, will encompass the gingival end of the male contact plate, making a nicer finished surface when the male attachment and the framework are soldered together. Tacky liquid, made by dissolving pieces of plastic pattern in acetone, is painted over the surfaces that will receive the wax pattern. Baseplate wax is then placed on the reproduced surface plate of the male attachment. This becomes the upright strut. Wax is flowed along the lingual and gingival areas of the male surface plate. The other steps in the partial denture wax-up are essentially the same as those used for any other partial denture with this type of configuration (Fig. 16-77).

## INVESTING, BURNOUT, AND CASTING

The wax pattern is sprued and painted with a surface tension reducer.* A new mix of cristobalite model investment* is painted over the entire surface of the wax pattern to a depth of 1/4 inch (0.8 cm) thick. The ratio of this mix will be 16 ml of water to 50 gm of powder, vacuum mixed. When this paint-on investment sets, a heavier mix of cristobalite model investment will be used to embed the cast with the paint-on investment in the casting ring. For the large size Kerr casting flask, 128 ml of water to 400 gm of model investment will be ample.

The mix should be hand mixed with a whipping motion to incorporate as many air bubbles as possible. This creates tracts for the escape of air in the mold—a venting effect in the more porous outer layer. The casting ring is allowed to set for a minimum of 30 minutes. A slow burnout, 3 hours to reach 1300° F (704.5° C), will reduce cracks in the mold and subsequent fins in the casting. The mold should be heat soaked at this temperature for 30 minutes. Use a good partial denture casting gold such as Ney G-3† or Baker extra hard.‡ The casting ring with the casting completed is allowed to bench cool 12 to 15 minutes. This will prevent warpage of

---

*J. F. Jelenko & Co., Chicago, Ill.

*Kerr Manufacturing Co., Romulus, Mich.
†The J. M. Ney Co., Bloomfield, Conn.
‡Baker Dental Division, Engelhard Industries, Carteret, N.J.

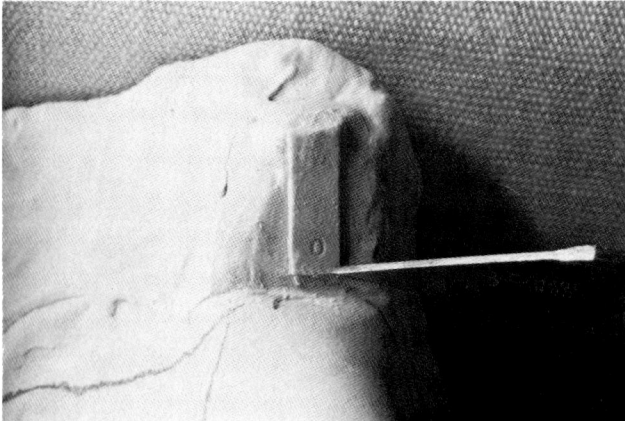

Fig. 16-76. Area gingival to male attachment trimmed to receive wax.

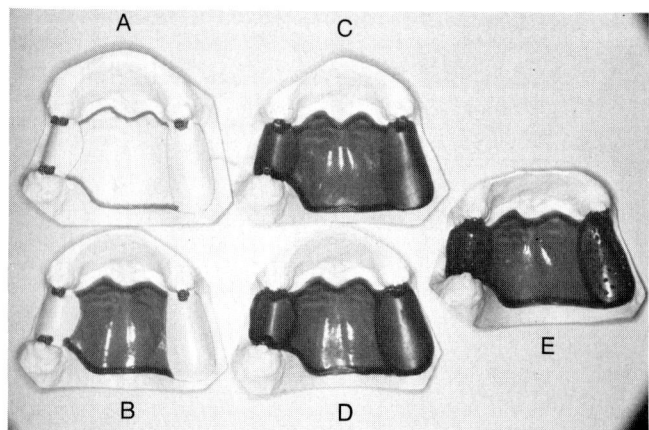

Fig. 16-77. Steps in waxing precision partial denture framework. A, Struts and beading. B, Palate. C, Saddles waxed. D, Finishing lines for acrylic added. E, Retention beads for acrylic.

the casting while it is still going through its congealing crystallization state.

The casting is recovered, cleaned up, pickled, and the sprues cut off. Large nodules are removed at this time. Generation of heat during machining operations of metal will cause proportionate distortion. Slow speeds, coolants, and frequent interruptions will reduce this effect.

## FITTING THE FRAMEWORK

The casting must fit the master cast before further steps can be accomplished.

Examination under a good light with magnification will frequently reveal small nodules and/or fins. These are removed with stones and burs. Unidentified imperfections must be detected and removed. The following three methods are commonly used:

1. Flow disclosing wax* on the entire tissue surface of the framework, and then place it on the master cast with pressure. Areas in need of adjustment are readily identified (Fig. 16-78). Repeated testing is usually necessary. Clean casting of wax by warming it in a flame and immediately blasting it with air. This should be followed with a wax solvent.

2. Paint pattern ink or layout† ink on the surface of the casting, allow it to dry, and then carry it to place, and test it for rock and movement. The areas of impingement or binding will show up on the casting as shiny spots where the imperfection has rubbed off the transfer ink (Fig. 16-79). This transfer ink comes in two different colors—blue and red. Trial and error will determine which color is more readable to the technician. Remove the material with Dykem solvent or methyl alcohol. Repeat this procedure until the casting fits the master cast.

3. Sandblast the tissue surface of the casting. Gently place the casting on the master cast. Imperfections will be indicated by small amounts of stone being picked up on the casting. Repetition is necessary until the casting fits. Obviously accuracy is not completely possible, since some of the cast is removed with each trial fitting.

On fitting the major framework casting to the master cast, the next step is to make sure that there is no binding against the abutment retainers, using one of the previously described disclosing procedures. Then it becomes necessary to fit the upright strut against the proximal surface of the male attachment. Dykem layout or pattern ink is most useful in fitting the male attachment to this strut. The surface of the strut is painted and allowed to dry (Fig. 16-80). The

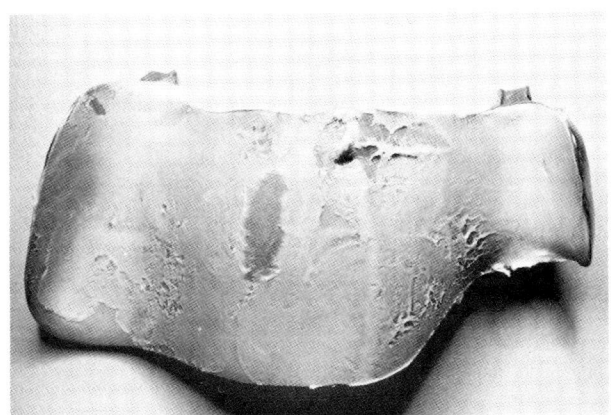

**Fig. 16-78.** Disclosing wax reveals imperfections in fit of framework.

*Kerr Manufacturing Co., Romulus, Mich.
†Dykem Co., St. Louis, Mo.

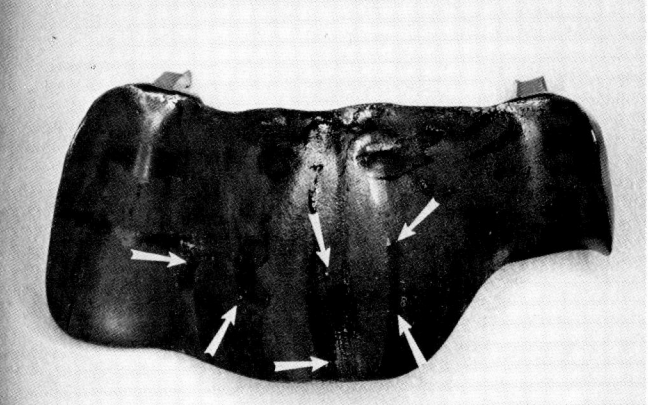

**Fig. 16-79.** Dykem reveals imperfections in fit of framework (arrows).

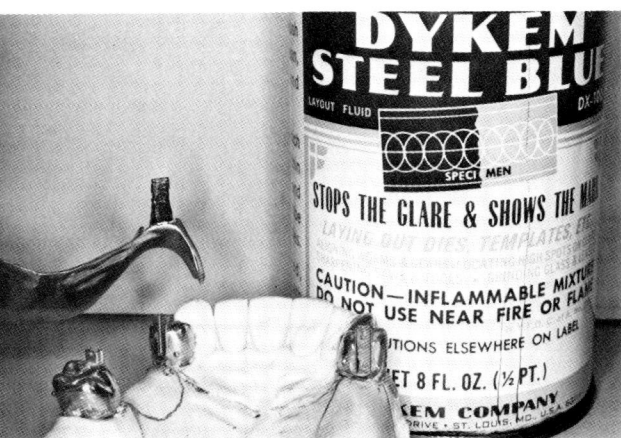

**Fig. 16-80.** Upright struts painted with Dykem.

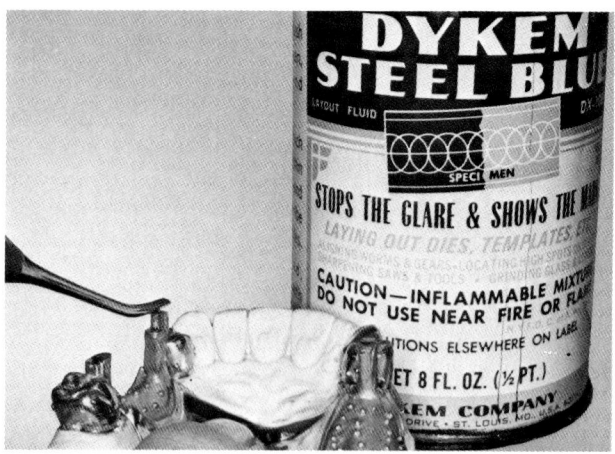

**Fig. 16-81.** Male attachment inserted in female until binding occurs.

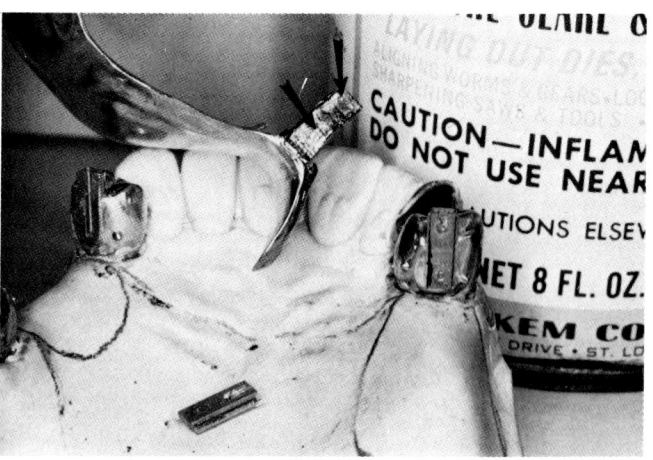

**Fig. 16-82.** Shiny spots reveal areas of impingement (arrows).

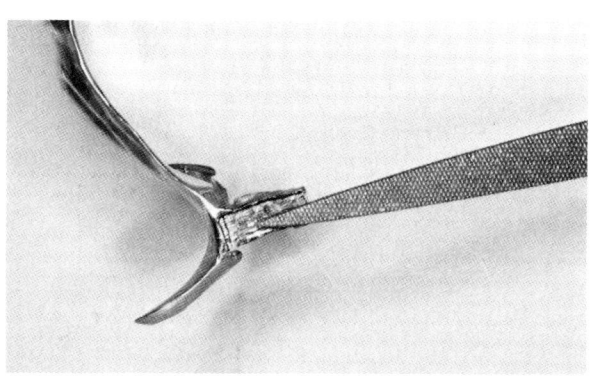

**Fig. 16-83.** Removal of imperfections.

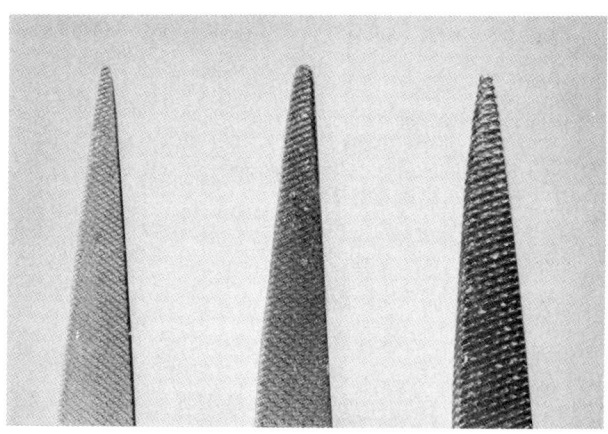

**Fig. 16-84.** Swiss pattern files.

framework is then placed on the master cast and held firmly in place with the fingers. One of the male attachments is inserted into the female attachment using a slight amount of pressure until binding is encountered (Fig. 16-81). When the male attachment and the framework are removed from the cast, the shiny spots showing the binding between the upright strut and the male attachment are obvious (Fig. 16-82). This can be dressed down by use of stones, burs, or, preferably, die sinkers files or Swiss pattern files (Fig. 16-83). These files come in various grades of coarseness (Fig. 16-84). This process is repeated for each one of the male attachments in its respective female in the abutment tooth until all of the male attachments will slide easily to place without any impingement on the upright struts of the partial denture framework. It is essential that there will be no binding in any position in any location between the attachments and the upright truss (arm). This prevents soldering a male attachment to the framework in a nonparallel position.

## FRAMEWORK AND MALE ATTACHMENT ASSEMBLY

Once the male attachments have been fitted, the transfer cast is realigned on the survey table. This is most easily accomplished by sight. Nonalignment between the mandrel and the male and female attachment is shown in Fig. 16-85. By tipping the survey table and sighting, parallelism can be achieved in this plane (Fig. 16-86). Similarly, the mediolateral parallelism can be checked (Fig. 16-87) and altered until it is parallel. The anteroposterior posi-

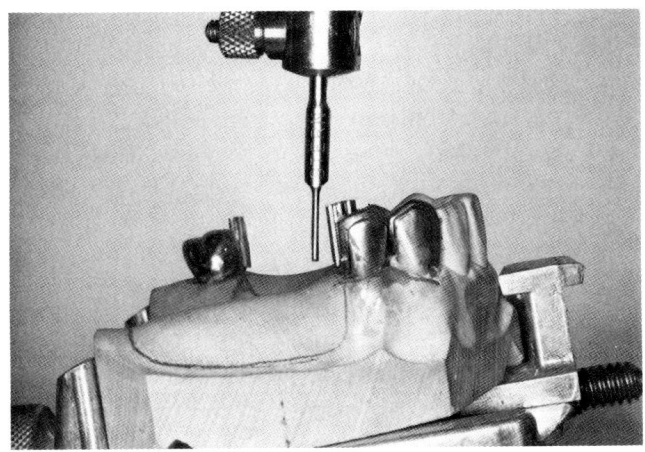

**Fig. 16-85.** Transfer cast on survey table. Path of insertion is not parallel.

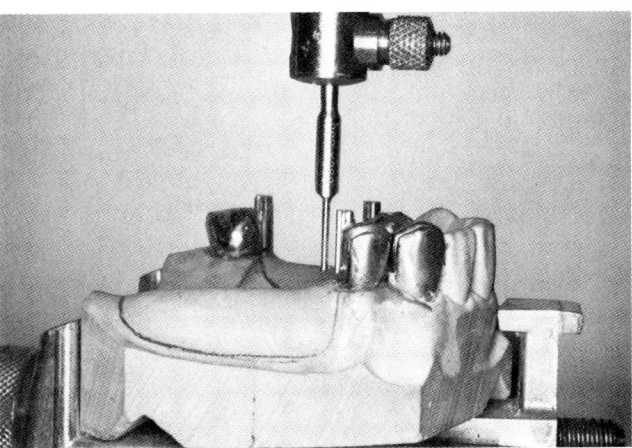

**Fig. 16-86.** Transfer cast on survey table. Parallelism has been reestablished by sight in anteroposterior dimension.

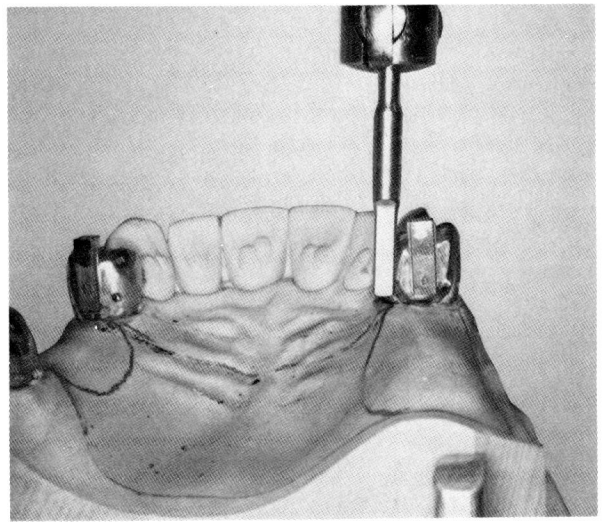

**Fig. 16-87.** Not parallel in mediolateral dimension.

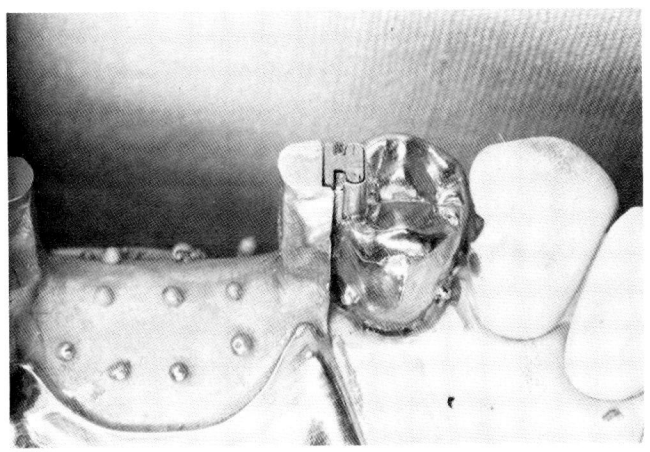

**Fig. 16-88.** Fit of strut and male attachment.

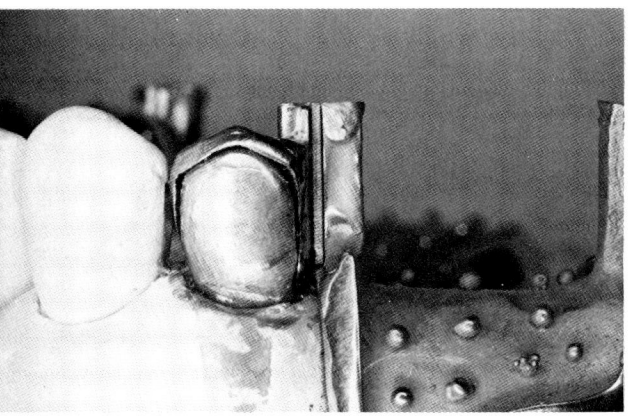

**Fig. 16-89.** Minimal space exists between strut and male attachment.

tion should be rechecked again. When this has been accomplished, the mandrel should drop into the female attachment without any binding, and it should float all the way to the bottom of the female attachment.

Fig. 16-88 illustrates the close adaptation of the upright strut against the proximal surface of the male attachment. Careful fitting between the strut and the male attachment is essential. Not only should there be no binding but there also should be no excessive amount of space. The fit should be very close. This reduces the amount of solder necessary to assemble the two parts and consequently reduces the amount of potential shrinkage that may occur as the solder congeals. In Fig. 16-89 there is scarcely any space at all. This is ideal.

The upright strut of the partial denture framework should be cut with a Dedeco NM thin disk* from the anterior to posterior side all the way to the gingival surface (Fig. 16-90). This will be a flowgate for the solder in order to get the solder to flow all the way to the gingival extent of the male contact plate and the strut of the partial denture framework.

The strut of the partial denture framework is now cut off to approximately the level of the occlusal table. The previously removed silver rods are now reassembled on the proximal surface of the male contact plate with a dot of solder (Fig. 16-91).

### Tissue support

The dentist will have determined from palpation just how much tissue support is needed. This may vary from 0 to 0.004 or 0.005 inch; the exact amount will be indicated on the prescription. An appropriate thickness of platinum foil is placed in the gingival seat of each female attachment. This shim prevents the male attachment from "bottoming out" prior to assembly to the framework. In the mouth the tissues will be stimulated under occlusal loading.

The male attachments with their reassembled silver rods are now placed in the female attachments

*Dental Development & Manufacturing Corp., Brooklyn, N.Y.

(Fig. 16-92). The silver rods attached to the male attachments are then bent over until they almost contact the partial denture framework (Fig. 16-93). Actual contact is not advisable, since it may cause a malposition of the partial denture framework or the male attachment. When all silver rods have been bent over to almost contact the partial denture framework, they are sticky waxed to the partial denture framework. The casting is held in place while the sticky wax congeals. Additional sticky wax is applied at the junction of the male attachment and the upright strut of the partial denture framework (Fig. 16-94). A large undercut gauge is inserted in the vertical shaft of the surveyor (Fig. 16-95). This undercut gauge is dropped down to contact the center of the palatal surface of the framework and is sticky waxed to the framework. Then, by lifting the vertical shaft of the surveyor, the entire framework with the sticky-waxed male attachments, may be removed without distortion or breaking (Fig. 16-96). A hard, brittle sticky wax is the choice of material at this time. It is better to know if there is distortion that would cause the breakage of the sticky wax rather than go through a soldering operation and subsequently have to break the solder joint and reassemble the parts.

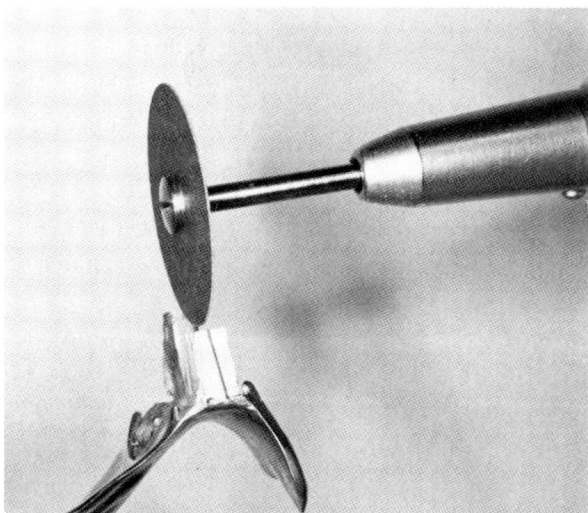

**Fig. 16-90.** Soldering sluiceway cut in strut to gingival extent of upright strut.

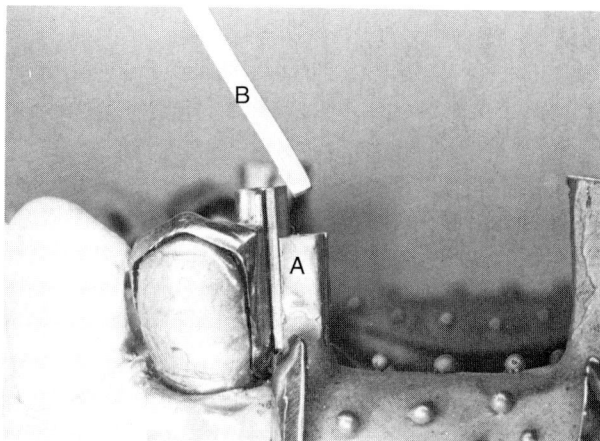

**Fig. 16-91.** *A,* Strut cut short of occlusal table. *B,* Silver rod resoldered to surface plate of male attachment.

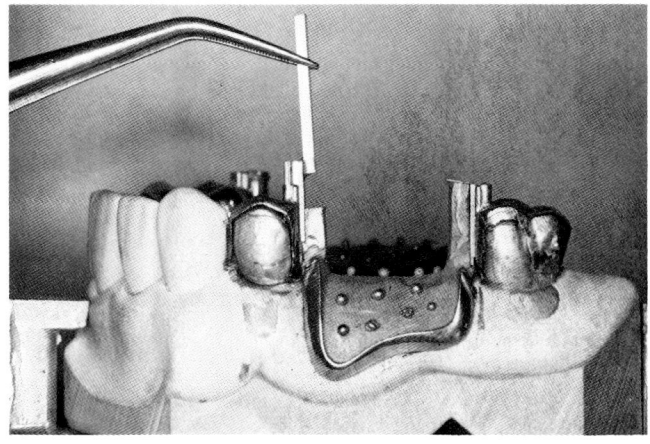

**Fig. 16-92.** Male attachments ready for assembly.

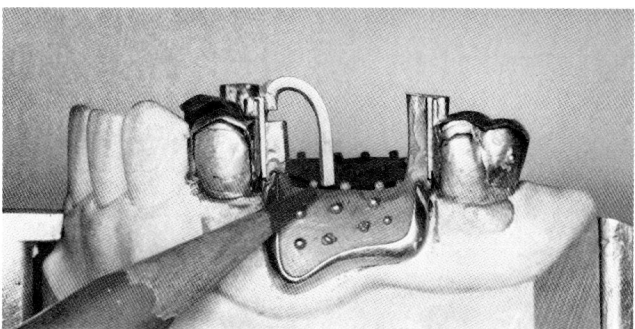

**Fig. 16-93.** Silver rod almost touches framework.

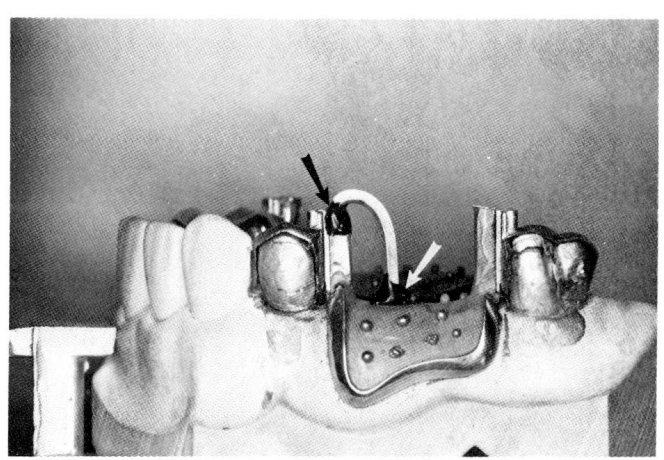

**Fig. 16-94.** Silver rod sticky waxed to framework (arrows).

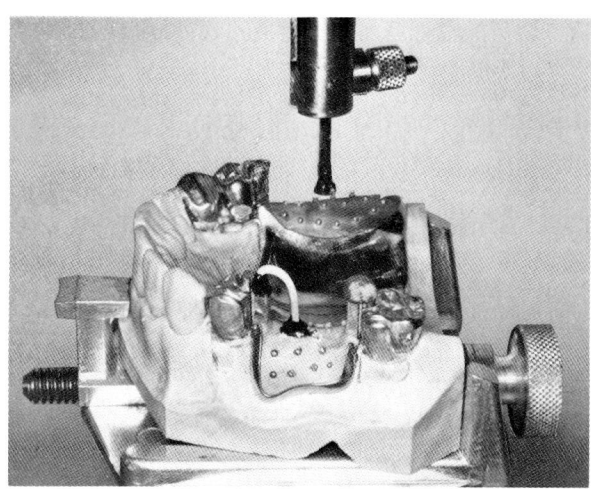

**Fig. 16-95.** Large undercut gauge in vertical shaft of surveyor.

**Fig. 16-96.** Sticky-waxed assembly removed in parallel path of insertion.

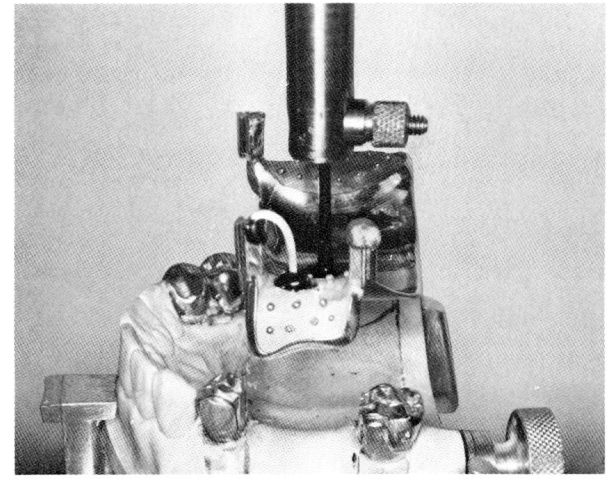

### ALTERNATE ASSEMBLY PROCEDURE NO. 1

An electric soldering machine* is used to spot weld the occlusal ends of the male attachment and the upright truss arm of the partial denture framework (Fig. 16-97). The partial denture framework is locked down to the cast by means of plaster or stone (Fig. 16-98). The occlusal ends of the truss arm and the male attachment should be ground level with each other. A slot is cut down the center of the truss arm in an anteroposterior direction. A silica flux is used rather than the conventional gold flux. The master cast is then immersed in water to a level just below the area to be spot welded (Fig. 16-99). This procedure will allow dissipation of the heat rapidly and will prevent the melting of the low-fusing metal supporting the retainer castings. Even though this is done under water, there is no danger of electrical shock. The metal pole is attached to the metal framework at some position. The carbon rod pole should be very flat so that it contacts both surfaces at exactly the same time. By using this procedure, the male attachment is tacked to the occlusal end of the strut of the partial denture framework and eliminates the possibility of distortion when removing the framework and the male attachments from the master cast preparatory to soldering. Experimentation with a casting button will show the proper setting for the particular soldering machine.

*SWest, Inc., Dallas, Tex.

### ALTERNATE ASSEMBLY PROCEDURE NO. 2

In this alternative method, DuraLay* is painted over the occlusal ends of the male attachment and the strut of the partial denture framework. Care should be taken that the cast is inverted so that the DuraLay does not run down into the female attachment and lock it into place (Fig. 16-100). On the premolar in Fig. 16-100, the silver rod is sticky waxed to the partial denture framework. Again, the use of the undercut gauge and the vertical shaft of the surveyor to remove the partial denture framework is useful to avoid breaking the male attachment loose from the upright strut and for checking the parallelism (Fig. 16-101).

Regardless of the method used to tack the male attachment to the upright strut of the partial denture framework, the entire circumference of the area to be soldered must then be sticky waxed (Fig. 16-102). This prevents investment from getting into the areas where solder is desired (Fig. 16-103). A rope of 10-gauge wax is placed at the gingival end of the male attachment (Fig. 16-104). This will become an aerodynamic sluiceway during the soldering operation.

*Reliance Dental Manufacturing Co., Chicago, Ill.

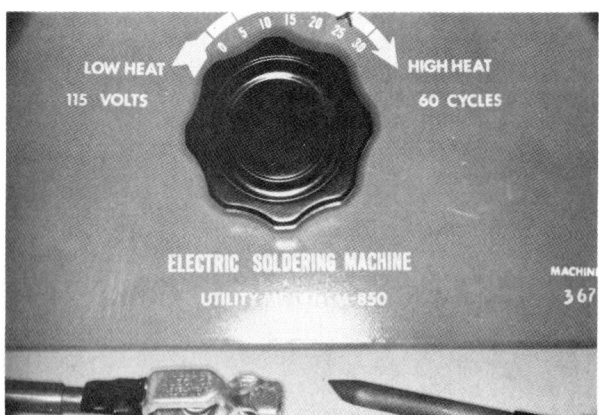

**Fig. 16-97.** Electric soldering machine.

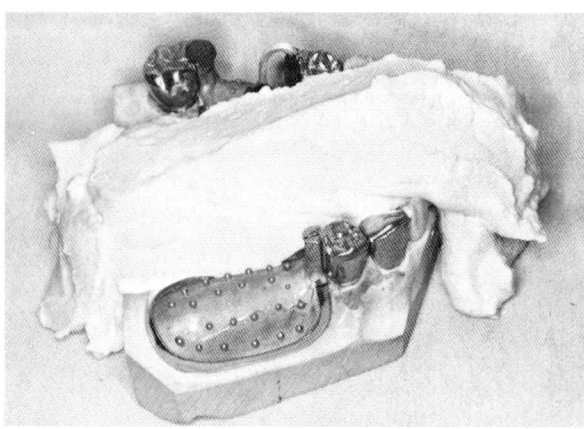

**Fig. 16-98.** Framework secured to cast with plaster or stone.

## Frictional wall precision attachment partial prosthesis 479

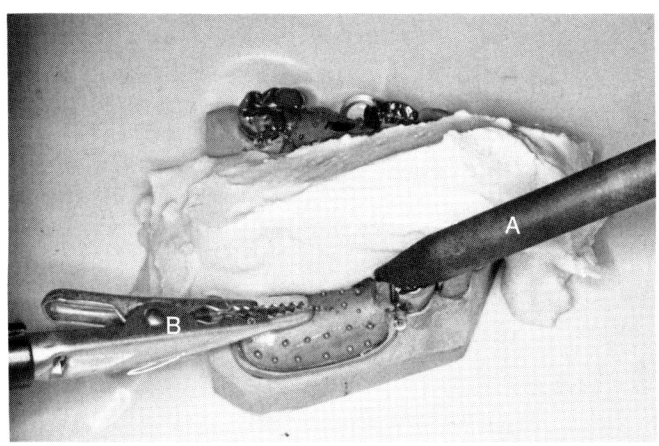

**Fig. 16-99.** Electric soldering setup. *A,* Carbon electrode. *B,* Metal electrode.

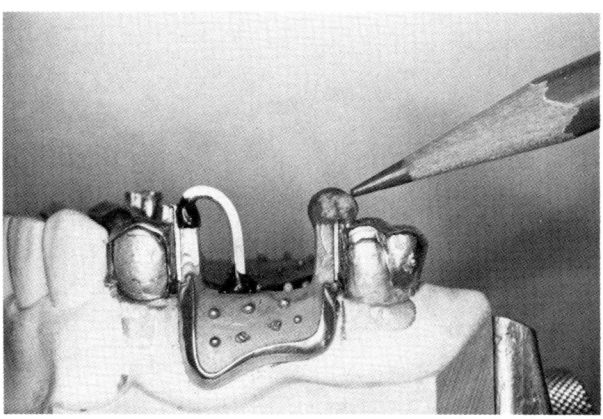

**Fig. 16-100.** DuraLay joins molar male attachment to upright strut.

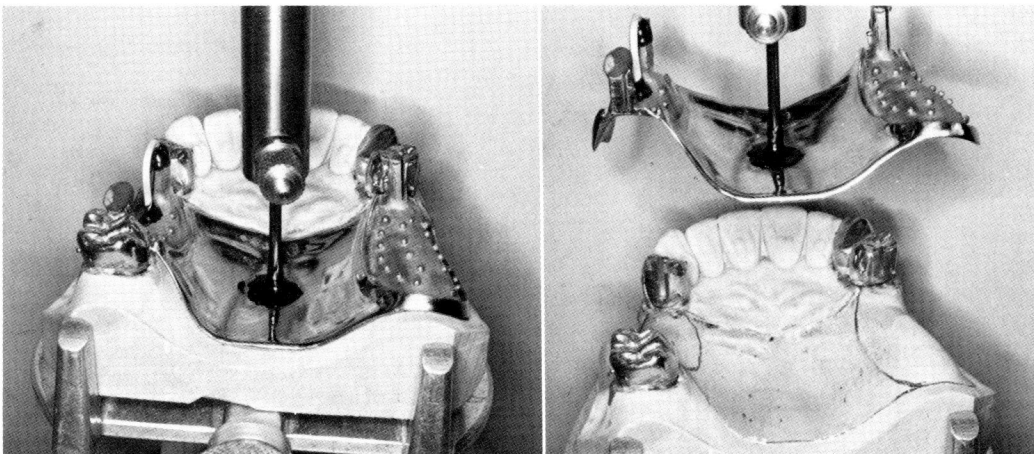

**Fig. 16-101.** Vertical shaft of surveyor used for lifting assembly.

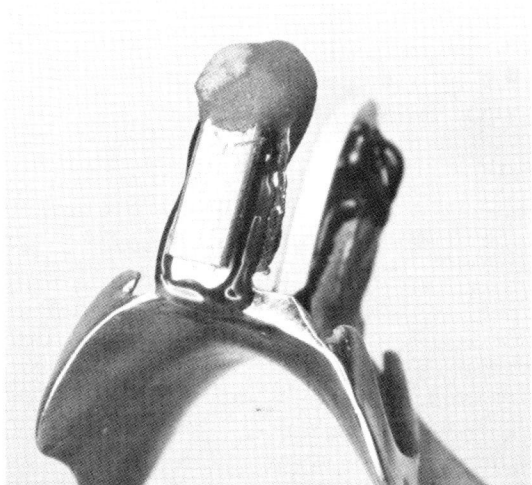

**Fig. 16-102.** Male attachment sticky waxed around entire circumference of joint (lingual oblique view).

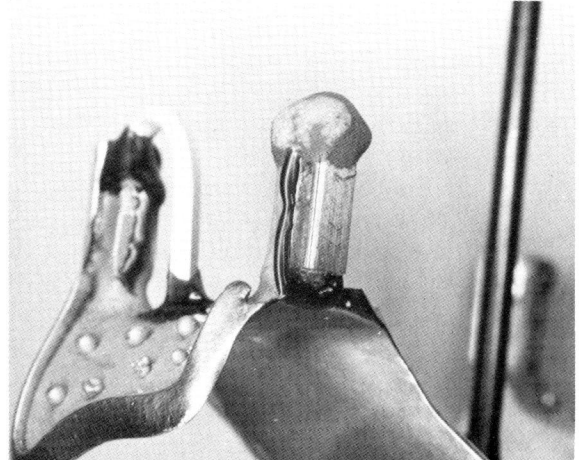

**Fig. 16-103.** Male attachment sticky waxed around entire circumference of joint (buccal oblique view).

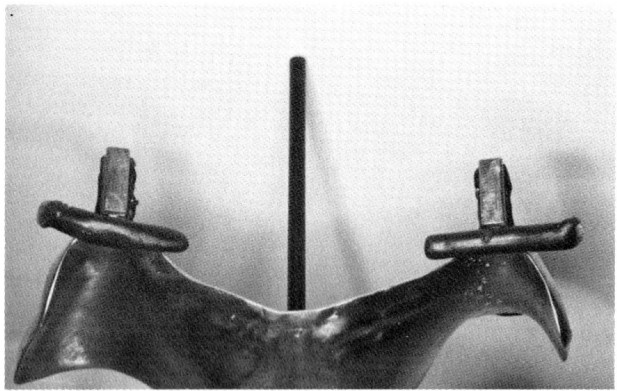

Fig. 16-104. Rope of 10-gauge wax placed at gingival end of male attachment.

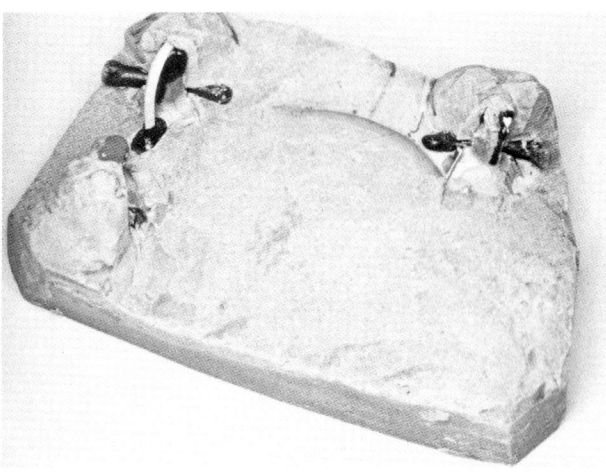

Fig. 16-105. Refractory cast trimmed for ease of soldering.

### ALTERNATE ASSEMBLY PROCEDURE NO. 3

A major partial denture framework is waxed with an additional 14-gauge upright strut close to the attachment area. This upright strut should be as nearly parallel to the female attachment as possible. The wax-up is invested, cast, recovered, cleaned, and fitted.

With the male attachment and the fitted framework in place, a housing around the male attachment is waxed or created with DuraLay. Extending from this nest around the male attachment are feet that surround the 14-gauge upright post and contact the surface of the framework. This pattern is invested, cast, recovered, cleaned up, and very carefully fitted to the male attachment and the framework. With a casting that fits like an inlay, it can be soldered freehand to the male attachment. A sluiceway cut in the casting in the area of the male contact plate will materially aid the soldering procedure.

This assembly is refitted to the framework. If the parts fit precisely, they can be riveted together. The upright strut is shortened to 1 mm over the extension. Crossed slots are cut in the strut with a jeweler's 6/0 saw blade. The strut is carefully peened down over the strut while the framework is held firmly in place. The parts may also be spot welded for lifting and subsequently reinforced with solder. Alternately, these parts may be assembled with DuraLay.*

### INVESTING AND SOLDERING

The partial denture framework with the male attachments sticky waxed into place or tacked into place by alternate method No. 1 or No. 2 is embedded in a good grade of soldering investment. Just prior to the time of the final set of the soldering investment, the refractory cast should be trimmed to allow the maximum benefit of aerodynamics (Fig. 16-105). The sticky wax is flushed out, the joints fluxed, and the refractory cast heated either in a rapidly-ascending oven or by gas-air blowpipe. As it approaches the proper temperature, the solder holding the silver rods to the male attachments will flow, and the silver rods can be readily removed (Fig. 16-106). The heat from the torch should be directed to the gingival end of the upright strut in all instances, and .650 fine solder should be fed from the occlusal end and down the previously cut slot. This will ensure that solder will flow all the way to the gingival extent of the upright strut and the male attachment (Fig. 16-107). The cast is allowed to cool for 10 minutes before immersing in water. Refractory material is cleaned off of the casting, and it is pickled.

It now becomes necessary to check the accuracy of the soldering operations. The partial denture framework itself is checked on the master cast without the retainers in place to assure that no warpage has occurred during the soldering operation (Fig. 16-108). Then one retainer casting is placed on the transfer cast, and the partial denture framework is seated in that retainer casting to check for possible distortion during soldering (Fig. 16-109). The retainer casting is removed, and another retainer casting is placed on the transfer cast. The partial denture framework is then inserted in the female retainer to check for possible distortion of soldering (Fig. 16-110). And, similarly, each subsequent retainer casting is placed on the cast individually to

---
*Lucia, V. O.: Personal communication, 1981.

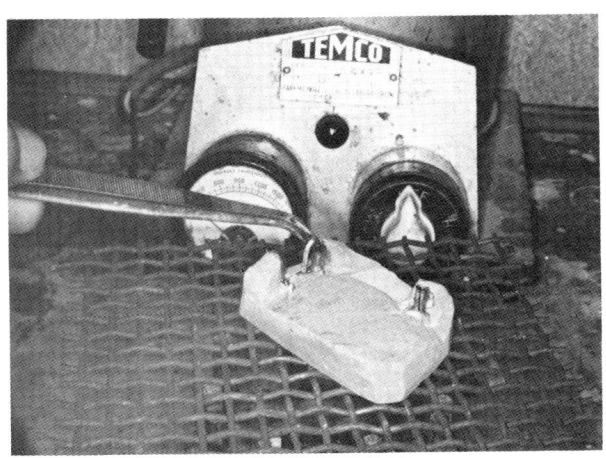

**Fig. 16-106.** Silver rods removed as cast reaches soldering temperature.

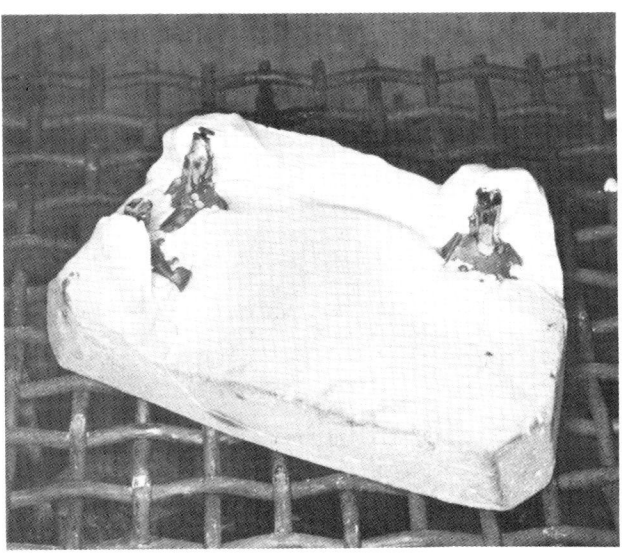

**Fig. 16-107.** Soldering completed.

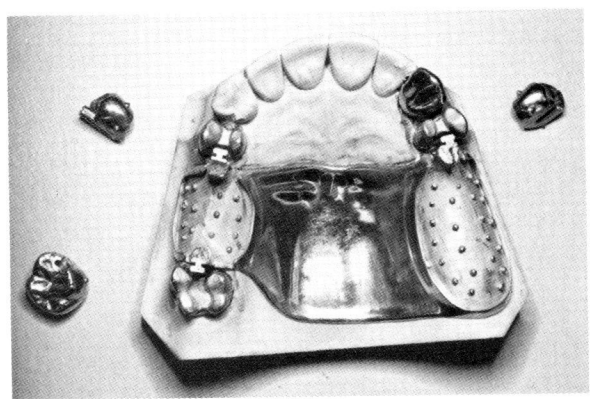

**Fig. 16-108.** Soldered framework checked for accuracy on master cast.

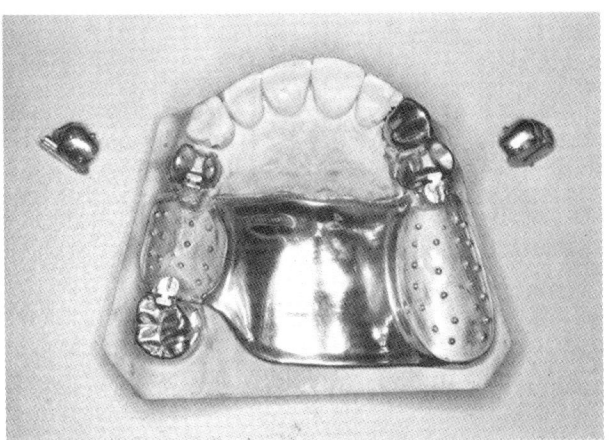

**Fig. 16-109.** Soldered framework checked for accuracy on master cast with one retainer in place.

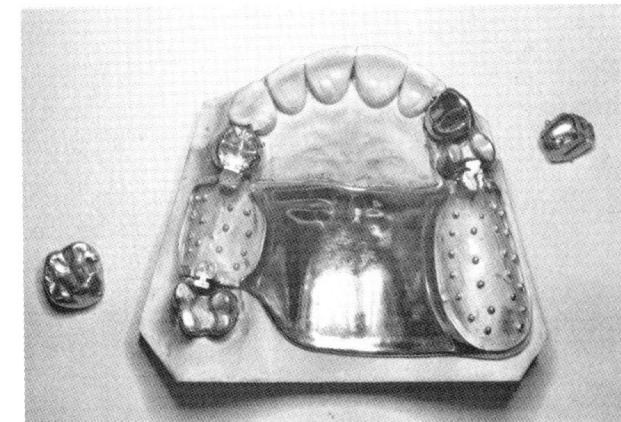

**Fig. 16-110.** Check accuracy of alternate retainer casting.

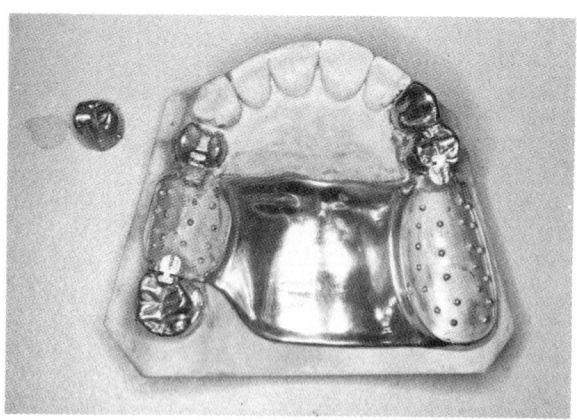

Fig. 16-111. Check accuracy with pair of retainers.

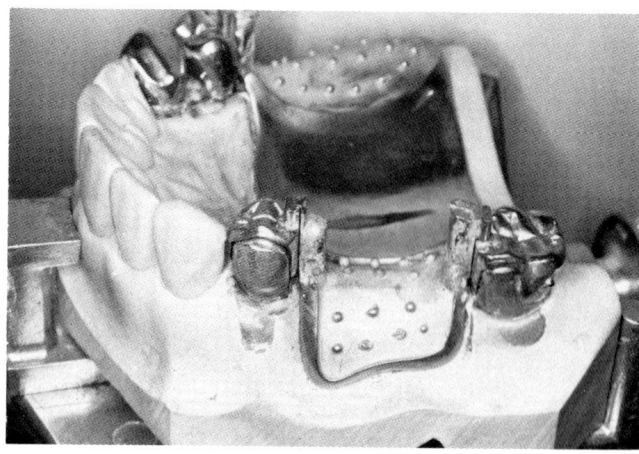

Fig. 16-112. Fit of soldered male attachment to retainer casting (buccal view).

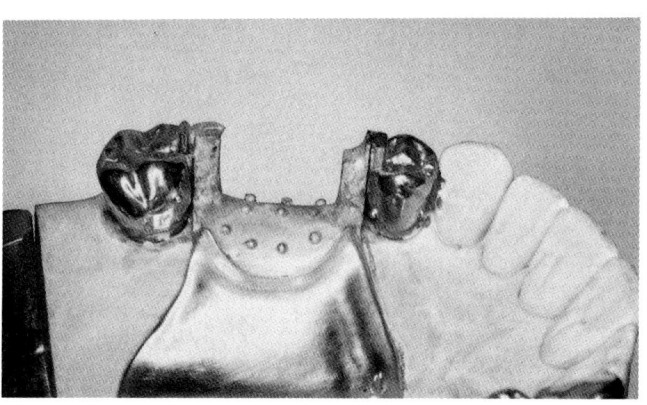

Fig. 16-113. Fit of soldered male attachment to retainer casting (lingual view).

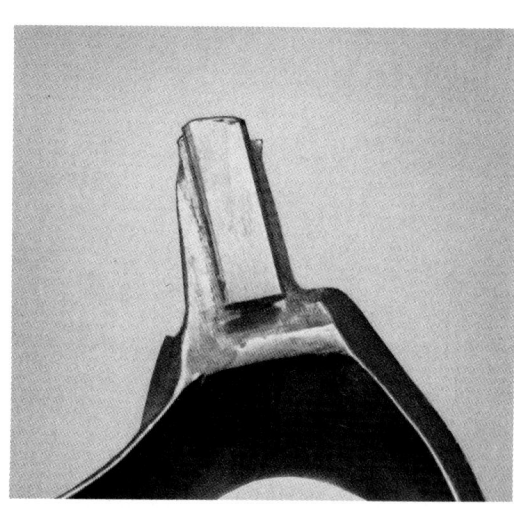

Fig. 16-114. Solder joint between male attachment and upright strut.

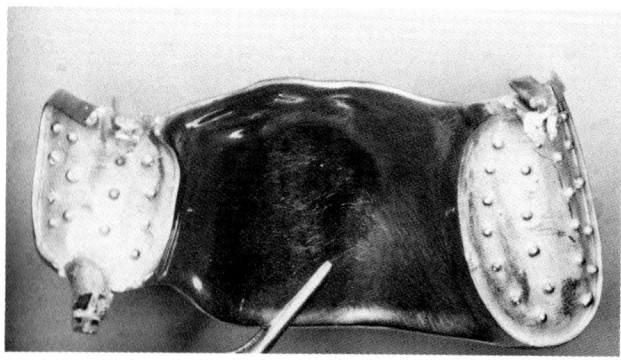

Fig. 16-115. Framework polished.

check for parallelism of the male soldering procedure to the upright strut. Then two retainer castings are placed on the transfer cast, and the partial denture framework is carried to place to verify the parallelism and the lack of soldering distortion between those two male attachments (Fig. 16-111). This is continued until all possible combinations between abutment castings have been accomplished. Then all abutment castings are put in place, and the partial denture framework is checked for parallelism between them all. At this time they should all fit nicely (Figs. 16-112 and 16-113). The soldered male attachments will have this appearance (Fig. 16-114) when the casting has been cleaned up. There should be a minimal amount of solder and very little refining necessary. The partial denture framework is finished to a high shine at this time (Fig. 16-115).

## REPLACEMENT TEETH

Different methods of restoring the occlusal surfaces on partial denture frameworks are available. Porcelain teeth may be arranged in the conventional fashion set up to the opposing occlusion and the tissue areas processed with acrylic. Processing errors necessitate correction before removal from the cast.

Gold occlusals are by far more accurate as far as occlusal function is concerned, and their fabrication is described in Volumes 1 and 2 of *Dental Laboratory Procedures*.

### ALTERNATE PROCEDURE FOR GOLD OCCLUSALS

Index V-shaped notches in several dimensions are cut in the occlusal end of the upright struts. Wax bases are built up to within 1 mm of the occlusal table. DuraLay is painted in a narrow band (approximately 2 mm wide buccolingually) anteroposteriorly. It is also painted into the struts that are indexed with V-shaped notches (Fig. 16-116). In an area of a free-end denture base a hole is cut into the wax down to the partial denture framework, and an index is made on two or three of the retentive areas so that a tripod effect in DuraLay may be accomplished (Fig. 16-117). If an upright strut is cast in the framework, the tripod can be created on its occlusal end. The occlusion is waxed over the DuraLay to the counterocclusion according to the prescription of the dentist (Fig. 16-118).

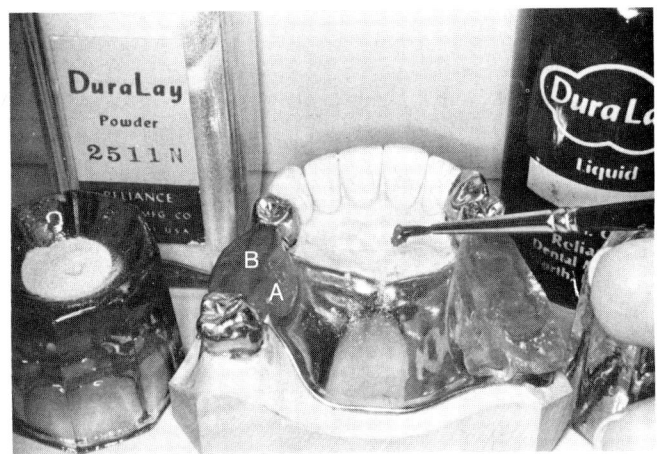

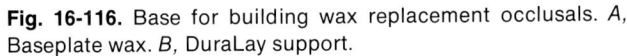
Fig. 16-116. Base for building wax replacement occlusals. *A*, Baseplate wax. *B*, DuraLay support.

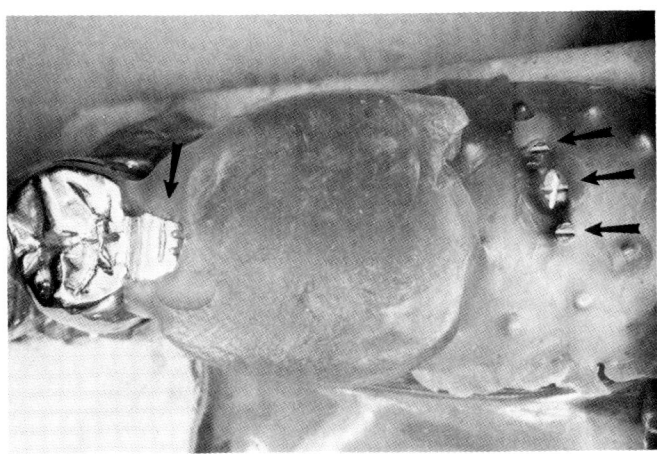
Fig. 16-117. Index notches for wax occlusals (arrows).

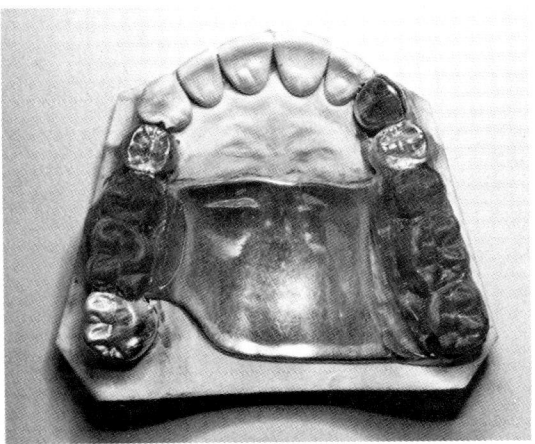
Fig. 16-118. Occlusion waxed to prescription of dentist.

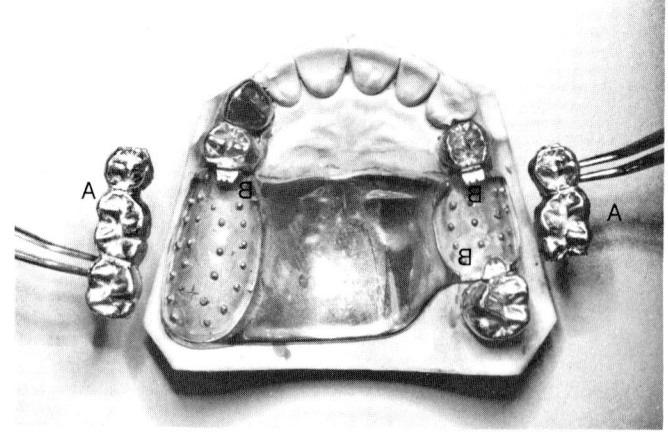

**Fig. 16-119.** Gold occlusals are ready to be seated in indices on framework. *A*, Gold occlusals. *B*, Indices on upright struts.

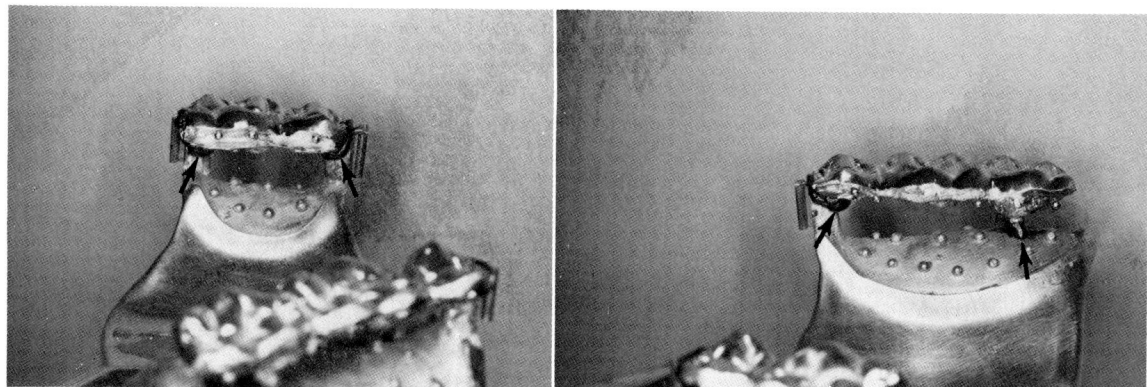

**Fig. 16-120.** Gold occlusals sticky waxed to framework (arrows).

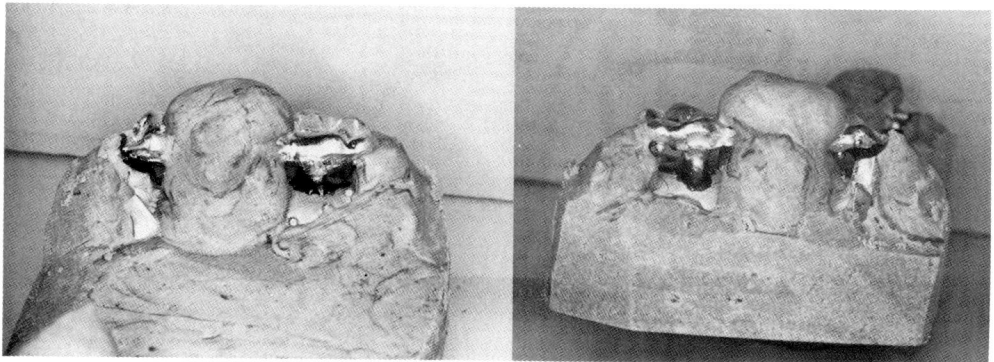

**Fig. 16-121.** Refractory cast trimmed.

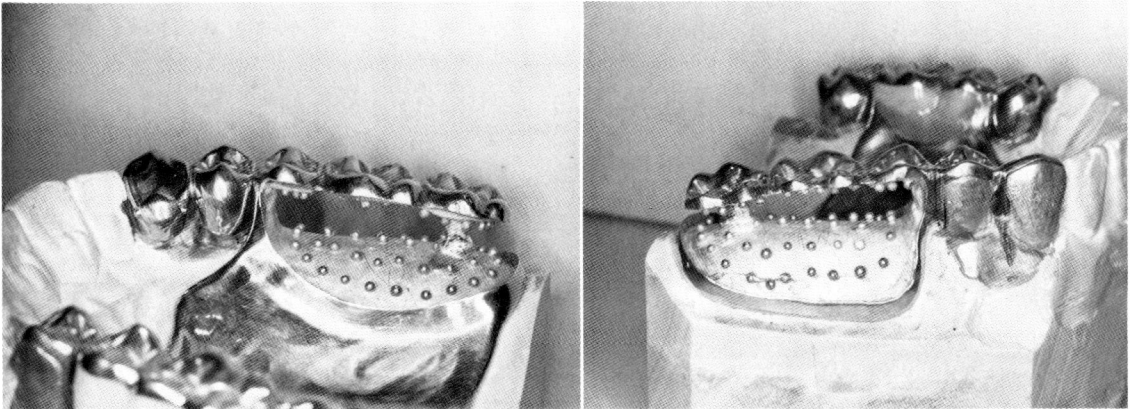

**Fig. 16-122.** Gold occlusals soldered to partial denture framework.

A thin stone index is made over the occlusal surface of the wax pattern to avoid distortion during handling. The baseplate wax is carved from beneath or gingival to the inlay wax patterns. It is carved up to the level of the DuraLay. The DuraLay gives rigidity to the wax patterns. They are separated away from the partial denture framework, invested, cast, and recovered. The recovered castings will now fit into indices cut in the upright struts and on a tripod in the retention areas (Fig. 16-119). These gold occlusals accurately indexed are now sticky waxed around their periphery (Fig. 16-120). The framework with the sticky-waxed gold occlusals is then embedded in a soldering investment, leaving wide-open sluiceways to take advantage of aerodynamics (Fig. 16-121). The sticky wax is flushed out, the cast is fluxed, and the gold occlusals are soldered to the partial denture framework (Fig. 16-122). With this method, no processing errors can occur from the acrylic manipulation. The gold occlusals are rigidly attached to the partial denture framework.

At this point the steps should be repeated to assure that no distortion has occurred during the process of soldering the gold occlusals to the partial denture framework. That is, the framework should be checked against the master cast without any retainer castings in place. Second, each retainer in succession should be checked with the partial denture framework to eliminate the possibility of error and then all pairs of alternate retainers should be checked. Finally, all retainers should be checked with the partial denture framework.

## ACRYLIC INSERTS

There are several methods of processing the acrylic in place between the gold saddles and the gold occlusals. None of the methods is completely satisfactory. A double processing procedure can be used in which the pink saddle material is processed first with heat-curing acrylic and deflasked. Areas are cut out for the tooth-colored material and rewaxed and reflasked and processed. Alternatively, the tooth-colored material can be processed in its entirety and the pink material processed subsequently. There is a side opening flask in which the double processing procedures can be combined into one procedure, first packing with pink acrylic and then cutting out for the tooth-colored material and processing it.

A simpler method is to wax up the buccal and lingual aspects of the areas to be reproduced in acrylic and make buccal and lingual cores. These cores are then removed and the wax eliminated. Either pour acrylic or autopolymerizing acrylic is placed in the areas to replace the wax. Before the acrylic sets, the area to be replaced with tooth-colored material can be cut out and these packed with a material such as Biolon* or an autopolymerizing acrylic. The completed casting is on the transfer cast with the plastic processed on one side only (Figs. 16-123 and 16-124) and on the technique typodont that represents the patient.

## ALTERNATE PROCEDURE FOR GOLD OCCLUSALS

Porcelain teeth are set up and processed onto the saddles. All acrylic processing errors are now current. The occlusal surfaces of the porcelain teeth may be prepared to receive onlay-type restorations. These are waxed, invested, cast, recovered and cleaned up, fitted, and cemented to the porcelain teeth. Several teeth should be made together rather than single teeth to prevent the possibility of the castings becoming dislodged from the porcelain teeth. One obvious problem in this procedure is the possibility of fracture of the porcelain teeth during their preparation. Another source of error is the overheating of the plastic during the preparation of the porcelain teeth.

These problems can be overcome by setting up the porcelain teeth in an extrahard baseplate wax. Each tooth is removed in turn from the wax without destroying its basal seat. The tooth is prepared and returned to its proper place and rewaxed to position. The saddles with prepared teeth are processed to the framework. Processing errors are now overcome, and wax patterns for gold occlusals can be created with a high degree of accuracy.

*The L. D. Caulk Co., Milford, Del.

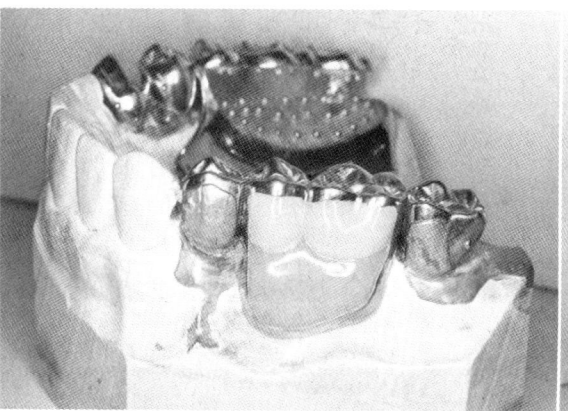
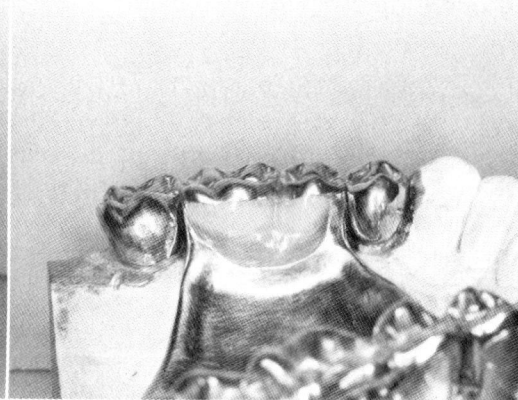
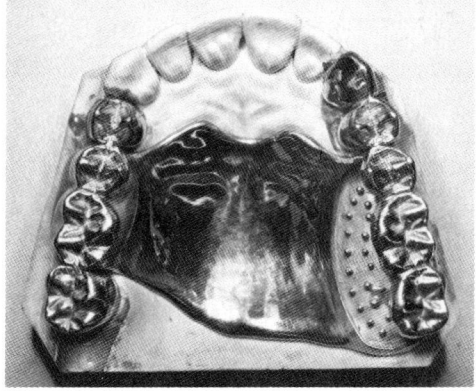

**Fig. 16-123.** Completed casting on master transfer cast showing several views. Plastic was not processed on left side to show retention details.

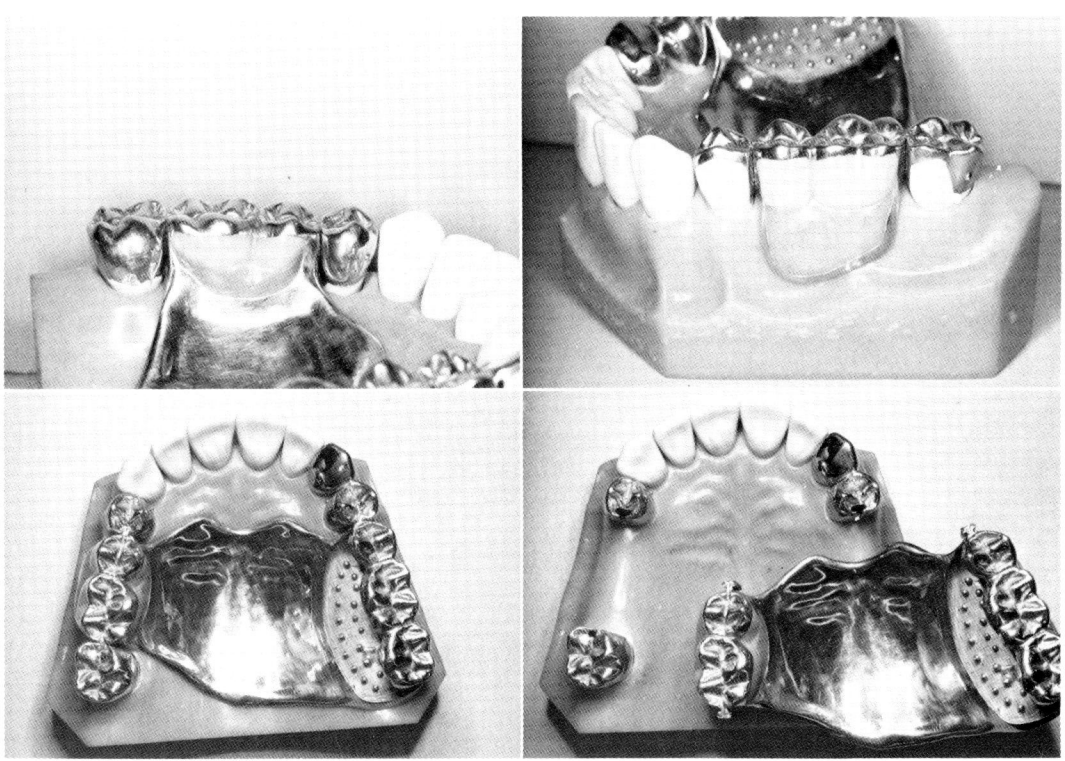

**Fig. 16-124.** Views of technique frictional wall precision attachment partial denture on typodent, which represents patient. Plastic denture base and tooth material processed on right side of partial denture. Left side shows details of fabrication.

**Table 16-1.** Fabrication of precision attachment partial denture

| Problem | Probable cause | Solution |
| --- | --- | --- |
| Female not within normal tooth contour | Inadequate preparation | Reprepare tooth |
| Hole in retainer casting | Inadequate preparation<br>Female recess cut too deep | Reprepare tooth; solder hole using platinum foil over gap, refit casting |
| Nonparallel females | Excessive pressure between cast and vertical shaft of surveyor<br>Uneven excessive space between recess and female attachment<br>Females not sighted for parallelism after sticky waxing | Paint thin mix of cristobalite in female, and insert carbon rod; break solder joint, mill recesses, and reassemble |
| Tight females | Excessive space between recess and female attachment, allowing too much solder, which contracts as it congeals | Lap with coarse, medium, or fine optical grinding powder |
| Solder over contact plate of female attachment | Inadequate investment procedure | Disclose area with Dykem and remove with stones, disks, and pattern files |
| Incomplete solder joint around female attachment | Failure in principles of soldering—clean, hot, proximity of parts, gravity, access | Freshen area, reinvest, and add lower fusing solder (.560 fine) |
| Distortion from male soldering | Excessive space between upright strut and male attachment, allowing too much solder, which contracts as it congeals<br>Binding between upright strut and male attachment at time of sticky waxing | Break joint and refit parts before reassembly<br>May need to shim excessive space with piece of casting gold |

## SUGGESTIONS FOR THE DENTIST

The precision attachment partial denture should be fitted to the mouth by itself. The prosthesis should be checked with each abutment casting singly and then with alternate pairs of abutments until all combinations have been exhausted. Remounting may be indicated to perfect the occlusion.

The abutment restorations should be cemented one at a time with all other abutments in place. A liberal application of petroleum jelly to the male and female attachments will prevent these from being cemented together. As soon as the abutment being cemented is carried to place, the prosthesis is seated and allowed to remain in position until the cement has set.

The patient should be *instructed* in removal and insertion of the prosthesis on the day of cementation. However, the patient should be advised not to attempt removal until the next day. It is good practice management for the dentist to see the patient on the following day for any minor adjustments and psychological reinforcement.

### PROBLEM AREAS

The most frequently encountered difficulties during fabrication of this type of prosthesis, along with causes and solutions, are covered in Table 16-1. With patient usage, difficult problems can occur. Their causes and possible solutions are described in Table 16-2.

## SUMMARY

This chapter describes in detail the step-by-step technical procedures required to fabricate an intracoronal rigid frictional wall precision attachment partial denture. Alternative procedures, where ap-

Table 16-2. Patient use of precision attachment partial denture

| Problem | Probable cause | Solution |
| --- | --- | --- |
| Broken male attachment | Wear, incomplete solder joint, abuse | Fit new male attachment to existing partial denture; pick up in mouth with DuraLay and/or plaster; resolder parts and replace plastic |
| Broken female attachment, or abutment resotration needs replacement | Improper retainer design initially | Redesign tooth preparation; master impression should incorporate partial denture wax abutment with proper recess; invest, cast, and fit casting in mouth; transfer impression, proceed with procedure as outlined in chapter |
| Broken tooth | Devital tooth, elderly patient, gingival erosion, excessive tooth preparation | Redesign tooth preparation; master impression should incorporate partial denture; wax abutment with proper recess; invest, cast, and fit casting in mouth; transfer impression, proceed with procedure as outlined in chapter |
| Lack of retention | Attachment length designed incorrectly, need more than half length of attachment | Add wrought wire gold clasp to engage lingual undercut |
| | Wear | Spread wings of attachment |
| | Broken leaf on male attachment partial denture designed with path of insertion same as arc of opening | Replace male attachment (see above) Complete redesign of partial denture is only satisfactory solution; lingual wrought gold wire clasp arms may be added but results will be questionable |

plicable, have been presented. Minor modifications with some ingenuity will allow the student/dentist/technician to adapt these procedures to most types of precision attachments. As with any phase of dentistry, attention to the minutiae is critical to a successful restoration.

**ACKNOWLEDGMENTS**

I would like to thank Dr. E. Evan Moore and the members of the Texas Gnathological Society for their valuable assistance in preparation of this chapter.

**REFERENCE**

Goodkind, R. J., and Baker, J. L.: Status report on precision attachments, Council on dental materials and devices, J. Am. Dent. Assoc. **92**:602-603, March, 1976.

**BIBLIOGRAPHY**

Applegate, O. C.: Essentials of removable partial denture prosthesis, ed. 2, Philadelphia, 1959, W. B. Saunders Co.

Augustin, A. G.: Removable bridge construction: inlays with male and female attachments, Dent. Digest **30**:109-111, 1924.

Barishman, H.: Accuracy in partials with internal attachments, N. Y. State Dent. J. **23**:141-143, 1957.

Barishman, H.: Technical procedures in the construction of a removable partial denture prosthesis with internal attachments, N.Y. State Dent. J. **30**:248-252, 1960.

Bartlett, A. A.: Duplication of precision attachment partial denture, J. Prosthet. Dent. **16**:1111-1115, 1966.

Bauer, A., and Gutowski, A.: Gnathology: introduction to theory and practice, Berlin, 1976 Buch- und Zeitschriften—Verlag.

Baum, L.: Advanced restorative dentistry, Philadelphia, 1973, W. B. Saunders Co.

Blatterfein, L., Klein, I. E., and Miglino, J. C.: A loading impression technique for semiprecision and precision removable partial dentures, J. Prosthet. Dent. **43**:9-14, 1980.

Brecker, S.: Clinical procedures in occlusal rehabilitation, Philadelphia, 1973, W. B. Saunders Co.

Brodbelt, R. H. W.: A simple paralleling template for precision attachments, J. Prosthet. Dent. **27**:285-288, 1972.

Cecconi, B. T.: Effect of rest design on transmission of forces to abutment teeth, J. Prosthet. Dent. **32**:141-151, 1974.

Chayes, H. E. S.: Bridgework conducive to health and the instruments for constructing it, Dent. Items Interest **37**:415-439, 1915.

Chayes, H. E. S.: A broad consideration of the principles involved in fixed and removable bridgework: the parallelism of abutments and attachments, and instruments for obtaining the same, Dent. Cosmos **57**:783-805, 1915.

Chayes, H. E. S.: Technique for a simple bridge, Dent. Items Interest **38**:8-24, 1916.

Cohn, L. A.: The physiologic basis for tooth fixation in precision attached partial dentures, J. Prosthet. Dent. **6**:220-244, 1956.

Diamond, M.: Twenty years with Chayes bridgework, Dent. Items Interest **56**:614-626, 688-696, 1934.

Doxtater, L. W.: Removable bridge attachments for vital and pulpless teeth, Parts 1 and 2, Dent. Items Interest **45**:265-271, 343-351, 1923.

Dressell, R. P.: Precision attachments and their practical application, Northwest Dentistry **32**:7-10, 1953.

Eich, F. A.: The role of removable partial dentures in the destruction of the natural dentition, Dent. Clin. North Am., pp. 717-731, 1962.

Evans, G. A.: Practical treatise on crown and bridgework, ed. 9, Philadelphia, 1922, P. Blakistons Sons & Co.

Gilson, T. D., Asgar, K., and Peyton, F. A.: The quality of union formed in casting gold to embedded attachment metals, J. Prosthet. Dent. **15**:464-473, 1965.

Granger, E. R.: Practical procedures in oral rehabilitation, Philadelphia, 1962, J. B. Lippincott Co.

Grosser, D.: The dynamics of internal precision attachments, J. Prosthet. Dent. **3**:393-401, May, 1953.

Grubb, H. D.: Partial dentures with precision attachments, J. Am. Dent. Assoc. **42**:154-162, 1951.

Hollenbach, G. M., and Oaks, S.: Role of the precision attachment in partial denture prosthesis, J. Am. Dent. Assoc. **41**:173-182, 1950.

Hudis, M. M.: Dental laboratory prosthodontics, Philadelphia, 1977, W. B. Saunders Co.

Hugel, I. M.: Geriatrics and dental service, J. Prosthet. Dent. **1**:295-300, May, 1951.

Kornfeld, M.: Mouth rehabilitation: clinical and laboratory procedures, ed. 2, vol. 2, St. Louis, 1974, The C. V. Mosby Co.

Leff, A.: Precision attachment dentures, J. Prosthet. Dent. **2**:84-91, 1952.

Lorencki, S. F.: Planning precision attachment restorations, J. Prosthet. Dent. **21**:506-508, 1969.

Lucia, V. O.: Modern gnathological concepts, St. Louis, 1961, The C. V. Mosby Co.

McCall, J. O., and Hugel, I. M.: Movable removable bridgework, Brooklyn, 1950, Dental Items of Interest Publishing Co., Inc.

Mensor, M. C., Jr.: Classification and selection of attachments, J. Prosthet. Dent. **29**:494-497, May, 1973.

Miller, C. J.: Intracoronal attachments for removable partial dentures, Dent. Clin. North Am., pp. 779-789, 1963.

Morrison, M. L.: Internal precision attachment retainers for partial dentures, J. Am. Dent. Assoc. **64**:209-215, Feb., 1962.

Nally, J. N.: The use of prefabricated precision attachments, Int. Dent. J. **11**:196-216, 1961.

Ney Attachment Manual, Bloomfield, Conn., 1970, The J. M. Ney Co.

Ney Chayes Technic, Bloomfield, Conn., 1961, The J. M. Ney Co.

Peeso, F. A.: Crown and bridgework for students and practitioners, Philadelphia, 1916, Lea & Febiger.

Preiskel, H. W.: The use of internal attachments, Br. Dent. J. **121**:564-566, 1966.

Preiskel, H.: Precision attachments for free-end saddle prosthesis, Br. Dent. J. **127**:462-468, 1969.

Preiskel, H. W.: Precision attachments in dentistry, ed. 3, St. Louis, 1979, The C. V. Mosby Co.

Ray, G. E.: Precision attachments, ed. 2, Bristol, England, 1978, John Wright & Sons, Ltd.

Ripol, C.: Prostodoncia: conceptos generales, Mexico, 1976, Promoción y Mercadotecnia Odotológico, S.A. de C. V.

Robinson, W. J.: Bridge attachments permitting conservation of the pulp and tooth, Dent. Cosmos. **61**:1409-1414, 1920.

Schuyler, C. H.: An analysis of the use and relative value of the precision attachment and the clasp in partial denture planning, J. Prosthet. Dent. **3**:711-714, 1953.

Schweitzer, J. M.: Restorative dentistry, St. Louis, 1947, The C. V. Mosby Co.

Singer, F.: Improvements in precision-attached removable partial dentures, J. Prosthet. Dent. **17**:60-72, 1967.

Singer, F., and Schon, F.: Partial dentures, London, 1966, Henry Kimpton, Publishers, Ltd.

Steiger, A. A., and Boitel, R. H.: Precision work for partial dentures, Zurich, 1959, Buchdruckerei.

Stern Dental Co.: Precision attachment work. Part 1: Introduction to attachments: chair procedures, Mt. Vernon, N.Y., 1964, Sterndent Corp.

Stern Dental Co.: Precision attachment work. Part II: Laboratory procedures, Mt. Vernon, N.Y., 1964, Sterndent Corp.

Sterngold/APM: Procedure manual, Mt. Vernon, N.Y., 1975, Sterndent Corp.

Terrell, W. H.: Specialized frictional attachments and their role in partial denture construction, J. Prosthet. Dent. **1**:337-350, 1951.

Tsuka, T., Hamada, T., and Yamado, S.: Casting a gold alloy to embedded precision attachment metals, J. Prosthet. Dent. **42**:262-270, 1979.

Tylman, S. D., and Malone, W. F. P.: Tylman's theory and practice of fixed prosthodontics, ed. 7, St. Louis, 1978, The C. V. Mosby Co.

Weaver, S. M.: Comparison of bone structure under movable and nonremovable restorations, J. Am. Dent. Assoc. **15**:645-653, 1928.

Weaver, S. M.: Physiologically functioning saddles with precision attachments, Parts 1, 2, and 3, Dent. Items Interest **57**:39-45, 132-140, 214-221, 1935.

Weinberg, L. A.: Lateral force in relation to the denture base and clasp design, J. Prosthet. Dent. **6**:785-800, 1956.

Weinberg, L. A.: Atlas of removable partial denture prosthodontics, St. Louis, 1969, The C. V. Mosby Co.

Williams, A. G.: Technique for provisional splint with attachment, J. Prosthet. Dent. **21**:555-559, 1969.

Wilson, W. H., and Lang, R. L.: Practical crown and bridge prosthodontics, New York, 1962, McGraw-Hill Book Co.

# CHAPTER 17

# SWING-LOCK

JOE J. SIMMONS

**labial bar** The anterior metal portion of a Swing-Lock prosthesis that is connected to the lingual metal section by means of a precast metal hinge attachment. The end opposite the hinge attachment contains the latch attachment that closes and frictionally locks into the latch recess groove of the lock attachment, which is incorporated into the lingual metal section.

**labial opening arc (LOA)** The labial bar opens along an arc in a plane that is approximately 90 degrees to the lingual path of insertion (LPI), and its vertical axis of rotation is centered in the long axis of the hinge cylinder barrel.

**labial veneer (labiogingival tissue acrylic veneer)** Labial veneer is processed onto the labial bar. The combination veneer and bar are also referred to as the *Swing-Lock labial flange.*

**labial veneer wax try-in** A wax-up of the proposed labial veneer made of pink baseplate wax on the diagnostic cast or master cast to aid the dentist, patient, and technician in determining if a labial acrylic veneer is indicated esthetically and mechanically.

**lingual path of insertion (LPI)** A path determined by the tilt of the survey table with respect to the stylus of the surveyor as in the case of clasped partial dentures.

**lingual section** The metal lingual or palatal major connector of an S/L prosthesis and the attached saddle areas and minor connectors (if the teeth are to be replaced). The S/L hinge and lock attachments are attached mechanically to the lingual section during metal casting.

**lip-support wax index** A wax try-in made of pink baseplate wax that aids the technician in developing the correct thickness of the labial flange of the completed prosthesis to enhance lip contour and facial esthetics.

**maximum lip extension (line)** Line recorded by the dentist and marked on the diagnostic cast or master cast to show the maximum upper and lower lip extension. The upper line indicates the highest position of the upper lip during smiling. The lower lip position is obtained phonetically.

**retention loops** Metal projections in a retentive form (loop or mesh) on the labial bar that are attached during the wax-up. They serve the same purpose as the retentive mesh in the saddle area. Retention loops secure the processed acrylic labial veneer to the labial bar.

**S/L** Abbreviation for Swing-Lock.

**S/L attachments** The two types of S/L attachments are (1) the original and (2) Mini-hinge and Flat-back lock. They are available precast in metal or in hard plastic form to be cast.

**S/L hinge** The S/L hinge consists of two parts: (1) the hinge attachment (precast in metal) is embedded in the lingual wax-up and mechanically locked into this section during casting and (2) the labial bar portion of the hinge that is waxed over the hinge cylinder barrel of the precast metal attachment, which is cast into metal. The parts do not fuse together because a separating oxide is formed during burnout.

**S/L lock** This portion consists of two components: (1) the S/L lock precast metal attachment that is waxed into the lingual section and mechanically locked into this section during casting, and (2) the latch portion (lock-latch) that is waxed into the latch recess groove or the precast metal lock attachment and is cast into metal.

**struts** The rigid metal projections from the labial bar that engage the tooth apical to the greatest curvature (contour line) to provide retention. Struts can be placed in a deep undercut and provide retention and stability for the prosthesis. Struts usually are designed as T, I, and L types.

**Swing-Lock (S/L) partial denture** A removable partial denture that incorporates a hinged and locked (but releasable) labial bar that reciprocates with its lingual section to form a stable and rigid framework for replacing teeth and gingival tissues. The retention is such that unless the labial bar is manually unlocked, it cannot be dislodged by any combination of function or masticatory loads.

**thumb release groove (TRG)** A groove waxed into the labial bar near the latch attachment (always toward the hinge) that allows the patient to use a thumbnail or an instrument to disengage the latch from the lock to permit removal of the partial denture.

**thumb release projection (TRP)** The projection (away from the hinge) at the end of the labial bar used by the patient in unlocking and removing the partial denture.

**try-in struts** Struts placed either from the labial bar or incisally from a retention loop into an undercut area of an abutment tooth that ultimately will receive a full labial acrylic veneer to stabilize the framework for try-in. If the acrylic veneer would be too thick at this point after processing, the try-in strut would be temporary and removed after the framework try-in.

The Swing-Lock (S/L)® concept* adds a new dimension to removable partial dentures. The basic structure in all S/L appliances uses preformed metal hinge and lock precision attachments in a single casting. The resultant cast metal framework has a labial section that is movably hinged and locked to the lingual section (Figs. 17-1 and 17-2). These prostheses provide a number of advantages in prosthodontics, including excellent retention, positive removable splinting, and esthetic gingival tissue replacement (Swing-Lock Clinical Manual, 1969). Depending on the esthetic requirements, labial metal struts or a labial acrylic veneer is designed to passively engage all abutments. When forces are applied, such as in mastication, then all the abutments share the load.

---

*Swing-Lock® is the registered trademark of Idea Development Co., Inc., 5510 Abrams Rd., Dallas, Tex. 75214. U.S. patents 3,271,858 and 3,486,230; Canada, 809,917; France, 1,486,335; Great Britain, 1,131,948; Italy, 781,668; West Germany, P1541228.9; Japan, 44199/1966.

Framework rigidity has resulted in fewer pressure spot adjustments, which may be due to a reduction in the lateral displacement of the denture bases under functional load. Since there appears to be more uniform tissue loading vertically, the need for rebasing occurs less frequently. The S/L prosthesis can also be used to splint mobile abutments.

Since both metal struts and labiogingival veneer do not spring over an abutment to engage major undercuts, there has been little noticeable wear on abutments in properly designed prostheses. Test frameworks have been cycled, opened, and closed to the equivalent of 30 years of use without noticeable wear of the lock or hinge attachments (Swing-Lock Imagineering Design and Technique Manual, 1969).

Oral hygiene is facilitated, which improves the prognosis for retention of remaining teeth. There are no critical abutments in an S/L prosthesis, and the procedures required to replace any tooth lost at any time after delivery can be accomplished easily. S/L appliances have proved successful in a wide variety of applications: minimal or mobile abutments; unilateral abutments; tilted or irregular abutments; cleft palates; accident victims and patients receiving postcancer treatment; with crowns, jackets, and copings; replacement of lost gingival tissue; lip and facial recontouring; splinting of mobile teeth with or without tooth replacements; and esthetic replacement of lost gingival tissue due to recession or sur-

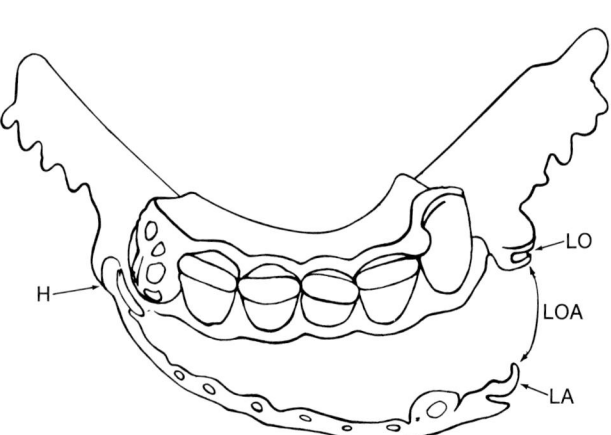

**Fig. 17-1.** S/L metal framework: *H,* hinge; *LO,* lock (in lingual section); *LA,* latch (on labial bar); *LOA,* labial opening arc.

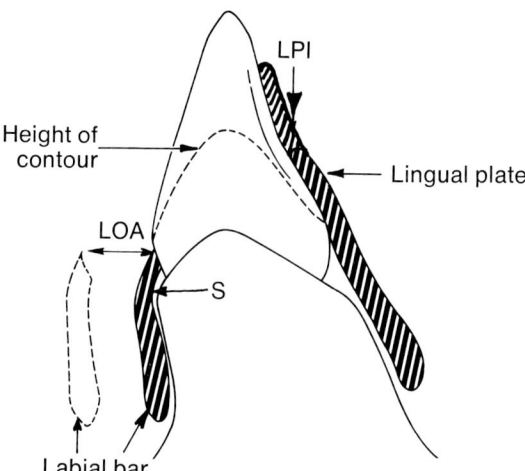

**Fig. 17-2.** Cross section of left canine abutment area showing details: appliance has been inserted along lingual path of insertion *(LPI),* with labial bar in position of dotted lines. Then, labial bar was closed and locked along *LOA* so strut *(S)* engages deep undercut apical to height of contour (survey line).

gery (Simmons, 1963; Swing-Lock Clinical Manual, 1969; Simmons, 1975; Antos, Renner, and Foerth, 1978).

## DENTIST AND DENTAL TECHNICIAN COOPERATION

To construct an S/L appliance, it is essential that the dentist and the laboratory technician understand as much as possible about the other's role and responsibility. Without this understanding, the results will not be as satisfactory. For instance, if the dentist does not know the requirements for the buccal undercut depth and design of a T strut to engage a casting, insufficient space or extension beneath the gingival tissue may be provided during tooth preparation. As a result, the technician may be unable to use it as an S/L abutment. Also, if the fixed partial denture technician is unaware of the metal design requirements of S/L abutments, the resulting crown may be technically unacceptable for use as an abutment in S/L partial denture construction. Obviously, there should be more than just a casual awareness between the various departments of the dental laboratory (design, metal finishing, fixed partial denture, ceramic, acrylic processing, and others) to avoid costly errors and remakes. If the technician does not know the reasons for the dentist using the recommended impression procedure or how to recognize a distorted frenum on the master cast, the S/L prosthesis will not fit as well (Swing-Lock Impression Technique Folder, 1969). There are many other reasons for technical and clinical failure that can be minimized through interdisciplinary cooperation. The Swing-Lock technique is one of the more advanced prosthetic techniques and requires considerable attention to detail by the dentist and dental technician if a satisfactory prosthesis is to be obtained (Sprigg, 1971).

## DIAGNOSTIC CASTS AND PRELIMINARY DESIGN

A stock tray and a plastic syringe are used to make an alginate impression, including the labial surfaces of the teeth and labial vestibule for diagnostic casts. The preliminary design is then outlined in pencil on the diagnostic cast. The dentist and technician(s) should communicate in planning the preliminary design. It is sometimes helpful to visualize placement of the attachments by placing them (either metal or plastic) on the outlined cast (Figs. 17-3 and 17-4). This cast is important to all who will be engaged in its design, fabrication, and clinical application. For instance, the S/L Mini-hinge plastic pattern can be placed on the cast to show the setup and acrylic finishing technicians that the attachment will be within the acrylic denture base and will not require any additional bulk. If bubbles occur on the master cast as occurred on the diagnostic cast in Fig. 17-4, a new master cast would be required. Fig. 17-3 shows the outline of the labial bar retention and

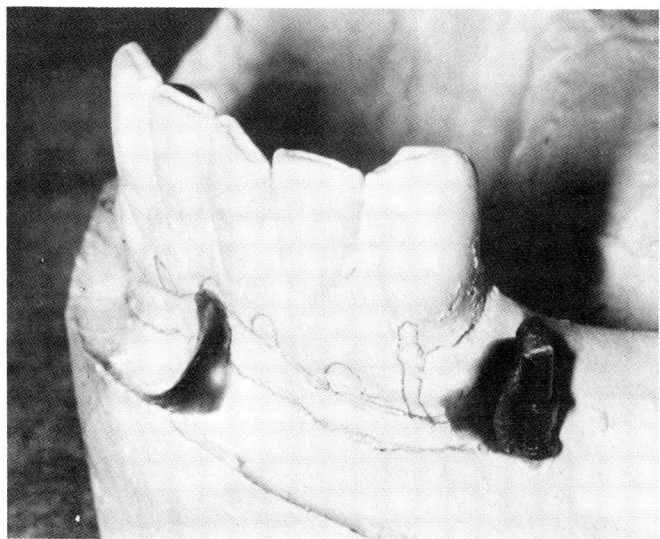

**Fig. 17-3.** Diagnostic cast with pencil outline of design and plastic Flat-back lock attachment positioned.

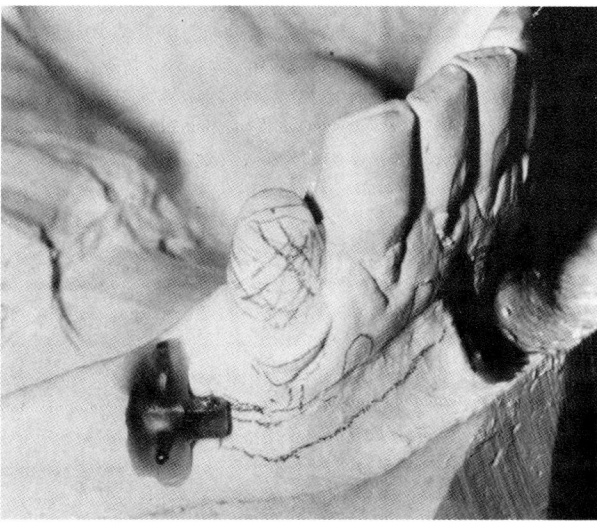

**Fig. 17-4.** Diagnostic cast with pencil outline of design, plastic Mini-hinge attachment positioned.

an I strut on the left canine. This I strut on the left canine is a try-in strut and will be cut off after the framework try-in and the jaw registration have been completed and before processing the labiogingival tissue acrylic veneer (Swing-Lock Technique Sheet Supplement to Swing-Lock Imagineering Design and Technique Manual for Veneering a Swing-Lock Partial, 1981). The plastic Flat-back lock attachment is waxed into a position that will require some wax relief on the master cast so as not to impinge the tissue on the canine eminence when the labial bar is closed and locked (Fig. 17-2). Note the wax over the midline labial frenum. Here, again, the dentist and dental technician must communicate with one another. If the frenum is heavy and very active, adequate relief should be provided. Less relief is needed for frena that are smaller and less active. No relief is required if frena are very weak or nonexistent.

## IMPRESSION TECHNIQUE PROCEDURE

The impression technique required for a successful S/L prosthesis is *absolutely essential* and different from that customarily used for a clasp-type partial denture. The essential difference between the two types of impression techniques is the need for accurately registering the interproximal spaces, labial vestibule, and frenum areas. Various impression techniques have been tried for making the master cast. Only one, however, will consistently produce a master cast with the unique requirements necessary for proper S/L prosthesis fabrication (Swing-Lock Impression Technique Folder, 1969). The recommended impression method involves the use of a large syringe to inject a heavy-bodied alginate into a custom acrylic tray. The impression registers with least distortion the full extension of the buccal vestibule, relaxed and undistorted midline and lateral frenum, and interproximal spaces. It also accurately registers the surfaces of the remaining teeth, crowns, or copings, including the labial and buccal surfaces adjacent to the gingival tissues.

## REQUIREMENTS OF MASTER CAST

It is mandatory that the master cast include the following essential requirements over those required for casts for other types of removable partial dentures:
1. An accurate impression of the labial and lingual surfaces of the teeth, including the interproximal spaces.
2. An accurate impression of the entire labial vestibule and frenum attachments in slight extension but not stretched or distorted beyond normal functional ranges.

### PROCEDURE

1. Make a diagnostic cast impression with a stock tray, taking care to inject with a plastic syringe or wipe with a finger into the labial vestibule areas. After separation and trimming of this cast, overlay 2 mm thickness of wet nonasbestos casting ring liner or paper towels of the same thickness on the remaining teeth and denture-bearing areas.
2. Form an autopolymerizing resin* with an adequate handle over the covered areas of this diagnostic cast. When it is set, wash out the relief or paper toweling thoroughly, and trim it to the approximate outline. Try the tray in the mouth, and trim the tray if indicated.
3. Spray or paint a coating of alginate adhesive† inside the thoroughly dried tray, and dry it with blasts of compressed air for 30 to 45 seconds. An alginate adhesive eliminates the necessity of perforating the tray for retention and greatly increases accuracy.
4. Use a heavy-bodied alginate,‡ mixed according to the manufacturer's instructions with a cool water mix to gain longer working time. Inject the alginate with a large plastic syringe§ or wipe it thoroughly into the interproximal spaces both labially and lingually and also into the labial vestibule and frenum areas to exclude most of the air entrapment. The prefilled acrylic tray is now inserted, carefully aligning the frenum notches. After the tray is seated, use light, upward on the lower, downward on the upper, finger pressure on the lip to border mold (similar to border molding with a complete denture impression). It is impossible to properly border mold the lips if a stock alginate or hydrocolloid tray is used.
5. Allow the impression to set up 1 or 2 minutes longer than usual, then grip the tray handle firmly with pliers, and remove it with one quick motion. Try not to rock or distort impression on removal.

---

*Fast Tray, Harry J. Bosworth Co., Skokie, Ill.; Tray Plastic, Coe Laboratories, Inc., Chicago, Ill.; Formatray, Kerr Manufacturing Co., Romulus, Mich.
†Hold, Getz-Opotow Division, Teledyne Dental Products Co., Elk Grove Village, Ill.
‡Super-Gel, Harry J. Bosworth Co., Skokie, Ill.; Jeltrate, The L. D. Caulk Co., York, Pa.
§Monoject, 35 ml, Sherwood Medical Industries, Inc., St. Louis, Mo.

## POURING THE MASTER CAST

### PROCEDURE

1. Immediately examine the impression, and reposition with cotton pliers any torn or distorted interproximal impression material tears. (With a heavy-bodied alginate, these interproximal tears can be fitted back together accurately.) Lightly sticky wax these repositioned tears.

2. After rinsing saliva from the impression, remove excess water and pour the impression immediately. If immediate pouring is not possible, store it in a humidor, and pour it within 10 minutes. If pouring is delayed longer than 10 minutes, gross distortions continue to such a degree that the dentist will have to remake the impression. Use an improved stone and vacuum mix if possible. Proportion the stone by weight according to the manufacturer's recommendations, mix it with water, and vibrate it carefully into the impression. Use the two-pour techniques as described in Chapter 4. The resulting quality and accuracy of the casts obtained by following these suggestions will be well worth the additional time required.

It is essential to the success of an S/L prosthesis that a high-quality master cast be used. The impression technique outlined is the only recommended proven technique to ensure an accurate master cast for an S/L prosthesis.

The use of reversible hydrocolloids is not recommended because of possible distortion caused by the stock water-cooled tray. Rubber base and silicone impression materials have not proved as useful as alginates because of the stretching and distortion that occurs in the interproximal spaces when they are removed, resulting in inaccuracies at the more critical areas for the S/L construction.

## EXAMINING THE MASTER CAST

First, examine the cast for any major distortion, bubbles, or chalky areas anywhere on the cast (Figs. 17-5 and 17-6). Remove small bubbles, and fill minor distortions in the denture-bearing areas. Next, examine the remaining teeth, copings, and crowns, paying particular attention to the lingual surfaces, gingival third, and interproximal spaces (if a labiogingival tissue veneer is contemplated). Very minor bubbles and irregularities may be removed. Major distortions, bubbles, voids, or fractures would necessitate a new impression and new master cast. Examine the entire labial vestibule (where the labial bar will be) for all of these defects, plus carefully note the position and possible distortion of the midline, labial frenum, and the lateral frenum (near the canines if present). If the recommended impression technique was followed, these frena will be undistorted and relaxed and the depth of the vestibule will be at its maximum.

### PROBLEM AREAS

If the proper impression technique is not used, the problems that will be present are too short a labial vestibule and a strained or distorted frenum. Not pouring the impression immediately or not vacuum mixing the stone carefully will result in

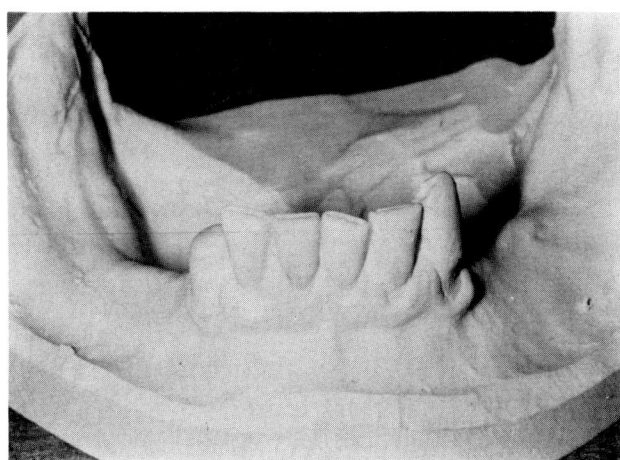

**Fig. 17-5.** Examine master cast carefully for distortions, bubbles, or chalky areas.

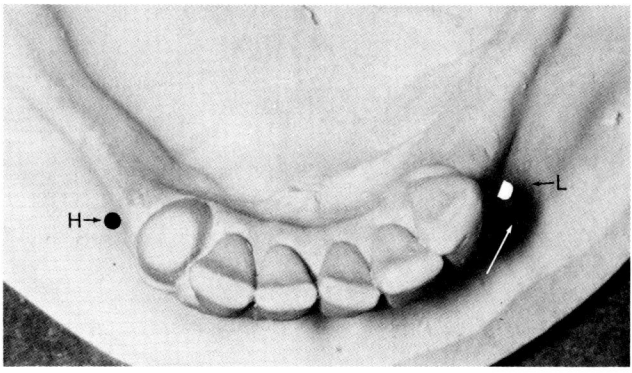

**Fig. 17-6.** Master cast with future hinge *(H)* and lock *(L)* position diagrammed.

**Table 17-1.** Examining the master cast

| Problem | Probable cause | Solution |
| --- | --- | --- |
| Labial vestibule short—not much space for labial bar (Fig. 17-67, A) | Master impression made in stock tray instead of custom tray; wrong impression material—probably hydrocolloid, silicone, or rubber base | Read this chapter or Swing-Lock Impression Technique Folder (1969) for proper requirements; remake impression by correct technique; pour cast immediately |
| Strained or distorted frenum | Same as above | Same as above |
| Distortions, bubbles, or imperfections in interproximal spaces on lingual or labial gingival third of teeth | Same as above or used correct impression technique but failed to pour master cast immediately and carefully | Same as above |
| Master cast looked good but finished appliance does not fit mouth well | Dentist followed recommended impression technique but failed to pour master cast immediately | Remake impression using recommended impression procedures, and use custom tray; pour master cast immediately after it is taken |
| Small bubbles and voids | Air entrapment from not using vacuum mix of stone; not carefully hand mixing and pouring stone | Remove small bubbles and fill small voids that are not in critical area (labiogingival third of teeth); use vacuum mix next time if at all possible; otherwise, hand mix, and pour cast immediately |

distortions, bubbles, or imperfections in the interproximal spaces. The cast will look good, but the finished appliance will not fit the mouth well. Use of the wrong impression material or a stock tray will make it impossible for the finished appliance to fit properly. These problems and their solutions are discussed in Table 17-1.

## DUPLICATE CAST

At least one stone duplicate cast should be made prior to blockout of the master cast and duplication to make the refractory cast. Two duplicate stone casts should be made if a labial veneer is contemplated.

## CASTING THE PLASTIC PATTERNS INTO METAL

Both the original S/L attachments and the Mini-hinge and Flat-back lock attachments can be purchased precast in Vitallium I,* eliminating this step.†

Fig. 17-7 shows the plastic patterns of the original hinge and lock. Several can be attached to the sprues of regular castings going through fabrication, or quite a number can be attached to a center sprue with auxiliary sprues and cast by themselves. During the investment phase, either vacuum or pressure invest or carefully hand paint your regular investment or Sepcoat* around the hinge cylinder barrel and into or over the dimples on either end. Also, hand paint into the latch recessed groove (LRG) in the lock attachment opposite the tail section (Fig. 17-12, B) and the recess groove in the Flat-back lock. The latch recess groove is where the latch attachment on the labial bar will be waxed later. Fig. 17-8 shows how the new Flat-back lock attachment patterns are received. The ten lock attachment patterns are already sprued and are ready for attaching to the main sprue of another casting. Examine the groove on the back of the Flat-back lock attachments (Fig. 17-9, right), and be sure it is clear of plastic flashing (Fig. 17-9, left). Plastic flashing can be removed with a sharp instrument. The new Mini-hinge attachment patterns are shipped with a plastic multiple sprue tray. All that is re-

---

*Vitallium I, Howmedica, Inc., Chicago, Ill.
†Precast attachments, Swing-Lock, Division of Idea Development Co., Inc., Dallas, Tex.

*Sepcoat, Howmedica, Inc., Chicago, Ill.

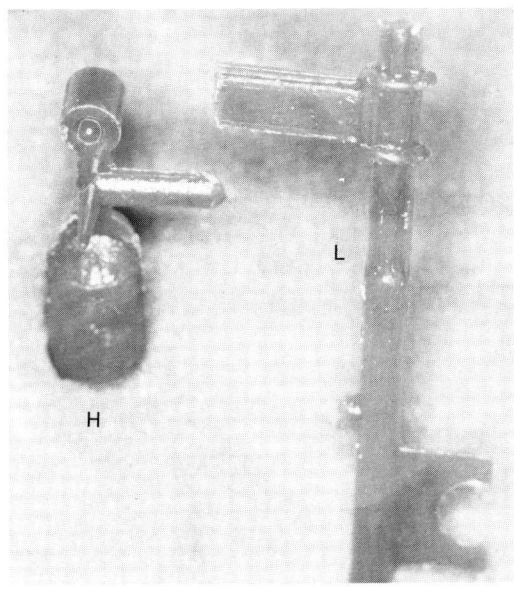

**Fig. 17-7.** Original S/L hinge *(H)* and lock *(L)* plastic patterns.

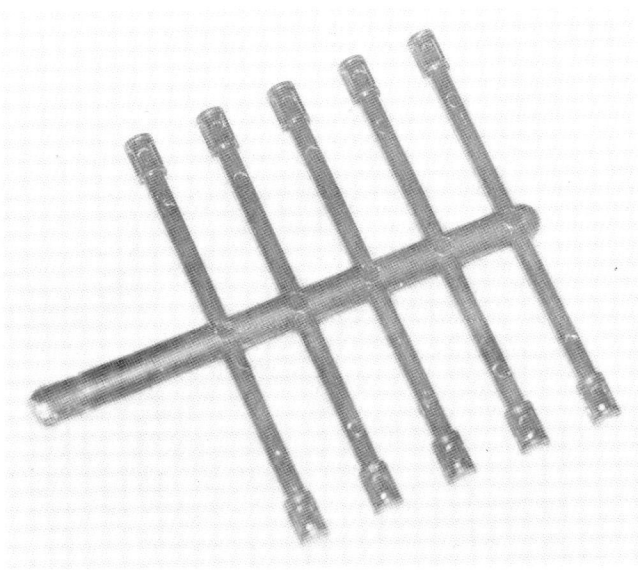

**Fig. 17-8.** S/L Flat-back lock attachment plastic patterns already sprued for investing.

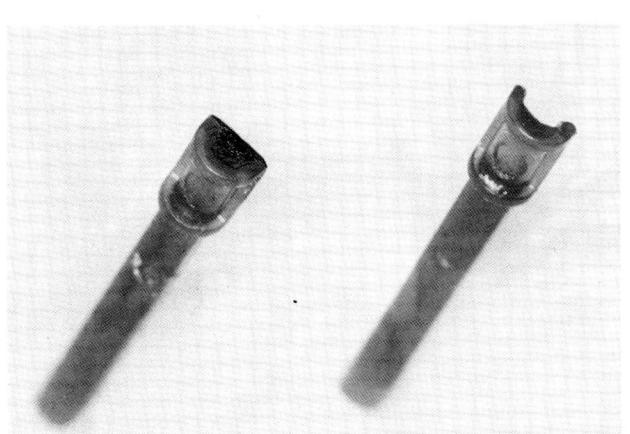

**Fig. 17-9.** Flat-back lock attachment pattern recess groove should be clear of flashing.

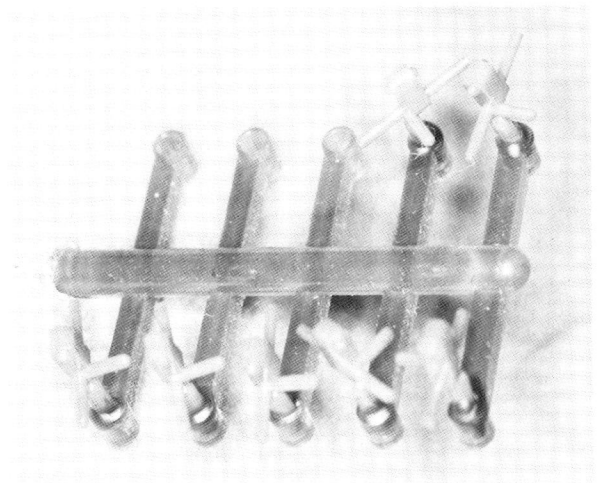

**Fig. 17-10.** Mini-hinge plastic patterns sticky waxed into sprue tray.

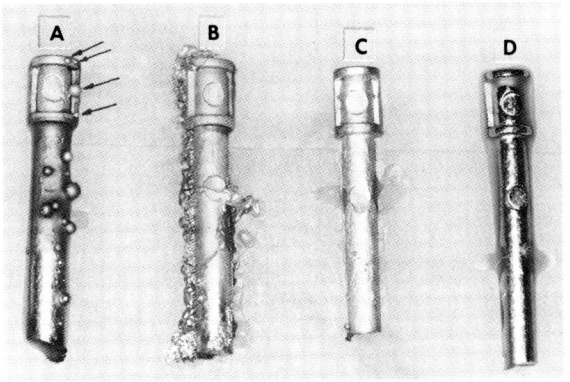

**Fig. 17-11.** Flat-back lock attachment castings.

quired is to place the round sprue ends of the ten Mini-hinges into the cups on the multiple sprue tray and lightly tack with wax (Fig. 17-10), with seven hinges placed and tacked in the tray cups. This multiple-hinge sprue tray can either be invested along with a regular casting or by itself. NOTE: Sometimes the burnout of a great many hard plastic patterns and sprues cracks the investment mold and causes a flashing around the castings (Fig. 17-11, *B*). If this happens, reduce the number of patterns being cast or lengthen the burnout time and raise the temperature very slowly.

## EXAMINING THE ATTACHMENT CASTINGS

Carefully examine your castings or those purchased precast in metal. It is advisable to use some type of magnification (3 to 8 power). Fig. 17-12, A, shows an original lock attachment casting that was improperly invested, and the resulting casting is unusable. Fig. 17-12, B, shows a proper casting after the tail section has been cut off and electropolished. If any small bubbles occurred in the only critical area of the lock, the latch recess groove (LRG), they can be removed if it can be done without changing the contour of the recess groove. Otherwise, the attachments should be returned for free replacement.* Fig. 17-12, C, shows a further refinement of the original lock attachment that allows tighter placement against the ridge. The tail section has been removed by cutting it off in the plastic pattern stage, and a groove has been cut in the metal attachment with a disk in the side away from the latch recess groove. This hand-modified design was so useful that it ultimately resulted in the newer Flat-back lock attachment (Fig. 17-11). The three original hinge castings in Fig. 17-13 are unusable. The one on the left has a bubble inside the hinge cylinder dimple. If incorporated into a final S/L prosthesis, the labial bar could not be opened. Hand finishing to remove this bubble must be extremely precise, or an odd egg shape will result. This also can cause freezing of the labial bar. The other two hinges have pitted areas on the hinge cylinder barrels and should never be used in a prosthesis. The only critical areas of either type of hinge (original or Mini-hinge) are the hinge cylinder barrel and the end dimples (either concave in the original or convex in the Mini-hinge). Bubbles elsewhere, such as in Fig. 17-14, will not make any difference in the completed framework and need not be discarded or returned for exchange.

The Flat-back lock attachment casting in Fig. 17-11, A, could be salvaged by removing only four small bubbles from the latch recess groove and the upper and lower flanges. The other bubbles on the alignment and investment retaining rod would not interfere in any way in waxing the cast attachment into the framework wax-up. In the attachment casting shown in Fig. 17-11, B, the flashing can be removed from around the latch recess groove and upper and side flanges, and it too can be used. If there is any doubt, however, it is best to return the miscast attachment for exchange. Fig. 17-11, C, shows a much better casting sandblasted. In Fig. 17-11, D, the attachment has been electropolished. Fig. 17-14 shows a Mini-hinge plastic pattern on the left and a

---

*Return to Swing-Lock, Division of Idea Development Co., Inc., Dallas, Tex., for exchange at no charge.

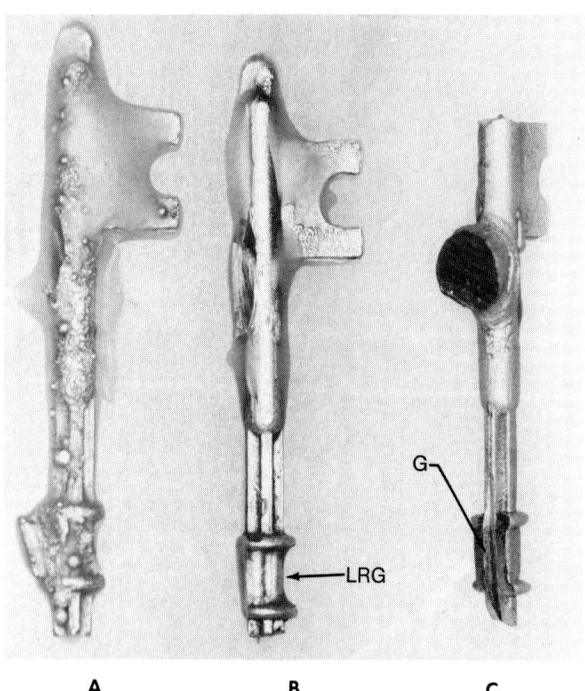

**Fig. 17-12.** Original lock attachment castings and suggested hand modifications for tighter placement against ridge. *LRG,* Latch recess groove; *G,* groove.

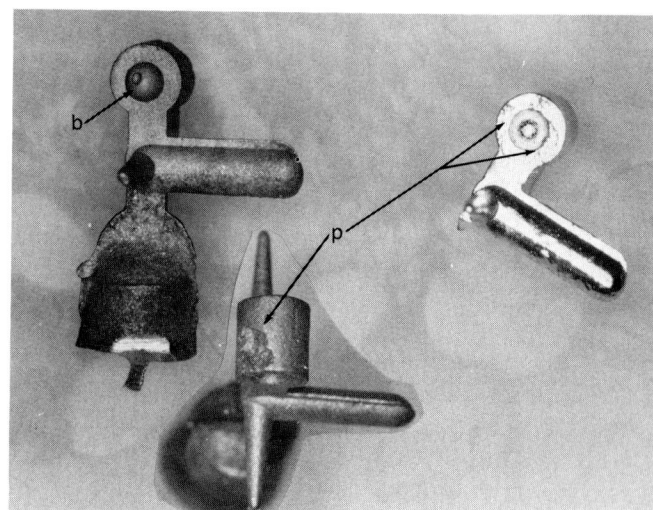

**Fig. 17-13.** Original hinge attachment investing and casting failures: *b,* bubble; *p,* pitted areas.

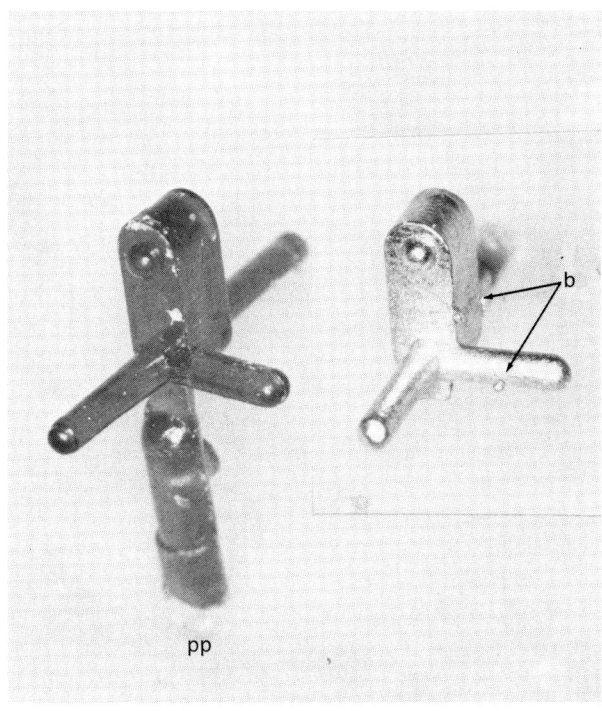

**Fig. 17-14.** Mini-hinge attachment plastic pattern *(pp)* and metal casting: *b*, bubbles.

completed and perfectly usable metal attachment on the right that has no defects in the only critical areas (around the hinge cylinder barrel and upper and lower convex projections). The bubbles on the investment retaining rod and body section of this attachment will not interfere in any way.

### PROBLEM AREAS

The most common mistakes in casting the attachments are failure to hand paint the investment material in and around the critical areas of the hinge and lock, too high a metal temperature, or too fast a burnout. Table 17-2 should be consulted for solutions to these problems.

**Table 17-2.** Examining the attachment castings

| Problem | Probable cause | Solution |
|---|---|---|
| Many bubbles on casting (Figs. 17-11, A, and 17-12, A) or in critical areas (Fig. 17-13, B) | Pressure or vacuum investing was not used; painting investment in and around critical areas was not done | Vacuum or pressure invest or hand paint investment into critical areas of both hinge and lock attachments |
| Flashing on attachment (Fig. 17-11, B) | Too fast burnout or too many plastic patterns invested at one time | Longer, slower burnout; put fewer plastic patterns with regular castings going through investing; reduce number of plastic patterns invested by themselves in one mold investment |
| Pitted castings (Fig. 17-13) | Defective plastic patterns; too high metal temperature; improper spruing during casting, causing shrink-back porosity | Carefully examine plastic patterns with magnification before investing; carefully sprue and do not cast with too hot a metal |
| Bubbles or defects in noncritical areas (Fig. 17-14) | Minor air entrapment | Not a problem; OK to use attachment |

## PLACEMENT OF ATTACHMENTS

An already discussed excellent method to visualize where to place the hinge and lock attachments is to use either the precast metal attachments or the plastic patterns used in Figs. 17-3 and 17-4. The plastic hinge pattern is luted with wax in the approximate position near the right canine coping. Note that the lower investment retaining rod was removed to obtain a closer fit against the ridge area. The tentative outline of the prosthesis has been drawn with pencil on the diagnostic cast. This pencil design shows the approximate position of the labial bar, T strut into the right canine coping undercut, retention loops (to hold the acrylic gingival veneer), amount of wax relief over the midline frenum (moderately muscled and active), and I strut into the left canine undercut. The Flat-back lock attachment plastic pattern is luted with wax in its proper position distal to the left canine. In this position, it will be within the normal confines of the finished acrylic resin denture base area and will not cause any additional bulk. If, however, this attachment was waxed into the wrong position (Figs. 17-17 and 17-20), it would work but would require additional bulk in the denture base acrylic resin and make an unnecessary bulge in this location for the patient. Carefully study the position of the lock attachment in Fig. 17-3. It is not waxed directly to the ridge and touching it. There is a small mound of wax approximately 0.5 mm thick between the back of the attachment and the ridge. It is necessary to review the fundamentals of S/L design to understand why. The labial bar in this case will pivot around the hinge cylinder, which is the forwardmost position of the plastic hinge attachment shown on the diagnostic cast in Fig. 17-4. In Fig. 17-6, looking down on the master cast, the dot distal to the right canine coping is the axis of rotation around the hinge cylinder barrel. The labial bar will pivot from this axis and swing toward the lock attachment (the white semicircle distal to the left canine). If this attachment were placed touching the ridge, the labial bar would contact the gingival tissue below the I strut on the left canine in opening and closing the prosthesis. The prosthesis would be a technical success but a clinical failure! To prevent this from happening, it is essential that a slight ridge of wax be made on the master cast (Fig. 17-15) before duplication and pouring of the refractory cast (Fig. 17-16).

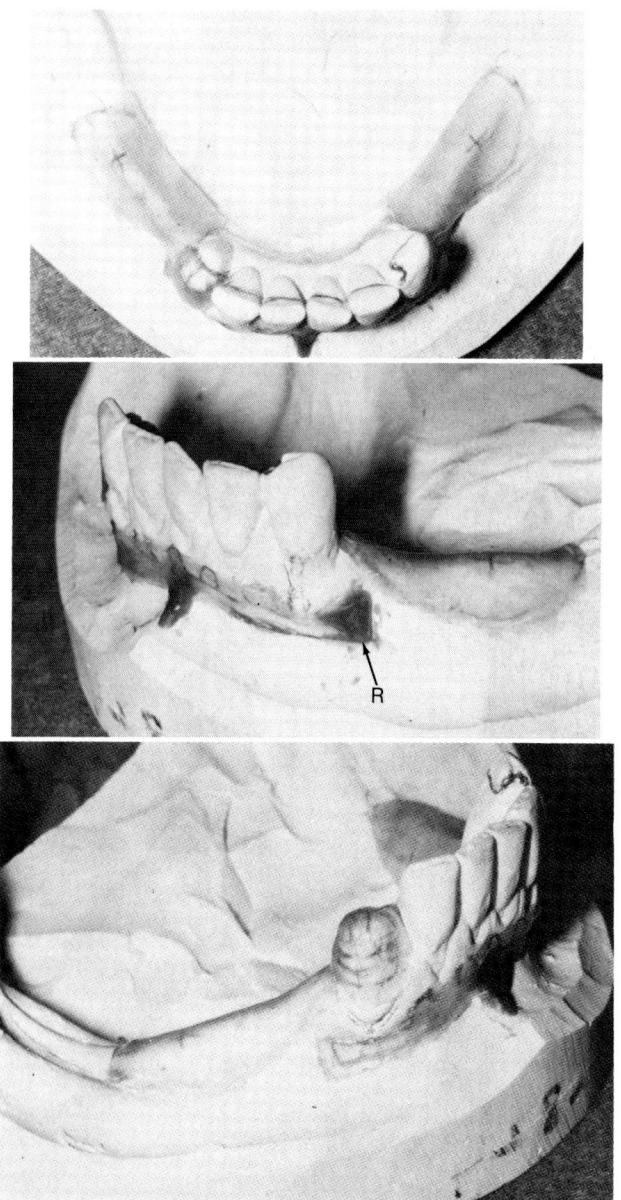

Fig. 17-15. Wax relief on master cast detailed.

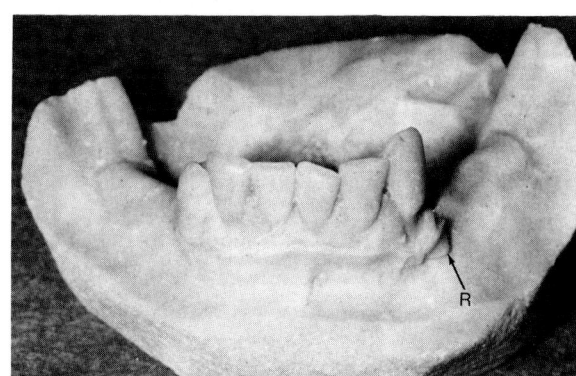

Fig. 17-16. Refractory cast. *R,* Relief area.

## PROBLEM AREAS

Improper placement of the attachments can cause impingement of the tissues in closing the labial bar and difficulty in opening and closing the labial bar (Table 17-3).

**Table 17-3.** Placement of attachments—waxing—spruing and investing—burnout and casting—freeing labial bar

| Problem | Probable cause | Solution |
| --- | --- | --- |
| Labial bar cannot be opened by any of suggested methods | Most common cause is heat-deformed hinge cylinder barrel (Fig. 17-23); use of deformed or out-of-round hinge attachment | Reduce casting metal temperature 50° to 75° Carefully examine plastic attachment before casting into metal; again examine metal attachment before waxing into lingual aspect |
|  | Bubble removal by hand in critical area of hinge resulted in out-of-round attachment | Do not attempt to hand finish any portion of critical area in hinge attachment, either original or Mini-hinge (send them back for free replacement) |
|  | Labial wax-up portion over hinge cylinder barrel covered too much of cylinder, would not allow for opening | Leave room in labial wax-up around hinge cylinder barrel for labial bar opening as detailed in Swing-Lock Imagineering Design and Technique Manual (1969) and Technique Sheet on Mini-hinge and Flat-back Lock Attachments (1977) |
|  | Labial and lingual wax-up not separated or fused together on casting with flashing between | If this is only reason for failure to open, cut metal apart where it is connected between labial and lingual sections; then open |
|  | Lock was set with too much locking action, making labial bar very hard to open (Fig. 17-43, 2) | If this is only reason labial bar will not open, then carefully grind away little at time, most distal portion of latch attachment (portion on labial bar) until labial bar can be opened |
| Labial bar opens with difficulty | Not long enough span in labial bar | Make labial bar design at least minimum span equal to four tooth widths; if shorter than this, there is not enough flexibility to allow latch to release from lock |
|  | Lock attachment set with too much locking action | Grind off some of most distal portion of latch attachment, little at time, to reduce functional locking action |
|  | Both labial and lingual section made too thick | Design and wax-up technicians should realize that S/L framework with its dual labial and lingual sections has tremendous inherent rigidity (I-beam effect) that allows both labial and lingual aspects to be much thinner than other types of frameworks |

*Continued.*

**Table 17-3.** Placement of attachments—waxing—spruing and investing—burnout and casting—freeing labial bar—cont'd

| Problem | Probable cause | Solution |
| --- | --- | --- |
| Labial bar has too much play | Hinge cylinder barrel underwaxed; too long burnout before casting allowing excess oxide formation | Remake and rewax hinge cylinder barrel as suggested in Swing-Lock Imagineering Design and Technique Manual (1969) and Technique Sheet on Mini-hinge and Flat-back Lock Attachments (1977); reduce burnout time |
| Porosity in labial bar | Too much heat and/or wrong sprue placements | Reduce metal casting temperature, and sprue wax-ups as in Figs. 17-60 and 17-62 and as outlined in Swing-Lock Imagineering Design and Technique Manual (1969) |
| Labial bar opens too easily | Latch not waxed completely into latch recess groove in lock attachment | Try simple adjustment procedure outlined in Swing-Lock Clinical Manual (1969) to increase locking action; sometimes groove can be milled into most distal portion (away from hinge) of latch recess groove of lock attachment and latch slightly bent so that frictional retention is improved; recast only labial bar portion of framework on duplicate investment cast |
|  | Lock attachment set without enough retention (Figs. 17-20 and 17-43, 3) | Try milling groove as suggested, then if enough retention is obtained, stop; if not, deepen groove and section away labial bar and try recasting labial bar; if this fails, then framework will have to be completely remade, but with proper setting of lock attachment for retention |
|  | Lingual plate or bar so thin that lateral displacement occurs and allows lock-latch combination to release (rare) | In remake, strengthen lingual section |
|  | Labial bar so thin that its excessive flexibility allows it to release under function (rare) | In remake, strengthen labial bar |
| Labial bar rubs against tissue part of stone cast when closing | No wax relief was used (Fig. 17-15) | Visualize where labial bar will swing along labial opening arc, and design lock attachment placement slightly away from ridge so labial bar will not rub against the cast (Fig. 17-6) |

## BLOCKOUT OF THE MASTER CAST

Fig. 17-15 shows the completed relief waxing on the master cast, top, right, and left labial views. Except for the labial frenum and the previously explained ridge of wax for the lock attachment, the remainder of the wax on the labial section is thin (30 gauge or less). The saddle areas are waxed as usual. The coping has 30-gauge wax relief. The lingual section is as usual, except less lingual tissue relief is applied because there is much better stability and less settling and movement of the lingual plate or bar than a clasp-type partial denture. Note that half of the occlusal and lingual surface of the coping is not relieved. This acts as an occlusal stop and a lingual brace for try-in. No wax relief is given to the lingual aspect of the teeth or interproximal spaces. The completed refractory cast (Fig. 17-16) has been coated with refractory cast dip and is now ready for waxing.

## WAXING THE FRAMEWORK

Fig. 17-17 shows the refractory cast with the lingual wax-up as originally completed and the metal precast Mini-hinge and Flat-back lock attachment waxed into this lingual portion. Even though this framework could now be completed by waxing and finishing the labial bar section, it probably would be functional, but neither the hinge nor the lock attachment are in their best possible positions. The axis of the hinge cylinder barrel (Fig. 17-17, dashed line) is not parallel with the vertical alignment rod of the lock attachment (solid line). Only one investment retaining rod is available to help hold the hinge attachment into the mold investment (Fig. 17-18). The lower rod has been properly removed but the upper one is completely embedded in the lingual wax-up. If the hinge were left at this angle, the labial bar would swing upward in opening but would probably still function. The attachments do not have to be exactly parallel in order to function. In fact, there is about a 15-degree variable in which function will not be seriously hampered. A more symmetrical and better functioning prosthesis is obtained when the labial bar swings in a plane more parallel to the plane of occlusion.

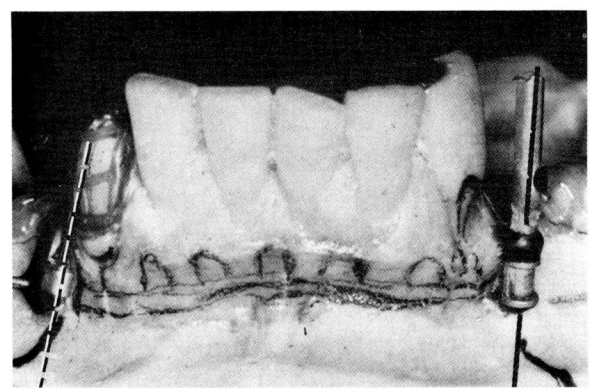

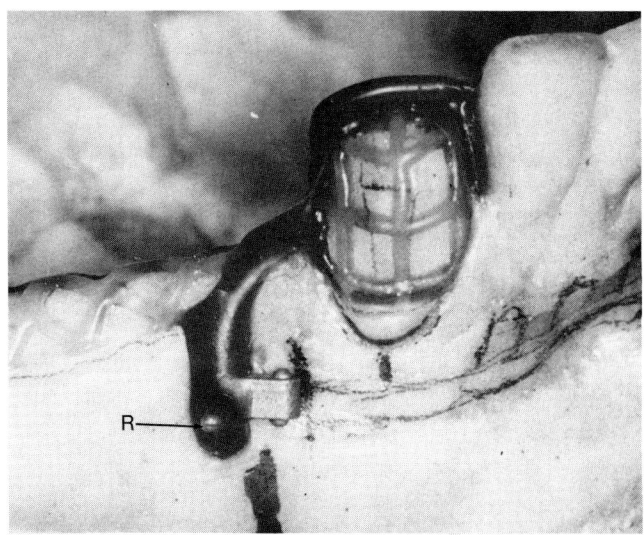

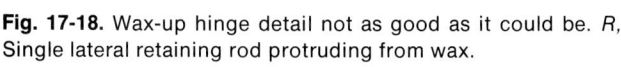

**Fig. 17-17.** Completed lingual wax-up showing poor placement of both hinge and lock attachments.

**Fig. 17-18.** Wax-up hinge detail not as good as it could be. *R*, Single lateral retaining rod protruding from wax.

**504** *Dental laboratory procedures: removable partial dentures*

## SPRUING AND INVESTING

Place at least two 8- to 10-gauge sprues to the lingual portion and two 10-gauge sprues to the labial section. The labial section sprues should be as close to the attachments as possible and enter the labial section at approximately 90 degrees with a slight wax thickening added to the area where it enters the labial section (Figs. 17-60 and 17-62). Hand paint investment or Sepcoat between the labial and lingual wax-ups around the hinge and lock attachments. Complete the mold investment in the usual manner.

Usually, a technician can "eyeball" the alignment much closer than the 15 degrees allowable. Fig. 17-19 shows the recommended correction in the wax-up of the hinge attachment. The hinge cylinder barrel is now parallel with the vertical alignment rod of the lock attachment. Two of the investment retaining rods on the hinge are sticking out of the lingual wax that will better secure this attachment in the mold investment and prevent slippage during burnout and casting. In Figs. 17-17 and 17-20, the lock attachment is improperly set two ways: (1) it is not set in the same position as was the plastic pattern on the diagnostic cast (Fig. 17-3) and (2) it is a little too far forward and will not fit inside the normal contours of the finished acrylic saddle outline (Fig. 17-20, dashed line). The flat-back portion of the lock attachment is not set correctly in respect to the labial bar at this location (solid line). If this framework was completed with this improper setting of the flat-back portion of the lock attachment, then the latch (the portion on the completed labial bar) may not have enough frictional or undercut action to allow locking of the labial bar, or it may engage slightly but be easy to unlock during functional loads. The flat-back portion should always be at least parallel to the labial bar wherever it is placed. Fig. 17-21 shows the new recommended position of the lock attachment. To assure good locking action, the flat-back portion of the lock attachment has been set so the lines are converging anteriorly about 5 degrees. Fig. 17-19 shows both the hinge and lock in their new changed positions ready to receive the labial bar portion of the wax-up. Fig. 17-22 shows details of the completed labial bar wax-up.

### PROBLEM AREAS

In waxing the framework, great care must be taken in proper placement and setting of the attachments; otherwise, a number of problems can occur, such as a frozen labial bar or one that will not lock (Table 17-3).

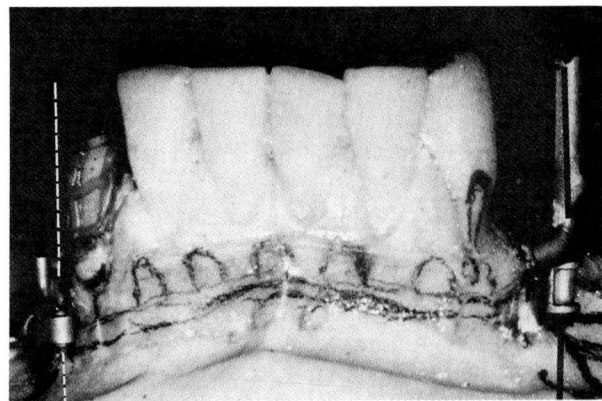

**Fig. 17-19.** Completed lingual wax-up with proper placement and alignment of both hinge and lock attachments.

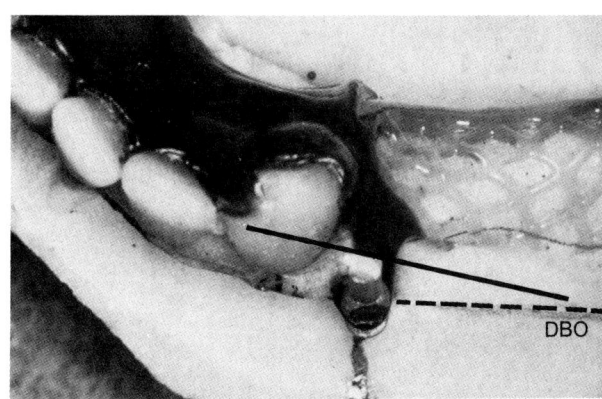

**Fig. 17-20.** Wax-up lock detail—improper setting for locking action. *DBO*, Denture base outline.

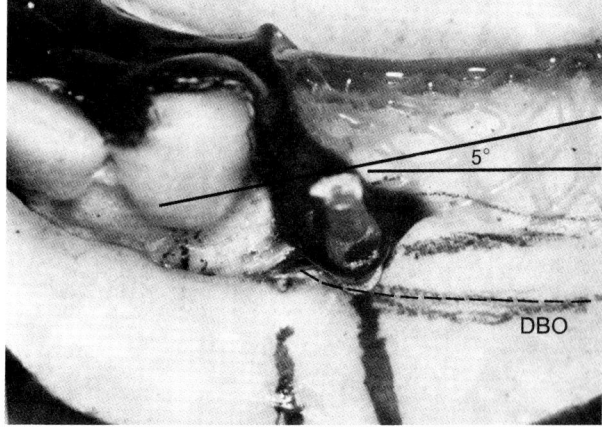

**Fig. 17-21.** Wax-up lock detail—corrected setting of flat portion of lock attachment. Now it is within normal denture base outline *(DBO)*.

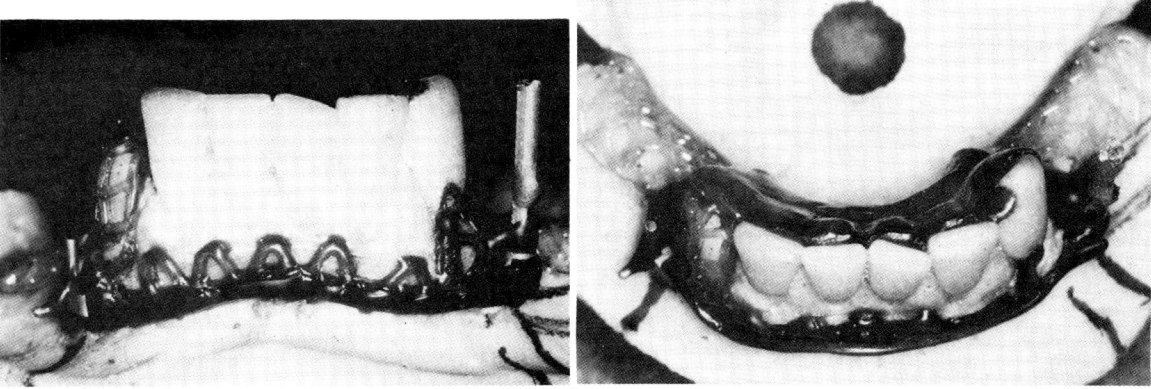

Fig. 17-22. Completed lingual and labial bar wax-up.

## METAL REQUIREMENTS

The ideal metal for S/L construction is one that has the following characteristics (chromium-cobalt metals meet all these requirements):
1. Rigidity. Allows for an ultrathin framework.
2. Nonflexibility. Flexibility is not necessary, since engaging any undercut for retention in an S/L prosthesis does not require a flexible arm (clasp action).
3. Extreme hardness. Resists wear or burnishing of the attachments that could result in labial bar looseness.

## S/L SINGLE CASTING TECHNIQUE

The S/L single casting technique requires only one refractory cast, one mold investment, and one casting to create both labial and lingual sections of an S/L metal framework. Both are cast simultaneously. Over 97% of S/L prostheses are cast using this technique.

## S/L DOUBLE CASTING TECHNIQUE

The S/L double casting technique requires two refractory casts, two mold investments, and two separate castings to create the labial and lingual sections of an S/L prosthesis. The lingual section is cast first, and the labial bar is waxed to the cast metal lingual section on a duplicate refractory cast and cast last. The first wax-up of the lingual section incorporates either metal or plastic hinge and lock attachments or a combination of both metal and plastic.

## BURNOUT AND CASTING

In general, all S/L framework mold investments should be brought to proper oven temperature and cast as soon as possible with little or no heat soaking. This applies to all types of metals and heating

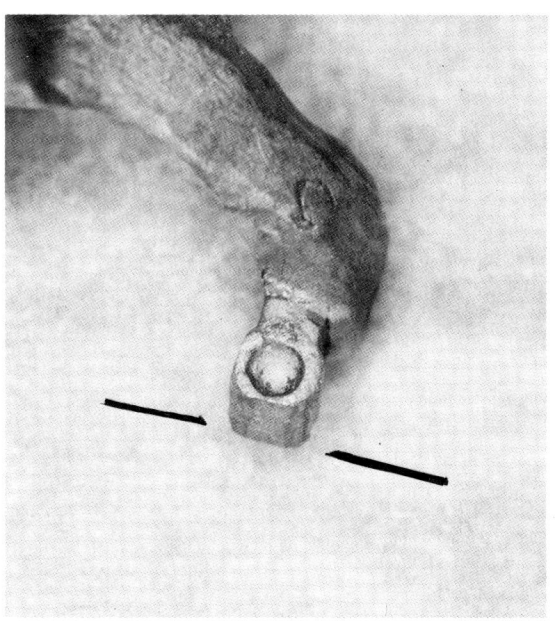

Fig. 17-23. Deformed hinge attachment cylinder due to excessive temperature of casting metal.

ovens. A long slow burnout with a long soaking time will produce excessive oxidation on the precast attachments and can possibly result in a loose labial section, both at the lock and hinge attachments. Plan to cast S/L castings first if a number of castings are to be done at one time. Laboratories using high-heat cobalt-chromium metals such as Vitallium* should be especially cautious not to exceed the burnout temperature of 2150° F (1176.5° C) and should also be careful not to heat the metal any more than necessary to cast. Failure to do so can result in a deformed hinge cylinder and the inability to open the casting (Fig. 17-23). If a frozen cast-

---
*Vitallium, Howmedica, Inc., Chicago, Ill.

ing is encountered, it is always wise to dissect the labial bar carefully away from the hinge attachment and see if this type of heat distortion of the hinge cylinder has occurred. If so, reduce the casting temperature of the metal at least 50° to 75° F on the next casting. To keep the near perfect tolerances ($\pm 0.003$ inch) of these cylinders, it is also strongly recommended that the hinge attachment patterns be vacuum invested or pressure invested and never hand finished.

## FREEING ATTACHMENTS—OPENING THE LABIAL BAR

Sandblast, electropolish, and cut sprues and flashings on castings that may cross over between the labial and lingual aspect around the hinge and lock attachments before attempting to open the prosthesis (Fig. 17-60). The following methods will free the attachments:
1. Use an oxide-cutting penetrating oil liberally around both the hinge and lock attachments.
2. Use a "knocker" such as an off-center lathe chuck.
3. Spot reheat with an alcohol torch or soldering iron the latch and labial portion of the hinge attachment.
4. Use an instrument to pry open the lock-latch combination.

Favorite methods will ultimately be selected that will become routine. If any difficulty is encountered on the first few castings, be sure to read and study Table 17-3.

### PROBLEM AREAS

When there is difficulty opening the labial bar, the most common cause is a heat-deformed hinge cylinder barrel, but it can also be caused by problems associated with too much wax over the hinge cylinder barrel, improper waxing of the labial and lingual areas, improper setting of the lock, or hand modification of the hinge in the critical area of the cylinder barrel. Also, if there is not enough of a span in the labial bar or if the labial and lingual section are too thick, there will be difficulty in opening the labial bar.

Porosity in the labial bar is caused by overheating the metal during casting or the wrong sprue placements. If the labial bar opens too easily, the latch may have not been waxed completely into the latch recess groove of the lock attachment or the lock attachment was improperly set. Although it is rare, lateral displacement can occur if the lingual plate or bar is too thin, allowing the lock-latch combination to release during function. If wax relief is not properly used, it can cause the labial bar to rub against the tissues (Table 17-3).

## FINISHING AND POLISHING

For finishing and polishing techniques, refer to Chapter 11.

## COMPLETED FRAMEWORK (PREFITTED ON THE CAST)

After the metal framework has been finished and polished and fitted back on the original master cast, any interference on the lingual aspect should be relieved before trying to close and lock the labial bar on the master cast. Figs. 17-24 and 17-25 show top views of the completed framework opened for insertion and closed and locked on the master cast. Figs. 17-29 and 17-30 show the framework opened and closed and locked off the model but from the underside. Fig. 17-26 is a detailed magnification of the hinge side, and Figs. 17-27 and 17-28 show similar views in detail of the lock side opened and closed and locked.

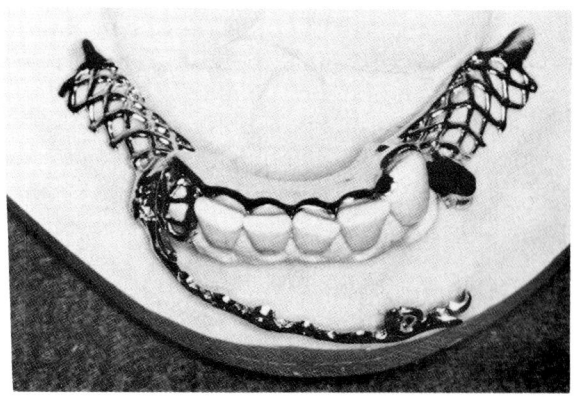

**Fig. 17-24.** Completed metal framework inserted on master cast, along lingual path of insertion with labial bar open.

Swing-Lock

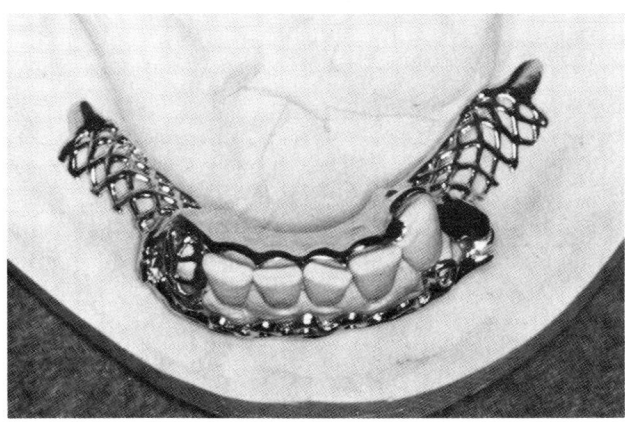

Fig. 17-25. Completed metal framework inserted on master cast, and labial bar closed and locked.

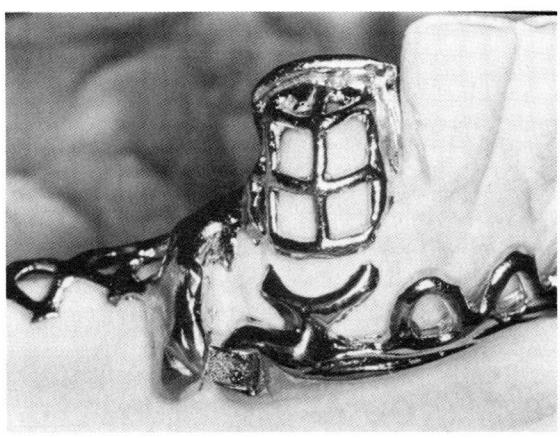

Fig. 17-26. Details of hinge side of framework on master cast—labial bar closed and locked.

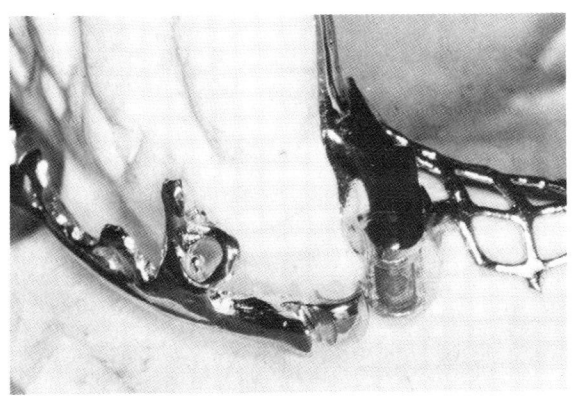

Fig. 17-27. Details of lock side of framework on master cast—labial bar open.

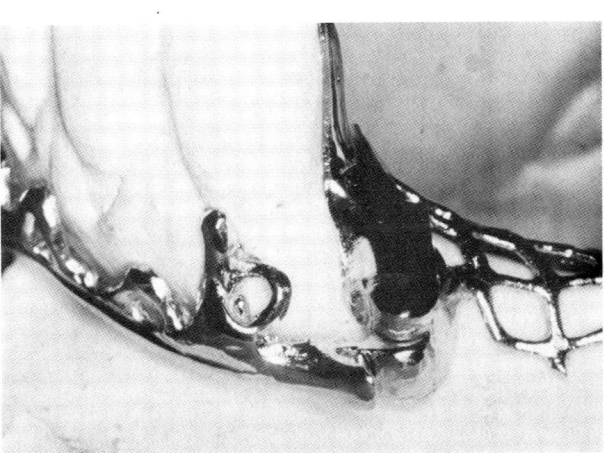

Fig. 17-28. Details of lock side of framework on master cast—labial bar closed and locked.

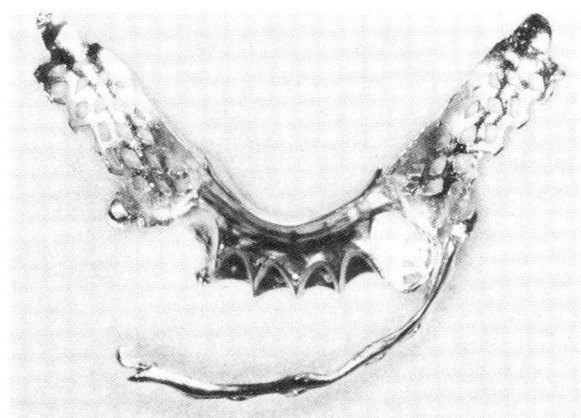

Fig. 17-29. Finished metal framework from underside—labial bar open.

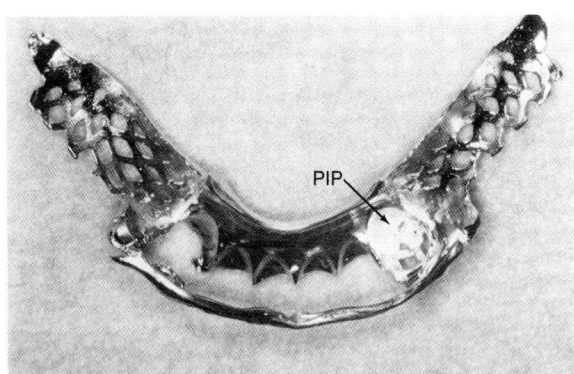

Fig. 17-30. Finished metal framework from underside—labial bar closed and locked. *PIP*, Pressure indicating paste.

## ADJUSTMENTS

Adjust struts of the framework for contact only, using no pressure, after making sure the labial bar will close and lock on the cast. When adjusting multiple struts for contact only, start with the one nearest the hinge and proceed to the lock. If the framework has too much or too little locking action between the lock-latch attachments, the very simple adjustment recommended in the Swing-Lock Clinical Manual (1969) should be tried.

## FRAMEWORK TRY-IN

The completed and adjusted (on the master cast) framework should now be sent to the dentist for try-in in the patient's mouth and for further adjustments if needed. The white pressure indicating paste (PIP)* was used in the overlay coping (Fig. 17-30) to indicate where it had to be relieved after try-in in the patient's mouth. This one high spot kept the lingual framework from seating perfectly and thus would not allow the labial bar to be completely closed and locked. Then the framework could be inserted into the patient's mouth, lingual portion first, seated all the way down, and the labial bar should be closed and locked (Fig. 17-31). This try-in in the patient's mouth should not be eliminated. It is important that the lingual framework be completely seated in the mouth. If it is not, the completed prosthesis will never be seated properly, and the labial bar will not lock or will lock so poorly that the prosthesis will open under functional loads.

### PROBLEM AREAS

If the framework does not seat properly on the cast and the labial bar will not close and lock, it is usually due to interferences in the lingual section or under the labial bar (Table 17-4).

---

*Mizzy, Inc., Clifton Force, Va.

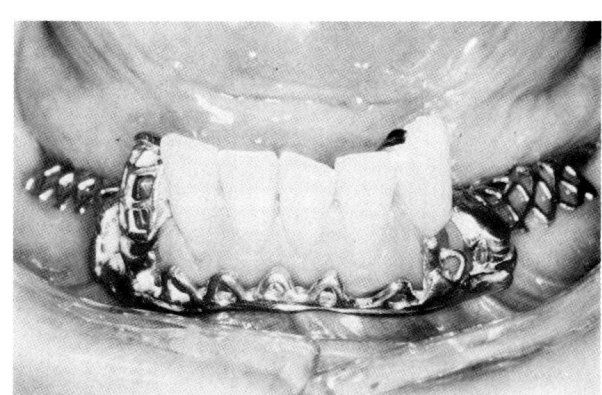

**Fig. 17-31.** Adjusted framework completely seated along lingual path of insertion and labial bar closed and locked.

**Table 17-4.** Completed framework prefitted on the cast

| Problem | Probable cause | Solution |
|---|---|---|
| Labial bar will not close and lock | Lingual framework not completely seated | Reduce all interferences in lingual section so it seats all the way down before attempting to close labial bar |
| | Lingual framework completely seated, but some interferences remain under labial bar preventing complete closure and locking | Reduce any interferences under labial bar, then close and lock with increasing pressure, starting at hinge and proceeding to lock. Check to be sure struts have contact only—no pressure |

## JAW RELATION REGISTRATION

The framework has been prefitted on the master cast by the technician and adjusted properly in the patient's mouth by the dentist. The metal framework can now be used as the best possible base for any type of final jaw relation registration (either functional or static). Fig. 17-32 shows where pink baseplate wax was luted to the lingual retention mesh and a bite registration was obtained using the excellent retention, rigidity, and stability inherent in the S/L framework.

## MOUNTING THE FRAMEWORK

The maxillary and mandibular casts are mounted in an articulator using the jaw relation registration that has been obtained using the S/L framework.

## SETUP AND FINISHING

The routine laboratory procedure is used in setting up and waxing the posterior teeth and saddle areas. It is advisable to try in this setup before processing and finishing the saddle area on one of the duplicate stone casts made before adding the wax relief on the master cast. It is always a good idea to try in the processed and finished saddle areas before processing and finishing the labiogingival tissue veneer on the second duplicate stone cast (Fig. 17-33). This try-in serves the following purposes:

1. It allows visual checking before the labial veneer is processed to the labial bar. This ensures that the completed lingual portion is completely seated and no interferences are present in the acrylic resin of the denture bases which would prevent complete seating along the lingual path of insertion.
2. Any pressure spots or sharp areas in the saddle acrylic can be relieved and marked for polishing at this stage, thus eliminating this step at delivery.
3. Adjustment of deflective contacts in the occlusion can also be accomplished now.

## CONSTRUCTING AND FINISHING LABIOGINGIVAL TISSUE ACRYLIC VENEER
### PROCEDURE

1. *Duplicate stone casts of the master cast.* If the master cast has not been duplicated twice, as suggested previously, it should be done now (after removing the wax relief). Use one stone cast duplicate to process the denture base areas. Use another stone cast duplicate, at least the tooth-bearing portion of it, in processing the labial veneer (Fig. 17-34).

2. *Outline the veneer on the cast.* Using a soft No. 2 lead pencil, outline the area where the acrylic will be to form the labiogingival tissue acrylic veneer. This soft pencil line will usually be trans-

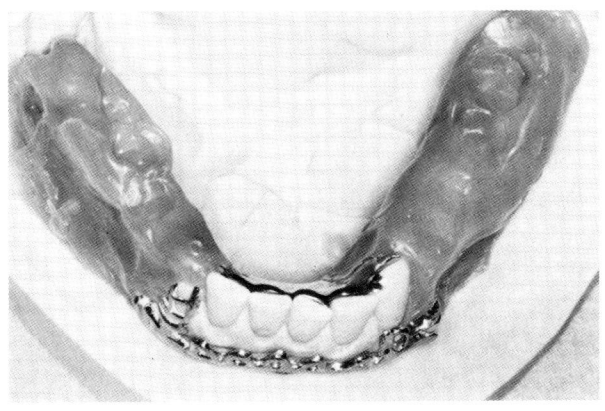

**Fig. 17-32.** Completed jaw relation record using rigid stable framework, locked on master cast for mounting.

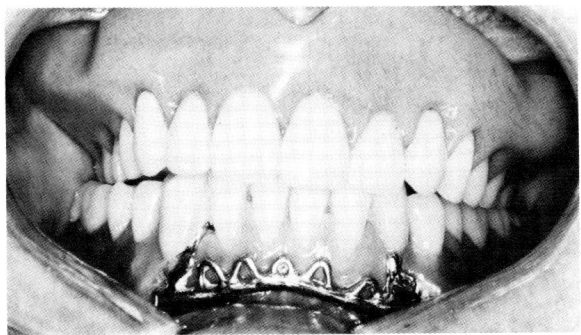

**Fig. 17-33.** Posterior section processed, finished, and tried in mouth before completion of labial gingival tissue veneer.

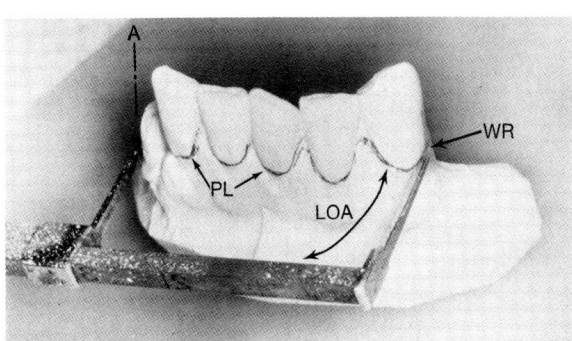

**Fig. 17-34.** Surveying for tooth undercuts on duplicate cast from labial opening arc. Pencil outline acts as trimming guide after processing of acrylic resin. *A,* Axis of rotation; *PL,* soft pencil line; *LOA,* labial opening arc (arrow); *WR,* wax relief.

ferred to the processed acrylic and can be helpful in trimming and finishing the acrylic veneer.

3. *Wax out undesirable undercuts.* The labiogingival tissue acrylic veneer will be swinging in an arc around the axis A (the hinge location) (Fig. 17-34). The paralleling instrument shown in Fig. 17-34 is also approximately the same plane as the labial bar swings. Other instruments that can be used in this survey of possible undercuts are a drafting compass or a Boley gauge. By holding this instrument with one end stationary at the approximate axis of rotation of the labial bar and then swinging it into each interproximal space one at a time (by shortening the distance between the parallel pointers), one can visualize where wax relief will be necessary before the acrylic is processed to the model. The area just distal to the left canine is the only place on this cast that requires wax relief. Note that such relief is always on the tooth side away from the hinge position, never toward it. If some area was not relieved at this stage, it should be done by trimming the acrylic veneer during prefitting back on the master cast.

4. *Make a final check of the labial bar before acrylic processing.* Check the acrylic retention loops or mesh for length, contour, and thickness. Allow at least ¼ mm of space under the retention loops toward the cast so that the acrylic completely encompasses these loops for retention. Remove the try-in struts that were used for the framework try-in in the mouth. Fig. 17-33 shows a try-in strut above the retention loop touching an undercut area on the left canine. Fig. 17-35 shows that this strut has been removed. If the strut were left in this location, the acrylic veneer would have to be excessively thick. Metal-to-tooth contact is not required or desired in this case. The entire labial bar has been sandblasted to enhance retention of the pink opaque material to be applied next.

5. *Opaque the labial bar.* To avoid any show through of metal in the acrylic veneer, carefully paint a thin coat of a pink opaque* on all areas of the labial bar framework that would show through the acrylic (Fig. 17-36). Obviously, only the front of the metal needs to be painted. Allow this opaque to dry while the next step is completed.

6. *Coat the duplicate cast with separator.* Place the completed framework with the processed and finished saddle areas back on the duplicate cast after tinfoil substitute† has been applied and the excess shaken off lightly (Fig. 17-37). Soak it for at least 5 minutes in cool water to thoroughly wet the cast.

7. *Coat the acrylic with a separator.* Fig. 17-37 also shows where a collodian acrylic separator‡ has been applied to the areas of the already finished acrylic, finished coping overlay on the right canine, right saddle flange, and left first premolar and saddle flange. This collodian separator is best applied

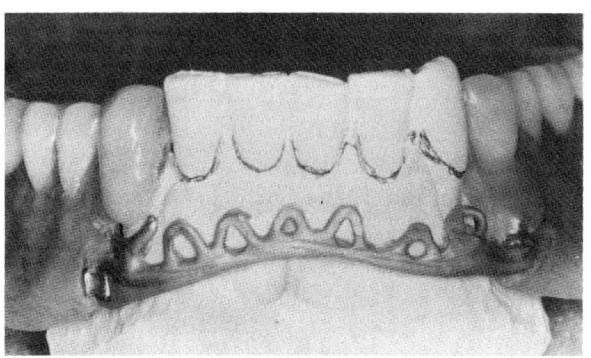

**Fig. 17-35.** Retention strut cut off, and labial bar sandblasted to help retention of opaque and acrylic resin.

---

*Vinyl Opaquer Pink No. 3527-13, Pink Opaque, Howmedica, Inc., Chicago, Ill.
†Modern foil, Modern Materials Manufacturing Co., St. Louis, Mo.
‡Luxene Vinyl Denture Base Separator (red) No. 3505-09, Howmedica, Inc., Chicago, Ill.

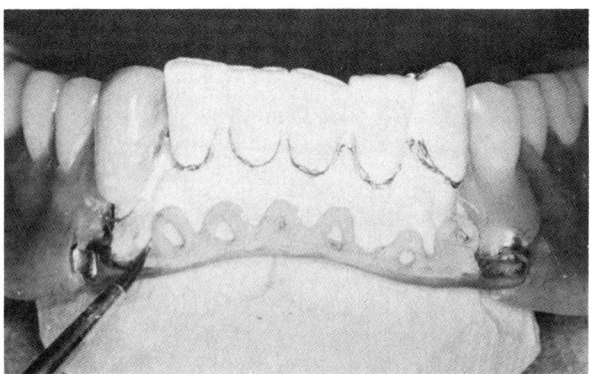

**Fig. 17-36.** Applying pink opaque to labial bar to help hide metal structure.

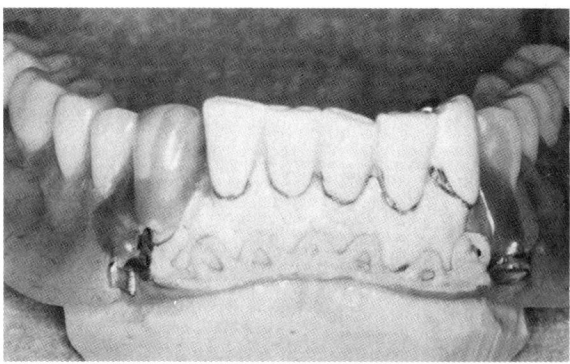

**Fig. 17-37.** Coating cast and finished acrylic resin with separators. Cast has been soaked in slurry water.

with a fine sable brush. Dip the brush into alcohol first, then into the separator, and paint the finished acrylic flanges and teeth wherever the labial acrylic veneer might possibly touch.

8. *Wax out the hinge and lock attachments.* In Fig. 17-38, pink baseplate wax has been applied to cover the hinge and lock-latch attachments. This is necessary to prevent freezing the labial bar by accidently processing acrylic into or around these attachments. Be sure also that there are no undetected undercut areas in the finished acrylic saddles that could mechanically lock the finished labial veneer to these areas, thus preventing the opening of the labial bar after processing. Also block them out if they exist.

9. *Add acrylic to the labial bar.* Using a salt and pepper technique and repair material,* alternately paint or drop on the liquid carefully, then powder around and under the retaining loops and into the blocked out interproximal spaces until a minimum thickness of 1 to 1.5 mm is obtained or until it is thick enough to build out for lip plumping if this is required. *Be sure to go slightly beyond the pencil line on the necks of the teeth* (Fig. 17-39).

10. *Processing and finishing.* Put the framework and duplicate cast into a pressure pot covered with warm water, 125° F (51.5° C), with at least 30 psi, long enough (approximately 15 minutes) to be sure that it is cured. Never boil veneer. Immediately, while it is still warm, open the labial bar, and carefully lift off the duplicate cast (Fig. 17-40). Then, put the processed restoration in a general purpose cleaner, and rinse it with clear water. Adjust the veneer with a rubber wheel or point to the pencil marked line. Round off the points in the interproximal areas to a natural look. Trim the veneer to the minimum thickness required, and stipple it with a No. 8 carbide bur. Pumice the denture base areas, if they are not already polished, but be very careful with the pumice on the veneer. Use a brush or rag wheel at low speed with a polishing compound* or equivalent material to polish the veneer. Put it into an ultrasonic cleaner, and rinse and dry it. Fit the processed restoration back on the duplicate cast, and check it to be sure the veneer fits up against the teeth correctly (Fig. 17-41).

---

*Repair material, The L. D. Caulk Co., Milford, Del.

*Creshine, Crescent Dental Manufacturing Co., Lyons, Ill.

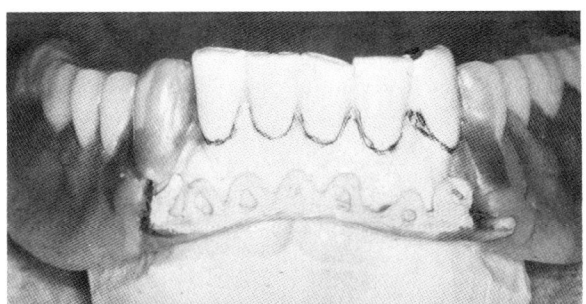

**Fig. 17-38.** Wax blockout of hinge and lock latch attachments to protect them when acrylic resin is added.

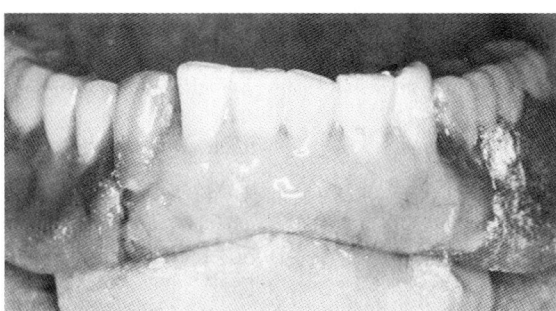

**Fig. 17-39.** Adding acrylic by "salt and pepper" method. Be sure to go beyond pencil line on cast.

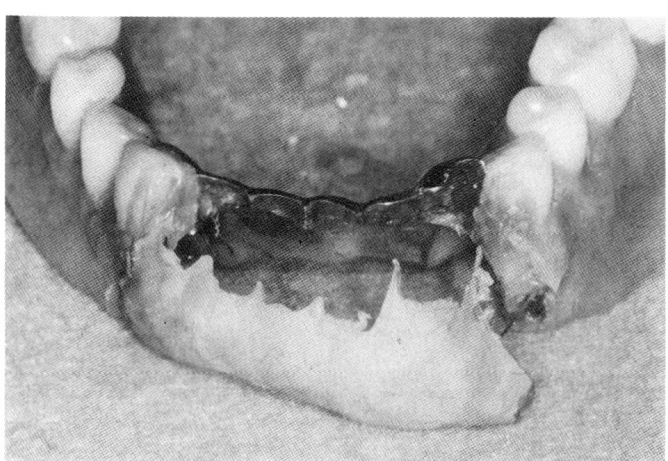

**Fig. 17-40.** Open labial bar while it is still warm and lift off cast.

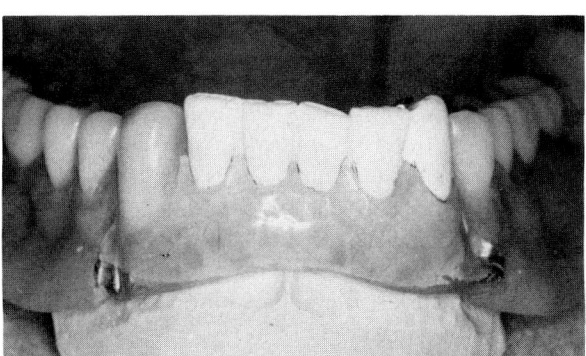

**Fig. 17-41.** Trimming, finishing, and polishing completed. Swing-Lock partial denture is fitted back on duplicate master cast.

### Table 17-5. Labiogingival tissue veneer

| Problem | Probable cause | Solution |
| --- | --- | --- |
| After processing labial bar, it will not open away from stone cast | Not enough undercuts were waxed out (Fig. 17-34) and new acrylic locked into stone undercuts | Cut, break away, or dissolve model (stone and investment remover in ultrasonic cleaner) |
| | Not enough tinfoil substitute separator was used | Same as above |
| | Not enough collodian separator was used to prevent labial acrylic from processing to saddle acrylic | Examine and remove labial acrylic that is causing labial and lingual sections to lock together |
| | Not enough wax was placed around hinge and lock attachments, and extra labial acrylic will not allow clearance for opening | Same as above |
| Retention loops or retained struts show through | Not enough pink opaque was used, or it was removed during process of adding acrylic | Repair these areas or redo entire veneer |
| Some gaps or spaces exist between labial veneer, saddle areas, and/or teeth | Not enough acrylic was added, or it shrank during processing | Make simple repair with new acrylic in these areas |

### PROBLEM AREAS

If the labial bar will not open away from the stone cast, either there were not enough undercuts waxed out and the new acrylic locked into the stone undercuts, or there was not enough tinfoil substitute or acrylic separator used. Failure of the labial bar to open can be caused by not placing enough wax around the hinge and lock attachments before adding the acrylic. If the retention loops or retained struts show through, not enough pink opaque was used, or it was removed during the process of adding the acrylic. If there are gaps or spaces between the labial veneer, denture base areas, and the teeth, not enough acrylic was added, or it shrank during processing (Table 17-5).

### OTHER S/L PROCEDURES (SIMPLE TO COMPLEX)
#### Mandibular struts (interrupted)

Fig. 17-42 shows a lower interrupted strut-type prosthesis in the completed wax-up on the refractory cast with seven anterior and one posterior remaining teeth. The patient's maximum lower lip line extension is shown in this illustration as a dashed line. None of the labial bar or any portion of the three struts on the canines and right first premolar would ever show.

Since perfect retention will be provided by the three struts from the labial bar, a stabilizing-only

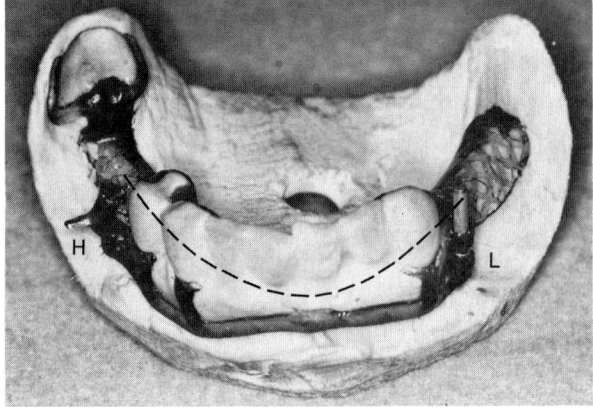

Fig. 17-42. Completed wax-up of struts only—interrupted Swing-Lock, lower four anteriors are not needed for abutments. Maximum lower lip extension (dashed line). H, Hinge; L, lock.

clasp could be designed for the right second molar if there was some mobility of this abutment. If not, then some retentive arms can be designed as in this situation. This clearly illustrates that it is not necessary to encompass all remaining teeth as abutments with struts from the labial bar. If mobility had existed on the lower four anterior teeth and the dentist had relayed this information to the technician (stone casts do not exhibit this clinical characteristic), then splinting of the mobile teeth could have been accomplished with small retention loops on the labial bar and a gingival tissue acrylic veneer. The veneer would have been brought up to the cementoenamel junction. No struts would be needed underneath. The reasons for not using metal-to-tooth contact are as follows:

1. Since there is no pressure of acrylic against the tooth (either enamel or root surfaces) and there is no functional movement up or down, then wear does not occur.

2. If a strut were placed on the tooth and an acrylic veneer processed over it, then it would make the gingival tissue veneer much thicker than necessary because pink opaque, plus the acrylic, would have to be added over the metal strut thickness. An acrylic thickness of only 1 mm is sufficient. With a strut remaining underneath, this would be at least 2.5 mm thick, and, unless a great deal of tissue recession had occurred, it would be much thicker than necessary and not as well tolerated by the patient.

Fig. 17-43 shows the completed wax-up on the refractory cast from the top. The cross section of the Flat-back lock attachment is distinct. The proper alignment of the flat-back portion of this cross section (solid line) is set for proper locking retention of the latch attachment on the labial bar. Note the definite separation of the labial and lingual wax-up on the hinge side. The shiny metal portion of the hinge cylinder tail section is completely clear of wax. The flat-back portion of the lock attachment should be parallel to the labial bar as shown by the solid line. If it were set to the dotted line, there would be too much locking action. If it were set to the dashed line, there would be too little or no locking action, and the bar would open too easily during function or would never lock at all.

The completed framework back on the master cast with the labial bar still opened is illustrated in Fig. 17-44. The investment retaining rods on both attachments have been removed. Note the thumb release groove on the labial bar just mesial to the latch attachment. In certain cases, it is better that a thumb release projection be on the other side of the latch attachment as is illustrated here. Both attachments will be well within the normal acrylic resin denture base outline areas (dashed lines). Fig. 17-45 shows the completed framework on the master cast with the labial bar closed and locked.

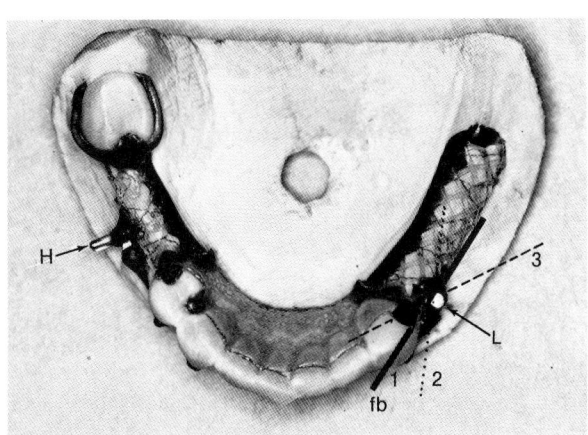

**Fig. 17-43.** Completed wax-up (top view) showing correct and other settings of flat-back portion of lock attachment. *H,* Hinge; *L,* lock; *fb,* flat back; *1,* correct setting; *2,* too much locking action; *3,* too little locking action.

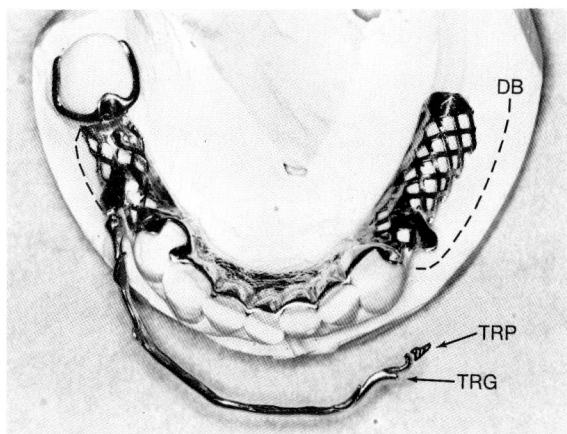

**Fig. 17-44.** Completed metal framework showing designs to be of help to patient in opening labial bar. Both attachments are well within confines of denture base outlines *(DBO). TRG,* Thumb release groove; *TRP,* thumb release projection.

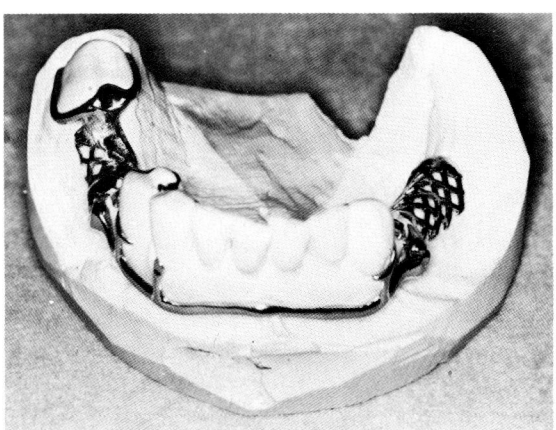

**Fig. 17-45.** Completed metal framework on master cast with labial bar closed and locked on master cast.

## Maxillofacial prosthesis—unilateral abutments

Fig. 17-46 is a resin model indicating a maxillofacial prosthesis. An S/L prosthesis was constructed as in Figs. 17-47 and 17-48 that used all the remaining abutment teeth in the left maxilla. When the prosthesis was closed and locked in place, it provided normal facial contours, a near normal smile and speech characteristics, and comfortable chewing.

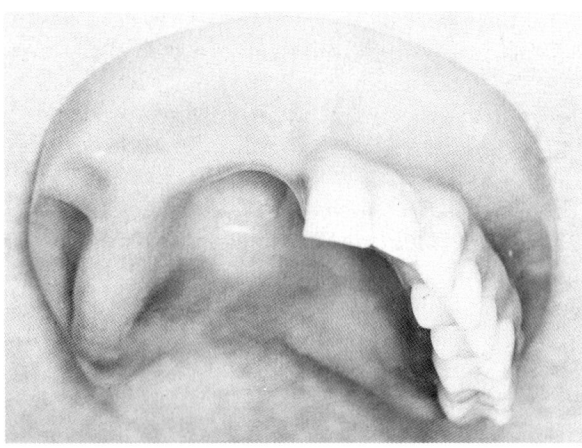

**Fig. 17-46.** Demonstration model of actual cast after patient had cancer surgery. Only unilateral abutments remain, and large palatal defect is present.

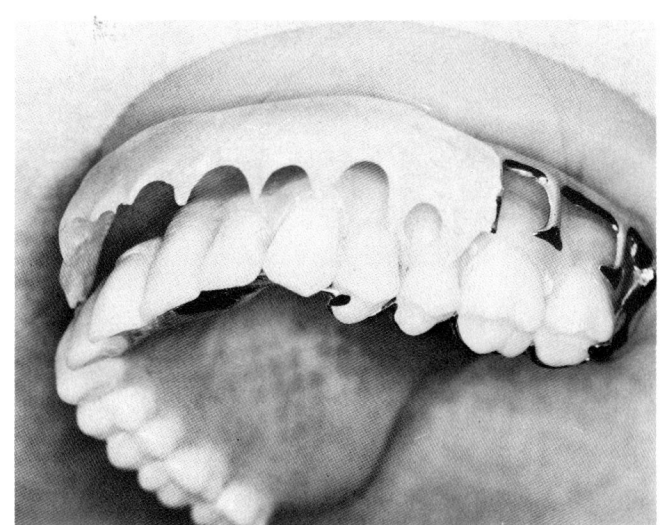

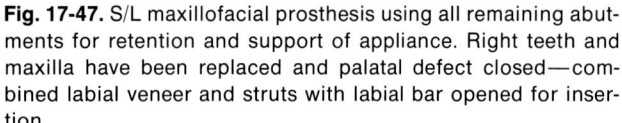

**Fig. 17-47.** S/L maxillofacial prosthesis using all remaining abutments for retention and support of appliance. Right teeth and maxilla have been replaced and palatal defect closed—combined labial veneer and struts with labial bar opened for insertion.

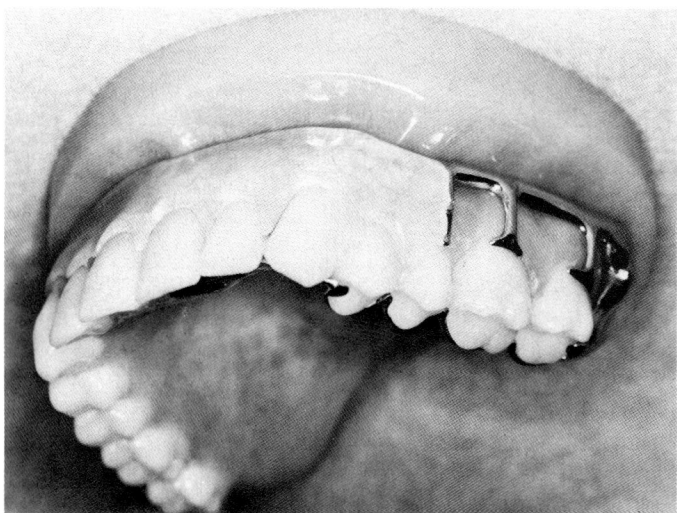

**Fig. 17-48.** Labial bar closed and locked. T struts on molars are above maximum upper lip extension and will not show. Esthetics uncompromised by any metal display.

## S/L complete denture

A number of S/L minimal abutment prostheses have been made with only one, two, or three teeth remaining in either arch. Most have been mandibular prostheses. A few S/L prostheses have been made for completely edentulous patients. The ridge was severely undercut as in Fig. 17-49. The S/L complete denture was constructed (Fig. 17-50). The denture is designed to be inserted lingually to the crest of the ridge and is seated by moving it downward and forward (Fig. 17-51). When the labial flange is closed, it engages the bony undercut and locks the denture securely in place without harm to the patient (Fig. 17-52).

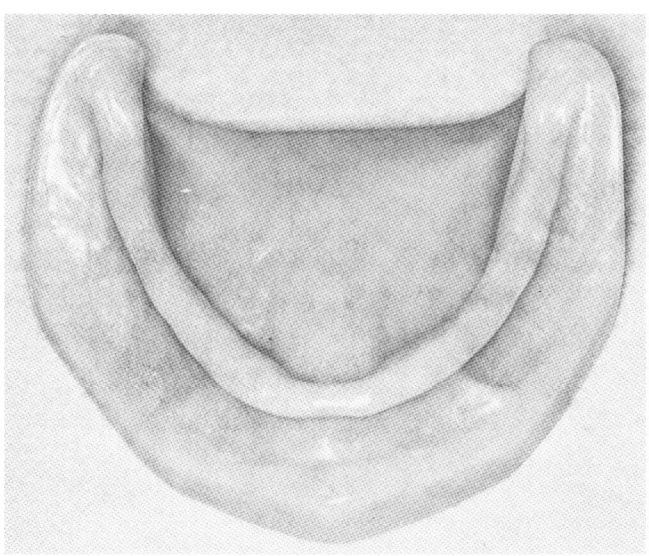

**Fig. 17-49.** Demonstration model with deeply undercut ridge.

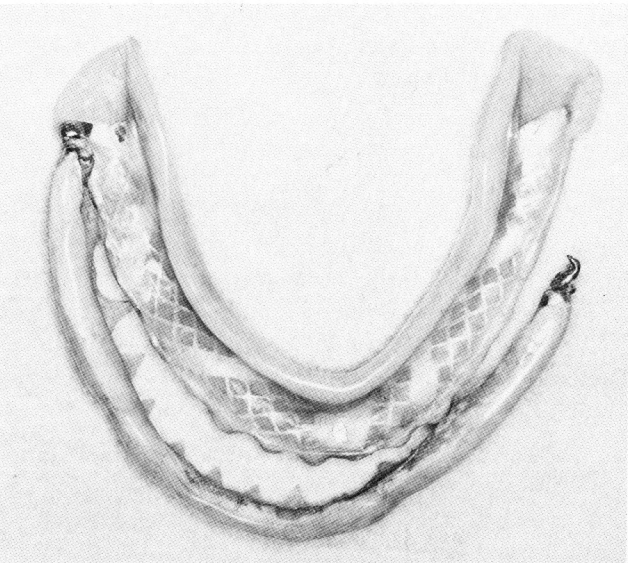

**Fig. 17-50.** S/L mandibular denture open. Labial bar completely embedded within labial flange. Metal framework in lingual section provides reinforcement.

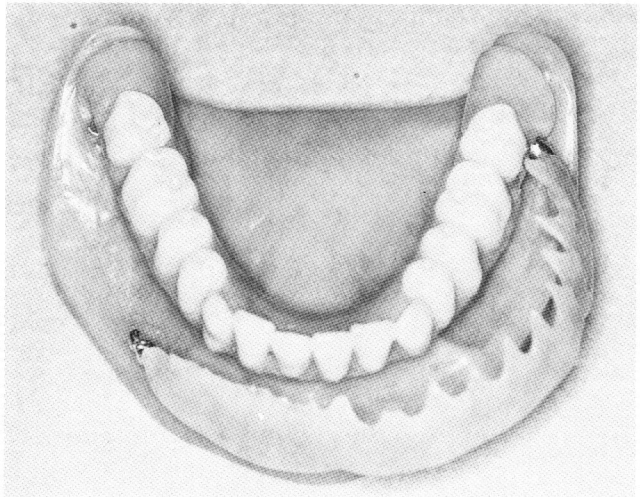

**Fig. 17-51.** S/L mandibular denture seated along lingually tilted lingual path of insertion. Labial flange open.

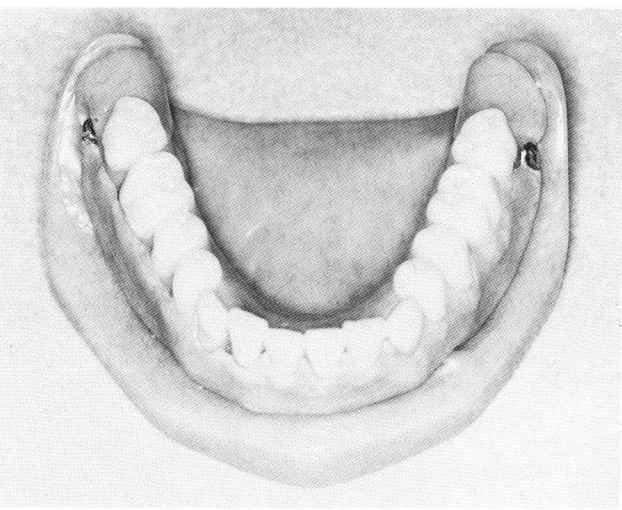

**Fig. 17-52.** S/L mandibular denture using tissue undercuts for retention. Labial flange closed and locked.

In Fig. 17-50, note the metal framework in the lingual section is made fairly strong to prevent breakage, and, the labial bar, except for the hinge and latch and thumb release groove, is completely embedded in the acrylic. To accomplish this, the master cast was relieved with one thickness of pink baseplate wax throughout the entire length of the labial bar design (except at the attachments) before the master cast was duplicated and the refractory cast made.

### Double bars, double hinges, single lock, pure periodontal splint, full arch labial gingival veneer

Fig. 17-53 is an acrylic demonstration model and appliance of a double bar with both labial bars opened. Fig. 17-54 is the same prosthesis with only the right labial bar closed. In Fig. 17-55 notice how the closed right labial bar carries the lock attachment at its end and the latch attachment and thumb release groove in the end of the still opened left labial bar. Note the extreme amount of tissue loss and root exposure on the anterior teeth. In Fig. 17-56 the left labial bar has been closed and locked.

### Maxillary coping overdenture

Fig. 17-57 shows the top view of an acrylic demonstration model of a clinical situation involving four copings. The patient has successfully worn a similar S/L overdenture replacement for 17 years (Fig. 17-61). Shortening the teeth and relining the original clasp appliance to cover the coping preparations improved the clinical mobility of these teeth (Miller, 1958; Larkin, 1973). Notice the extreme tissue undercut that exists in the labial and buccal vestibule from approximately the right second premolar to the left first molar area. If a regular overdenture had been constructed for this patient, either all the anterior teeth would have to be butted, or the resulting denture flange would have to be relieved (Fig. 17-71, A). This could create a food trap and would provide too much support for the entire upper lip.

When additional lip support is desirable, such as for a cleft palate, accident, or hemisection, the dentist must furnish the technician with a wax lip index that has been tried in the patient's mouth and modified to the correct thickness. This wax lip index can then be used to complete the labial bar design, the placement of retention loops, and to determine whether there will be sufficient thickness to completely bury the labial bar within the labial flange

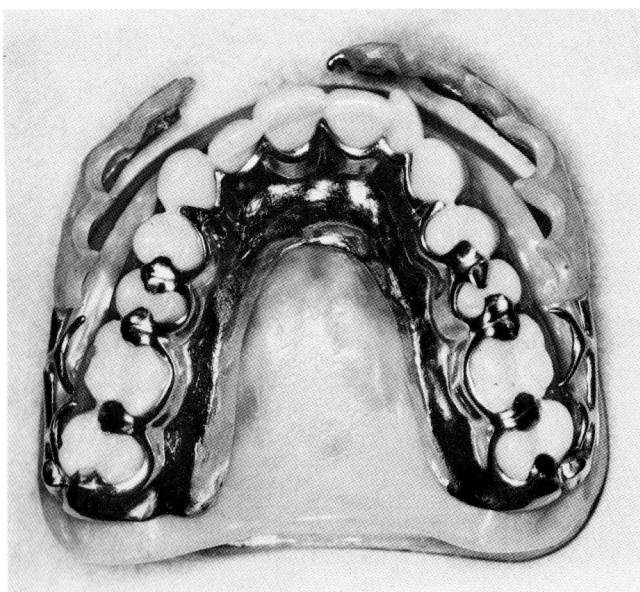

**Fig. 17-53.** Double-hinge single-lock pure periodontal splint. Both labial bars are open.

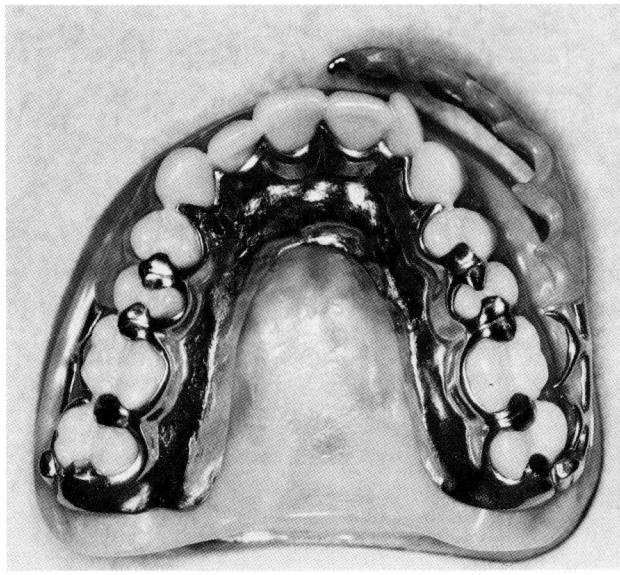

**Fig. 17-54.** Periodontal demonstration S/L partial denture. Right labial bar has to be closed first.

**Fig. 17-55.** Lock attachment at end of right labial bar, latch attachment at end of left labial bar, thumb release groove mesial to latch.

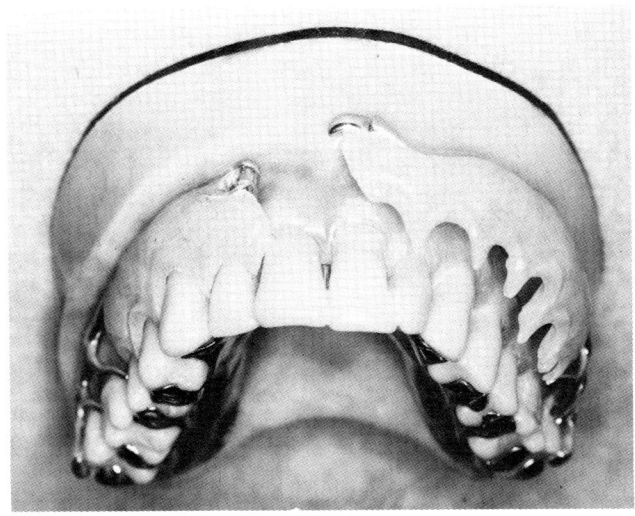

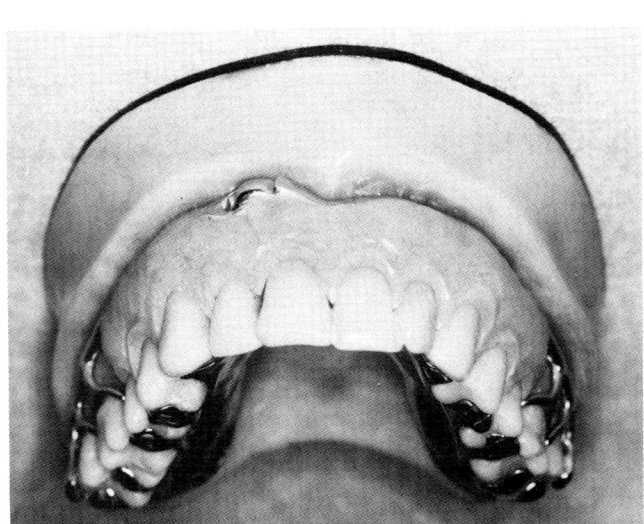

**Fig. 17-56.** Left labial bar has been closed and locked. This S/L partial denture demonstrates removable periodontal splinting and esthetic replacement of lost gingival tissues.

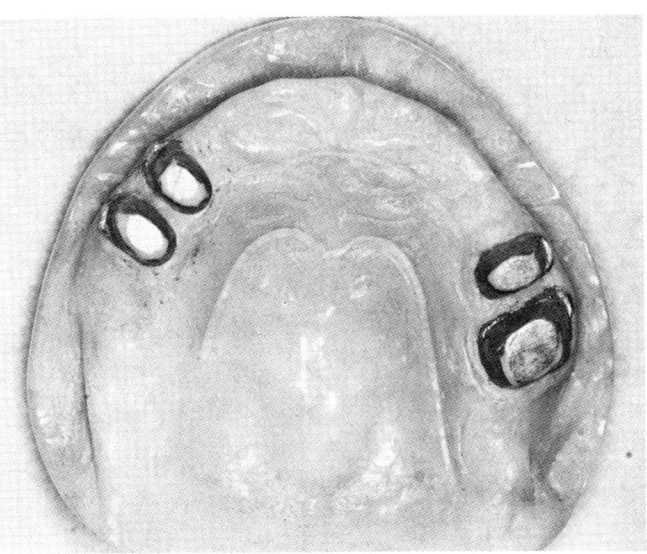

**Fig. 17-57.** Acrylic demonstration model with four copings and severe labial tissue undercut.

as shown in Fig. 17-50. Figs. 17-58 and 17-59 show details of the original hinge and lock S/L attachments in the completed wax-up on the refractory cast. Notice how several millimeters of the vertical x member of the lock attachment have been left protruding from the wax-up in order to secure the lock attachment into the investment mold and prevent its slippage during subsequent burnout and casting. Likewise, two investment retaining rods, which also serve as heat dissipating rods, have been left protruding from the wax-up on the hinge attachment. Where space permits, it is better to use the larger original hinge attachment in longer span labial bars such as this one or in situations where extra heavy labial bars are required like cleft palate appliances. Either type lock attachment can be used with either type hinge attachment.

The retention for the acrylic gingival veneer is made by one row of retention mesh squares continuously around the long-span labial bar. As in most upper S/L prostheses, it is not necessary to completely cover the palate, thus leaving the patient with more tongue room, less gagging, and a better sense of taste and feel in this sensitive region of the mouth. The following are reasons for not completely covering the palate or using a palatal strap:

1. The rigidity of the S/L prosthesis obtained by the I-beam effect makes possible a thinner lingual section and less coverage of the palate. When the labial bar with the processed acrylic (Fig. 17-61) is closed and locked into the undercuts of the copings and into the interproximal spaces of the teeth, it creates a very rigid structure. It cannot be made to flex across the posterior saddle areas; therefore no palatal strap to connect these two areas to improve rigidity is required.

2. Retention and stability are more than adequate in this type of prosthesis and therefore additional coverage of the palatal areas to enhance retention or to resist lateral displacement is usually not required. The exception to this general rule of palatal coverage is for congenital defects, accidents, or hemisections where closure of a palatal defect is required. Palatal coverage would usually be desirable also where only unilateral abutments remain.

### Sprue placement

Fig. 17-60 shows the completed casting still attached to the casting button with only the two major sprues to the labial bar cut before opening. Note how the sprues to the labial bar are connected near each attachment. Sometimes a small auxiliary sprue from the labial bar to the lingual portion, about the midline, is also used. This 18-gauge auxiliary sprue has been cut off. The stump where it was cut is at the midline of the labial bar. Similar auxiliary sprues are still connected from the loops around the copings to the lingual palatal portion. There are three major sprues still connected from the button to the lingual portion of this casting.

Fig. 17-61 shows a completed demonstration S/L overdenture. The right side of the restoration remains metal framework only. The left side has been completed. The labial bar remains open. The T struts were not cut off during acrylic processing because there was enough thickness required in the labial flange in this area so that unnecessary thickness by leaving these struts was not a problem. As previously explained, however, acrylic to coping or tooth contact is perfectly permissible and even desirable in certain situations where the labial acrylic tissue veneer must be as thin as possible. The esthetics in the final appliance were totally uncompromised by any metal display. The mobility of the coping abutments was further reduced only a few weeks after delivery of the S/L appliance, and they have remained stable (Antos, Renner, and Foerth, 1978; Gomes et al., 1980; Gomes, Renner, and Bauer, 1980).

### Double labial bar

In Fig. 17-62 a double-hinge (original size S/L hinge) double-lock (original), double–labial bar casting with button and casting sprues still attached is depicted. Note the two sprues to each labial bar near each attachment and the four sprues to the lingual section. The original lock attachments were designed with an indexing tab attached to the vertical alignment rod that was useful in setting the lock attachment. The alignment rod was used to align the lock attachment more or less parallel to the hinge attachment with a vertical hinge alignment tool. A vertical hinge alignment tool is included with all original attachment patterns. Its use is illustrated in the *Swing-Lock Imagineering Design and Technique Manual* (1969). The indexing tab is used to set the proper degree of locking action at almost 90 degrees to the labial bar in a horizontal direction. This indexing tab was useful for the first few attachment placements, while the technician was becoming familiar with the S/L concept. As more insight is developed in designs and waxing of the attachments by the more experienced technician, this entire upper vertical rod was cut off a few millimeters above the lock attachment, exposing an x member cross section that was used as in the present Flat-back lock attachment in setting proper locking action (Figs. 17-59 and 17-62).

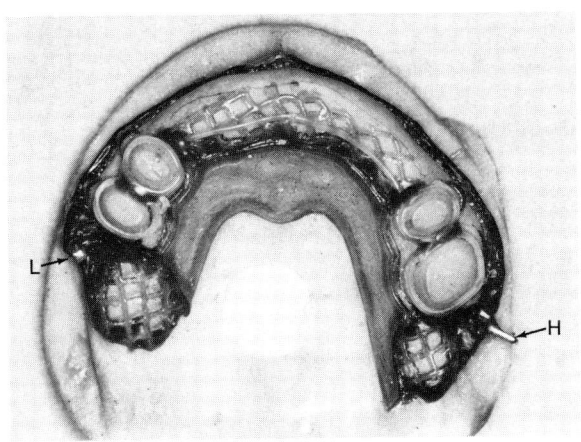

**Fig. 17-58.** Completed wax-up on refractory cast with original lock *(L)* and hinge *(H)* positions indicated.

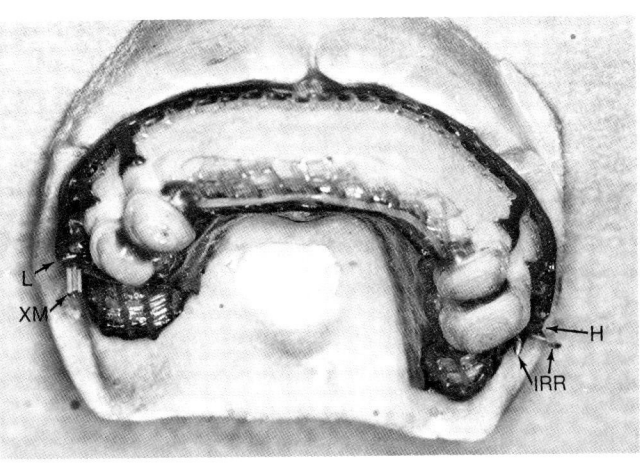

**Fig. 17-59.** Completed wax-up showing investment retaining rods *(IRR)* on hinge *(H)* and x member *(XM)* on lock *(L)* attachments.

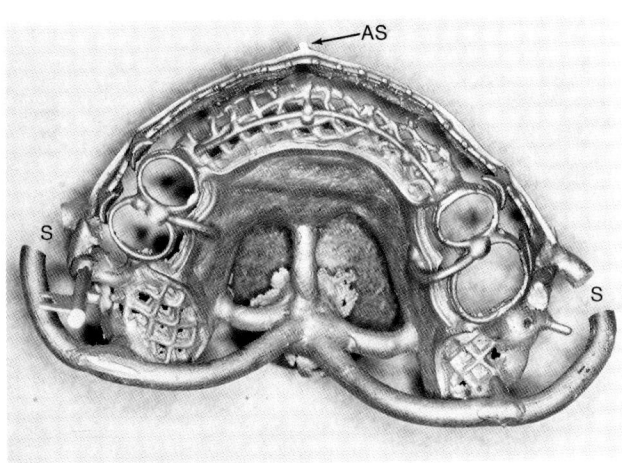

**Fig. 17-60.** Metal casting with major labial bar sprues *(S)* cut into. Lingual sprues are still attached *(AS,* auxiliary sprue).

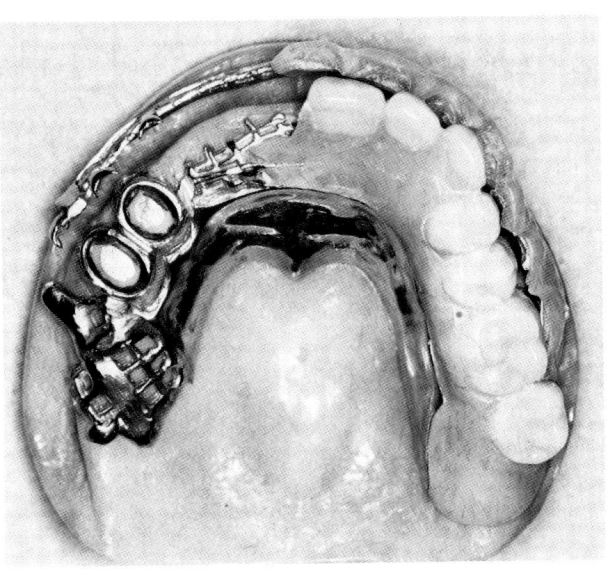

**Fig. 17-61.** Demonstration S/L overdenture, left side completed. Right side, framework only.

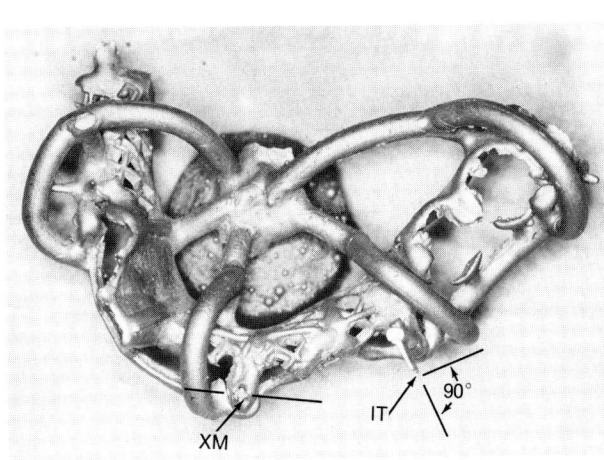

**Fig. 17-62.** Double labial bar, and double hinge and lock casting with all sprues still attached. *IT,* Indexing tab; *XM,* x member (original lock attachments).

The hinge alignment tool was useful in training but is not needed after a few S/L appliances have been completed. "Eyeballing" the vertical hinge placement can be accomplished by using only the hinge cylinder barrel. Fig. 17-63 shows the top view of the complete demonstration model and appliance right and anterior sides finished, and the left posterior sides, framework only. Both labial bars are opened to permit seating along a common lingual path of insertion. There are, however, two separate and distinct labial opening arcs. Fig. 17-64 shows an angled front view. Note the groove in the anterior acrylic resin into which the anterior teeth have been processed. When closed and locked in, the plain portion of the labial bar fits into this groove. If such a bar is used, it must have a slight downward angle on the top. If this were reversed, the labial bar could not be unlocked after acrylic processing.

Both labial bars are open in Fig. 17-64 and closed and locked in Fig. 17-65. One labial bar could have been designed to encompass both molars and the three teeth on the right, but would not have produced as much rigidity as did the double labial bars.

## PROBLEM AREAS

The original S/L partial denture constructed for the patient illustrated in the first part of this chapter was deficient in design, construction, and desired esthetics (Fig. 17-66). The partial denture lifted up slightly during mastication even with the labial bar closed and locked. This caused considerable wear on the teeth. The partial denture fit the master cast well, but the technician had to make the labial bar too high up on the labial gum tissue because there was not enough room on the master cast to make it lower. Too much metal showed, the labial bar was too thick, and when the patient smiled, the lower lip got caught under the metal bar. There was excessive fullness in the cheek areas. The patient had soreness of the tissues under the labial bar due to movement of the bar during mastication and tongue action. Causes for these problems and procedures to correct them during the redesign and remake of the partial denture are discussed in Table 17-6.

Swing-Lock 521

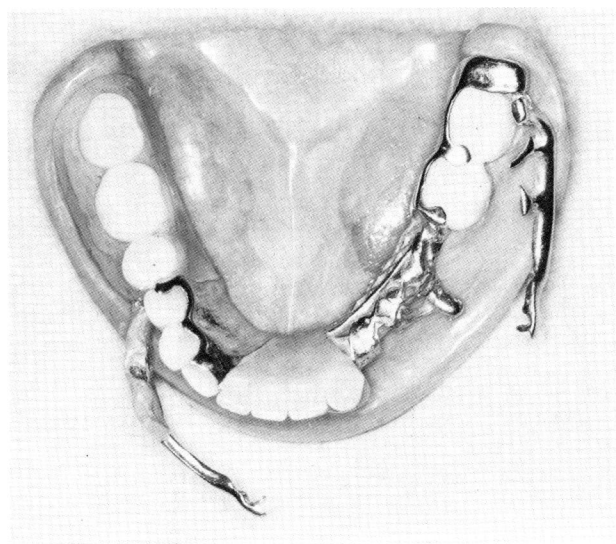

**Fig. 17-63.** Demonstration S/L partial denture with both labial bars open.

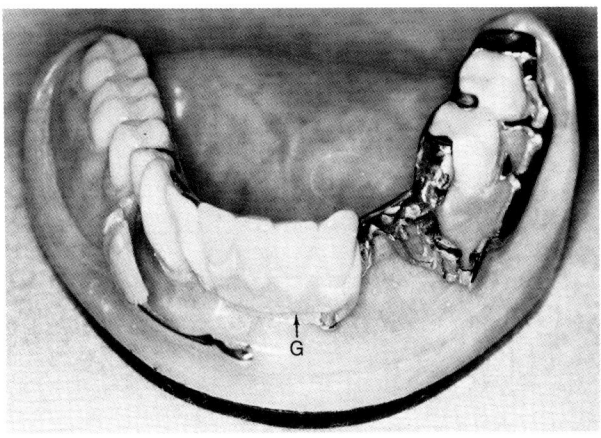

**Fig. 17-64.** Right labial bar has combination labial veneer and labial bar that will close into anterior acrylic groove *(G)*. Left labial bar has struts only. Both bars have thumb release projections for opening.

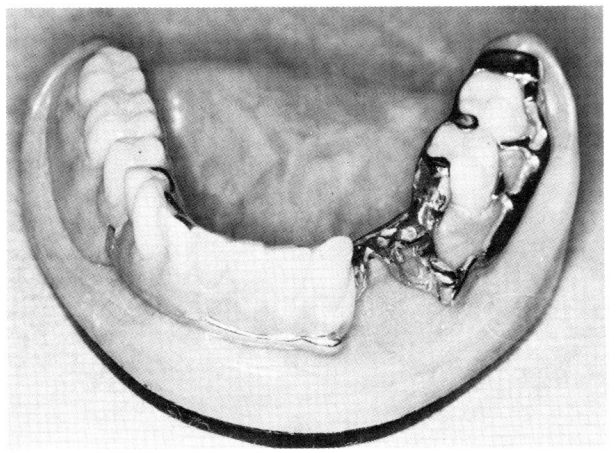

**Fig. 17-65.** Both right and left labial bars closed and locked. Right labial bar flush with anterior acrylic resin.

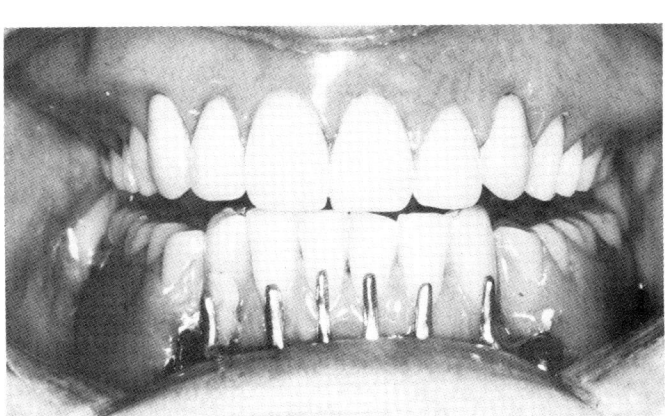

**Fig. 17-66.** Original S/L design. What is wrong?

### Table 17-6. Design and construction

| Problem | Probable cause | Solution |
| --- | --- | --- |
| After closing and locking labial bar, appliance lifted up during mastication | As in Fig. 17-67, A, there were no undercuts engaged by labial struts to resist this dislodging force; minimum retention allows partial denture to move upward during function or tongue action, causing wear in enamel (Fig. 17-4) | Redesign and remake appliance so that struts or labial veneer engage major undercuts below dotted survey lines (Fig. 17-67, B); dislodging force is resisted |
| Appliance completed and fit master cast well; labial bar had to be made high up on labial part of cast and gum tissue because there was not enough room to make it lower; patient had three complaints: too much metal shows, labial bar feels too thick, "when I smile real big, my lower lip gets caught under metal bar" | Master cast was made with wrong impression technique, hydrocolloid impression using stock water-cooled tray; result was beautiful master cast, but lip was pulled out and distorted to about dotted line (LRL) (Fig. 17-67, A); this resulted in master cast that did not have full extent of labial vestibule; therefore technician had to place thickest portion of labial bar higher than it should have been (Fig. 17-67, B), which caused feeling of thickness and lip catching under metal bar; proper strut designs far below survey line could have eliminated much metal display (Fig. 17-68) | Simple procedure can help determine whether struts or labial veneer is indicated; using pink baseplate wax, contour it to diagnostic or master cast to approximately outline of labial acrylic veneer (Fig. 17-69); have dentist try this in patient's mouth so they both can preview potential esthetic results<br>Take impression with recommended technique, then redesign appliance as in Fig. 17-67, B, or with full labial gum tissue veneer (Fig. 17-70) |
| Patient complains of excessive fullness in cheeks | Hinge and lock attachments were set out away from ridge (Figs. 17-17 and 17-20), resulting in unnecessary bulk in saddle areas | Use Mini-hinge and Flat-back lock attachments where possible and set in position that will be within normal saddle outline (Figs. 17-19, 17-21, and 17-44) |
| In lower S/L coping overdenture appliance using only two remaining copings as abutments, labial bar caused sore spots in various places under it; also, appliance could be dislodged by tongue action without opening labial bar | If wrong coping designs for S/L overdenture are used, like Fig. 17-71, W, rounded incisal design allows overdenture to rotate; it can be rotated enough that dislodgment can occur; tissue irritation due to binding of labial bar will also occur | Use proper design for copings that will be under S/L overdenture (Fig. 17-71, P); slightly tapered walls of coping will resist these rotating forces and prevent dislodgment and irritation under labial bar |

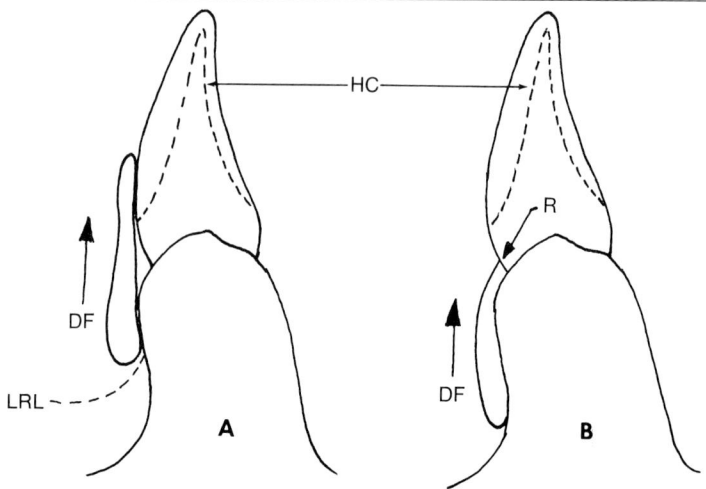

Fig. 17-67. Diagrams of original and redesigned strut placement. (Cross section of central area.) **A,** Original improper strut placement and labial bar design. Labial made above lip reflection line *(LRL)*. Strut placement on and above height of contour *(HC)*, providing little resistance for dislodging forces *(DF)*. **B,** Correct redesign of struts or veneer and labial bar. Labial bar placed well down in labial vestibule, and strut or veneer placed into deep undercut below height of contour *(HC)*, providing major resistance *(R)* to dislodging forces *(DF)*.

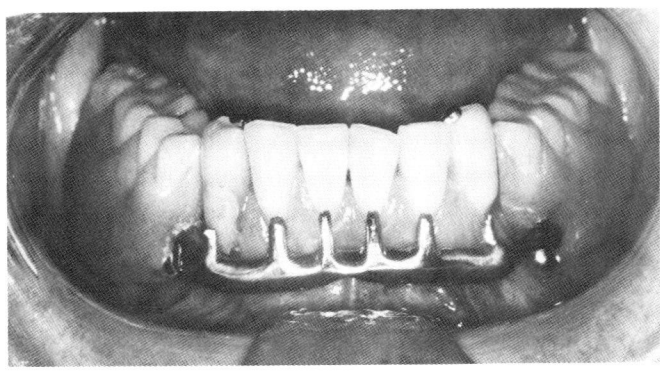

**Fig. 17-68.** Proper strut length—better, but not best, design.

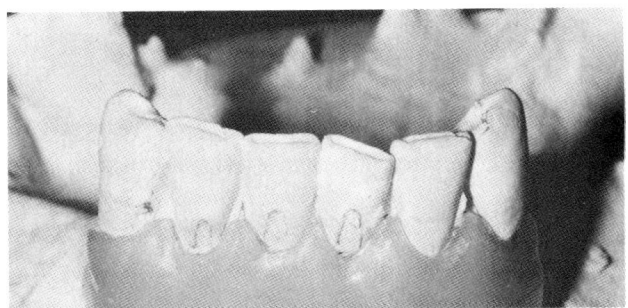

**Fig. 17-69.** Pink baseplate wax try-in fabricated on diagnostic cast. Provides preview of what labiogingival tissue acrylic resin veneer will look like. Pencil lines on central and right lateral incisors show original poor esthetic strut placement.

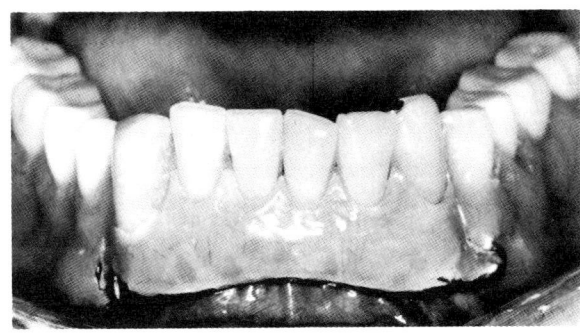

**Fig. 17-70.** Redesigned and completed S/L appliance with esthetic labial veneer instead of struts.

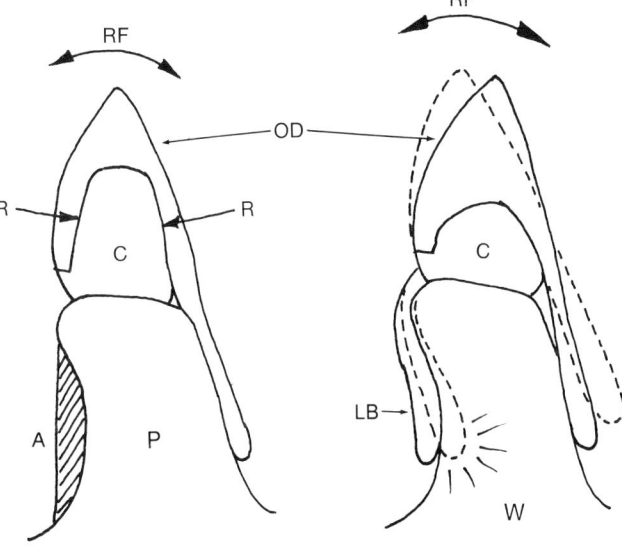

**Fig. 17-71.** Rotational forces *(RF)* influence coping *(C)* designs. *P*, Cross section showing proper design for S/L overdenture; *A*, tissue undercut; *R*, resistance to rotational forces; *OD*, overdenture; *W*, improper design, showing lack of resistance to rotational forces that permits labial bar *(LB)* to impinge on soft tissue.

## SUMMARY

The various steps for redesigning and constructing an S/L mandibular partial denture properly are discussed in this chapter. In the last portion of the chapter, other simple and complex variations are presented. The requirements for the clinical success of an S/L partial denture are exacting for both the dentist and the dental laboratory technician. Mutual cooperation and understanding between all involved contribute to a successful prosthesis.

## REFERENCES

Antos, W. E., Jr., Renner, R. P., and Foerth, D.: The Swing-Lock partial denture: an alternative approach to conventional removable partial denture service, J. Prosthet. Dent. **40:**257-262, 1978.

Gomes, B. C., Renner, R. P., Antos, W. E., Jr., Carlsson, G. E., and Bauer, P. N.: A longitudinal study of the periodontal status of abutment teeth supporting Swing-Lock removable partial dentures, J. Prosthet. Dent. **44:**566, 1980.

Gomes, B. C., Renner, R. P., and Bauer, P. N.: Periodontal considerations in removable partial dentures, J. Am. Dent. Assoc. **101:**496-498, 1980.

Simmons, J. J.: Swing-Lock stabilization and retention, Tex. Dent. J. **81:**10-12, 1963.

Simmons, J. J.: Swing-Lock overdentures: the impossible cases made possible (unpublished data), 1975.

Sprigg, R. H.: Six-year clinical evaluation of the Swing-Lock removable partial denture, Anglo-Continental Dental Society J. pp. 15-27, 1971.

Swing-Lock Clinical Manual: Dallas, 1969, Swing-Lock, Divison of Idea Development Co.

Swing-Lock Imagineering Design and Technique Manual: Dallas, 1969, Swing-Lock, Division of Idea Development Co.

Swing-Lock Impression Technique Folder: Dallas, 1969, Swing-Lock, Division of Idea Development Co.

Swing-Lock Technique Sheet on the S/L Mini-hinge and Flatback Lock Attachments: Dallas, 1977, Swing-Lock, Division of Idea Development Co. (Supplement to Swing-Lock Imagineering Design and Technique Manual.)

Swing-Lock Technique Sheet for Veneering a Swing-Lock Partial: Dallas, 1981, Swing-Lock, Division of Idea Development Co. (Supplement to Swing-Lock Imagineering Design and Technique Manual.)

## BIBLIOGRAPHY

Larkin, J. D.: Tooth supported complete dentures, Twenty-seventh Year of Observation, Tex. Dent. J. **91:**26-30, 1973.

Miller, P. A.: Complete dentures supported by natural teeth, J. Prosthet. Dent. **8:**924-928, 1958.

CHAPTER 18

# REINFORCED FACINGS AND METAL BACKINGS

WILLIAM B. AKERLY

## INDICATIONS FOR METAL BACKINGS

Fabrication of metal backings requires precise planning on the part of the dentist and meticulous technical work in the laboratory. The decision to use metal backings will often be based on one or more of the following conditions:
1. Occlusion of opposing natural teeth is the only factor to prevent extrusion.
2. Occlusal guidance will be restored by the prosthesis.
3. Rapid wear or repeated breakage of previous dentures.

Failure to use metal backings under these conditions often results in a compromise of the prosthesis (Fig. 18-1).

## TECHNIQUES FOR METAL BACKINGS

Several techniques can be used to fabricate metal backings. The most common method uses conventional flatback facings (Fig. 18-2). These facings are called flatback facings because of the flat surface that accommodates a preformed plastic backing. The plastic backings are modified by grinding and adding wax to meet individual requirements. Flatback facings are especially useful for replacing single or isolated teeth, especially when there is minimum resorption of the residual ridge. A disadvantage of flatback facings is the limited mold selection. In addition, the flatback design limits the

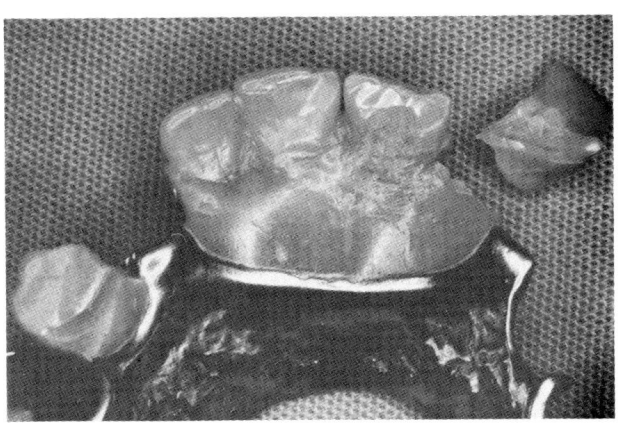

Fig. 18-1. Breakage and abrasion of resin prosthesis cause aggravating situation that may endanger health of remaining teeth.

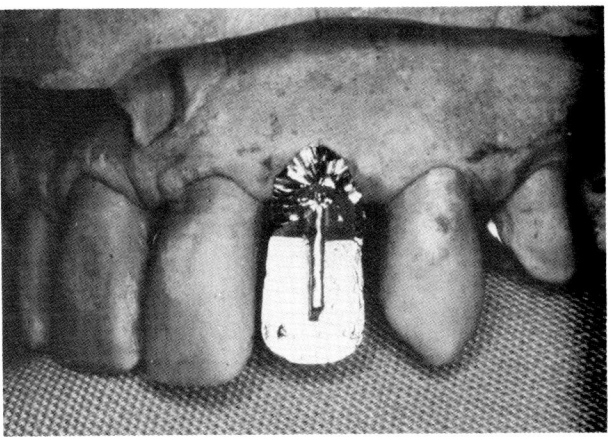

Fig. 18-2. Example of flatback metal backing.

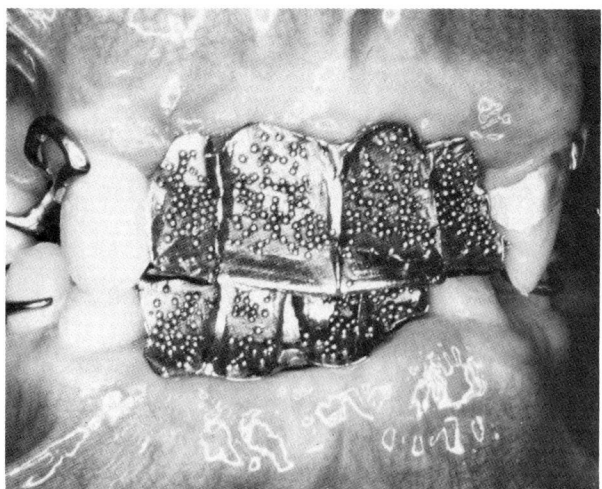

Fig. 18-3. Metal beads used for retention of resin denture teeth.

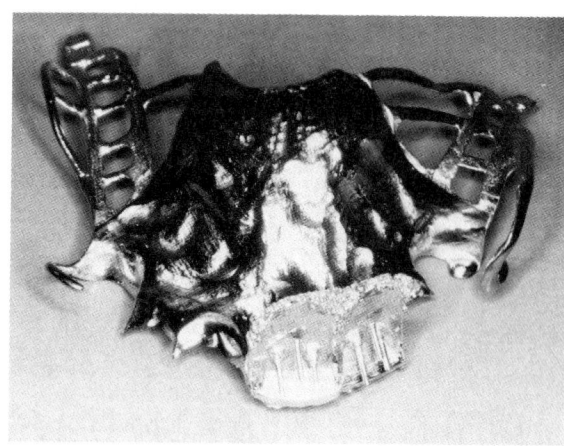

Fig. 18-4. Metal pins used for retention of resin denture teeth.

possibilities of arrangement and amount of modifications in all dimensions of the facing.

Denture teeth offer advantages in both mold selection and arrangement. Individual molds can be modified and arranged to meet esthetic requirements. When indicated, metal backings should be fabricated in conjunction with the use of denture teeth to provide and protect the desired occlusion of a prosthesis. Metal backings will also prevent the opposing teeth from extruding and will improve the strength and durability of the restoration.

The lingual surfaces of denture teeth can be retained to metal backings by the use of beads or pins (Figs. 18-3 and 18-4). The bead retention technique is especially useful in situations of extreme vertical overlap or where excessive loss of the residual ridge has occurred. The bead retention method will be discussed later with alternate approaches.

The reverse-pin technique, originated by Shooshan (1959), provides a simple and reliable method of attaching denture teeth to fixed partial dentures. The principles and technique of fabricating reverse-pin facings for removable partial dentures will be described in detail. With slight modifications, these concepts can be applied to any method of making metal backings for a more durable and successful prosthesis. Although porcelain teeth can be used, the choice of resin teeth is suggested for both economics and practicality in fabricating the removable prosthesis.

## Technique for reverse-pin facings
### PROCEDURE

1. Survey the edentulous ridge and the teeth adjacent to the edentulous area (Fig. 18-5). The survey will determine the compatibility of the selected mold and provide the basis for necessary modifications of the natural teeth, if recommended. The tilt should be modified to minimize the amount of undercut of either the tooth or edentulous ridge. The height of contour of the edentulous area generally determines the extension of the flange. In instances of extensive ridge loss with no undercut, the flange may extend to any desirable limit.

2. Select and arrange resin denture teeth of the proper width and length. A divider or Boley gauge is useful in selecting the proper size mold (Fig. 18-6). Avoid selecting teeth that are excessively tapered to prevent unsightly spaces adjacent to the abutment teeth. Incisal translucency will be altered by the type of metal backing. Modify the tooth form as desired but do not characterize completely until the teeth have been tried in the mouth or until the final selection has been decided (Fig. 18-7). First alter the incisal edge of the selected teeth and then the gingival collars. Try-in of the selected teeth is advised to confirm mold and shape selection, adequacy of tooth modifications, and room for occlusion.

3. Adapt a shellac baseplate form to the cast. If the ridge is not excessively resorbed, do not extend

*Reinforced facings and metal backings* **527**

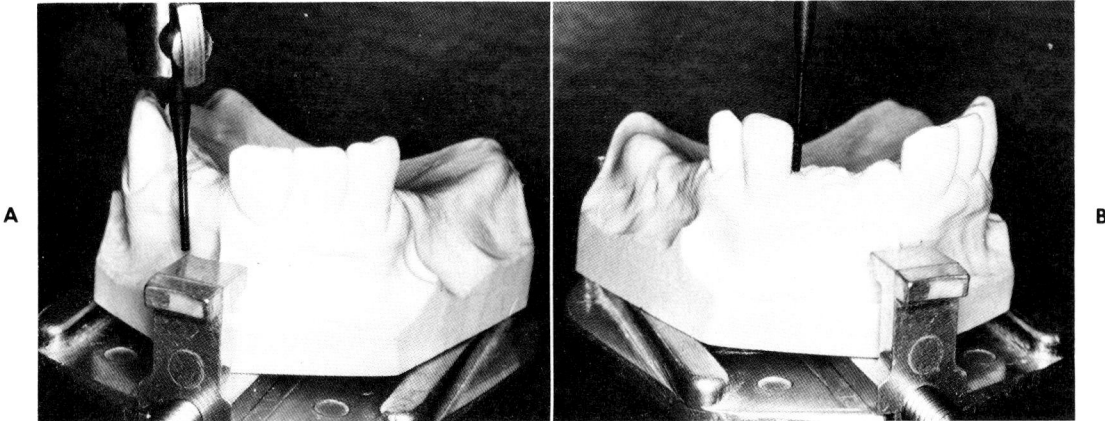

**Fig. 18-5. A,** Survey of edentulous area affects design of labial flange. **B,** Proximal surfaces of abutment teeth are surveyed to determine best path of insertion and need for selective modification.

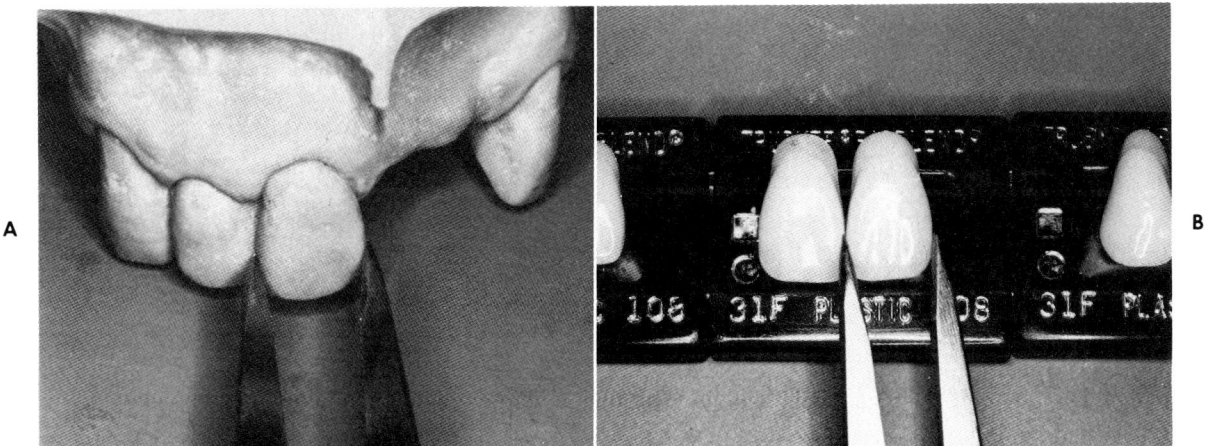

**Fig. 18-6. A,** Divider or modified Boley gauge is used to determine exact tooth size. **B,** Measurement of actual tooth size can be compared to selected teeth or mold guide.

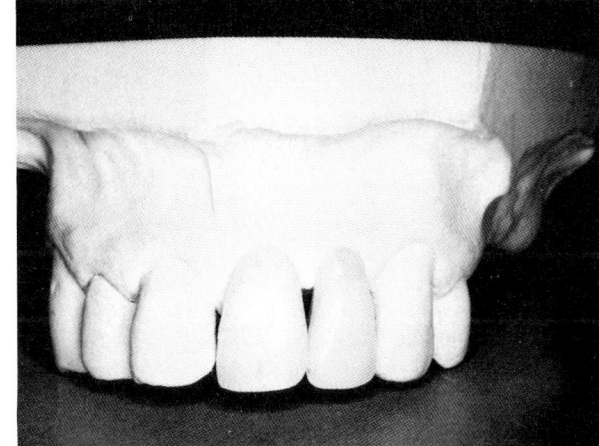

**Fig. 18-7.** Modifications are limited to those necessary for try-in arrangement.

the baseplate subjacent to the collars of the artificial teeth (Fig. 18-8). Attach the teeth to the baseplate from the lingual side (Fig. 18-9). Wax on the labial side or gingival to the collars is not usually necessary and promotes excessive tooth modifications prematurely. With moderate or excessive resorption, apply tinfoil, and do a complete waxing. It is important to note the amount of room available for the metal backing (Fig. 18-10). In some instances, modifications of the opposing teeth may be necessary especially if the opposing teeth have extruded or become malpositioned.

4. Trim and index the border of the cast subjacent to the edentulous area (Fig. 18-11). The stone core should include the indexed area, artificial teeth, and relate to part of the labial surfaces of the adjacent abutment teeth. Paint these areas with separating fluid prior to making the stone core.

5. Block out the labial undercuts on the mucosal areas of the master cast (Fig. 18-12). These undercuts should be blocked out prior to making the stone core to ensure that the stone core will fit accurately on the refractory cast. The same blockout should remain in place for duplicating and making the refractory cast.

6. With the artificial teeth in the desired position, a stone core is made (Fig. 18-13). A small quantity of ground stone or a mixture of slurry can be added when mixing the stone to accelerate the setting reaction.

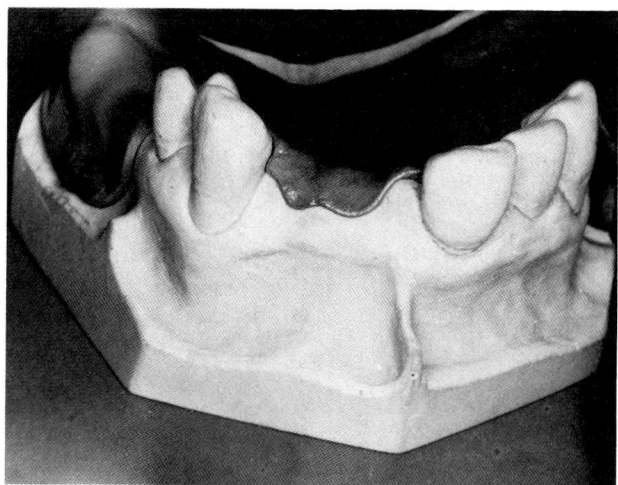

**Fig. 18-8.** Shellac baseplate form is adapted short of teeth for try-in purposes.

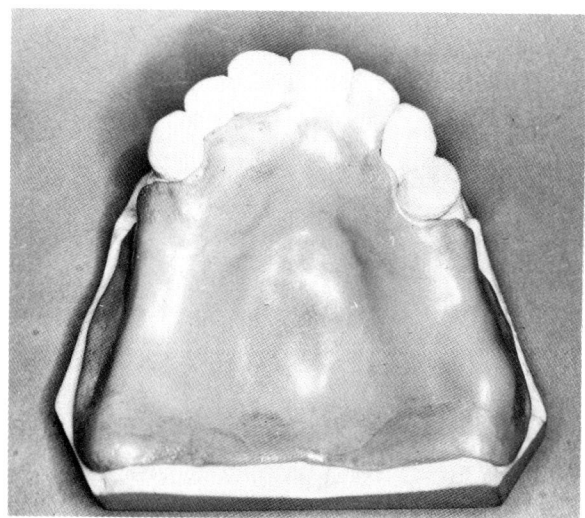

**Fig. 18-9.** Teeth are attached lingually with baseplate wax.

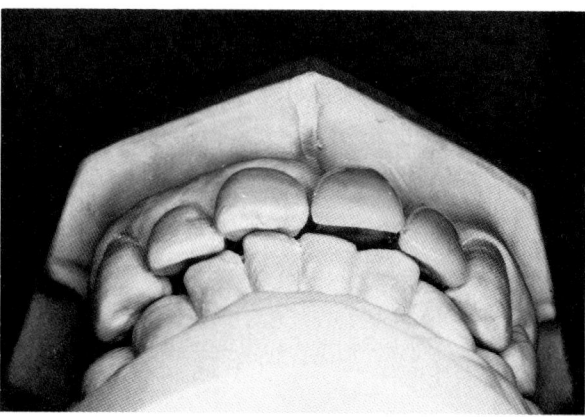

**Fig. 18-10.** Note amount of room available for metal backings. Tooth can be reduced only 1 mm to provide necessary space for backing.

## Reinforced facings and metal backings 529

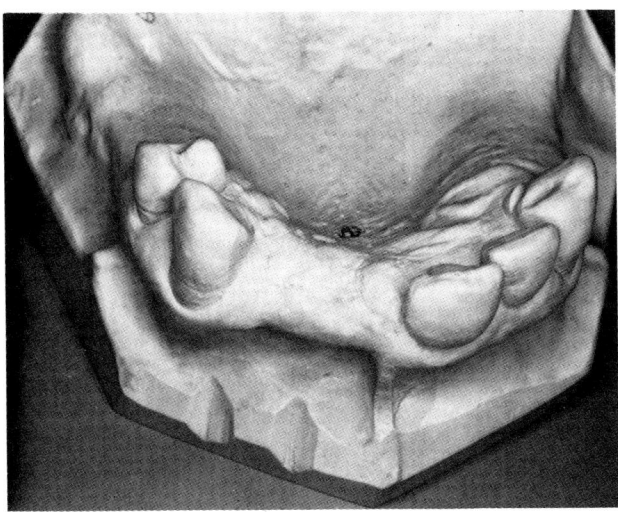

**Fig. 18-11.** Border of master cast is indexed for positive relation of stone core.

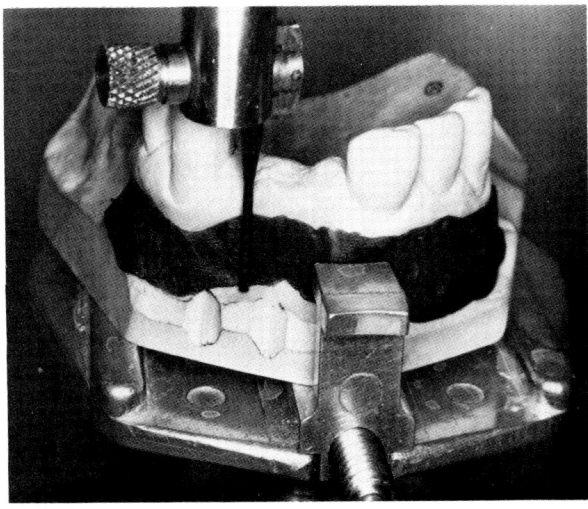

**Fig. 18-12.** Blockout of mucosal undercut areas in preparation for making stone core and later duplication of master cast.

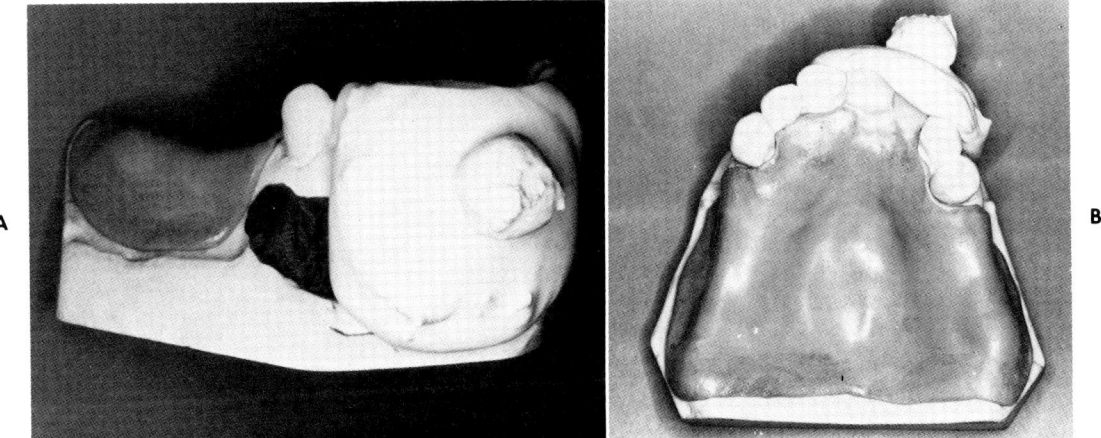

**Fig. 18-13. A,** Stone core fabricated to relate facings to border of cast and adjacent teeth. **B,** Approximately half of labial surfaces of adjacent teeth should be included by core.

7. Prepare the lingual surfaces of the denture teeth to provide room for the metal backings (Figs. 18-14 and 18-15). Mark the incisal finishing line approximately 1 mm from the incisal edge (Fig. 18-16). If more translucency is desired, place the incisal finishing line more than 1 mm from the incisal edge.

8. Use a separating disk to reduce the lingual surface and create the finishing line (Fig. 18-17). Smooth this preparation with a mounted green stone wheel, and sharpen the finishing line with a sharp instrument such as a straight chisel (Figs. 18-18 and 18-19). The lingual reduction should be a minimum depth of 1 mm. Carry the proximal reductions to a line just short of the interproximal contacts (Fig. 18-14, A). The actual extent of reductions will depend on the amount of space between the artificial teeth and the opposing teeth or residual ridge (Fig. 18-14, B).

9. Mark the location for the pinholes (Fig. 18-20). The holes should be centrally located in the body of the tooth and approximately 2 mm from proximal surfaces. Three holes are recommended for retention of maxillary anterior teeth, whereas two holes are sufficient for mandibular anterior teeth.

10. Prepare recesses for the pinholes with a No. 8 round bur (Fig. 18-21). The recesses will provide a strong union between the pin and the backing, especially while working with the wax pattern.

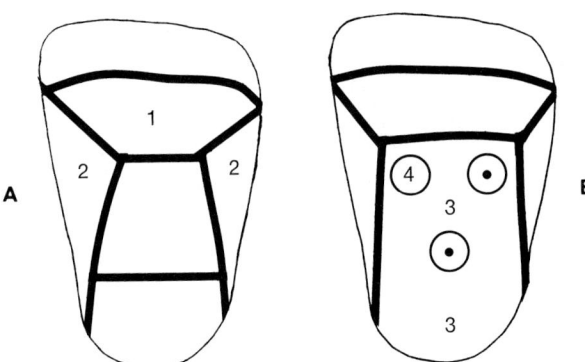

**Fig. 18-14. A,** Initial incisal reduction *(1)* and proximal reduction *(2)* outlined on lingual surface of resin denture tooth to provide 1 mm space for metal backing. **B,** Reduction of body of lingual surface *(3)*, leaving at least 3 mm for pinholes. Recesses prepared with No. 8 round bur *(4)* for strong union of resin pin in wax pattern.

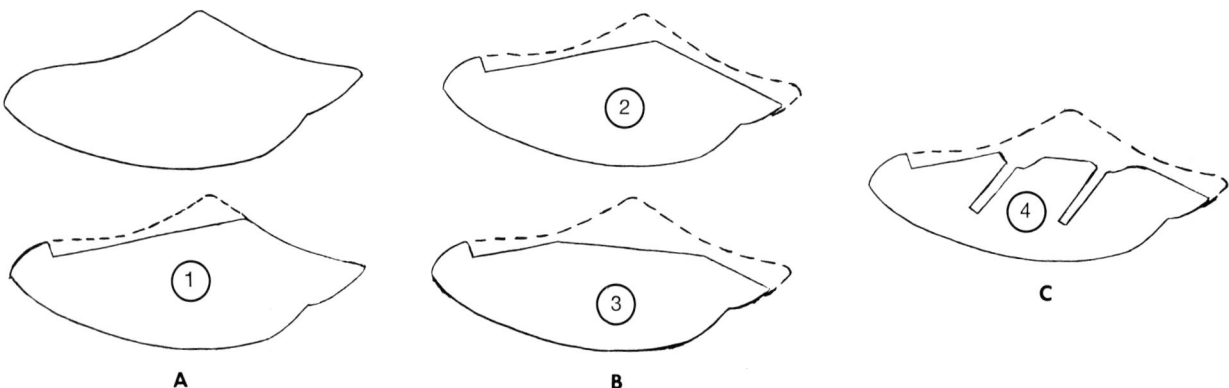

**Fig. 18-15. A,** Incisal reduction *(1)* may vary according to mold and thickness of tooth. **B,** Reduction of body of tooth *(2 and 3)*. **C,** Direction and depth of pinholes *(4)* that are directed incisally.

*Reinforced facings and metal backings* **531**

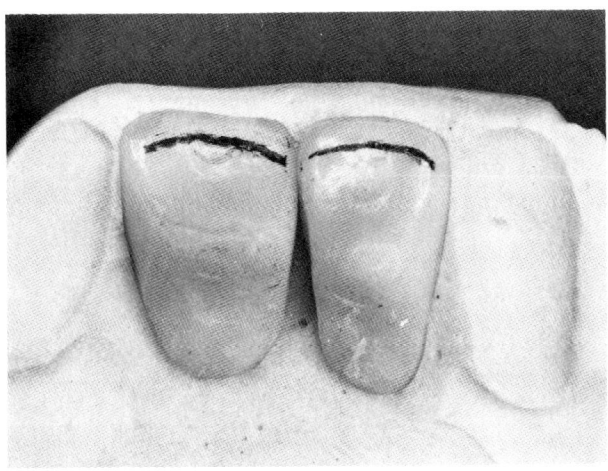

**Fig. 18-16.** Incisal finishing line marked 1 mm from incisal edge.

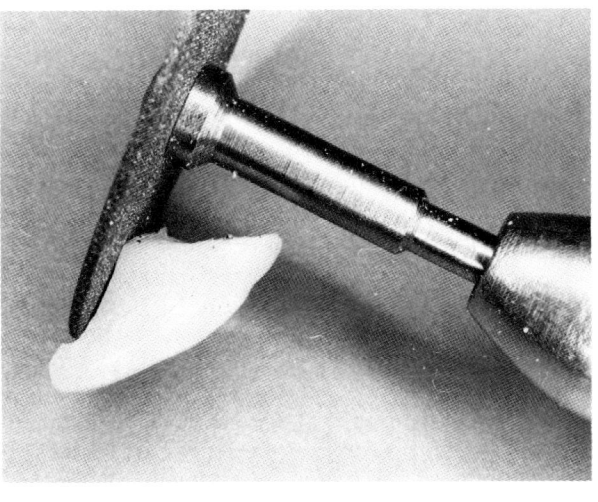

**Fig. 18-17.** Separating disk is first used to create finishing line and slightly reduce lingual surface.

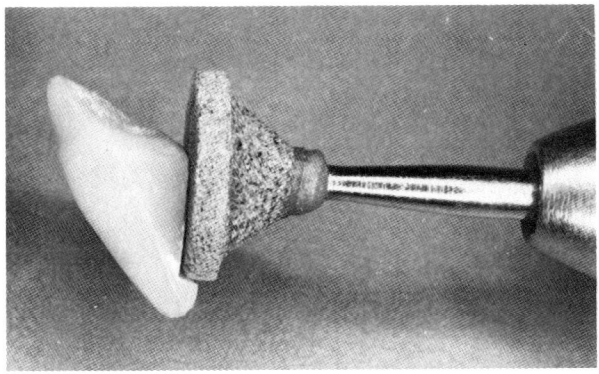

**Fig. 18-18.** Green stone is used to smooth incisal margin.

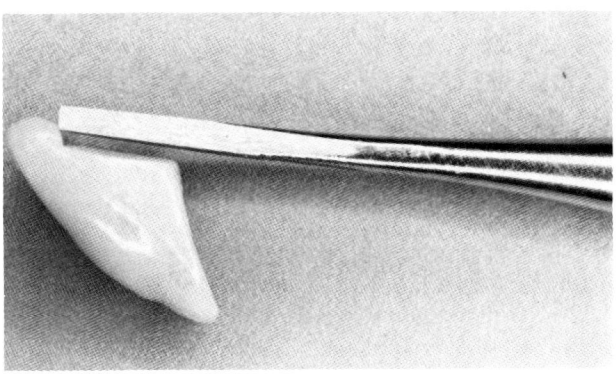

**Fig. 18-19.** Sharp instrument is used to finish margin of preparation.

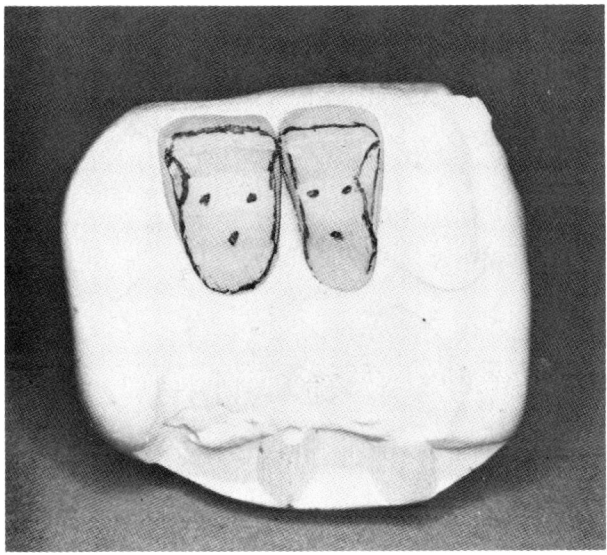

**Fig. 18-20.** Location of pinholes.

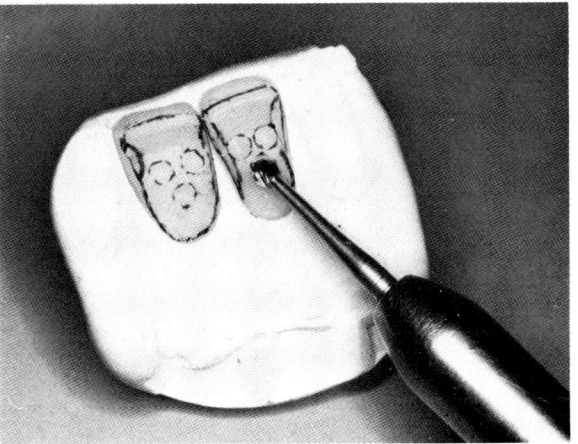

**Fig. 18-21.** Recesses for pinholes and to ensure strong wax pattern.

11. Return the teeth to the master cast, and confirm that the proximal and gingival reductions are adequate (Fig. 18-22). Also confirm that adequate space exists for the metal backings (Fig. 18-23).

12. Embed the labial surfaces of the teeth in a patty of plaster. After the plaster sets, place the patty on a surveyor (Fig. 18-24). Tilt the facings at an angle of 45 degrees to the base of the surveyor.

13. Drill the holes with a 0.027-inch twist drill in a straight handpiece secured parallel to the vertical arm of the surveyor by a handpiece holder* (Fig. 18-25). Drill presses are ideal for this operation, if available. The pinholes in each tooth will be parallel. There is no requirement for precise parallelism between facings because the facings will be cemented individually. The pinholes should be approximately 3 mm in depth from the bottom of the recess.

---

*Handpiece holder, The J. M. Ney Co., Bloomfield, Conn.

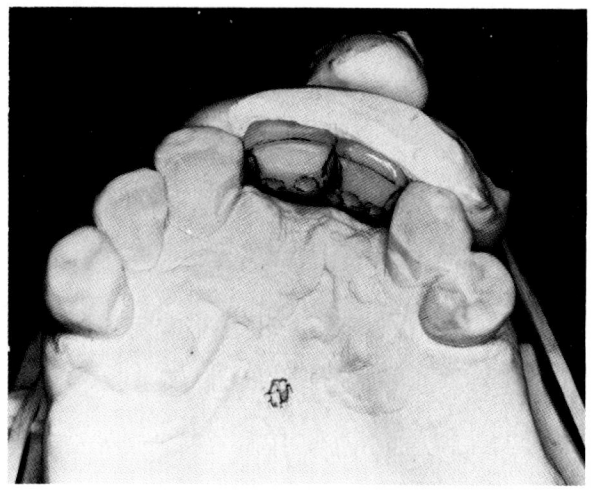

**Fig. 18-22.** Confirm that proximal and gingival reductions are adequate.

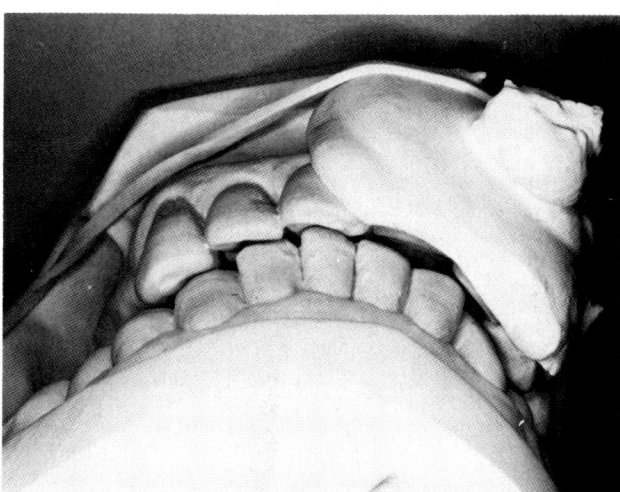

**Fig. 18-23.** Confirm that adequate space exists for metal backings.

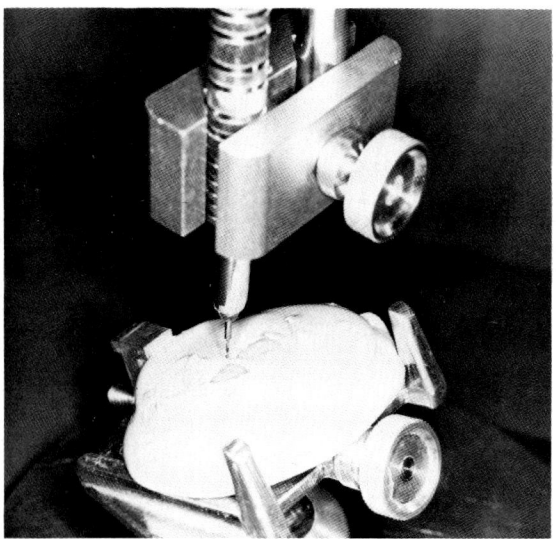

**Fig. 18-24.** Facings at 45-degree angle on surveyor in patty of plaster.

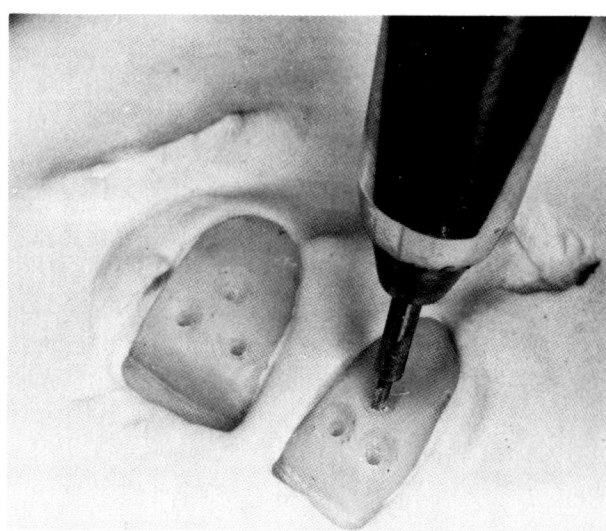

**Fig. 18-25.** Pinholes are drilled using 0.027-inch twist drill.

14. Prepare the master cast for duplication in the conventional manner (Fig. 18-26). Before duplicating, it is wise to check the fit of the stone core on the master cast. Confirm the fit of the core on the refractory cast (Fig. 18-27).

15. Perlon or nylon pins or nylon fishing line segments of approximately 0.023 inch in diameter are cut to extend from the pinhole 2 mm. The nylon pins should fit freely in the pinholes. Cut the end of the pin that will be inserted in the hole with a scalpel or razor blade on a piece of wood or vinyl to ensure a smooth cut. Cut the pin to the proper length with a wire cutters (Figs. 18-28 and 18-29).

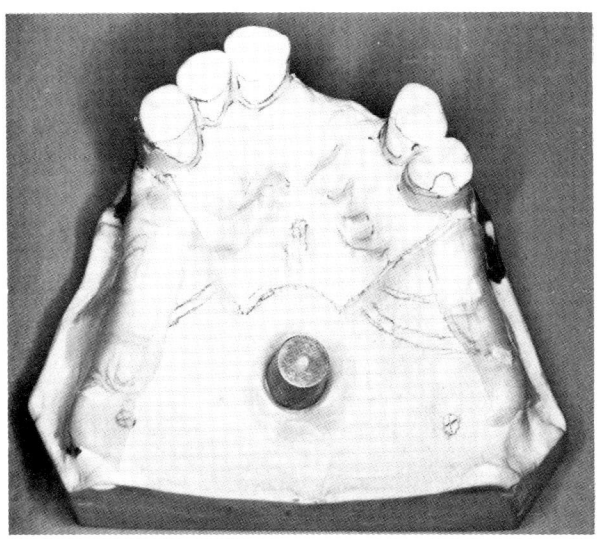

**Fig. 18-26.** Master cast ready for duplication.

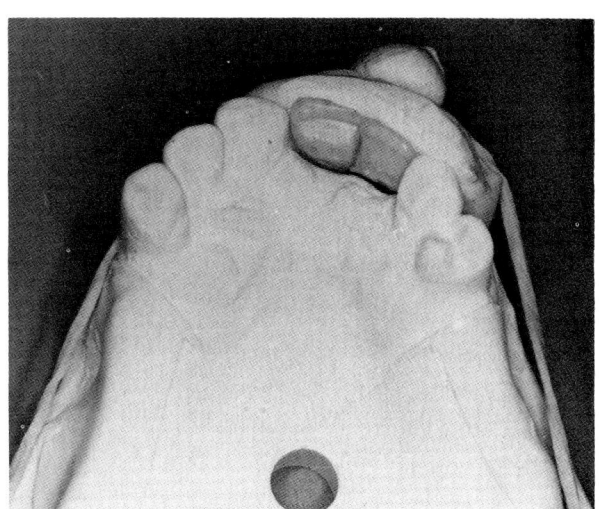

**Fig. 18-27.** Core and teeth on refractory cast.

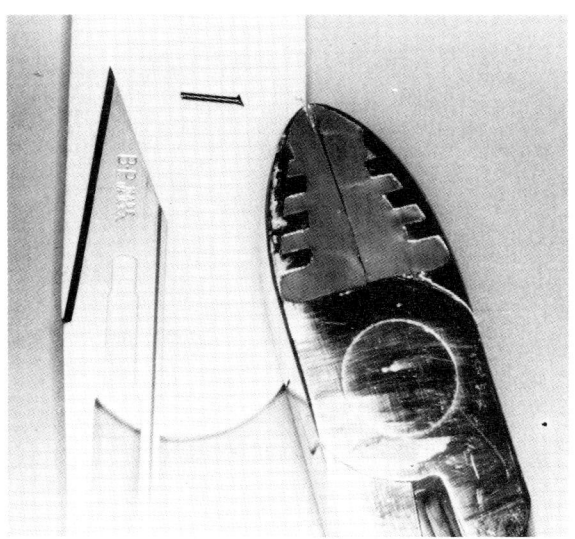

**Fig. 18-28.** Sharp blade gives smooth cut. Wire cutters are used for cutting to proper length.

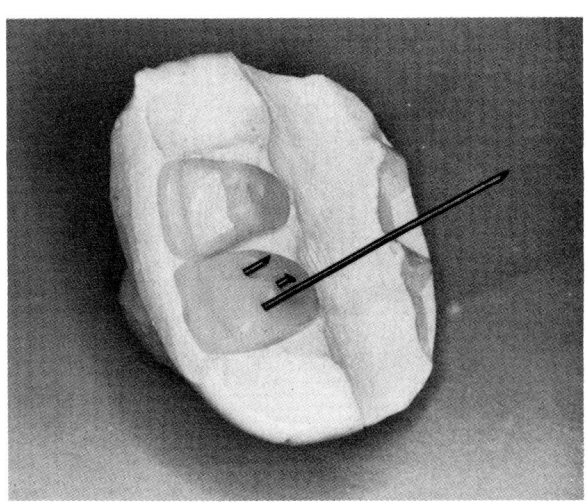

**Fig. 18-29.** Pins in holes with two cut to proper length.

16. Flatten the ends of the pins with a hot burnisher or spatula to the level of the recesses (Fig. 18-30).

17. Lubricate the facings with a suitable wax pattern and die separating liquid (Fig. 18-31).

18. Insert the pins in the pinholes, and flow hot wax around the heads of the pins in the recesses to form a strong union (Fig. 18-32).

19. Wax up the individual backings, and inspect their position in the stone core (Fig. 18-33). Dust wax powder* on the wax prior to checking the fit of the wax backings to the refractory cast.

20. Relate the facings to the refractory cast, and adjust the wax as necessary until the stone core fits accurately (Fig. 18-34). At this point the wax backings should be attached to the wax pattern on the refractory cast.

21. Remove the core and the facings, remembering the direction of the pins. Note the areas where the backings are not sealed to the master cast (Fig. 18-35).

22. Replace the facings, and seal the gingival edges of the wax pattern to the refractory cast (Fig. 18-36).

*Almore International, Inc., Portland, Ore.

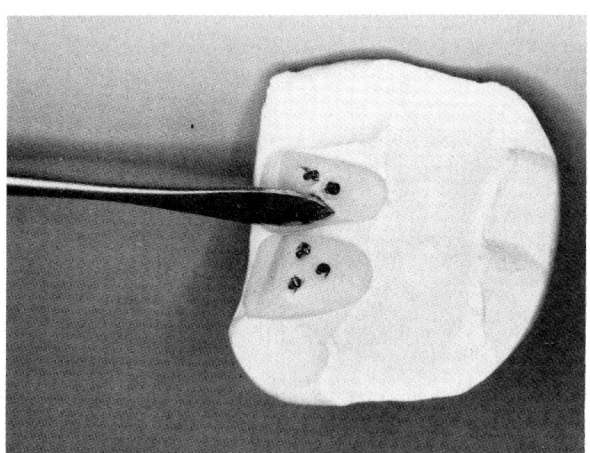

Fig. 18-30. Ends of pins flattened to ensure retention in wax.

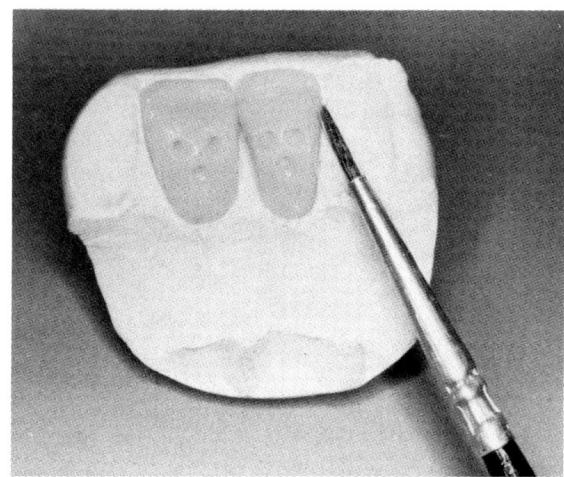

Fig. 18-31. Facings lubricated for making wax pattern.

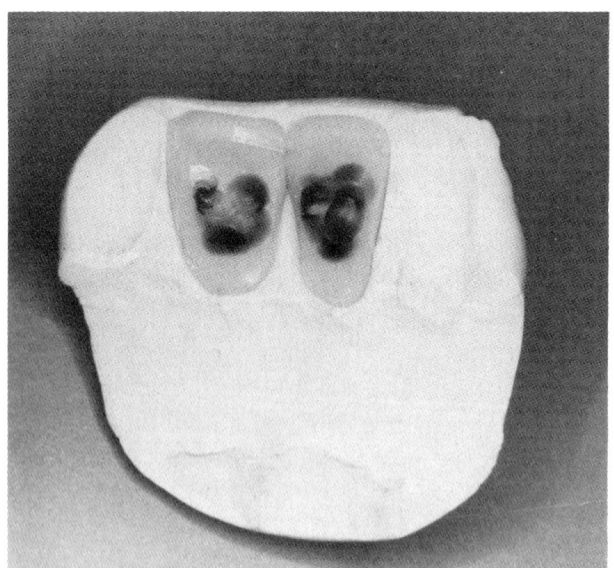

Fig. 18-32. Hot wax is flowed into recesses.

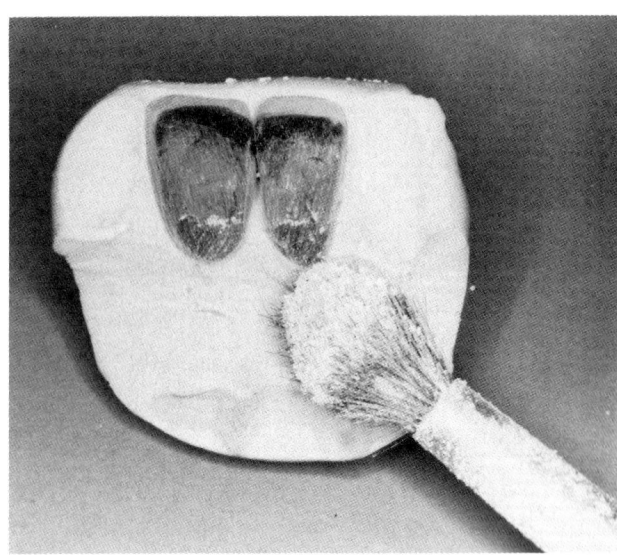

Fig. 18-33. Backings are waxed and dusted with wax powder and accurately placed in stone core.

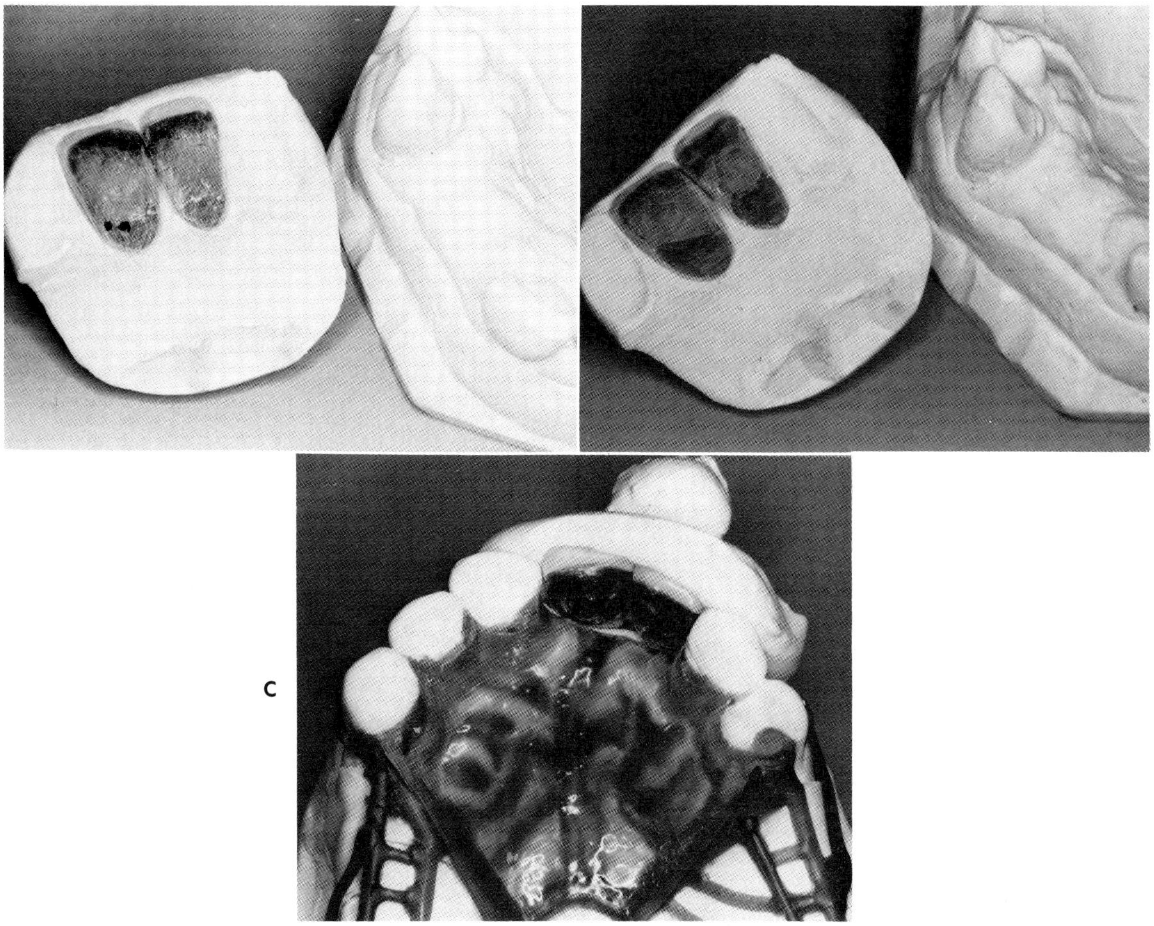

Reinforced facings and metal backings **535**

**Fig. 18-34. A,** Patterns fitted to refractory cast. **B,** Gingival portion of pattern fitted to refractory cast. **C,** Wax pattern ready for union to each other.

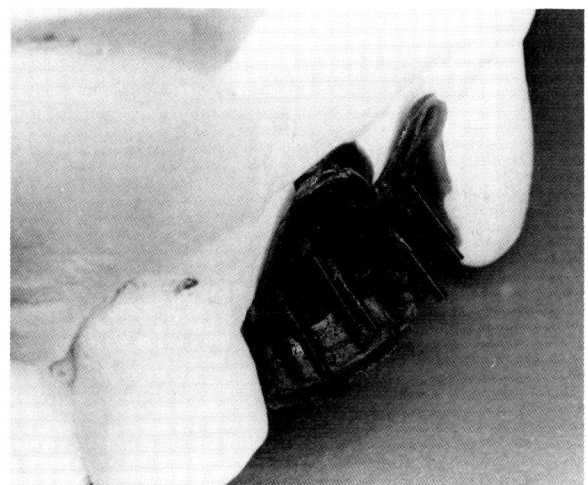

**Fig. 18-35.** Defects noted in gingival edges of wax pattern.

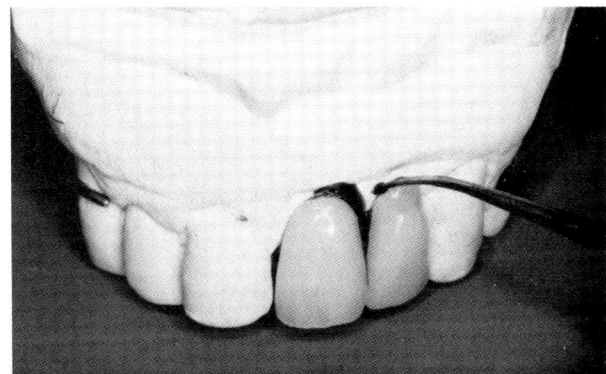

**Fig. 18-36.** Gingival edges sealed to refractory cast.

23. Carve away any excess wax from the interproximal or gingival areas (Fig. 18-37). The wax can be extremely thin gingivally and can be reduced in bulk as much as desired as long as the pins are not disturbed. Apply crystals for retention of tissue-colored resin to the wax that is gingival, lateral, and interproximal to the facings (Fig. 18-38).

24. Articulate the refractory cast, if necessary, and mount it in an articulator. Lubricate the base of the refractory cast with a separating medium to ensure ease of separation (Fig. 18-39).

25. Adjust the condylar guidance with an interocclusal record or prescription and set the incisal guidance according to the function of the remaining natural teeth. It is generally most favorable for the incisal guidance to be equal or less than the condylar guidance (Fig. 18-40).

26. The incisal guidance can often be made more favorable by reducing the amount of vertical overlap or increasing the amount of horizontal overlap. Adjust the opposing teeth as necessary, and wax the backings to restore occlusion (Fig. 18-41).

27. Apply wax powder to the wax pattern, and alter the wax-up or opposing teeth to restore the desired occlusion (Fig. 18-42).

28. Move the articulator into eccentric position, and refine the shape of the lingual concavity for optimum occlusal guidance (Fig. 18-43). Use cloth articulating ribbon to mark areas of opposing teeth that require modification (Fig. 18-44). The labial

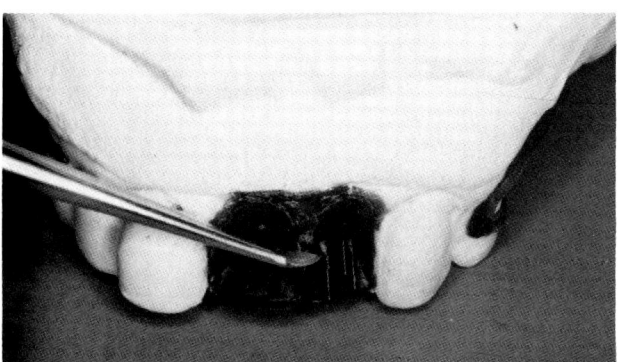

**Fig. 18-37.** Excess wax is carved away from interproximal and gingival areas.

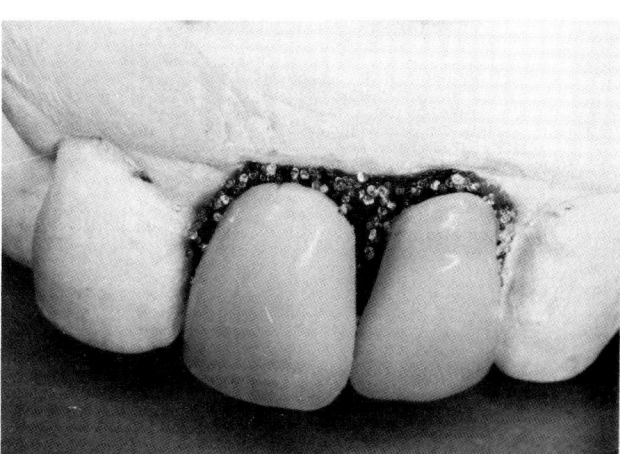

**Fig. 18-38.** Resin crystals applied to wax for retention.

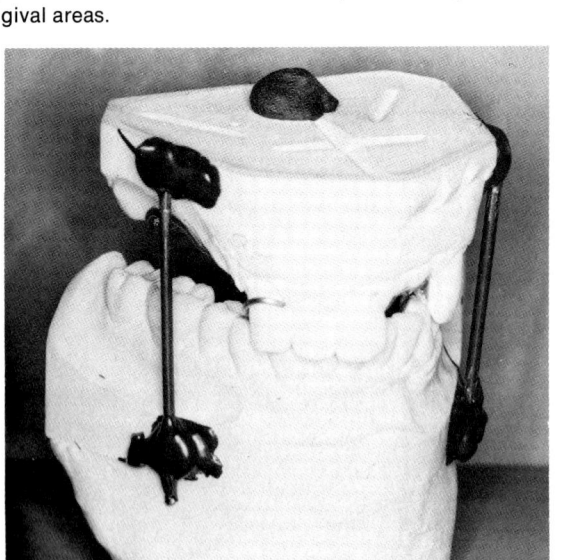

**Fig. 18-39.** Refractory cast prepared for articulation.

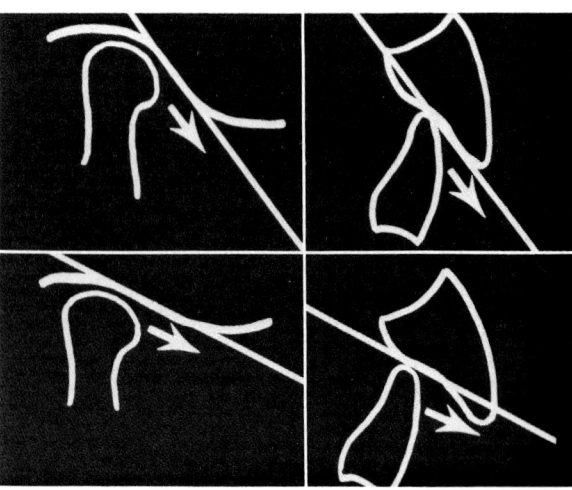

**Fig. 18-40.** Incisal guidance should generally be similar to condylar guidance.

## Reinforced facings and metal backings 537

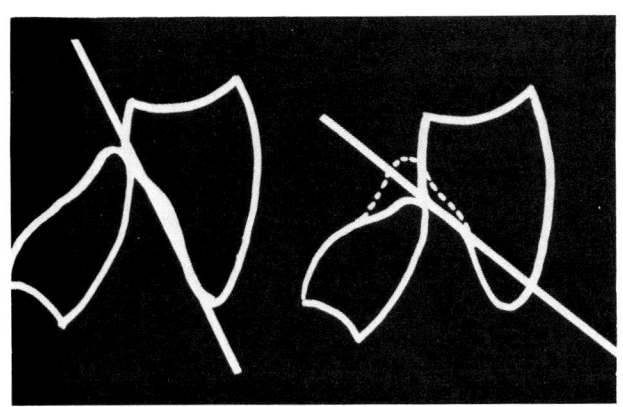

**Fig. 18-41.** Adjustment of opposing incisal edges can provide more optimum guidance.

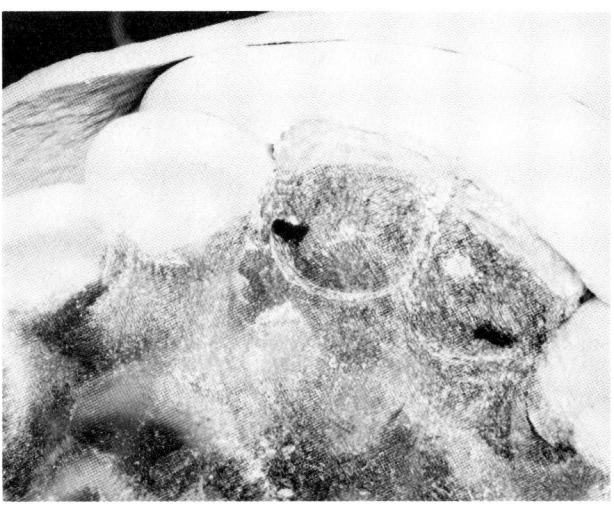

**Fig. 18-42.** Wax powder used to disclose occlusion.

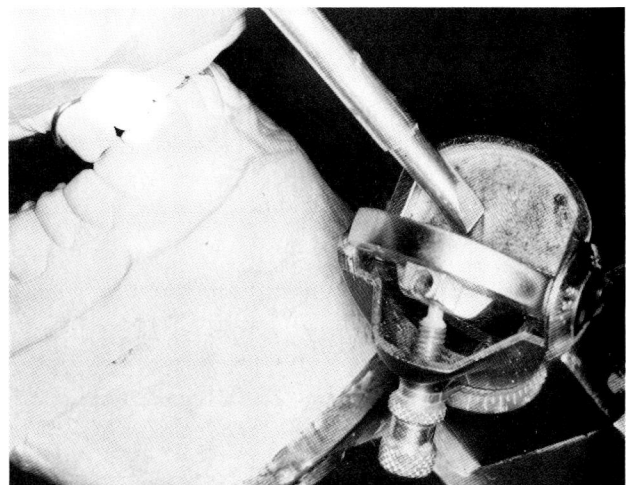

**Fig. 18-43.** Eccentric movements are examined.

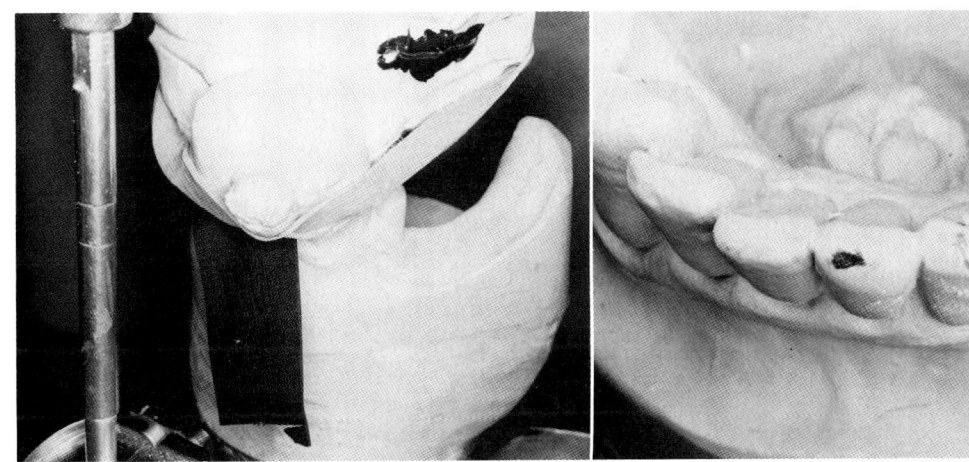

**Fig. 18-44. A,** Articulating ribbon used to mark areas to be altered on opposing teeth. **B,** Area to be reduced is marked off as plan for adjustment of natural teeth.

surfaces of the opposing teeth can often be selectively modified to provide more horizontal overlap and decrease the angle of incisal guidance (Fig. 18-45, *A*). Reshaping of this nature changes the position of the incisal edge and requires rewaxing in centric occlusion. Indicate modifications clearly on the altered teeth (Fig. 18-45, *B*). Apply wax powder, and develop the wax pattern as necessary to complete the contour of the lingual concavity (Fig. 18-45, *C*).

29. Invest and cast the removable partial denture framework. Adjust the metal casting to fit the master cast. Remove nodules or fins around the pin with small burs (Fig. 18-46, *A*). Round off the ends of the pins with a tapered stone (Fig. 18-46, *B*).

30. Return the master cast to the articulator, and make any necessary occlusal adjustments. Set up the remaining artificial teeth. Process the posterior teeth to the metal casting by the method desired. If the metal casting is invested in plaster, the metal backings and pins should be protected with block-out compound.

31. Remount the master cast, and make occlusal corrections for changes that occurred during processing. Clean the facings, pins, and metal backings with resin monomer (Fig. 18-47).

32. Mix an extremely thin mix of a dark, tooth-colored resin. Place the resin around the pins and in the pinholes with a Lentulo spiral* or a fluted or fissure bur (Fig. 18-48). Seat the facings quickly and forcefully. Remove excess resin from the surface of the facings, and spread some resin over the crystals of the metal casting to serve as a masking agent. Seat no more than one or two facings at a time. The polymer particles can be pulverized, if desired, to reduce the amount of pressure required for accurate cementation.

33. Add a fibered repair resin of the desired shade to restore the form of mucosal and gingival tissues (Fig. 18-49, *A*). Place the cast in a pressure

---

*Union Broach Corp., Long Island City, N.Y.

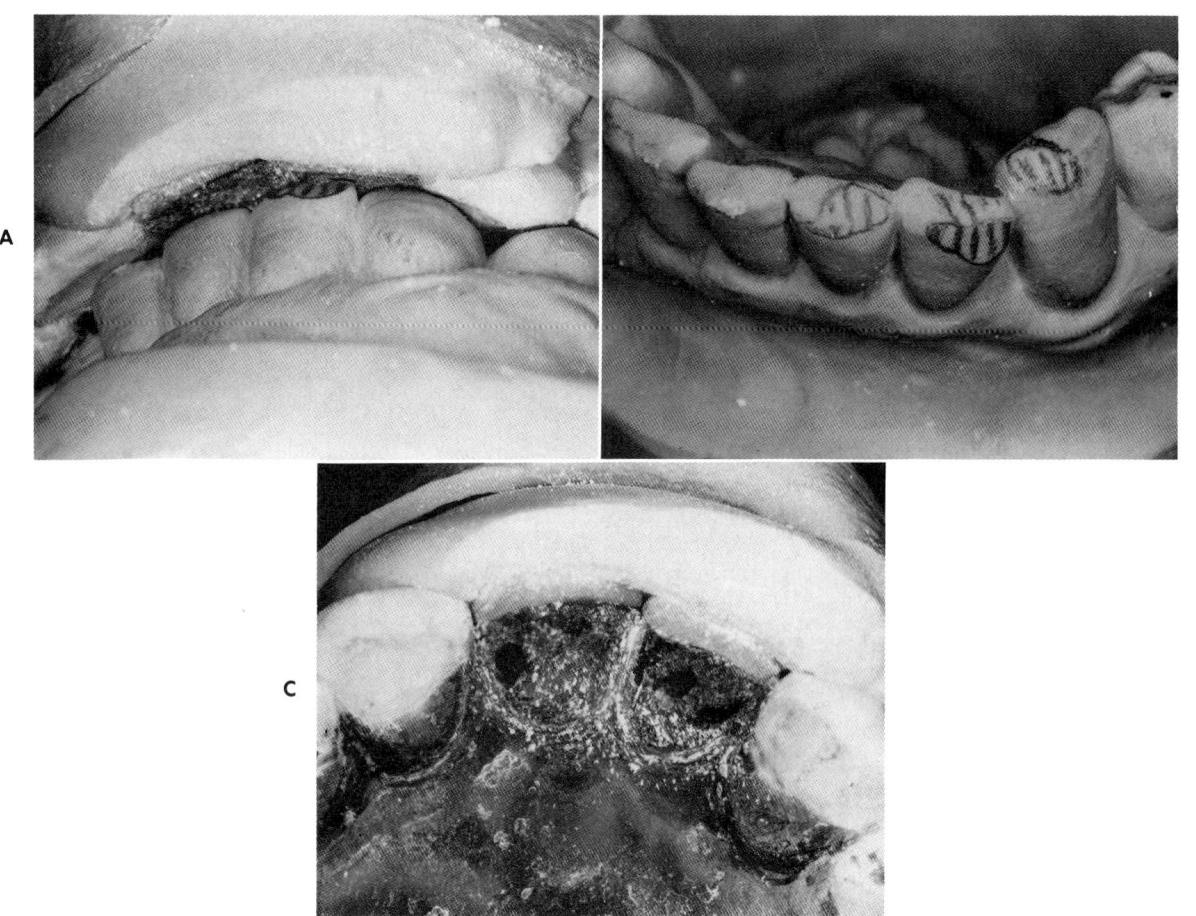

Fig. 18-45. **A,** Reduction of labial surface to provide more horizontal overlap. **B,** Marks to guide proper adjustment of teeth in mouth. **C,** Desired occlusion and guidance are confirmed.

### Reinforced facings and metal backings 539

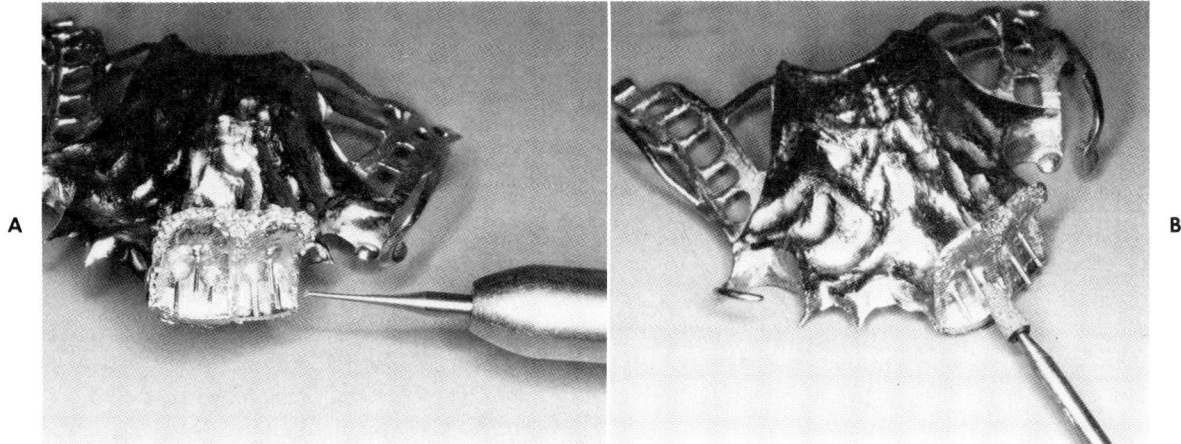

**Fig. 18-46. A,** Nodules or fins removed with carbide bur or stone. **B,** Ends of pins rounded to facilitate complete seating of facings.

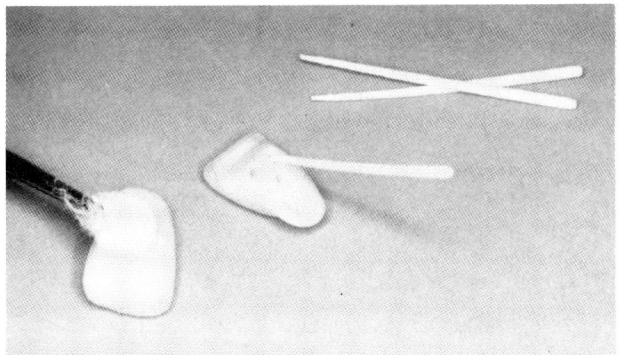

**Fig. 18-47.** Resin facings are cleaned with resin monomer prior to cementation.

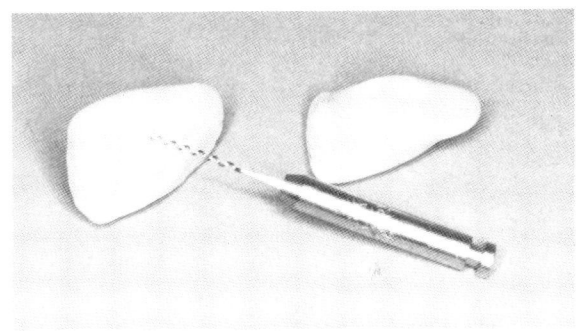

**Fig. 18-48.** Thinly mixed resin of dark shade is placed in pinholes with a Lentulo spiral.

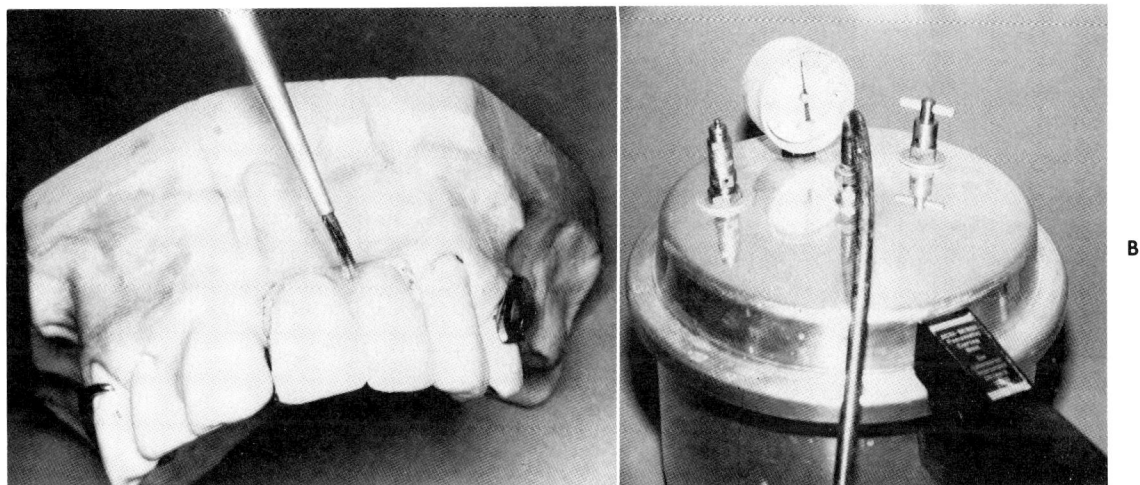

**Fig. 18-49. A,** Tissue-colored and chemically accelerated resin is applied to restore gingival and mucosal tissues. **B,** Resin is processed in pressure pot at 110° F (43.5° C) at 30 psi for 15 minutes.

pot at 110° F (43.5° C) at 30 psi for 15 minutes (Fig. 18-49, *B*). The resin can be placed around the cemented facings on the master cast or on a duplicate cast before or after processing of the remaining teeth. Avoid carrying the resin into undercut areas to prevent the possibility of breaking the master cast. For this reason, it is usually desirable to complete the mucosal portion of the restoration on a duplicate of the master cast with blockout in place.

34. Finish the restoration with fine stones and burs. Polish the resin with a mixture of water and pumice. Polish around the teeth with a rubber cup in a straight handpiece. Use extreme care in polishing with wheels to avoid abrasion of the resin. The finished anterior resin restoration should restore gingival and mucosal contours and blend evenly with the metal casting (Fig. 18-50).

## Alternative approaches
### Flatback facing technique

Flatback facings are most useful when individual teeth are to be replaced and when characterization or incisal translucency is not an important consideration. The procedures are essentially the same as with pin facings (Figs. 18-51 to 18-54). A common misconception is that excessive loss or ridge form is a contraindication for facings and metal backings. The only technical modification is to apply wax at the gingival level. Carve the wax thin, and then apply crystals to facilitate the retention of resin.

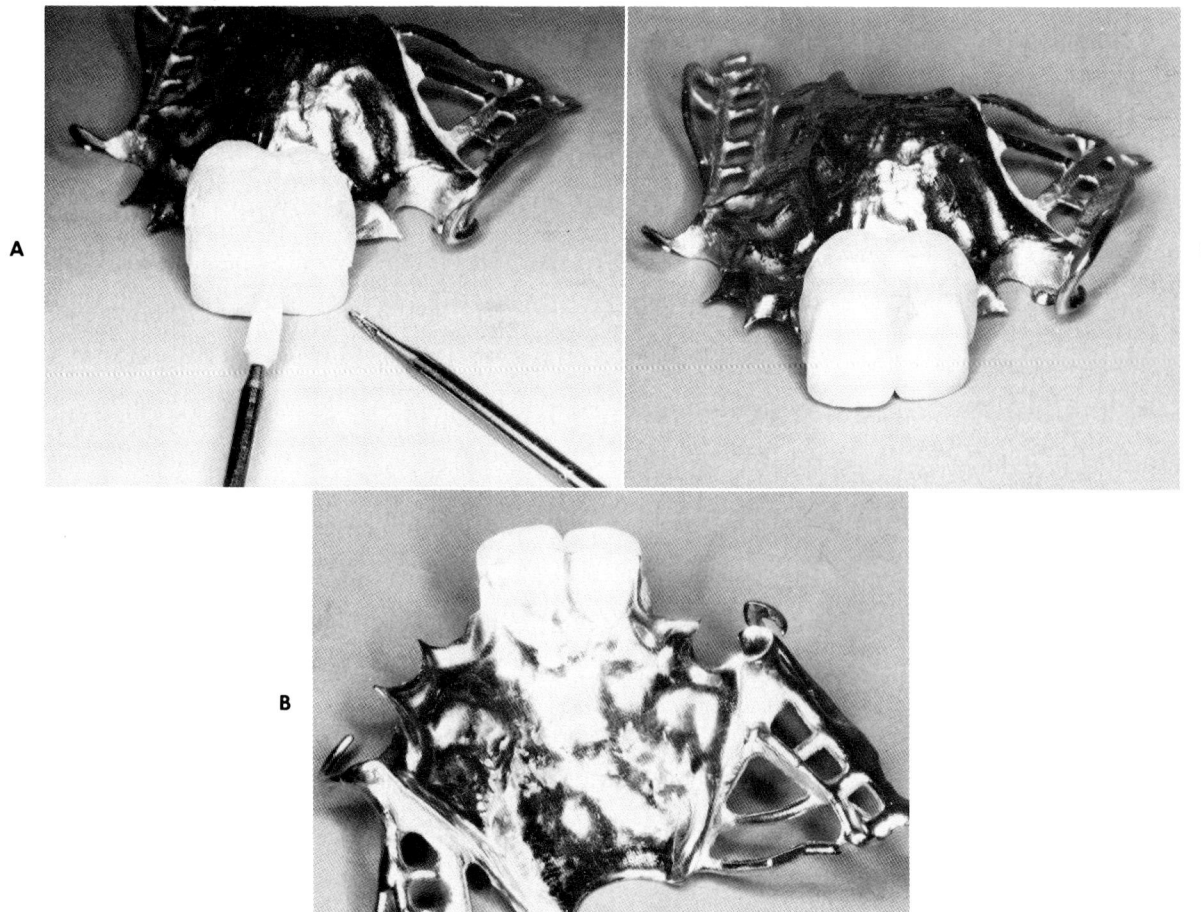

**Fig. 18-50. A,** Tissue-colored resin is finished with burs, stones, and polished with rubber cup and flour of pumice. **B,** Missing gingival and mucosal tissues are replaced with tissue-colored resin. **C,** Metal backing restores occlusion and guidance and provides strong durable restoration.

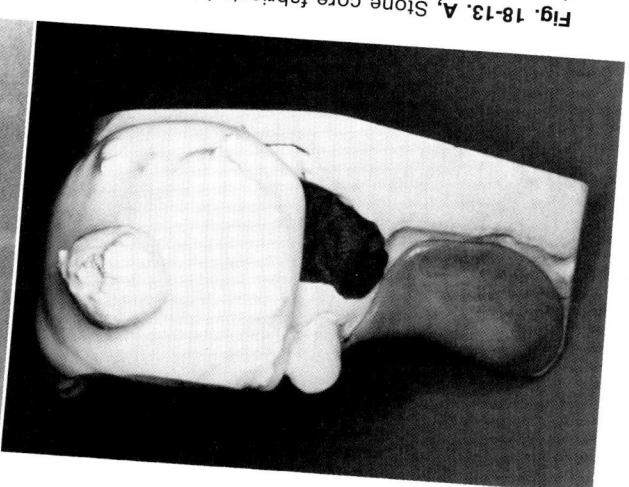

**Fig. 18-11.** Border of master cast is indexed for positive relation of stone core.

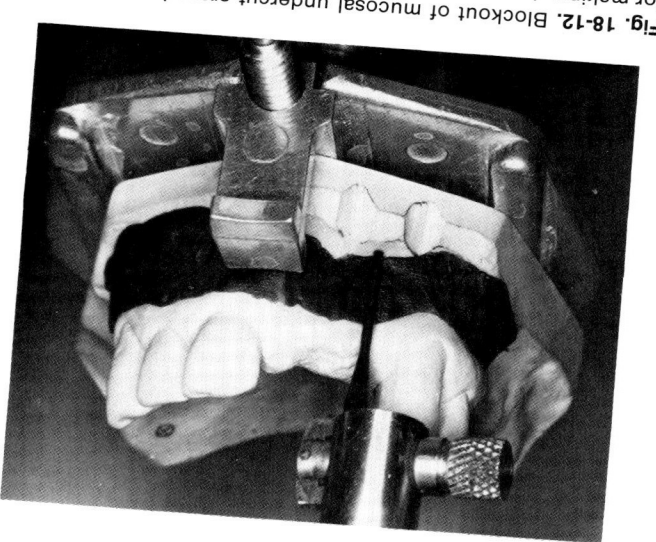

**Fig. 18-12.** Blockout of mucosal undercut areas in preparation for making stone core and later duplication of master cast.

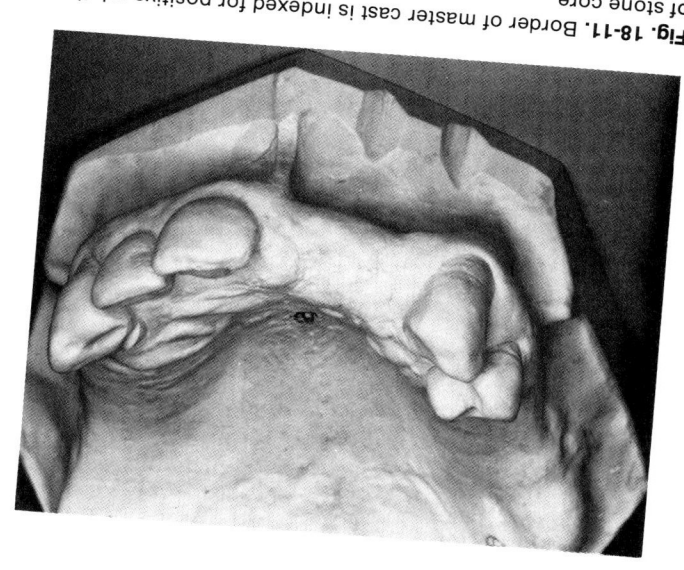

**Fig. 18-13. A,** Stone core fabricated to relate facings to border of cast and adjacent teeth. **B,** Approximately half of labial surfaces of adjacent teeth should be included by core.

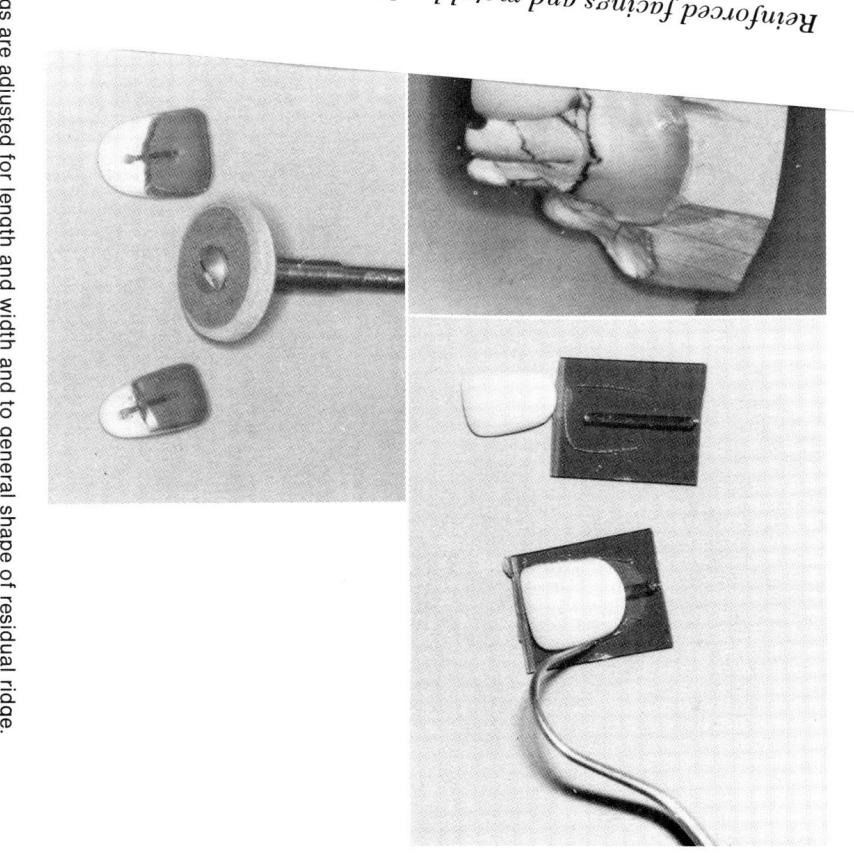

**Fig. 18-52. A,** Facings are adjusted for length and width and to general shape of residual ridge. **B,** Resin backings are marked for trimming to shape of facing. **C,** Backing is trimmed with disk or stone wheel.

**542** Dental laboratory procedures: removable partial dentures

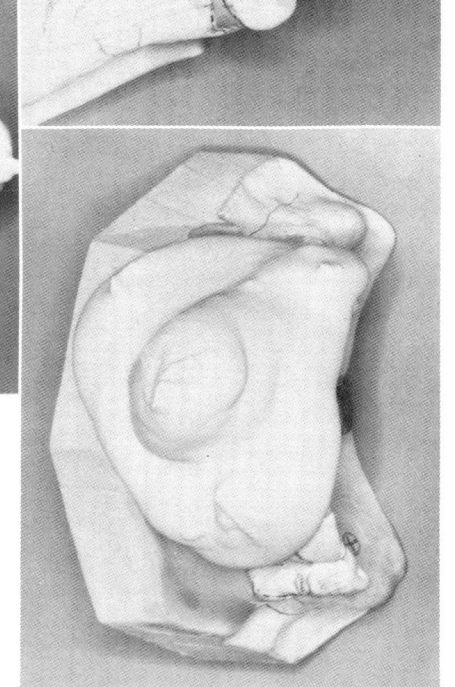

**Fig. 18-53. A,** Facings positioned with aid of blockout compound for making stone core. **B,** Stone core is related to adjacent teeth and base of cast after master cast is blocked out for duplication. **C,** Facings related to refractory cast.

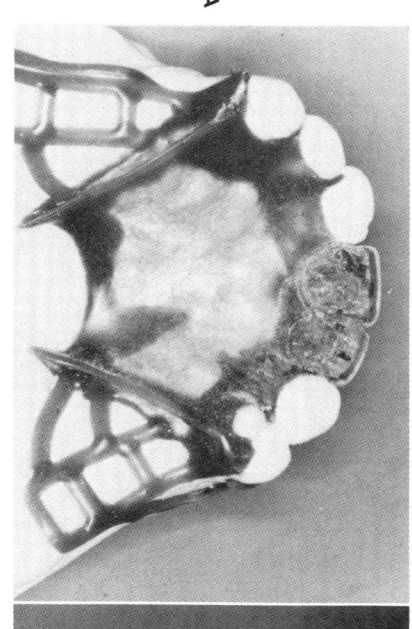

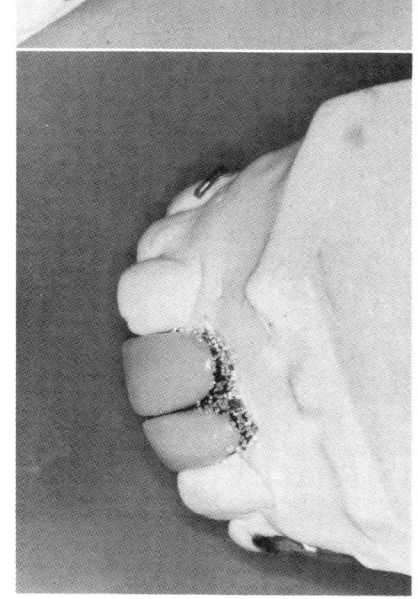

**Fig. 18-54. A,** Lingual anatomy waxed for proper occlusion and guidance. **B,** Resin crystals applied gingival to facings for retention of tooth-colored resin.

sharp instrument such as a ... (18 and 18-19). The lingual reduction should be a minimum depth of 1 mm. Carry the proximal reductions to a line just short of the interproximal contacts

...pecially while working with the...

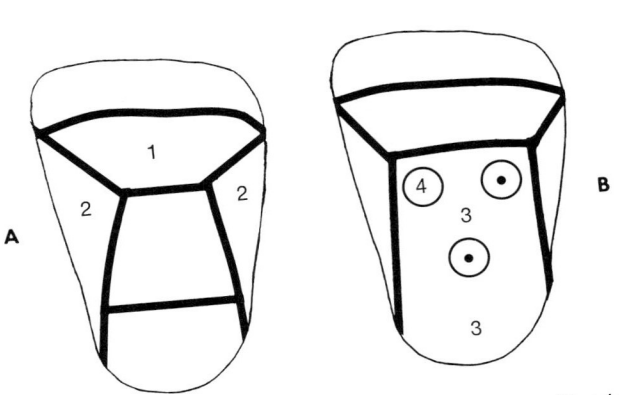

**Fig. 18-14. A,** Initial incisal reduction *(1)* and proximal reduction *(2)* outlined on lingual surface of resin denture tooth to provide 1 mm space for metal backing. **B,** Reduction of body of lingual surface *(3)*, leaving at least 3 mm for pinholes. Recesses prepared with No. 8 round bur *(4)* for strong union of resin pin in wax pattern.

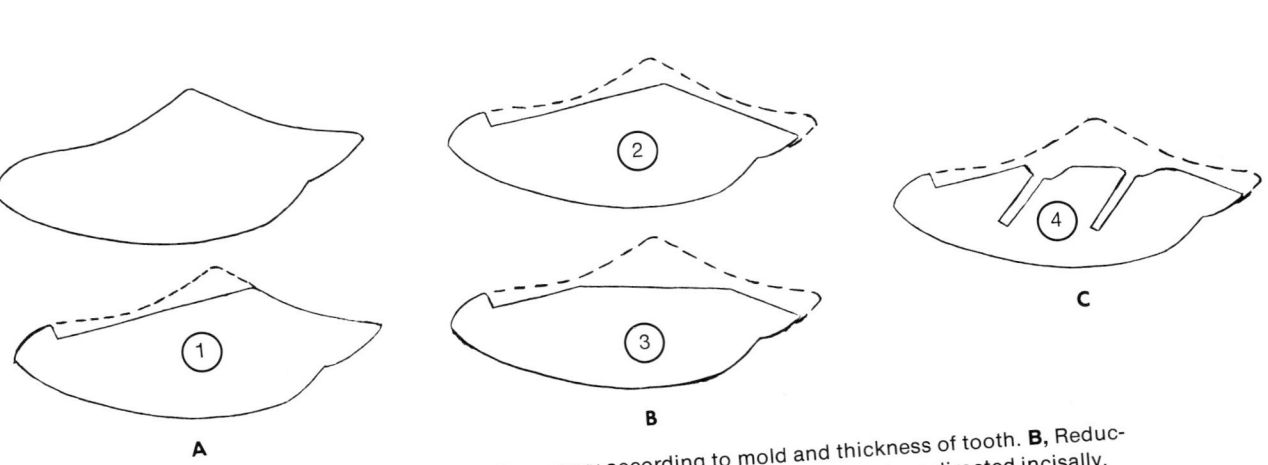

**Fig. 18-15. A,** Incisal reduction *(1)* may vary according to mold and thickness of tooth. **B,** Reduction of body of tooth *(2 and 3)*. **C,** Direction and depth of pinholes *(4)* that are directed incisally.

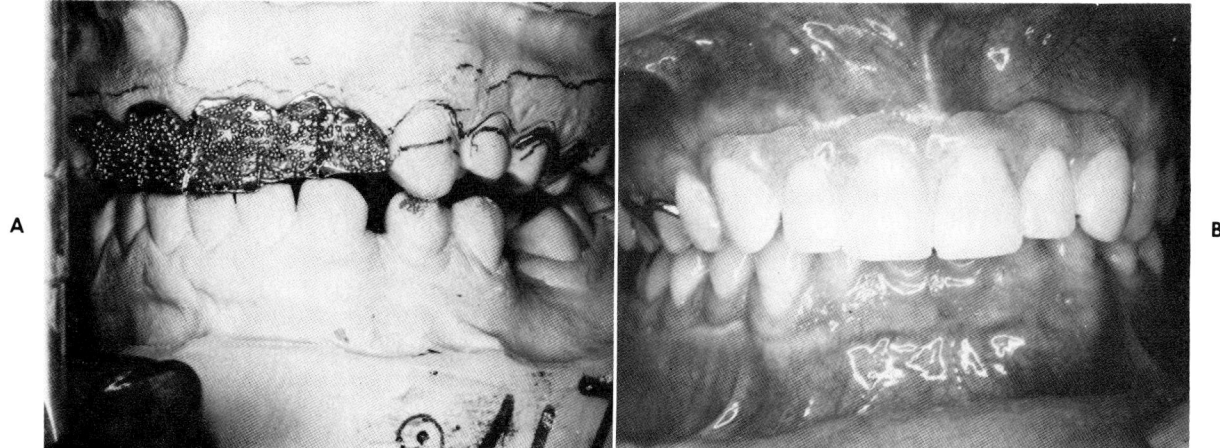

**Fig. 18-55. A,** Metal backings for long-span partially edentulous situation. Attention must be given to occlusal guidance and application of beads for retention of facings. **B,** Finished partial denture in mouth. Facings were processed with resin in flask in this situation.

### Bead or crystal retention technique

The bead or crystal retention method of retaining resin facings can be successfully employed if several steps are followed carefully (Fig. 18-55). Do not relieve the teeth excessively thin prior to cementation of the facings, or the color of the teeth will be altered. Some space must be provided just prior to cementation to compensate for the addition of resin crystals or beads to the wax pattern. The facings must be seated with the core for their final relief and during cementation. The beads must be carefully applied to the wax pattern with a minimum amount of adhesive so the undercuts will not be obliterated. Finally, special care must be used in investing the wax pattern so the beads will not be dislodged.

### Reinforced anterior pontic technique

The reinforced anterior pontic (RAP) is fabricated with a resin denture tooth that has been altered to accommodate a vertical reinforcement of the metal casting. The RAP technique provides a stronger union than single teeth supported by mesh. The RAP has a resin occlusal surface rather than a metal backing and thus should not be used where metal backings are indicated. Resin will not provide durable occlusal guidance, and, if wear occurs, the opposing teeth may extrude. The RAP is an esthetic and strong replacement when factors such as occlusal guidance and extrusion are not of major concern in the treatment of a prosthodontic patient. The important steps in fabricating an RAP are illustrated in Figs. 18-56 to 18-60.

The selection, adjustment, and positioning of denture teeth are essentially the same as for reverse-pin facings (Fig. 18-56). It is best to select a tooth mold that is thick labiolingually. The teeth are prepared on the lingual surface to accommodate an 8-gauge half-round wax form (Fig. 18-57). With the core in accurate position on the refractory cast, the vertical wax form is attached to the wax pattern (Fig. 18-58). The vertical reinforcements of the metal casting are slotted to increase retention with a separating disk (Fig. 18-59). The facings are related to the metal casting and attached by applying chemically accelerated resin (Fig. 18-60) and cured in a pressure pot at 30 psi for 15 minutes. The anatomy and occlusion are developed on the lingual surface of the pontics.

**544** *Dental laboratory procedures: removable partial dentures*

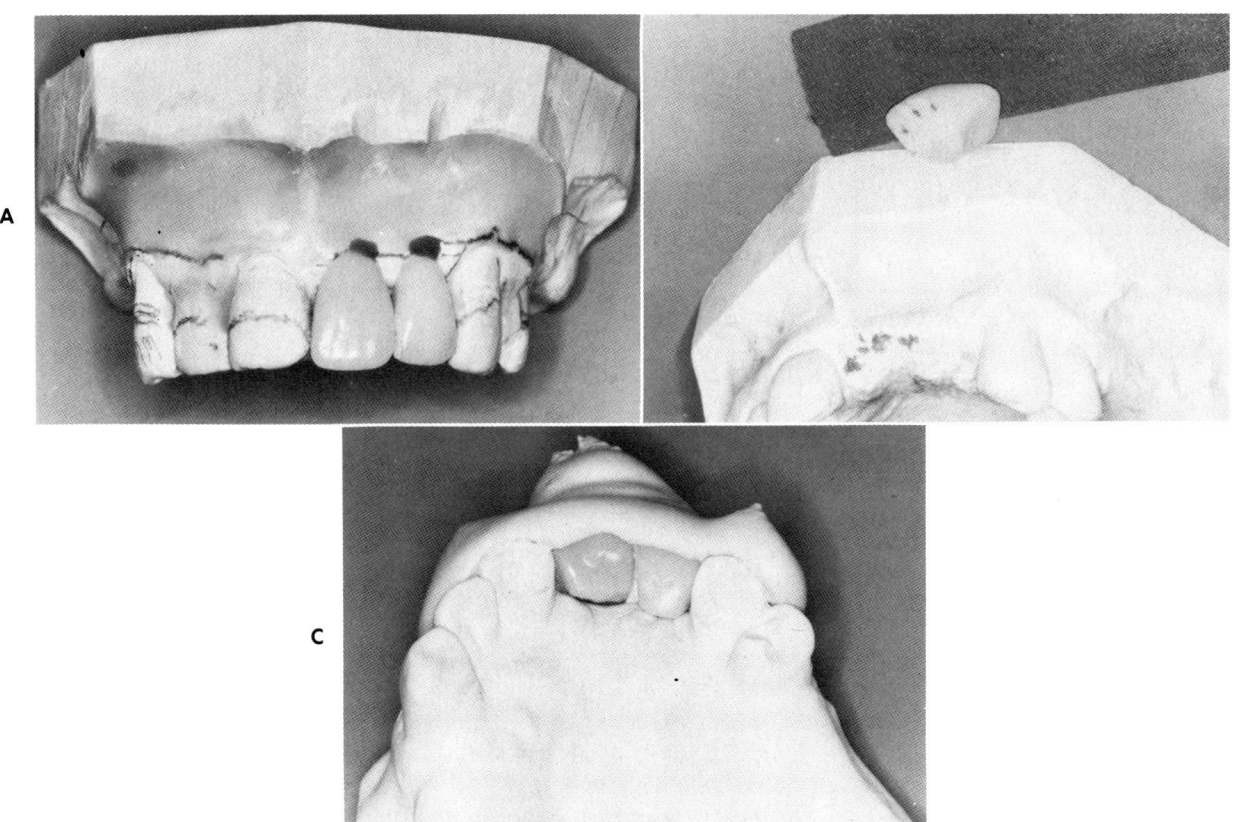

**Fig. 18-56. A,** Denture teeth positioned on master cast. **B,** Articulating ribbon is used to adjust denture tooth to residual ridge. **C,** Stone core is made on master cast, and accuracy of fit is verified on refractory cast.

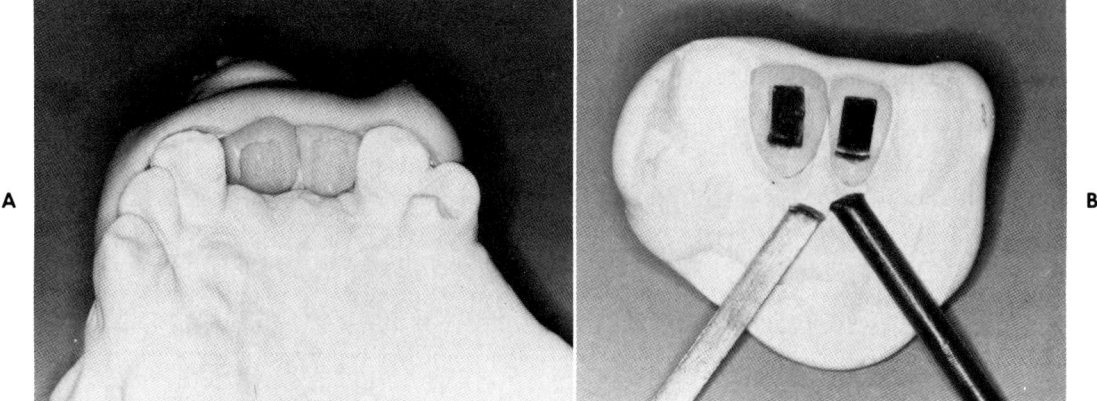

**Fig. 18-57. A,** Lingual surface prepared for 8-gauge half-round wax form. **B,** Wax form related to preparation.

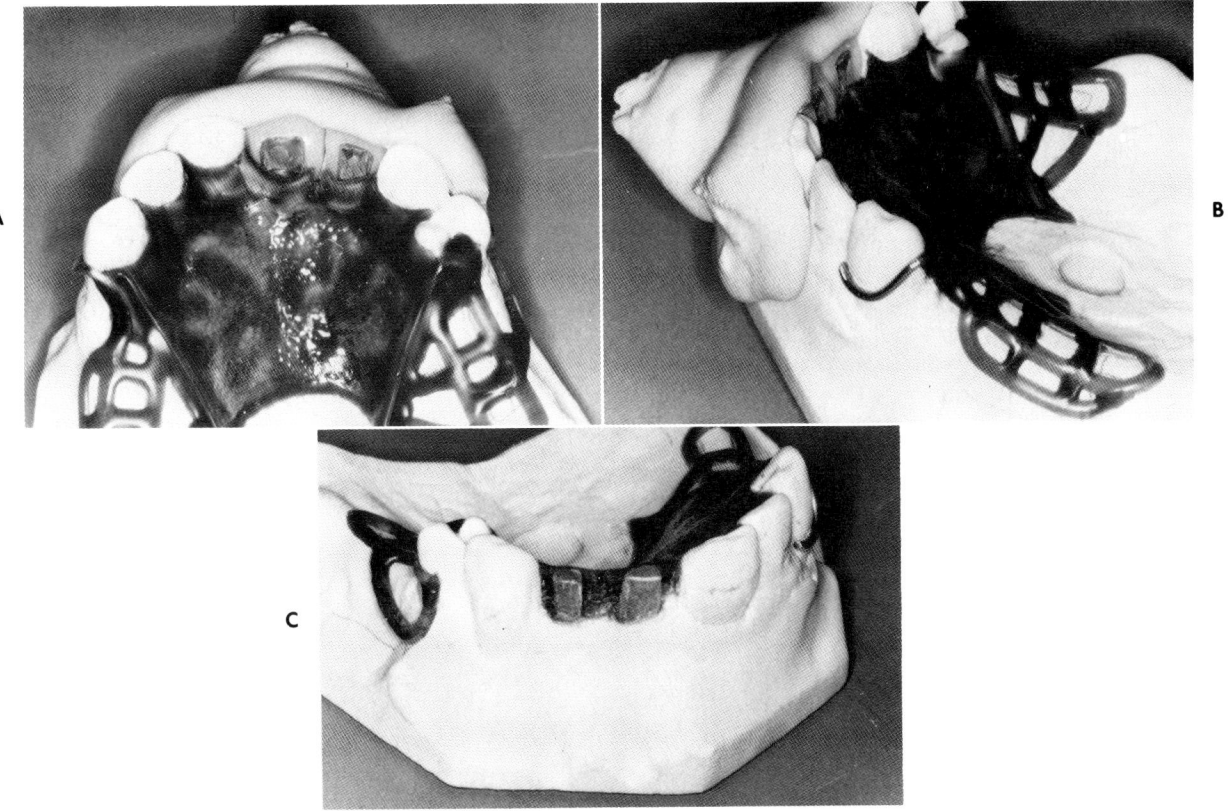

**Fig. 18-58. A** and **B,** Denture teeth related for waxing to wax pattern. **C,** Vertical reinforcements on wax pattern ready for investing.

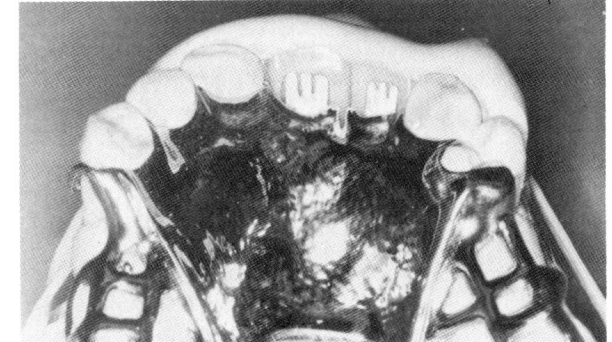

**Fig. 18-59.** Slots prepared in vertical reinforcements with separating disk.

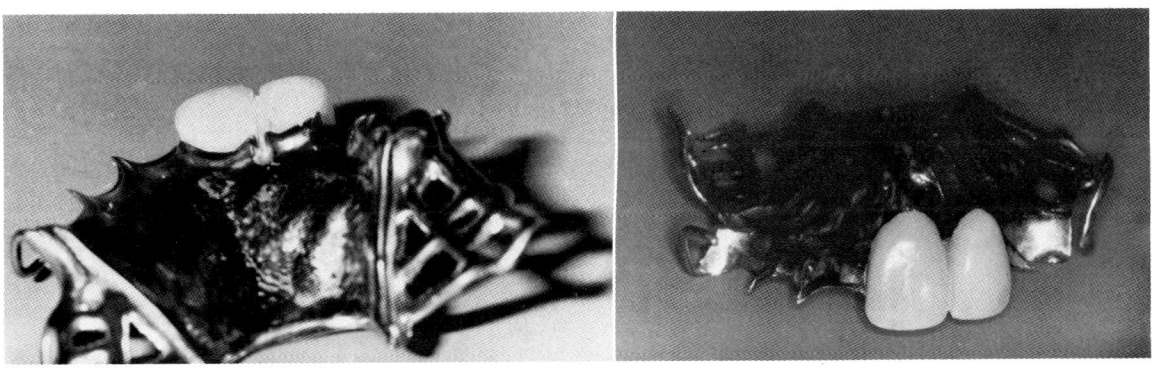

**Fig. 18-60.** Denture teeth attached to metal casting with chemically accelerated resin.

**Table 18-1.** Fabrication of metal backings

| Problem | Probable cause | Solution |
| --- | --- | --- |
| Inability to remove stone core | Separating medium not applied; core locked around arch | Apply separating medium to all areas of contact with stone; make two or more stone cores |
| Inability to relate stone core to refractory cast | Master cast blocked out after fabrication of core; refractory cast inaccurate; refractory cast index ground away | Block out master cast before making core; avoid inaccurate duplication procedure |
| Display of metal objectionable at interproximal space | Proximal reduction of facing carried too far labially | Mark area of extension and observe teeth core before preparation |
| Pins too short for adequate retention | Teeth prepared too extensively; holes not drilled to proper depth | Prepare teeth to accommodate no more than 1 mm of metal; Drill holes to depth of 3 mm at 45-degree angle |
| Pins dislodged from wax backings | Recesses not prepared prior to drilling pinholes; wax not hot enough to flow into recesses around pins | Drill recesses with No. 8 round bur; flow extremely hot wax into recesses; repair by perforating wax, and reseal with core in place |
| Metal shows through facings | Pinholes drilled too deep or perforated; tooth reduced excessively; pins not drilled at 45-degree angle | Reduce lingual surface only to provide room for metal; drill at 45-degree angle in body of facing |
| Metal shows through resin gingival to facings | Metal excessively thick; beads are too large for limited space | Carve wax very thin gingival to facings; use small crown and bridge crystals |
| Poor junction between facing and metal backing | Wax-up properly adapted; rough pins or nodules on casting; thick mix of resin used for cementation; insufficient pressure during cementation | Wax should be precise and neat; round ends of pins, and remove surface roughness; use extremely thin mix of resin for cementation; cement facings individually using heavy pressure |

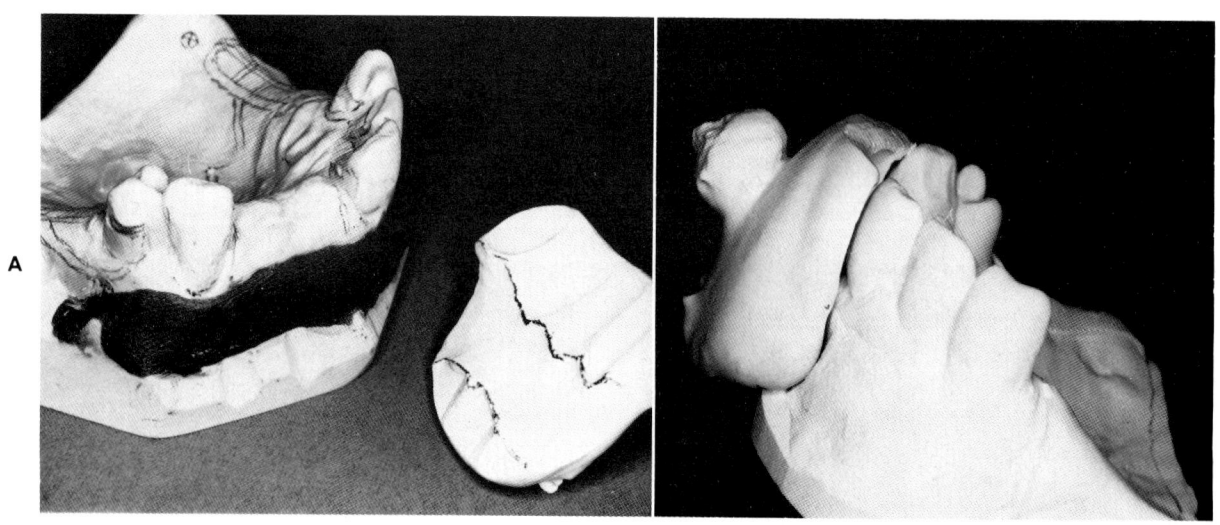

**Fig. 18-61. A,** Master cast blocked out prior to duplication and making of stone index. **B,** Stone index does not fit refractory cast due to blocking out after making stone core. One or other must now be relieved, or facings will be malpositioned.

## PROBLEM AREAS

Problem areas may be encountered during fabrication of metal backings. Metal backing techniques are often avoided because of difficulties encountered in the laboratory or dental office. Precise planning and meticulous efforts will minimize most problems. Possible problems and probable causes and solutions are presented in Table 18-1.

1. The core will not relate accurately to the refractory cast. This is a frequent problem and usually results from inadequate blockout prior to making the core. If the master cast is blocked out later or to a greater extent when the core was originally made, then the core will not fit the refractory cast (Fig. 18-61). If this occurs, then the mucosal surface of the core must be relieved until it fits the refractory cast accurately.

2. Multiple facings that continue around the arch often require more than one core (Fig. 18-62). Multiple cores are easier to relate and will often prevent breakage of abutment teeth.

3. Unnecessary display of metal may be objectionable to some patients. This can result if proximal preparations are carried too far labially (Fig. 18-63). If provision of a diastema is necessary for esthetics, it should be wide enough to be self-cleansing (Fig. 18-64, A). The proximal extension can be limited on the side of tooth adjacent to the diastema. The diastema should be entirely open from the gingival to incisal edge to avoid food retention (Fig. 18-64, B).

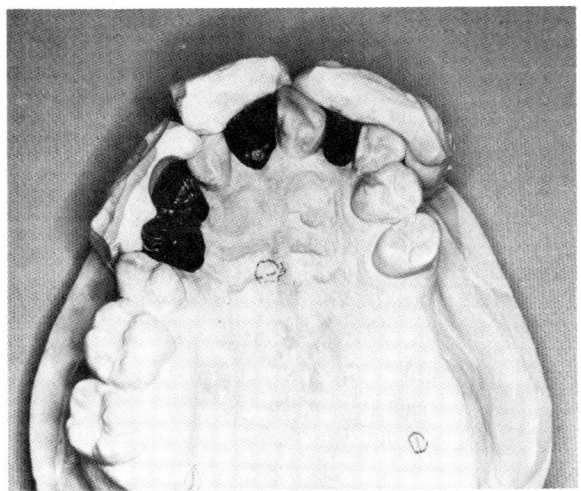

Fig. 18-62. Multiple stone indices due to curved arch form.

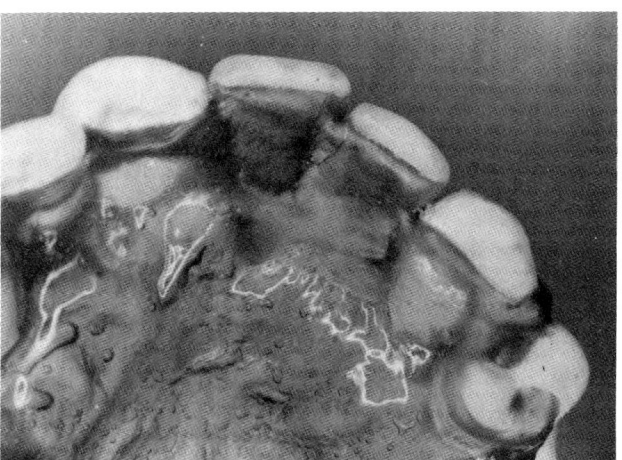

Fig. 18-63. Unnecessary display of metal due to excessive preparation of rotated proximal surfaces.

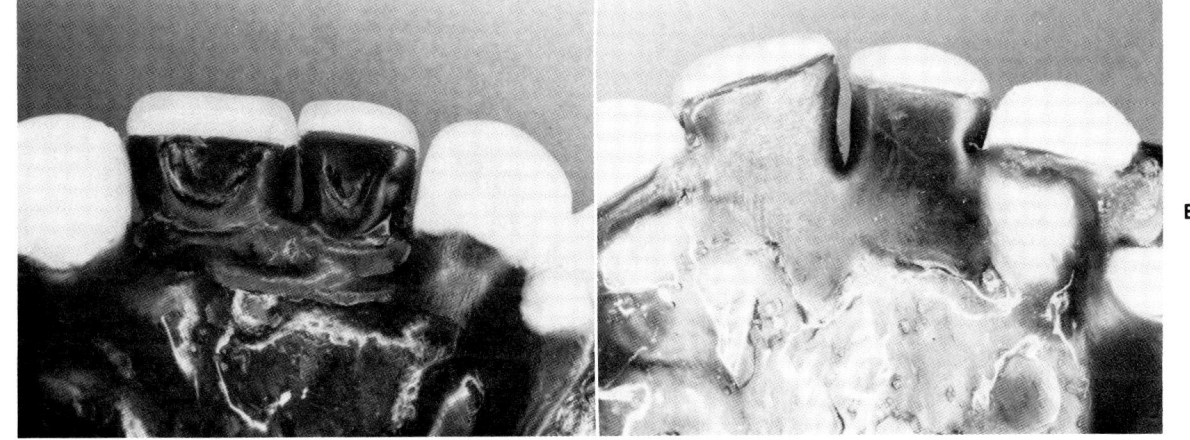

Fig. 18-64. **A,** Poorly formed diastema that is not self-cleansing. **B,** Properly formed diastema.

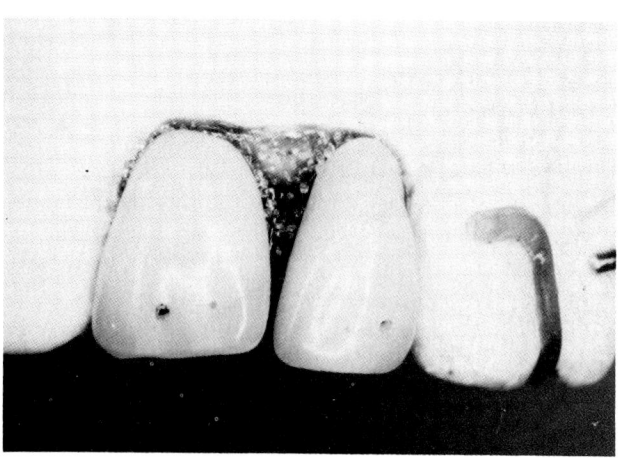

**Fig. 18-65.** Perforation of denture teeth due to drilling too perpendicular or excessively deep.

4. If the pinholes are drilled carelessly, the artificial teeth may be perforated (Fig. 18-65). Avoid excessive reduction of the lingual surface, and drill the pins at a 45-degree angle to prevent this problem. When visible, the pin can be shortened before cementation to allow resin to fill the void.

5. The wax will not flow around the pinheads in the recesses if it is not sufficiently hot. A discrepancy in the bond of a pin may be repaired before finishing the wax-up (Fig. 18-66). Perforate the wax backing with a round bur. Place pins in the pinholes, and position the facings with the core. Melt wax in the area that was reamed out with a hot spatula.

6. Large beads should not be used for retention of resin gingival to the beads (Fig. 18-67). Small crown and bridge–type crystals are indicated in areas of limited space. Large beads are difficult to mask, especially when using translucent resin.

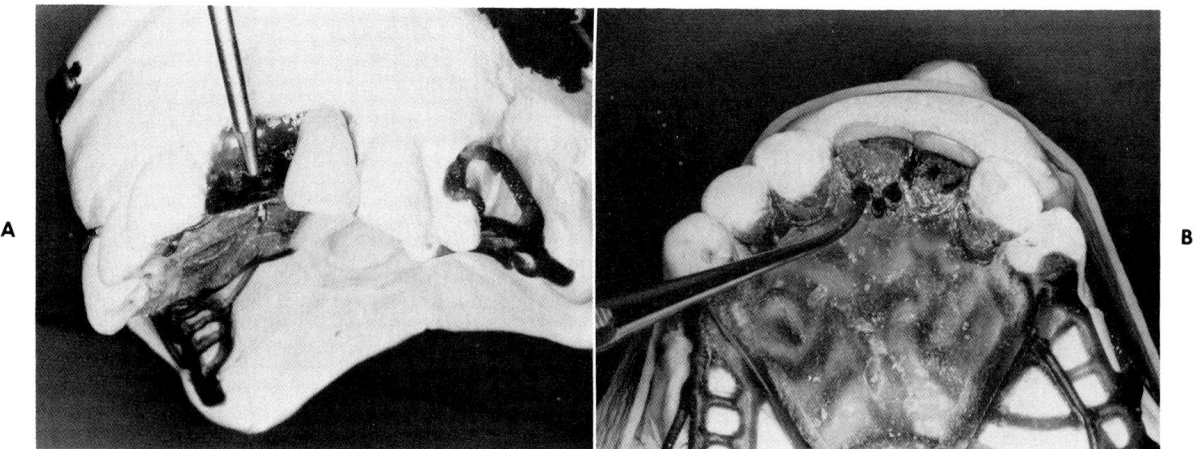

**Fig. 18-66. A,** Wax backing perforated for repair. **B,** Repair of wax backing by addition of wax with hot instrument.

**Fig. 18-67.** Small crystals should be used for retention of resin rather than large heads.

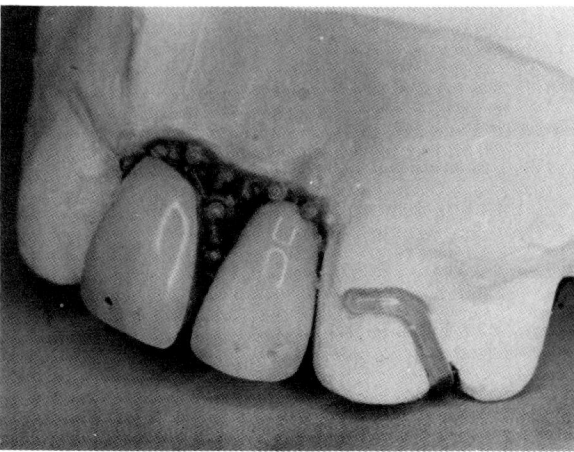

## SUMMARY

The successful replacement of missing anterior teeth with a removable prosthesis requires special planning. Several techniques have been described to meet the needs of most clinical situations. If occlusal guidance is provided by the prosthesis or the opposing teeth have extruded, then metal backings may be indicated. In these instances or when individual teeth are replaced, metal backings will provide maximum strength and durability.

Ideally, anterior teeth should be selected in advance and viewed in the mouth at the time of preparation and final impressions. Careful planning and coordination of laboratory procedures will assure efficient delivery and future maintenance of the prosthesis.

## REFERENCE

Shooshan, E. D.: The reverse pin porcelain facing, J. Prosthet. Dent. 9(2):284-301, 1959.

# CHAPTER 19

# ATTACHMENTS FOR OVERDENTURES

MERRILL C. MENSOR, Jr.

## TELESCOPE CROWNS AND ATTACHMENTS

There is general agreement that the overdenture patient should receive an interim transitional or immediate overdenture before the remote telescope crown or attachment-supported overdenture is considered (Brewer and Morrow, 1980). This is done to allow for the period of healing after endodontic and surgical procedures.

**immediate overdentures** Immediate, or transitional, overdentures are partial or complete denture units constructed for insertion following the removal of natural teeth where one or more residual clinical crowns or root elements remain for support.

**remote overdentures** Remote overdentures are overdentures other than immediate overdentures constructed for insertion at some time "remote" from the removal of hopeless natural teeth and may or may not carry a metal base. The metal base of the remote overdenture reinforces the overdenture, makes it resist dimensional changes, and improves the health of the critical gingival areas immediately adjacent to the supporting abutments (Brewer and Morrow, 1980).

**telescope crown** The telescope crown is a prosthodontic retainer for a fixed or removable prosthesis and usually consists of the conical preparations with a like casting and a secondary telescope casting that is embedded in a prosthesis or is an abutment or crown itself. It is a system used to stabilize an overdenture where 4 mm or more of clinical crown is available.

The telescope crown, according to Körber (1975) and Brewer and Morrow (1980), has been used as a method of overdenture fixation since 1861. Telescope tooth preparation requires a conical taper to provide space for fabrication of a coping with a selected taper (Fig. 19-1).

The retention of the telescope crown, according to Körber (1975), varies as to the included angle taper (Fig. 19-2). It is most retentive at 1 degree, dropping to zero retention at 9 degrees. The telescope crown concept can be used with a clinical crown preparation that provides the retentive taper followed by fabricating an overdenture which is to fit over the prepared tooth. This method is the least expensive but requires a high polish of the denture surface, flouride maintenance, and assiduous attention to the hygiene. Many times a single casting is fabricated with the desired taper and provides the support element, whereas the true telescope or double crown will provide the additional features as stated for the metal base remote overdenture. The advantage of the telescope crown or telescope preparation over the standard overdenture is the increased stabilization and retention of the denture while using remaining vital or nonvital teeth without dowels or screws.

## TELESCOPE CROWN (SINGLE CROWN)

A diagnostic preparation and survey should be made on a diagnostic cast before the telescope

# Attachments for overdentures

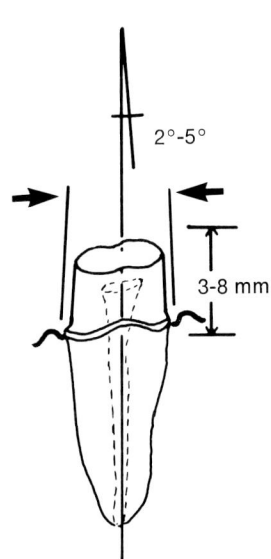

**Fig. 19-1.** Telescope preparation should have occlusal reduction of 3 mm and occlusogingival height of 3 to 8 mm. Make sure included rententive angle is 2 to 5 degrees, measured opposite from each other (horizontal arrows). Preparation may vary, but two opposing sides of stated degrees are necessary for retention.

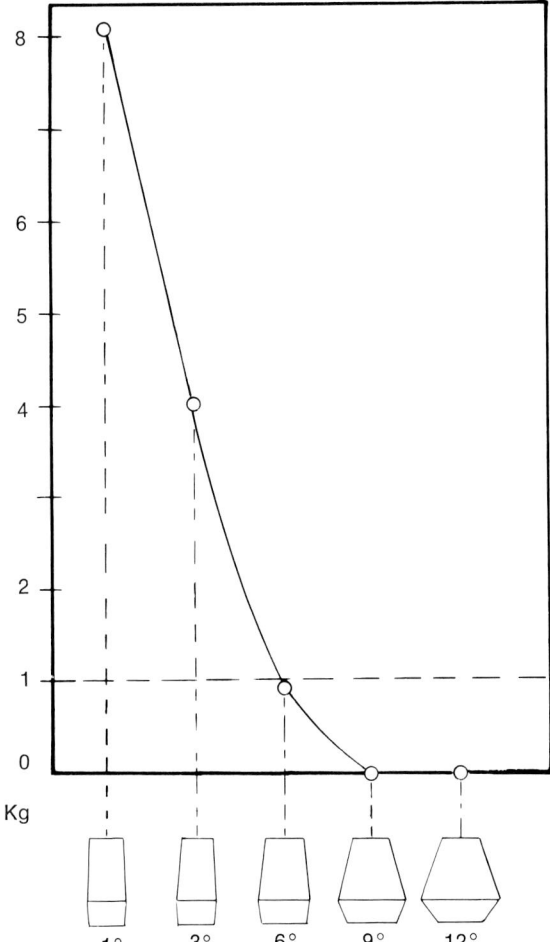

**Fig. 19-2.** Ordinate represents load in kilograms necessary for separation of one telescope element from other, given included angle on abscissa. Graph represents separation of one cast metal coping from primary cemented cast metal coping.

preparations are made on the patient. This will considerably reduce the chair time for the dentist and provide the exact reductions for the technician to produce a retentive telescope system. If necessary, a preparation jig such as used in the Pankey-Mann technique can be provided for the dentist (Fig. 19-3).

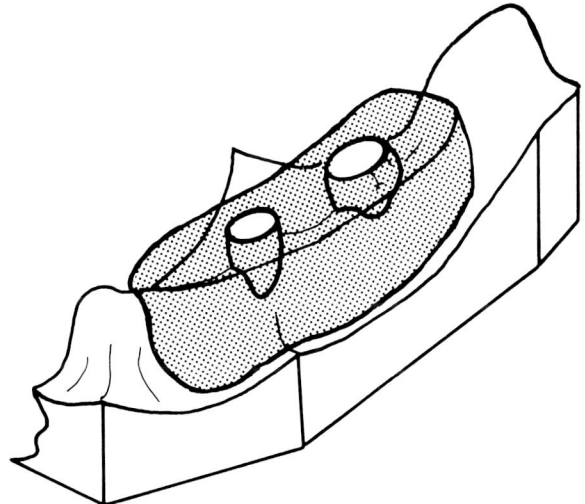

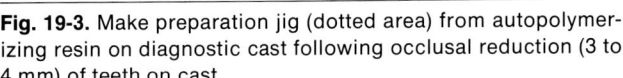

**Fig. 19-3.** Make preparation jig (dotted area) from autopolymerizing resin on diagnostic cast following occlusal reduction (3 to 4 mm) of teeth on cast.

**PROCEDURE**

1. Cast the master impression, and place the resultant master cast on a tiltable survey table such as the Ney* or Bachmann.† The master cast is ideally oriented by using a parallelometer to determine the preparation shed (Fig. 19-4).

2. Begin the wax-ups either using an Omnivac‡ coping material, 0.020 gauge, to form a primary coping, or make a coping wax-up.

---
*Ney Surveyor, The J. M. Ney Co., Bloomfield, Conn., or equivalent.
†Bachmann Parallelometer, Cendres & Metaux, S. A., Biel, Switzerland, or equivalent.
‡Omnivac coping, Omnidental Corp., Harrisburg, Pa., or equivalent.

3. Establish the selected included angle using a wax knife Konometer* (Fig. 19-5), or using a wax knife with a given blade angle in the parallelometer to establish the taper.

4. Sprue the copings at their thickest point, and place two secondary sprues 1 mm short of the margin to ensure a complete cast.

5. Finish the casting in the usual manner, and machine finish the sides to the same degree using carbide milling burs† matching the same degree angulation as the wax knife of the Konometer.

6. Elevate the crowns on the dies by either using 12-μm plastic film‡ or temporary cementation§ and

---
*Konometer, HUG GmbH, Freiburg i.Br., Germany.
†Milling burs, Brassler U.S.A., Inc., Lombard, Ill.
‡Mylar film leader Tape, 3M Co., Minneapolis, Minn.
§ProTem, Professional Products Co., San Diego, Calif., or equivalent.

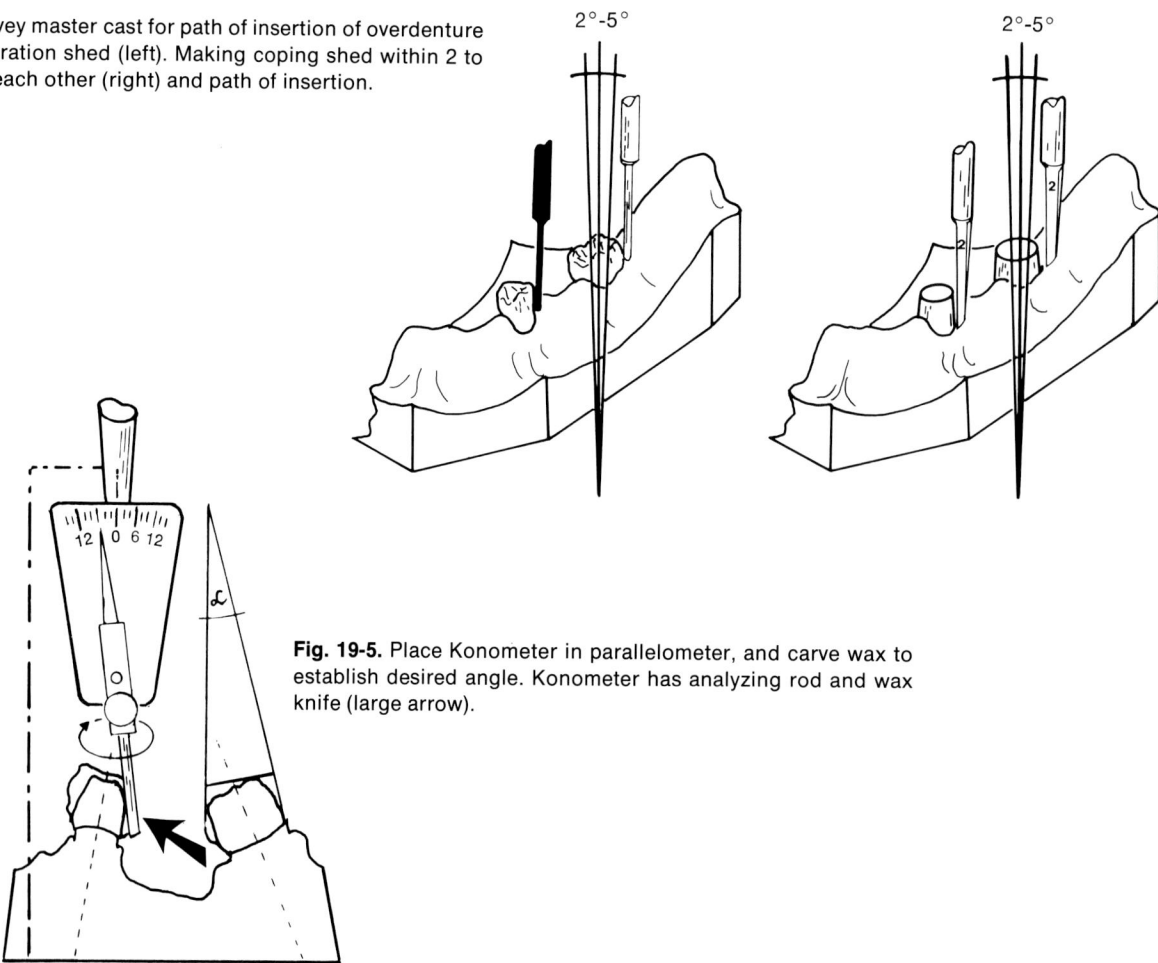

**Fig. 19-4.** Survey master cast for path of insertion of overdenture and for preparation shed (left). Making coping shed within 2 to 5 degrees of each other (right) and path of insertion.

**Fig. 19-5.** Place Konometer in parallelometer, and carve wax to establish desired angle. Konometer has analyzing rod and wax knife (large arrow).

some crown and bridge cement powder of choice (this is done to correct for the cement elevation of the crowns on final placement). Alternately the crown can be returned to the mouth for a master impression in situ with the same type of temporization.

7. Block out the undercut areas about the copings and gingival to the preparation with stone or undercut wax, and pour a duplicate fabricating cast (Fig. 19-6).

8. If fabrication is done on the master cast, paint a silicone release agent* over the metal. Fabrication is done with the resin of choice.

9. Use pressure indicator paste† or Occlude‡ to check the clearance of the overdenture to the castings.

---

*Dow Corning No. 7, Dow Corning Corp., Midland, Mich., or equivalent.
†Pressure indicator paste, Mizzy, Inc., Clifton Forge, Va., or equivalent.
‡Pascal Co., Inc., Bellevue, Wash.

## ALTERNATE PROCEDURE (DOUBLE CROWN)

Steps 1 to 5 are carried out as for the single crown.

1. Wax up the secondary coping using DuraLay, the method of choice, or an Omnivac coping with wax added to provide retention in the resin of the overdenture (Fig. 19-7).

2. Fit the secondary coping to the primary using a deplater on the secondary casting for about 10 seconds and an indicator of choice to locate any interferences.

3. Place the copings on the master cast as given in step 6 of the single crown procedure, and seat the secondary coping with a silicone release agent.

4. Block out undercuts with stone or crown and bridge cement.

5. Process the overdenture on the master cast.

6. Return the overdenture to the articulator for occlusal control before removing it from the master cast.

7. The overdenture will either release from the master cast or will require a combination of sectioning and shellblasting.

8. Remove the primary copings using a compressed air nozzle, and finish the telescope overdenture in the usual manner.

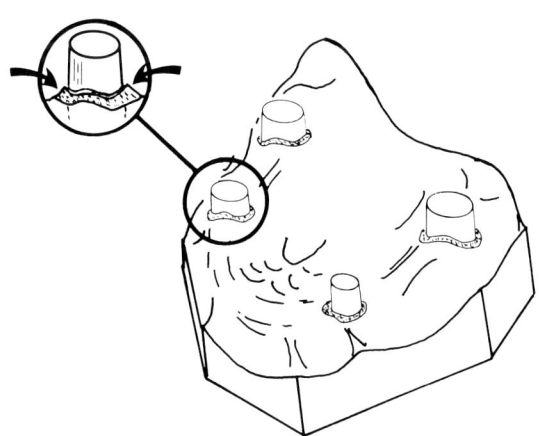

**Fig. 19-6.** Block out undercut areas below height of contour of telescope crown with stone, crown and bridge cement, or undercut wax. Duplicate cast for fabrication (inset).

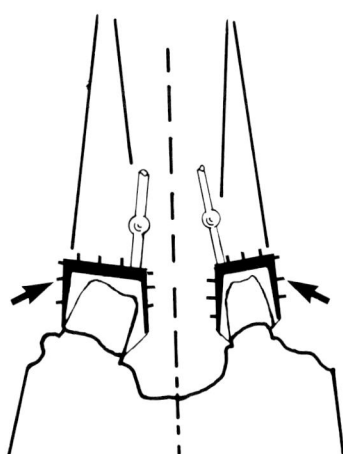

**Fig. 19-7.** Wax-up secondary copings 0.5 to 1 mm in thickness. Make sure to provide retention tangs (arrows) for fixation in resin of overdenture.

## ATTACHMENTS

Attachments are classified as precision or semiprecision as discussed in Chapter 11 of *Dental Laboratory Procedures: Fixed Partial Dentures.* They are generally prefabricated or partially prefabricated male or female elements that are used to join a prosthesis to a cemented retainer carrying the opposite attachment member. They provide orientation, retention, stability, and as near normal function to the wearer as possible. For overdentures, stud, bar, and auxiliary attachments of groups III, IV, and V are used (Mensor, 1973).

**stud attachments** Stud attachments are any of a series of stud or pressure buttons consisting of two or more parts, one of which becomes part of a dowel-supported coping and the other, part of the prosthesis. They may be rigid or resilient (Fig. 19-8).

**bar attachments** Bar attachments usually consist of two parts, the bar and some form of retentive rider or clip. Bars are further classified into bar joints, those which have movement, and bar units, those without any movement. The bar is attached to two or more screw or dowel-supported copings or crowns, and the rider clip is a part of the removable prosthesis (Fig. 19-9). Bar systems provide splinting as well.

**auxiliary attachments** Auxiliary attachments used for overdenture support consist of the various types of spring-loaded pawl connectors (Fig. 19-10), bolts, and other customized retaining devices used to secure the overdenture. Most auxiliary attachments are used to provide additional retention on a modified telescope crown or implant stud.

NOTE: All attachment procedures are complementary to standard overdenture laboratory techniques. They do require a dowel or screw fixation (Brewer and Morrow, 1980), preferably with a cylindrical dowel of sufficient length to resist dislodg-

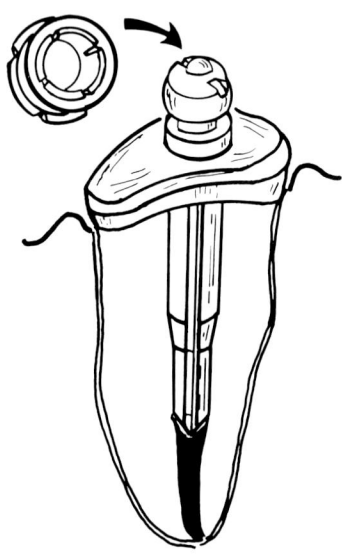

**Fig. 19-8.** Ancrofix attachment represents typical stud system. Male stud is part of coping dowel assembly. Retention cap (female) fits over male stud (arrow) and is retentive part of overdenture.

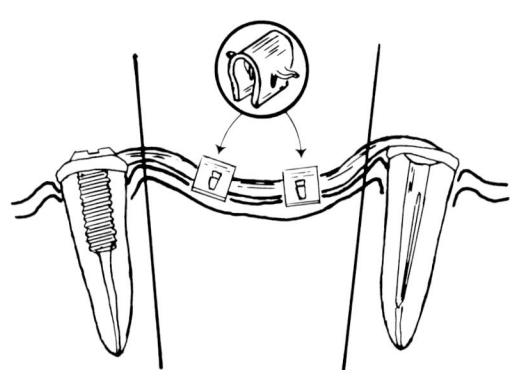

**Fig. 19-9.** Ackermann clip (inset) is representative of rider clips used on bar joints or units. Illustration shows typical splinting problem with divergent teeth. Bar joint is bent to be bar unit and is part of dowel coping system on right and open coping on left. Open coping on left is secured with Kurer coping retaining screw.

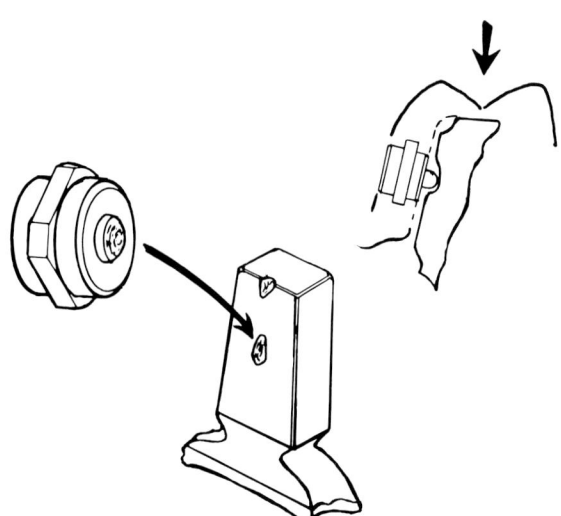

**Fig. 19-10.** Mini-Presso-matic (left) represents typical spring-loaded pawl connector used for auxiliary retention of telescope crowns and overdentures. Attachment is either part of resin overlay or cast secondary retainer. Plunger engages notch of implant (curved arrow) as illustrated above right (sectional view).

ment and attachment orientation in harmony with the insertion path of the overdenture.

Any metal framework must clear the attachments by 1 mm and under no circumstances touch the attachments to provide space for repositioning the attachments as well as bulk of resin for retention of the attachments.

## Stud attachment use

Stud attachments are the most popular systems used for overdenture fixation. Each one is a self-contained support unit independent of other similar units. They can be used singly or in multiples bilaterally usually on canine or premolar roots. The greatest stability is seen with this application, although they may be used anywhere in the mouth.

Selecting the stud attachment is a critical point. Not only is the occluded clearance a factor, but the coping height must also be considered in the overall height measurement. This additional height is usually 1 mm for the occlusal thickness of the coping. The characteristics of function of most stud and bar attachments are noted on the EM Attachment Selector* or in the manufacturer's perspectus, and they are a determinate of selection.

The shortest of the stud attachments is the Rothermann,† measuring only 1.1 mm (Fig. 19-11) in the nonresilient form and 1.7 mm in the resilient form.

The next shortest attachment is the Mini-BK,† 1.8 mm, followed by the frictive Baer,‡ 2.2 mm, and the retentive Baer, which is 2.6 mm (Fig. 19-12).

The Sandri§ attachment is available with a stainless steel housing. It is 2.5 mm as a ball unit (Fig. 19-13, *A*) and may be shimmed to be a tissue-resilient unit (Fig. 19-13, *B*). It is a practical attachment because of its adjustability, size, and replaceable parts.

---

*EM Attachment Selector, Bell International, Inc., San Mateo, Calif.
†Mini-BK, Bell International, Inc., San Mateo, Calif.
‡APM-Sterngold, Stamford, Conn.
§Sandri, Bell International, Inc., San Mateo, Calif.

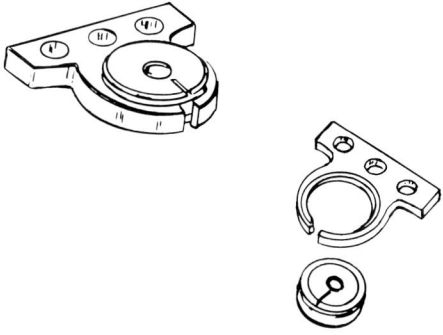

**Fig. 19-11.** Rothermann attachment is stud type with built-in solder core. Female is machined retention bar with open retention clip. Loading is eccentric, and overall height is 1.1 mm in nonresilient form.

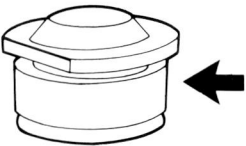

**Fig. 19-12.** Retentive Baer attachment is stud type with horizontal open retention clip covered by polyvinyl chloride ring (arrow) to provide flexion. Height is 2.6 mm.

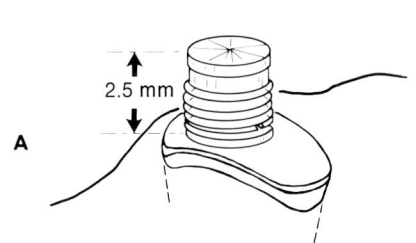
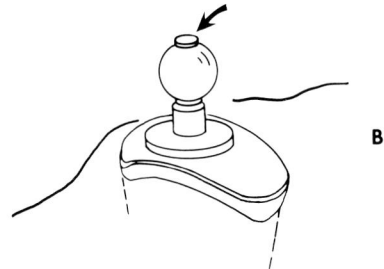

**Fig. 19-13.** Sandri is practical stud attachment 2.5 mm in height with metal-to-resin retention. All component parts are replaceable and retention adjustable **(A)**. Shim (arrow) on top of stud provides tissue-controlled vertical resilience **(B)**.

The Dalla Bona cylinder,* 3.7 mm, and the Dalla Bona ball anchor,* 4 mm (Fig. 19-14), have the longest use in the United States next to the Gerber attachment. The assembly for the Dalla Bona is representative of the Baer, Dalla Bona, Ancrofix,† and the housing part of the Kurer Press-Stud‡ (Ancrofix). The Ancrofix is very similar to the Dalla Bona and has the function of both types of Dalla Bona studs plus the replaceable male stud. It measures 3.2 mm vertically (Fig. 19-15).

The Gerber* rigid attachment with a stainless steel housing is 4 mm, and the resilient form is 4.7 mm. It provides the most sophisticated and yet one of the easiest maintained systems with the largest in-service record in the United States (Fig. 19-16).

The Ceka* attachment (Fig. 19-17) enjoys a similar popularity with the Gerber and Dalla Bona and comes in two heights. A similar type, the König† anchor, is also available.

The Press-Stud‡ is a hybrid attachment that is available in two sizes, 2.5 and 3.6 mm. It is a unique combination of the Kurer-Anchor with the Ancrofix in a molybdenum–stainless steel alloy that can either use a coping to seal the radicular section or bypass a coping completely (Fig. 19-18).

---

*APM-Sterngold, Stamford, Conn.
†Ancrofix, Degussa, Placentia, Calif.
‡Kurer Press-Stud, Union Broach Co., Inc., Long Island City, N.Y.

*J. F. Jelenko & Co., New Rochelle, N.Y.
†König Anker, Karl König, KG, Meinerzhagen 1, Germany.
‡Kurer Press-Stud, Union Broach Co., Inc., Long Island City, N.Y.

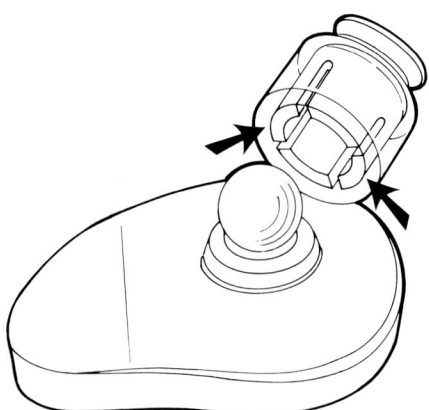

**Fig. 19-14.** Dalla Bona ball anchor is simple stud anchor 4 mm in height. Retention is provided by adjustable lamellae (arrows).

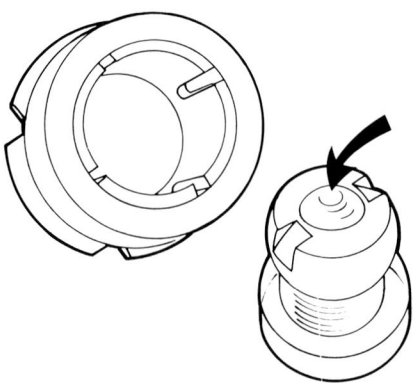

**Fig. 19-15.** Ancrofix is similar to both Dalla Bona studs. Hemisphere (arrow) may be flattened to convert attachment to cylinder type. Male stud is interchangeable; height is 3.2 mm.

# Attachments for overdentures

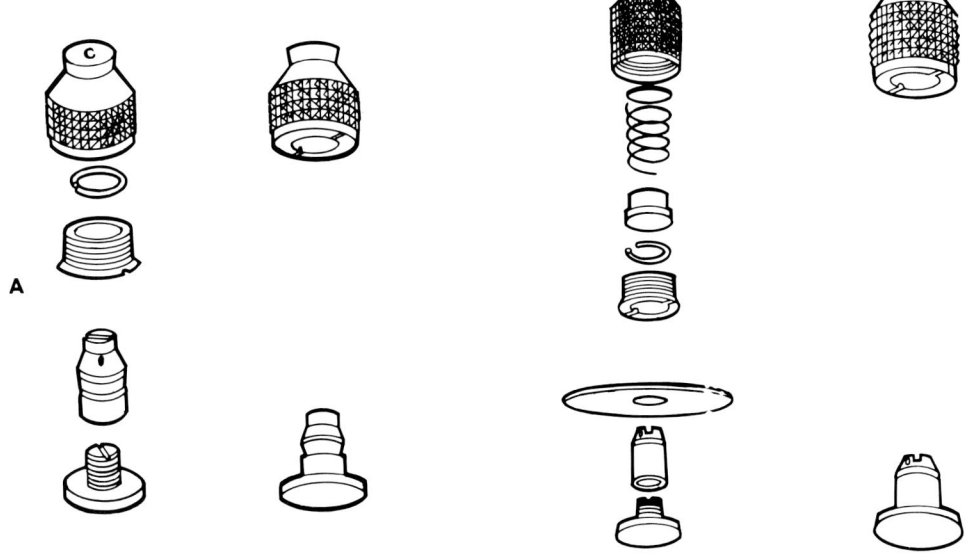

**Fig. 19-16.** Gerber rigid attachment **(A)** is nonresilient. Housing is tent shaped, has no coil spring, C-clip retention, and solder base common to resilient Gerber **(B)**. Height is 4 mm. Gerber resilient attachment has cylinder housing with coil spring, repulsion ring, and C-clip retention. Height is 4.7 mm.

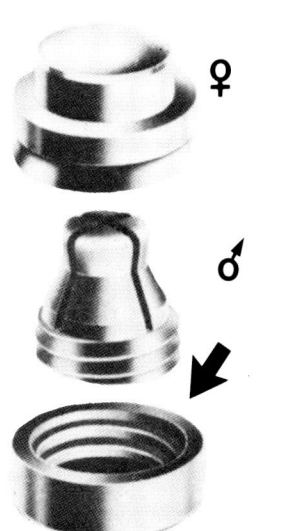

**Fig. 19-17.** Ceka is much copied adjustable stud attachment and is simple to use with good wear characteristics. Split-leaf retention screws extend into coping base (arrow) and engage female housing. Height is 4.1 mm.

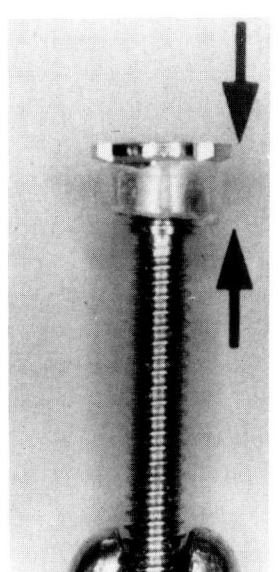

**Fig. 19-18.** Kurer Mini Press-Stud is combination Kurer-Anchor and Ancrofix attachment in molybdenum–stainless steel alloy. Height is 2.5 mm (arrows).

## Rothermann rigid attachment

The Rothermann rigid attachment consists of two parts, the adjustable split ring in Elasticor* alloy and the grooved OSV* anchor plate with a 1470° F (799° C) solder core incorporated (Fig. 19-19). The anchor plate has an occlusal index notch that indicates the opening position for the split ring. The Rothermann does not require exact parallelism, and one may diverge from the other by ± 10 degrees.

---

*Special attachment alloy, Cendres &Metaux, S. A., Biel, Switzerland

### PROCEDURE

1. Make the trial setup of the dentures, and cast a positional stone index of the facial relation of the denture teeth about the attachment area (Fig. 19-20).

2. Cast a master impression of the dowel coping preparations, and make the wax-up to provide no less than 0.8 mm of thickness at the occlusal surface.

3. Notch the dowel at the interphase where the coping joins the dowel to provide both a mechanical and metallurgical bond.

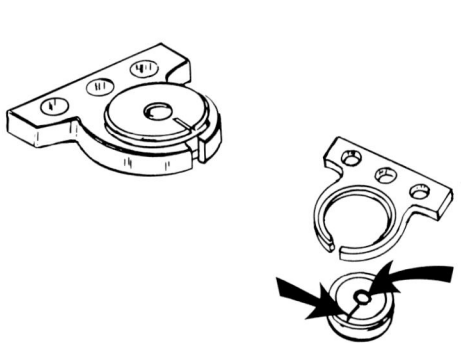

Fig. 19-19. Rothermann male stud attachment has solder core (curved arrow) and orientation notch (straight arrow). Align attachment with retention bar to lingual side of crest of ridge. Scribe open section of clip on coping, and set orientation notch to facial side (toward opening of C ring).

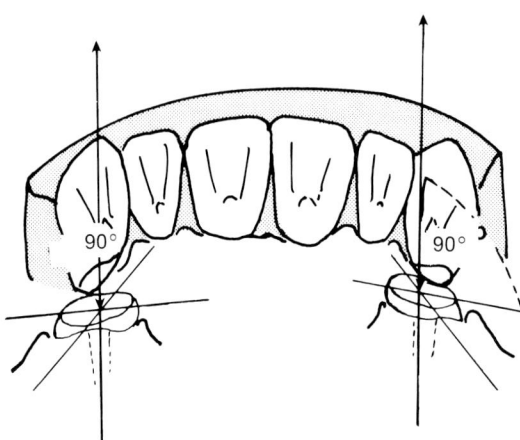

Fig. 19-20. Make stone key index on setup cast after wax-up try-in. Note relative position of attachments to lingual side of crest of ridge, parallel to path of insertion of overdenture, and parallel to each other.

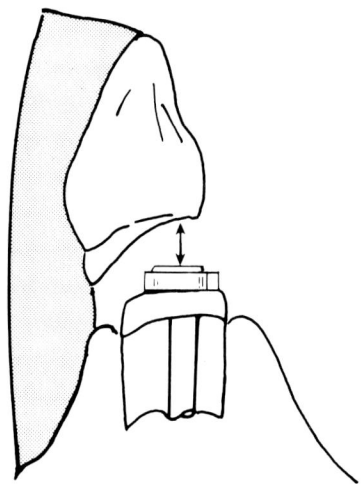

Fig. 19-21. Check attachment position and clearance. Replace porcelain denture tooth with resin denture tooth if space is limited.

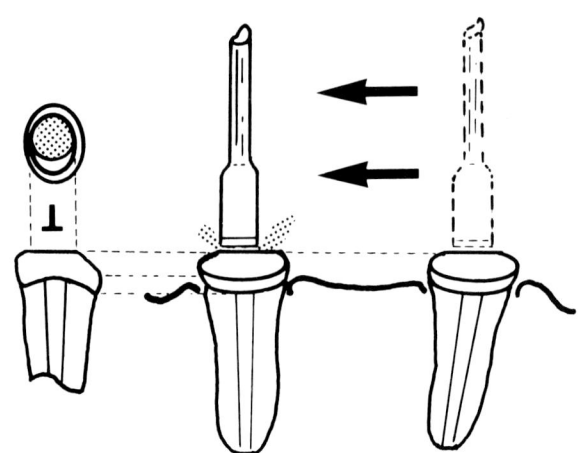

Fig. 19-22. Rothermann attachment requires flat surface on coping. To simplify wax-up for all attachments, determine partial denture or overdenture path of insertion, and then cut multiple wax-ups flat with end cutting wax knife as illustrated from right to left. This procedure can reduce need for parallelometer mandrel. Arrow indicates activity of wax knife from right to left.

4. Invest and cast the dowel coping with a mold temperature of 1350° F (732° C) to ensure a metallurgical bond of the dowel and coping.

5. Finish the dowel coping in the usual manner and return it to the master cast.

6. Place the stone index on the model with the teeth in place, and check the assembled attachment for clearance (Fig. 19-21).

7. Mark the position of the attachment for orientation and soldering.

8. The Rothermann attachment requires a flat surface, and the anchor plate index position is marked on the gold coping (Fig. 19-22).

9. Check the split-ring retention for clearance with adjacent teeth, and reduce it where necessary (do not bend it because the split ring may become distorted).

10. Position the attachment with the index mark up opposite the scribed line, and hold it with a pair of quartz-tip soldering pliers (Fig. 19-23).*

11. Hold the assembly in a Bunsen burner flame until the solder melts. Pickle and finish it in the usual manner. (The OSV anchor plate has a black oxide surface and is best cleaned using a fiberglass brush.)

12. Heat treat the dowel coping attachment in an oven at 850° F (454° C), and drop the temperature to 450° F (233° C) for ½ hour before quenching the attachment in water.

13. Final polish the unit for assembly with the overdenture.

14. Temporarily cement the dowel coping with ProTem and crown and bridge cement powder of choice to compensate for the final cement elevation of the coping.

15. Place the split ring with the retention to the lingual aspect and the opening opposite the index.

16. Cover the ring spring area with a 1-mm thickness of crown and bridge cement or an equivalent thickness of Rubber Sep* to provide for the spring flexion. Do the same about the undercut of the coping to prevent bottle-opener dislodgment of the coping by the prosthesis (Fig. 19-24).

17. Process the overdenture in the usual manner.

18. Remove the cement or Rubber Sep, and prepare the attachment overdenture for delivery.

*Degussa, Placentia, Calif.

*APM-Sterngold, Stamford, Conn., or equivalent.

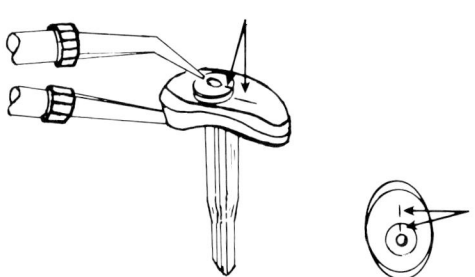

**Fig. 19-23.** Hold attachment with quartz-tipped soldering pliers. Freehand solder attachment to dowel coping. Keep index opposite scribe mark on coping (arrows).

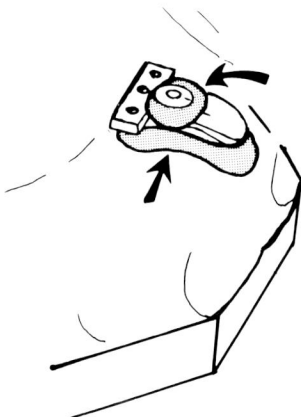

**Fig. 19-24.** Place Rubber Sep about coping and clip arms (arrows).

#### ALTERNATE PROCEDURE I

Complete steps 1 to 14.

1. Take the trial base to the mouth, clear about the attachment, and make an impression in the trial base with Impregum.*

2. Substitute a processing jig (Fig. 19-25) for the attachment, and complete steps 15 to 18.

#### ALTERNATE PROCEDURE II

Complete steps 1 to 14.

1. Fabricate the overdenture, and prepare a lingual window in the overdenture about the attachment area (Fig. 19-26).

2. Place the split ring, check it for clearance, and block it as in step 16.

3. Make a resin pick-up of the attachment by wetting the attachment area with monomer, placing some wet self-curing resin in the attachment space of the overdenture, and seating the overdenture.

4. Add extra resin to ensure the relation and the jaws are closed in a centrically related occlusion.

5. After the initial set, remove the overdenture with the dowel coping in place.

---

*Impregum, Espe, GMBH, West Germany; Premier Dental Products Co., Philadelphia, Pa., or equivalent.

6. Add extra resin, and complete a pressure pot curing.

#### REBASING—ATTACHMENT REPLACEMENT

Rubber Sep or Impregum is painted over the outside of the spring arms, a silicone release agent is applied to the cavity, and the rebase impression is made.

1. Insert a processing jig, and pour the rebase cast.

2. Rebase the overdenture in the usual manner.

3. If the split ring is to be replaced or repositioned, then follow steps 15 to 18 of the procedure for the rigid Rothermann attachment.

Retention activation is performed after delivery and is usually a chairside procedure.

### Rothermann resilient attachment

The Rothermann resilient attachment has the same split ring with a 1.7-mm male element and two processing spacers to provide for the 0.6-mm vertical movement clearance about the attachment (Fig. 19-27). The nonparallelism is more critical with the resilient Rothermann and requires a tolerance of ±5 degrees.

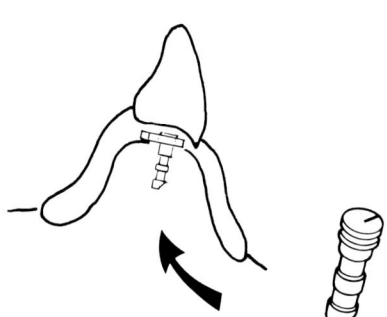

Fig. 19-25. Substitute processing jig for attachment (arrow) and cast impression.

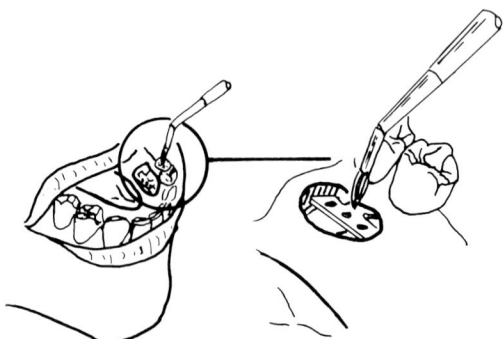

Fig. 19-26. Prepare lingual window about attachment area, check clearance, and relate attachment to overdenture with self-curing resin placed with brush.

## PROCEDURE

The assembly procedure follows steps 1 to 14 of the rigid system.

1. Adapt the mounting spacer over the coping (Fig. 19-28).
2. Place the split ring over the male, and cement the occlusal spacer to the male stud with cyanoacrylate cement (Fig. 19-29).
3. Place crown and bridge cement or Rubber Sep to the thickness of 1 mm around the ring springs to join the occlusal surface of the male spacer (Fig. 19-30).
4. Process in the usual manner.
5. Remove the cement or Rubber Sep, and prepare the attachment overdenture for delivery.

Alternate methods, rebasing, and replacement all follow the standard technique with the additions noted here.

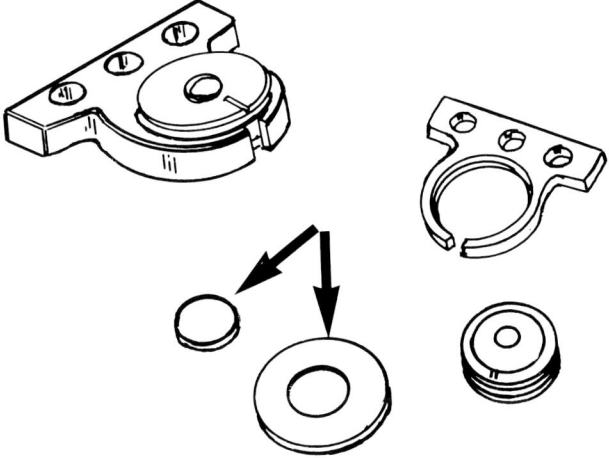

**Fig. 19-27.** Resilient Rothermann attachment has two spacers, 0.6 mm (arrows), to provide for resilience. Height is 1.7 mm.

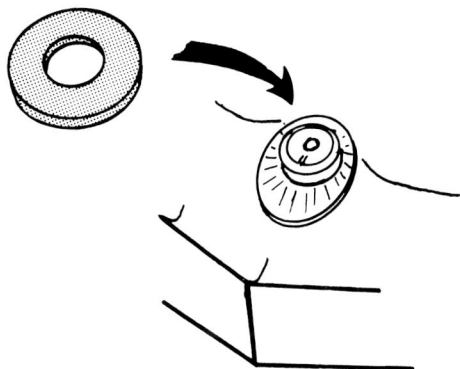

**Fig. 19-28.** Adapt mounting spacer over coping (arrow).

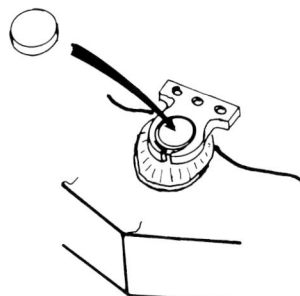

**Fig. 19-29.** Place female over assembly (arrow), and cement occlusal spacer on male stud with cyanoacrylate cement.

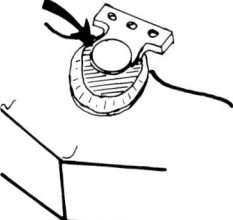

**Fig. 19-30.** Place Rubber Sep to thickness of 1 mm around ring clip, and blend with spacer (arrow).

### Baer, Dalla Bona, Ancrofix, and the Kurer Press-Stud housing attachments, including the basic assembly for Sandri and Gerber

The assembly procedures for these attachments are identical with minor exceptions. The Dalla Bona cylinder is most representative of the miniature prefabricated telescope systems.

#### PROCEDURE

1. Carry out steps 1 to 7 of the Rothermann rigid procedure.
2. Use a special parallelometer mandrel to position the attachments. The orientation must not only be parallel to each other, but also the path of insertion of the overdenture.
3. Sticky wax the attachment base to place (Fig. 19-31).
4. Embed the dowel coping attachment in a soldering investment, and solder it (Fig. 19-32). In the case of Ancrofix, Sandri, and Gerber attachments, a special soldering mandrel protects the threaded portion and holds the attachment base in position (Fig. 19-33).
5. Heat treat the attachments in a furnace at 850° F (450° C), drop the temperature to 450° F (233° C) in 1/2 hour, quench them in water, and clean and polish them.
6. Return the dowel coping assembly to the master cast, and temporarily cement it in place with a mixture of ProTem cement and crown and bridge cement powder of choice.
7. Block out the papilla area about the coping with crown and bridge cement (Fig. 19-34, arrows).
8. Fit either the tin mounting spacer or 0.4 mm of

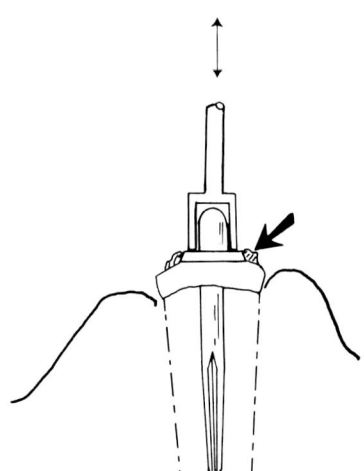

Fig. 19-31. Place attachment in position with parallelometer mandrel, and sticky wax to place (large arrow).

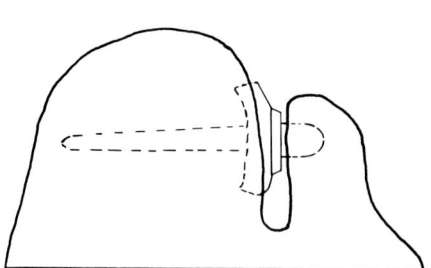

Fig. 19-32. Invest assembly in soldering investment, boil out sticky wax, and solder in usual manner.

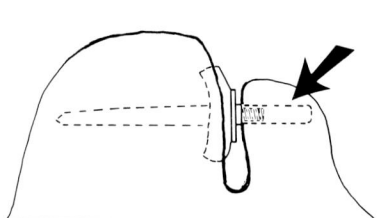

Fig. 19-33. Sandri, Ancrofix, and Gerber attachments use special soldering mandrel (arrow).

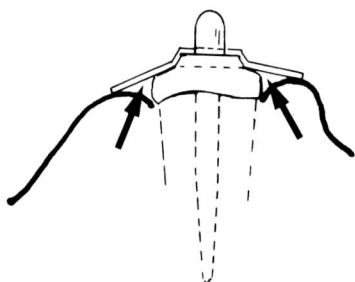

Fig. 19-34. Block out papilla area (arrows) with crown and bridge cement, and fit spacer or aluminum foil over coping. Assemble female housing.

aluminum foil* about the coping to provide space in the overdenture for the translation (Fig. 19-34). In the case of the rigid Baer, Gerber, or Dalla Bona attachments, a thin sheet (0.05 mm) of aluminum foil will protect the coping.

9. Lubricate the attachment housing with a polyvinylchloride ring on the inside with a silicone release agent,† and place it on the stud (the resilient Gerber attachment requires placement of the processing shim in the housing before final assembly).

10. Complete the overdenture processing in the usual manner to include the attachments.

11. After processing and checking for occlusion, carefully remove the dowel coping assembly using cotton-protected pliers (Fig. 19-35), and clear the cement and metal spacers from about the attachments.

12. Prepare the overdentures for delivery without activation (Fig. 19-36). In the case of the Gerber attachments, the C locking springs are removed for initial placement.

### Ancrofix
#### PROCEDURE

The procedures are the same as Dalla Bona except the male stud is replaceable and must be secured in the base with Gun Lock* or Lock 'N Seal.† The male may be converted from a rotational attachment function to a cylindrical function by reducing the hemisphere top (Fig. 19-37).

---

*Household kitchen foil may be folded to thickness, cut, and rubber dam punched for hole size.
†Dow Corning No. 7, Dow Corning Corp., Midland, Mich., or equivalent.

*Gun Lock, Master Lock, Milwaukee, Wis.
†Lock 'N Seal, Loctite Corp., Newington, Conn., or equivalent.

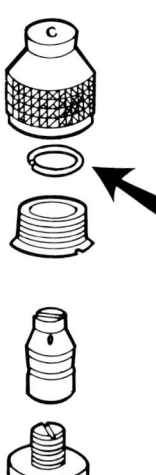

**Fig. 19-35.** Test fit of attachment assembly.

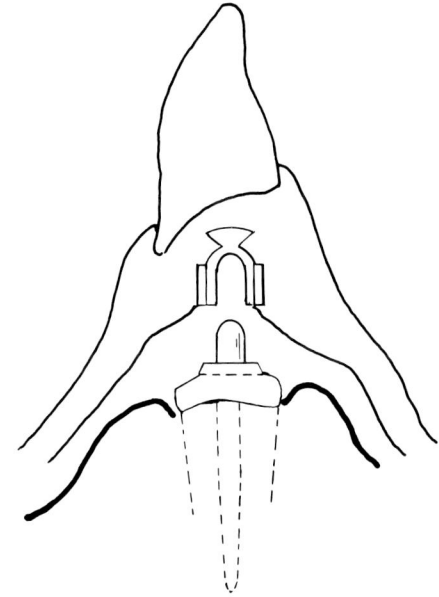

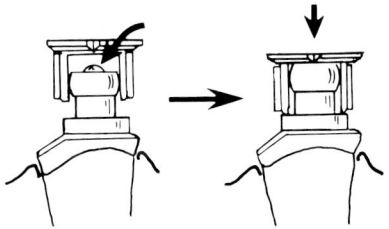

**Fig. 19-36.** Remove retention elements before delivery of overdenture. With Gerber attachments, remove C clip (arrow); with others, do not activate, follow manufacturer's suggestions.

**Fig. 19-37.** Convert Ancrofix from rotational to cylinder type by flattening hemisphere (curved arrow).

### Sandri

**PROCEDURES**

The procedures are the same as the Dalla Bona attachment except the parallelometer mandrel is also used as a soldering mandrel. The steel retention ball is screwed onto the male thread, and the height of the thread is reduced to mechanically "lock" the ball in place (Fig. 19-38).

The female housing consists of three parts: (1) threaded housing, (2) split-ring retention cylinder, and (3) housing cap. Once the housing is processed, the housing cap remains in the prosthesis while the threaded housing may be unscrewed to service or replace the split-ring retention cylinder (this procedure is similar to the replacement of the C spring in the Gerber technique and uses the Gerber screwdriver).

### Gerber

**PROCEDURES**

Both rigid and resilient Gerber attachments share the same solder base. The procedures are the same as the Dalla Bona attachment except for the soldering mandrels. The resilient housing requires the presence of the housing shim to deactivate the resilient spring. Access to the housing of both types of Gerber attachments is by means of a special spring-loaded screwdriver.

NOTE: Rebasing replacement or resin pickup procedures follow the same techniques as outlined for the Rothermann attachments.

### Kurer Press-Stud

The Kurer Press-Stud* attachment is a hybrid of the Group III attachment systems in that the retentive dowel and stud is a single unit.

**PROCEDURES**

1. Transfer the dowel space and preparation details to the laboratory by the master impression using a coping transfer dowel (Fig. 19-39).
2. Complete the coping wax-up, and flatten the occlusal surface by placing the root facer wax knife over the transfer dowel and rotating to mill the wax surface. The coping must be thin (0.8 mm) to maintain the vertical space (Fig. 19-40).
3. Make the casting in the usual manner, and test it to clear the transfer dowel.
4. Send the coping to the dentist for cementation and have him make the master impression (the dentist must be instructed to temporarily block out the screwdriver notches on the stud head with crown and bridge cement before making the master

---

*Union Broach Co., Inc., Long Island City, N.Y.

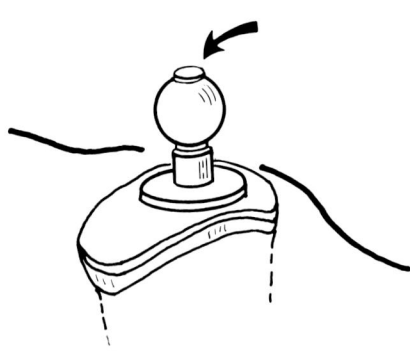

**Fig. 19-38.** Reduce height of thread, and burnish to ball (arrow).

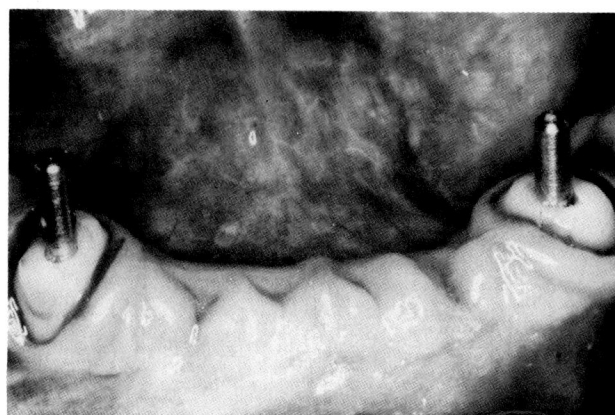

**Fig. 19-39.** Make master impression with No. 1 transfer dummy dowels, and cast master impression. No. 1 transfer dummies are shown in situ.

impression, or the stud transfer dowels will not seat in the impression) (Fig. 19-41).

5. Seat the stud transfer dowels in an elastomeric impression* material (preferable) or heavy-body hydrocolloid,† and cast the impression in dental stone (Fig. 19-42).

6. Fill in the papilla area about the coping with crown and bridge cement, and cement a layer of aluminum foil over the coping area. If vertical resilience is required, then insert a shim of the same thickness as the relief material between the stud and the housing.

7. Fill the housing with a silicone release agent, and assemble it with a slight tilt when necessary to clear the denture teeth using the trial setup index. (See Rothermann rigid procedure, step 6, Fig. 9-21.)

8. When necessary, substitute a resin tooth for the porcelain tooth, and then grind it to clear the attachment housing.

9. Block out the housing between the lower border of the housing using the metal foil with plaster or crown and bridge cement to block entry of the resin and stabilize the position of the attachment providing space for insertion of the stud (Fig. 19-43).

---
*Impregum, Premier Dental Products Co., Philadelphia, Pa., or equivalent.
†Van R Dental Products, Inc., Los Angeles, Calif.

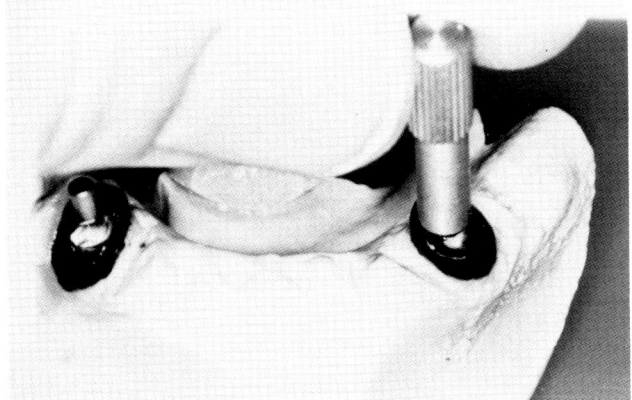

Fig. 19-40. Place root facer wax knife over transfer dowel, and rotate to produce flat surface.

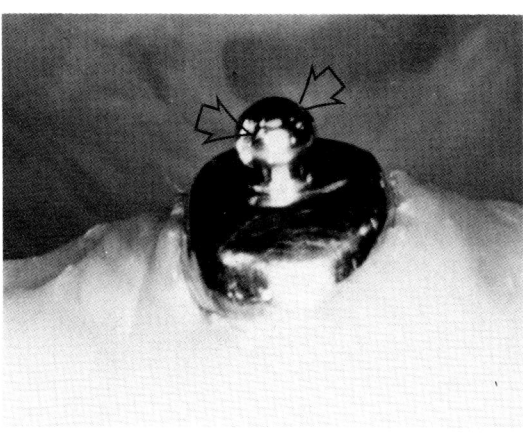

Fig. 19-41. Have dentist block out notches (arrows) with temporary cement before making impression.

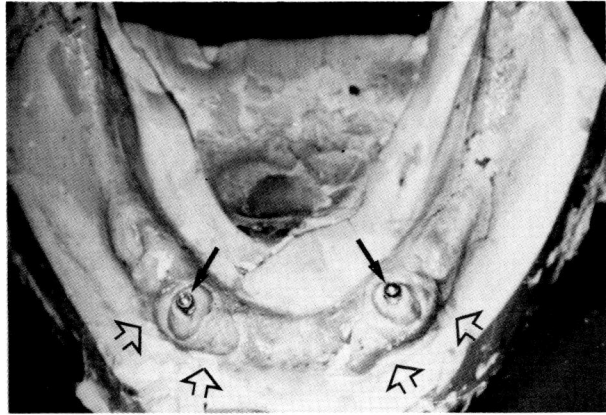

Fig. 19-42. Place No. 2 transfer dummies in impression, and cast in dental stone. Transfer dummies represent exact attachment position in mouth (solid arrows). Block out undercut areas with dental stone before processing overdenture (open arrows).

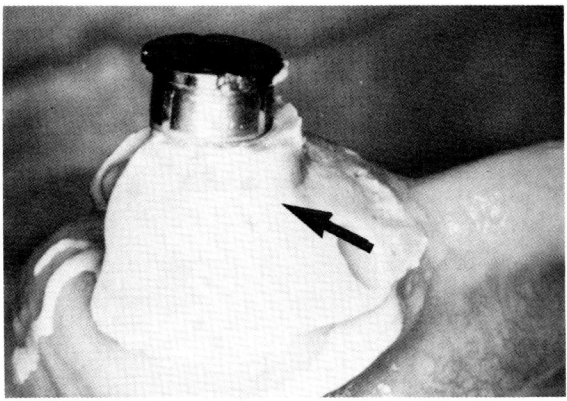

Fig. 19-43. Block out space between attachment and coping with dental stone, crown and bridge cement, or Rubber Sep. Illustration shows Impregum blocking same space in mouth preparatory to resin pickup (arrow).

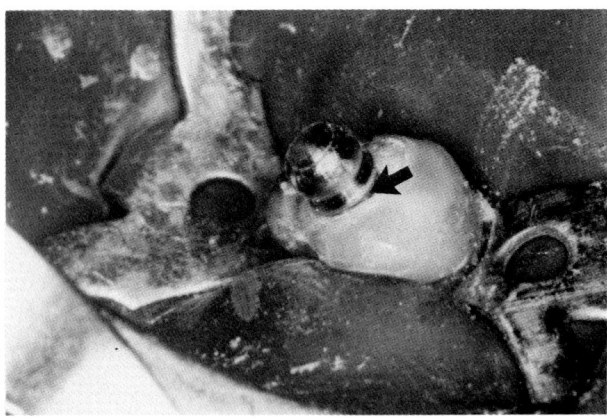

**Fig. 19-44.** Kurer Press-Stud used without coping. Root surface must be highly polished, and root facer must be used in dowel space to provide seal of Press-Stud collar (arrow).

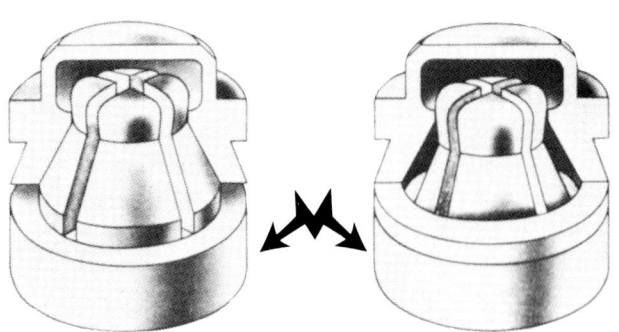

**Fig. 19-45.** Ceka stud attachments have common cast-to-base (arrows) for rigid (left) and resilient (right). Height, including base, is 4.2 mm.

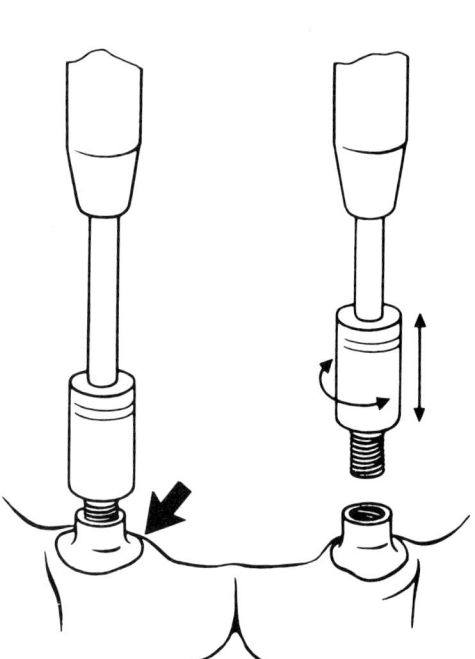

**Fig. 19-46.** Locate base (arrow) as far lingual as possible, sticky wax to position, and unscrew parallelometer mandrel.

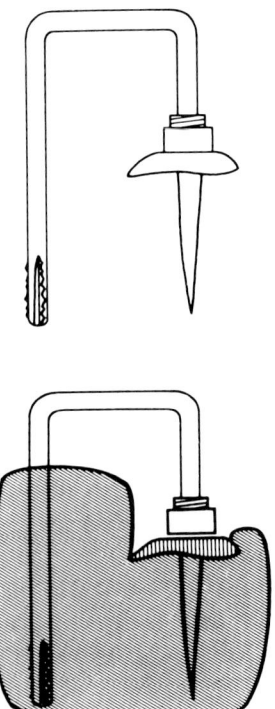

**Fig. 19-47.** Replace parallelometer mandrel with soldering accessory H-4, and invest for soldering.

### RESIN PICKUP

Resin pickup or replacement of the attachment may be accomplished as outlined for the Rothermann system. Care must be taken to ensure that the overdenture is seated in a terminal hinge centrically related occlusion, or the attachment-over denture position will be incorrect.

NOTE: The coping procedure steps 1 to 4 may be omitted if the root surface is to remain bare. If this is the case, the surface should be highly polished, the area adjacent to the dowel space should be milled with a root facer to engage the shoulder of the stud (Fig. 19-44), and the exposed area should be maintained with a stannous fluoride gel.

## Ceka
### PROCEDURE

The Ceka resilient and rigid stud attachments have a common base ring into which the resilient or rigid spring pins are threaded. Both spring pins provide retention; the resilient unit provides vertical and rotational movement, while the rigid allows absolutely no movement (Fig. 19-45). The Ceka is provided in three alloys: Pallax 1 and Orax 1 for soldering and Ceramax 1 for direct casting procedures.

### SOLDERING PROCEDURE

1. Carry out steps 1 to 8 of the Rothermann procedure.
2. Thread the parallelometer mandrel P-4 into base D, locate the attachments in the middle facially and as far lingually as possible, and sticky wax them to place (Fig. 19-46).
3. Replace the parallelometer mandrel by the soldering accessory H-4 (Fig. 19-47), and invest the dowel coping attachment base for soldering.
4. Heat treat the soldered unit, finish it in the usual manner, and it is ready for the processing phase.

### DIRECT CASTING PROCEDURE (CERAMAX 1)

1. Carry out steps 1 and 2 of the Rothermann rigid procedure.
2. Set the base with the parallelometer mandrel using the stone setup index, and wax it into the coping flush to the upper surface (Fig. 19-48).
3. Elective: Wax 20-gauge wax loops onto the coping to act as pickup loops for the master cast impression transfer.
4. Complete steps 3 to 5 of the Rothermann rigid procedure; note that investment should be hand painted onto the threaded section before investing to limit the gold from that area.
5. The castings are finished and ready for the processing phase.

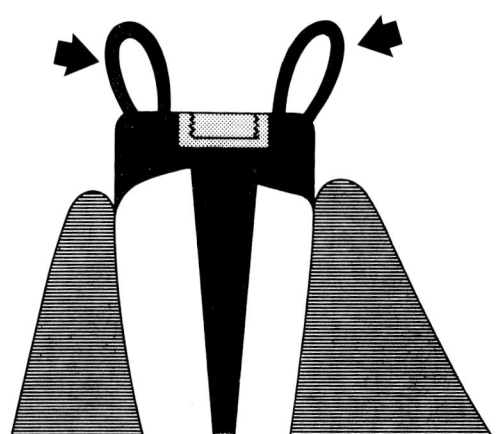

**Fig. 19-48.** Cast-to procedure: wax coping flush to occlusal surface of base. Include temporary pickup loops (arrows) in wax-up.

### DIRECT PROCESSING PHASE OF THE RESILIENT CEKA

1. Thread the spring pin into the base (Fig. 19-49).
2. Place the spacer ring over the stud, and lock it with the retention cap (Fig. 19-50).
3. Place the perforated space maintainer over the anchor assembly, and adapt it over the coping to extend 1 to 1.5 mm over the gingival margin (Fig. 19-51).
4. Make a duplicate master cast, and process the overdenture on this cast.
5. Cut lingual or palatal windows out about the attachment area.
6. Use indicator wax to check the clearance of the Ceka attachments to the prosthesis on the master cast.
7. Deliver the Ceka overdentures assembly to the dentist for resin pickup procedures.
8. The dentist temporarily cements the dowel copings, places the spacer or equivalent thickness of aluminum foil over the coping, and seats the overdenture.
9. The dentist paints a monomer wet resin into the window area (Fig. 19-52) and guides the patient to firm closure, retaining this position until the resin is set.
10. The dentist returns the overdenture and dowel copings to the laboratory for additional resin, and completes the processing by a pressure pot technique.

### INDIRECT PROCESSING PHASE OF THE RESILIENT CEKA

1. Thread processing pins into the base instead of the spring pins.
2. Place the spacer ring over the processing stud and lock it with the retention cap.
3. Place the perforated spacer over the anchor assembly, and adapt it over the coping to extend over the gingival area.
4. Transfer the stud assemblies to the processing cast, and lightly cement them with crown and bridge cement. (If the master cast is used for processing, then cement the dowel copings on the master cast.)
5. Complete and finish the setup in the usual manner.

### DIRECT PROCESSING PHASE OF THE RIGID CEKA

The steps are exactly the same as the resilient attachment except for steps 2 and 3 in which the spacers are omitted. The coping should be temporarily cemented and covered with one layer of household aluminum foil, using a rubber dam punch to make the stud hole, and extended at least 1 to 1.5 mm over the gingival margin. Seating the overdenture will burnish the foil. (This prevents resin from locking into the undercut of the coping or impinging the tissue.)

### INDIRECT PROCESSING PHASE OF THE RIGID CEKA

The blockout of the gingival margin can be handled the same as for the direct technique.

### RIVETING THE CEKA SPRING PIN

Riveting the pin prevents it from coming unscrewed.

1. Replace processing studs with resilient or rigid spring pins.
2. Place riveting tool H-6a for the resilient attachment or H-6b for the rigid system, and rivet with a sharp blow (Fig. 19-53).
3. If the riveted stud needs removal, it is done by using a laboratory key H-5.

### REBASING CEKA OVERDENTURES

1. Use the overdenture as an impression tray, and return an elastomeric impression to the laboratory. Use spacers if the attachment is resilient.
2. Screw the corresponding resilient or rigid Ceka spring pin into the auxiliary tool H-3 (Fig. 19-54), snap it into the housing (spacers must be used

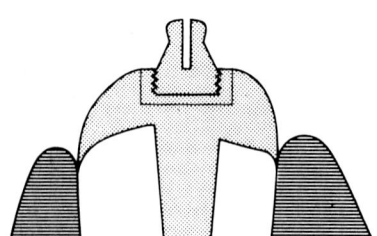

**Fig. 19-49.** Screw spring pin into base.

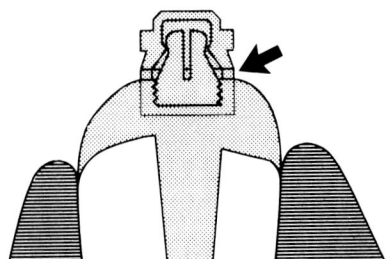

**Fig. 19-50.** Place spacer ring (arrow) over stud, and secure with retention cap.

ing it with a paint-on resin pickup in the mouth with the processing completed by the laboratory.

3. Sometimes the overdenture will seat and the attachment will not engage due to too much cement elevation prior to processing. This is usually the result of the cement being mixed too thick and too dry. A wet mix is most suited for laboratory assembly.

4. Retention factors are usually the perogative of the dentist, but the attachments are generally fabricated with some retention. If the retention problem exists with the Rothermann attachment, it is due to improper positioning of the male as it relates to the spring ring. The orientation groove of the male should always be facial and designate the spring opening of the ring spring.

5. Lack of retention may also be due to a broken arm, which may be the result of overbending and metal fatigue. The problem is solved by replacing the retention ring.

6. The Baer attachment retention is minimal unless it is laboratory processed or picked up in the mouth with a brush resin technique. When the polyvinyl chloride ring deteriorates, the housing overloads its retentive ability, and it becomes loose or comes out of the overdenture. This problem is rectified by replacing the housing or replacing the polyvinyl chloride ring and using a paint-on resin pickup technique.

7. The Sandri attachment presents only two problems over the other systems. The first is that the male thread was cut down so the attachment housing rides on the male. This is simply controlled by reducing the height to the ball. Second, the ball loosens or is lost. This requires cutting the thread down and burnishing the threaded section over the ball.

8. The Dalla Bona resilient and nonresilient and the Ancrofix attachments can hold the overdenture off-ridge contact if the cement elevation of the dowel coping is not considered, and, in the case of the resilient attachments, the shims are not used. Cement elevation of the copings on final placement is accomplished by using a wet mix of crown and bridge cement to secure the dowel copings to the processing model. In addition, the resilient shims are placed between the housing and the coping to ensure the resilient potential after delivery.

9. If the lack of resiliency is due to maximum contact of the denture base to the supporting tissue, there is no problem and this can be verified by having the dentist use pressure indicator paste.

10. Retention is usually a mechanical problem of simply bending the lamellae slightly inward using a sharp pointed instrument between the lamellae and the polyvinyl chloride ring (Fig. 19-55).

11. If the Dalla Bona retention lamellae are broken to the point of severe retention loss (usually two to three lamellae), then the housing is replaced. The breakage is usually the result of overbending and metal fatigue.

12. If the Dalla Bona housing is loose in the overdenture, it can be the result of insufficient resin contacting the retention or an overload on the retention due to the breakdown of the polyvinyl chloride ring. The solution is to remove and pick up the housing again with resin or remove, replace the polyvinyl chloride ring, and pick up the housing with resin.

13. The Ancrofix has essentially the same problems as the Dalla Bona. In addition, it has a problem with the male post coming unthreaded. This is resolved by seating the male post with a resin lock (Gun Lock).

14. The hemisphere elevation on the stud may be reduced to change from a resilient to rigid attachment, but to convert from rigid to resilient requires the placement of a new male stud for the Ancrofix system.

15. The Gerber rigid and resilient attachments experience identical problems with few exceptions. If the retention is good and there is no tissue contact of the denture base, several things could be involved. One, no provision was made for cement elevation of the dowel coping after placement. Two, the male was not seated all the way to the solder base. Cement elevation is a standard problem, but the male post not seating is a technical problem that requires checking before processing.

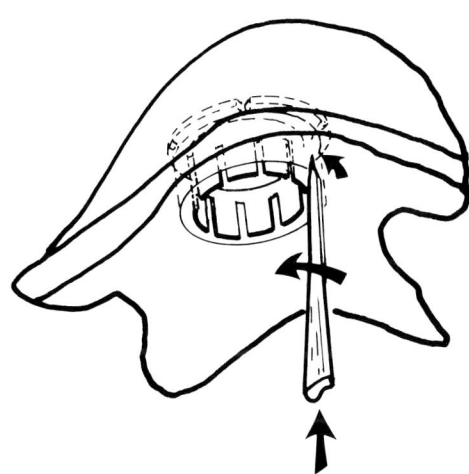

**Fig. 19-55.** Place point of sharp instrument between lamellae and resin base, and bend in slightly to increase retention.

16. Where there is no retention, the C spring may be missing, the C spring may be broken, or it may be fatigued, and the solution in all cases is to replace the C spring.

17. If there is no resiliency, the shim may still be in the housing, and it should be removed by disassembly and reassembly.

18. If the lack of resiliency is due to a broken or fatigued coil spring or the absence of the spring, resiliency can be restored by placing a new coil spring.

19. If all these steps are correct and there is still no resiliency, then the resin base is contacting the coping. This can be cleared to be flush with the base of the attachment housing or the housing can be removed and replaced with a shim between the housing and coping using the resin pickup technique.

20. If the housing is loose, there is insufficient resin contact, and the contents of the housing are replaced with a heating rod to remove the housing by applying a soldering iron to the rod to soften the resin. The attachment housing is removed, reassembled, and picked up with resin by the paint-on technique.

21. The Ceka attachment retention depends on having the correct spring pin to match the housing, resilient or rigid, and also the need for activation of the spring leaves.

22. If the retention loss is due to a broken spring, the spring is replaced by unscrewing and replacing the spring pin.

23. If there is no resiliency with the resilient Ceka attachment, it could be because a shim was not used for processing, or if a shim was used, none was used over the coping. It is necessary to remove the housing and repeat the resin pickup assembly procedure to correct the problem.

24. A loose Ceka housing in the overdenture is usually the result of insufficient resin in contact with the retention flanges. The housing has to be removed and the assembly procedure repeated by the paint-on resin pickup technique. If cylindrical-type dowels or screws are used for coping retention, there is seldom a failure of this part of the system. Definite chamfer margins, inlay seat, and an antirotation tent preparation reduce the possibility of coping failure (Fig. 19-56).

### Bar attachments

Bar attachments consist of prefabricated sections, resin pattern forms, and round or rectangular extrusions. Most bars have some form of clip retention, and they provide splinting as well as rigid and re-

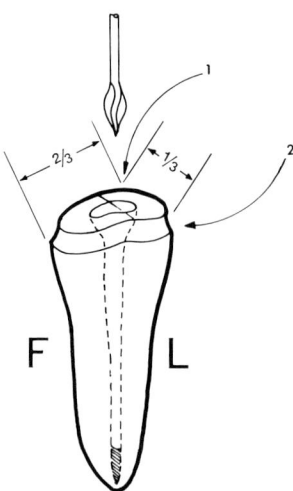

**Fig. 19-56.** Copy this illustration for dentist. Preparation for attachment retained overdenture: *F,* facial; *L,* lingual; occlusal reduction, two thirds facial, one third lingual (orientation reduction to provide space for replacement tooth and prevent rotation of coping): *1, inlay seat; 2* chamfer margin; Gates-Gliden bur used to prepare dowel space.

silient units. The best known bar system is the Dolder rigid and resilient followed by the Ackermann and Hader. The clips that can be used interchangeably with all the systems are the Ackermann and C. M. clip, and they are used to replace the resin training clips of the Hader system.

The Dolder bar unit* consists of a rider section with a retention mesh and the church window profile bar. It is used for splinting as an overdenture support in both anterior and posterior sections. The Dolder bar unit requires 3.5 to 4.5 mm of space for use.

### Dolder bar unit
**PROCEDURE**

1. Telescope crown or dowel coping preparations are required. Cast the impressions, section the dies, and cast the copings or telescope crowns.

2. Set up denture teeth on a trial base, and make a stone key to relate these teeth to the attachment.

3. Cut a section of the bar to fit the space, position the bar using the special parallelometer mandrel, staying away from the denture teeth that are set in the stone key, and then sticky wax it to place (Fig. 19-57).

4. Pick up the assembly, and invest it in solder-

---
*Dolder with mesh retention, APM-Sterngold, Stamford, Conn.; Dolder Standard, Degussa, Placentia, Calif.

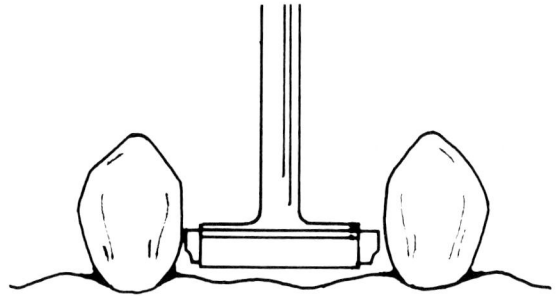

**Fig. 19-57.** Section Dolder bar unit to fit space. Use parallelometer mandrel to position bar, and sticky wax to place. Keep lingual to denture teeth and stone key.

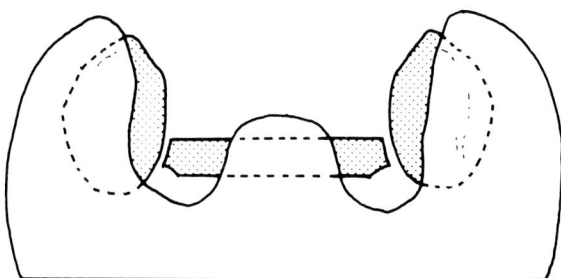

**Fig. 19-58.** Invest and solder bar to copings.

ing investment. Solder it with .650 solder followed by heat treatment (Fig. 19-58).

5. Temporarily cement the copings to the cast, and cut the rider to fit the bar section (Fig. 19-59).

6. Fill the free space between the bar and the gingiva, as well as the flexion area (Fig. 19-60), with dental stone to provide flexion adjustment of the rider.

7. Wax the denture teeth to the assembly, using the plaster index, and process in the normal manner.

8. After processing, remove the blockout stone or Rubber Sep and activate the attachment retention flanges with a sharp pointed instrument (Fig. 19-61).

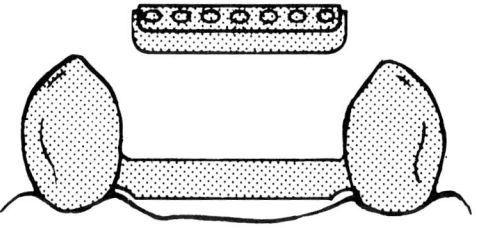

**Fig. 19-59.** Temporarily cement coping assembly to cast, and cut rider to fit bar section.

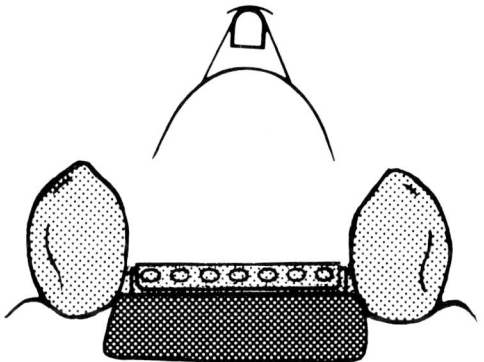

**Fig. 19-60.** Fill free space between bar and gingiva as well as flexion areas.

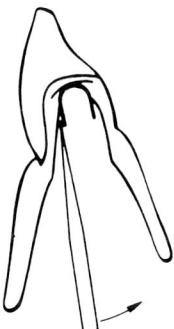

**Fig. 19-61.** Finish overdenture, remove blockout material, and activate retention flanges with sharp pointed instrument in direction of arrow.

## REBASING

1. Wash the base with the impression material of choice.
2. Section a processing jig to fit the rider, and invest it in the retentive section (Fig. 19-62).
3. Cast the impression, and set up the rebase by keying the denture teeth with stone occlusally and facially and stripping the case down to remove the rider clip.
4. Reposition the clip, or replace it with a new clip, and rebase in the usual manner.

### Dolder bar joint

The Dolder bar joint* consists of the same rider as the bar unit, a spacer to provide resiliency, and an egg-shaped bar to provide rotation in straight sections—any bending of the bar converts it from a bar joint to a bar unit.

---

*Dolder with mesh retention, APM-Sterngold, Stamford, Conn.; Dolder Standard, Degussa, Placentia, Calif.

## PROCEDURE

1. Prepare dowel copings, and use an overall master inpression to transfer the copings and the ridge detail.
2. Cast the model, and take a trial setup to the mouth.
3. Index the trial setup with a stone key, and establish the orientation of the bar joint section (Fig. 19-63).
4. Sticky wax the bar in place, and solder, heat treated, and finish it (Fig. 19-64).
5. Section the rider to fit (Fig. 19-65).
6. Place the rider over the bar with a spacer between them (Fig. 19-66).
7. Cover and fill in the flexion area and space between the bar and ridge as well as the coping with dental stone or Rubber-Sep.
8. The Dolder overdenture wax-up is completed using the stone keys and processing in the usual manner.
9. Remove the stone or Rubber-Sep along with the spacer, and bend the flanges in very slightly for retention.

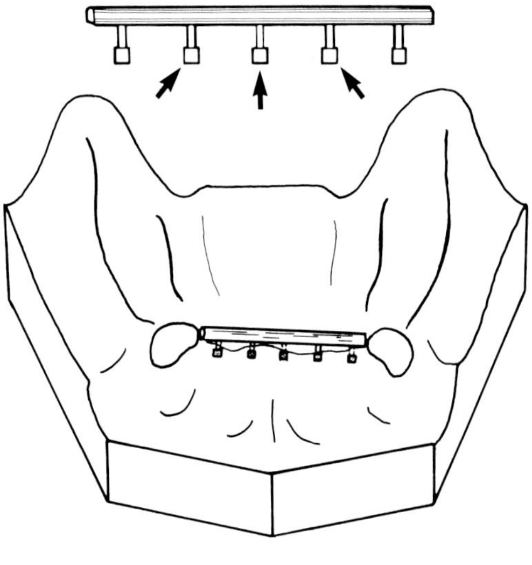

**Fig. 19-62.** Section processing jig to fit rider, insert it in rebase impression, and cast in stone. Retention tangs (arrows) hold processing jig in stone.

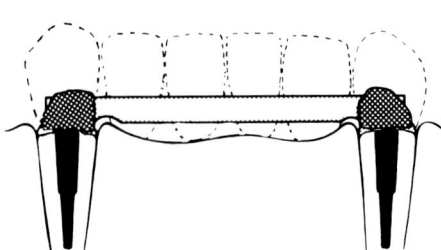

**Fig. 19-63.** Position bar to lingual side of stone key index to allow space for rider.

## REBASING

Rebasing requires placement of a spacer using sticky wax before washing the base. Processing is done as for the Dolder bar unit.

NOTE: The Dolder bar can be bent to conform to the ridge, and the rider should be segmented to fit the straight sections (Fig. 19-67).

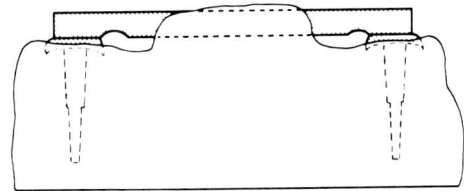

**Fig. 19-64.** Invest bar and coping assemblies and solder.

## The Hader bar

The Hader bar* consists of a keyhole-shaped male bar resin pattern, Teflon fabricating rider, and female nylon rider clip (Fig. 19-68). The rider clips work best in a metal framework and are least effective in a resin base. In a resin base they are routinely replaced with metal riders such as Ackermann clips† and C. M. clips.*

The apron of the male pattern allows contouring to fill gross tissue defect areas, whereas if the space is limited to just 3 mm, it is sometimes better to use a 13-gauge (1.8-mm) plastic rod to provide the bar section.

---

*Hader bar, C. M. clips, APM-Sterngold, Stamford, Conn.
†Ackermann clips, Degussa, Placentia, Calif.

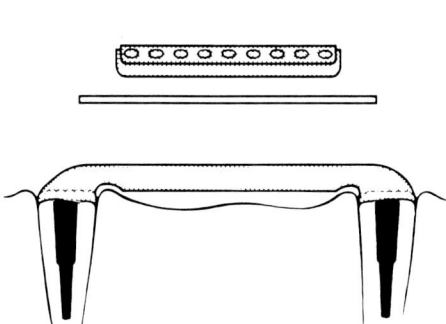

**Fig. 19-65.** Section rider and spacer to fit.

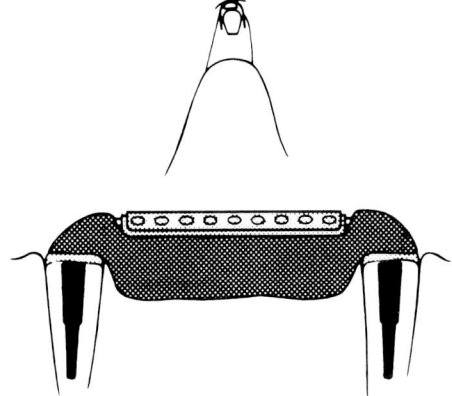

**Fig. 19-66.** Place rider and spacer over bar, and block out flexion areas with stone or Rubber Sep for processing.

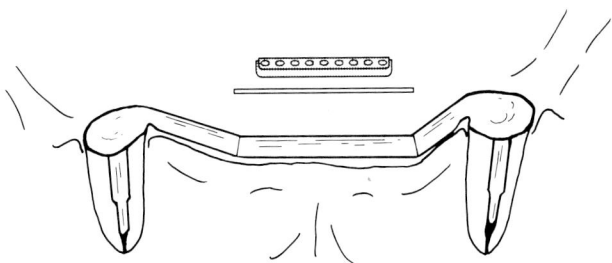

**Fig. 19-67.** Bend bar to conform to ridge. Segment rider to fit straight sections.

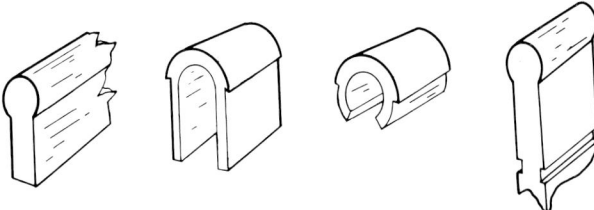

**Fig. 19-68.** Hader bar (left to right): keyhole-shaped male bar resin pattern, Teflon fabrication rider, female nylon rider clip, and insertion tool.

## PROCEDURE

1. Cast dowel-copings, and then transfer them in a master impression.
2. Pour a master cast, and make the overdenture trial setup.
3. Make a stone key of the anterior setup, and use it to position the plastic male pattern.
4. Shape the male pattern by dipping it in boiling water to curve and then cooling it in cold water. Establish the contour by using an acrylic bur (Fig. 19-69).
5. Place the plastic riders on the bar pattern to check the clearance of the teeth and the occlusion.
6. The bar can be cast separately and soldered to the copings or cast as a part of the dowel coping complex. Resin patterns require positive spruing with sticky wax and 1 hour extra burnout time to ensure complete vaporization of the resin pattern. After casting, heat treat the metalwork, and give it a high polish, preferably using electropolishing, and then temporarily cement it on the cast. (Spruing should be on the apron side rather than the bar.)
7. Set two or more riders on the bar, and wax out the undercut areas (Fig. 19-70) as well as rider undercuts.
8. Make a duplicate cast by placing the fabricating riders in the depression of the plastic riders and casting the impression (Fig. 19-71). The extension of the fabricating riders holds them in the stone.
9. Complete the setup using the stone index, and process it in the usual manner.
10. After processing, remove the fabricating riders with a pair of pliers (Fig. 19-72).
11. Insert the plastic riders with a plastic seating tool.

### Metal base procedure

Carry out steps 1 to 8 of the procedure for the Hader bar.

1. Make a second duplicate of the first duplicate cast.
2. Vacuum form Omnidental* coping material, .020, over the second duplicate cast (Fig 19-73), and then cast it in gold or Vitallium.
3. Complete the metal frame, then set it on the first duplicate processing cast (Fig. 19-74), and carry out steps 9 to 11 of the procedure for the Hader bar.

---

*Omnidental Corp., Harrisburg, Pa., or equivalent.

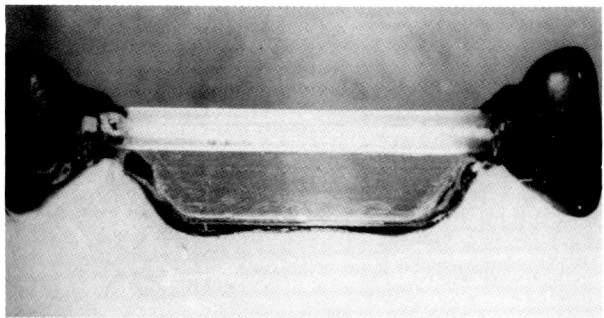

**Fig. 19-69.** Contour plastic bar to fit space.

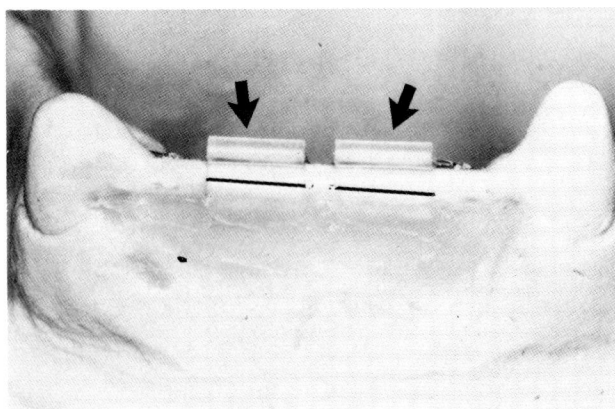

**Fig. 19-70.** Place riders (arrows) on bar or duplicate cast, wax out undercut areas to include height of contour of rider (black lines).

Attachments for overdentures 579

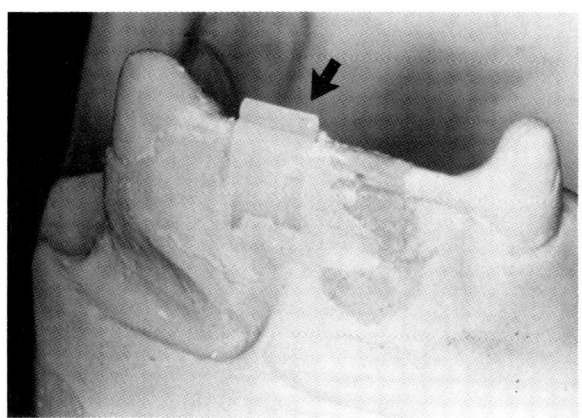

Fig. 19-71. Replace plastic rider with fabrication rider (arrow) in depression of duplication medium, and cast in stone.

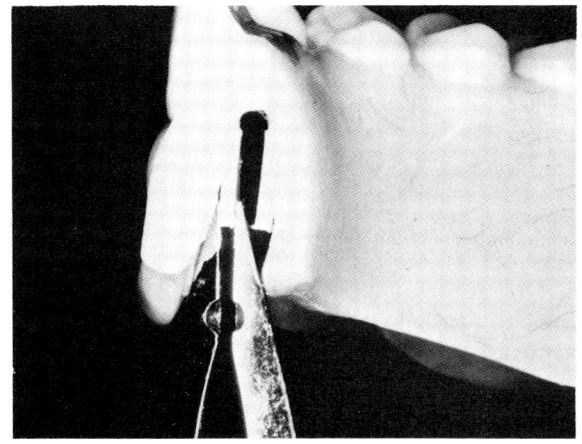

Fig. 19-72. Remove fabrication riders with pair of pliers.

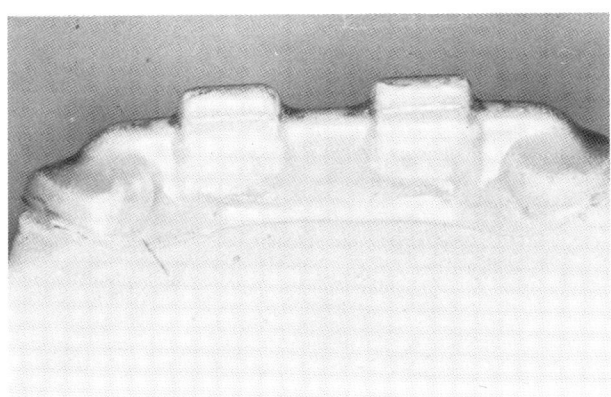

Fig. 19-73. Trim plastic coping material to fit cast, add retention with wax beads, and sprue for investment.

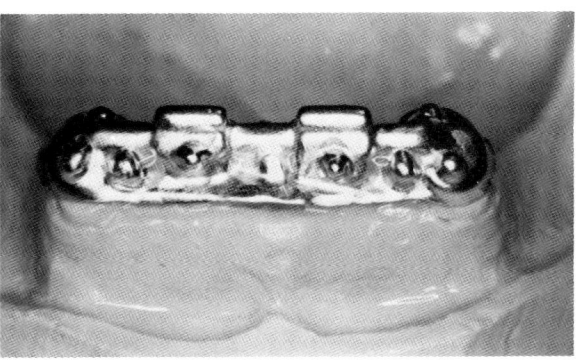

Fig. 19-74. Finish metal frame, and place on first duplicate processing cast.

### Rebasing procedure

1. Wash the overdenture base with a material of choice, and then return it to the laboratory.
2. Remove the existing plastic riders, and replace them with the fabricating riders.
3. Cast a model, make an index, and strip down the overdenture to provide new resin about the attachments.
4. The rebasing procedure follows steps 9 to 11 of the procedure for the Hader bar.

#### METAL RIDER REPLACEMENT

Either the Ackermann (Fig. 19-75) or C. M. riders (Fig. 19-76) may be used. Where there is a short occlusal space, the Ackermann rider is preferable because of its facial and lingual retention. The C. M. rider is ideal for the Hader system because the retention units are occlusal and may be bent down, occupying the same space as the original Hader riders.

#### PROCEDURE

1. Replace the old plastic riders with fabricating riders, and cast a model.
2. Cut lingual or palatal windows about the riders, and then deepen the space occlusally and to both sides of the rider space to provide room for the retention flanges.
3. Give the C. M. riders with the spacer (if vertical resilience is required) to the dentist.
4. The dentist checks the clearance of the clips to the prosthesis and paints out the gingival two thirds of the C. M. clips (Fig. 19-77) with Impregum as well as any adjacent undercut area.
5. The dentist picks up the clip wings with a wet paint-on resin technique and returns the overdenture to the laboratory for pressure pot processing and finishing.
6. Remove the Impregum after processing, and the overdenture is ready to be delivered to the dentist.

### C. M. rider

The C. M. rider is an advanced design of the Gilmore, Ackermann, and Baker clip systems and is available in small and large sizes. The combined bar/rider height is 2.7 mm for both sizes. The C. M. rider system consists of the C. M. clip in Elitor,* a brass spacer for assembly, and a round bar, 1.9 mm, in OSV or Protor 3* alloy (Fig. 19-78). The spacer provides vertical movement of 0.5 mm. The clips are available separately and may be used with customized 12- or 13-gauge resin pattern bar forms (Hader) or 13-gauge round bar systems. If employed on a straight anterior section, axial rotation and vertical resilience are available (bar joint). If the bar is bent, then only vertical movement is available, and the system becomes a bar unit.

#### PROCEDURE

Complete steps 1 to 4 of the procedure for the resilient Dolder.

1. Place the small clips and spacer (if resilience is desired) on the bar, bending the retention wings down if necessary and making sure the denture teeth clear the outer rider surface (use index with teeth in place for checking) (Fig. 19-79).

---

*Elastic alloy, bar alloys for soldering, Cendres & Metaux, S. A., Biel, Switzerland; Protor 3 is self-annealing, APM-Sterngold, Stamford, Conn.

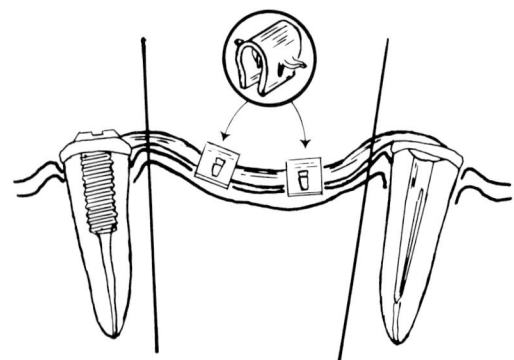

**Fig. 19-75.** Ackermann rider has faciolingual retention tabs (inset). Note divergent teeth and bar secured with Kurer screw (left).

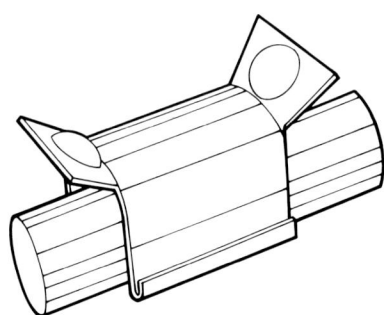

**Fig. 19-76.** C. M. rider or clip has retention tabs parallel to bar. Height is 2.7 mm.

Attachments for overdentures 581

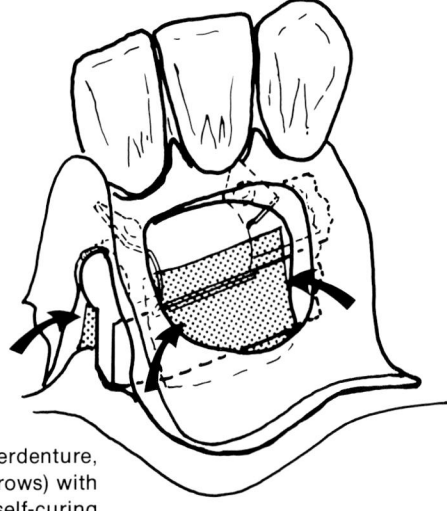

**Fig. 19-77.** Have dentist check clearance of clips to overdenture, paint out undercut areas below height of contour (arrows) with Impregum, and relate C. M. rider to overdenture with self-curing resin.

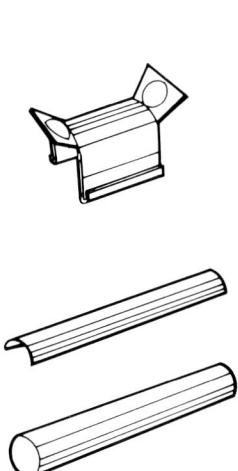

**Fig. 19-78.** C. M. rider system (top to bottom): C. M. clip; brass spacer, 0.5 mm; and round bar in wrought gold, 1.9 mm in diameter.

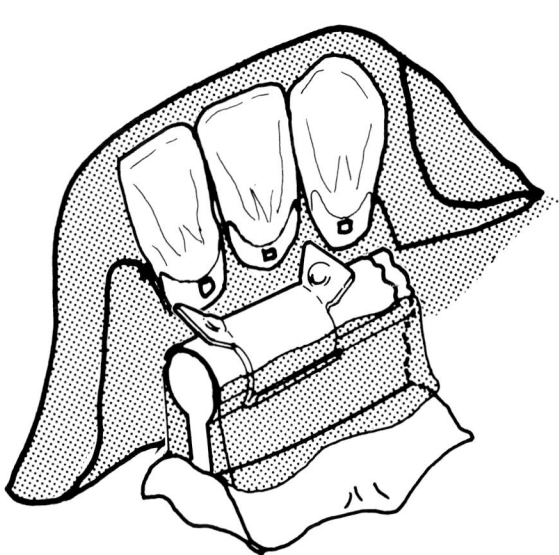

**Fig. 19-79.** Use index with teeth in place. Check clip for clearance. Bend retention wings down if necessary. Dotted area with teeth (stone index) and dotted area about attachment (Rubber Sep).

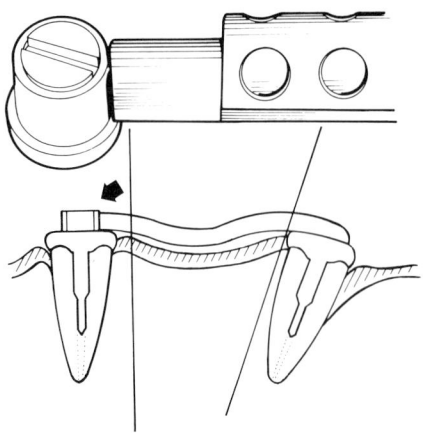

**Fig. 19-80.** Use Schubiger screw system to join divergent teeth. Ring of Schubiger system (arrow) is soldered to bar and then screwed onto stud base on coping. Stud base is identical to Gerber and allows for conversion to stud. Top is Schubiger with Dolder bar.

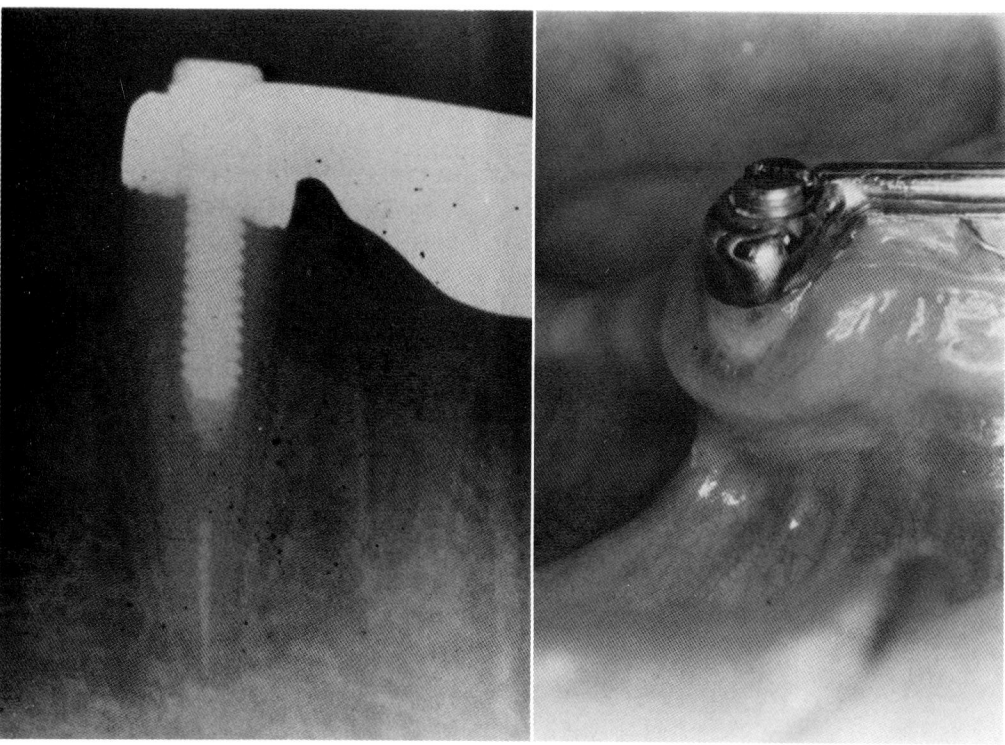

**Fig. 19-81.** Kurer screw and coping system follow same technique as Kurer Press-Stud. Join bar to Kurer coping, and secure with Kurer screw.

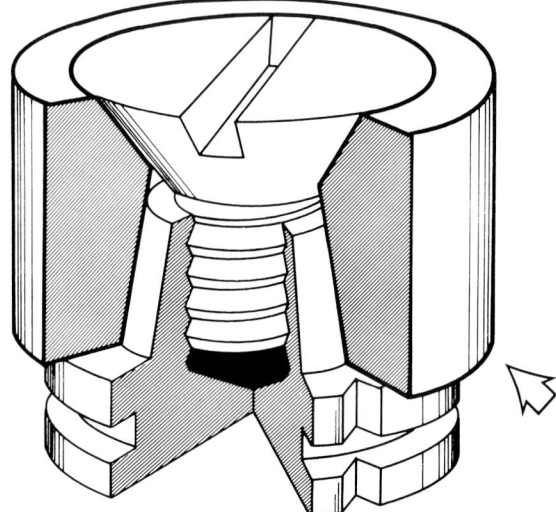

**Fig. 19-82.** BZ-75 is similar to Schubiger. Double conical cylinder (arrow) provides positive locking of ring-bar units.

## REBASING

Rebasing can be simplified by casting a processing bar with retention to fit the riders and follow the Dolder procedure.

NOTE: Any bar system can be used with divergent abutments by use of screw systems such as the Schubiger* (Fig. 19-80), Kurer Screw† (Figs. 19-75 and 19-81), or BZ-75‡ (Fig. 19-82), using a screw fixation on both ends, or soldering the weaker abutment coping to the bar and fixing the anchorage by means of a screw on the stronger abutment.

## PROBLEM AREAS

The problem areas for the bar attachments and clips appear to be common with few exceptions. The Dolder, Hader, and C. M. riders have no real problems with the bar, except in casting of the Hader bar. The problems exist with the metal clips or with the nylon riders. The problems, their probable causes, and solutions are presented in Table 19-2.

---

*Schubiger, APM-Sterngold, Stamford, Conn.
†Kurer Screw, Union Broach Co., Inc., Long Island City, N.Y.
‡BZ-75, Bell International, Inc., San Mateo, Calif.

1. The metal clips do not hold unless they are activated by bending inward with a sharp pointed instrument placed between the resin and the metal rider.

2. If the clip contact is present without tissue contact, the copings were not temporarily cemented to the fabricating cast before processing. This can be rectified by rebasing or by replacing the riders with a resin pickup technique.

3. If the prosthesis is to be resilient and there is no resiliency, several things could be wrong. One, no spacer was used between the bar and the rider, and two, no relief was provided over the copings. This can be solved by relieving the coping area to a fixed depth by using a No. 33½ inverted cone bur for depth in the coping space and removing the resin to this depth with an acrylic bur. Place a spacer between the bar and rider, and reline the overdenture except for the coping area.

4. If the Dolder rider separates from the overdenture, the retention weld is broken and the rider must be replaced either by the reline method or resin pickup method in the mouth.

5. If the overdenture will not seat in the mouth or master cast, the undercut areas were not sur-

**Table 19-2.** Bar attachments

| Problem | Probable cause | Solution |
|---|---|---|
| **Dolder, Hader, and C. M. rider** | | |
| Retention clip does not hold | Clip not activated | Use sharp instrument between rider and plastic and bend in slightly |
| Clip contacts, but overdenture does not contact ridge | Copings were not temporarily cemented to cast before processing | Replace clip by resin pickup technique or reline if freeway space is available |
| No resiliency | No spacer was used between bar and rider | Replace clip by resin pickup technique, or reline if freeway space is available; reline with spacer |
| No resiliency | Spacer was used, but coping area was not relieved | Use pressure indicator paste for control; use No. 33½ inverted cone bur for depth cut in coping space, and remove balance with acrylic bur |
| **Dolder** | | |
| Clip separated from retention | Retention weld broken | Replace riders |
| Overdenture will not seat in mouth or master cast | Undercut areas not blocked out in path of insertion | "Eyeball" path of insertion on denture with one eye closed, verify with pressure indicator paste, and remove interference; *caution:* block out undercuts before processing |

*Continued.*

**Table 19-2.** Bar attachments—cont'd

| Problem | Probable cause | Solution |
| --- | --- | --- |
| **Hader** | | |
| Retention clips do not hold | Resin pickup of clips, free monomer attacks clips | Replace clips |
| Retention clips bent; overdenture will not seat | Forced insertion, distorted clips | Replace clips |
| Retention clips do not hold | Water sorption softens clip | Replace clips |
| Clips will not engage bar | Clips were used for processing instead of fabricating riders, no flexion space available | Remove clips, flare out clip area, insert fabricating rider, and flow in resin to contact rider; remove fabricating riders, and insert new retention clips |
| Retention clips will not stay in receptacle | Undercut blockout was carried to retention area; fabricating rider spread in receptacle before pouring | *Caution:* keep blockout below retention, remove clip, place fabricating rider in space, hold rider extensions together with alligator clip, and flow wet resin between fabrication rider and overdenture; process, remove, and place new clip |
| New clips will not go into place | Fabricating rider damaged before processing | Clear receptacle area, tap resin release hole to lingual or palatal, shorten fabrication side, clip at gingival margin, paint wet resin in overdenture and seat with fabrication clip; process, remove, and place new retention clip |
| Clip will not go into place | Calculus and water sorption swelling of denture base | Use sonic scaler and cleaner to remove debris; if still will not seat, treat as previous section |
| Clips will not hold | Bar overfinished or tongue too active | Convert to metal cliplike C. M. rider |
| Clips wear | Nonprecious metal bar not smooth, acts like file | Fine finish with rubber wheels |
| Incomplete casting | Improper spruing or incomplete burnout | Larger sprues required for nonprecious metals; sticky wax sprues into place, and hold investment burnout for 1 hour extra time to ensure burnout of resin pattern |
| Casting miscast bar to abutment | Insufficient wax to hold in place | Use adequate wax and sticky wax to join parts |
| Casting miscast bar to abutment | Excessive vibration during investment | Invest carefully with minimum vibration |
| Difficult insertion and removal of overdenture | Undercut retentive area not related to insertion path | *Caution:* survey cast coincident with insertion path; block out undercuts before processing, remove riders, reduce undercut areas, use resin pickup with fabrication riders to reposition riders |

veyed to coincide with the path of insertion, and they were not blocked out prior to processing. The insertion path has to be examined with one eye closed. The first interference is verified with pressure indicator paste, and this excess is reduced on the tissue side of the overdenture until there is complete insertion.

6. Hader clips present the greatest problems with the system and are viewed as "training clips" according to Brewer and Morrow (1980). The retention clips will not hold if free monomer is present, or they were resin picked up for processing. The solution is to replace the clips.

7. If the Hader overdenture will not seat, the retention clips are usually bent from forced insertion, and the clips must be replaced.

8. If the Hader retention clips do not hold the prosthesis, it can be due to water sorption and softening of the nylon clip, which requires clip replacement.

9. When the clips fail to engage the bar, clips were used for processing instead of the Teflon fabrication riders, and no clip flexion space was available. This problem can be solved by removing the clips, flaring the resin to the retention notches in the receptacle, and inserting the Teflon fabricating riders. Hold the rider extensions together with an alligator clip, and flow wet resin between the base and the fabrication riders. Remove the fabrication riders, and insert new clips.

10. When the clips fail to stay in the receptacles, the undercut blockout was carried up to the retention extensions so that the fabricating riders spread in the impression transfer before the cast was poured, producing too large a receptacle. This can be avoided in the processing by keeping the blockout below the retentive area (Fig. 19-83, arrow). It

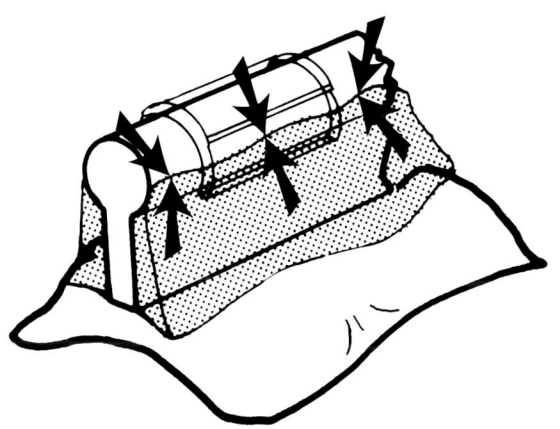

**Fig. 19-83.** Keep blockout below retentive area (arrows), or clips will not hold.

can be corrected by inserting a fabrication rider in the receptacle and flowing wet resin between the fabrication rider and the base. The extensions of the fabrication rider must be held together with an alligator clip to prevent the problem from reoccurring.

11. If a new clip will not seat following fabrication, it is most likely due to damage of the fabrication rider before processing. This is best handled by tapping a resin release hole lingually or palatally from the receptacle and widening the receptacle. A shortened fabrication rider (1 mm longer occlusogingivally than the clip) is fitted to the overdenture and bar and is then resin related to the overdenture by half filling the receptacle with a wet mix of resin and seating the prosthesis. After curing, the fabrication rider is replaced by a Hader nylon clip.

12. If a new clip will not go to place, it can also be because of calculus, debirs, and water sorption swelling of the denture base. An ultrasonic cleaner can remove the calculus and debirs; if the clip will not seat, it must be treated as for the damaged fabrication rider.

13. When the nylon clips will not hold, it can be due to an overactive tongue or an overfinished bar, and a metal clip, such as the C. M. rider, must be used to provide retention.

14. Nylon clips usually wear, particularly with nonprecious metal that has not been finished, due to a file action. The wear can be reduced by fine finishing with abrasive rubber wheels, such as Shofu* rubber finishing points.

15. Casting problems, such as an incomplete cast, result from improper spruing and insufficient burnout time. Sprues must be of the proper dimension (10-gauge for nonprecious metals), and they must be sticky waxed to place. Resin patterns, especially large units, require at least 1 hour extra burnout time to totally remove the resin pattern.

16. Miscast bars or bars to abutments are due to insufficient wax to hold the components and sprues to place. It can also be due to excessive vibration during investing, which requires careful investment procedures with minimal vibration.

17. Insertion and removal are common problems because the master cast was not surveyed in relation to the path of attachment insertion, and undercut blockout was not done before processing. It can be corrected by viewing the insertion path in the overdenture base with one eye closed, noting the undercut areas, and, with pressure indicator paste verification, the excess can be removed. Avoidance

---

*Shofu Dental Corp., Menlo Park, Calif.

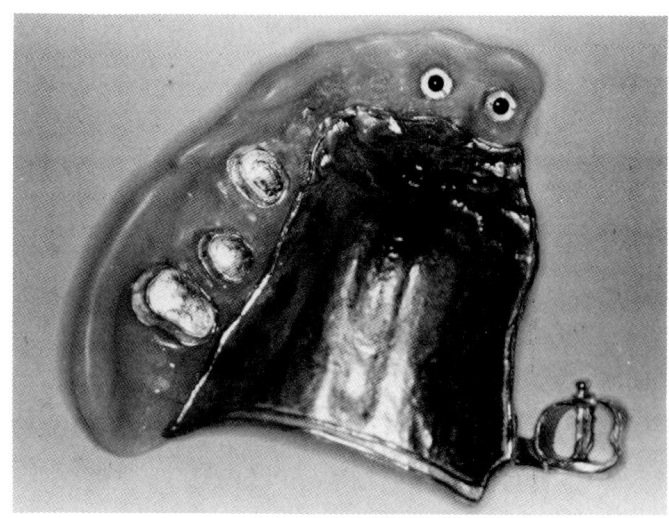

Fig. 19-84. Use overdenture concept as combined removable partial denture and overdenture. Left side, maxillary, three telescope crowns: anterior, Sandri stud attachments; right side, posterior, fixed bridged with telescope ring retained by auxiliary Mini-Presso-Matic.

is the best method, and this can be accomplished by surveying the path of overdenture insertion coincident with the attachment insertion pathway and blocking out the undercuts before processing.

The overdenture concept with or without attachment fixation may be used in combination with partial dentures where one side of the arch may have a normal clinical crown configuration (Fig. 19-84). The concept reduces the torque on questionable teeth and provides a predictable method of treating an area of the mouth that might normally be committed to extraction.

## REFERENCES

Brewer, A. A., and Morrow, R. M.: Overdentures, ed. 2, St. Louis, 1980, The C. V. Mosby Co.

Körber, K.: Zahnartliche Prothetik, Bd II, Stuttgart, 1975, Georg Thieme, Verlag.

Mensor, M. C.: Classification and selection of attachments, J. Prosthet. Dent. **29**(5):494-497, 1973.

CHAPTER 20

# ORTHODONTIC PROCEDURES

WILLIAM C. BERLOCHER and BRETT H. MUELLER

PART ONE

## Interceptive orthodontic appliances

**fixed interceptive orthodontic appliance** An intraoral apparatus that is cemented directly onto the teeth and is used in the treatment of incipient malocclusions.

**removable interceptive orthodontic appliance** An apparatus that is retained in the oral cavity by metal clasps and is used in the treatment of incipient malocclusions.

Developing malocclusions are observed in children of almost any age. If these irregularities are recognized and corrected in their formative stages, a major malocclusion can sometimes be averted. The dentist will often use an interceptive orthodontic appliance for the treatment of a developing occlusal problem. This chapter will attend to the technical skills necessary for fabrication of the interceptive orthodontic devices as well as describe the construction of some of the more commonly used appliances.

## Section 1: COMPONENTS OF THE INTERCEPTIVE ORTHODONTIC APPLIANCE

### ORTHODONTIC WIRE

A significant portion of an interceptive orthodontic appliance is wire. This wire is used for clasps and springs and to connect the various components of an appliance. The majority of orthodontic wire in use today is stainless steel. Stainless steel wire is available from a number of manufacturers in a variety of diameters, lengths, and tempers. Choice of the appropriate wire is in part determined by how it will be employed in appliance construction.

### Preactivated wire

The ideal wire for an orthodontic spring is one that is capable of distributing an adequate force for tooth movement over a considerable distance for a long period of time. The wire that comes closest to fulfilling these criteria was developed in 1962 by an Australian metallurgist to be used in Begg fixed orthodontic therapy. This wire has excellent resilience, or ability to regain its original shape after being deflected, and is strong enough to withstand the forces exerted upon it in the oral cavity without distortion or failure.

### Annealed wire

Generally, the larger in diameter a wire becomes the stiffer it is. For this reason, a large-gauge wire is indicated for the portions of an appliance that need to be rigid or resistant to flexion. However, large-diameter stainless steel is difficult to bend. To facilitate bending, this type wire is sometimes marketed in an annealed form, which makes the wire soft and easy to manipulate.

Although annealed wire is easy to bend, it does have certain disadvantages in appliance construction. Because it is soft, it is easily distorted. The annealing process also removes most of the elasticity from the wire so it has little use in spring construction. Hardness and elasticity can be returned to an annealed wire by a heat treatment process. This is accomplished by gently heating the wire with a small flame or electric heating unit until an amber or straw-colored appearance is attained in the metal. Overheating a wire will destroy its physical properties. Therefore care must be taken to avoid heating the wire until it glows red.

## ORTHODONTIC PLIERS

The number of orthodontic pliers available for wire bending is almost limitless, and choice of an appropriate pliers is often a matter of operator preference. Two pliers, however, the Nos. 139 and 200, provide excellent results and are applicable in the construction of most interceptive orthodontic appliances.

The No. 139, or bird-beak, pliers is probably the most versatile of all wire-bending pliers (Fig. 20-1). The pliers have a square beak that can be used to bend angles and a round beak that is used for curves and loops. The two jaws also taper from a large-diameter area close to the hinge, which has the strength needed to work with large-gauge wire, to a very small end that is capable of fine manipulations in thin wire.

The No. 200, or three-prong, pliers is useful in appliance construction not for its versatility but because of its application in specific situations (Fig. 20-2). Most orthodontic pliers require either a rotation of the pliers or finger pressure away from a stationary pliers to produce a bend. The design of a No. 200 pliers allows it to exert considerable force on a wire simply by squeezing the pliers. This makes the No. 200 pliers particularly effective when working in confined areas or bending sharp angles in large-diameter wire.

## WIRE BENDING

Bending a wire into a prescribed form would seem like a simple maneuver, requiring nothing more than orthodontic pliers and the wire itself. Nevertheless, wire bending can acquire a fairly complex character easily and become quite frustrating unless certain guidelines are established. Sim (1977) lists the following general rules for wire bending:

1. Orthodontic wire must be of the proper size and temper. It is better to have a wire that is too large and too soft than too small and too highly tempered.
2. Appropriately shaped pliers must be used to make the proper bends.
3. Wire should be bent around the pliers by firm pressure with the thumb or index finger, with the pliers used as a more or less stationary vise.
4. Bend the wire in one plane (dimension) at a time.
5. When a long complex series of bends is to be made, with configurations at both ends of the wire, it is usually best to start at the middle and work toward the ends.
6. When bending shorter springs and clasps, start by bending the complicated section of the wire first; then bend the easier sections.

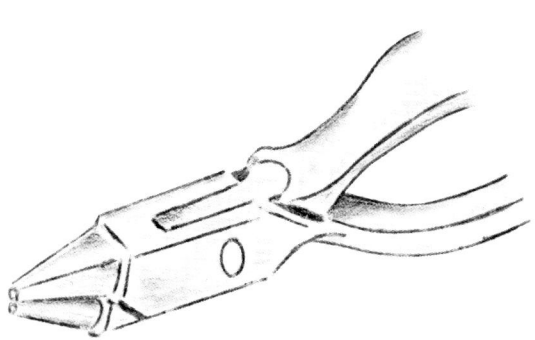

**Fig. 20-1.** No. 139, or bird-beak, pliers. Square beak can be used to bend angles, and round beak is used for curves and loops. Pliers are applicable for both large- and small-diameter wire.

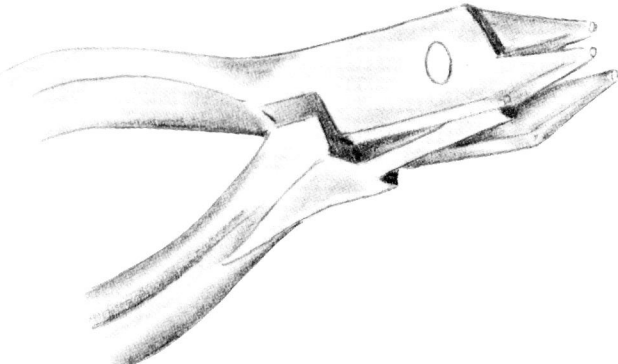

**Fig. 20-2.** No. 200, or three-prong, pliers. Design of these pliers allows them to exert considerable force on wire by simply squeezing them. They are particularly effective when working in confined areas or bending sharp angles in large-diameter wire.

## WIRE-BENDING PROCEDURES

There are a number of basic wire-bending maneuvers. Of these bends the semicircle, helix, closed end loop, right angle, deflection, zigzag, and smooth curve are especially useful in the construction of interceptive orthodontic appliances.

### Semicircular bend

**semicircle** A wire bent into the shape of a half circle (Fig. 20-3).

#### APPLICATION

The semicircle is employed most often when spring action in a wire is needed. The simple finger, simple helix, dumbell and labial bow spring all use a semicircle bend in their fabrication.

#### PROCEDURE

1. Position a No. 139 pliers with the working end facing you and the square beak pointing up. Then grasp the wire firmly with the pliers. The size of the semicircle will depend on the position of the wire in the jaws of the pliers. The end of the jaws will produce the smallest semicircle, and the area closest to the hinge will produce the largest semicircle (Fig. 20-4).

2. Stabilize the pliers, and turn the wire around the round beak of the pliers with finger pressure to complete the semicircle (Fig. 20-5).

### Helical bend

**helix** A coil formed by turning wire around a uniform cylinder (Fig. 20-6).

#### APPLICATION

The helix, like the semicircle, is used in spring construction. It is the preferred method of adding a spring action to wire because it allows for light force application with a long duration of action.

#### PROCEDURE

1. Adjust the wire in the jaws of a No. 139 pliers until the desired diameter of the helix is attained. Make sure the working end of the pliers is facing you and the square beak is pointing up (Fig. 20-7).

Fig. 20-3. Semicircular bend.

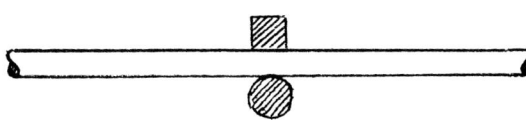

Fig. 20-4. Position No. 139 pliers facing you with square beak pointing up.

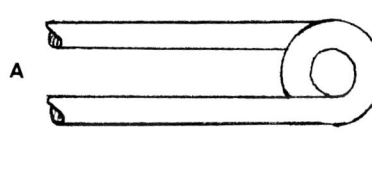

Fig. 20-6. **A,** Helical bend. **B,** Rotated view of helical bend.

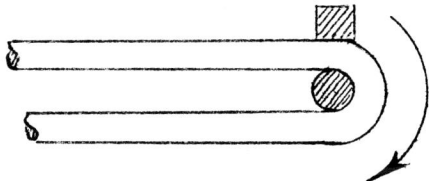

Fig. 20-5. Stabilize pliers, and turn wire around round beak of pliers (arrow) with finger pressure to complete semicircle.

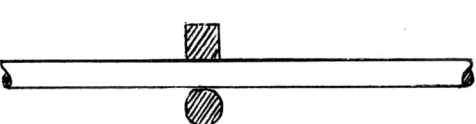

Fig. 20-7. With working end of pliers facing you and square beak pointing up, adjust wire in jaws of No. 139 pliers until desired diameter of helix is attained.

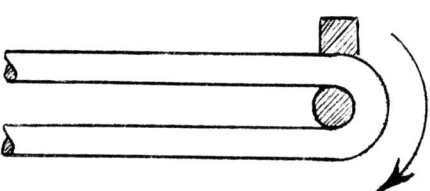

**Fig. 20-8.** Using finger pressure, turn wire around round beak of pliers (arrow) to form semicircle.

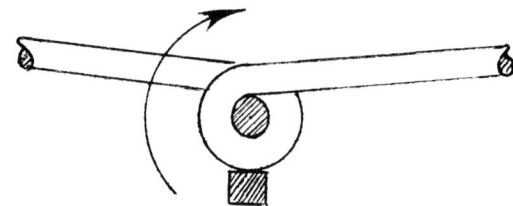

**Fig. 20-9.** Rotate pliers 180 degrees, and bend wire around round beak to form loop (arrow).

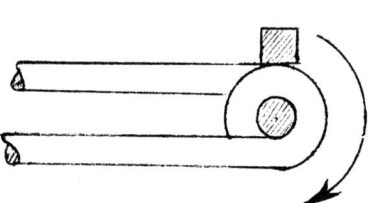

**Fig. 20-10.** Again invert pliers 180 degrees, and turn wire to complete helix (arrow).

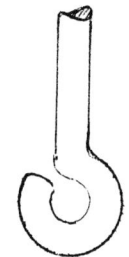

**Fig. 20-11.** Closed end loop.

2. Turn the wire around the round beak of the pliers to form a semicircle (Fig. 20-8).

3. Invert the pliers 180 degrees until the round beak is facing up, and bend the wire to form a loop (Fig. 20-9).

4. Again invert the pliers 180 degrees, and turn the wire to complete the helix (Fig. 20-10).

### Closed end loop

**closed end loop** A complete ring or circle at the end of a segment of wire (Fig. 20-11).

#### APPLICATION

The closed end loop is used primarily to provide mechanical retention for clasps. A small loop can be retained in undercut areas of the dental arch, or a large loop can be used on the end of wire extensions that are to be embedded in acrylic. The closed end loop can also serve as a means of attaching elastic material to an appliance.

#### PROCEDURE

1. With the No. 139 pliers in the proper position, take hold of the end of a piece of wire (Fig. 20-12).

2. Hold the pliers stationary, and use finger pressure to form the wire into a tight circle (Fig. 20-13).

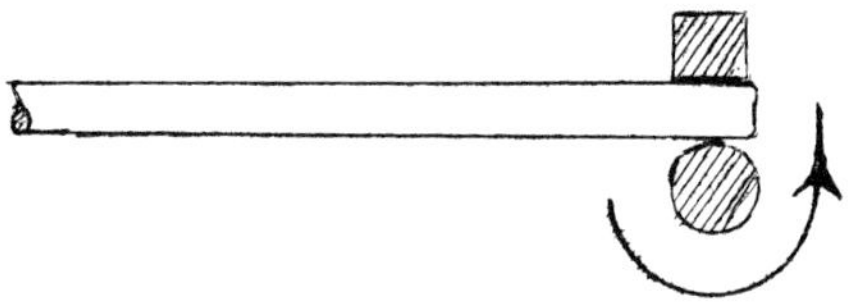

**Fig. 20-12.** No. 139 pliers are used to make this bend. Take hold of end of piece of wire. Wire will be pulled around pliers to make bend (arrow).

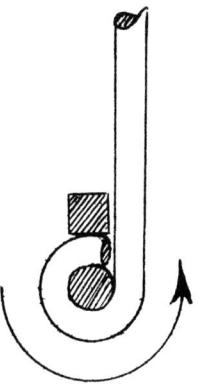

**Fig. 20-13.** Hold pliers tightly, and carefully pull wire into tight circle (arrow).

3. Rotate the square end of the pliers until it is directly across the wire from its previous position (Fig. 20-14).

4. Again, hold the pliers stationary, and complete the procedure by bending the wire coming off of the circle down approximately 45 degrees (Fig. 20-15).

### Right-angle bend

**right angle** A wire that is bent to form an angle such that the two lines produced are perpendicular to each other (Fig. 20-16).

#### APPLICATION

Many times during the fabrication of springs and clasps the direction of the wire must change abruptly. A right-angle bend is particularly adept at affecting this change.

#### PROCEDURE

1. With the working end of a No. 200 pliers facing you and the middle prong point up, grasp the wire (Fig. 20-17).

2. Squeeze the pliers with one hand, and apply finger pressure to the wire with the other hand until a 90-degree angle is formed in the wire (Fig. 20-18).

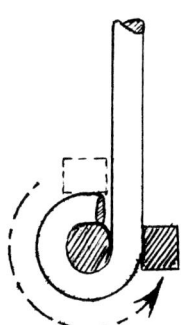

Fig. 20-14. Rotate square end of pliers until it is directly across wire from its previous position (arrow).

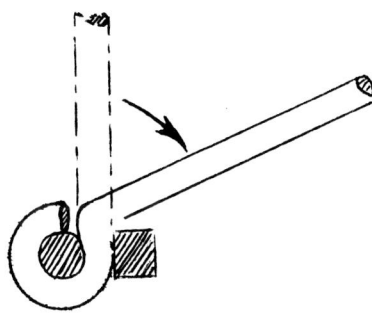

Fig. 20-15. Closed end loop is completed by once again holding pliers as stationary as possible and bending wire coming off circle (arrow) down approximately 45 degrees.

Fig. 20-16. Right-angle bend.

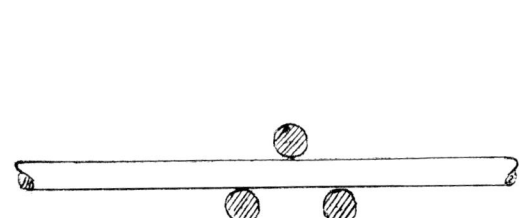

Fig. 20-17. Position working end of No. 200 pliers with middle prong pointing up. Open jaws, and grasp wire in middle of beaks.

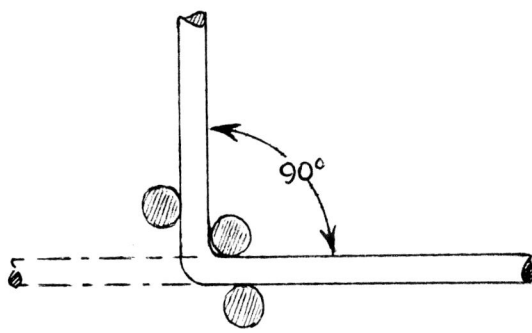

Fig. 20-18. Squeeze pliers with one hand while applying finger pressure to wire with other hand. Continue this motion until 90-degree angle is formed in wire.

## Deflection bend

**deflection** A wire that is bent to deviate slightly from its original direction (Fig. 20-19).

### APPLICATION

The deflection bend is used when subtle changes must be made in the direction of a wire. Isolated tooth contact with a wire, clearing a spring or clasp from interfering contact with opposing teeth, and close adaptation of a wire to the tooth surface are situations in which this bend is useful.

### PROCEDURE

1. Take hold of a segment of wire with the outer third of the jaws of a No. 139 pliers (Fig. 20-20).
2. On one side of the pliers bend the wire slightly downward with finger pressure (Fig. 20-21).
3. With the pliers in the same position, move to the other side of the jaws, and bend the wire very slightly upward until the two angles formed are equal (Fig. 20-22).

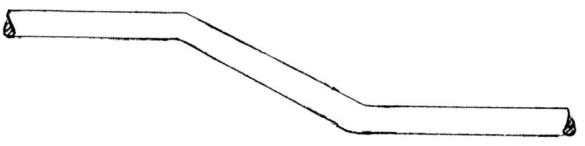

**Fig. 20-19.** Deflection bend.

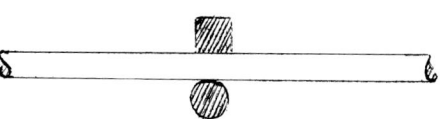

**Fig. 20-20.** Hold segment of wire with outer third of jaws of No. 139 pliers.

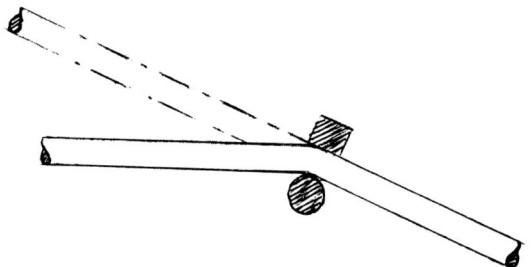

**Fig. 20-21.** Hold pliers as tightly as possible, and, with finger pressure, bend one side of wire slightly downward.

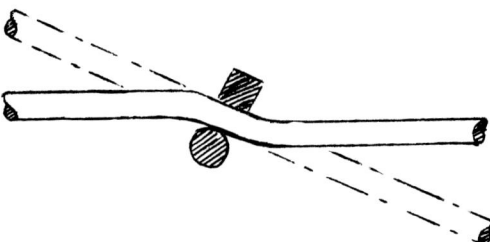

**Fig. 20-22.** Continue to hold pliers tightly, move to other side of jaws, and bend wire slightly upward until two angles formed are equal.

## Zigzag bend

**zigzag** A wire having a series of short turns or angles (Fig. 20-23).

### APPLICATION

Any spring or clasp that will be placed in an acrylic base requires some form of mechanical retention. The zigzag bend is an effective method of providing this retention.

### PROCEDURE

1. With a No. 200 pliers facing you and with the middle prong pointing up, firmly grasp the wire (Fig. 20-24).
2. Squeeze the pliers to produce a bend of approximately 135 degrees (Fig. 20-25).
3. Invert the pliers 180 degrees, and take hold of the wire about 10 mm from the bend (Fig. 20-26).
4. Squeeze the pliers to produce a second bend of approximately 135 degrees (Fig. 20-27).
5. Repeat these procedures until the desired length of zigzag pattern is attained (Fig. 20-28).

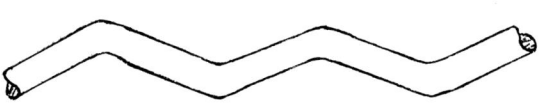

**Fig. 20-23.** Zigzag bend.

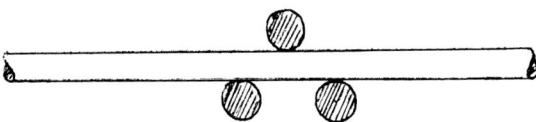

**Fig. 20-24.** With No. 200 pliers in position similar to one used for right-angle bend, firmly grasp wire.

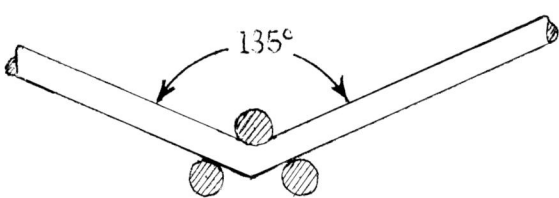

**Fig. 20-25.** Squeeze pliers gently until bend of approximately 135 degrees is produced.

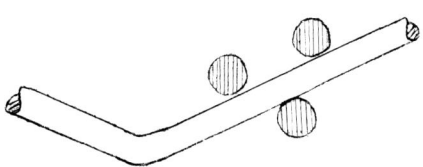

**Fig. 20-26.** Invert pliers 180 degrees, and take hold of wire about 10 mm from bend.

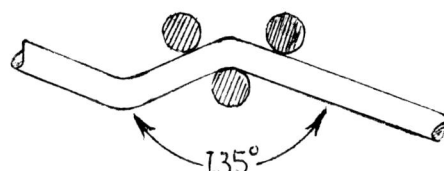

**Fig. 20-27.** Again squeeze pliers to produce second bend of approximately 135 degrees.

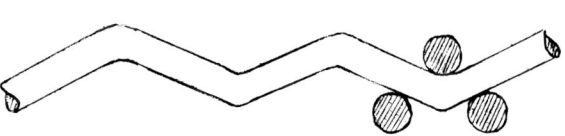

**Fig. 20-28.** Pattern is continued until desired length of zigzag is obtained.

## Smooth curve bend

**curve** A wire that turns from a straight line without sharp bends or angularity (Fig. 20-29).

### APPLICATION

The curve is used primarily to adapt wire to soft tissue and teeth. It is used on most springs and clasps as well as major connecting wires.

### PROCEDURE

1. Using a No. 139 pliers, take hold of the end of a long segment of wire in the area of the jaws closest to the hinge (Fig. 20-30).
2. Slowly apply finger pressure around the round beak of the pliers to form a smooth curve (Fig. 20-31).

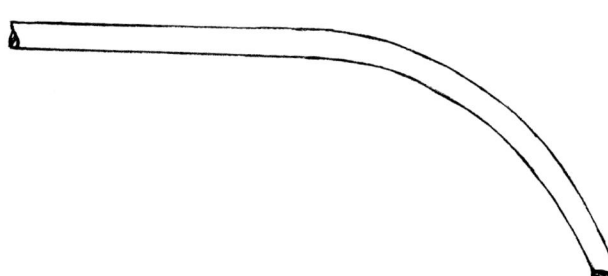

**Fig. 20-29.** Smooth curve bend.

## ORTHODONTIC SPRINGS

**orthodontic spring** A length of wire attached to an orthodontic appliance that serves as a lever to apply force to a tooth or teeth.

There are many times during the course of interceptive orthodontic therapy when tooth movement is needed. The dentist can accomplish this movement with some sort of spring-activated appliance. Some of the more common springs used for this purpose are the simple finger, helical finger, labial bow, dumbell, and slingshot.

## Simple finger spring

The simple finger spring's action originates from the incorporation of one or more semicircle bends into a wire. It is usually employed for the movement of a single anterior or posterior tooth, although it is capable of moving multitooth segments. Most often the simple finger spring is used on the removable-type interceptive orthodontic appliance (Fig. 20-32).

WIRE TYPE AND SIZE. Use 0.020-inch preactivated wire.

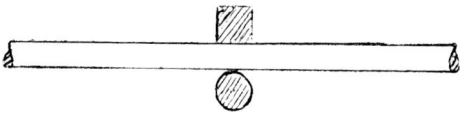

**Fig. 20-30.** With No. 139 pliers correctly positioned, take hold of wire in area of jaws closest to hinge.

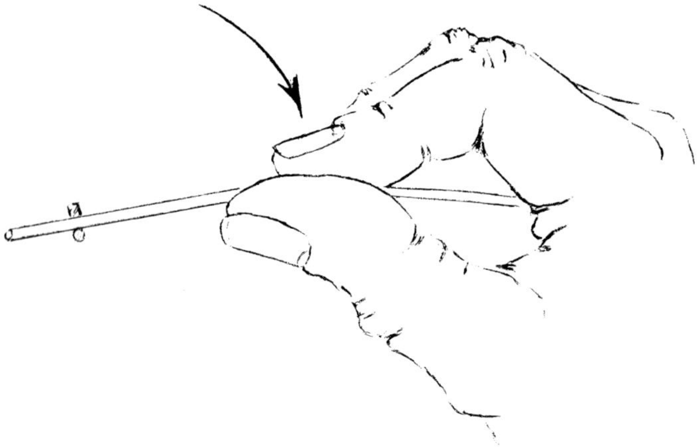

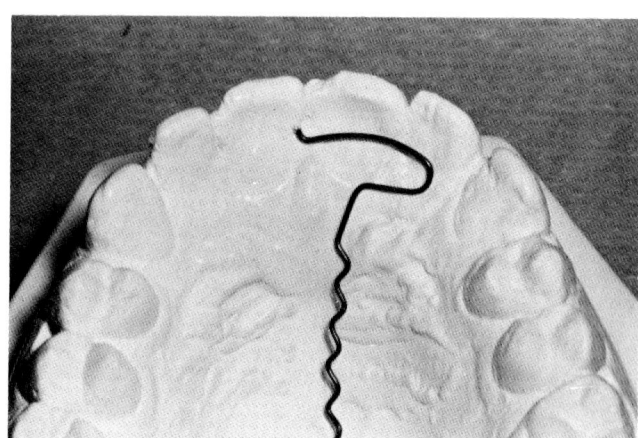

**Fig. 20-31.** Apply finger pressure away from pliers (arrow) to form smooth curve.

**Fig. 20-32.** Simple finger spring.

## PROCEDURE

1. Starting with a 2-inch (5-cm) length of wire, form a medium-size semicircle about ½ inch (1.3 cm) from one end (Fig. 20-33).
2. Contour the short end of the wire to the lingual surface of the tooth (Fig. 20-34).
3. At the middle of the tooth make a bend perpendicular to the tooth surface on the long end of the wire, and adapt the remaining length of wire to the soft tissue behind the tooth. There should be approximately 0.5 mm of clearance between the soft tissue and the wire (Fig. 20-35).
4. To facilitate retention of the spring in an acrylic base, bend a zigzag pattern in the wire extension (Fig. 20-36).

### Helical finger spring

The helical finger spring's action originates from the incorporation of one or more helical bends into a wire. The indications for the helical spring are identical to the simple finger spring. However, the helical spring is usually the better choice because the addition of a helix provides more effective action than a semicircle (Fig. 20-37).

WIRE AND TYPE SIZE. Use 0.020-inch preactivated wire.

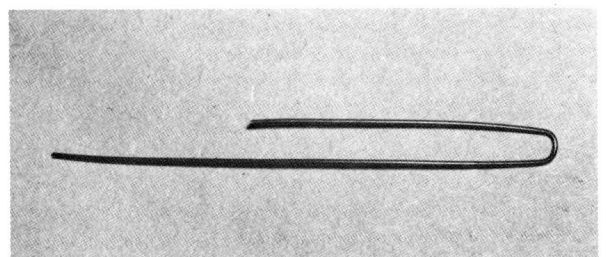

**Fig. 20-33.** Semicircle is formed in 2-inch (5-cm) length of wire about ½ inch (1.3-cm) from one end.

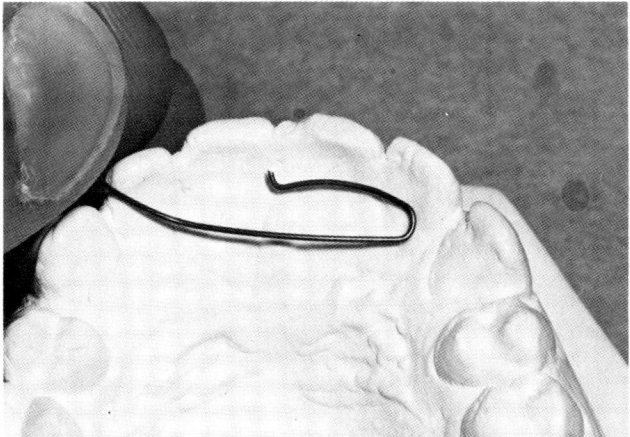

**Fig. 20-34.** Contour short end of wire to lingual surface of tooth.

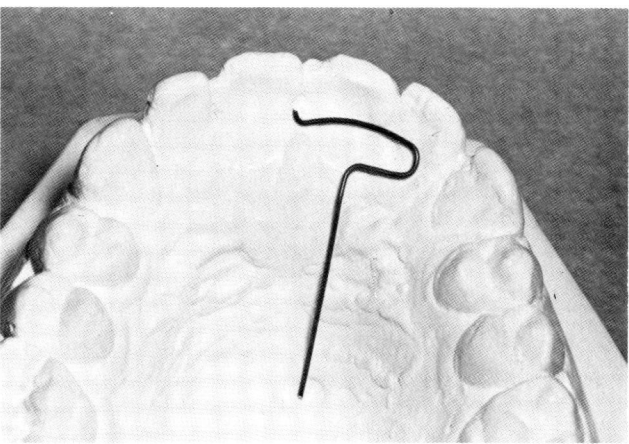

**Fig. 20-35.** At middle of tooth bend long end of wire until it is perpendicular to tooth surface. Then adapt long end of wire to soft tissue behind tooth.

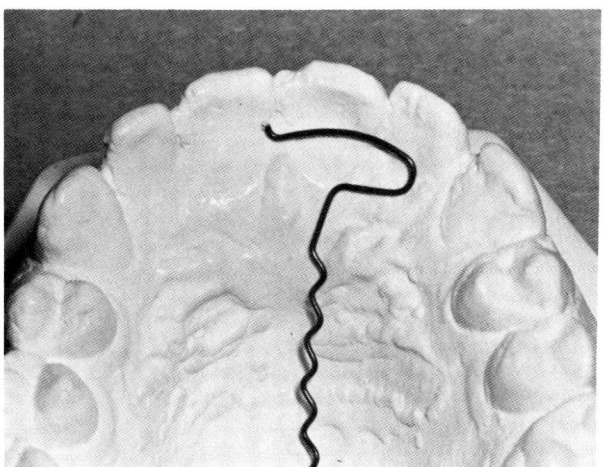

**Fig. 20-36.** Zigzag pattern in wire extension will facilitate retention of spring in acrylic resin base.

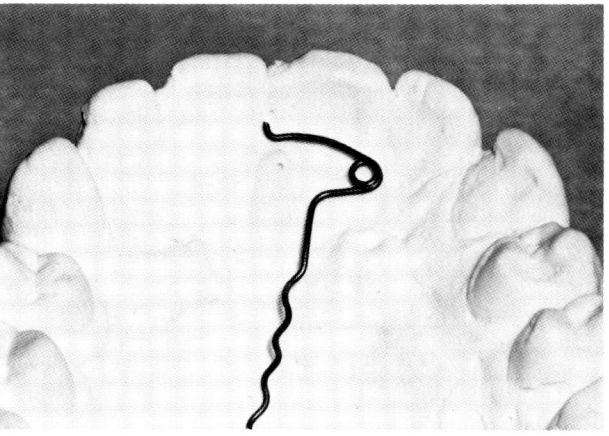

**Fig. 20-37.** Helical finger spring.

**PROCEDURE**

1. On a 2-inch (5-cm) piece of wire, bend a small helix about ½ inch (1.3 cm) from the end. Completion of the helical finger spring then follows the same steps as the simple finger spring (Fig. 20-38).

2. Adapt the short end of the wire to the lingual surface of the tooth (Fig. 20-39).

3. Make a bend perpendicular to the tooth surface on the long end of the wire. Adapt this portion of the wire to the soft tissues (Fig. 20-40).

4. Complete the spring with a series of zigzag bends on the soft tissue extension (Fig. 20-41).

## Labial bow spring

The labial bow spring is designed to include multitooth segments of the anterior dental arch with a spring action coming from loops at each end of the assembly. The labial bow spring has a number of uses including correction of minor rotations, closing of spaces, and, when used in combination with a lingual finger spring, to position anterior teeth labiolingually. It can also be used as a clasp when retention in the anterior region is required (Fig. 20-42).

WIRE TYPE AND SIZE. Use 0.028- to 0.034-inch Elgiloy* or stainless steel.

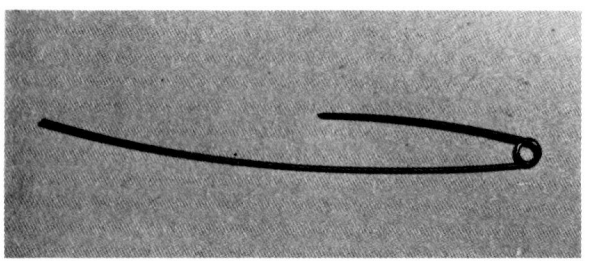

**Fig. 20-38.** Helical finger spring follows same steps as simple finger spring with helical bend substituted in place of semicircle.

*Rocky Mountain Dental Products, Denver, Colo.

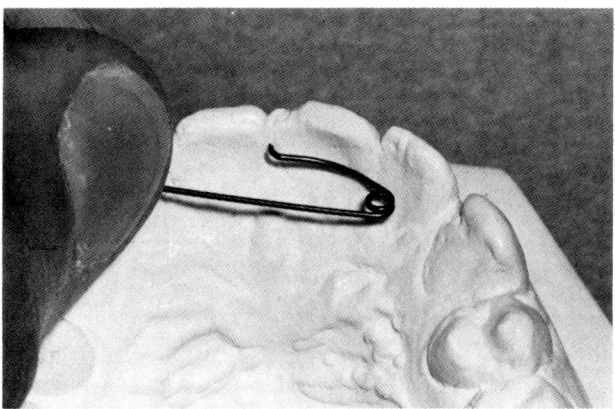

**Fig. 20-39.** Contour short end of wire to lingual surface of tooth.

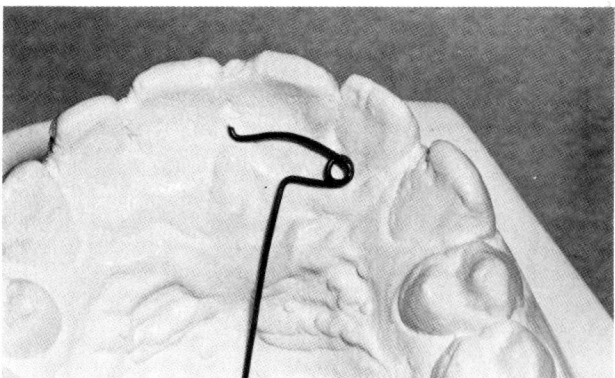

**Fig. 20-40.** At middle of tooth, bend long end of wire until it is perpendicular to tooth surface. Then adapt long end of wire to soft tissue behind tooth.

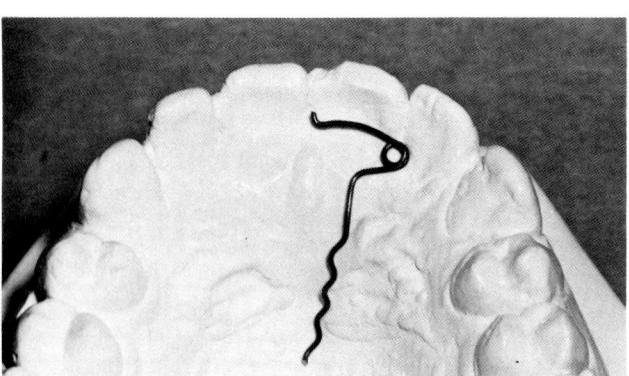

**Fig. 20-41.** Zigzag pattern in wire extension will facilitate retention of spring in acrylic base.

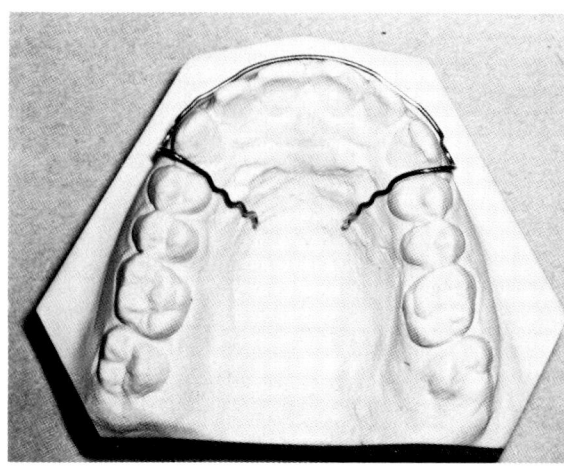

**Fig. 20-42.** Labial bow spring.

## Orthodontic procedures

### PROCEDURE

1. Starting at the midline and working distally, curve a 5-inch (12.5-cm) length of wire around the six anterior teeth (Fig. 20-43). The wire should contact the teeth on the middle half of the labial surface (Fig. 20-44).

2. Using deflection bends, adapt the wire until all anterior teeth are in contact (Fig. 20-45).

3. Form a spring loop at each end of the anterior segment (Fig. 20-46). This loop should begin at the middle of the canine and end at the distal marginal ridge of the same tooth. The loop should extend approximately 2 mm past the free gingival margin (Fig. 20-47).

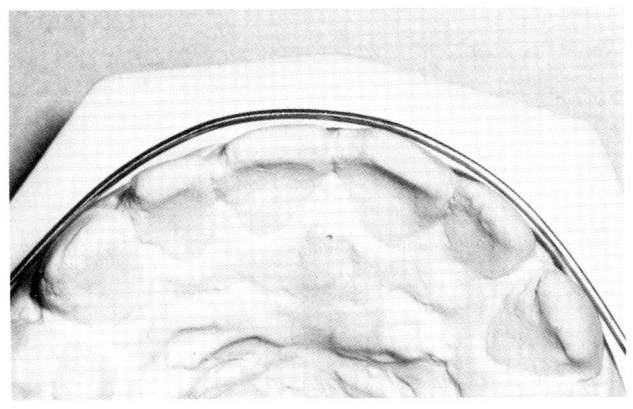

**Fig. 20-43.** Curve 5-inch (12.5-cm) piece of wire around six anterior teeth.

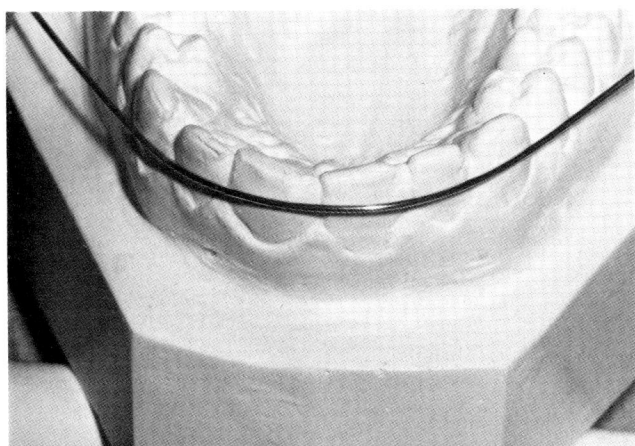

**Fig. 20-44.** Wire should contact teeth in middle half of labial surface.

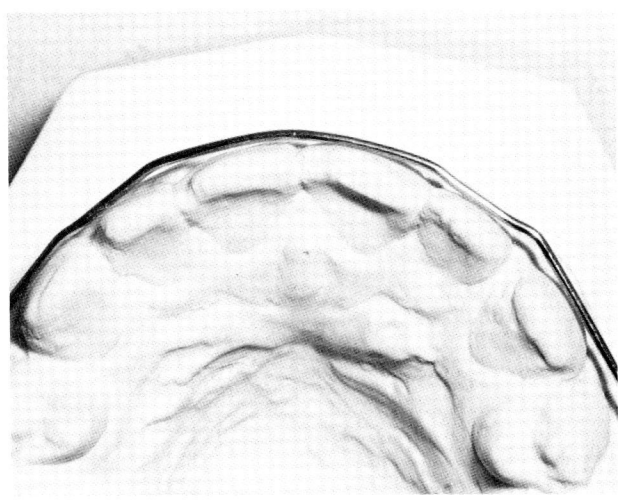

**Fig. 20-45.** Adapt wire until all anterior teeth are in contact.

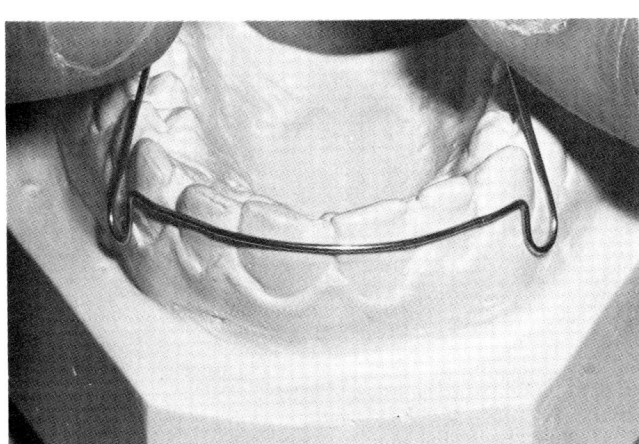

**Fig. 20-46.** Omega loop is formed at each end of anterior segment.

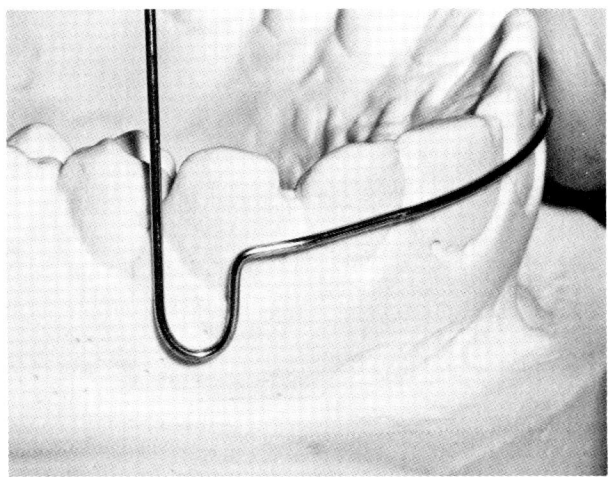

**Fig. 20-47.** Note that omega loop begins at middle of canine and ends at distal marginal ridge of same tooth. Loop should extend approximately 2 mm past free gingival margin.

4. Bend each end of the spring over the marginal ridge and onto the soft tissue area (Fig. 20-48).

5. Complete the spring by adding zigzag retention patterns to these extensions (Fig. 20-49).

### Dumbbell spring

The dumbbell spring gets its name and its action from connected wire loops on either side of the dental arch. The spring has only limited application to interceptive orthodontic therapy because an edentulous area in the arch form is required for its placement. It is usually employed in the child who has lost primary teeth because of ectopic eruption, ankylosis, or rampant dental caries and needs a procedure to regain lost arch perimeter (Fig. 20-50).

WIRE TYPE AND SIZE. Use 0.028- to 0.034-inch Elgiloy or stainless steel.

#### PROCEDURE

1. Bend a semicircle in the middle of a 4-inch (10-cm) length of wire (Fig. 20-51).

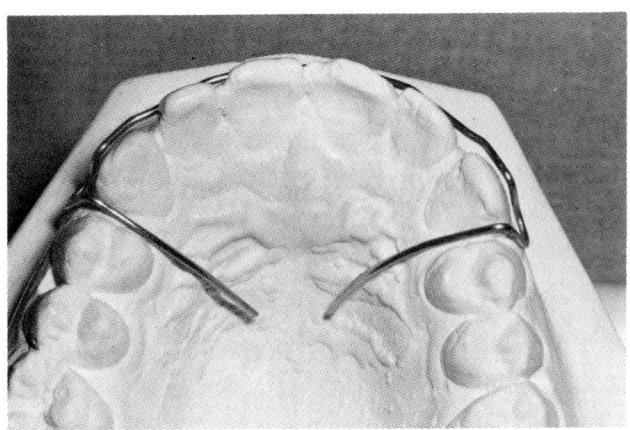

Fig. 20-48. Adapt each end of wire coming from omega loops over marginal ridge and onto soft tissue area.

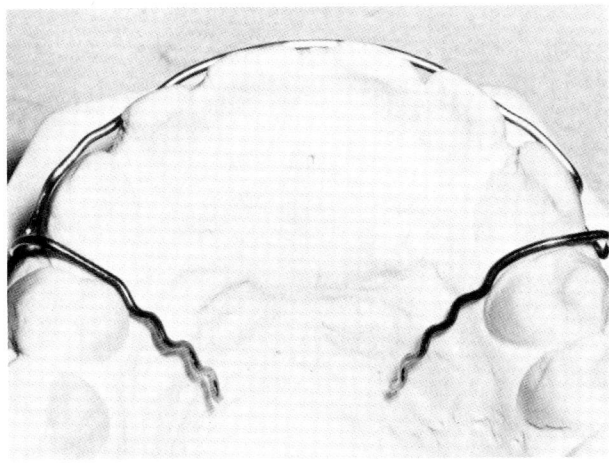

Fig. 20-49. Zigzag retention pattern is added to these extensions to complete spring.

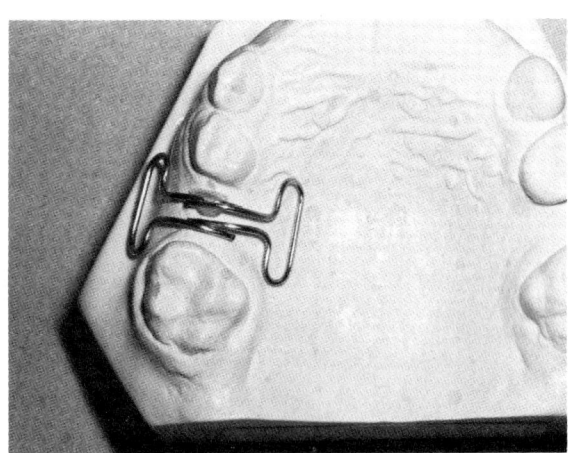

Fig. 20-50. Dumbbell spring.

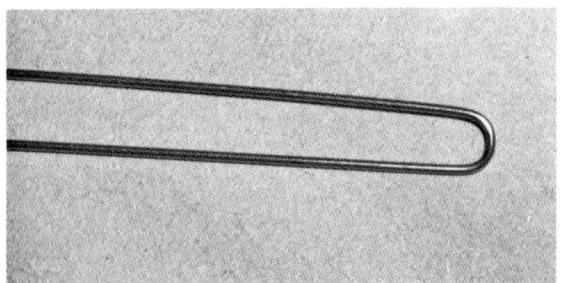

Fig. 20-51. Bend semicircle in middle of 4-inch (10-cm) length of wire.

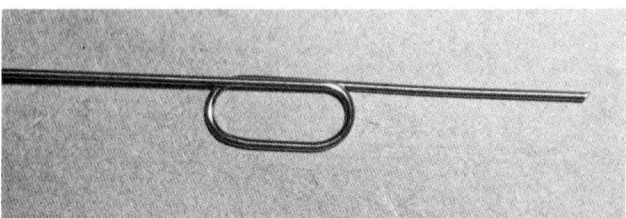

Fig. 20-52. About ½ inch (1.3-cm) from initial semicircle make another semicircle coming back in opposite direction.

2. About ½ inch (1.3 cm) from the initial semicircle, form another semicircle coming back in the opposite direction (Fig. 20-52).

3. Bend extensions from these two semicircles to form 90-degree angles (Fig. 20-53). A loop with parallel wire extensions coming off the loop approximately ⅛ inch (0.3 cm) apart will be formed.

4. Make another wire loop identical to the one described in steps 1 to 3.

5. Adapt one loop to the buccal anatomy and one loop to the lingual anatomy of the gingival tissues, and contour the wire extensions over the edentulous area (Fig. 20-54). There should be about 0.5 mm of clearance from the wire to the gingiva.

6. Complete the spring by soldering the two loops together to form one unit. Seat the wire extensions in the acrylic base of a removable appliance (Fig. 20-55).

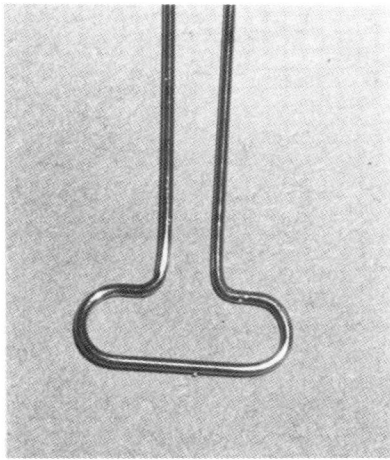

**Fig. 20-53.** Bend wire extensions coming from these two semicircles to form 90-degree angles.

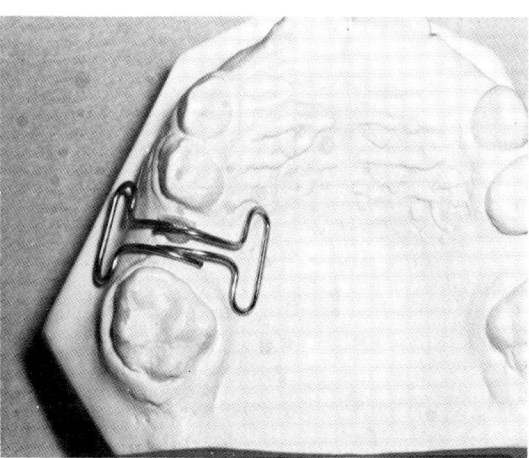

**Fig. 20-54.** Adapt one loop to buccal anatomy and one loop to lingual anatomy of gingival tissues, and contour wire extensions over edentulous area.

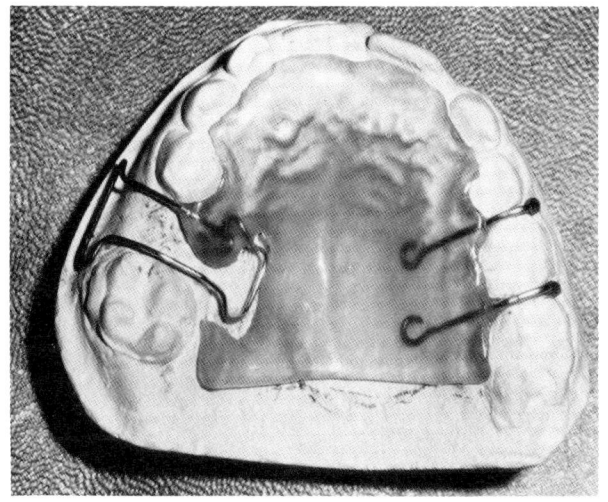

**Fig. 20-55.** Dumbbell spring is completed by soldering two loops together to form one unit and seating assembly in acrylic base of removable appliance.

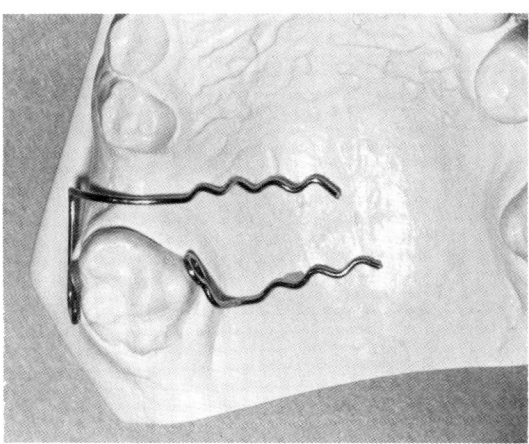

**Fig. 20-56.** Slingshot spring.

## Slingshot spring

The slingshot spring is a unique apparatus that uses elastic material supported by a wire assembly as the source of its spring action. Much like the dumbbell spring, the slingshot spring is indicated when distal movement of a posterior tooth is needed to regain lost arch length (Fig. 20-56). The spring may also be used in the anterior region to close spaces and move teeth lingually.

WIRE TYPE AND SIZE. Use 0.030-inch Elgiloy or stainless steel.

### PROCEDURE

1. Form a closed end loop in a 3-inch (7.5-cm) length of wire (Fig. 20-57).

2. Position the closed end loop on the buccal surface of the tooth and slightly distal of the marginal ridge. Using two right-angle bends, redirect the wire down and forward toward the anterior teeth (Fig. 20-58).

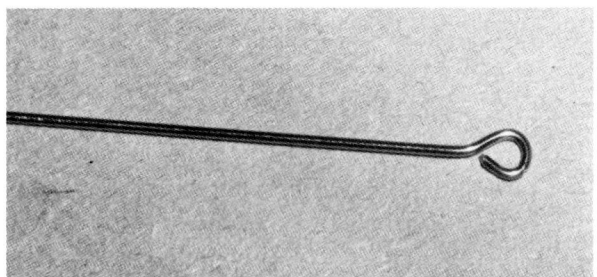

**Fig. 20-57.** Form closed end loop in 3-inch (7.5-cm) length of wire.

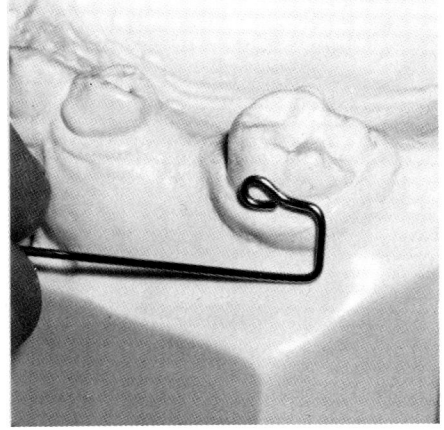

**Fig. 20-58.** Closed end loop is positioned on buccal surface of tooth and slightly distal of marginal ridge. Two right-angle bends are used to redirect wire down and forward toward anterior teeth.

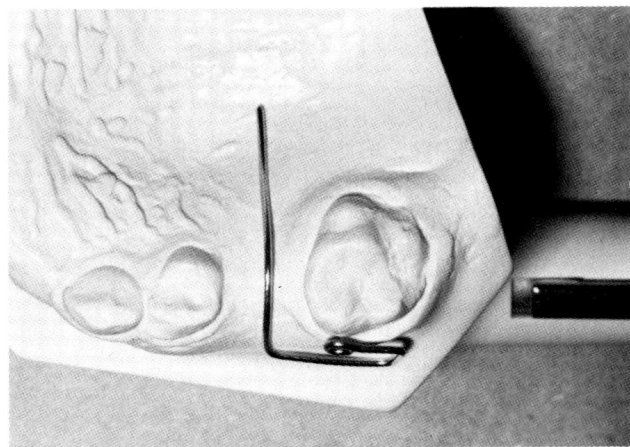

**Fig. 20-59.** Contour wire over edentulous area and onto soft tissue.

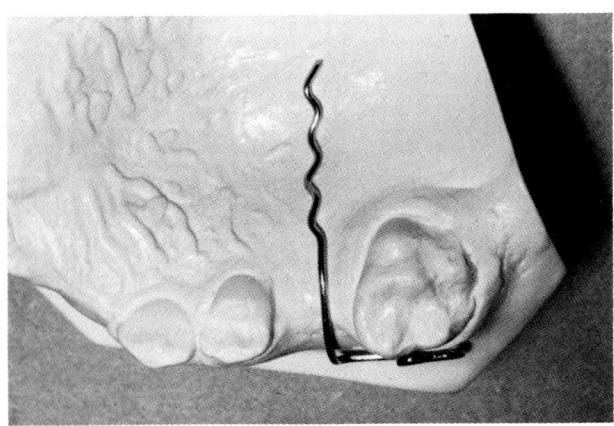

**Fig. 20-60.** Complete extension with zigzag bends.

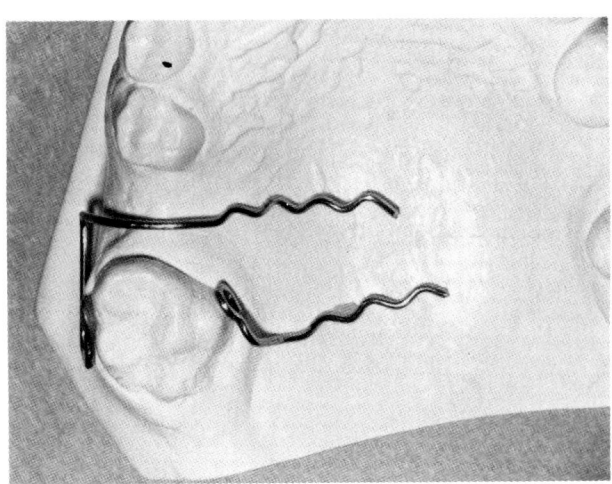

**Fig. 20-61.** Make lingual elastic attachment following outlined steps to complete spring.

3. Contour the wire over the endentulous area and onto the soft tissues of either the palate or mandible (Fig. 20-59).

4. Complete the extension by adding a series of zigzag bends (Fig. 20-60).

5. Following steps 1, 3, and 4, construct a lingual elastic attachment. To complete the spring, the wire extensions are embedded in an acrylic base, and the elastic material is suspended from the tire hooks (Fig. 20-61).

**PROBLEM AREAS**

The principal problem associated with the fabrication of orthodontic springs is the failure of the finished spring to supply sufficient force for tooth movement (Table 20-1). If annealed wire is used in fabrication, a heat treatment is necessary to return hardness and elasticity to the wire. Care must be taken during heat treatment not to overheat the wire and destroy its physical properties permanently. A preactivated wire that does not need heat treatment is the preferred wire for spring construction.

**Table 20-1.** Orthodontic springs

| Problem | Probable cause | Solution |
| --- | --- | --- |
| Weak force supplied by completed spring | Not heat treating annealed wire<br>Overheating wire during heat treatment | Use preactivated wire<br>Be careful when heat treating annealed wire |

## ORTHODONTIC CLASPS

**orthodontic clasp** A wire device that retains and stabilizes an orthodontic appliance in the oral cavity by contacting or partially surrounding an abutment tooth.

The removable interceptive orthodontic appliance requires a mechanical retention system so that the appliance can be inserted into and removed from the mouth at the patient's or dentist's discretion. Wire clasps made to fit into undercut areas of the dental arch serve this purpose well. Four useful wire clasps in interceptive orthodontic therapy are the circumferential, ball, arrowhead, and Adams.

### Circumferential clasp

The circumferential clasp is probably the most widely used of all wire clasp designs. It is easily formed and can be adapted to all primary and permanent teeth. It does not, however, provide excellent retention in young children because many of the teeth will be partially erupted. Therefore the circumferential clasp should be used only as an auxiliary clasp (Fig. 20-62).

WIRE TYPE AND SIZE. Use 0.028- to 0.034-inch Elgiloy or stainless steel.

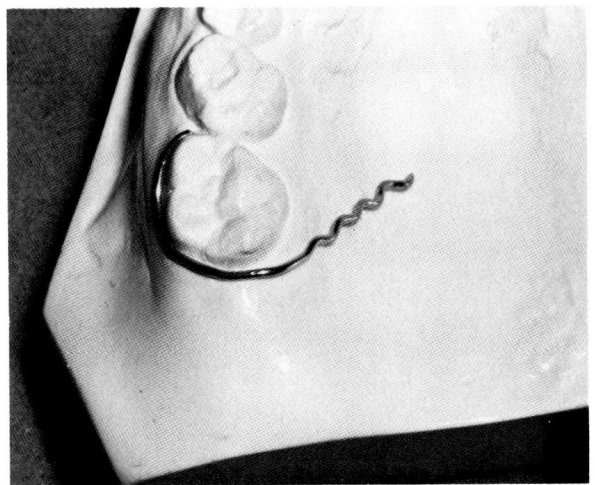

**Fig. 20-62.** Circumferential clasp.

#### PROCEDURE

1. Contour one end of a 2-inch (5-cm) piece of wire to the buccal anatomy of the tooth. Keep the wire slightly above the free gingival margin, and extend it around the mesiobuccal and distobuccal line angles, ending in the interproximal embrasure (Fig. 20-63).

2. Adapt the long end of the wire around the proximal surface of the tooth and onto the lingual or palatal surface (Fig. 20-64). If the clasp is being constructed for a tooth with proximal contacts on both ends, adapt the wire over the marginal ridge area.

3. Complete the clasp by adding a zigzag retention pattern to the long end of the wire (Fig. 20-65).

### Ball clasp

There are times when an appliance for a young child must have maximum retention. The ball clasp is excellent for this purpose because it requires little time for fabrication and can be adapted to almost any area of the dental arch (Fig. 20-66).

WIRE TYPE AND SIZE. The ball clasp may be fabricated with either 0.025- to 0.040-inch preformed clasp material or a length of 0.025- to 0.040-inch Elgiloy or stainless steel wire with a ball of solder at one end.

#### PROCEDURE

1. Use a wax spatula or round bur to create a depression in the embrasure area of the working cast, and seat the ball end of a 1½-inch (3.8-cm) piece of clasp material into the depression (Figs. 20-67 and 20-68).

2. Bend the wire over the marginal ridge area, and extend it onto the lingual or palatal area (Fig. 20-69).

3. Make a zigzag retentive pattern into this extension to complete the clasp (Fig. 20-70).

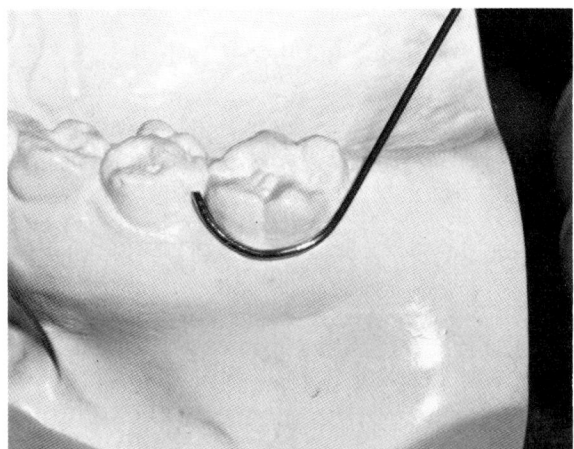

**Fig. 20-63.** A 2-inch (5-cm) piece of wire is contoured to buccal anatomy of tooth. Wire is positioned above free gingival margin and is extended into interproximal embrasure.

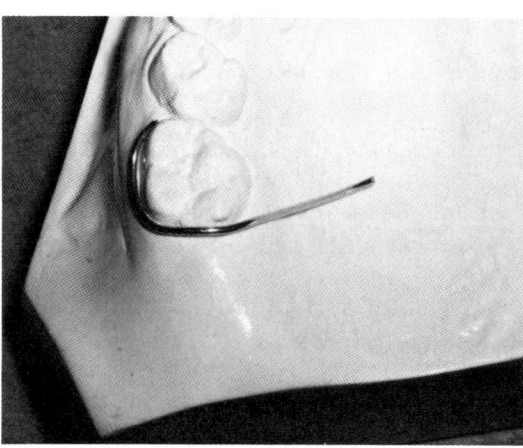

**Fig. 20-64.** Long end of wire is adapted through proximal surface and onto lingual or palatal tissue.

## Orthodontic procedures 603

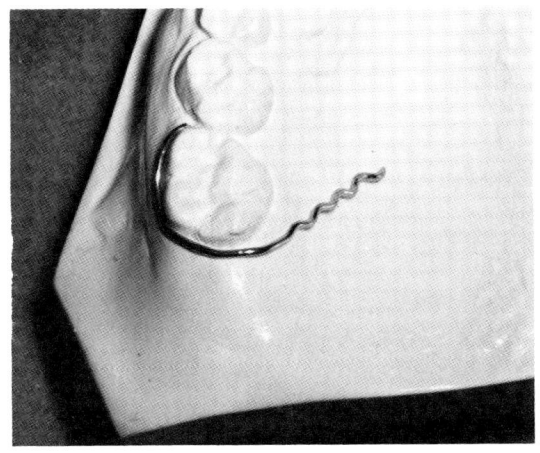

Fig. 20-65. Complete extension with zigzag bends.

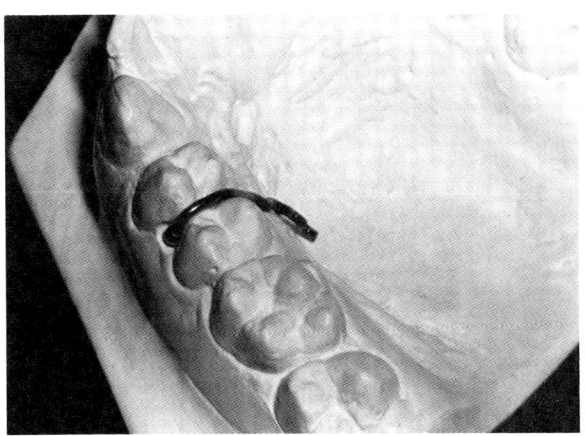

Fig. 20-66. Ball clasp.

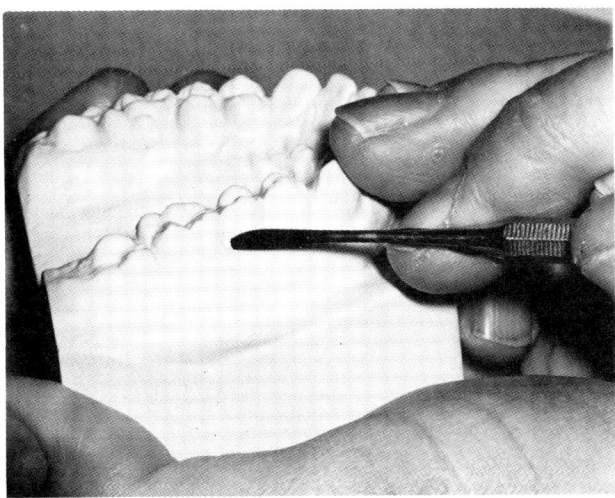

Fig. 20-67. Use wax spatula or round bur to create depression in embrasure.

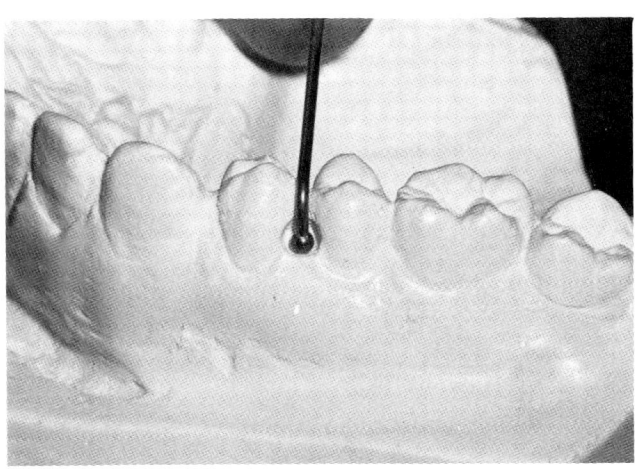

Fig. 20-68. Seat ball end of clasp into depression, and contour long end through embrasure.

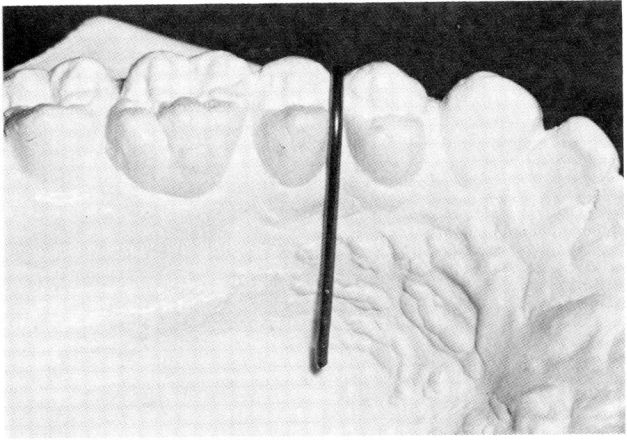

Fig. 20-69. Carry extension onto lingual or palatal tissues.

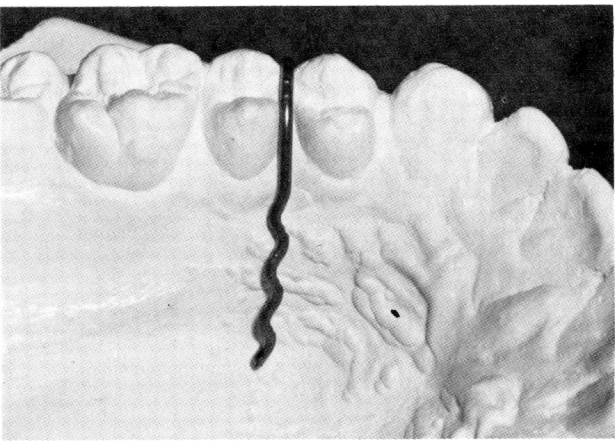

Fig. 20-70. Complete extension with zigzag bends.

## Arrowhead clasp

A suitable alternative to the ball clasp is the arrowhead clasp. This clasp provides excellent retention and requires neither the manufactured clasp material nor the laboratory procedure needed to add solder to the end of a segment of wire (Fig. 20-71).

WIRE TYPE AND SIZE. Use 0.025- to 0.034-inch Elgiloy or stainless steel.

### PROCEDURE

1. Begin by bending a small closed- end loop in a 1½-inch (3.8-cm) segment of wire. Completion of the arrowhead clasp then follows the same steps as the ball clasp.
2. Adapt the closed end loop into a depression created in the interproximal area of the working model (Fig. 20-72).
3. Contour the wire over the marginal ridge areas and onto the lingual or palatal soft tissue area (Fig. 20-73).
4. Complete the clasp by adding a zigzag retentive pattern (Fig. 20-74).

## Adams clasp

The Adams clasp is similar to the ball and arrowhead clasps because interproximal areas of the dental arch are used for retention. Unfortunately, the clasp is complicated in design, and, even though a prefabricated clasp is available, proper adaptation to the tooth surface is difficult. The clasp does have excellent retentive properties and is an acceptable choice when maximum retention is necessary (Fig. 20-75).

WIRE TYPE AND SIZE. Use 0.025- to 0.030-inch Elgiloy or stainless steel.

### PROCEDURE

1. Using a 3-inch (7.5-cm) segment of wire, bend a small semicircle approximately one third down the length of the wire. Then crimp this semicircle together (Fig. 20-76).
2. On the long end of the wire, form a right angle going away from the crimped semicircle (Fig. 20-77).
3. On a working model that has been prepared with depressions in the interproximal areas, seat the crimped semicircle in the mesial depression, and conform the long end of the wire to the buccal surface of the tooth (Fig. 20-78).

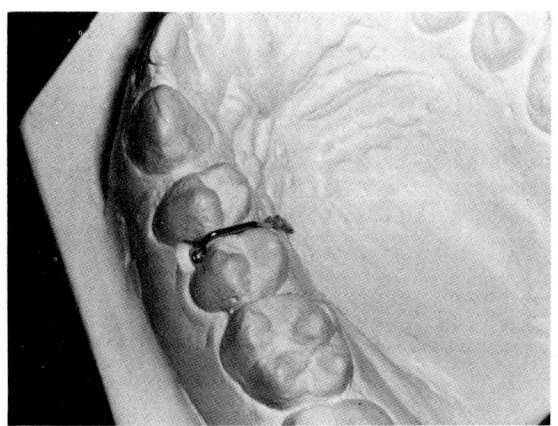

**Fig. 20-71.** Arrowhead clasp.

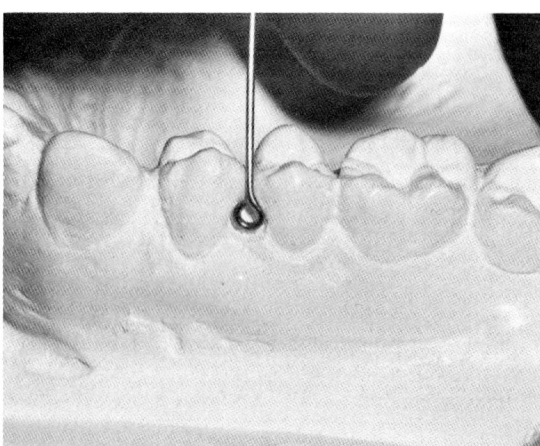

**Fig. 20-72.** Bend small closed-end loop in 1½-inch (3.8-cm) segment of wire, and adapt closed-end loop into depression created as with ball clasp in interproximal area.

# Orthodontic procedures 605

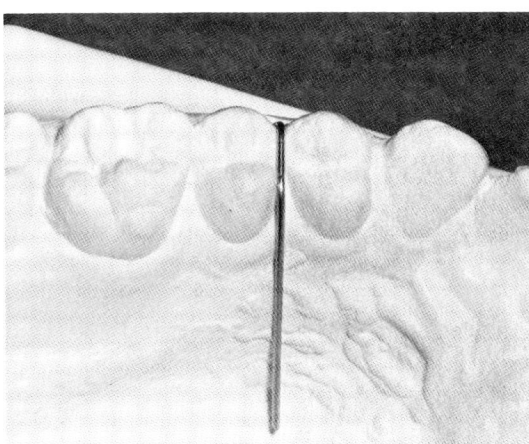

**Fig. 20-73.** Contour wire through marginal ridge area onto lingual or palatal tissues.

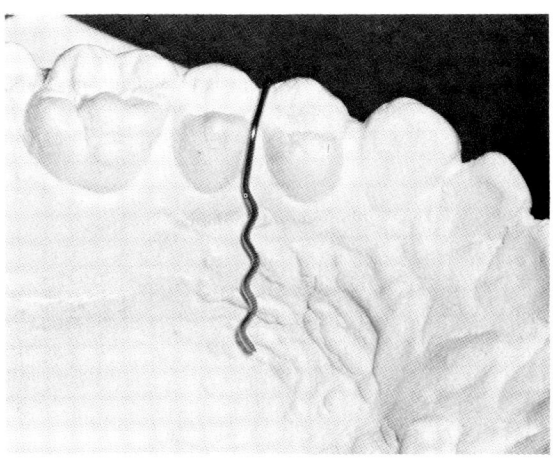

**Fig. 20-74.** Complete extension with zigzag bends.

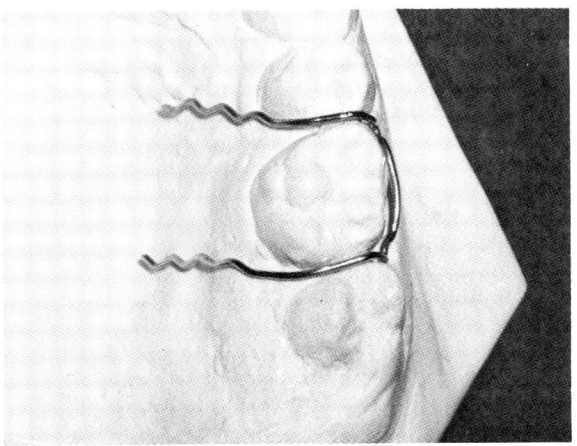

**Fig. 20-75.** Adams clasp.

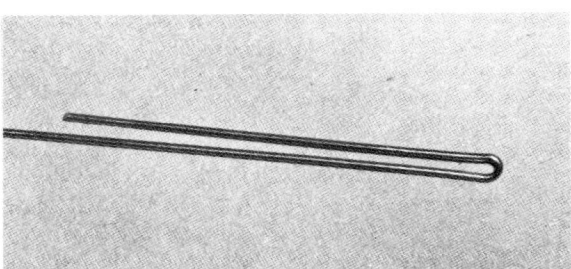

**Fig. 20-76.** Bend semicircle approximately one third down length of 3-inch (7.5-cm) piece of wire, and then crimp this semicircle.

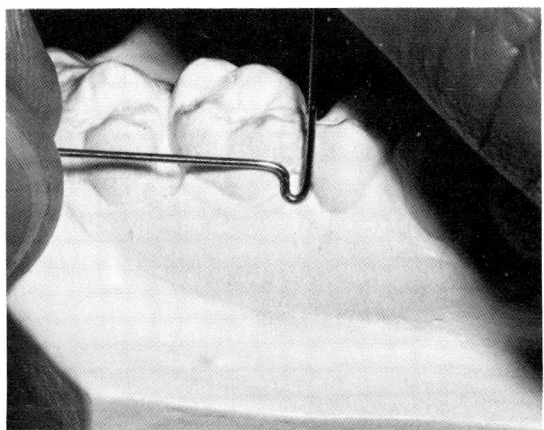

**Fig. 20-77.** Form right angle going away from crimped semicircle with long end of wire.

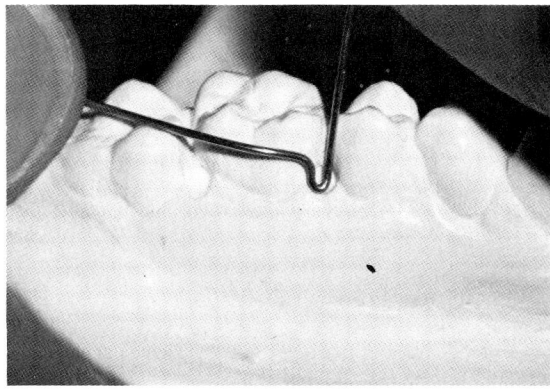

**Fig. 20-78.** Seat crimped semicircle in mesial depression, and contour long end of wire to buccal surface of tooth distally.

4. In the distal depression form a small crimped semicircle similar to the one in the mesial interproximal area (Fig. 20-79).

5. Contour both ends of the wire over the marginal ridge areas and onto the lingual or palatal surface of the working model (Fig. 20-80).

6. Complete the clasp by adding a zigzag pattern to both of these extensions (Fig. 20-81).

### PROBLEM AREAS

The two problems most frequently encountered in the construction of orthodontic clasps are failure of the clasp to adequately retain the appliance and interference of normal occlusal function because of inappropriate clasp placement (Table 20-2). Retention problems usually result from placing the clasp in areas of insufficient undercut and can be corrected with careful clasp design. A well-designed clasp will also have enough elasticity to deflect over the convex tooth surface and into the undercut areas without permanently distorting the wire. To ensure this elasticity, the careful wire manipulation that is important for spring construction is equally important for clasps. A consideration of normal maxillary-mandibular cusp-fossa relationships when planning where to place clasps will usually preclude any problems with the opposing dentition.

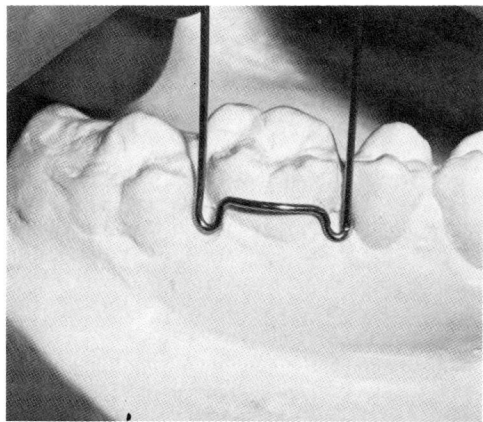

**Fig. 20-79.** Form small crimped semicircle in distal interproximal area.

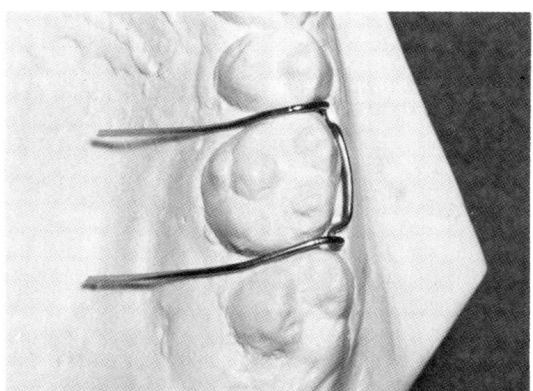

**Fig. 20-80.** Contour both ends of wire through embrasures onto palatal tissues.

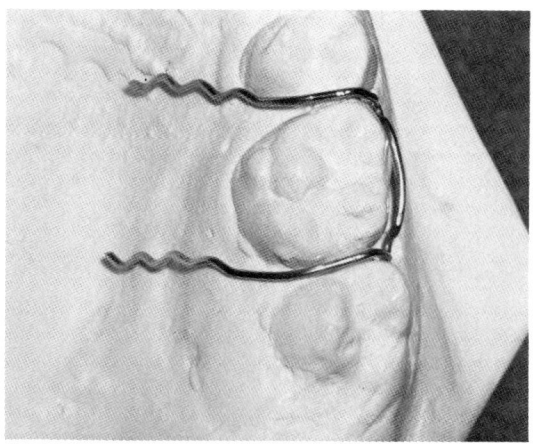

**Fig. 20-81.** Complete extensions with zigzag bends.

**Table 20-2.** Orthodontic clasps

| Problem | Probable cause | Solution |
|---|---|---|
| Inadequate retention | Clasp placed in area of insufficient undercut | Design clasp so it will fit in area of maximum undercut |
| | Inappropriate handling of wire | Properly heat treat and manipulate wire |
| Wire interferes with occlusion | Wire is placed in areas of tooth contact | Carefully consider mandibular-maxillary cusp-fossa relationship |

# STAINLESS STEEL SOLDERING

**solder** To unite pieces of metal using a metal or metallic alloy in a fusible state (Fig. 20-82).

Joining two or more pieces of stainless steel with solder is a procedure that has a number of applications in orthodontic appliance fabrication. Soldering is used to attach small-diameter wires and clasps to larger wires, add auxiliary support wires to major connecting wires, and fasten completed wire frameworks to orthodontic bands. Whereas soldering with precious metals allows for a true union of the metal and solder, soldering with stainless steel results in only an intimate contact of the metal and solder. Proper technique is therefore critical to ensure a union of sufficient strength to withstand normal oral forces. This discussion will present the materials and method necessary to produce a clinically acceptable solder joint.

## Materials
### Heat source

The soldering technique centers around the production of a small area of high-intensity heat that can be generated by an open flame or with electrical current. An open flame is the simplest and most versatile heat source for soldering. The bench top orthodontic blowpipe is probably the most common instrument used for flame soldering (Fig. 20-83). The blowpipe's flame is easy to control, reasonably well concentrated, and of sufficient intensity for soldering stainless steel. More sophisticated flame soldering instruments, such as the HydroFlame,* produce an extremely well-concentrated flame from a hand-held torch. The HydroFlame is an excellent alternative to the orthodontic blowpipe (Fig. 20-84).

*Unitek Corp., Monrovia, Calif.

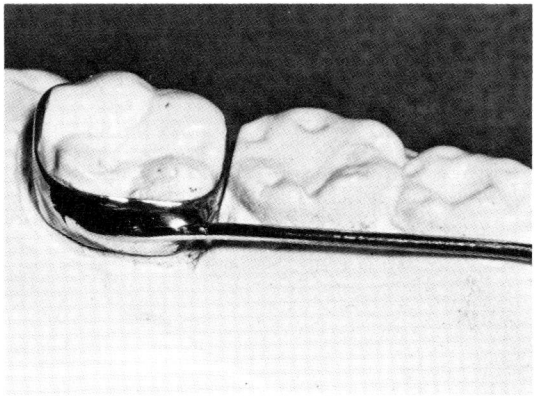

**Fig. 20-82.** Orthodontic band and orthodontic wire that have been joined with solder.

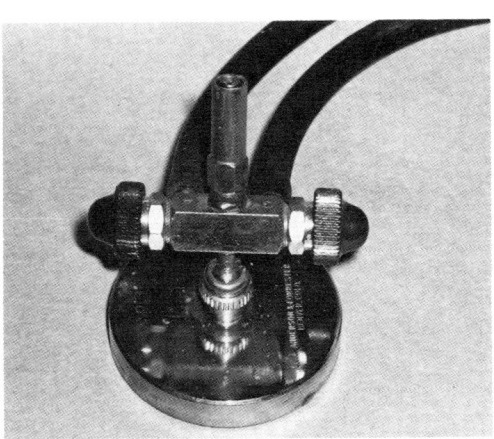

**Fig. 20-83.** Bench top orthodontic blowpipe.

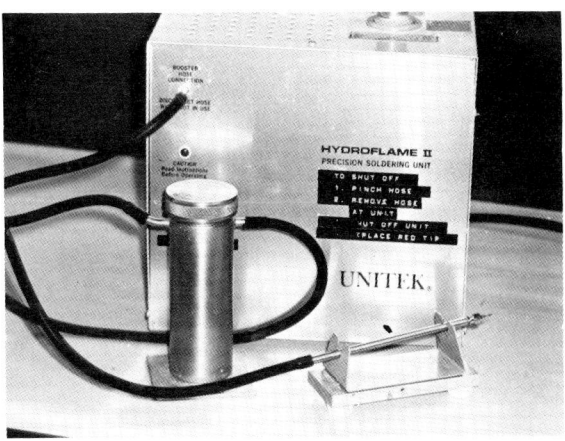

**Fig. 20-84.** HydroFlame soldering instrument.

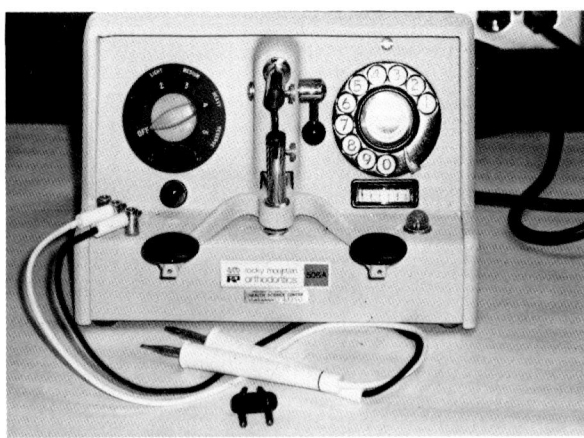

Fig. 20-85. Electric welding unit with carbon-tipped electrodes and extension cables providing heat suitable for soldering.

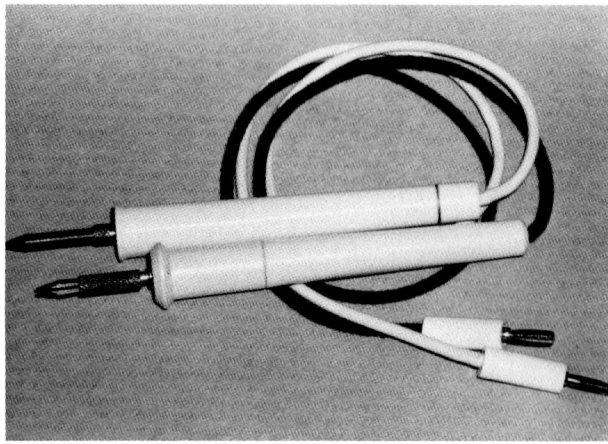

Fig. 20-86. Extension cables used with electric welding unit.

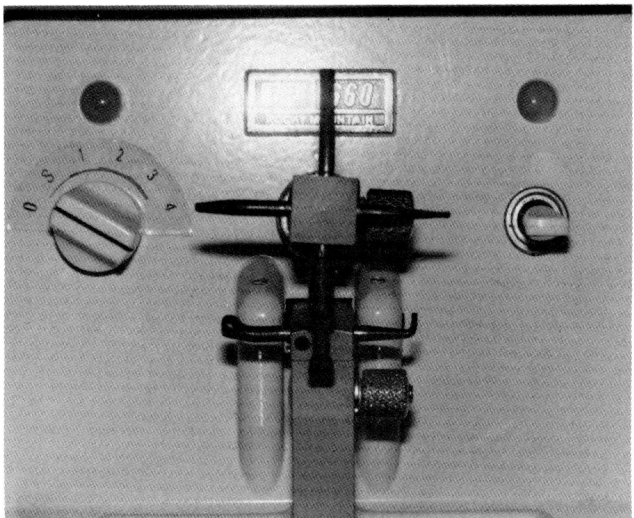

Fig. 20-87. Soldering jack used with electric welding unit.

Many electric welding units have soldering capabilities. Carbon-tipped electrodes mounted directly on the unit or connected to the unit by extension cables provide heat suitable for soldering (Fig. 20-85). Because of their versatility, extension cables are the preferred method of soldering with the electric unit (Fig. 20-86). The soldering jack mounted directly to the unit is cumbersome and difficult to use properly (Fig. 20-87).

### Silver solder

Solder used to connect stainless steel wire has certain properties that set it apart from precious metal solder. To facilitate handling, the solder has a low melting point. For this reason it is important that stainless steel wire must not be heated to an extreme temperature. Overheating will cause porosity in the hardened solder and excessive softening of the orthodontic wire. Also, the melting range must be small so the solder joint will harden promptly when the heat is removed. Most solders used for stainless steel wire are alloys of copper and zinc to which varying amounts of silver have been added to increase the tarnish resistance and decrease the melting point.

### Soldering flux

As mentioned earlier, the best possible stainless steel solder joint is only a close approximation of the stainless steel and solder. To provide the best results, the areas of wire to be jointed should be free of any oxides or impurities. A solder flux applied to the wire prior to heating is used for this purpose. Soldering flux used for stainless steel contains boric acid, boric glass, and silica. Some form of fluoride is also included to dissolve the passivating film supplied by the chromium in the stainless steel wire.

### Soldering

Although there are a number of ways to produce an acceptable stainless steel–solder joint, a detailed discussion of each method is not the purpose of this section. The technique that will be presented is a basic one, using the HydroFlame precision soldering instrument as a heat source.

## PROCEDURE

1. Approximate the surfaces that are to be soldered until metal-to-metal contact is acquired (Fig. 20-88).

2. After making sure the surfaces to be joined are as clean as possible, flow soldering flux over the solder joint area. Then unroll a 3-inch (7.5-cm) length of silver solder, and form it into a straight segment (Fig. 20-89).

3. Gently heat the fluxed solder joint area for about 15 seconds, making sure that the area is not overheated. The metal should not be allowed to glow to a red color. Place the length of solder into the solder joint area, and quickly heat it until the solder melts and begins to flow (Fig. 20-90).

4. When the solder has flowed sufficiently to cover all of the metal surfaces of the solder joint area, discontinue the flame, and immediately cool the metal (Fig. 20-91).

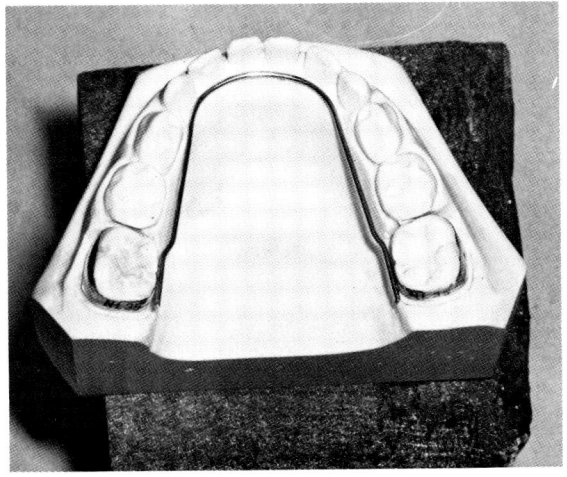

**Fig. 20-88.** Approximate two metal surfaces that are to be soldered.

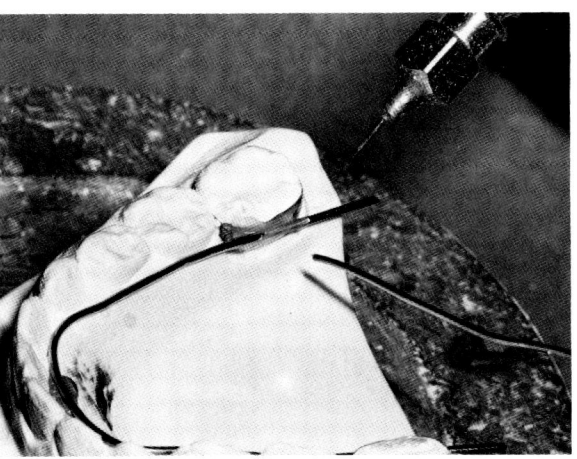

**Fig. 20-89.** Flow soldering flux over soldering joint area, and unroll 3 inches (7.5 cm) of silver solder, and form it into straight segment.

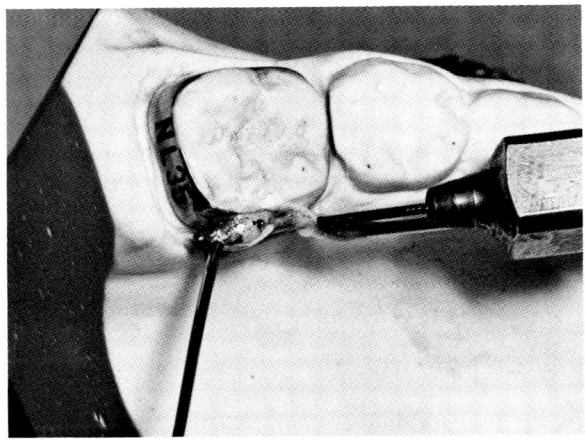

**Fig. 20-90.** Gently heat solder joint area and increase heat until solder melts and begins to flow. Add solder as needed at this time.

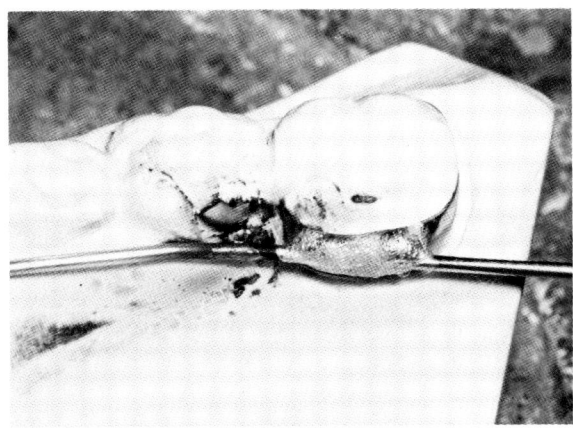

**Fig. 20-91.** Allow heated solder to flow, covering all of metal surfaces, and then discontinue flame, and allow metal to cool.

**610** *Dental laboratory procedures: removable partial dentures*

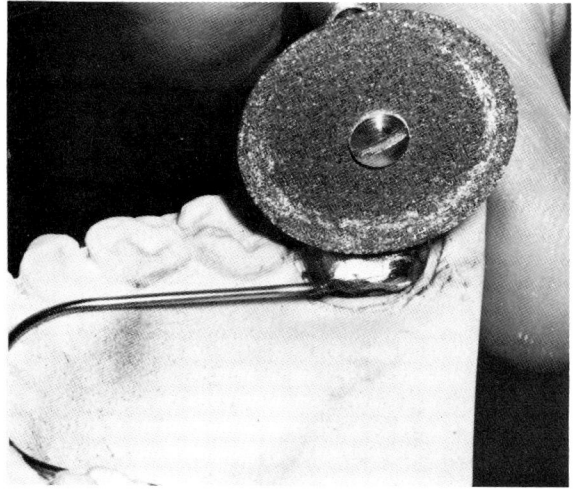

**Fig. 20-92.** Reduce excess solder in solder joint area with appropriate materials, making sure that margins come to fine feather edge.

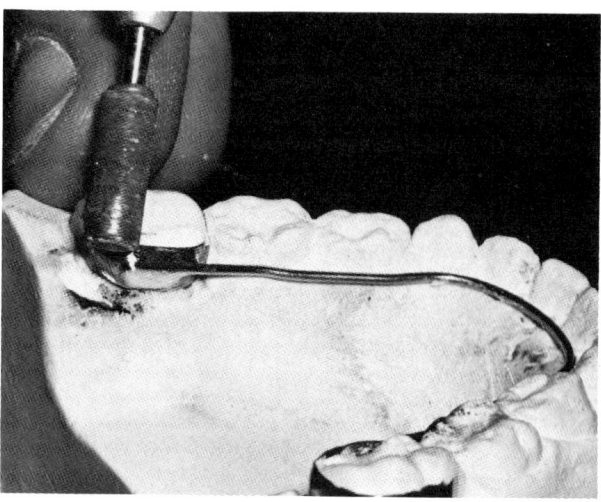

**Fig. 20-93.** Smooth roughed out solder joint with rubber wheel.

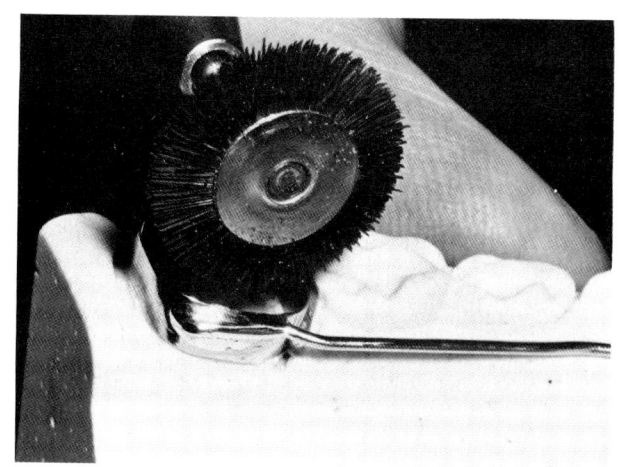

**Fig. 20-94.** Finish and polish solder joint with bristle or chamois wheel.

**Table 20-3.** Stainless steel soldering

| Problem | Probable cause | Solution |
| --- | --- | --- |
| Melted solder will not flow | Impurities on wire surface | Use sufficient amount of soldering flux |
| Porosity in solidified solder | Overheating solder | Carefully apply heat to solder and wire |
| Clinical failure of solder joint | Poor union of solder to metal | Liberally apply flux to remove surface impurities |

5. Reduce the excess solder with an abrasive stone or wheel, tapering the solder from the center of the solder joint to fine feather edges at the solder joint margins (Fig. 20-92).

6. Smooth the roughed out solder joint with rubber abrasive points or wheels (Fig. 20-93).

7. Complete the solder joint by applying polishing compound with a mounted brush or felt wheel (Fig. 20-94).

#### PROBLEM AREAS

The principal problems associated with soldering stainless steel are failure of the melted solder to flow over the solder joint area, porosity in the solder after it solidifies, and weakness in the finished joint, resulting in a clinical failure of the union (Table 20-3).

Impurities on the wire surface will result in both the inability of the melted solder to flow and a weakened completed joint. A liberal application of stainless steel soldering flux will usually resolve these problems. Porosity is due to overheating the solder and can be controlled by careful heat application to the solder and wire.

### ACRYLIC RESIN PREPARATION

**autopolymerizing acrylic resin** An acrylic resin that can be polymerized without the use of external heat by addition of an activator or a catalyst.

Cold-curing acrylic resin is used in a substantial number of removable interceptive orthodontic appliances. Acrylic resin provides a means of securing springs and clasps to appliances as well as connecting the various appliance components. The material is well tolerated by the oral tissues, can be processed easily with minimal equipment, can be modified readily in its processed form, and is sufficiently strong to withstand the forces that will be encountered in the oral cavity.

#### Materials

1. Autopolymerizing acrylic resin, liquid and powder
2. Acrylic resin processing unit
3. Assortment of acrylic burs
4. Rag wheel and coarse pumice
5. Chamois wheel and acrylic resin polishing compound

#### PROCEDURE

1. Make sure that appliance wires are adapted securely to the working cast. If adaptation is a problem, sticky wax will provide sufficient adhesion of these wires to the cast (Fig. 20-95).

2. Soak the working cast in water for at least 10 minutes. Soaking eliminates the need for a separating medium between the acrylic resin and cast; however, a separating medium may be used if desired. After blowing excess moisture from the model, build up the acrylic resin to a thickness of approximately 3 mm (Fig. 20-96). Adding powder to the liquid monomer (salt and pepper) is the preferred method.

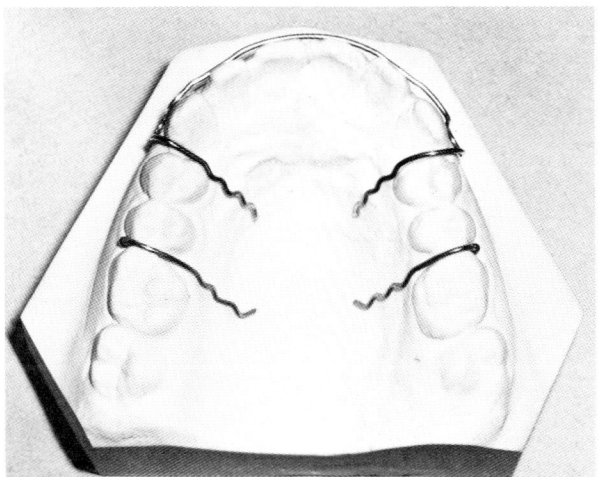

**Fig. 20-95.** Adapt and secure wires for appliance.

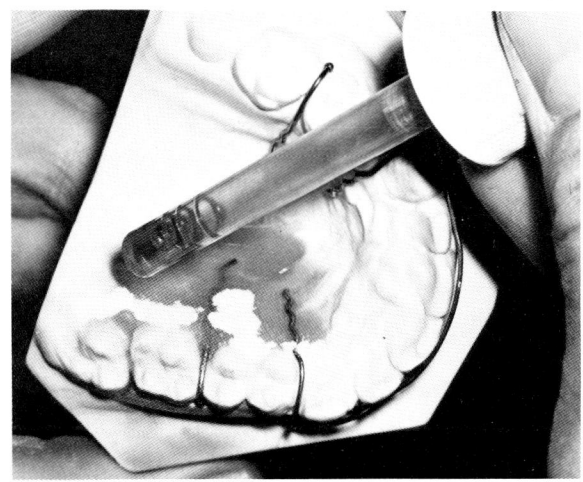

**Fig. 20-96.** After either soaking cast or placing separating medium, build up autopolymerizing acrylic resin to thickness of 3 mm. It is easier to build up half of acrylic resin base at time.

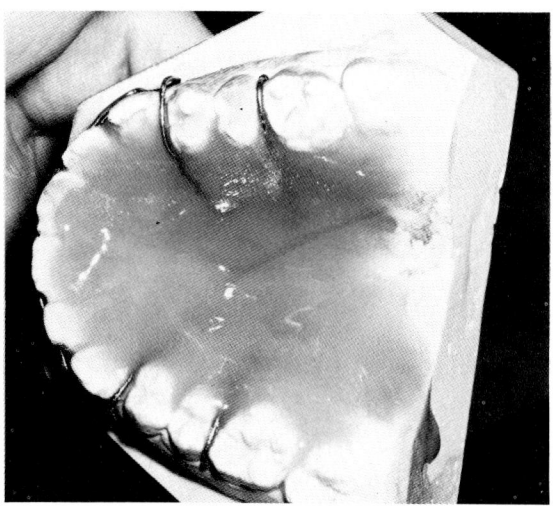

Fig. 20-97. Extend resin, making sure outline form of appliance and all wires are covered.

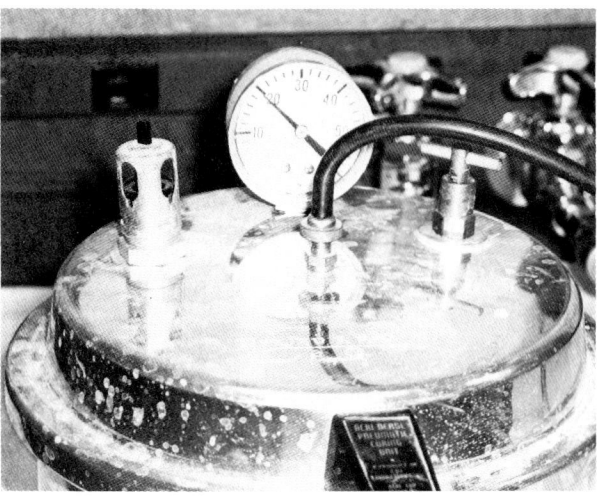

Fig. 20-98. Pressure cooker is used to complete polymerization of resin. Resin is cured for 20 minutes at 20 psi.

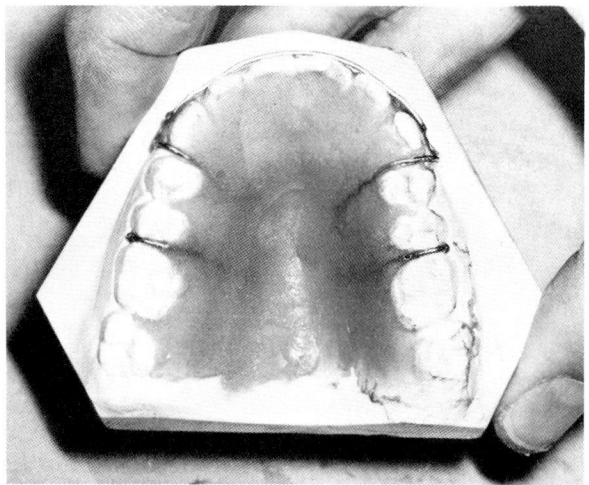

Fig. 20-99. Polymerized resin immediately after removal from pressure cooker.

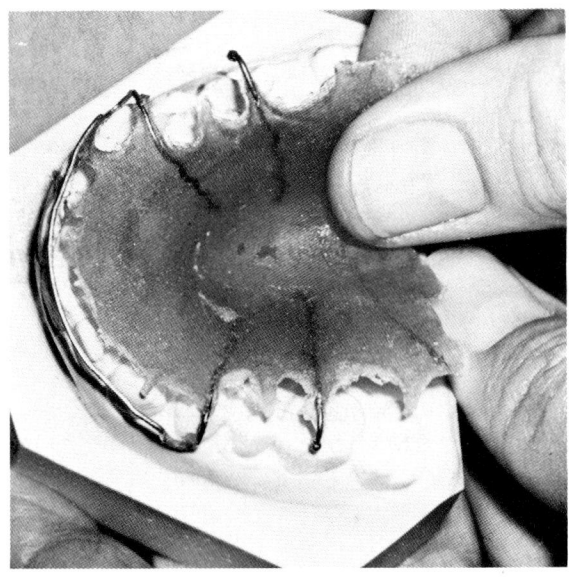

Fig. 20-100. Cured appliance is gently removed from working cast.

3. Extend the resin slightly past the outline form of the appliance, making sure all of the wires to be retained are covered (Fig. 20-97).

4. Immediately place the acrylic resin in a processing unit. Set the pressure to 20 psi, and let the resin cure for 20 minutes (Fig. 20-98). Processing under pressure allows for a more dense polymerization by reducing unwanted porosity.

5. Remove the cured resin from the unit, and gently lift the appliance off the working cast (Figs. 20-99 and 20-100).

6. Using an assortment of acrylic resin burs,

## Orthodontic procedures 613

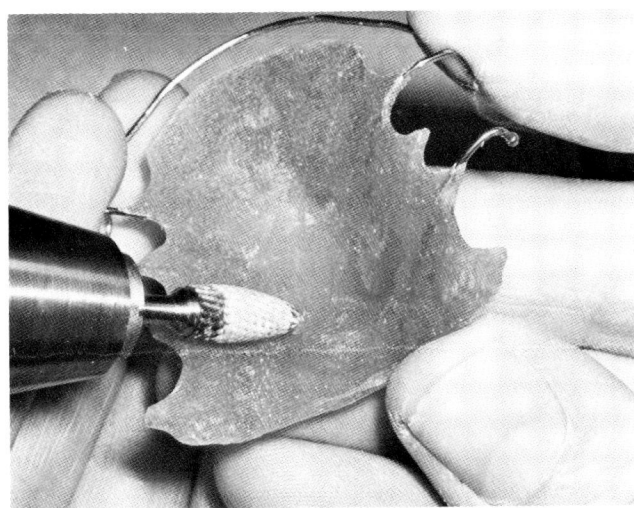

**Fig. 20-101.** Rough out outline form of appliance using acrylic burs, making sure no embedded wires are exposed by overreduction of acrylic resin.

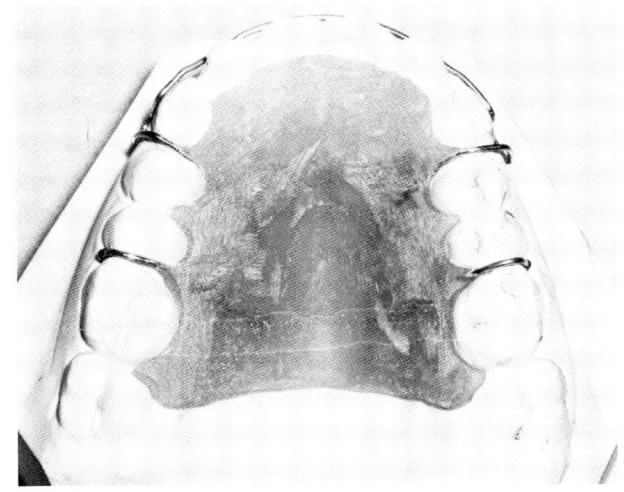

**Fig. 20-102.** Completed roughed out appliance.

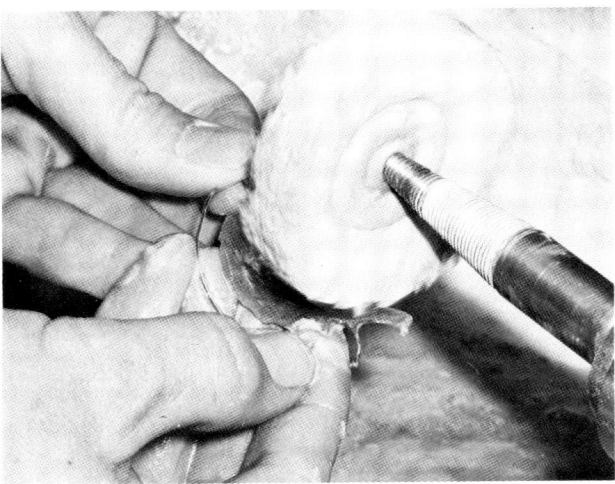

**Fig. 20-103.** Use coarse pumice to smooth acrylic resin surface. Make sure both internal and external surfaces are smoothed.

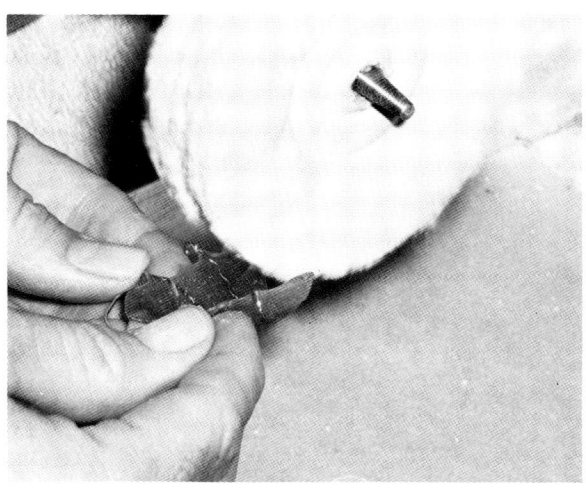

**Fig. 20-104.** Complete procedure by using polishing compound on rag wheel to produce smooth high-luster finish.

rough out the final form of the appliance. Take care not to expose an embedded wire by overfinishing at this point (Figs. 20-101 and 20-102).

7. Polish the roughed out acrylic with a coarse pumice compound on a rag wheel. Make sure that both the internal and external surfaces of the acrylic resin are smooth (Fig. 20-103).

8. Complete the polishing procedure using a fine polishing compound on a chamois wheel (Fig. 20-104). This leaves a high luster finish that is well tolerated by the oral tissues and easy to clean (Fig. 20-105).

**Fig. 20-105.** Finished acrylic resin procedure.

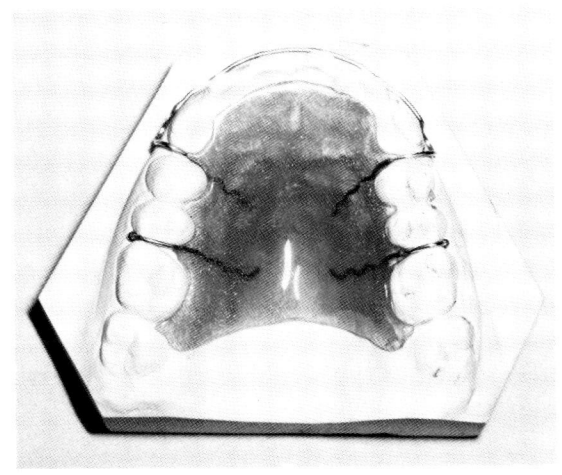

**Table 20-4.** Cold-curing acrylic resin

| Problem | Probable cause | Solution |
| --- | --- | --- |
| Poor appliance fit | Distortion of processed resin during finishing | Apply coolant during polishing<br>Use light polishing pressure |
| Gingival irritation under acrylic | Porosity in acrylic<br>Rough surface finish | Polymerize acrylic using pressure cooker<br>Use proper finishing procedures |

## PROBLEM AREAS

Two problem areas commonly encountered in appliances constructed with autopolymerizing acrylic resin are poor appliance fit and gingival irritation (Table 20-4). Excessive heat produced during finishing can permanently distort acrylic resin. Light polishing pressure and an adequate coolant will help keep finishing temperatures at an acceptable level. Gingival irritation is usually a result of either porosity within the acrylic resin or a poor finishing technique that leaves the acrylic surface rough. Polymerizing the acrylic resin in a pressure cooker will control porosity and leave a dense, well-processed resin that, with proper finishing procedures, is well tolerated by the gingival tissues.

## Section 2: FABRICATION OF INTERCEPTIVE ORTHODONTIC APPLIANCES

Fabrication of the various types of interceptive orthodontic appliances uses and combines all the previous mentioned material in this chapter. A properly constructed orthodontic appliance occurs as a result of a planned sequence of events. This sequence should include an accurate diagnosis, an adequate working cast, a descriptive prescription of the desired appliance, and proper appliance construction.

### ACCURATE DIAGNOSIS

A thorough and proper diagnosis is essential for successful orthodontic therapy. If a dentist is not confident in his diagnositic ability, knowledge should be increased through continuing education courses, study group participation, and working directly with other dentists who treat children's orthodontic problems during the primary and mixed dentition. Hoping an appliance will accomplish an impossible task becomes frustrating to the patient and dentist.

### WORKING CAST

The initial step in appliance fabrication is acquiring an accurate impression of the dental arch. An accurate impression is predicated on good tray size selection, proper impression material manipulation, and good patient management during the impression procedure. The impression material may be either alginate or red compound. If the appliance is to be retained with orthodontic bands, they are adapted to the teeth prior to making the impression. After the impression is taken, the bands are removed from the patient carefully and inserted into the impression. If alginate has been used, the bands should be pinned to place before pouring the impression. If red compound is used, the bands should be waxed to place and the impression poured. In both cases, the dentist should check the working cast for proper band placement and impression accuracy prior to the construction of the appliance.

### PRESCRIPTION

If the appliance is to be fabricated by a laboratory technician, a prescription is required. A good prescription includes the patient's name and age and the referring dentist's name, address, registration number, and telephone number. A descriptive drawing of the desired appliance and a written outline for appliance construction should be included.

A phone call to the laboratory technician might possibly prevent an error in construction if the appliance varies significantly from the usual design. Once the working cast and prescription are in the hands of the laboratory technician, it is his responsibility to check that no discrepancies exist in any of these sequences.

### APPLIANCE CONSTRUCTION

The final step of constructing the appliance is made easier if the steps just mentioned have been followed. The majority of problems in appliance

## Orthodontic procedures

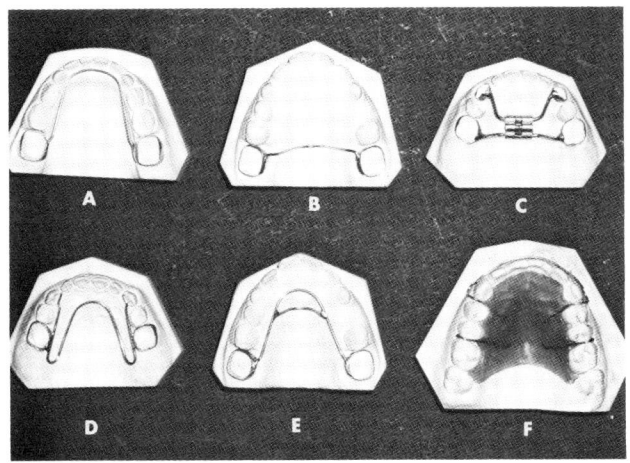

Fig. 20-106. *A*, Lingual arch; *B*, transpalatal; *C*, rapid palatal expander; *D*, W arch; *E*, modified Nance; *F*, Hawley.

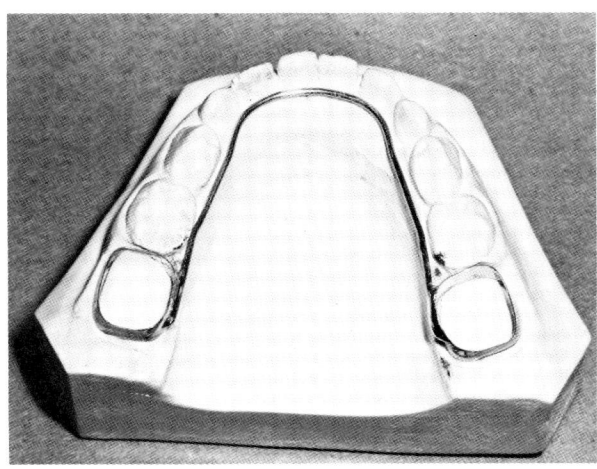

Fig. 20-107. Lingual arch appliance.

construction usually arise because of faulty communication rather than technical error. The following discussion will expand on this subject and develop a step-by-step procedure for appliance construction.

The construction of six appliances will be demonstrated in this section: the lingual arch, transpalatal, modified Nance, rapid palatal expander, W-arch, and Hawley (Fig. 20-106). The first five appliances are of the fixed variety and the last is a removable type. The appliances will be presented in their most basic form. It should be understood that modification of these appliances is always possible. The addition of activating springs, activating loops and hooks, etc., will increase the versatility of each device. Modification allows the dentist to accomplish expanded treatment goals, provided that a correct diagnosis and appliance limitations are considered.

### Lingual arch appliance

**lingual arch** A heavy-gauge orthodontic wire adapted to the lingual surfaces of mandibular teeth and fastened to orthodontic bands on the terminal teeth of the arch form (Fig. 20-107).

#### APPLICATION

The lingual arch appliance is used to prevent mesial shift of the mandibular posterior teeth. It is applicable to the child who has adequate space in the primary arch perimeter for the permanent teeth but who has lost or will lose primary posterior teeth prematurely. The lingual arch appliance is also indicated for the child who has a mild arch space discrepancy, and in whom an arch guidance protocol is planned.

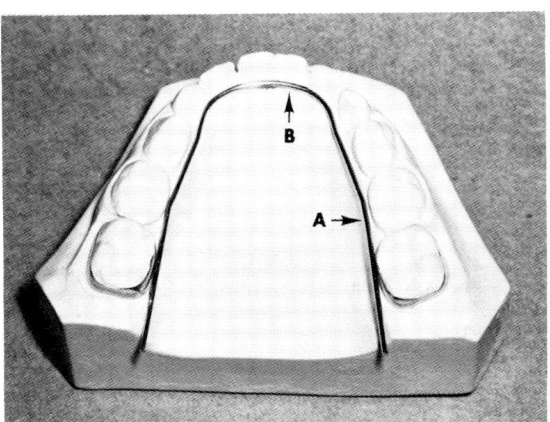

Fig. 20-108. Adapted wire fitting passively on lingual side of mandibular arch form. Correctly positioned wire fitted slightly above gingival margin at posterior molar area *(A)*. Wire positioned on cingula of lower incisors in anterior area *(B)*.

ORTHODONTIC BANDS. Mandibular primary second molars or mandibular permanent first molars.

WIRE SIZE. 0.036- to 0.040-inch Elgiloy or stainless steel.

#### PROCEDURE

1. Adapt the wire so that it will fit passively on the lingual side of the mandibular arch form. The wire should extend 4 or 5 mm past the banded teeth. Make sure that as many teeth as possible contact the wire. The wire should be positioned slightly above the gingival margin for the posterior teeth (Fig. 20-108, arrow A) and on the cingula of the lower incisors (arrow B).

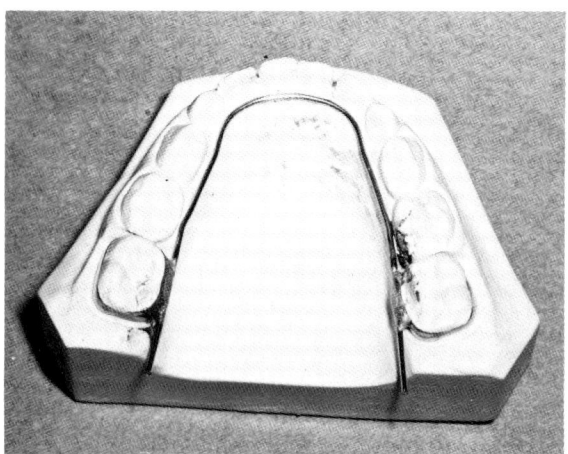

**Fig. 20-109.** Completed solder joints on lingual arch appliance.

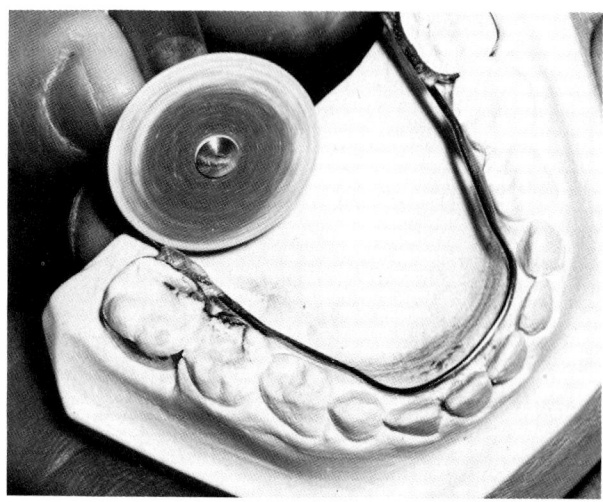

**Fig. 20-110.** Finishing of appliance is accomplished with stones, wheels, and compound prior to removal of appliance from cast.

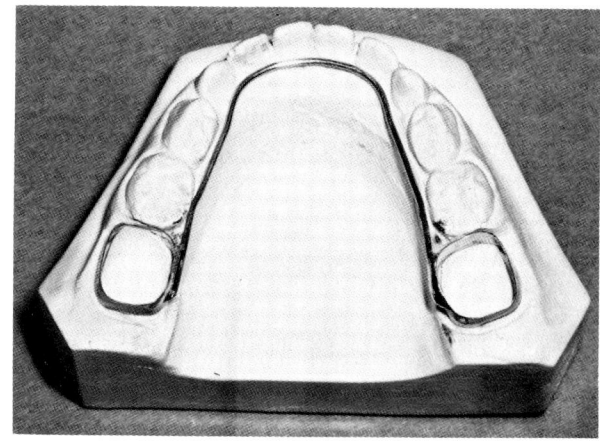

**Fig. 20-111.** Completed lingual arch ready for patient delivery.

**Table 20-5.** Lingual arch appliance

| Problem | Probable cause | Solution |
|---|---|---|
| Gingival irritation around orthodontic band after cementation | Pressure necrosis due to faulty placement of solder joint | Place solder joint in incisal third of orthodontic band |
| Expansion of permanent molars after cementation of appliance | Wire has become active rather than passive | Properly manage wire during bending and finishing to decrease possibility of activation<br>Heat treat wire to release any potential stresses if it is stainless steel and to maximize resiliency if it is Elgiloy |

2. Stabilize the arch wire in its proper position using alligator clips, soldering putty, or dental stone, and solder the wire to the orthodontic bands. Care should be taken to keep the solder joint in the incisal third of the band. Proper solder joint position will prevent gingival irritation when the appliance is cemented in place (Fig. 20-109).

3. Finish and polish the solder joints using stones, wheels, and polishing compound (Fig. 20-110).

4. To complete the lingual arch, remove the plaster inside the bands with a large round acrylic bur. Carefully lift the appliance from the working cast and clean off any finishing debris. Check the appliance for distortion expansion and correct any that is present (Fig. 20-111). Make sure to heat treat the wire at this point if annealed wire was used in construction.

### PROBLEM AREAS

1. Placing the solder joint too low on the orthodontic band and causing gingival irritation after cementation.

2. The possibility of the appliance being active rather than passive due to wire expansion in the molar area. Expansion in the molar area is usually a result of faulty wire manipulation and finishing (Table 20-5).

3. Failure to heat treat the wire to release any potential stresses. If Elgiloy wire is used in construction, the wire must be heat treated to activate the wire to maximum resiliency.

### MODIFICATIONS

1. Auxiliary springs in the anterior region to help align ectopically positioned incisors.

2. Activating loops mesial to the permanent molars can be used to flare the anterior teeth.

## Transpalatal appliance

**transpalatal arch** A heavy-gauge orthodontic wire adapted directly across the palate and attached to orthodontic bands on contralateral maxillary posterior teeth (Fig. 20-112).

### APPLICATION

The transpalatal appliance is used to prevent mesial shift of the maxillary posterior teeth. The appliance is applicable to the child who has adequate space in the primary arch perimeter for the permanent teeth but who has lost or will lose primary posterior teeth prematurely. The maxillary transpalatal appliance is also indicated for the child who has a mild arch space discrepancy and an arch guidance protocol is planned.

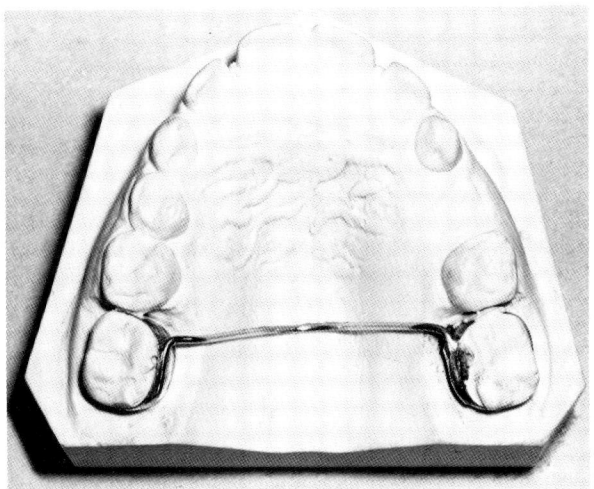

**Fig. 20-112.** Transpalatal arch.

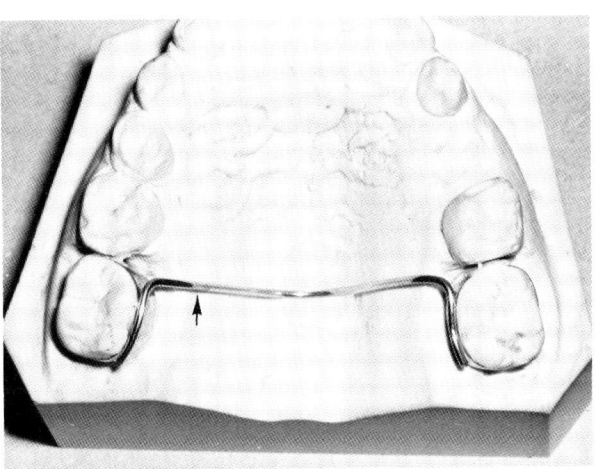

**Fig. 20-113.** Adapted wire fitting passively across palate from mesial surface of one banded tooth to mesial surface of opposite banded tooth. Approximately 1 mm of clearance is provided from palatal tissues (arrow). Wire is bent distally across banded teeth in incisal third for proper fit.

ORTHODONTIC BANDS. Maxillary primary second molars or maxillary permanent first molars.

WIRE SIZE. 0.036- to 0.040-inch Elgiloy or stainless steel.

### PROCEDURE

1. Adapt the wire directly across the palate from the mesial surface of one banded tooth to the mesial surface of the opposite banded tooth. Make sure the wire has approximately 1 mm of clearance from the palatal tissues (arrow A). Bend the wire distally to cross each banded tooth in its incisal third, and conform the wire to the lingual morphology of the tooth (arrow B) (Fig. 20-113).

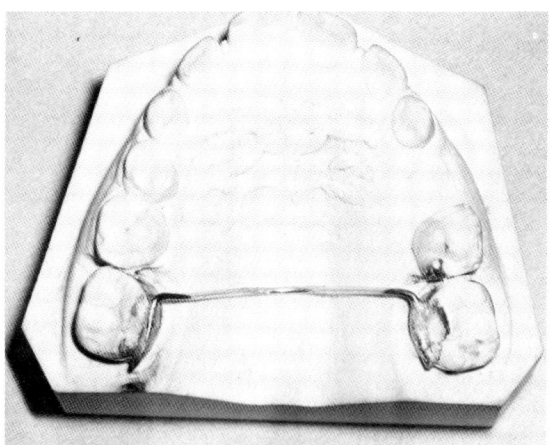

**Fig. 20-114.** After stabilization, wire is soldered to two bands.

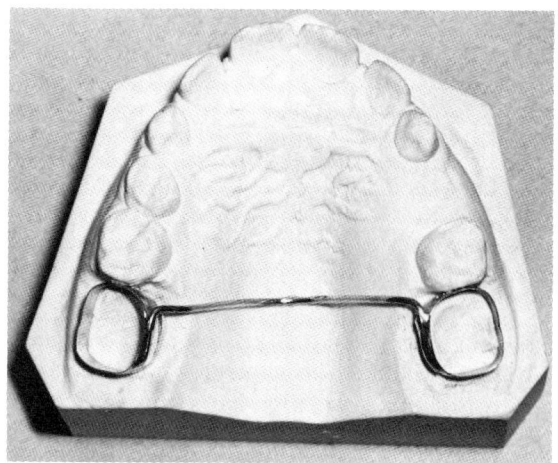

**Fig. 20-115.** Finished and polished appliance ready for patient delivery.

**Table 20-6.** Transpalatal appliance

| Problem | Probable cause | Solution |
| --- | --- | --- |
| Pressure necrosis in or around solder joint or transpalatal wire | Faulty impression giving inaccurate tissue definition or plaster breaking away from orthodontic band in gingival sulcus area, allowing wire to be placed into tissue | Provide relief in area adjacent to banded teeth |

2. Stabilize the arch wire using sticky wax, soldering putty, or dental stone, and solder the wire to the bands (Fig. 20-114).

3. Finish and polish the appliance on the cast prior to appliance removal from the cast. The appliance is then removed from the working cast using a round acrylic bur, and any finishing debris is cleaned off (Fig. 20-115).

#### PROBLEM AREA

Not providing enough relief for the area adjacent to the banded teeth. Many times plaster will break away from this area, and the wire will be placed in close approximation to the plaster. Pressure necrosis can occur after cementation (Table 20-6).

#### MODIFICATION

The transpalatal appliance can be used in the primary arch to hold the primary second molars instead of the permanent 6-year molars.

### Modified Nance appliance

**modified Nance** A heavy-gauge orthodontic wire traversing across the anterior portion of the palate and fastened to contralateral maxillary posterior teeth with orthodontic bands (Fig. 20-116).

#### APPLICATION

The modified Nance appliance has the same applications as the transpalatal arch. Many clinicians, however, believe that a transpalatal arch does not prevent the mesial migration of the permanent molars when bilateral loss of the second primary molars has occurred. For this reason, the modified Nance is usually the appliance of choice when multiple dental units have been lost or their loss is anticipated.

ORTHODONTIC BANDS. Maxillary primary second molars or maxillary permanent first molars.

WIRE SIZE. 0.036- to 0.040-inch Elgiloy or stainless steel.

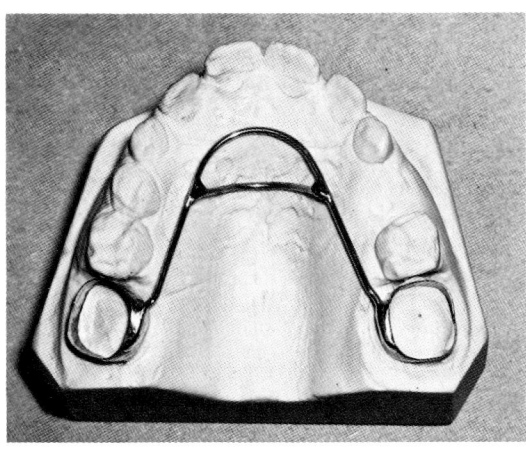

**Fig. 20-116.** Modified Nance appliance.

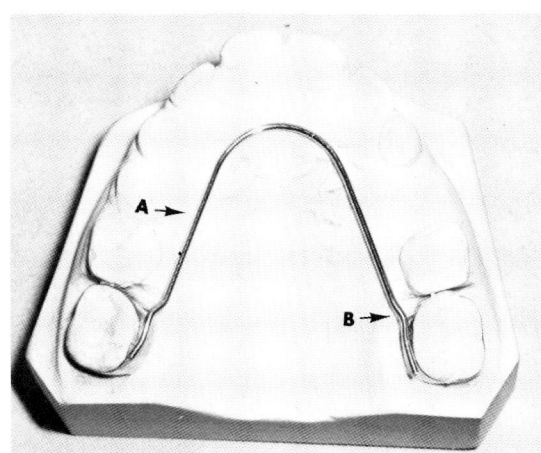

**Fig. 20-117.** Adapted wire fitting passively from banded molars to anterior palatal vault area. Wire fitted correctly in anterior palatal vault area, leaving 3 to 5 mm of space between wire and teeth *(A)*. Bayonet bend used to get desired relief from lingual surfaces of maxillary teeth *(B)*.

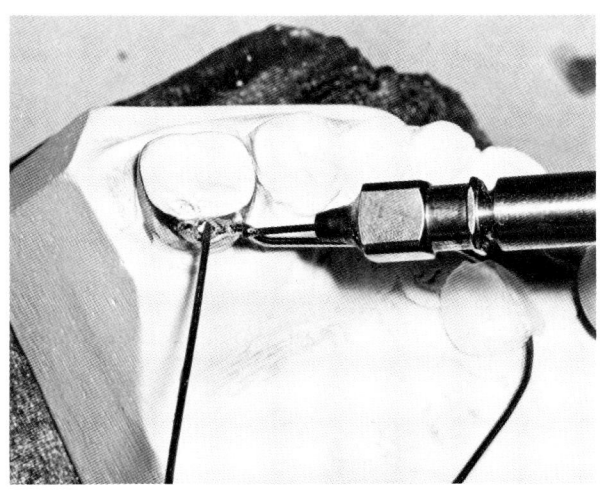

**Fig. 20-118.** Adapted wire being soldered in incisal third of band.

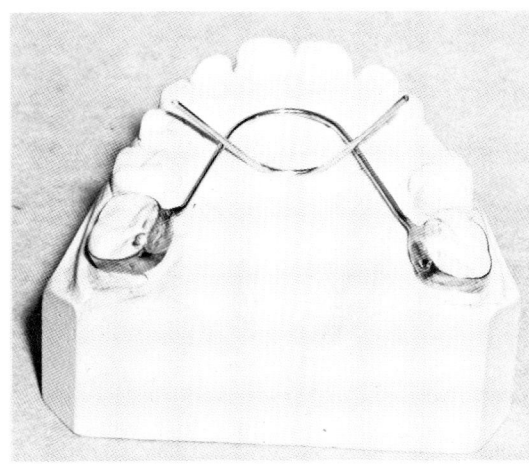

**Fig. 20-119.** Another wire of same diameter is adapted to depth of palatal vault and extends past soldered wire.

**PROCEDURE**

1. Form a smooth curve of wire that will fit passively in the anterior palatal vault area. Extend this curve mesially to the canine area and distally past the banded teeth, leaving about 3 to 5 mm of space between the wire and the lingual surfaces of the maxillary teeth (Fig. 20-117, arrow A). Use bilateral bayonet bends to get the desired relief from the lingual surfaces of the maxillary teeth (arrow B). Relieve the wire approximately 1 mm from the palatal tissues (Fig. 20-117).

2. Stabilize the arch wire, and solder the adapted wire to the bands (Fig. 20-118).

3. Adapt a piece of the same diameter wire near the anterior bow in the canine area of the arch. Extend this wire to the depth of the palatal vault with about 1-mm clearance of the palatal tissues (Fig. 20-119).

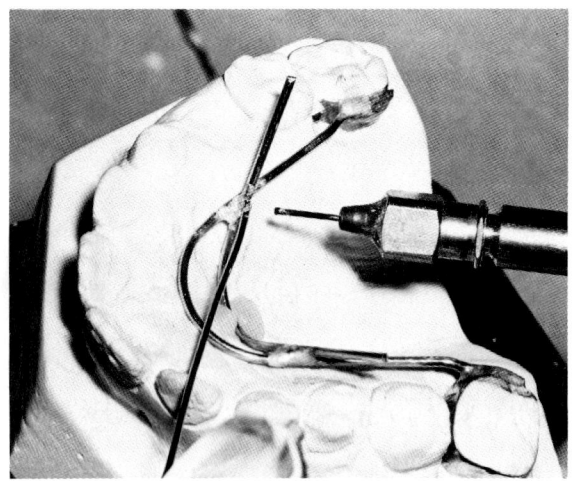

**Fig. 20-120.** After stabilization with soldering putty, auxiliary wire is soldered to main arch wire.

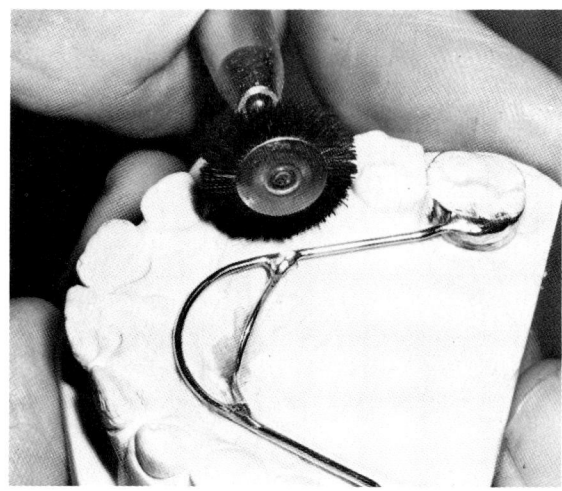

**Fig. 20-121.** Polishing is accomplished prior to removal from working cast.

4. Stabilize this wire, and solder it to the main arch wire that has already been fastened to the orthodontic bands (Fig. 20-120).

5. The solder joints can be finished with the appliance still on the working cast. Use an acrylic bur to remove the appliance from the stone cast (Fig. 20-121).

### PROBLEM AREAS

The problem areas for the modified Nance appliance are the same as described for the transpalatal arch appliance.

### MODIFICATION

The addition of a crib in the anterior bow area can be used on a patient with an active thumbsucking habit.

## Rapid palatal expansion appliance

**rapid palatal expander** An apparatus consisting of two rigid units connected with a separating screw, each unit being attached by orthodontic bands to separate sides of the dental arch (Fig. 20-122).

### APPLICATION

The rapid palatal expander is used to correct posterior functional crossbites in the primary and early mixed dentition. This appliance also can be used for orthodontic rehabilitation of the cleft palate patient.

ORTHODONTIC BANDS. Maxillary primary second molars or maxillary permanent first molars. Maxillary primary canines or maxillary permanent canines.

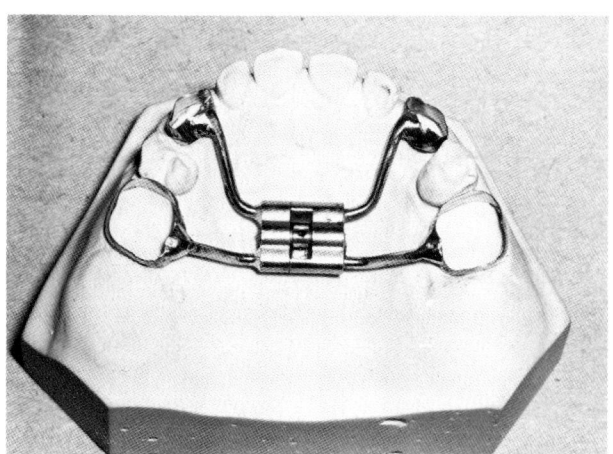

**Fig. 20-122.** Rapid palatal expansion appliance.

WIRE SIZE. Preformed Hyrax* wire expansion screw.

### PROCEDURE

1. Fit a Hyrax expander into the palatal vault with the expansion screw lined up so it can be activated from the front of the mouth to the back of the mouth (Fig. 20-123, arrow A). The unit should be adapted so that the expansion screw is located in the middle of the palatal area with the four attachment wires extending to the banded teeth. Make sure the expansion screw and the wires have sufficient relief from the palatal tissues (Fig. 20-123, arrow B).

*OIS/Orthodontics, Wilmington, Del.

## Orthodontic procedures 621

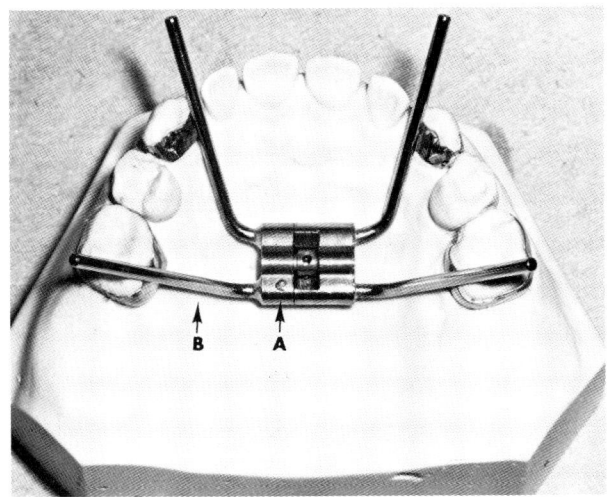

**Fig. 20-123.** Hyrax expander positioned into palatal vault with extending lateral arms positioned for correct soldering technique. Dot on expander should be placed distally so that activation occurs front to back of mouth *(A)*. Correct relief from palatal tissues is desired *(B)*.

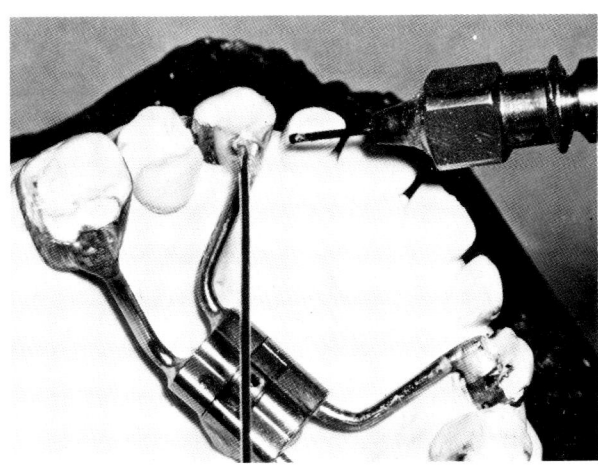

**Fig. 20-124.** Soldering extending arms to bands in incisal third of orthodontic bands.

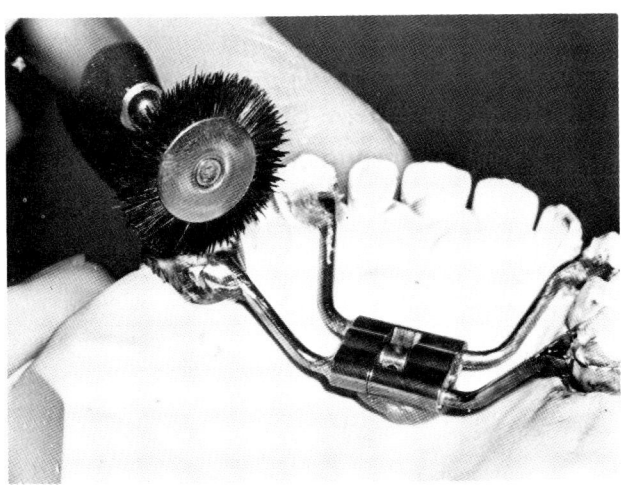

**Fig. 20-125.** Polishing four solder joints prior to removal from working cast.

2. After the Hyrax expansion screw is fit properly, stabilize it in the usual manner, and solder the wire extensions to the four banded teeth (Fig. 20-124).

3. Polish the four solder joints using an assortment of wheels, stones, and polishing compound, and remove the completed appliance from the cast (Fig. 20-125).

**PROBLEM AREAS**

1. Insufficient relief from palatal tissues. Food and debris will accumulate and make cleaning difficult for the patient.

2. Placing the expansion screw so that it turns backward. If the expander is made to work in this manner the entire procedure must be done by feel and this is a very difficult procedure to accomplish (Table 20-7).

**Table 20-7.** Rapid palatal appliance

| Problem | Probable cause | Solution |
| --- | --- | --- |
| Food and debris getting caught under appliance | Insufficient relief between connecting wires and expander and palatal tissues | Make sure sufficient relief is allowed for during appliance construction |
| Expander placed backwards in palatal vault, resulting in need to activate back to front at turning mechanism | Faulty placement of expander | Open and close expanding mechanism prior to placement and soldering to ensure proper placement for use |

**622** *Dental laboratory procedures: removable partial dentures*

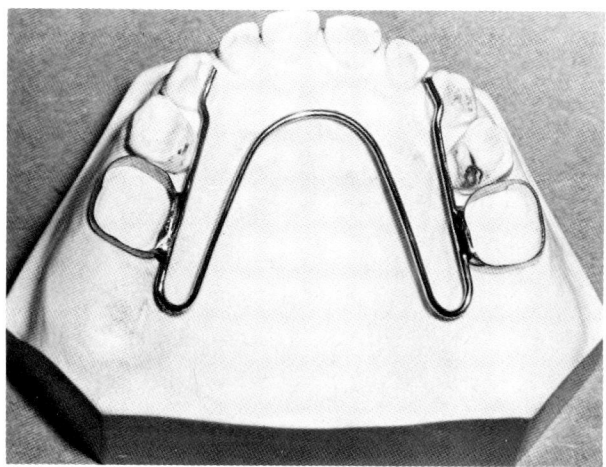

**Fig. 20-126.** W-arch appliance.

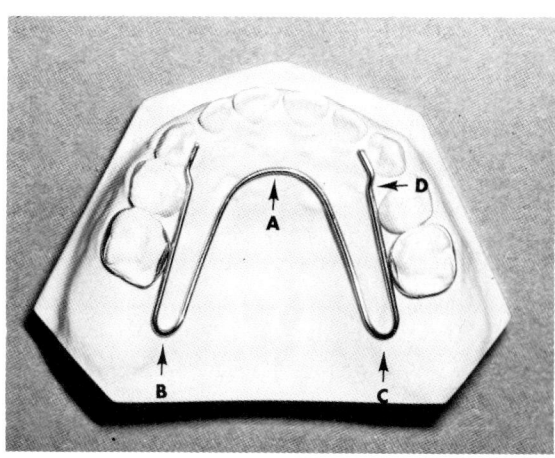

**Fig. 20-127.** Completed W arch fitting passively into palatal contour. Large smooth curve is bent initially in 8-inch (20-cm) segment of wire into anterior palatal area *(A)*. Then smaller curves are bent to bring wire forward *(B* and *C)*. Anterior extending arms are then formed to make contact with teeth. Bayonet bends are used in canine area so that this can be achieved *(D)*.

#### MODIFICATION

Use an expansion screw that is embedded in acrylic rather than suspended by wire extensions. The acrylic should be relieved, and tissue pressure points should be checked for prior to cementation. An acrylic palatal expander is harder to clean and sometimes difficult for a child to tolerate.

### W-arch appliance

**W-arch** An activated orthodontic wire molded into the shape of a W, fit into the palatal vault, and soldered to bands on the posterior teeth (Fig. 20-126).

#### APPLICATION

The W-arch appliance is used for the correction of posterior functional crossbites in the primary and early mixed dentition.

ORTHODONTIC BANDS. Maxillary primary second molars or maxillary permanent first molars.

WIRE SIZE. 0.030- to 0.036-inch Elgiloy or stainless steel.

#### PROCEDURE

1. Initially, form a smooth curve in the middle of an 8-inch (20-cm) segment of wire so the curve will fit passively into the anterior palatal area. This curve should extend mesially to a line formed by connecting the mesial surfaces of the maxillary canines (Fig. 20-127, arrow A). On each distal extension of the wire, bend a smaller curve so the wire will come forward (arrow B). These anterior extensions should make contact with the palatal surface of the maxillary teeth (arrow C). Using finger pressure, adapt the wire configuration to the palatal contour until there is a 1-mm clearance with the soft tissues (Fig. 20-127).

2. Stabilize the assembly, solder the wire to the orthodontic bands, and finish the solder joints in the usual manner (Figs. 20-128 and 20-129).

3. After the finishing and polishing has been completed, remove the appliance from the working cast using an acrylic bur (Fig. 20-130). Prior to cementation, activate the appliance by spreading the W shape laterally approximately 3 to 5 mm.

#### PROBLEM AREA

Placement of the distal extending loops too far distally, causing pressure necrosis or gagging problems (Table 20-8).

#### MODIFICATION

Helical coils may be added to the intramaxillary wire assembly in place of the semicircle bends. The coils add to the effectiveness of the expansion force.

## Orthodontic procedures

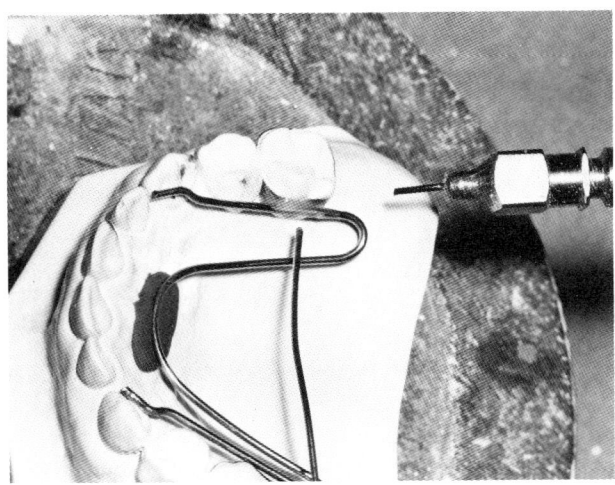

**Fig. 20-128.** After stabilization, wire is soldered to orthodontic bands.

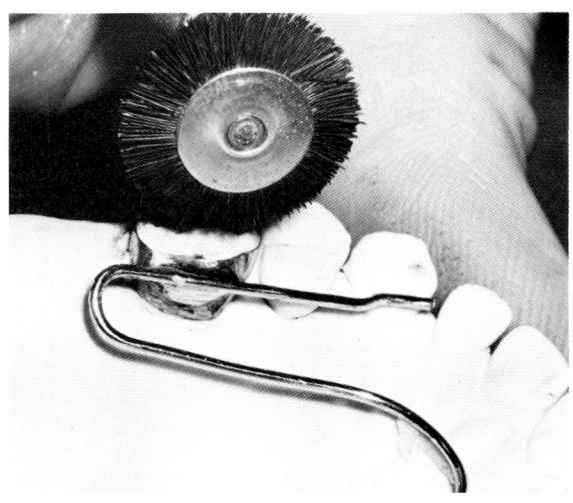

**Fig. 20-129.** Finishing and polishing are accomplished prior to removal from working cast.

**Fig. 20-130.** W-arch appliance replaced on working cast and ready for patient delivery.

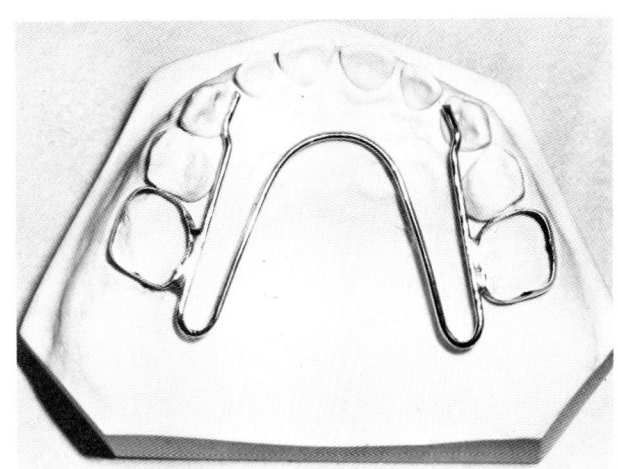

### Table 20-8. W-arch appliance

| Problem | Probable cause | Solution |
|---|---|---|
| Pressure necrosis around U bend of distal extending wire arch | Improper relief from palatal tissues or wire placement into tissue area due to false impression | Proper relief is important from accurate working cast |

## Hawley appliance

**Hawley appliance** An acrylic framework that fits into either the maxillary palatal area or mandibular lingual area and is retained in the oral cavity by wire clasps (Fig. 20-131).

### APPLICATION

The Hawley appliance is probably the most widely used interceptive orthodontic device. It has enjoyed considerable success in space maintenance, space regaining, crossbite correction, closure of interdental spaces, tipping of teeth, retention, and habit control. However, because of its ease of construction and wide range of applicability, it also carries the distinction of being the most widely misused appliance.

ORTHODONTIC BANDS. Wire size for labial bow: 0.030- to 0.036-inch Elgiloy or stainless steel. Wire size for ball clasps: 0.024- to 0.040-inch preformed clasp material.

### PROCEDURE

1. Construct a labial bow spring following the prescribed method. Make sure the omega loops do not extend too far into the facial vesti-

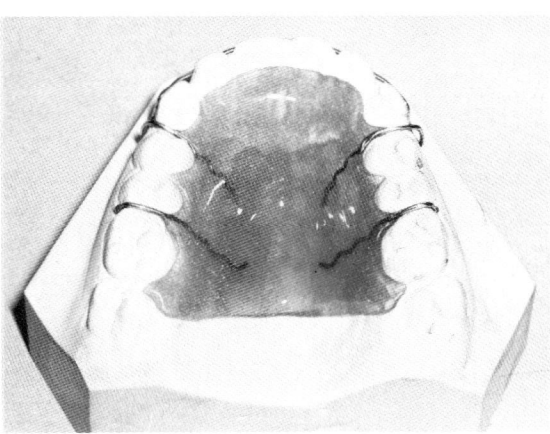

Fig. 20-131. Hawley appliance.

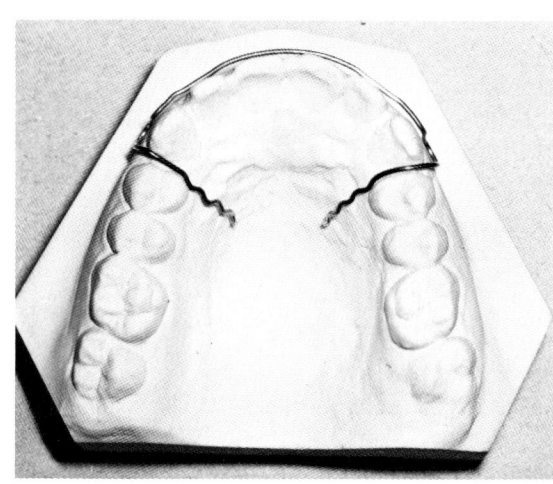

Fig. 20-132. Anterior labial bow fitting passively on anterior segment of working cast.

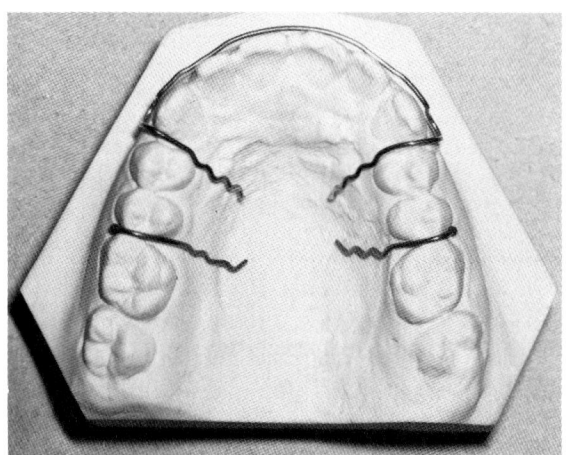

Fig. 20-133. Adapt ball clasps to embrasure area of posterior teeth.

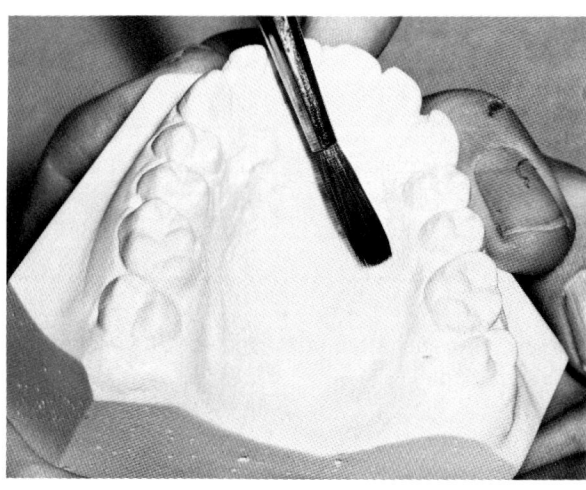

Fig. 20-134. Separating medium applied prior to autopolymerizing acrylic resin technique.

bule where they could irritate the mucosa (Fig. 20-132).

2. Adapt ball clasps to the embrasure areas of the posterior teeth. Usually one or two clasps on either side of the arch will provide sufficient retention (Fig. 20-133).

3. Soak the working cast for 10 minutes before applying the resin or painting on separating liquid. Extend the medium over all of the teeth and soft tissues that will be covered by the acrylic resin (Fig. 20-134).

4. Build up the acrylic in the palatal area using a sprinkle-on technique. The acrylic should extend to the distal surface of the most posterior teeth in the arch and to the lingual surface of all maxillary teeth. The acrylic should be approximately 3 mm in thickness (Fig. 20-135).

5. Polymerize the resin in the pressure cooker, remove it from the working cast, and trim it to its final form using arbor bands, acrylic burs, and wheels (Figs. 20-136 and 20-137).

6. The appliance is completed by applying polishing compound with a chamois wheel to produce a high-luster finish (Fig. 20-138).

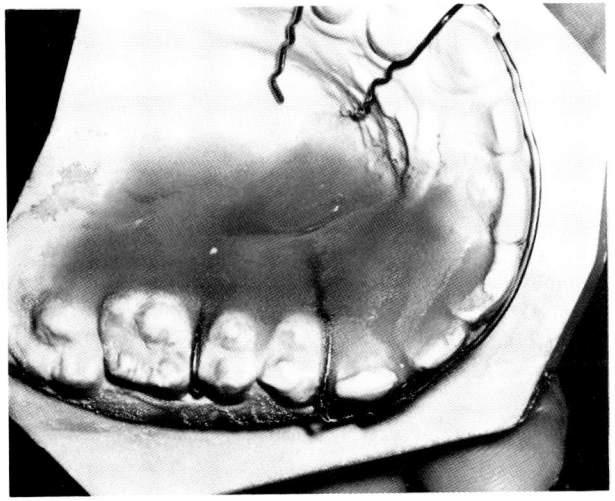

Fig. 20-135. Acrylic resin built up on one side of cast after first making sure that palate, teeth, and wires are covered with at least 3 mm of acrylic resin.

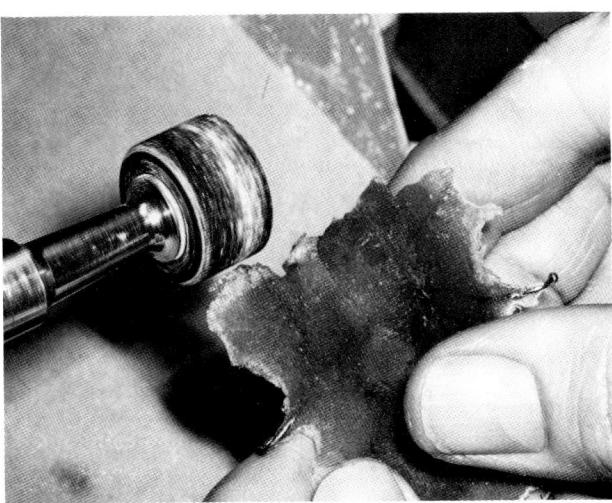

Fig. 20-136. Arbor band used to rough out outline form of appliance.

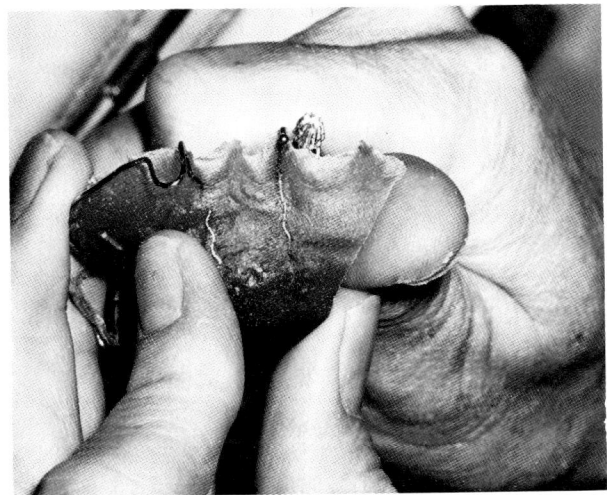

Fig. 20-137. Acrylic bur is used to complete outline form of appliance and produce suitable finish for final polishing.

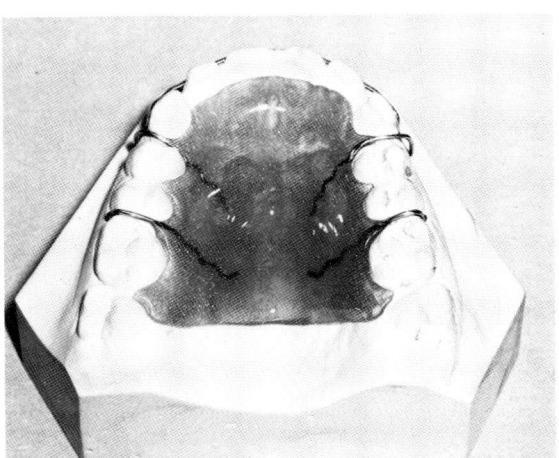

Fig. 20-138. Completed Hawley appliance.

**Table 20-9.** Hawley appliance

| Problem | Probable cause | Solution |
| --- | --- | --- |
| Occlusion problems and displacement problems around embrasure area | Incorrect placement, usually too high placement of wire through embrasure | Place wire as close as possible to embrasure as it passes from buccal position to palatal side |
| Speech problems, gagging, and difficulty in finishing | Acrylic too thick to begin with | Control technique by first doing one side and allowing it to gain some polymerization and then contralateral side |
| Acrylic porosity | Improper acrylic manipulation | Keep polymer wet with monomer at all times; try to always add powder to liquid |
|  | Nonuse of pressure cooker | Allow resin to polymerize in pressure cooker for 15 minutes under 20 psi |
| Acrylic distortion | Overheating of cured resin during finishing and polishing | Take care during finishing and polishing phase not to get acrylic too hot |

### PROBLEM AREAS

1. Incorrect placement of the wire through the embrasure areas. Wires placed too high in these areas will cause problems with the occlusion and result in the displacement of the appliance.
2. Making the acrylic too thick when using the salt and pepper technique. If one side is completed and then the other, this will help keep the thickness under control.
3. Improper acrylic polymerization. Porosity is always a potential problem with cold-curing acrylic resin, and a pressure cooker will help reduce this.
4. Distorting the appliance when finishing and polishing. Cured acrylic resin is still susceptible to heat. Make sure that the acrylic resin does not get too hot during the finishing and polishing phase (Table 20-9).

### MODIFICATIONS

1. Adding springs or elastics for aligning teeth or correcting cross-bites.
2. Adding acrylic resin to the occlusal portion of the teeth for bite opening purposes.
3. Incorporating a tongue crib in the palatal area for habit control.
4. A dumbbell spring or slingshot spring may be added to distalize posterior teeth.

PART TWO

# Preparation of diagnostic casts

DAVID L. KING

Diagnostic, or study, casts are plaster models of the maxillary and mandibular dental arches of a patient. The usual purpose in securing study casts is to aid in diagnosis and treatment planning, but they serve several other useful purposes as well. Many dentists find diagnostic casts invaluable as visual aids in explaining problems and treatment objectives to patients. Also, serial diagnostic casts of a patient provide an effective means of evaluating and demonstrating anatomic changes brought about by growth and development or treatment intervention. Finally, as a particularly tangible part of a patient's records, diagnostic casts may function as evidence in litigational or forensic areas.

### REQUIREMENTS FOR STUDY CASTS

There are two components to a finished study cast; the anatomic portion and the base, or art, portion (Fig. 20-139).

The anatomic portion of a diagnostic cast must include an accurate and complete reproduction of the dentition and adjacent supporting structures. This depends largely on events such as impression mak-

*Orthodontic procedures* **627**

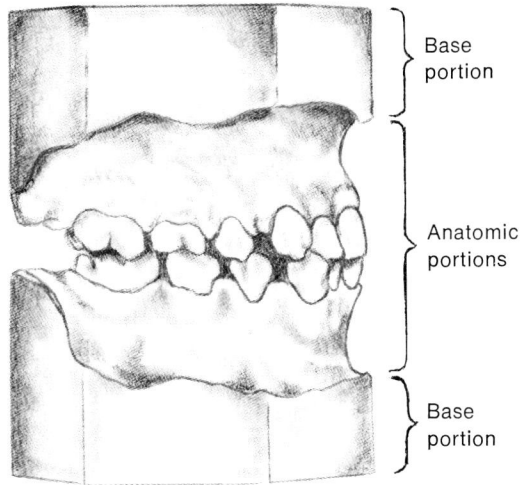

**Fig. 20-139.** Relative proportions of base and anatomic portions are shown. Note that top and bottom surfaces are parallel to each other and that back surfaces (heels) of each cast are flush when casts are articulated properly.

ing and pouring, which have taken place prior to the procedures discussed in this chapter.

The base, or art, portion of diagnostic casts should be prepared in a precise, sequential manner. There are a number of published descriptions of base preparation, no two of which will be found to agree completely on methodology. These differences arise partly because of variations in the type of equipment used and partly because there are aspects to base preparation that are arbitrary and subject to personal preference. All methods will arrive at much the same end if the prescribed rules are followed.

Diagnostic cast preparation, for the most part, requires that a series of cuts or facets be made on the base portion of the casts (Fig. 20-140). These cuts are made in a certain sequence and at certain angles to each other. There are various ways of making these cuts, depending on the equipment available. It will be assumed here that a motor-driven cast

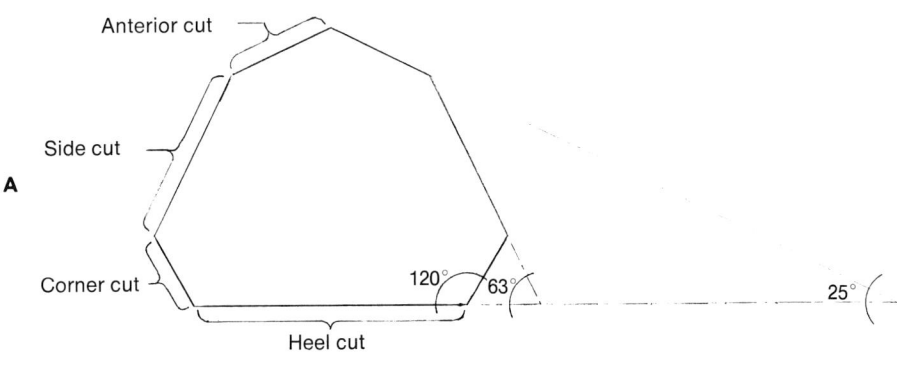

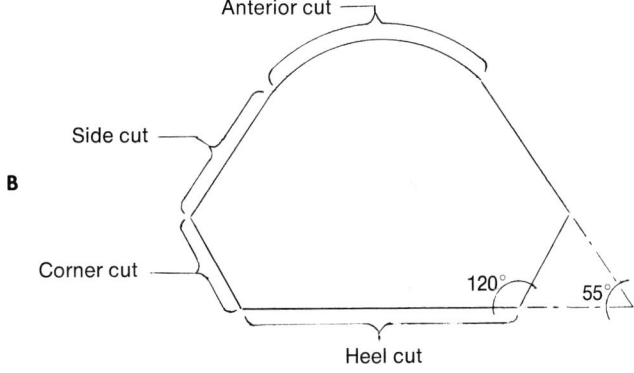

**Fig. 20-140. A,** Angular relationship of various cuts on maxillary cast base. **B,** Mandibular cast base.

trimmer with angular table markings is available; however, the directions may be adapted to more sophisticated cast trimmers with table attachments specifically designed for diagnostic cast preparation.

It is important to begin with plaster base pours that are oversize in thickness and peripheral extent to ensure an adequate amount of material for the finishing cuts (Fig. 20-141). Large base molds are available for this purpose.*

All plaster "bubbles" on the occlusal surfaces of the teeth must be removed so that the casts may be related accurately in occlusion during certain trimming and finishing steps. Ideally, the tongue area of the mandibular impression should have been filled in with alginate or some puttylike material before the plaster pour to have a flat, smooth surface in this area. If this has not been done, excess plaster may be carved away later to produce such a surface.

**PROCEDURE**

1. Rough trim the periphery of the maxillary and mandibular casts only enough so that their bases are able to fit within the "window" of the cast trimmer and contact the abrasive wheel. In accomplishing this step, an effort should be made to trim peripheral areas farthest away from those anatomic portions of the cast which must be preserved when the final cuts are made. Avoid trimming any closer than ½ inch (1.3 cm) from the vestibular areas. Posteriorly, keep at least ¾ inch (1.9 cm) away from the pterygomaxillary notch areas of the maxillary cast and the retromolar pad areas of the mandibular cast (Fig. 20-142).

2. Place the maxillary cast, teeth down, on a thin piece of baseplate wax, which in turn has been placed on a flat, smooth bench area. With a compass opened to 1½ inches, scribe a pencil line around the periphery of the cast. Take care to keep the compass points vertically oriented so that the line always will be 1½ inches (3.8 cm) from the bench surface. The teeth should be in maximum contact with the wax during this step so that the pencil line will be parallel with the occlusal plane (Fig. 20-143).

3. *Base cut.* Trim the top of the maxillary cast to line scribed around the periphery (Fig. 20-144).

4. *Heel cut.* With the base of the cast on the trimming table, make the heel cut at a right angle to the base. This cut should be perpendicular to the palatal midline (median raphe) and stopped about ¼ inch (0.6 cm) distal to the deepest point of the pterygomaxillary notch area on either side (Fig. 20-145).

5. *Side cuts.* Make the side cut on the maxillary cast at an angle of 63 degrees to the heel cut. Keep the heel cut lined up with the appropriate angle marking on the trimming table, and stop trimming when the cut first reaches the vestibular sulcus (Fig. 20-146). Repeat the procedure for the opposite side.

6. *Anterior cuts.* Make these cuts at angles of 25 degrees to the heel cut (or alternatively, 142 degrees to the side cut). Stop trimming when the angle formed by the anterior and side cut lies over the canine eminence region (Fig. 20-147). In some instances it may be necessary to trim less than this to avoid damage to the anterior teeth.

7. At this time, examine the maxillary base for symmetry. Ideally, corresponding cuts on either side should be equal to each other and form identical angles with the base. The point formed anteriorly by the anterior cuts should fall on an imaginary

---

*TP Laboratories, Inc., LaPorte, Ind.

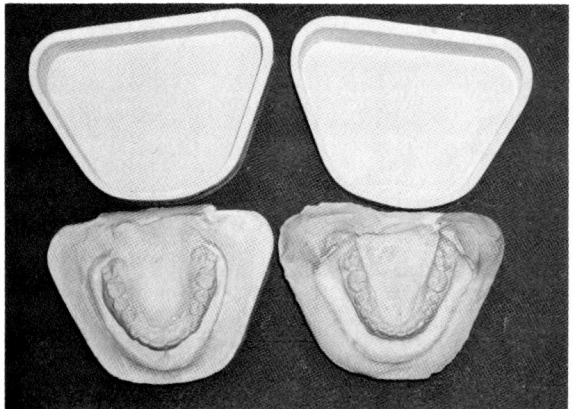

**Fig. 20-141.** Maxillary and mandibular casts have been removed from their respective base molds.

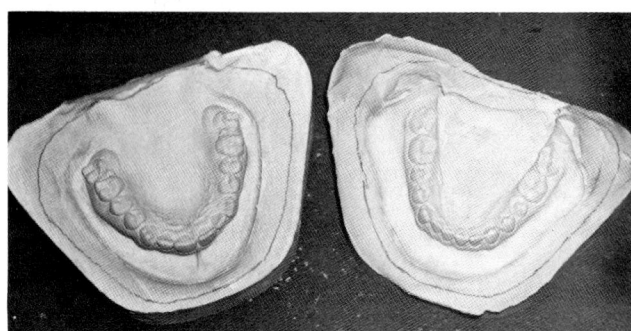

**Fig. 20-142.** Pencil line indicates approximate amount of plaster to be removed for rough peripheral trim.

*Orthodontic procedures* **629**

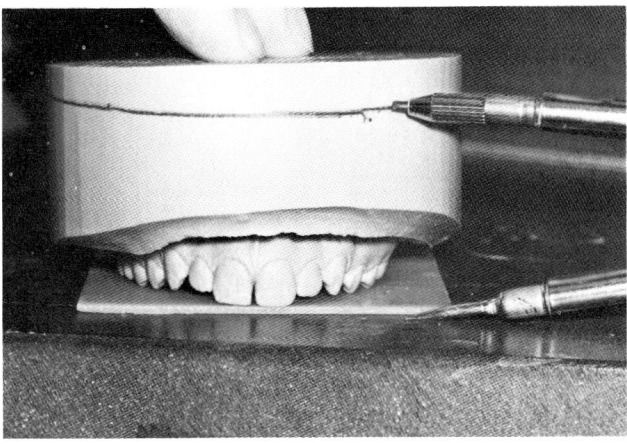

Fig. 20-143. Pencil line scribed around periphery of maxillary cast as guide for base cut.

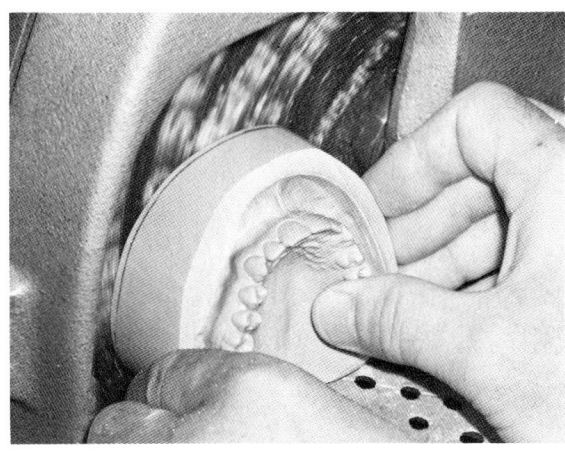

Fig. 20-144. Base cut on maxillary cast is made to pencil line.

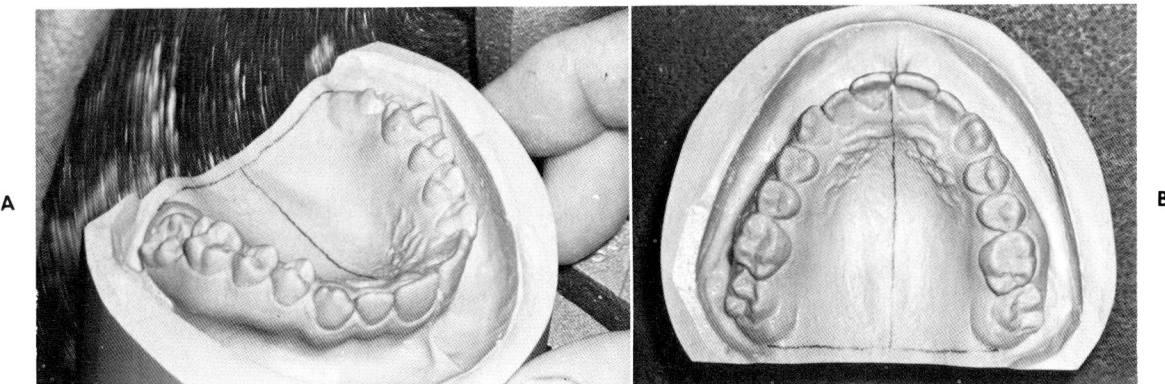

Fig. 20-145. **A,** Heel cut on maxillary cast is made parallel to line through pterygomaxillary notch area and perpendicular to palatal midline. **B,** Heel cut should stop about 1/4 inch (0.6 cm) short of pterygomaxillary notch area.

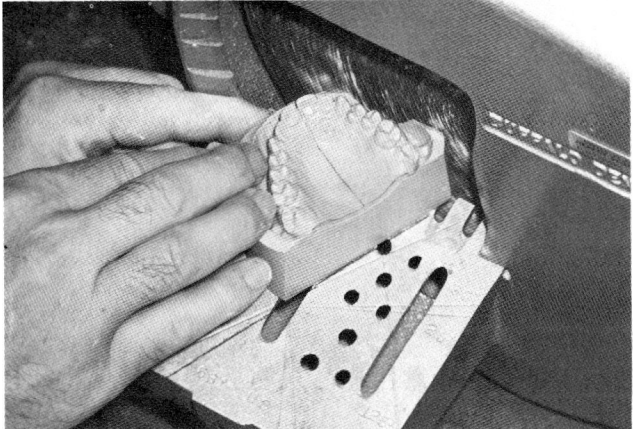

Fig. 20-146. Side cuts on maxillary cast are made with heel aligned at 63 degrees to cutting wheel.

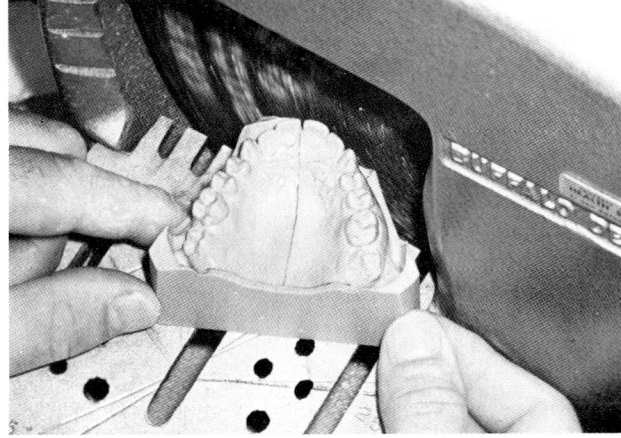

Fig. 20-147. Anterior cuts on maxillary cast are made at 25 degrees to heel cut. Point formed by anterior cuts should lie along imaginary extension of palatal midline.

**630** *Dental laboratory procedures: removable partial dentures*

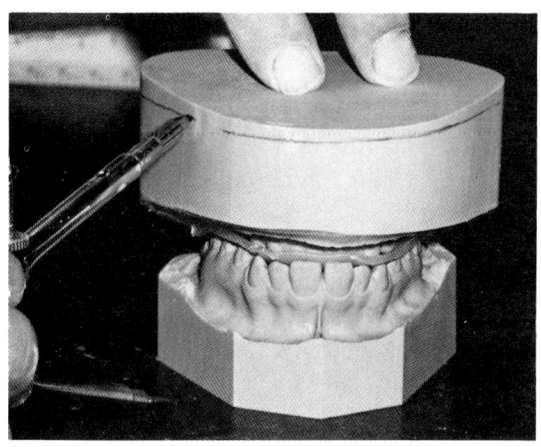

**Fig. 20-148.** Guideline for the mandibular base cut is scribed. Note that despite relatively thick base pour, there is little material to remove for base cut.

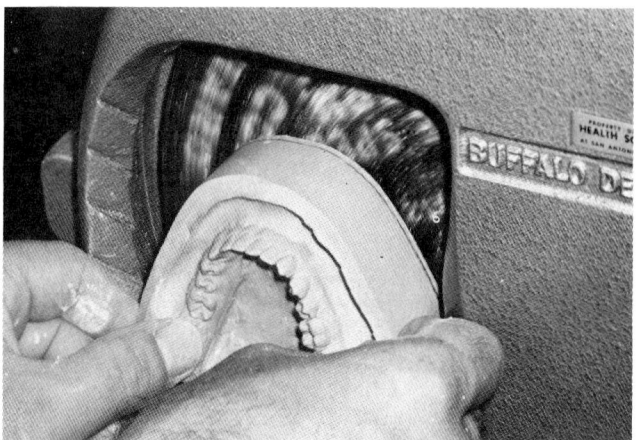

**Fig. 20-149.** Base cut on mandibular cast is made to pencil line.

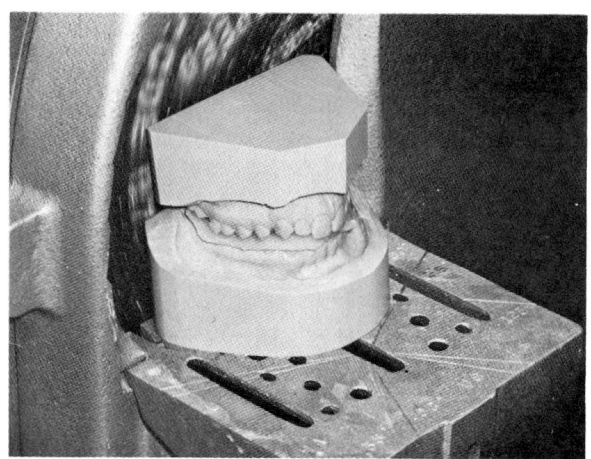

**Fig. 20-150.** Mandibular heel cut is made with casts articulated. Slight amount of maxillary heel is removed during this step also to ensure that heel surfaces of both casts will be flush.

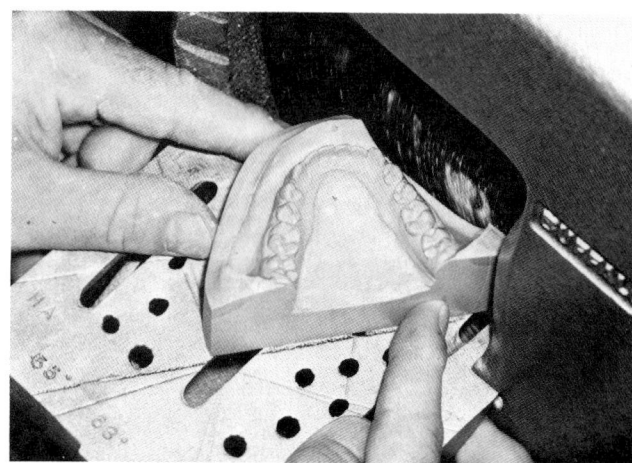

**Fig. 20-151.** Side cuts on mandibular cast are made with heel aligned at 55 degrees to cutting wheel.

line extending from the palatal midline (not necessarily the dental midline as this is frequently in error). Minor adjustments may be made to achieve symmetry by additional trimming on the side and anterior cuts, but a significant error in the heel cut is often irreversible.

8. Occlude the casts with the maxillary cast base down on the bench surface. Use the wax bite registration if such is available to avoid damage to the teeth for this step. With the compass opened to 2³⁄₄ inches (6.9 cm), scribe a pencil line as previously described around the base of the mandibular cast (Fig. 20-148).

9. *Base cut.* Trim the bottom of the mandibular cast to the line scribed around the periphery (Fig. 20-149).

10. *Heel cut.* With the casts occluded and the mandibular cast base on the trimming table, trim the heel of the mandibular cast while keeping the heel of the maxillary cast parallel to the abrasive wheel. Stop trimming when a slight amount (no more than ¼ inch; 0.6 cm) of the maxillary heel has been removed (Fig. 20-150). This step will make the heels of the two casts flush with each other when the casts are related in the patient's usual occlusion. Use extreme care in this step to avoid damage to the teeth during trimming, especially if a wax bite registration is not used.

11. *Side cuts.* Make the side cuts on the mandibular cast at an angle of 55 degrees to the heels. Use the appropriate angle marking on the trimming table, and stop trimming when the cut reaches the vestibule (Fig. 20-151).

12. *Anterior cut.* Make the anterior cut on the mandibular cast by simply rounding off this area by freehand trimming to parallel the anterior dental arch form and vestibule (Fig. 20-152).

13. *Corner cuts.* Reduce the sharp angles formed by the side and heel cuts by "corner" cuts. These are made by occluding the casts and trimming maxillary and mandibular bases simultaneously at an angle of 120 degrees to the heels. These cuts should be approximately ½ inch (1.3 cm) in width (Fig. 20-153).

14. *Finishing and polishing the casts.* Fill any small voids in the surface of the casts by smearing a fresh mix of plaster over the surface, using a spatula or finger. Soak the casts in clear slurry water prior to this step, and take care to wipe away all excess plaster after the voids are filled.

Marks from the coarse abrasive wheel can be removed from the cast bases with fine wet or dry sand paper (used wet) on a sanding block. Alternatively, a large fine Arkansas stone works well for this purpose. The heel and corner cuts of both casts should be smoothed simultaneously with the casts in proper occlusion. Sharp edges formed where the anatomic and base portions meet may be trimmed with a plaster knife.

After the casts have been allowed to dry thor-

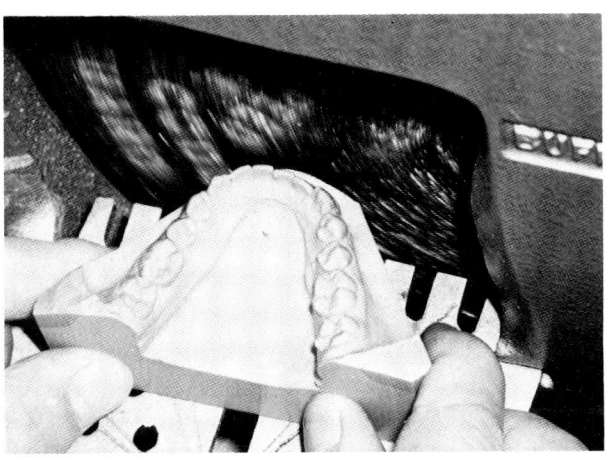

**Fig. 20-152.** Anterior cut on mandibular cast is rounded to parallel anterior arch form.

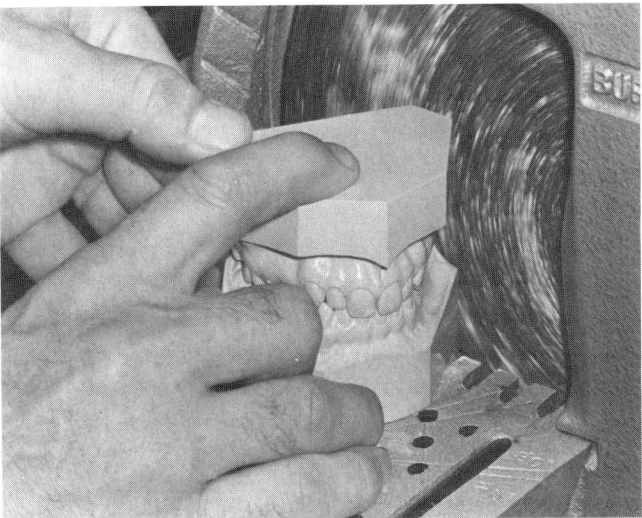

**Fig. 20-153.** Corner cuts are made at 120 degrees to heel cuts with casts articulated.

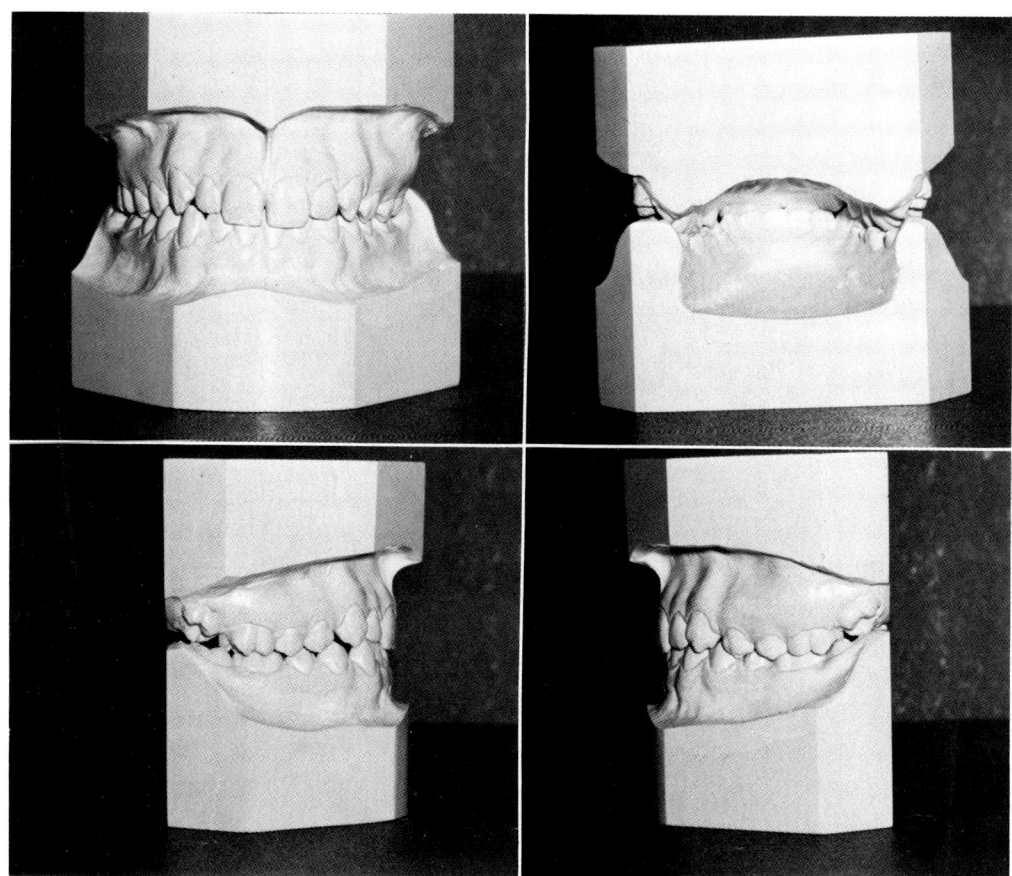

**Fig. 20-154.** Views of completed diagnostic casts.

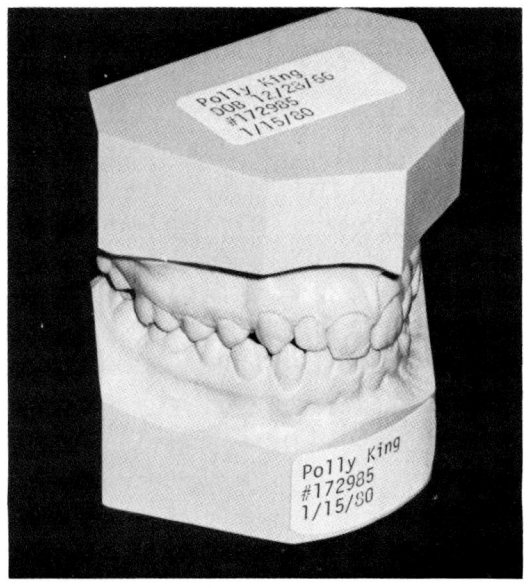

**Fig. 20-155.** Diagnostic casts are usually labeled with appropriate identifying information.

oughly, they may be immersed in clear liquid soap for about 30 minutes and rinsed and polished with a soft cloth to a high gloss. Fig. 20-154 depicts different views of the finished casts. Finally, the casts are usually identified with labels indicating such information as the patient's name, age, record or file number, and the date the impressions were taken (Fig. 20-155).

### PROBLEM AREAS

Most problems associated with the preparation of diagnostic casts arise from inadequate base pours, damaging anatomic portions of casts during trimming, or errors in the angulation or length of the different cuts. Careful planning and meticulous technique will minimize the occurrence of these problems (Table 20-10).

### SUMMARY

This chapter presents a relatively simple and efficient technique for the production of esthetic and

**Table 20-10.** Preparation of diagnostic casts

| Problem | Probable cause | Solution |
| --- | --- | --- |
| Inadequate material to finish bases properly | Not enough plaster used when impressions were poured, or too much plaster removed when periphery was rough trimmed | Add plaster to cast base in deficient areas |
| Fracturing or otherwise damaging teeth during trimming procedures | Wax bite registration not used whenever casts are occluded | Trim casts without wax bite if none is available, but use extreme care |
| | Plaster not allowed to harden completely | Allow sufficient time for plaster to set before beginning trimming procedures |
| | Abrasive wheel is dull and/or out of balance and vibrating | Replace wheel |
| | Casts are water soaked | Allow casts to dry, and avoid saturating with water during trimming procedure |
| Asymmetrically finished bases | Improper trimming angles or differing lengths of corresponding cuts that should be equal | Correct minor errors by appropriate trimming; correct major errors by taking impression of anatomic portions and repouring casts |

diagnostically accurate study casts. With some modification the method may be adapted to various types of cast trimmers.

### REFERENCE

Sim, S. M.: Minor tooth movement in children, ed. 2, St. Louis, 1977, The C. V. Mosby Co.

### BIBLIOGRAPHY

Finn, S. L.: Clinical pedodontics, ed. 4, Philadelphia, 1973, W. B. Saunders Co.

Graber, T. M.: Orthodontics—principles and practice, ed. 3, Philadelphia, 1972, W. B. Saunders Co.

McDonald, R. E.: Dentistry for the child and adolescent, ed. 3, St. Louis, 1978, The C. V. Mosby Co.

Moyers, R. E.: Handbook of orthodontics, ed. 3, Chicago, 1973, Year Book Medical Publishers, Inc.

Thurow, R. C.: Atlas of orthodontic principles, ed. 2, St. Louis, 1977, The C. V. Mosby Co.

Tweed, C. H.: Clinical orthodontics, vol. 2, St. Louis, 1966, The C. V. Mosby Co.

# CHAPTER 21

# THREE-DIMENSIONAL TEACHING AIDS

CONNIE A. REISBICK

**three dimensional visual aid** A model constructed from a suitable material for purposes of demonstration and instruction.

Commercial sources for various types of educational teaching aids are available; however, they often operate on a mass production level and may not be responsive to specific visual aid requests from individuals. As a result, visual aid companies usually market a specific line, and dentists must select from that line or develop their own construction capabilities. There are many advantages of having a fabrication facility: individual communication directly with the fabricator, changes can be made midstream, prototypes can be fabricated, duplicate models of existing teaching aids and/or prototypes can be modified, and the visual aids can often be made more economically.

Fabrication of three-dimensional teaching aids is an exciting and challenging aspect of dental education. Possibilities are virtually unlimited, and aids that can be constructed are limited only by the imagination. The ease of handling contemporary duplicating materials has made it possible to construct acceptable three-dimensional teaching aids simply and economically. In this chapter two methods for constructing flexible molds and a method of making epoxy resin models will be described.

## SILICONE ELASTOMER MOLDS

The Silastic elastomers* produce superior reproduction of master models, have a long shelf life, and are compatible with other materials used in dentistry (epoxy resin, gypsum products, acrylic resin waxes, and polyvinyl chloride). In addition, handling and mixing are easier, and there is greater batch consistency. The advantages of the Silastics for producing precise replications outweigh the disadvantage of increased cost. A significant advantage of silicones is they are color coded. Catalysts are different colors, which minimizes the possibility of using the wrong catalyst/base combination. For example, A catalyst is blue, E catalyst is clear, and J catalyst is green. Some of the catalysts and bases are interchangeable. Data brochures are available, or the dealer will furnish information on request.

### Constructing a silicone mold
*Preparing original model for silicone pouring*
**PROCEDURE**

1. Suggested instruments and materials for preparing the model are usually found in most dental offices (Figs. 21-1 to 21-3).

2. Clean the cast to be duplicated thoroughly by removing all traces of excess plaster or stone. Block out pits and holes with wax, and make the cast

---
*Dow Corning, Silastic Division, Midland, Mich.

## Three-dimensional teaching aids  635

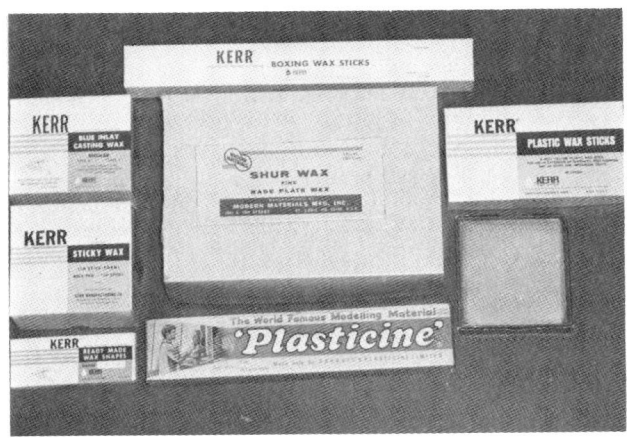

Fig. 21-1. Waxes used for constructing silicone molds.

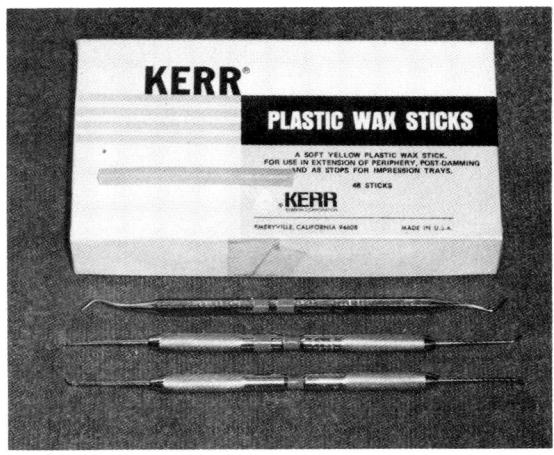

Fig. 21-2. Wax stick and carving instruments.

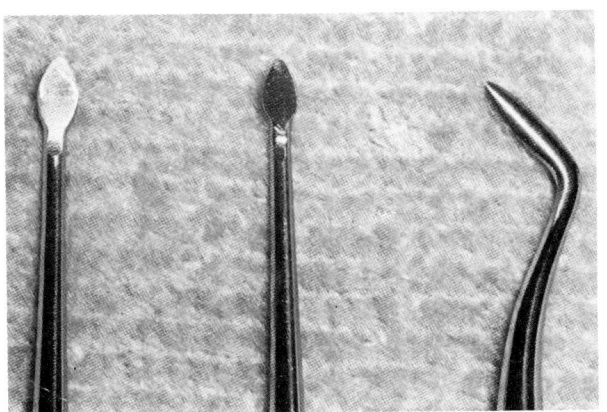

Fig. 21-3. Carvers used during fabrication of silicone molds.

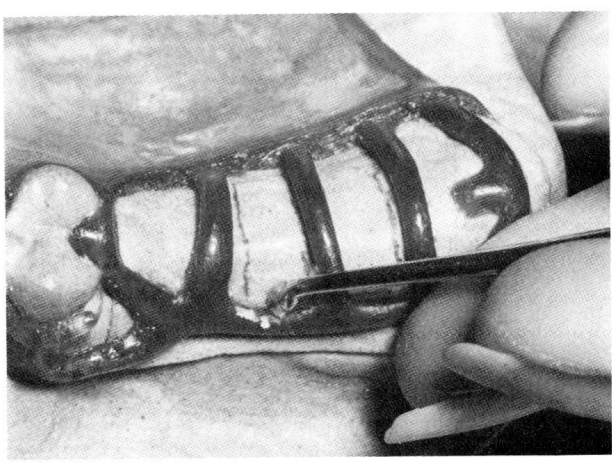

Fig. 21-4. Undercuts of removable partial denture framework wax-up are filled in prior to making silicone mold.

smooth. Remove any wax scrapings with a stream of air (Figs. 21-4 to 21-7).

3. Secure plastic type labeling* to the lower half of the boxing paper, and contour it (Figs. 21-8 and 21-9).

4. Spray stone or plaster models that are to be duplicated first with clear spray lacquer.† Three to four light coats of a clear lightweight lacquer are required.

5. It is extremely important to permit each coat to dry before applying the next coat.

6. Spray the casts evenly and lightly, taking care to cover the entire surface. Do not overspray, since

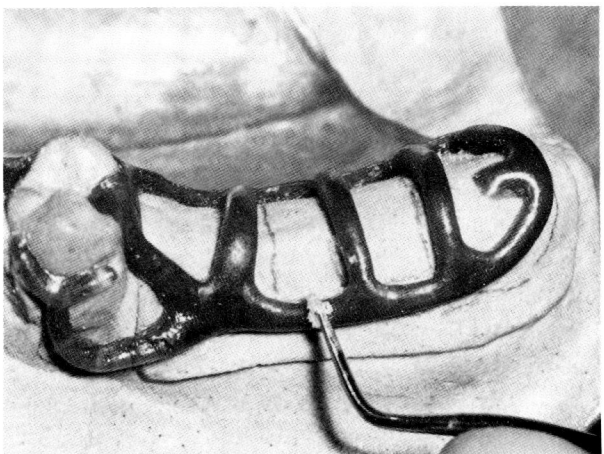

Fig. 21-5. It is important that patterns be clean and all traces of wax shavings removed.

---

*Dymo Tape Labeling Gun, Hacienda Heights, Calif.
†Pactra Clear Spray Lacquer, No. LS20, Pactra Industries, Inc., Los Angeles, Calif.

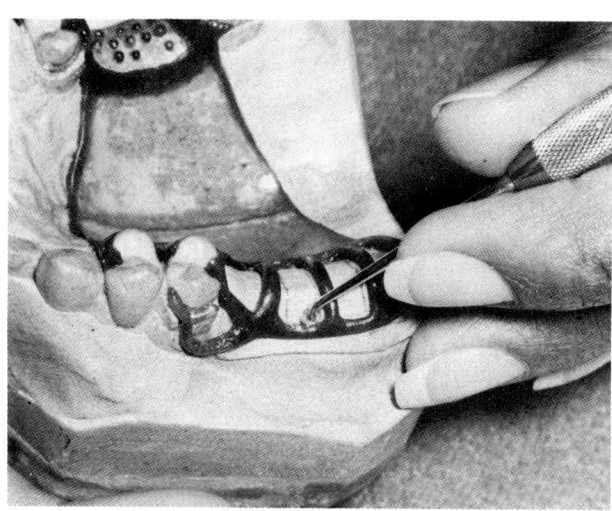

Fig. 21-6. Cleoid carver used to make sharp wax borders.

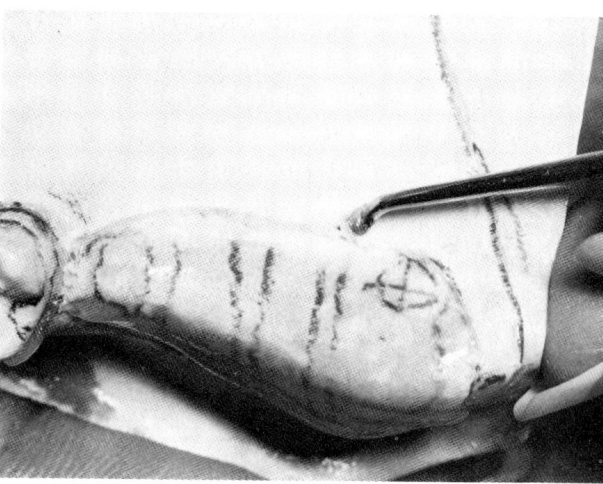

Fig. 21-7. Finish lines on model to be duplicated also must be sharp.

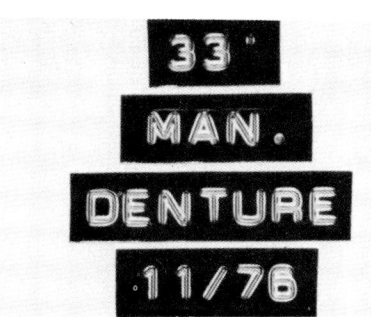

Fig. 21-8. Plastic labeling tape can be placed on lower half of boxing paper to identify resultant mold.

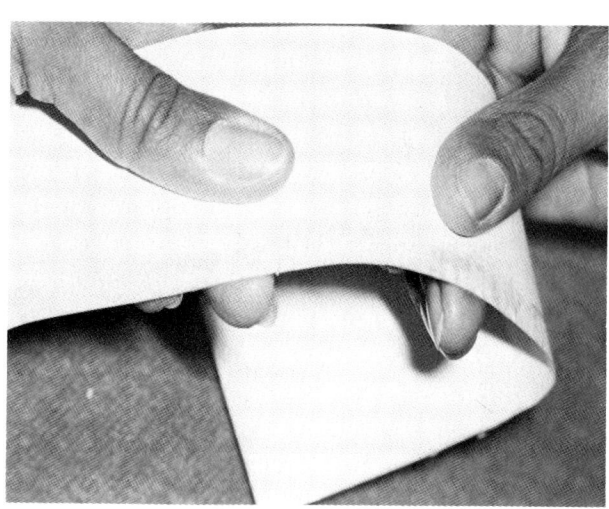

Fig. 21-9. Boxing paper is contoured to appropriate size.

pooling will change the contour and result in an inaccurate mold.

7. The thoroughly dried cast should now be ready for addition of a base and boxing.

8. It is normal for the lacquer to remain somewhat tacky where added wax has been coated, even though the rest of the cast is thoroughly dry.

9. Block out all undercuts with wax, and smooth them before spraying with lacquer.

### Base and boxing for silicone mold
**PROCEDURE**

1. Secure the sprayed cast to a cardboard base* with white Wilhold† glue. Only models made of gypsum materials are sprayed (Fig. 21-10).

---

*Crescent Poster Board, No. 601, white, 28 × 44, art supply stores.
†Wilhold Glues, Inc., Santa Fe Springs, Calif.

## Three-dimensional teaching aids 637

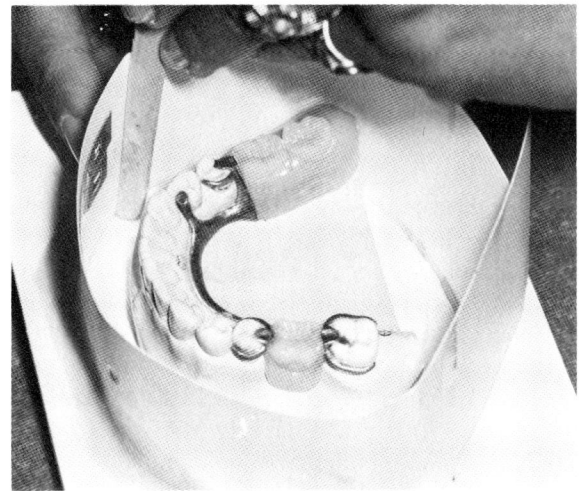

**Fig. 21-10.** Sprayed cast is cemented to cardboard base with white glue. It is important also to leave ¼- to ½- inch (10.6- to 1.3-cm) space between paper boxing and cast to be duplicated.

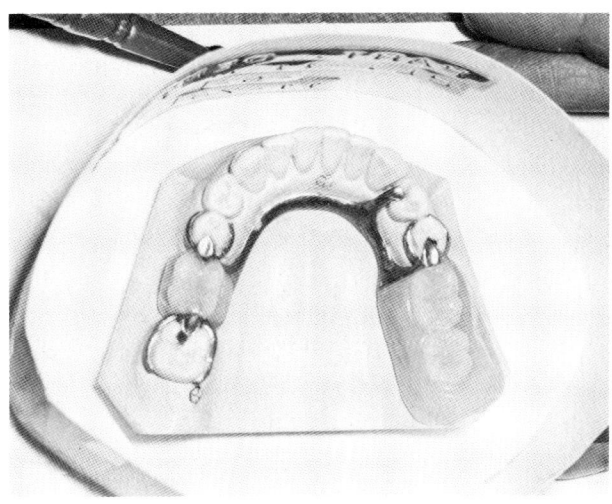

**Fig. 21-11.** Boxing paper is contoured to allow ¼- to ½-inch (0.6- to 1.3-cm) space between cast and boxing.

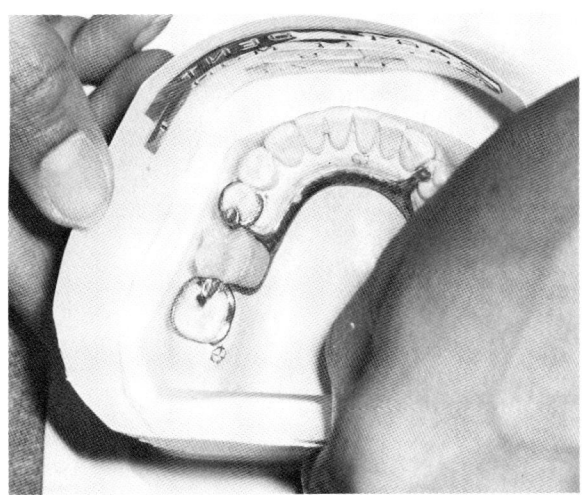

**Fig. 21-12.** Boxing paper is joined and overlapped at rear of cast.

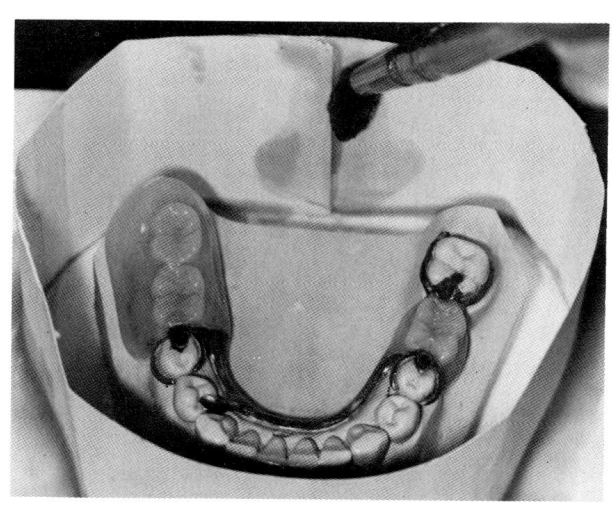

**Fig. 21-13.** Boxing paper is secured with hot liquefied wax using brush.

2. Use heavy paper* to box the mold, leaving ¼- to ½-inch (0.6- to 1.3-cm) space between the paper and cast. Wax-up wax† may be occasionally used for boxing. Time and experience will indicate which is more effective (Fig. 21-10).

*Strathmore Drawing Board, No. 72, white, 23 × 29, art supply stores.
†Miners Wax, S.S. White Dental Products, Philadelphia, Pa.

3. Form a boxing around the cast to be duplicated, following its contours. Use heavy paper, and seal it in place with hot wax with a thick brush, such as a No. 8 or 10 sable brush (Figs. 21-11 to 21-13).

4. Be certain that boxing paper is sealed securely prior to pouring the mold. The seal should be watertight to prevent leakage.

5. Construct the boxing so that it extends

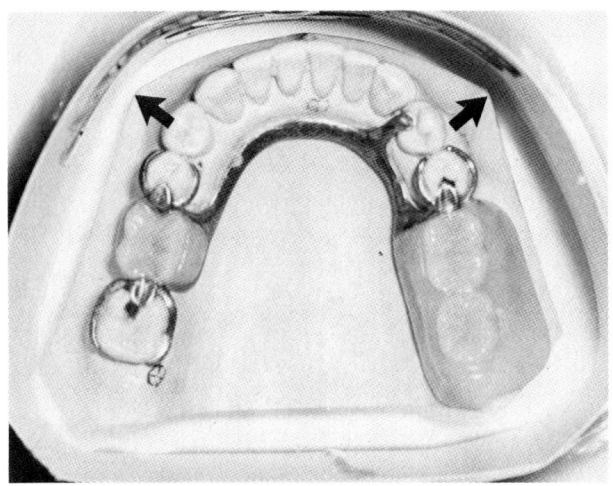

**Fig. 21-14.** Boxing paper adapted and sealed. Note there should be at least ¼-inch (0.6-cm) space between cast and boxing paper at narrowest point (arrows).

1½ inches (3.8 cm) above the highest point of the cast to be duplicated. Be sure that boxing paper is not closer than ¼ inch (0.6 cm) to the sides of cast base (Fig. 21-14).

6. Reinforce the larger cast boxing with wax strips. Secure the reinforcing wax to the paper and around the base about three fourths of the distance from the base (Figs. 21-15 to 21-18).

7. Form a bridge with cellophane tape or wax strips across the top of the boxing. These bridges are placed at stress points to minimize distortion of the mold during pouring and also resultant excess use of model material (Figs. 21-37 and 21-38).

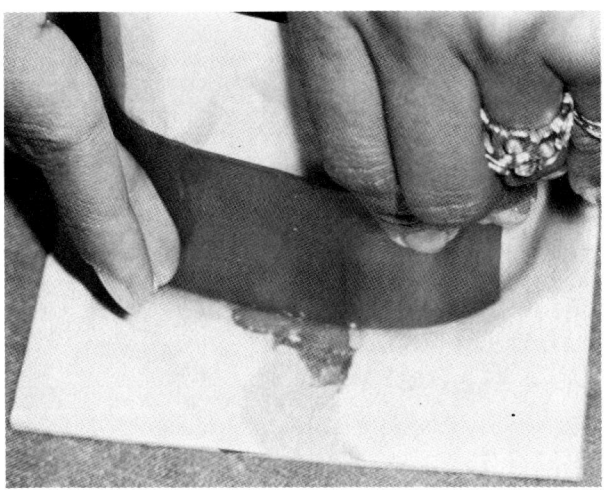

**Fig. 21-15.** Boxing wax can be used to reinforce paper boxing.

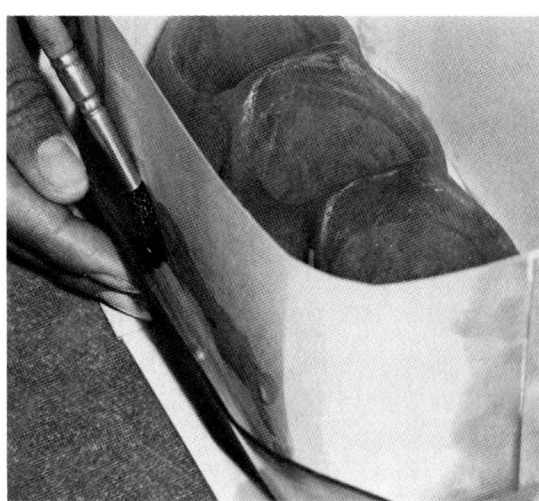

**Fig. 21-16.** Liquefied wax is painted onto boxing paper and boxing wax adapted to it.

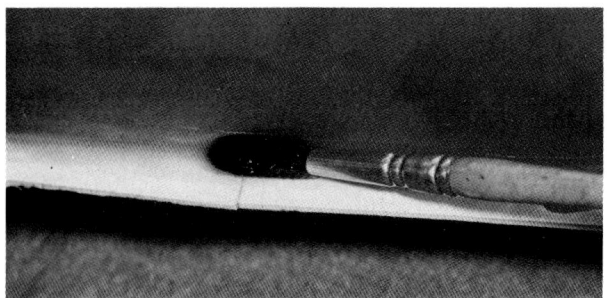

**Fig. 21-17.** Boxing wax strip is sealed with liquefied wax and brush along lower border.

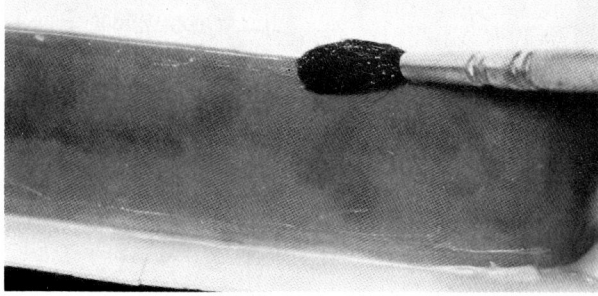

**Fig. 21-18.** Upper border of boxing wax is sealed to paper with brush and liquefied wax.

## Mixing Silastic mold material
**PROCEDURE**

1. Materials used to construct the molds are catalyst No. 1 RTV* and Silastic base RTV 3110* (Fig. 21-19).

2. Weigh the mixing container on a triple beam balance (Fig. 21-20).

3. Pour desired volume of Silastic base RTV 3110 into the container on the balance. Use a sufficient volume of Silastic base to fill the mold. This can best be determined through experience (Fig. 21-21).

4. Add the required amount of catalyst No. 1 RTV in the ratio of 10 gm of catalyst to 100 gm of the base material (Fig. 21-21).

---

*Dow Corning Corp., Silastic Division, Midland, Mich.

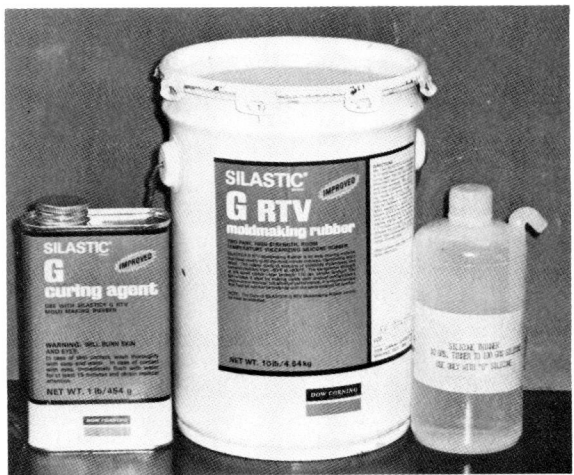

**Fig. 21-19.** Silastic RTV moldmaking rubber used for making flexible molds.

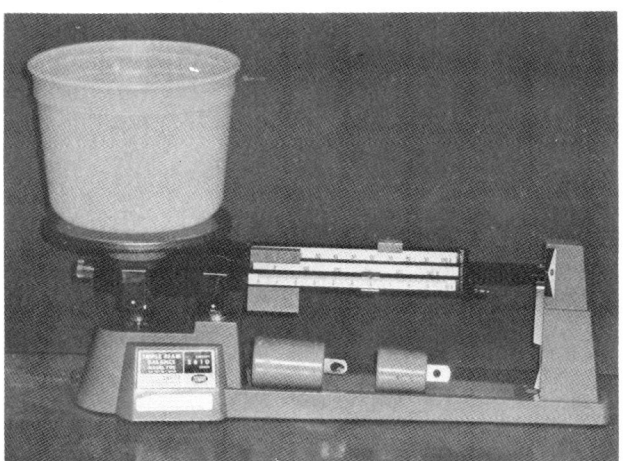

**Fig. 21-20.** Prior to proportioning silicone mold material, weigh mixing container on scale.

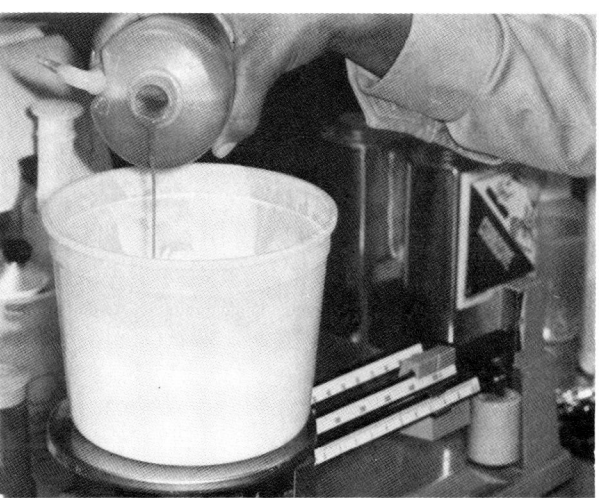

**Fig. 21-21.** Components are carefully proportioned by weight.

5. Spatulate the catalyst and base with a spatula* for approximately 60 seconds, taking care to scrape around the outer walls of the mixing material to assure complete incorporation of the catalyst and base (Figs. 21-22 to 21-24). A counterrotating electric mixer† is useful for mixing the material. Do not, however, mix longer than 2 minutes. Materials can be mixed by hand if an electric mixer is not available.

6. Using the 10 gm of catalyst to 100 gm of base ratio, the resultant mixture will require from 18 to 24 hours to set.

7. Thoroughly clean the lid, rim, and outer can of the materials prior to storing.

8. Never dip the used base mixing spatula into the catalyst container, or vice versa, because this will contaminate the materials.

### Silastic vacuum and pour methods
PROCEDURE

1. When pouring the silicone into the boxed mold, pour the silicone from one point only, permitting material to flow and fill around the boxed cast. Continue filling the mold until the level reaches the cervical line of the teeth on the boxed cast (Fig. 21-25).

2. Place the poured mold under a bell jar,* and reduce the atmospheric pressure.† Watch carefully that the material does not overflow the paper boxing. *Never* apply pressure to the top or sides of the jar during the vacuuming procedure (Fig. 21-26).

3. Striking the vacuum table base and/or releasing the vacuum will help prevent the mold material from overflowing (Figs. 21-27 to 21-29).

4. Release the vacuum, and remove the vacuumed model from the bell jar.

5. Place the container of remaining material under the bell jar and vacuum as described previously.

6. The material being vacuumed will bubble and rise quite rapidly, then fall back, and rise and fall again, gradually decreasing in height. After it has fallen back, continue vacuuming another 30 seconds.

7. Release the vacuum, remove the container, and finish pouring the boxed mold. Again pour silicone material into the mold from one point only, and place it aside for overnight setting.

8. An alternate method is simply to vacuum the entire mass of material as directed, and then pour directly into the boxed mold. The material is added at one point and permitted to flow and fill from only

---

*Buffalo dental spatula, Buffalo Dental Manufacturing Co., Inc., Brooklyn, N.Y.
†Brookfield Engineering Laboratory, Inc., Stoughton, Mass.

*Bell jar, 12 × 12; vacuum plate and mat, 356-14; plate/355-14 mat; Dick Ellis Co., Los Angeles, Calif.
†Vacuum pump. Duo-Seal, Van Waters & Rogers, Los Angeles, Calif.

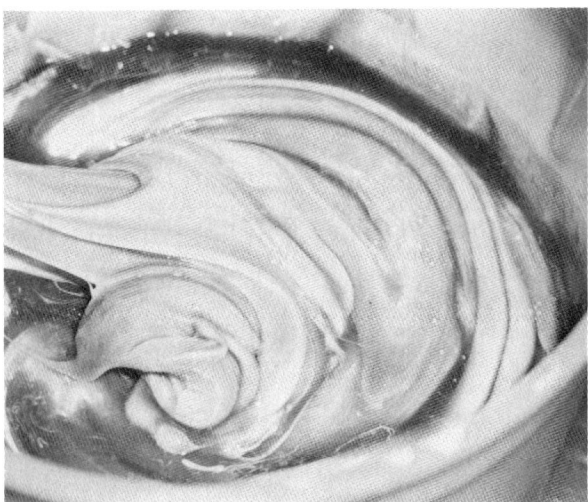

**Fig. 21-22.** Incorporated material is spatulated thoroughly to minimize noncatalization of some of material.

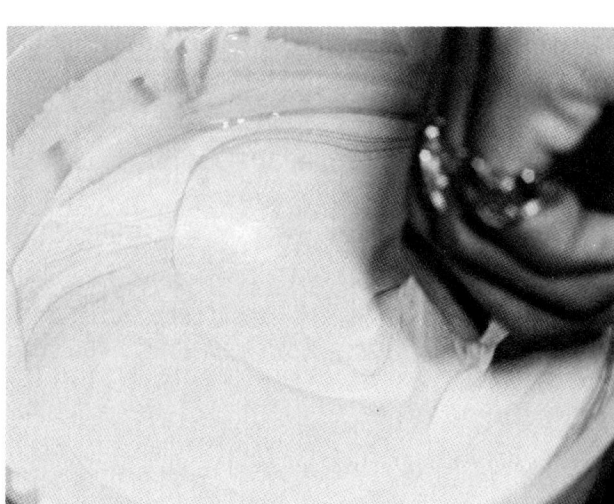

**Fig. 21-23.** Smooth mix of uniform color indicates that mold material has been thoroughly mixed with catalyst material.

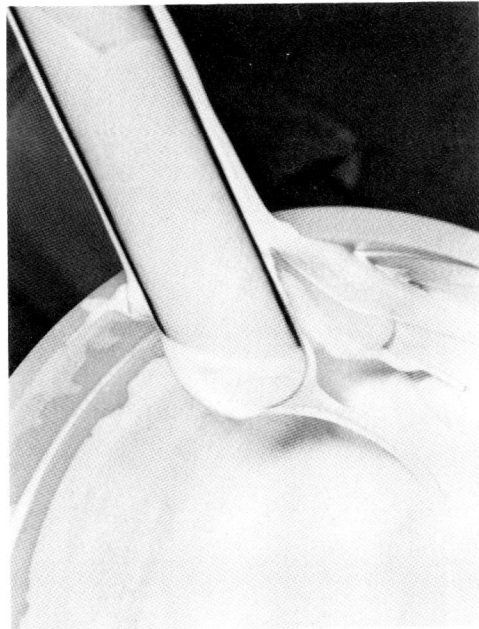

**Fig. 21-24.** Be sure to scrape inside of container to ensure that base and catalyst materials are well mixed.

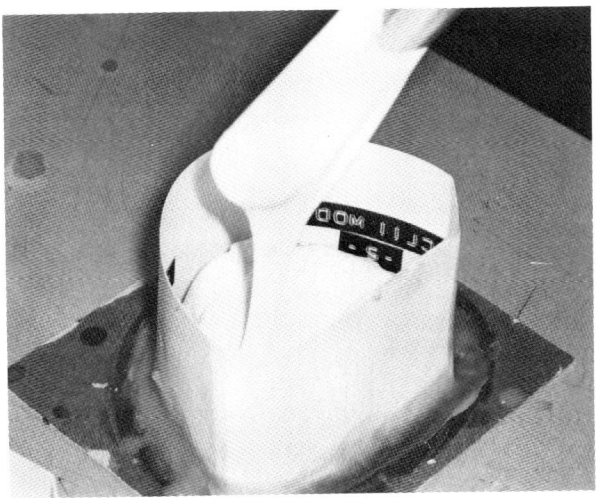

**Fig. 21-25.** Fill mold slowly from one point to level of cervical line on teeth of boxed cast.

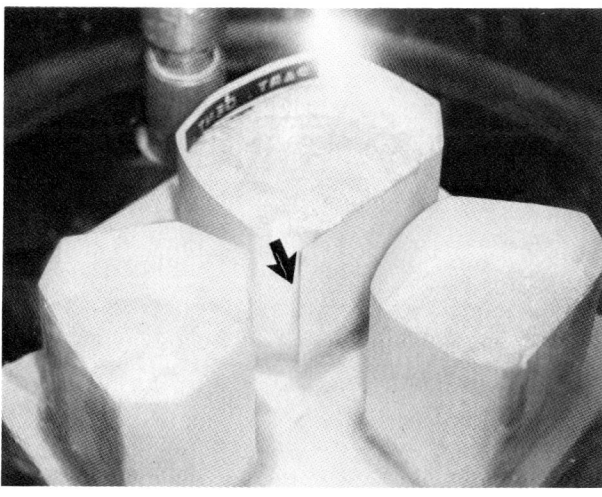

**Fig. 21-26.** Material will bubble vigorously when pressure is reduced in bell jar. Note mold boxing has been reinforced in center mold (arrow).

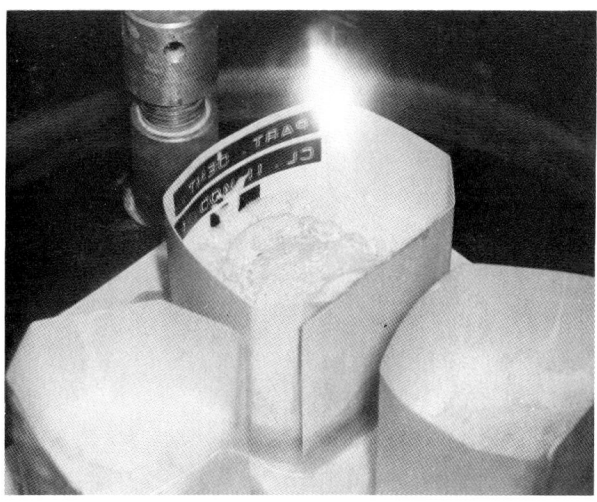

**Fig. 21-27.** Silicone material has fallen back as result of striking vacuum table base or releasing vacuum momentarily.

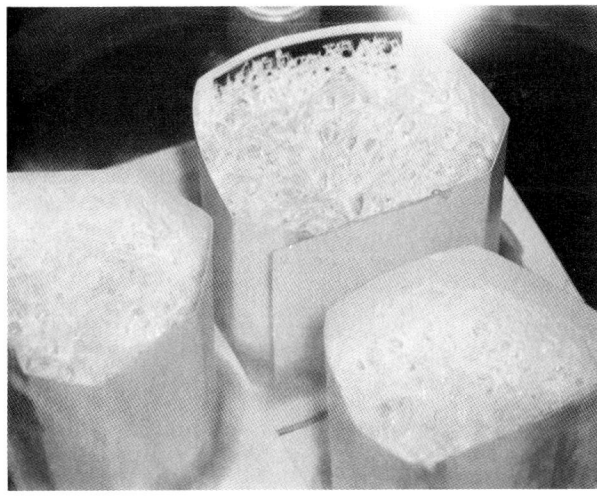

**Fig. 21-28.** Material begins to rise again and bubble vigorously.

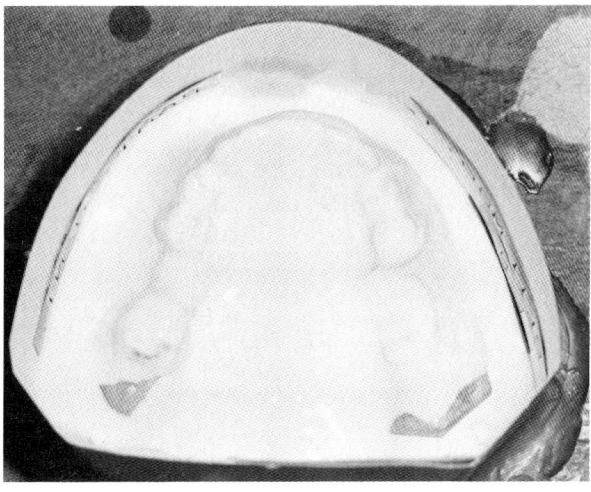

**Fig. 21-29.** After removing from bell jar, cast is covered with smooth mix of silicone material with few air inclusions.

one point. This method is not recommended if the boxed cast has severe undercuts.

9. Figs. 21-30 and 21-31 show the completed silicone mold and cast that is duplicated.

10. Alternate methods may be used for boxing as indicated in Figs. 21-32 to 21-41.

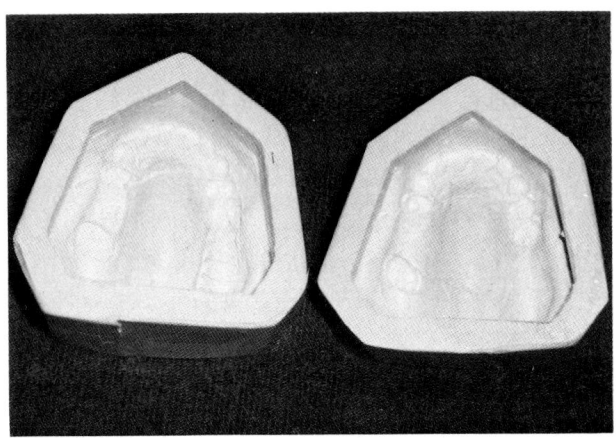

**Fig. 21-30.** Completed silicone molds are flexible and can be used to produce models from variety of materials.

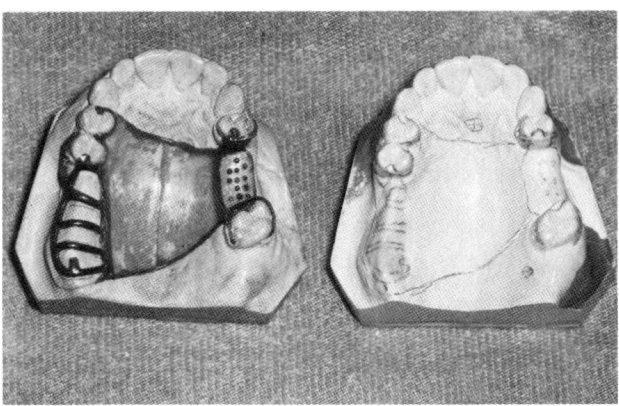

**Fig. 21-31.** Casts that were used to construct silicone molds. In this situation they are removable partial denture framework demonstration casts.

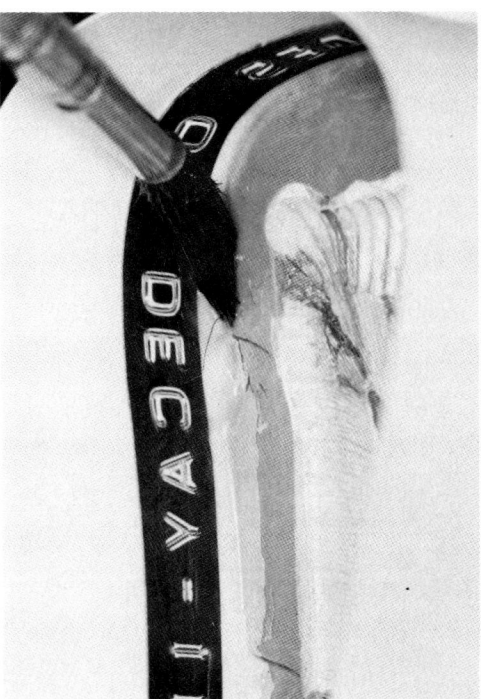

**Fig. 21-32.** Various models can be duplicated with silicone materials. Here section of molar tooth is being boxed for two-part mold.

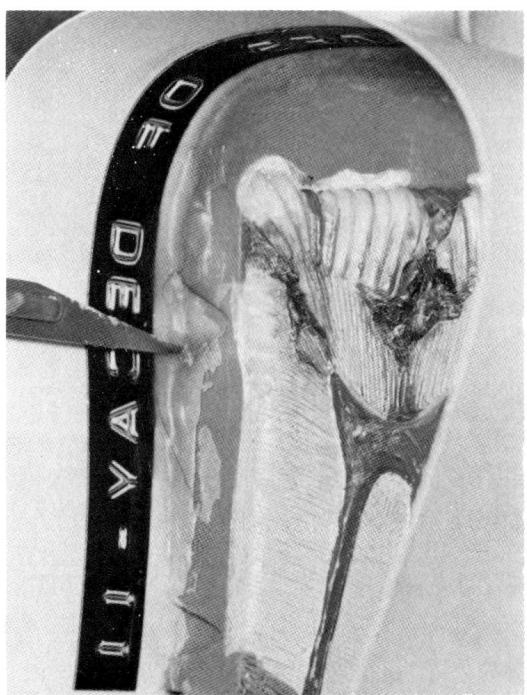

**Fig. 21-33.** Boxing wax is sealed to cardboard boxing and trimmed smooth.

Three-dimensional teaching aids **643**

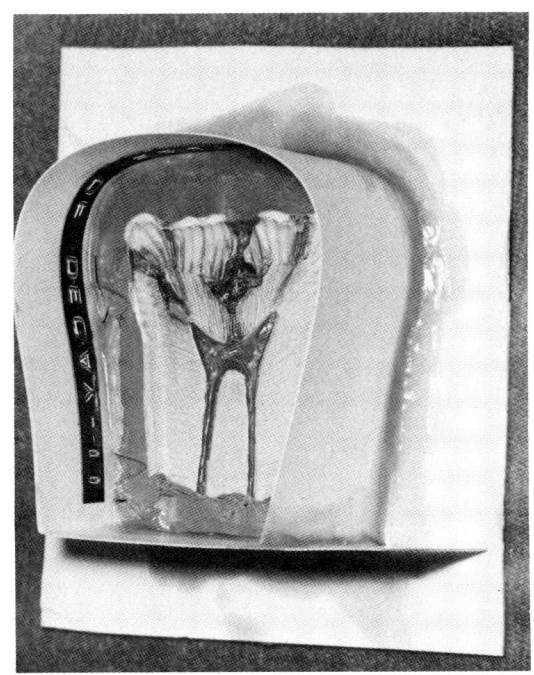

**Fig. 21-34.** Model boxed and ready to pour.

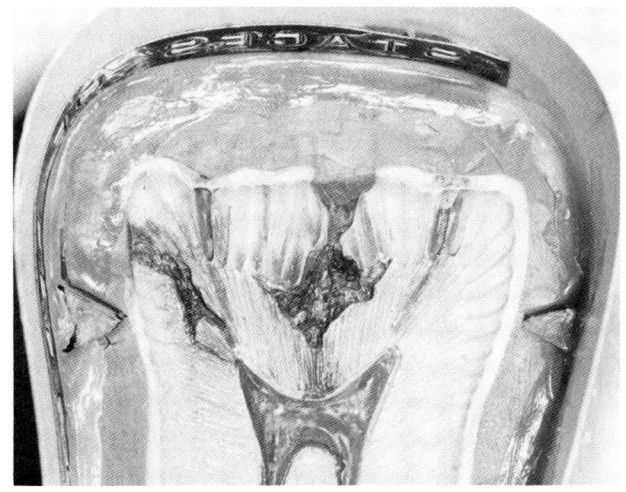

**Fig. 21-35.** Closeup of interior of boxed model. Note keyed notches for two-part mold.

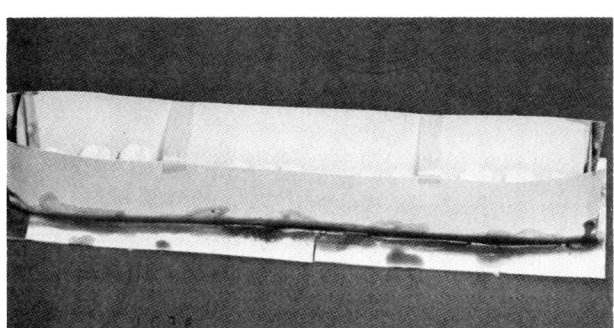

**Fig. 21-36.** Group of teeth being boxed in preparation of making flexible mold.

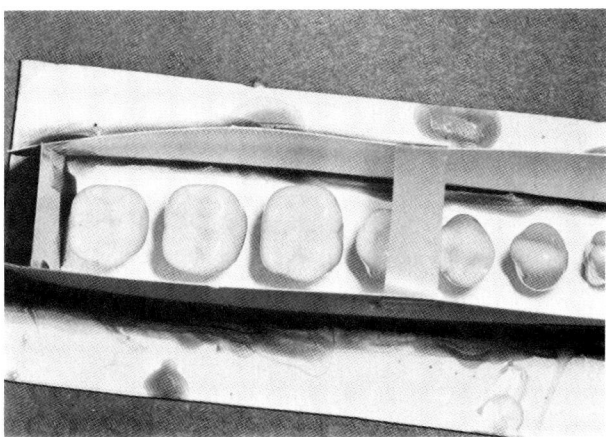

**Fig. 21-37.** Mold is reinforced across top with cellophane tape to prevent distortion.

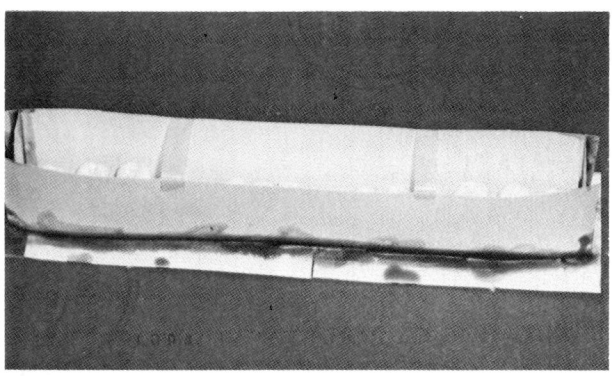

Fig. 21-38. Mold reinforced and ready to pour.

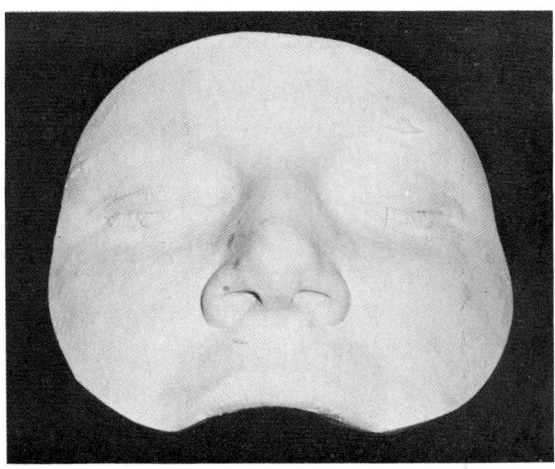

Fig. 21-39. Maxillofacial models can also be duplicated.

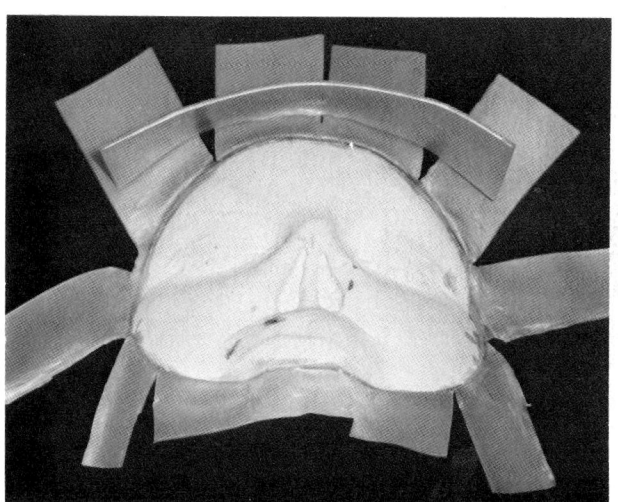

Fig. 21-40. Model being prepared for boxing.

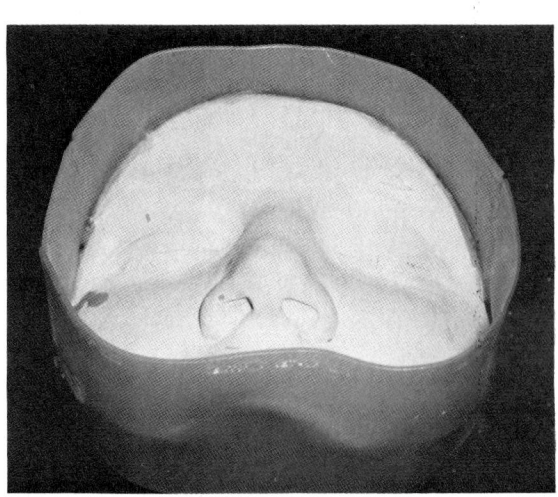

Fig. 21-41. Boxed model ready for construction of silicone mold.

### PROBLEM AREAS

Following are the principal problems associated with the construction of silicone molds: material does not set and remains tacky, mold material sticks to cast, and mold material leaks from the boxing (Table 21-1). Careful attention when proportioning and mixing the catalyst, coating the master cast with lacquer, and sealing the boxing paper with hot wax will significantly reduce these problems.

## CONSTRUCTING EPOXY RESIN MODELS

Caution should be taken when working with ivory epoxy resins. It is important to have proper ventilation in the working area and to wear protective glasses, a face mask, a plastic apron, and gloves. Since many chemicals can be harmful if used incorrectly, it is extremely important to follow exactly the manufacturer's recommendations concerning their proper manipulation and storage.

**Table 21-1.** Silicone elastomers

| Problem | Probable cause | Solution |
|---|---|---|
| Material not thoroughly set, tacky to touch | Not enough catalyst or not thoroughly mixed; chemical reaction between wax used for boxing and material | Weigh catalyst carefully; be sure base color of catalyst can no longer be detected after mixing |
| Set silicone sticking to model when breaking out of mold | Improper lacquer coverage of master model | Apply even coverage at least three or four times |
| Leakage | Boxing paper not properly secured with hot wax, or material in large pour breaking wax seal | Wax at least three times around outer side of boxing paper and once or twice on inside; reinforce outer side of boxing paper with strip of red boxing wax when pouring large models |

Ivory epoxy resin No. RF3503* is a three-part system consisting of a base material, ivory epoxy resin No. RF3503, plus a mixture of two catalyzing chemicals, triethylene tetramine (TETA) and methane diamine (MD). The ratio of each depends on whether a large model or a small model is to be constructed. A large model is considered to be anything larger than a natural dental arch form. A small model would be somewhat less than half the size of a natural dental arch. Ratios are changed as related to the size of the model to control curing shrinkage and drawback. Following are two ratios of catalyst that are often used:

1. For large models, 30 gm of TETA to 70 gm of MD.
2. Small models, 70 gm of TETA to 30 gm of MD.

The ratio of the mixed catalyst to the epoxy resin base material is 10 gm of catalyst to 100 gm of resin for large models. The ratio of catalyst for small models is 12 gm of catalyst per 100 gm of base. Models constructed of this material may be painted with water-soluble acrylic artist's colors; however, metallic colors may also be used. The model should be thoroughly cleaned with acetone prior to painting with a metallic color. It is equally important to determine that each coat is thoroughly dry before applying another coat of either acrylic color or metallic color. This is to prevent the coats from pulling away or separating, which would produce an uneven surface. The epoxy resin cast poured into the Silastic mold is cured at room temperature.

### Preparing silicone mold for epoxy pour
**PROCEDURE**

1. Clean all inner surfaces of the silicone mold with a gentle stream of air to remove all foreign objects.
2. Clean the surface of the silicone mold with a cotton swab and acetone. Be certain that all excess acetone is removed from the mold prior to pouring the model. It is important that the mold be thoroughly cleaned and dry before pouring.
3. Molds that have been cut on one or two sides to construct a sectional mold must be secured with rubber bands prior to pouring. Two, three, four, or more may be required to maintain mold integrity. Rubber bands should be just tight enough to hold the mold together.
4. Take care that the rubber bands are not too tight around the mold. This may produce distortion, which would provide an imperfect duplication.
5. Spray the cleaned, dried, and now banded molds lightly on the interior surface with Zip Silicone Lubricant No. D5100.* Make certain the entire interior surface is covered without pooling.
6. Remove excess lubricant from the mold with a stream of air. Place the mold upside down until ready for pouring.
7. All molds must be thoroughly cleaned, dried, and sprayed before making an epoxy resin model. It is not necessary, however, that all molds be banded.
8. Store all silicone molds after use upside down on a shelf or in a box that will not confine or distort the molds.

---

*E. V. Rogerts and Associates, Culver City, Calif.

*Zip Aerosol Products, Canoga Park, Calif.

### Mixing ivory epoxy resin No. RF3503

It is extremely important that the following necessary precautions for safety be taken prior to working with epoxy resins:
1. Protective glasses must be worn.
2. A face mask must be used.
3. A plastic apron and protective gloves should be used.
4. Proper ventilation should be available.

**PROCEDURE**

1. Materials used for the epoxy resin are indicated in Fig. 21-42.
2. If more than 24 hours have elapsed, since the resin has been used, stir it thoroughly prior to use (Fig. 21-43).
3. Proportion the MD and TETA, and mix them together in glass or plastic containers. This mixing is completed prior to adding to the No. RF3503 base. Premix an extra amount of catalyst so it can be available for use if needed (Fig. 21-44).
4. Spray the silicone mold with silicone lubricant as previously described to prolong mold life, and

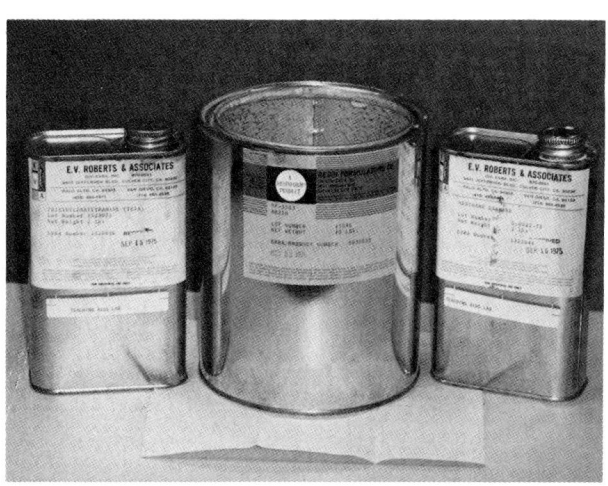

**Fig. 21-42.** Materials used for constructing epoxy resin casts.

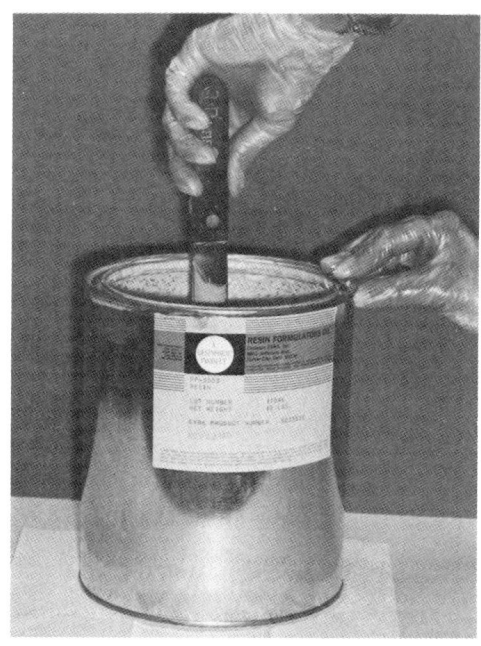

**Fig. 21-43.** Stir material thoroughly before use, particularly if it has not been used in 24 hours or longer.

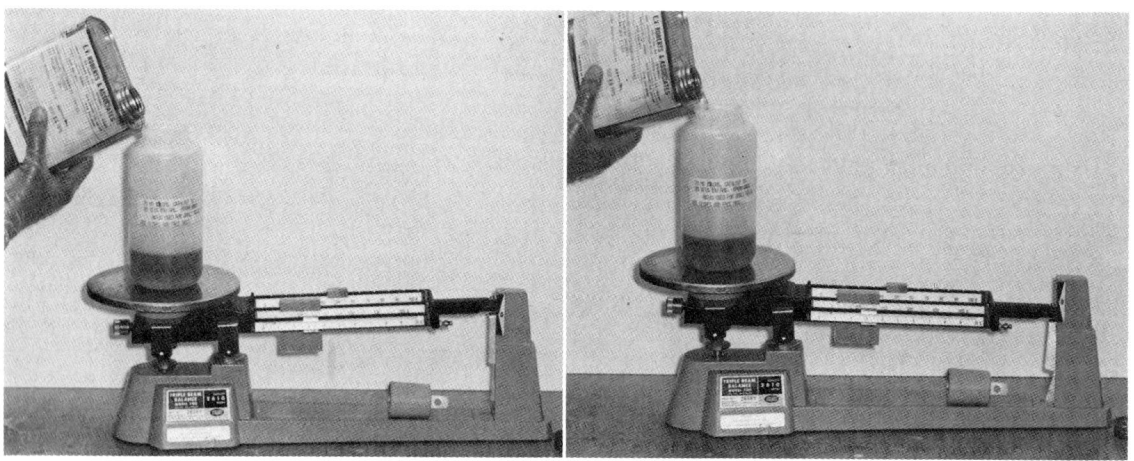

**Fig. 21-44.** Catalysts are proportioned by weight and mixed together in plastic containers prior to adding to base.

blow out the excess. Place the mold upside down until needed (Fig. 21-45).

5. The ratio of MD to TETA depends on the size of the mold being poured and whether fast or slow setting is desired: small molds, 30 MD to 70 TETA, using 12 gm of this mixture to 100 gm of the base; large molds, 70 MD to 30 TETA, using 10 gm of this mixture to 100 gm of the base.

6. To accurately determine the amount of material needed, weigh a duplicate cast if available to determine the exact amount of resin needed (Fig. 21-46). Carefully weigh a clean metal mixing container (coffee can or anesthetic Carpule can). Never use paper or cardboard cups. Paper cups absorb the catalyst and may inhibit setting of the resin (Fig. 21-47).

7. Weigh the can, and note the weight. Pour in the desired amount of epoxy base No. RF3503. Note the amount, and add the required amount of catalyst according to desired ratio and mix (Fig. 21-48).

8. Stir the No. RF3503 base and the MD-TETA catalyst mixture with a spatula. Take care to scrape the excess from around the sides of the container with a spatula.

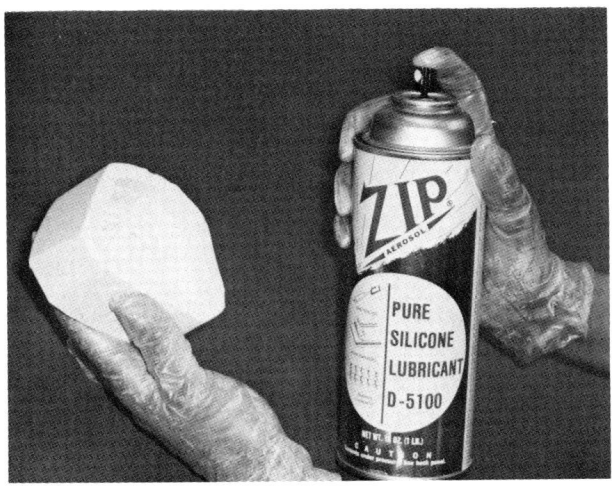

Fig. 21-45. Silicone mold is sprayed with pure silicone lubricant prior to constructing epoxy model.

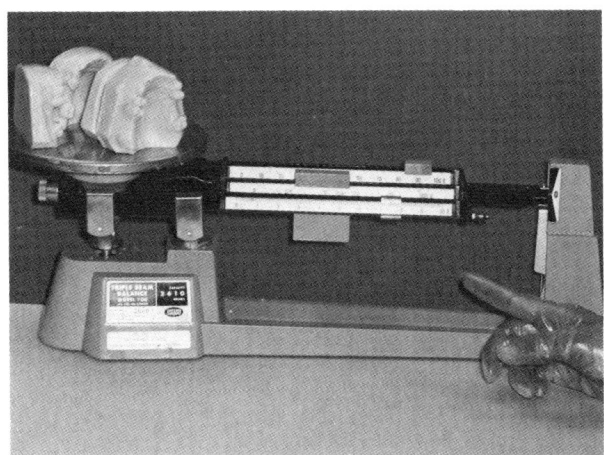

Fig. 21-46. Weighing resin models to be duplicated will help to determine volume of epoxy material required for pouring mold.

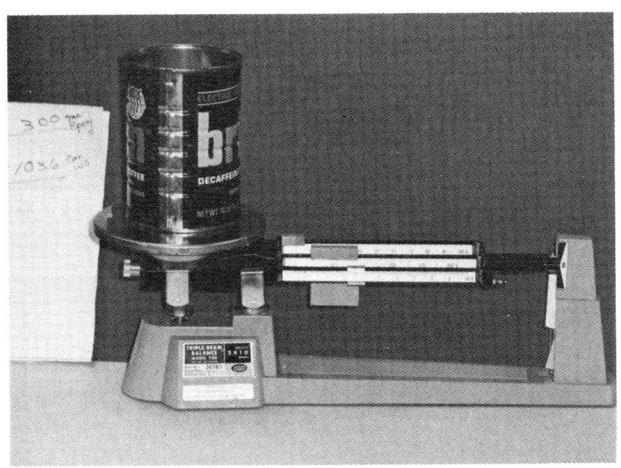

Fig. 21-47. Clean metal mixing containers such as coffee cans or anesthetic Carpule cans should be used, since they can be discarded after use.

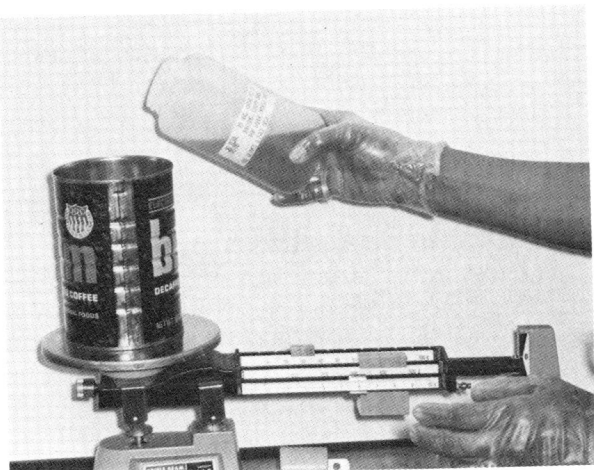

Fig. 21-48. Required amount of catalyst is proportioned by weight to assure accuracy.

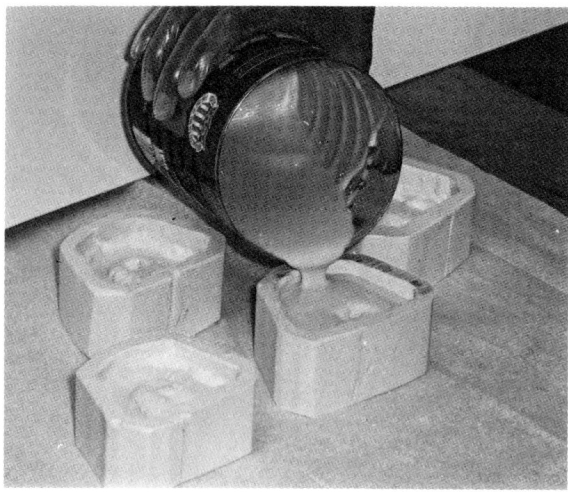

Fig. 21-49. To preclude air entrapment and resultant voids, pour material at one point on mold.

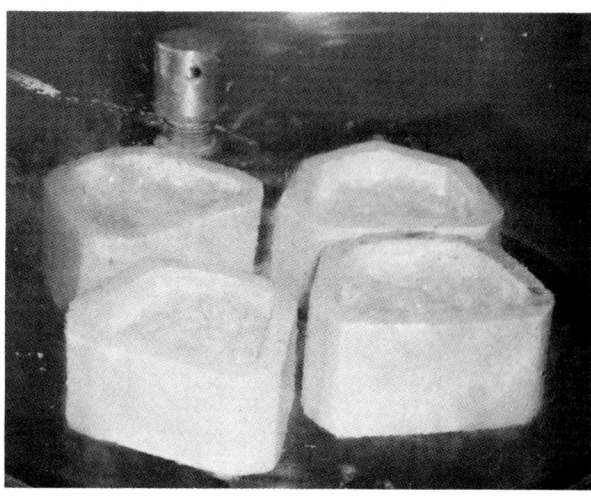

Fig. 21-50. Use care when vacuuming resin material to prevent overflow when under bell jar.

9. The base and catalyst must be thoroughly incorporated. Stir the mixture 60 to 90 seconds, prior to pouring in a prepared mold. Pour resin from one point only (Fig. 21-49).

10. Once the base and catalyst have been incorporated, setting action starts immediately. The working time depends on the quantity and ratio mixed.

11. Always mix in clean metal cans, and throw the can away after use.

12. Clean all spills and spatulas immediately following the completion of epoxy pouring. Once the material has set on any surface, it is next to impossible to remove without surface damage. Again, it is extremely important for safety to rigidly adhere to all safety precautions when using these materials. Follow the manufacturer's recommendations explicitly.

### Pouring the ivory epoxy model
#### PROCEDURE

1. Fill the prepared silicone mold to the ¼- to ½-inch (0.6- to 1.3-cm) level with the mixed epoxy resin. Pour the resin from one point, permitting the resin to flow throughout the mold (Fig. 21-49).

2. Place the partially filled mold under the bell jar as previously described, and reduce the atmospheric pressure. Observe the material carefully, since it rises rapidly and may overflow the mold (Fig. 21-50).

3. Reduce the pressure within the bell jar and note that the material will rise. A boiling-type motion with the development of small bubbles will be noted. Bubbles will become larger with rapid boiling motion, and the material will rise and fall several times. The object is to obtain a bubble-free mix.

4. Rapping the edge of the vacuum rubber mat–surfaced top will often help to prevent the epoxy from overflowing the mold. Reducing the amount of vacuum also may be necessary to prevent overflow.

5. Reduce the vacuum by opening the air valve, wait 2 to 3 seconds, close the valve, and continue the vacuuming procedure. Repeat if necessary.

6. Carefully remove the vacuumed mold from under the bell jar, and set it aside on a paper-protected surface.

7. Place the container of remaining resin material beneath the bell jar, and vacuum using steps 2, 3, and 4. Follow this procedure, and finish pouring the mold (Figs. 21-51 to 21-54).

8. The completed duplication model and mold are shown in Fig. 21-55.

9. It is important to remember to protect all working surfaces with paper, since epoxy resin is extremely difficult to remove.

10. Use at least two layers of paper beneath the molds, which are placed aside for curing. Immediately on completing work with epoxy, clean any spillage with cotton soaked in acetone. The outer rim of the container surface and the mixing spatula should also be thoroughly cleaned with cotton and acetone. It is important to not incorporate acetone in the base material.

11. An alternate procedure for pouring the mold is to vacuum all the epoxy mixture at one time. The

## Three-dimensional teaching aids 649

**Fig. 21-51.** Remaining resin material is placed under bell jar and subjected to vacuuming procedure as previously described.

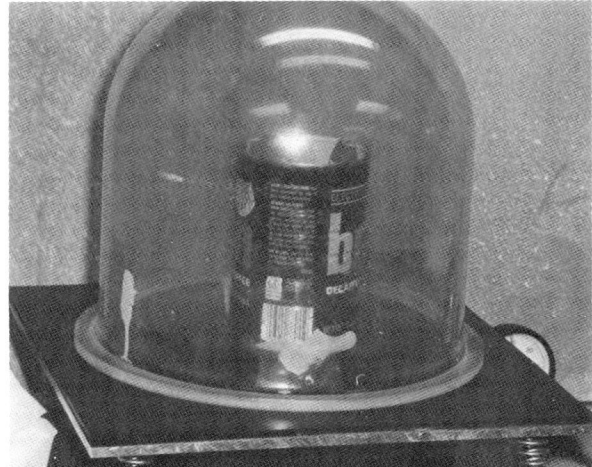

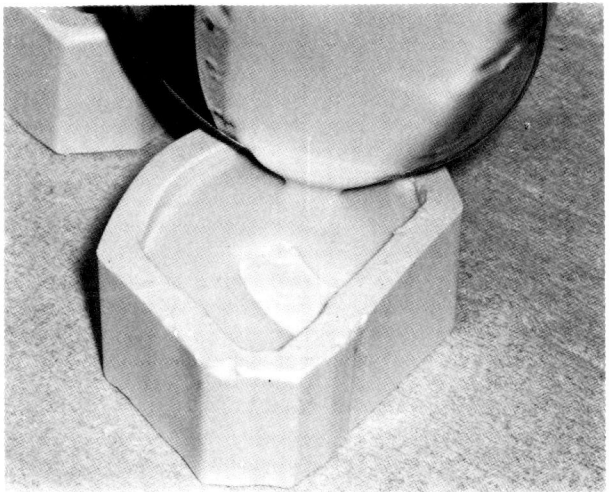

**Fig. 21-52.** Epoxy resin is poured into mold at one point on cast to permit material to flow throughout cast without forming voids.

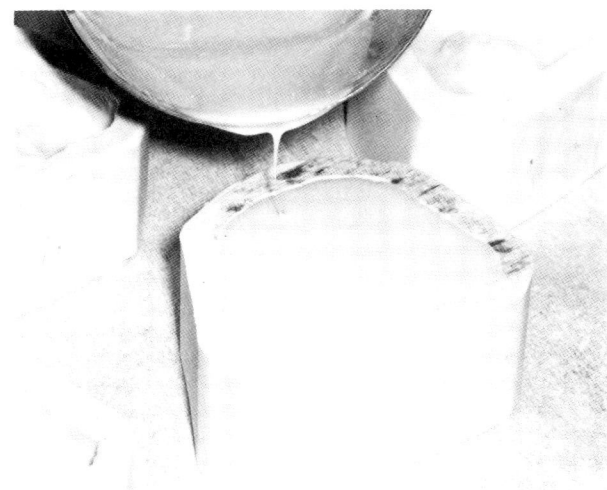

**Fig. 21-53.** Mold is completely filled with resin material.

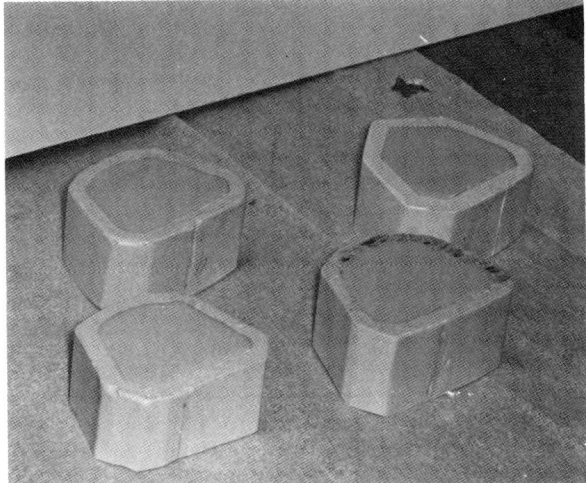

**Fig. 21-54.** Four molds have been filled with one mix of material.

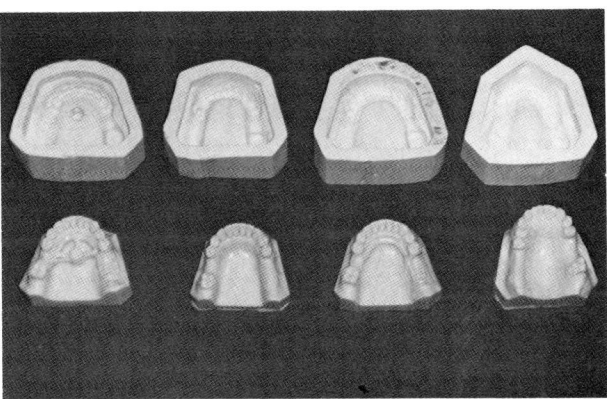

**Fig. 21-55.** Completed epoxy models after removing from silicone molds ready to be cleaned and painted.

**Table 21-2.** Epoxy resins

| Problem | Probable cause | Solution |
| --- | --- | --- |
| Mobility of set model; material not setting | Not enough catalyst or incorrect ratio used | Weigh catalyst carefully; check material before starting to work |
| Voids in set model | Improper vacuuming | Use enough pressure with pump; use proper seal between baseplate and bell jar |
| Cracking of copper epoxy model | Oven too hot or model too cold | Preheat model in oven at lower temperature for 1 hour or more; reset temperature, and allow cast to heat with oven |

mold is then poured with this mix of resin. Time and experience will indicate the preferred method of the individual technician.

12. The setting time will be 8 to 12 hours for small molds and 18 to 24 hours for large molds.

### PROBLEM AREAS

The principal problems associated with pouring epoxy models are as follows: the resin fails to set properly, voids are present in the duplicated model, and the model cracks (Table 21-2). Catalysts should be weighed accurately to facilitate the set, and resin should be vacuumed to prevent voids in the duplicated model. The oven-curing temperature and procedure should be closely monitored to avoid cracking the model.

## POLYVINYLCHLORIDE ELASTOMERS

Polyvinylchloride (PVC)* is a heat-cured material. It is a one-component system in that no chemical catalyst is required. Heat is used to cure the resin. Viscosities of PVC range from water thin to the thickness of paste. The PVC elastomers are cured at temperatures ranging from 200° F (93.5° C) to as much as 375° F (190.5° C). Curing can be accomplished in any of a number of standard heat-cure ovens. The Thelco model 28,† which is a larger oven, and the Thelco 16 or 19 are adequate for curing this material. Hardness and resiliency will vary with the specific PVC formulas, and dimensional change appears to be minimal.

The three PVC formulas discussed for reproduction of three-dimensional teaching aids in dentistry are PK5482FC, green; PK5483FC, green; and PK5484FC, green. PK5482FC is the most flexible, and PK5484FC is much harder and rigid. Other PVC elastomers are available, but for the purposes of three-dimensional visual aids, these three are well suited. PVC resins come in a variety of colors, including clear. The materials described here are industrial materials; however, medical grades are also available.

### Fabricating PVC duplicating molds
#### PROCEDURE

1. Construct a master silicone mold of the cast that is to be duplicated. The method for this has been described in the discussion on constructing a silicone mold (Fig. 21-55). It is important to remember that the silicone mold must be sprayed with a silicone lubricant before using with epoxy resin (Fig. 21-56).
2. Make a copper epoxy duplicate model of the master model. The silicone master mold is used for this purpose.
3. The copper epoxy model becomes the master model for fabrication of a PVC mold.
4. Materials used in order are: base—ivory epoxy No. RF3503 with Copper Fleck* and catalyst, which is the MD-TETA combination (Figs. 21-57 and 21-58).

---

*GCA/Precision Scientific Group, Chicago, Ill.
†Chemical Products Corp., Valencia, Calif.

*Nontarnish epoxy-coated sparkles, 0.008 x 0.00045-inch square; Copper AMP No. 49558, Atlantic Powder Metals, Inc., N. Y.

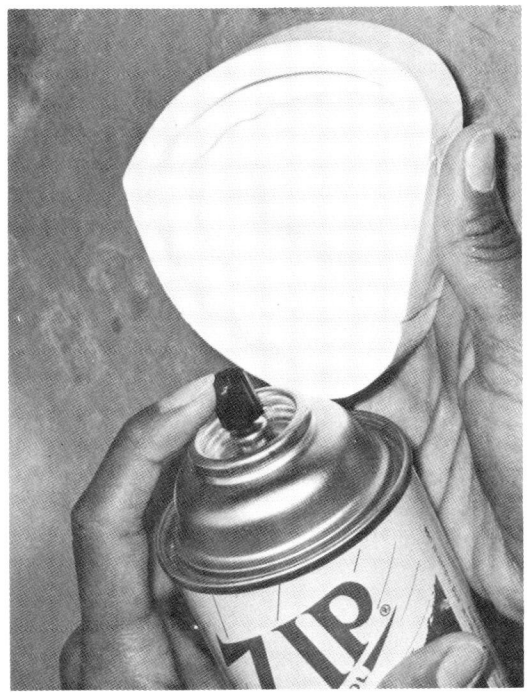

Fig. 21-56. Silicone mold is coated with silicone lubricant.

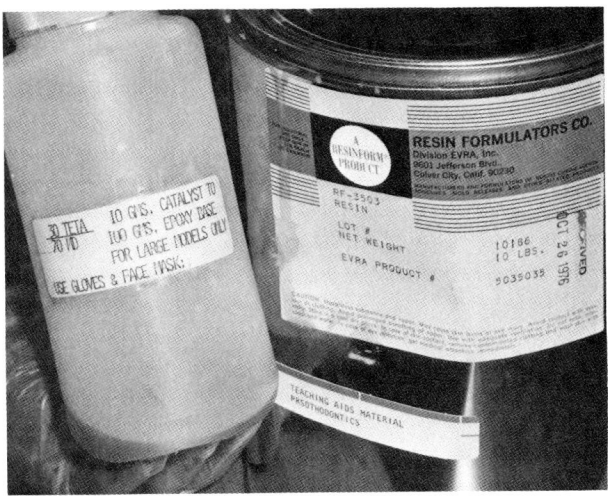

Fig. 21-57. Epoxy resin material used to fabricate master model.

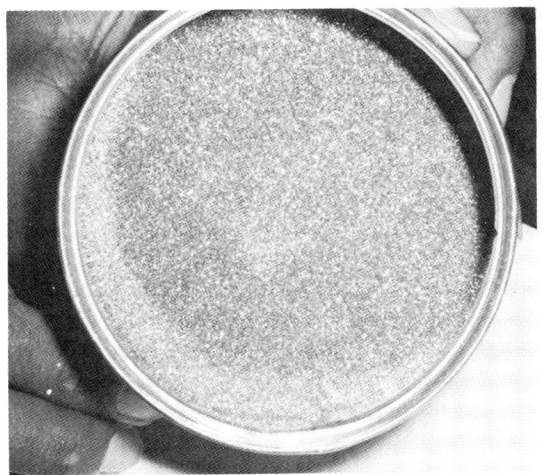

Fig. 21-58. Copper flecks that will be incorporated in epoxy resin material.

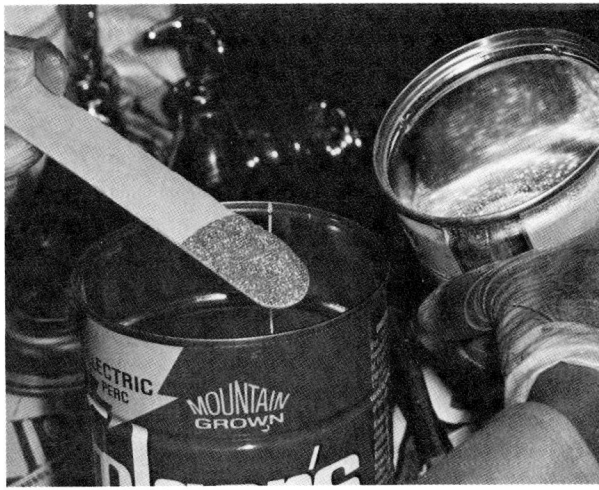

Fig. 21-59. Copper flecks being added to epoxy resin material before adding catalyst.

## Fabrication of copper epoxy models for PVC duplicating molds

### PROCEDURE

1. Mix and pour the material in the same manner as described for the ivory epoxy resin. The only difference is the addition of Copper Fleck to the base material before adding the catalyst. This should be incorporated prior to adding the required amount of catalyst to the entire mixture (Fig. 21-59).

2. The ratio of copper epoxy fleck is 10 gm to 100 gm of ivory epoxy. After this has been thoroughly incorporated, add and mix the catalyst mixture.

### 652 *Dental laboratory procedures: removable partial dentures*

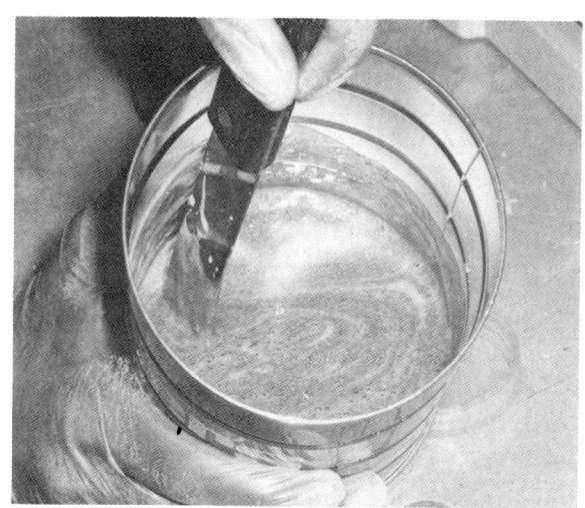

**Fig. 21-60.** Copper flecks are stirred thoroughly into epoxy resin material. Next add catalyst–MD-TETA mixture.

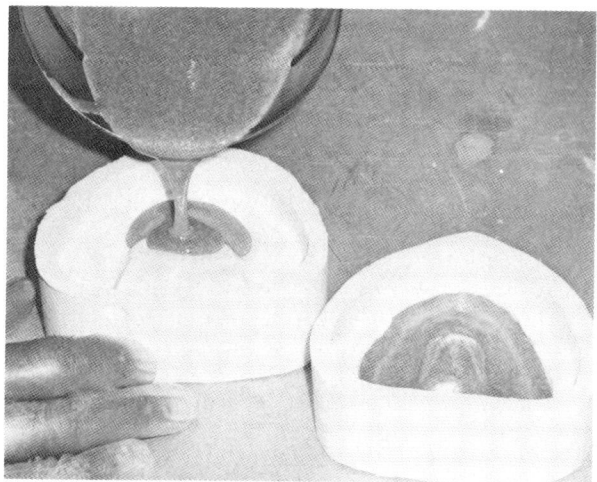

**Fig. 21-61.** Material has been vacuumed as previously described and is poured into mold.

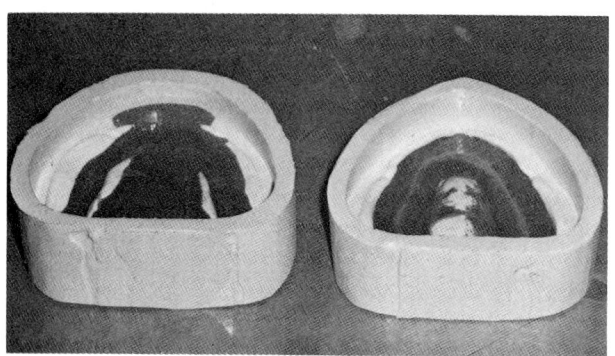

**Fig. 21-62.** Epoxy resin has been poured to cover mold.

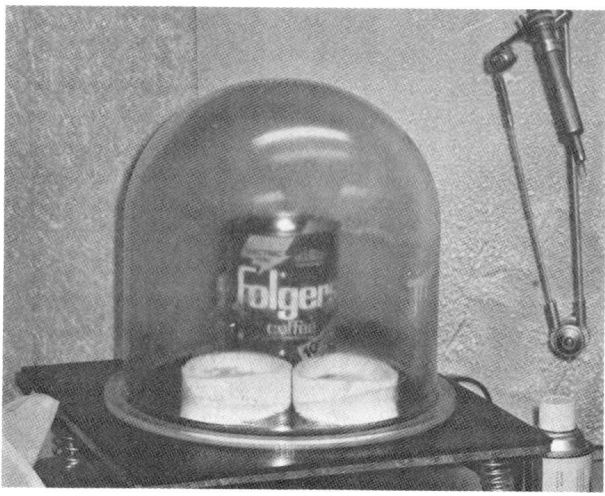

**Fig. 21-63.** Bulk of mixed resin and molds containing epoxy resin are placed in bell jar, and pressure is reduced.

Pour the resin, and vacuum as described for the ivory epoxy material (Figs. 21-60 to 21-67).

3. The material requires 24 hours to set. After setting, remove the copper model from the mold (Fig. 21-68). The copper epoxy model is placed in a cold oven for final curing. Set the oven temperature between 30° to 35° C, permitting the temperature to rise to the desired setting, and bake it before resetting the temperature for use with PVC.

4. The final curing temperature should be achieved in about 3 to 4 hours. Remove the model from the oven to cool, and store it if it is not needed immediately.

5. Never place a copper epoxy model in a hot oven without first preheating at a low temperature for 1 hour. The drastic change from room temperature to the hot oven will cause the material to crack and render it useless for duplicating.

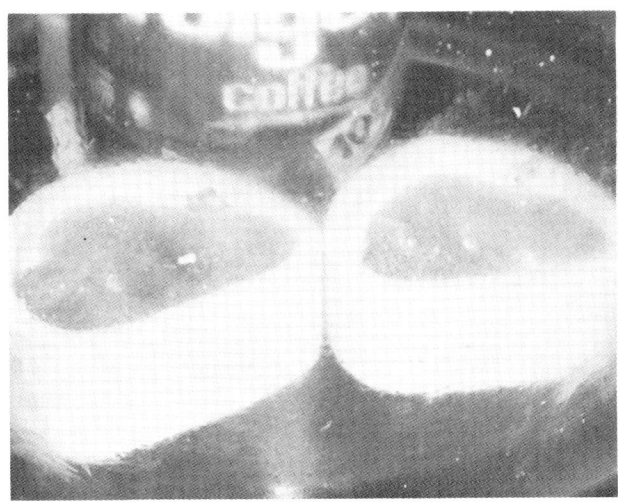

Fig. 21-64. Resin bubbles vigorously as pressure is reduced.

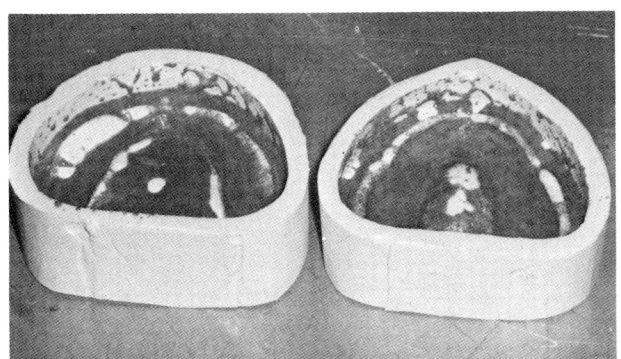

Fig. 21-65. When pressure is released, material will be free of bubbles.

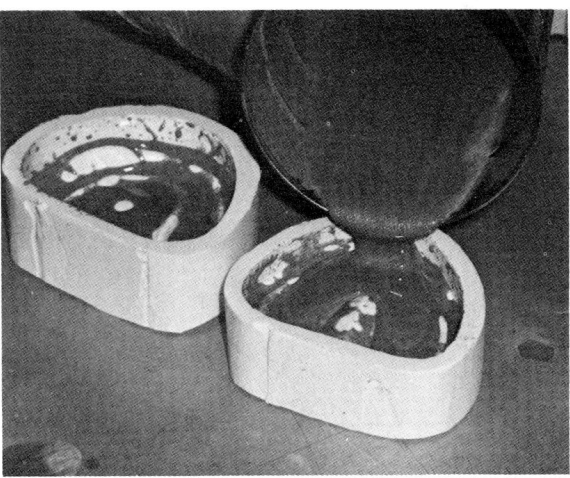

Fig. 21-66. Remainder of material is poured into mold.

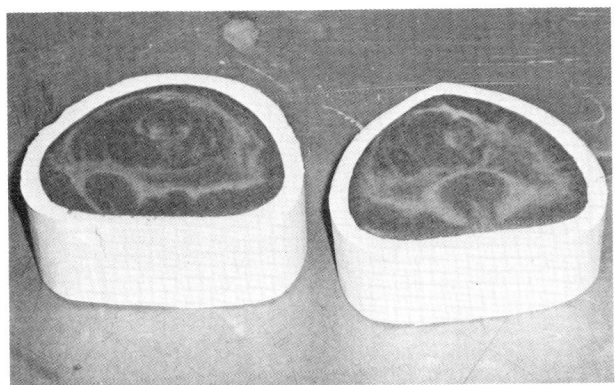

Fig. 21-67. Molds are completely filled with copper epoxy resin.

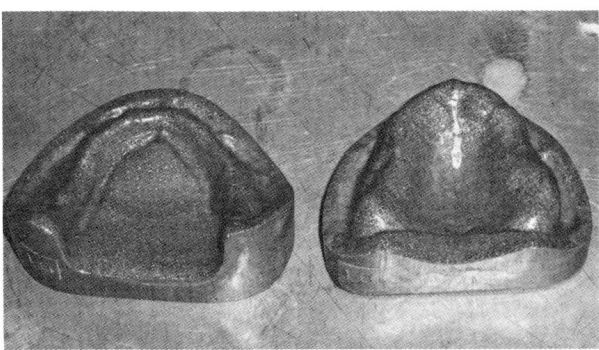

Fig. 21-68. Completed copper model after removing from mold.

## Fabricating PVC molds
### PROCEDURE

1. The material used to construct the PVC mold is PK5482FC, green; PK5483FC, green; and PK5484FC, green. Follow recommended safety precautions when handling these materials (Fig. 21-69).

2. Vacuum the material before using if 24 hours has elapsed since it was last used. Stir the mix thoroughly in an empty coffee can. Continue to vacuum as previously described until only one or two bubbles continue to rise. Incomplete vacuuming may produce voids during curing (Fig. 21-70).

3. Place the copper epoxy cast previously constructed on a sturdy 6 x 6-inch (15 x 15-cm) square plate of stainless steel. Box the cast with a contoured stainless steel holding reservoir (Figs. 21-71

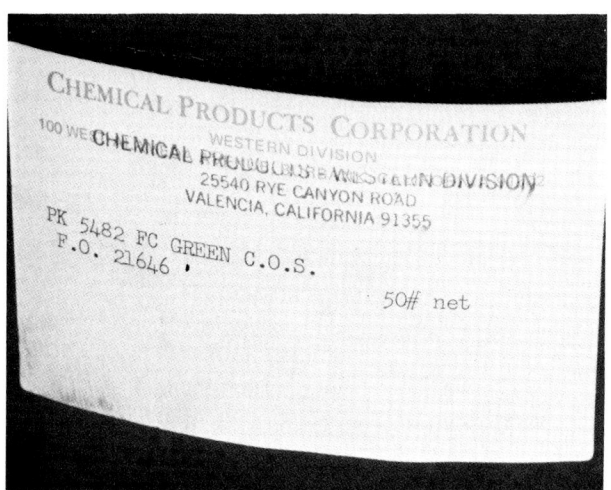

Fig. 21-69. One type of PVC used for construction of flexible molds.

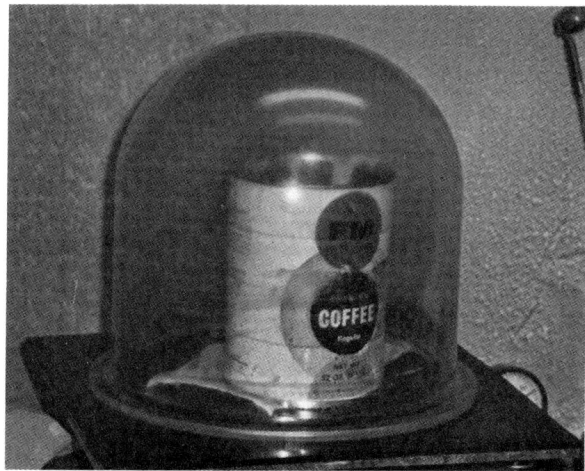

Fig. 21-70. Material being vacuumed beneath bell jar prior to use.

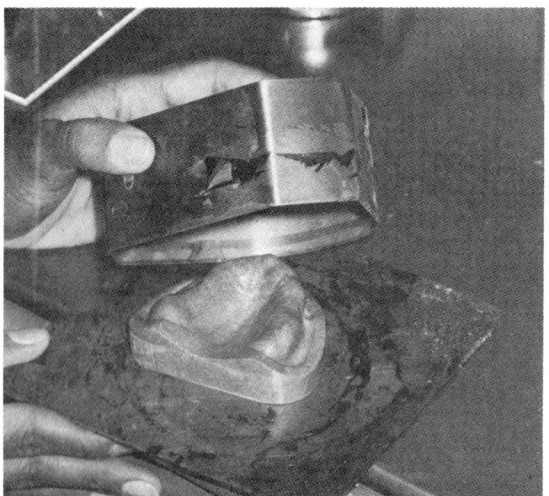

Fig. 21-71. Epoxy model is placed on stainless steel plate, and stainless steel boxing reservoir is placed around it.

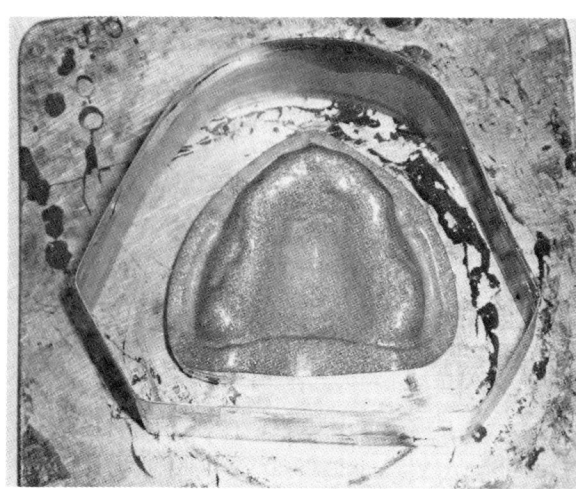

Fig. 21-72. Stainless steel boxing in position ready for pouring.

and 21-72). The boxing should be approximately 4 inches (10 cm) high and permit ¼-inch (0.6-cm) space between all sides of the model to be duplicated.

4. Preheat the boxed cast in a low-temperature oven, 30° C for 1 hour. Raise the setting to 90° to 95° C, and, when the oven has reached the second setting, remove the cast from the oven, and brush around the base with PVC to secure the cast to the base. Return it to the oven for curing. Cured PVC will be transparent (Figs. 21-73 to 21-75).

5. After curing, remove the based cast from the oven, and repeat the PVC brush-on procedure a second time. Secure the metal holding reservoir to the metal base in the same manner (Fig. 21-76).

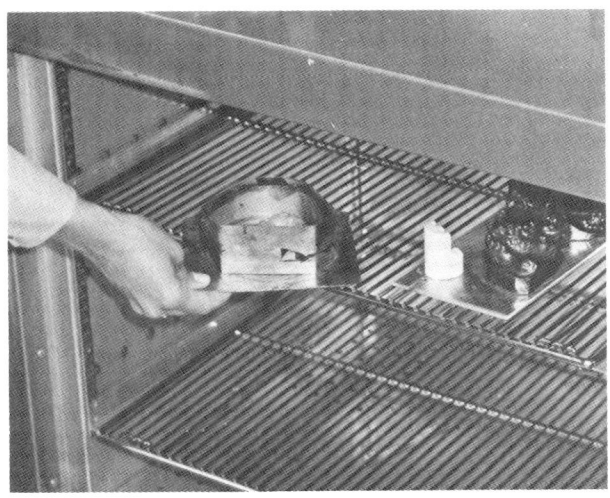

**Fig. 21-73.** Boxed model is preheated in oven as described previously.

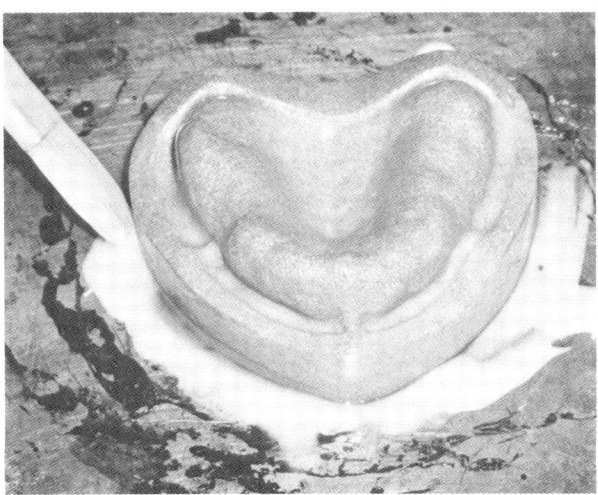

**Fig. 21-74.** PVC is painted around base of cast to secure base to metal plate.

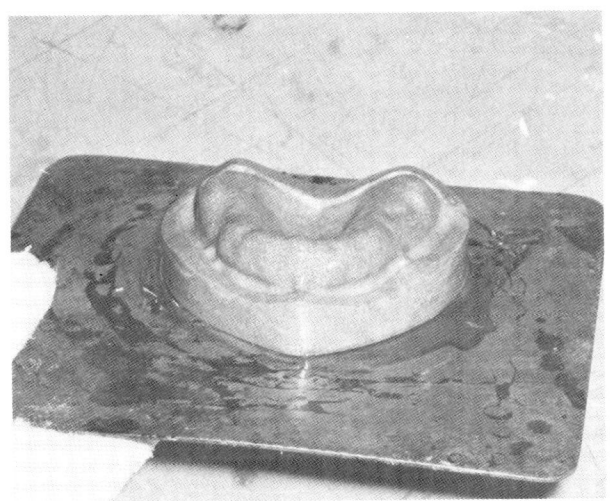

**Fig. 21-75.** After curing PVC is clear. Cast is sealed to plate with cured PVC.

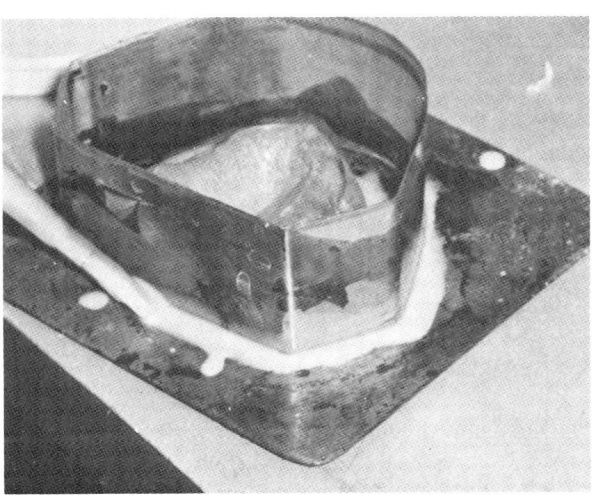

**Fig. 21-76.** Second coat of PVC is applied to seal boxing reservoir to metal plate and cured again in oven.

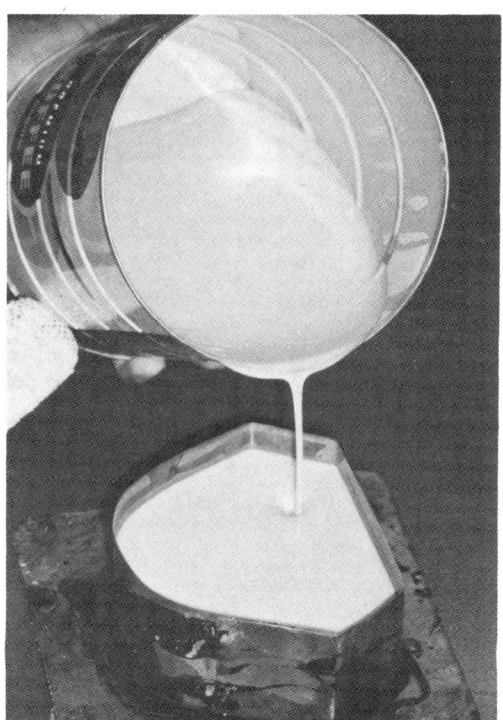

**Fig. 21-77.** PVC is poured into mold to within ¼ inch (0.6 cm) of top.

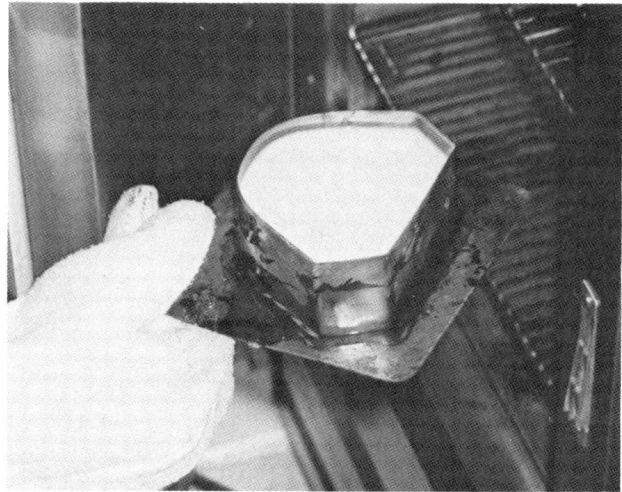

**Fig. 21-78.** Filled mold is placed into oven for curing.

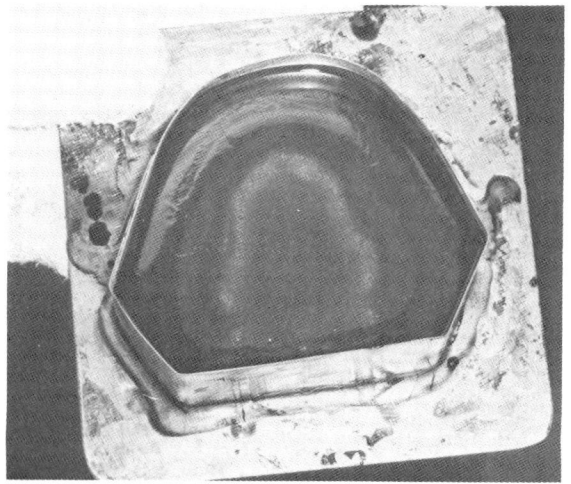

**Fig. 21-79.** Cured mold material is clear when properly processed.

6. Completely fill the holding reservoir with vacuumed PVC, return it to the oven, and cure it (Figs. 21-77 and 21-78).

7. Curing time should be at two temperature levels. First, start at a low setting of 50° C for about 25 minutes, reset to 90° to 95° C, and continue curing for another 20 to 30 minutes depending on the size of the cast. This should be checked about every 10 minutes.

8. The properly cured PVC mold will be clear (Figs. 21-75 and 21-79). Before curing, the material will be milky (Figs. 21-76 to 21-78).

9. Remove the cured mold from the oven, and set it aside to cool. The cooling time will depend on the size of the model being duplicated; however, the model should only be slightly warm to the touch before removing it from the mold.

### PROBLEM AREAS

The principal problems associated with the construction of PVC molds are that the material remains doughy and does not set and the material leaked beneath the cast when pouring (Table 21-3). Using the correct temperature curing cycle and applying a sealing coat of PVC to prevent leakage will usually solve these problems.

**Table 21-3.** Polyvinylchloride elastomers

| Problem | Probable cause | Solution |
|---|---|---|
| Hazy look to material; doughlike consistency | Not enough curing time, incorrect temperature, or both | Use timer; check temperature before starting to work with material |
| Cast sticking to metal base and leakage | PVC leaked under cast and out under metal boxing that was not properly sealed and cured | Apply sealing PVC, and cure two separate times to base and metal boxing reservoir |

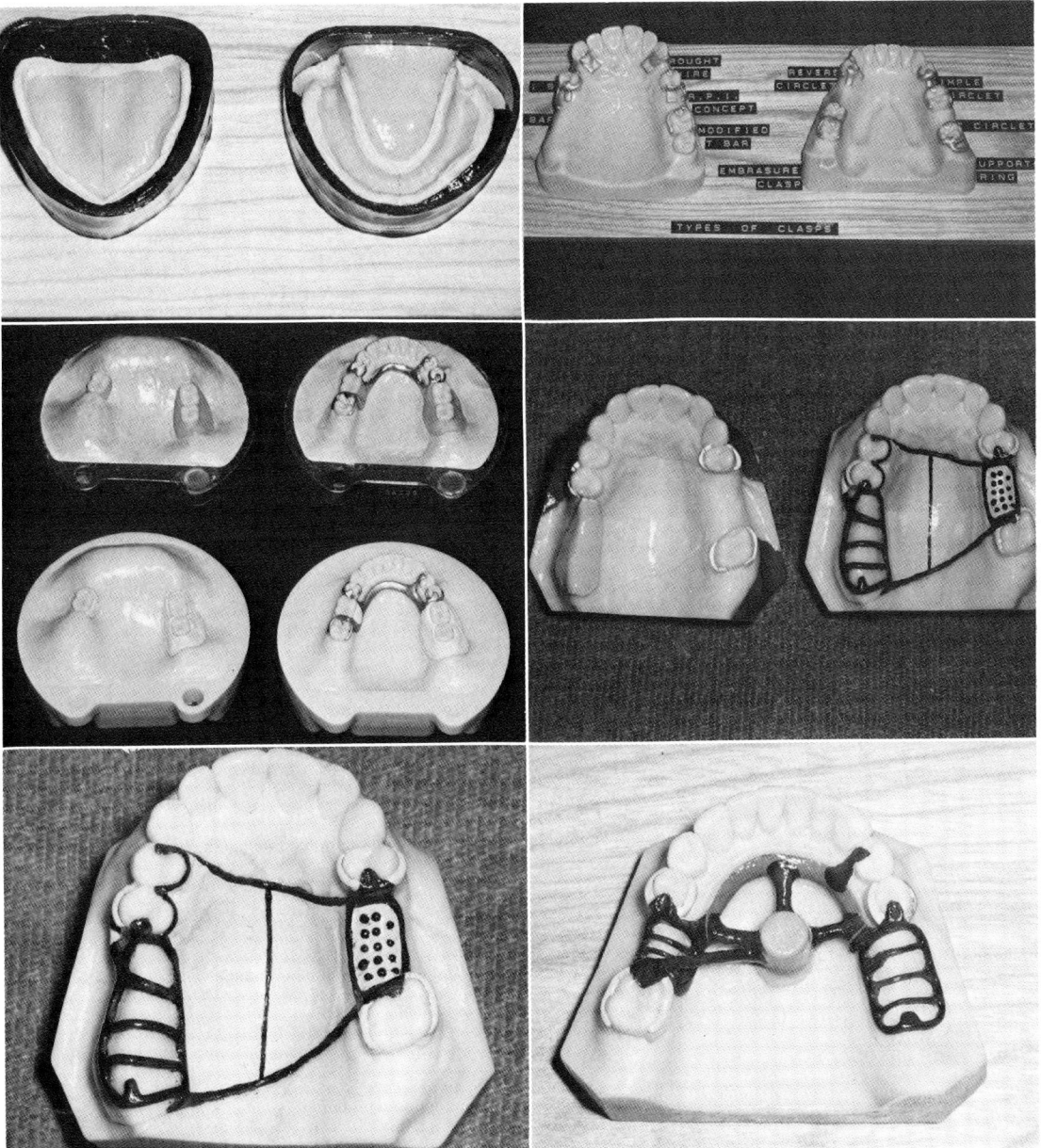

**Fig. 21-80.** Applications of methods described for producing three-dimensional visual aids are limited only by imagination of technician. Well-constructed visual aids can contribute to improved teaching.

*Continued.*

**658** *Dental laboratory procedures: removable partial dentures*

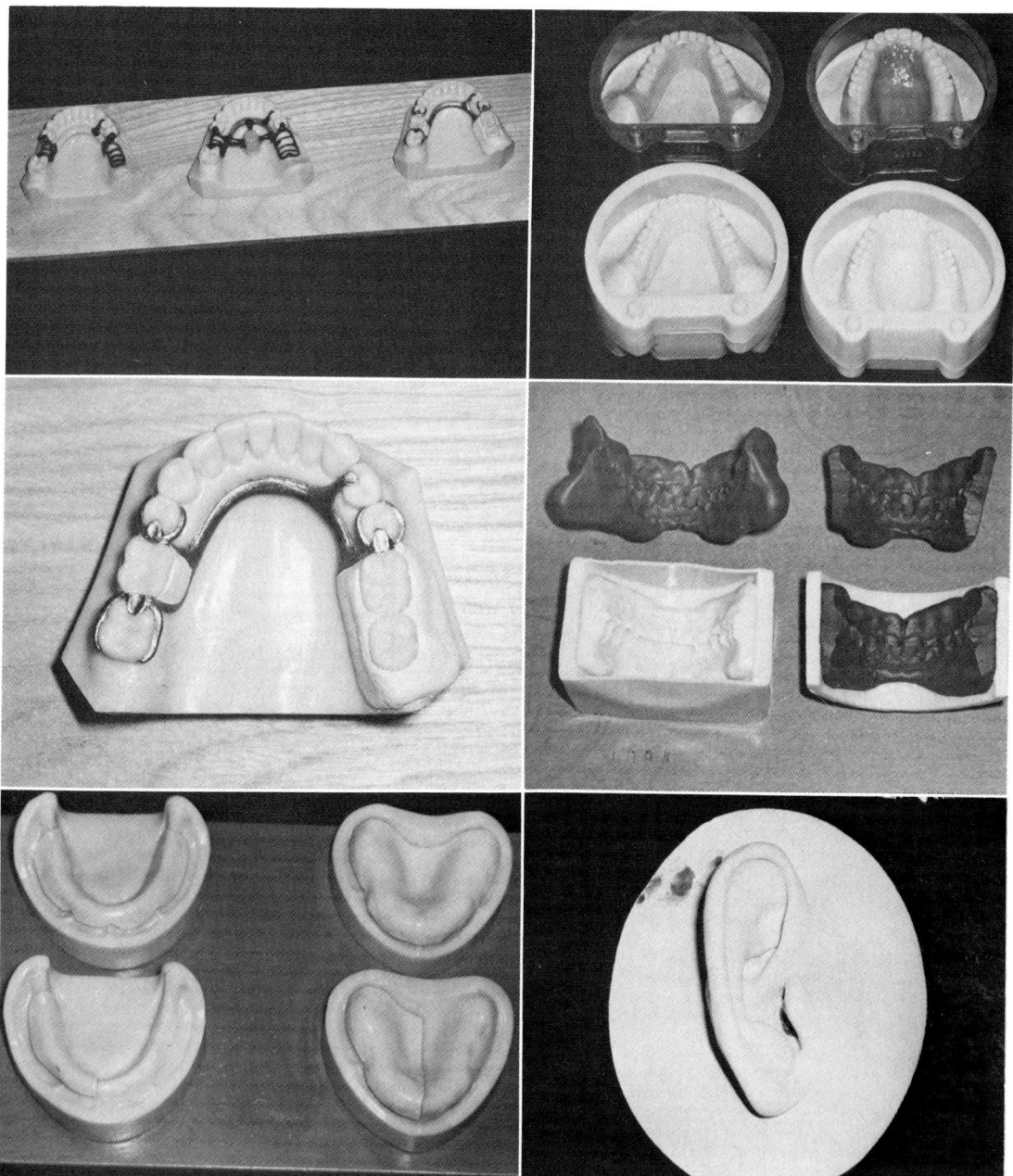

**Fig. 21-80, cont'd.** For legend see p. 657.

## SUMMARY

In this chapter two methods were described for making flexible molds that can be used to construct duplicate models. In addition, a method was described for constructing duplicate models from epoxy resin. The resultant epoxy models can be painted with water-soluble acrylic paint or with metallic paints to simulate dental prostheses. Although the boxing procedure will vary for the various types of casts to be duplicated, there are few original master casts that cannot be duplicated by one of the methods described (Fig. 21-80). The methods are uniquely suited in dentistry for construction of three-dimensional visual aids to increase teaching effectiveness.

# CHAPTER 22

# PACKING AND SHIPPING

JAMES D. BROWNING and SAM R. ADKISSON

When a dentist sends a case to the laboratory for fabrication of a prosthesis, the contents of the cast box represent a considerable investment of time, thought, effort, and no small amount of money. By the time the laboratory returns the finished prosthesis the investment is even greater. It is frustrating, time consuming, and expensive to all concerned—dentist, technician, and patient—if the cast is damaged in shipment.

Fortunately, these losses can be almost completely eliminated by careful packing and the use of appropriate containers. A small investment of time and money in procuring suitable packing materials and training and supervising someone in their use will pay great dividends. Most breakage occurs because the shipping containers are used incorrectly. Packing casts for shipment is an important part of prosthodontic service and as such should be closely supervised by the dentist and laboratory manager.

## PACKING MATERIALS

A satisfactory shipping container will be crushproof, shock resistant, and will prevent the contents from shifting. Packing boxes designed especially for shipping dental casts are available in a variety of shapes, sizes, and materials (Fig. 22-1). Cardboard boxes, some with corners reinforced by metal; polystyrene plastic boxes with detachable lids; and Styrofoam containers are among those currently in use. Some boxes have self-locking lids, slots for address cards, and other time- and labor-saving features.

Polyurethane foam inserts are avilable to fit most of these containers (Fig. 22-2). Loose packing material in many shapes and materials—Styrofoam beads, air-bubble plastic sheets, foam sheets—can make any container a cast shipping box (Fig. 22-3). With reasonable care and proper use these shipping containers last a long time and are well worth the initial cost.

One of the most satisfactory boxes for shipping dental casts is cardboard with foam inserts compartmented to hold one cast in each of two compartments (Fig. 22-4, A). If more than two casts, or casts plus something else, are to be shipped, two boxes should be used (Fig. 22-4, B). The two boxes should be wrapped together in paper and taped so they will not become separated in transit (Fig. 22-5). It is not advantageous to wrap more than two boxes into one package. Do not put tape directly on cardboard shipping boxes. When the tape is removed it destroys part of the box, thus shortening its useful life.

Some shipping boxes have foam inserts that are not compartmented (Fig. 22-6). These make it possible in some circumstances to ship more than two casts in each box, but great care is required in packing. When the casts are small, three casts may be shipped in such a box if they are carefully placed in position and then packed firmly so that position does not shift during transit (Fig. 22-7).

Larger shipping boxes or plain cartons with loose packing material have the advantage of allowing several items to be shipped in one box but require extreme care in packing (Fig. 22-8). Loose packing material has a tendency to move or shift position

**660** *Dental laboratory procedures: removable partial dentures*

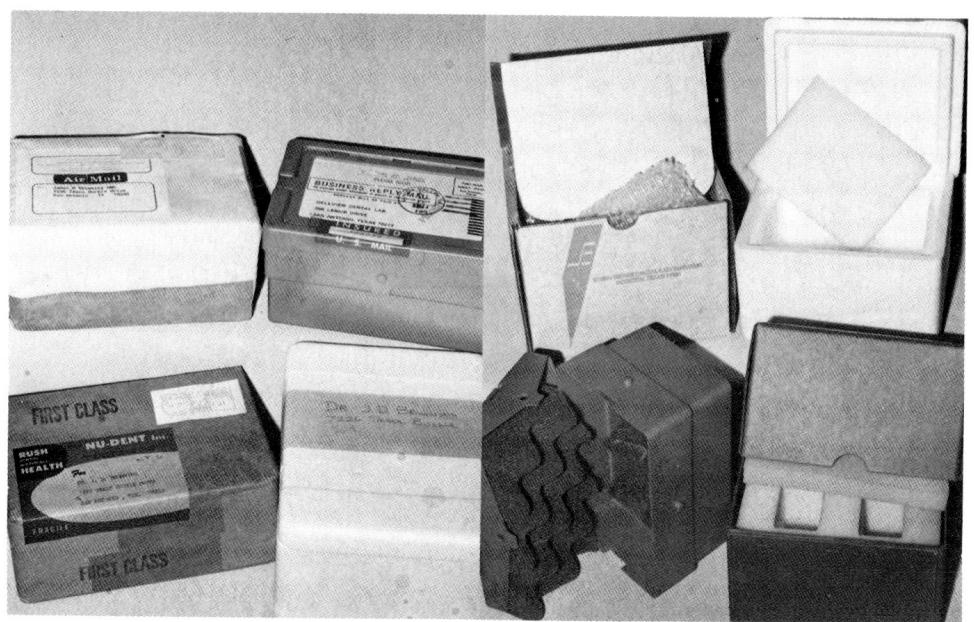

**Fig. 22-1.** Four types of dental shipping boxes.

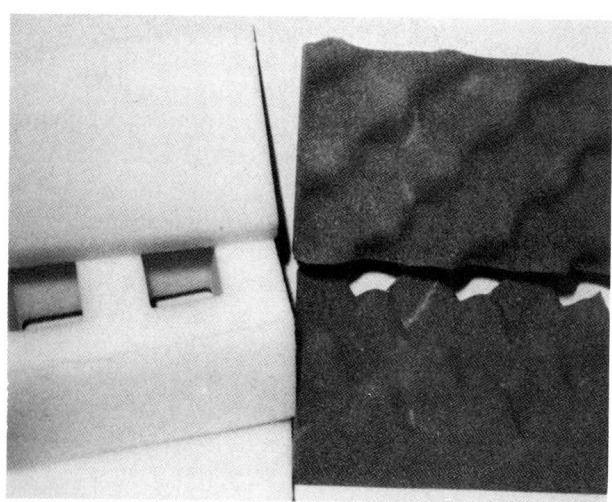

**Fig. 22-2.** Two types of foam inserts.

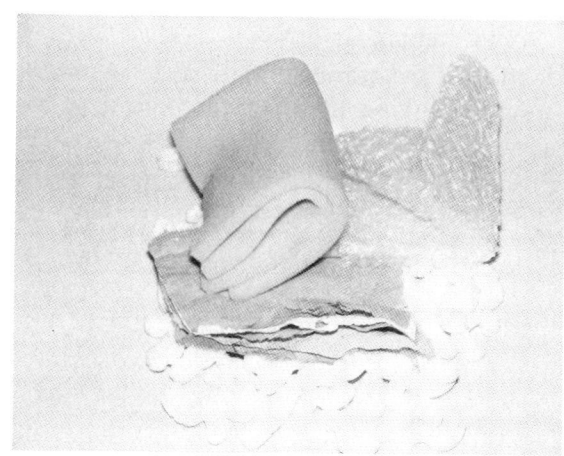

**Fig. 22-3.** Several types of loose packing materials.

*Packing and shipping* **661**

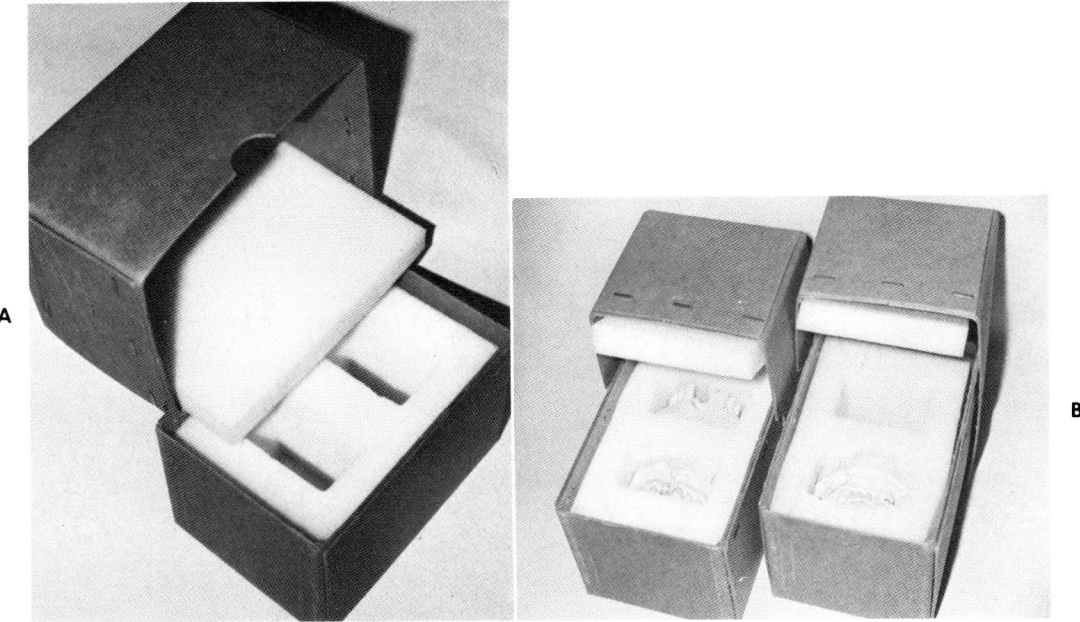

**Fig. 22-4. A,** Cardboard box with foam insert. **B,** Boxes packed with one item per compartment.

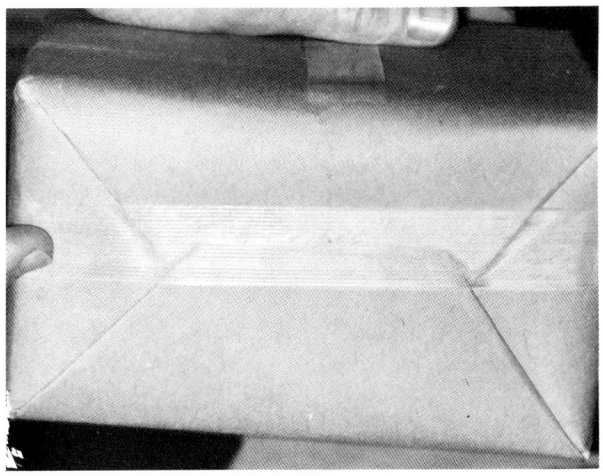

**Fig. 22-5.** Two boxes wrapped together for shipping.

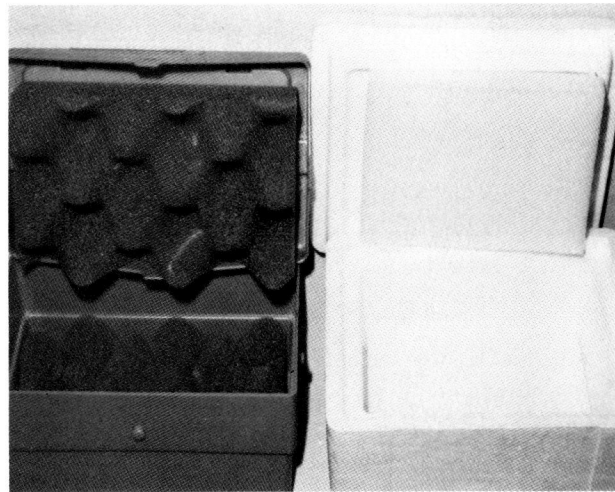

**Fig. 22-6.** Examples of uncompartmented foam inserts.

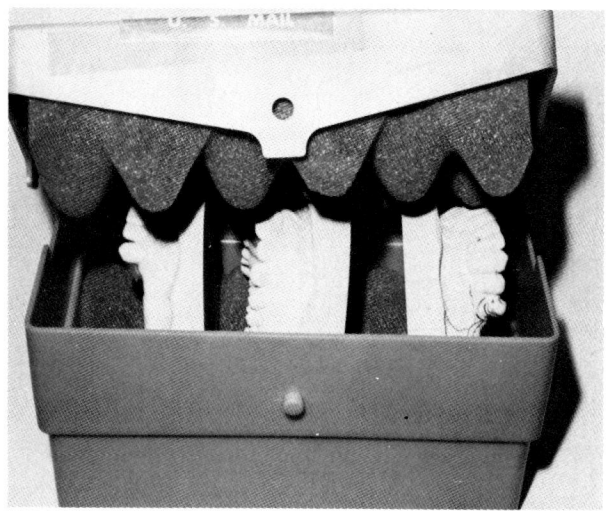

Fig. 22-7. Three items packed in uncompartmented foam.

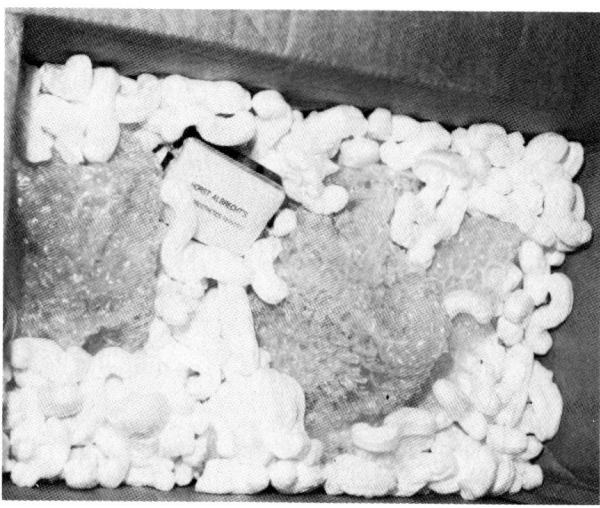

Fig. 22-8. Several items packed in loose packing materials.

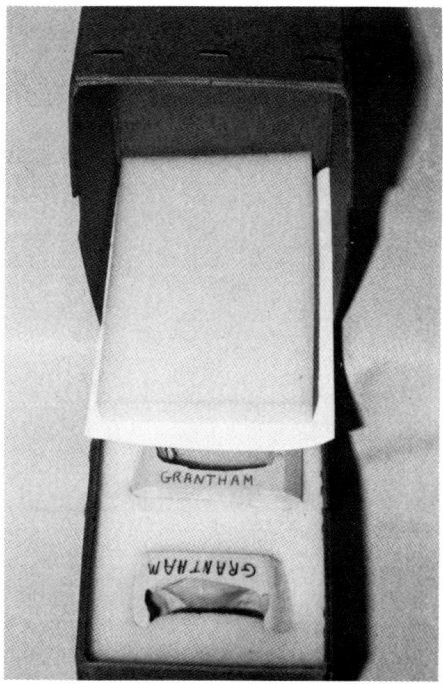

Fig. 22-9. Casts packed base to base. Note visible name.

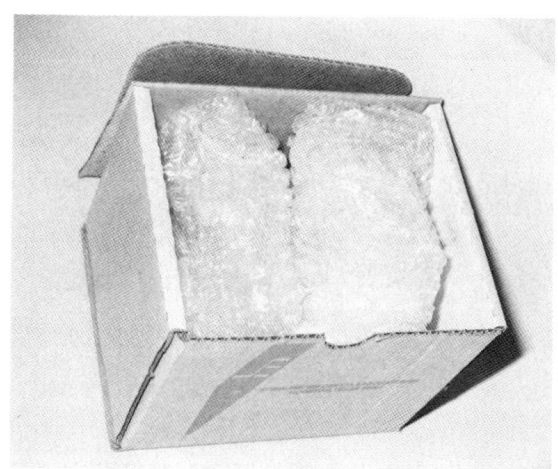

Fig. 22-10. Casts wrapped in bubble pack.

during shipment and can allow the casts to bang together. The small amount saved in shipping costs by placing several items in one box is more than lost if just one cast is damaged.

The choice of which shipping container to use depends on how it will be used. If the cast might be packed by someone who is in a hurry, or if the cast must be shipped in the mail or other commercial shipping service, containers especially designed for shipping casts are by far the best choice. Random cartons with loose packaging material can be recommended only if the dentist or laboratory manager packages the cast and delivery is made directly to the laboratory or office by dependable courier.

*Casts* should be packaged base to base, with no more than two casts in each compartmented box (Fig. 22-9). If compartmented containers are not used, each cast should be wrapped separately with a soft protective material such as thin foam sheets or air-bubble plastic sheets (Fig. 22-10). Bulk cotton

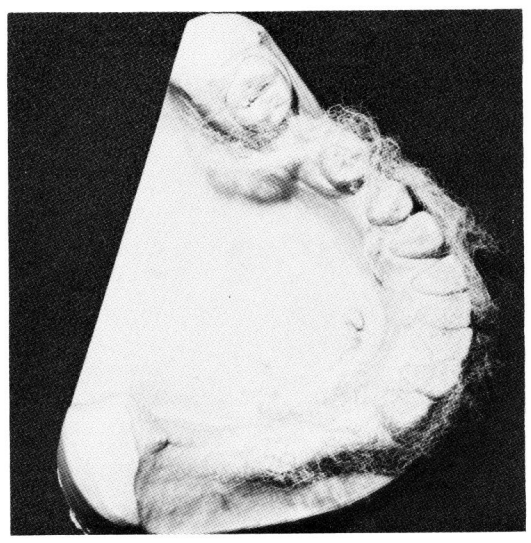

**Fig. 22-11.** Cotton adhering to cast due to dampness.

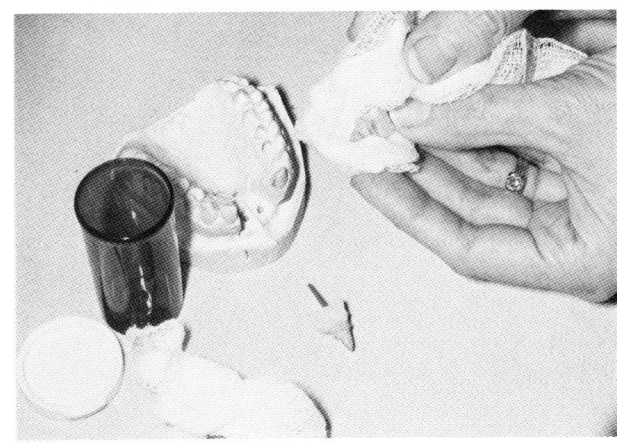

**Fig. 22-12.** Die wrapped in gauze for shipping.

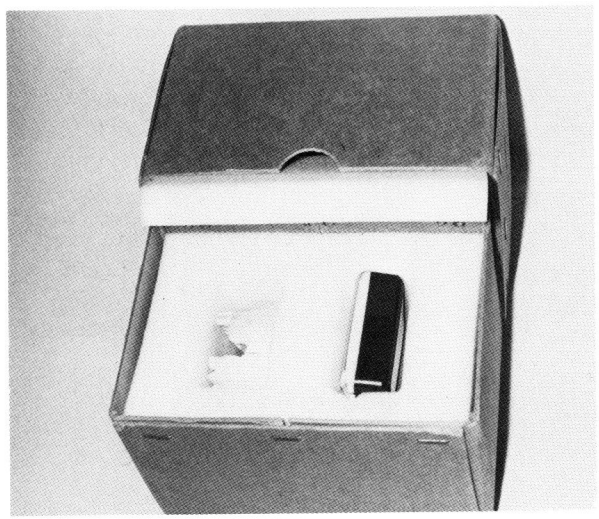

**Fig. 22-13.** Die container and master cast in shipping box.

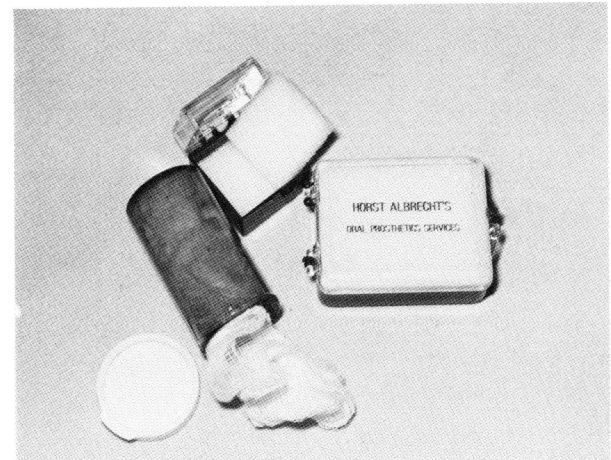

**Fig. 22-14.** Plastic containers suitable for shipping dies.

or soft paper patient napkins should be avoided because they may stick to the cast, especially if it is damp or becomes moist during transit (Fig. 22-11). Casts should be thoroughly dried before packaging and the patient's name placed on the base of each cast where the name can be seen after the cast is mounted on an articulator.

*Dies* should not be shipped as part of the master cast. Each die should be removed from the master cast, wrapped individually in gauze, and packed firmly into a small container so the dies cannot move (Fig. 22-12). This container should then be placed in one compartment of the shipping box (Fig. 22-13). Several kinds of small plastic boxes are sold for the purpose of packing dies for shipment; ordinary pill bottles serve the purpose very well (Fig. 22-14). When the restoration is completed, it can be shipped on the die, wrapped in gauze, and packed firmly into the same type of container.

Neither the master cast nor the dies should be

shipped in the original impression. Impressions can be distorted in shipment, and, if this occurs, the cast and dies will probably be damaged. Impression materials can score the dies and destroy accuracy. It is the responsibility of the dentist to trim the dies and mark the margins in red crayon pencil before shipment to the laboratory (Fig. 22-15).

*Jaw relation records* are so varied and are made of many different fragile materials that they require extra care in packaging for shipping. The materials of choice for registering jaw relations are those which set chemically and are not thermoplastic. Gypsum products, zinc oxide–eugenol pastes, and acrylic resin products survive shipment well if handled and packaged properly.

Wax cannot be used successfully as the registration medium, especially when the jaw relation record must be shipped. Wax experiences rather large dimensional changes when the shipping container undergoes temperature fluctuations during transit, and the wax jaw relation record usually arrives so distorted that it cannot be used to relate the casts precisely.

When the jaw relation record is made on a shellac baseplate, it should be placed on the master cast and both wrapped carefully together. Since shellac is easily deformed because of pressure, it will remain much more accurate when it is shipped on the cast.

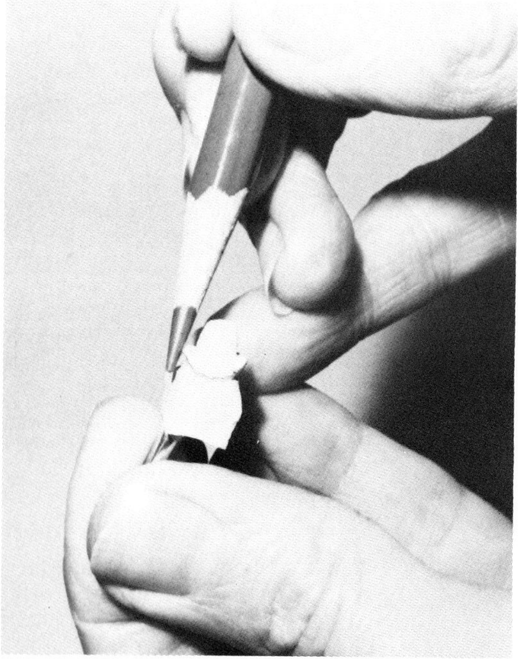

Jaw relation records made with acrylic resin baseplates may be wrapped in some form of soft packing material (Fig. 22-16), such as foam, and placed in a container of the proper size so that the record cannot shift during shipment.

Use minimum pressure to create a cushioning effect rather than a distorting force. Shellac baseplate records will not harm the cast, if they are wrapped securely to prevent movement. Other types of jaw relation records should be removed from the cast and packed in a separate container because frequently they will move during transit and score the cast, thus destroying its accuracy.

If the jaw relation record is small, such as a wafer covering only one tooth, it can be shipped in a pill bottle or one of the special boxes designed for shipping dies (Fig. 22-17). If the jaw relation record is larger, such as a full arch, anesthetic Carpule cans make good containers (Fig. 22-18).

Efforts to keep the record moist during shipment usually are not successful and frequently do more harm than good. It is much better to use registration materials that do not change dimensionally when dried.

*Articulated casts* are difficult to ship safely. No matter how carefully the articulator is packaged, the casts or the mounting or both are frequently broken on arrival. If the procedure must be used, the articulator should be taken apart and the upper and lower members packaged in separate boxes. Even when handled this way, a high percentage arrive broken.

**Fig. 22-15.** Marking margins on die with red pencil.

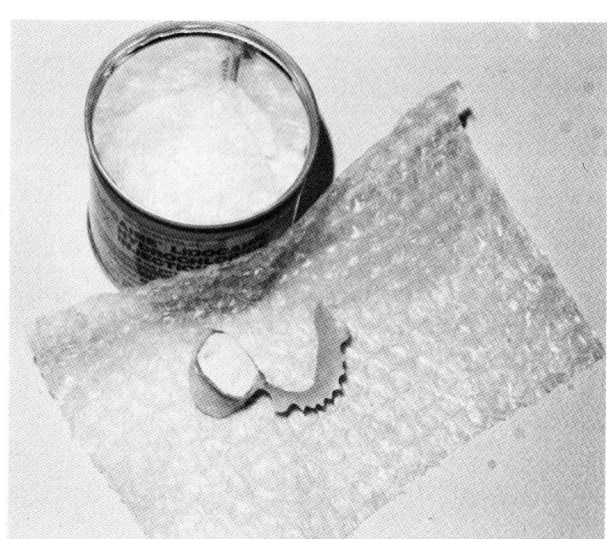

**Fig. 22-16.** Jaw relation record with bubble pack.

It is seldom necessary to place the casts on the articulator for shipment. The essential point is to send accurate casts accompanied by some precise means of relating master and opposing casts. This should be checked when the patient is present for verification.

Even when a face-bow or axis mounting is used to relate the casts to a particular type of articulator, it is not necessary to complete the mounting before shipping the cast. In that situation the following procedure can be used:

1. Key the maxillary cast and lubricate the base.
2. Mount the maxillary cast on the articulator using the appropriate relating method.
3. Remove the maxillary cast from the articulator still attached to the mounting ring or attachment.
4. Ship the maxillary cast with the mounting ring, together with the mandibular cast, the jaw relation record, and whatever information is necessary to program the articulator (Figs. 22-19 and 22-20).

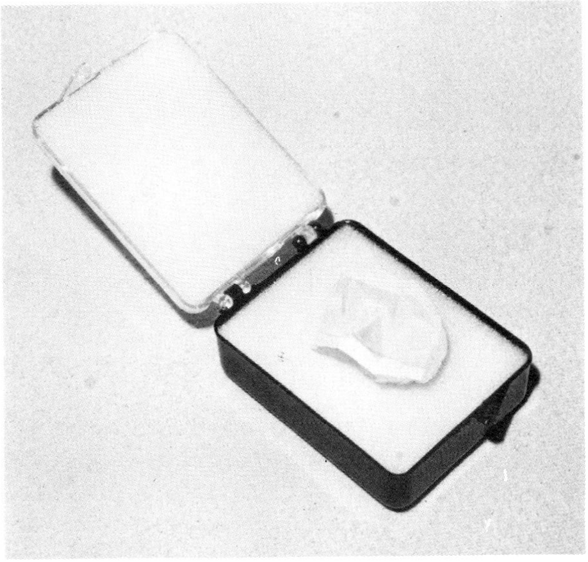

**Fig. 22-17.** Small jaw relation record packed in die box.

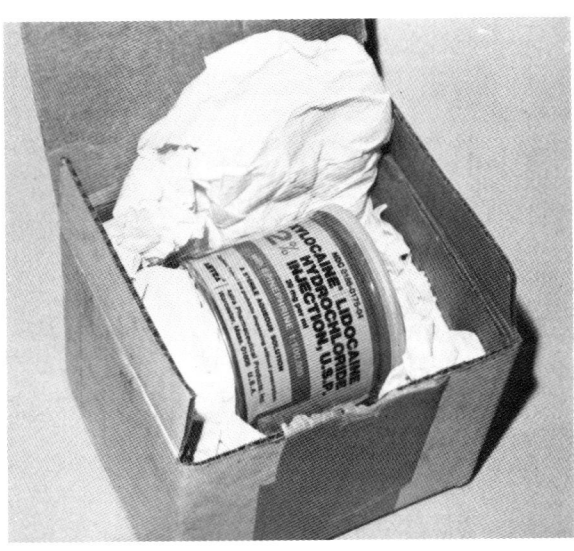

**Fig. 22-18.** Large jaw relation record packed in metal can.

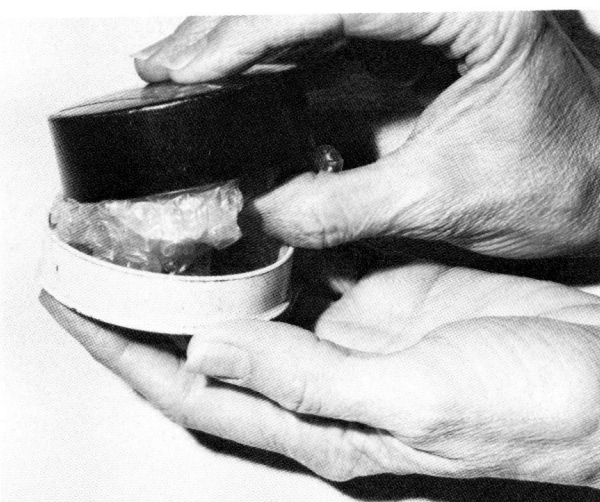

**Fig. 22-19.** Jaw relation record in bubble pack and small box.

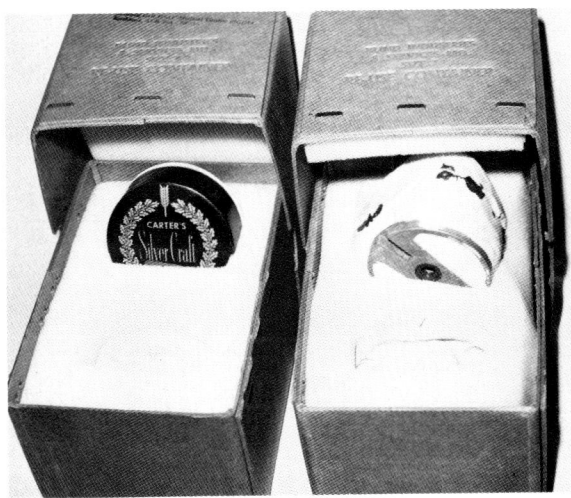

**Fig. 22-20.** Face-bow mounted cast ready for shipment.

**666** *Dental laboratory procedures: removable partial dentures*

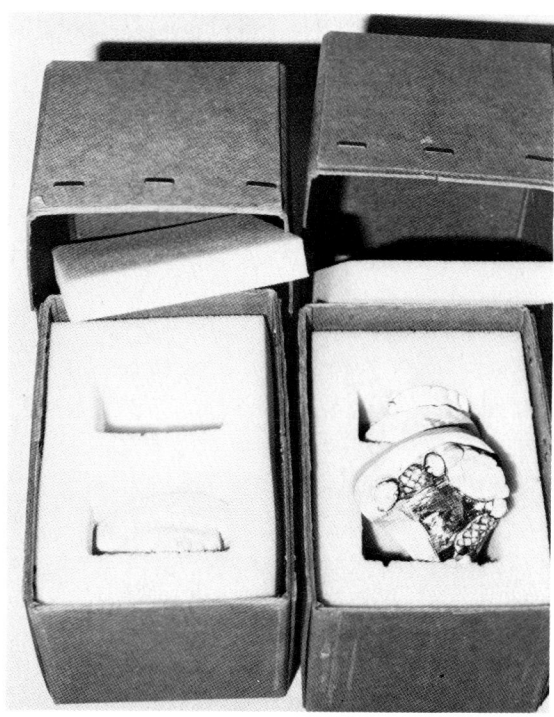

Fig. 22-21. Finished framework in compartmented box.

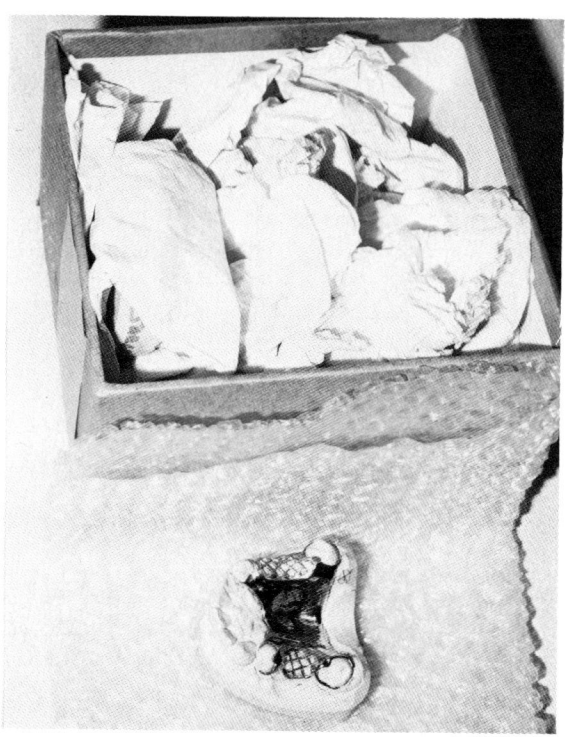

Fig. 22-22. Finished framework in uncompartmented box.

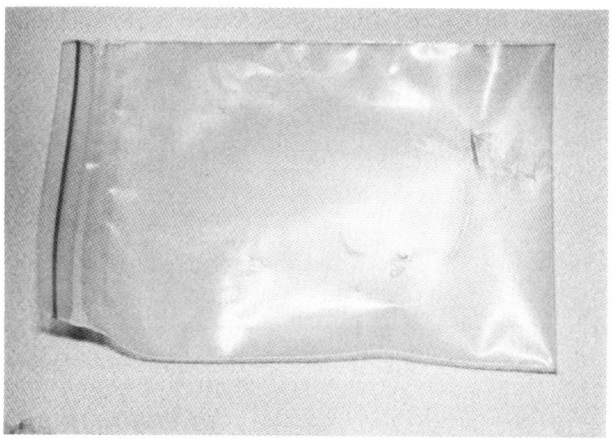

Fig. 22-23. Completed partial denture in plastic bag.

On arrival, place the maxillary cast and mounting attachment on an articulator similar to the original one and mount the lower cast using the jaw relation record. The control elements can then be used to set the new instrument. This simple technique is much preferable to shipping casts mounted on an articulator.

*Removable partial denture frameworks* should be shipped on the master cast or a duplicate master cast. The cast with the framework in place can be placed in one compartment of the shipping box (Fig. 22-21). If shipped in boxes that are not compartmented, the cast with the framework should be wrapped in foam or soft paper and packed firmly so that it cannot shift during transit (Fig. 22-22).

*Completed removable partial dentures and complete dentures* should be placed in a heat-seal or self-sealing plastic bag, with moist cotton or facial tissue, one restoration per plastic bag, and the bag sealed (Fig. 22-23). The plastic bag should then be wrapped in soft paper or foam and packed in a compartment of the shipping container (Fig. 22-24). If there are two restorations involved in the case they should be packed in separate plastic bags, wrapped separately, and each placed in a compartment of the shipping box. Any casts involved should be packed and shipped in separate boxes. It is important that the plastic bags be sealed so the moisture cannot escape during transit. If the plastic is allowed to dry out it may warp and destroy the fit.

*Completed full crowns* or *partial veneer crowns* should be placed on the original die and the dies handled for shipping in the manner previously described (Fig. 22-25).

*Fixed partial dentures* should not be shipped on the master cast, since any damage to the cast during

*Packing and shipping* **667**

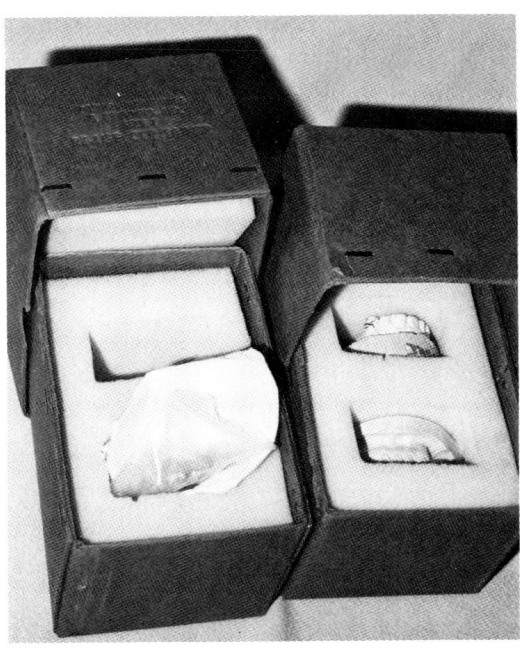

**Fig. 22-24.** Acrylic appliance in plastic bag packed in foam.

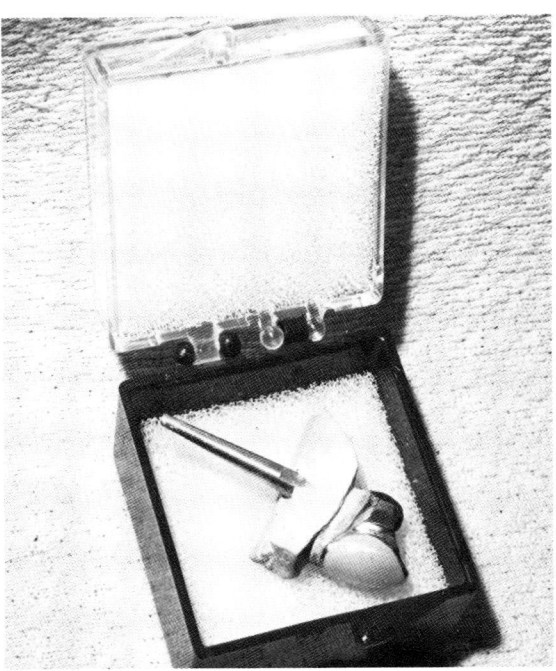

**Fig. 22-25.** Completed restoration on die, packed in foam.

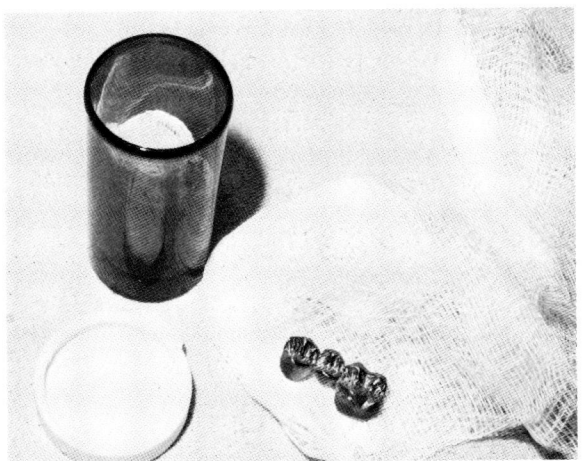

**Fig. 22-26.** Fixed partial denture with wrapping materials.

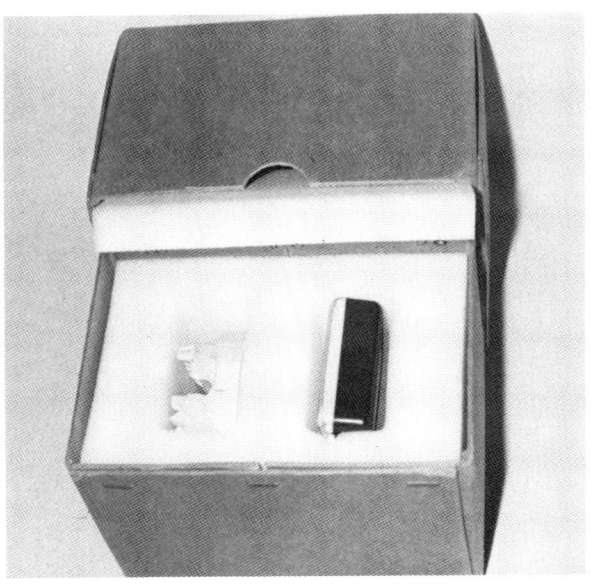

**Fig. 22-27.** Fixed partial denture and cast ready for shipping.

shipment could result in damage to the casting, requiring a remake. The completed fixed restoration should be wrapped, packed in a pill bottle or similar container so that it cannot move during shipment, (Fig. 22-26), and the container packed firmly in one compartment of the shipping box (Fig. 22-27).

*Impressions* should not be packed or shipped. The purpose of the impression is to obtain an accurate cast, and to do this, the impression should be poured as quickly as possible. An accurate cast is the only link between the dentist, the patient, and the technician.

## CHOOSING A CARRIER

The ideal way of shipping dental prosthetic casts in a limited geographical area is to have a responsible individual personally pick up and deliver the properly packaged shipping container. Some laboratories have employees who perform this service. Other possibilities are commercial services listed in the telephone directory under Delivery Service or Messenger Service. Delivery within the building or close by may not require packaging, but with even the best delivery service shipment should be made only after the cast has been properly packed.

If personal delivery of prosthetic casts is not feasible, several options are available. The United States Postal Service and commercial delivery services such as United Parcel Service each have advantages, depending on the circumstances. Many common carriers such as Greyhound and Trailways provide a package delivery service. It is worthwhile to experiment to see which is most satisfactory in terms of speed, dependability, cost, convenience, and careful handling.

## SUMMARY

Shipping of dental casts and prostheses is an important link in the dentist-laboratory relationship. Selection of appropriate packing materials, careful packing to avoid damage, and selection of the best carrier can yield a substantial saving in time, money, and frustration to both the dentist and laboratory.

# INDEX

## A

Acco No. 1 clamps, 73
Ackermann clip, 554, 577
Ackermann rider, 580
Acri-Dense Pneumatic Curing Unit, 74
Acrylic inserts, 486
Acrylic pontic, reinforced, 152, 154-155, 543-548
Acrylic resin
  autopolymerizing, 611
  cold-curing, 611-614
Acrylic resin denture base, 150, 151
Acrylic resin impression trays, 62-67
Acrylic resin preparation, 611-614
Acrylic veneer, labiogingival tissue, 491
Adams clasp, 280, 281
Agar, 1
Agar reversible hydrocolloid impression, 23-26
  care of, 23-24
  definition of, 1
  for duplication, 203-214
  pouring, 24-26
  water-cooled tray for, 59
Akers clasp, 136, 137
Alborium, 293, 313
Al-Cote, 374
Alginate, 1
Alginate irreversible hydrocolloid impression, 2-23
  artificial stone in, 7-17
  care of, 4-11
  definition of, 1
  over framework and relined bases, 402
  pouring, 12-18
  trimming, 19-23
Alloy
  cobalt-chromium, 214, 268
  gold, 214, 268
  heat softening of, 315-316
  heat hardening of, 315-316
  nickel-chromium, 268
  nonprecious metal, 268
  precious metal, 268
  wrought wire, 433-434

Altered cast, 30
Ancrofix stud attachment, 554, 556, 562-563, 572, 573
Annealed orthodontic wire, 587-588
Approach arm of clasp, 136
Aqueous impression materials, 1
Arbitrary blockout, 190, 191
Arrowhead clasp, 604
Articulated casts, packing and shipping, 664-666
Artic-U-Locs, 456
Artificial stone in alginate irreversible hydrocolloid impressions, 7-17
Asbestos, 294
Attachment
  Ancrofix, 554
  auxiliary, 554
  bar; *see* Bar attachment
  frictional, 448
  internal, 448
  key and keyway, 448
  male framework and assembly of, 474-480
  for overdentures, 550-586
  parallel, 448
  precision, 448
  S/L, 491
  slotted, 448
  stud; *see* Stud attachment
Attachment castings of S/L partial denture, 498-499
Autopolymerizing resin
  acrylic, 611
  record bases stabilized with, 109-113
  repairs of, 441
Autopolymerizing resin powder, soft-curing, 77
Autopolymerizing resin record bases, 73-96
Auxiliary attachments, 554

## B

Bachmann parallelometer, 552
Backing, metal; *see* Metal backing
Baer stud attachment, 555, 562-563, 571, 573

Ball clasp, 279-280, 602, 603
Bar
  Kennedy, 146, 147
    closed, 144
  labial; *see* Labial bar
  lingual, 144, 145, 146, 147, 250, 251, 252
  palatal; *see* Palatal bar
Bar attachment, 574-586
  C. M. rider, 580-586
  definition of, 554
  Dolder, 574-576, 583-584
  Hader, 577-578, 583-584
Bar clasp, 141, 190, 191, 197
Bar joint, Dolder, 576-577
Base
  denture; *see* Denture base
  and framework with reline impression, 400
  record; *see* Record base
  temporary, 72
  trial, 72
Baseplate, 72
Bead(ing), 194, 195
  boxing corrected cast impression with wax, 36-41
  for closed horseshoe connector, 200
  corrected cast impression with wax and two-stage pour, 42-49
  definition of, 181
  for double palatal bar, 200
  for full palate connector, 200
  for horseshoe connector, 200
  for palatal bar, 200
  retention, 234-235, 246, 543
Beading grip wax, 36
Bell jar, 640
Bench top orthodontic blowpipe, 607
Bending of orthodontic wire, 588-594
  closed end loop, 590-591
  deflection, 592
  helical, 589-590
  right-angle, 591
  semicircular, 589-590
  smooth curve, 594
  zigzag, 593

Bilateral distal extension removable partial denture, 130-131
Biolon, 486
Bird-beak pliers, 588, 589-591, 592, 594
Bite rim former, 124
Blockout
  arbitrary, 190, 191
  definition of, 181
  and duplication, 188-202
  parallel, 188, 189
  relief, beading, and design transfer, 181-202
  shaped, 190
Blockout wax, formula for, 194
Blow torch, 313, 314
Blowpipe, bench top orthodontic, 607
Boilout and packing, 381
Boley gauge, 527
Boxing corrected cast impression
  and beading with wax, 36-41
  with plaster/pumice mix and wax, 30-35
Boxing grip wax, 39
Boxing paper, 636-638
Boxing wax, 355, 356, 638, 642
Bridges, precision, 449
Buffalo dental spatula, 640
Burnout, 308-312, 319
  casting, and investing, 293-320, 472-473
  definition of, 293
  for S/L partial denture, 505-506

## C

Carborundum disk, 430
Carrier for dental prosthetic casts, 668
Cast clasp, repair of, 434-437
Cast framework, material for, 134
Cast impression, corrected; *see* Corrected cast impression
Cast(ing), 1-29, 313-318, 319
  accurate fit of record base of, 86, 91
  altered, 30
  articulated, packing and shipping, 664-666
  attachment, of S/L partial denture, 498-499
  cleaning, 316
  corrected, 30
  definition of, 293
  diagnostic; *see* Diagnostic cast
  investing, and burnout, 293-320, 472-473
  investment, 214-227
  mandibular, 161, 249-253, 254
  master; *see* Master cast
  maxillary, 233-249, 253, 254, 264
  metal, retention beads for, 246
  mounting, record bases and, 72-129
  orientation of, 160
  packing and shipping, 659-668
  path of insertion of, 164
  pickling, 318, 319
  preoperative, 72
  preparation of, for duplication, 188-202
  reconstruction, 425-426
  recovering, 315-316
  refractory; *see* Refractory cast
  requisites for, 1-2
  separation of record base from, 84-86, 91
  for S/L partial denture, 505-506
  study, 626-633
  tilting of, 160-169
Casting investment, 293
Casting machine, centrifugal force, 313

Ceka stud attachment, 556, 557, 566, 567-574
Centrifugal force casting machine, 313
Cingulum rest preparation, 134
Circlet clasp, 136, 137, 138-139, 190, 191, 197
Circumferential clasp, 136, 137, 270-273, 601-602
Clamp, Acco No. 1, 73
Clasp, 135-144
  Adams, 280, 281
  Akers, 136, 137
  approach arm of, 136
  arms of, 134, 135-136
  arrowhead, 604
  attachment of, to framework, 282-283
  ball, 279-280, 602, 603
  bar, 141
  body of, 135
  cast, repair of, 434-437
  circlet, 136, 137, 138-139, 190, 191, 197
  circumferential, 136, 137, 270-273, 601-602
  Class I, 136, 137
  Class II, 141
  cobalt-chromium alloy for, 268
  contouring of, 270-280
  definition of, 135
  double l, 144, 145
  E, 144, 145
  embrasure, 140, 141, 278-279
  fish hook, 138
  gold alloy for, 268
  half and half, 144, 145
  I, 143
  I-bar, 142, 143, 274-275
  infrabulge, 135, 141-144, 273-276
  L-bar, 276-277
  materials for, 268
  mesiodistal, 144, 145
  nickel-chromium alloy for, 268
  onlay, 139-141
  orthodontic; *see* Orthodontic clasp
  platinum-gold-palladium wire for, 268
  precious metal alloys for, 268
  push-type, 141
  repair of, 286-291, 433
  requirements of, 136
  ring, 144
  Roach, 141
  split, 144, 145
  stainless steel wire for, 268
  suprabulge, 135, 136-141
  T, 141-142, 276-277
  U, 144, 145
  wrought wire, 143-144, 267-292
Clasp attachment, 282, 283-286
Closed end loop of orthodontic wire, 590-591
Closed horseshoe major connector, 148, 149
Closed Kennedy bar, 144
Cloth wheel for lathe for polishing metal framework, 332-335
C. M. rider bar attachment, 580-586
Cobalt-chromium alloy, 214, 268
Coe-Flex, 107
Coe-Flo, 102
Coe-Soft, 73, 74
Coe Tray Plastic, 62, 88
Cold-curing acrylic resin, 611-614
Concentrate, slurry, 125

Connector, 144-148
  major, 144-146
    full palate, 148, 149, 200
    horseshoe, 148, 149
    maxillary, 146-148
    repair of, 430-431
  minor, 148, 149, 431-432
Copper epoxy resin, 651-653
Corrected cast, 30
Corrected cast impression
  beading and boxing with wax, 36-41
  beading with wax and two-stage pour, 42-49
  boxing with plaster/pumice mix and wax, 30-35
  definition of, 30
  North Carolina technique of pouring, 49-57
  pouring, 30-57
Crescent poster board, 636
Creshine, 511
Cristobalite model investment, 216, 472
Crown
  double, 553
  full or partial veneer, packing and shipping, 666
  single, 550-553
  telescope, 550-553
Crystal retention technique, 543
Curing unit, 380, 381
Custom impression tray; *see* Impression tray, custom

## D

Dalla Bona stud attachment, 556, 562-563, 571, 573
DAP rope caulk, 86
Debubblizer, 296, 370
Deflasking, 383-387
  definition of, 363
  finishing, flasking, and processing, 363-399
Deflection, 592
Deflection bend of orthodontic wire, 592
Dentsply Vacu-Press, 68, 69
Denture
  packing and shipping, 666
  removable partial; *see* Removable partial denture
Denture base, 150
  acrylic resin, 150, 151
  additions of, 445-446
  fractures of, repair of, 441-444
  metal, 150
  resin, 150, 156
  retention of, 150, 151
Denture teeth
  for anterior tooth replacement, 152, 154
  arrangement of, 344-352, 358-362
  metal occlusals of, for posterior tooth replacement, 156-157
  selection of, 339-343
Design
  definition of, 130
  and survey, 130-180
Design transfer, 181-186, 228
  blockout, relief, and beading, 181-202
  definition of, 181
Diagnostic cast, 178
  definition of, 72
  design of, for removable partial dentures, 170-178

Diagnostic cast—cont'd
  preparation of, 626-633
  for S/L partial denture, 493-494
Die Lube, 238
Dies, packing and shipping, 663-664
Dolder bar attachment, 574-576, 583-584
Dolder bar joint, 576-577
Dough method of autopolymerizing resin record base
  finger-adapted, 86-91
  wax-confined, 91-96
Drom-Flux, 284
Dumbbell spring, 598-599
Duplicate master cast, 398-399
Duplicating flask, 203
Duplication
  agar reversible hydrocolloid molds for, 203-214
  and blockout, 188-202
  definition of, 203
  preparation of cast for, 188-202
  and refractory casts, 203-227
DuraLay, 455, 479, 480, 483, 485
Dykem, 473
Dymo tape labeling gun, 635

### E

E clasp, 144, 145
Eagle drawing leads, 167
Elastomer
  polyvinylchloride, 650-656, 657
  silicone, 634-644, 645
Elastomeric impression, 26-28
Elastomeric impression material
  definition of, 1
  record bases stabilized with, 106-109
Electric solder, 428
Electric soldering machine, 478, 479
Electrosoldering
  in clasp attachment, 283-286
  in clasp repair, 290-291
EM Attachment Selector, 555
Embrasure clasp, 140, 141, 278-279
Epoxy resin
  copper, 651-653
  ivory, No. RF3503, 645, 646-650
Epoxy resin models, construction of, 644-650
Eraser, pencil, 101, 198

### F

Facing
  for anterior tooth replacement, 152-153
  flatback, technique of, 540-543
  reinforced, 525-549
  reverse-pin, technique for, 526-540
  Steele's, 152, 153
Fast Tray, 494
Fastcure, 73
Finger spring
  helical, 595-596
  simple, 594-595
Finger-adapted dough method of autopolymerizing resin record bases, 86-91
Finishing
  definition of, 363
  flasking, processing, and deflasking, 363-399
  framework, 321-338, 390-397
  S/L partial denture, 509
Finishing line, 437
Fish hook clasp, 138

Fixed interceptive orthodontic appliances, 587
Fixed partial dentures, packing and shipping, 666-667
Flasking, 368-380
  definition of, 363
  processing, deflasking, and finishing, 363-399
Flatback facing, technique of, 540-543
Flatback metal backing, 525
Flour of pumice, 394-397
Fractured denture base, repair of, 441-443, 444
Fractured and missing teeth, repair of, 444-445
Framework
  attachment of clasp to, 282-283
  and bases with reline impression, 400
  finishing, 321-338
  fitting, 473-474
  and male attachment assembly, 474-480
  packing and shipping, 666
  and relined bases, alginate impression over, 402
  sprinkle-on method with, for autopolymerizing resin record bases, 80-86
  waxing, 230, 472, 503
Frictional attachment, 448
Frictional wall precision attachment partial prosthesis, 448-490
Functional impression, 30

### G

Gerber stud attachment, 556, 557, 562-563, 564, 572, 573
Gold alloy, 214, 268
Gold occlusals, 483-485, 486
Gordon contouring plier, 268, 269
Gray investment, 215
Groove
  latch recess, 498
  thumb release, 491
Gun Lock, 563
Gypsum-bonded casting investment, 293

### H

Hader bar attachment, 577-578, 583-584
Half and half clasp, 144, 145
Hanau curing unit, 380, 381
Hanau flask ejector, 382, 383
Handpiece holder, 532
Handy Sandy sandblast machine, 317
Hawley appliance, 615, 624-626
Heat hardening of metal, 315-316
Heat softening of alloy, 315-316
Helical bend of orthodontic wire, 589-590
Helical finger spring, 595-596
High-speed lathe for polishing castings, 321
Hinge, S/L, 491
Hold, 494
Hooper duplicator, 402, 405
Horseshoe major connector, 148
  beading for, 200
  closed, 148, 149, 200
Hydrocal, 368, 402
Hydrocolloid
  definition of, 1
  irreversible; see Alginate irreversible hydrocolloid impression
  reversible; see Agar reversible hydrocolloid impression

HydroFlame soldering instrument, 607
Hyrax expander, 621

### I

I clasp, 143
I-bar clasp, 142, 143, 274-275
Immediate overdentures, 550
Impregum, 560, 565
Impression
  agar reversible hydrocolloid; see Agar reversible hydrocolloid impression
  alginate irreversible hydrocolloid; see Alginate irreversible hydrocolloid impression
  care of, 1-29
  corrected cast; see Corrected cast impression
  definition of, 58
  functional, 30
  packing and shipping, 667
  partial denture, 1
  preliminary, 1, 58
Impression cement, 458
Impression materials
  aqueous, 1
  elastomeric; see Elastomeric impression material
  rubber base, 106
Impression paste
  Opotow Standard ZOE, 73, 102
  zinc oxide–eugenol, 100-106
Impression tray
  custom, 58-71
    acrylic resin, 62-67
    thermoset vinyl, 68-71
    vacuum-adapted, 71
  definition of, 58
  perforated metal rim-lock, 59
  requirements for, 58
  solid metal rim-lock, 59
  stock, 58-71
    mandibular, 59
    maxillary, 59
    plastic, 60
  water-cooled, for reversible hydrocolloid impression, 59
Incisal rest preparation, 134
Infrabulge clasp, 135, 141-144, 273-276
Interceptive orthodontic appliance, 587-626
  accurate diagnosis in, 614
  components of, 587-614
  construction of, 614-615
  fabrication of, 614
  fixed, 587
  prescription of, 614
  removable, 587
  working cast for, 614
Internal attachment, 448
Interrupted mandibular struts, 512-513
Investing
  burnout, and casting, 293-320, 472-473
  definition of, 293
  S/L partial denture, 504
  and soldering, 480-483
  of sprued pattern, 293-308
Investment
  casting, 293
  outer, 293
  paint-on, 293
  phosphate-bound, 214
Investment cast, 214-227

Irreversible hydrocolloid; *see* Alginate irreversible hydrocolloid impression
Ivory epoxy resin No. RF3503, 645, 646-648

**J**

Jaw relation records, packing and shipping, 664, 665
Jelenko surveyor, 158-159
Jel-Pac, 318
Jeweler's rouge, 302, 315
Jig, reline, reline using, 402-413
Johnson's baby powder, 96

**K**

Kaoliner casting ring liner, 68
Kennedy bar, 144, 146, 147
Kennedy classification of removable partial dentures, 130-133
Kerr Permlastic, 73
Key attachment, 448
Keyway attachment, 448
Konometer, 552
Kurer Press-Stud, 556, 557, 562-563, 564-567, 572

**L**

Labial bar, 146, 147
 definition of, 491
 double, in S/L partial denture, 518-520
 opening, in S/L partial denture, 506, 507
Labial bow spring, 596-598
Labial opening arc (LOA), 491
Labial veneer, 491
Labiogingival tissue acrylic veneer
 constructing and finishing, 509-512
 definition of, 491
Laboratory plaster, 32
Latch recess groove (LRG), 498
Lathe, high-speed, for polishing castings, 321
L-bar clasp, contouring of, 276-277
Ledging, 190, 191, 197
Lingual arch appliance, 615
Lingual bar, 144, 145, 146, 147, 250, 251, 252
Lingual path of insertion (LPI), 491
Lingual plate, 144-146
Lingual section, 491
Lip extension, maximum, 491
Lip-support wax index, 491
Liquid monomer, 78
Liquid, tacky, 242, 247, 249
LOA; *see* Labial opening arc
Lock 'N Seal, 563
Lock, S/L, 491
Loop, retention, 491
LRG; *see* Latch recess groove
Lucitone denture base resin, 376
Luralite, 102
Luxene Vinyl Denture Base Separator, 510

**M**

Mandibular cast, 161, 249-253, 254
Mandibular stock impression tray, 59, 60
Mandibular struts, interrupted, 512-513
Mandrel, 322, 323
Masque, 88, 125
Master cast
 duplicate, 398-399
 relining, 400-403
 of S/L partial denture, 494, 495-496, 503
Maxillary cast, 233-249, 253, 254, 264

Maxillary coping overdenture, 516-518
Maxillary major connectors, 146-148
Maxillary stabilized record base, 105
Maxillary stock impression tray, 59
Maxillofacial prosthesis, S/L, 514
Mechanical spatulator, 12
Mesiodistal clasp, 144, 145
Metal
 heat hardening of, 315-316
 heat softening of, 315-316
 nonprecious, 268, 428
 precious, 268, 427-428
Metal backing
 fabrication of, 546
 flatback, 525
 indications for, 525
 and reinforced facings, 525-549
 techniques for, 525-548
Metal casting, retention beads for, 246
Metal denture bases, 150
Metal occlusals on teeth, 156-157
Metal pontics, 157
Metal repairs, 427-441, 447
Milling burs, 552
Miners wax, 637
Mini-hinge, 493, 497, 499, 503
Mini-Presso-Matic, 554
Missing and fractured teeth, repair of, 444-445
Model spray for refractory cast, 223-224
Modeling plastic occlusion rims, 128
Modern foil, 76, 510
Modification areas of Kennedy classification of removable partial dentures, 132, 133
Mold, silicone; *see* Silicone mold
Monoject, 494
Monomer, liquid, 78
Mounting, 72
Multiple circlet clasp, 139
Mylar film leader tape, 552

**N**

Nailhead retention, 234-235, 248
Nance appliance, modified, 615, 618-620
Ney surveyor, 158-159, 552
Ney undercut wax, 194
Nickel-chromium alloy for clasps, 268
Nonprecious metal alloys for clasps, 268
Nonprecious metal solders, 428
Nontarnish epoxy-coated sparkles, 650
North Carolina technique of pouring corrected cast corrections, 49-57

**O**

Occlusal rest preparation, 134
Occlusals
 gold, 483-485, 486
 metal, 156-157
Occlusion, functionally generated path, arranging artificial teeth to, 358-362
Occlusion rim
 definition of, 72
 modeling plastic, 128
 record bases with, 73
 wax, 124-128
Omnidental blockout compound, 114
Omnidental Omnivac, 68, 69
Omnilube spray silicone, 114
Omnivac baseplate material, 114
Omnivac coping, 552
Onlay clasp, 139-141

Open rentention
 with relief, 236-238
 without relief, 235-236
Opening arc, labial, 491
Opotow Standard ZOE impression paste, 73, 102
Orthodontic appliance, interceptive; *see* Interceptive orthodontic appliance
Orthodontic blowpipe, bench top, 607
Orthodontic clasp, 601-606
 contouring of, 279-280
 definition of, 601
 stainless steel, soldering of, 607-611
Orthodontic pliers, 588
Orthodontic procedures, 587-633
Orthodontic spring, 594-601
 definition of, 594
 dumbbell, 598-599
 helical finger, 595-596
 labial bow, 596-598
 simple finger, 594-595
 slingshot, 599, 600-601
Orthodontic wire, 587-588
 annealed, 587-588
 bending of; *see* Bending of orthodontic wire
 preactivated, 587
Outer investment, 293
Overdenture
 attachments for, 550-586
 immediate, 550
 maxillary coping, 516-518
 remote, 550
Overjet principle, 254-255, 259

**P**

Packing, 376-380
 and boilout, 381
 and shipping casts, 659-668
Pactra clear spray laquer, 635
Paint-on investment, 293
Palatal bar, 146-147
 anterior-posterior, 147-148
 beading for, 200
 double, 147, 200
 single, 146
Palatal strap, 146, 147
Paper, boxing, 636-638
Parallel attachment, 448
Parallel blockout, 188, 189
Parallelism, verifying, 469-471
Parallelometer, Bachmann, 552
Partial denture; *see* Removable partial denture
Partial prosthesis, frictional wall precision attachment, 448-490
Pencil eraser, 101, 198
Perforated metal rim-lock impression tray, 59
Permlastic, 107
PGP wire; *see* Platinum-gold-palladium wire
Phosphate-bonded casting investment, 293
Phosphate-bound investment, 214
Pickling casting, 318, 319
Plaster, laboratory, 32
Plaster/pumice mix and wax, boxing corrected cast impressions with, 30-35
Plastic, modeling, 128
Plastic repairs, 447
Plastic stock impression tray, 60
Plasticine, 201

Plate, lingual, 144-146
Platinum-gold-palladium (PGP) wire for clasps, 268
Pliers
 bird-beak, 588, 589-591, 592, 594
 orthodontic, 588
 three-prong, 588, 591, 593
 wire-bending, 268-269
Polishing and finishing framework, 321-338, 390-397
Polysulfide rubber, 106
Polyvinylchloride (PVC) elastomers, 650-656, 657
Pontic
 metal, 157
 reinforced acrylic, 152, 154-155, 543-548
Porcelain teeth processed to denture base for posterior tooth replacement, 156
Porosity of record base, 86
Powder, soft-curing autopolymerizing resin, 77
Preactivated orthodontic wire, 587
Precast attachments, 496
Precious metal alloys for clasps, 268
Precious metal solders, 427-428
Precision attachment
 definition of, 448
 frictional wall, 448-490
Precision bridges, 449
Preliminary impression, 1, 58
Preoperative cast, 72
Press-Stud, 556, 557, 562-563, 564-567, 572
Pressure indicator paste, 553
Pro Tem, 552
Process(ing), 380
 definition of, 363
 errors in, remounting and casting, 387-388
 flasking, deflasking, and finishing, 363-399
Prosthesis
 frictional wall precision attachment partial, 448-490
 S/L maxillofacial, 514
Pumice, 394-397
Push-type clasp, 141
PVC; see Polyvinylchloride (PVC) elastomers

R

Rag wheel for lathe for polishing metal framework, 332-335
RAP; see Reinforced acrylic pontic
Rapid palatal expansion appliance, 615, 620-622
Rebase(ing), 413-415
 definition of, 400
 and relining, 400-426
Recess preparation, 454, 455
Reciprocal clasp arm, 135
Reconstruction cast, 425-426
Reconstruction of removable partial denture, 425-426
Record base
 accurate fit of cast of, 86, 91
 autopolymerizing resin, 73-96
 chipping or breaking teeth during removal of, 91
 clinical application of, 72-73
 definition of, 72
 material for, 73
 and mounting casts, 72-129

Record base—cont'd
 with occlusion rims, 73
 porosity of, 86
 requirements for, 72-73
 rigidity of, 86
 separation of, from cast, 84-86, 91
 shellac, 96-113
 stabilized; see Stabilized record base
 uniform thickness of, 86, 91
 wax, 119-123
Record rim, 72
Refractory cast
 care of, 472
 definition of, 203
 and duplication, 203-227
 model spray for, 223-224
 preformed sprue hole in, 256-265
 treating, 222-227
 wax for, 225-227
Reinforced acrylic pontic (RAP), 152, 154-155, 543-548
Reinforced facings and metal backings, 525-549
Reinforcement wire, 106, 110, 121
Relief, 192-194, 198
 beading, design transfer, and blockout, 181-202
 definition of, 181
 open retention with, 236-238
 open retention without, 235-236
Relief wax, 199, 200
Reline impression, framework and bases with, 400
Reline jig, reline using, 402-413
Reline(ing), 400-413
 definition of, 400
 of master cast, 400-403
 and rebasing, 400-426
 using reline jig, 402-413
 resin for, 408, 409
Relined bases, alginate impression over framework and, 402
Remote overdenture, 550
Removable orthodontic interceptive appliance, 587
Removable partial denture
 anterior edentulous area of, 132
 bilateral distal extension of, 130-131
 classification of, 130-132
 components of, 134-157
 design of diagnostic casts for, 170-178
 fixed, packing and shipping, 666-667
 impression of, 1
 packing and shipping, 666
 reconstruction of, 425-426
 repairs of, 427-447
 Swing/Lock; see Swing/Lock partial denture
 unilateral distal extension, 131
Repair
 autopolymerizing resin, 441
 cast clasp, 434-437
 clasp, 433
 of denture base fractures, 441-443
 of fractured and missing teeth, 444-445
 major connector, 430-431
 metal, 427-441, 447
 plastic, 447
 of removable partial dentures, 427-447
 resin, 441-444
 resin retention, 437-441
 rest and minor connector, 431-432

Repair—cont'd
 with wrought alloys, 433-434
Replacement teeth for removable partial dentures, 483-485
Resin
 acrylic; see Acrylic resin
 autopolymerizing; see Autopolymerizing resin
 in clasp attachment, 282
 epoxy; see Epoxy resin
 for relines, 408, 409
 thermoplastic, 113-119
Resin denture base, 150
Resin impression tray, custom acrylic, 62-67
Resin record base, autopolymerizing, 73-96
Resin repair, 441-444
Resin retention repairs, 437-441
Resin teeth processed to denture base, 156
Rest preparation, 134
Rest, repair of, 431-432
Retention
 bead, 234-235, 246, 543
 crystal, 543
 nailhead, 234-235, 248
 open; see Open retention
 resin, repair of, 437-441
Retention hole, 107
Retention loop, 491
Retentive clasp arm, 135
Reverse approach circlet clasp, 138
Reverse-pin facing, 526-540
Reversible hydrocolloid; see Agar reversible hydrocolloid impression
Rider, Ackermann, 580
Right-angle bend of orthodontic wire, 591
Rim
 occlusion; see Occlusion rim
 record, 72
Rim-lock impression tray, 59
Ring clasp, 144
Roach clasp, 141
Rothermann stud attachment, 555, 570
 resilient, 560-561
 rigid, 558-560
Rouge, jeweler's, 302, 315
Rubber base impression material, 106
Rubber, polysulfide, 106
Rubber Sep, 559, 560, 561

S

Sandblaster, 316, 317, 318
Sandri stud attachment, 555, 562-563, 564, 571, 573
Semicircular bend of orthodontic wire, 589-590
Sepcoat, 496
Septisol solution, 328
Shaped blockout, 190
Shellac record bases, 96-113
Shellblaster, 316, 317, 318
Shipping and packing casts, 659-668
Silastic elastomer molds, 634-644
Silastic RTV moldmaking rubber, 639
Silicone elastomer, 645
Silicone mold
 base and boxing for, 636-638
 construction of, 634-644
 elastomer, 634-644
Silver solder, 428, 608
S/L; see Swing/Lock partial denture
Slingshot spring, 599, 600-601
Slotted attachment, 448

Slurry concentrate, 125
Smooth curve bend of orthodontic wire, 594
Snow White impression plaster No. 2, 458
Soft tissue undercuts, 166, 168, 201
Soft-curing autopolymerizing resin powder, 77
Solder, 438, 440
  in clasp attachment, 283-286
  in clasp repair, 290-291
  definition of, 607
  electric, 428
  hard, 427
  and investing, 480-483
  nonprecious metal, 428
  precious metal, 427-428
  silver, 428, 608
  soft, 427
  stainless steel, 607-611
  technique of, 428-430
Soldering flux for stainless steel wire, 608
Soldering machine, electric, 478, 479
Solid metal rim-lock impression tray, 59
Spatulator, mechanical, 7-12
Splint, transfer, 239
Split clasp, 144, 145
Spring, orthodontic; see Orthodontic spring
Sprinkle-on method of autopolymerizing resin record bases, 74-86
Sprue cones, 256-265
Sprue hole, preformed, in refractory cast, 256-265
Sprued pattern, investing, 293-308
Spruing, 254-266, 432
  definition of, 228
  multiple, 254
  placement of, in S/L partial denture, 518
  single, 254
  slingshot, 599, 600-601
  S/L partial denture, 504
  and waxing, 228-266
Stabilized record base, 73, 105
  with autopolymerizing resin, 109-113
  definition of, 72
  with elastomeric impression material, 106-109
  maxillary, 105
  shellac, 100
  with zinc oxide-eugenol impression paste, 100-106
Stainless steel soldering, 607-611
Stainless steel wire for clasp, 268
Stalite Sta-Vac, 114, 115
Steele's facings for anterior tooth replacement, 152, 153
Stock impression tray; see Impression tray, stock
Stone, artificial, in alginate irreversible hydrocolloid impressions, 7-17
Strap, palatal, 146, 147
Strathmore drawing board, 637
Strut, 148
  definition of, 491
  interrupted mandibular, 512-513
  try-in, 492
Stud attachment, 555-572
  Ancrofix, 554, 556, 562-563, 572, 573
  Baer, 555, 562-563, 571, 573
  Ceka, 556, 557, 566, 567-574
  Dalla Bona, 556, 562-563, 571, 573
  definition of, 554
  Gerber, 556, 557, 562-563, 564, 572, 573

Stud attachment—cont'd
  Rothermann, 555, 570
    resilient, 560-561
    rigid, 558-560
  Sandri, 555, 562-563, 564, 571, 573
Study cast, 626-633
Super-Gel, 494
Super-Sep separating fluid, 32, 356, 363, 367, 369, 371, 414, 459
Suprabulge clasp, 135, 136-141
Surface tension reducer, 472
Survey line, 130, 166, 167
Surveying
  definition of, 130
  and design, 130-180
  instruments for, 158, 159-160
  principles of, 158-169
Surveyor, 158-159, 160, 451
  definition of, 130
  Jelenko, 158-159
  Ney, 158-159
  Wills, 158
Swing/Lock complete denture, 515-516
Swing/Lock hinge, 491
Swing/Lock lock, 491
Swing/Lock (S/L) partial denture, 491-524
  adjustments to, 508
  attachment for, 491, 500-502
  attachment castings for, 498-499
  burnout and casting for, 505-506
  completed framework prefitted on cast of, 506, 507, 508
  definition of, 491
  design and construction of, 522, 523
  diagnostic casts and preliminary design of, 493-494
  double casting technique for, 505
  double labial bar in, 518-520
  framework try-in, 508
  freeing attachments of, 506
  impression technique for, 494
  jaw relation registration of, 509
  mandibular, 515-516
  master cast for, 494, 495-496, 503
  maxillofacial, 514
  metal requirements for, 505
  mounting framework of, 509
  opening labial bar in, 506, 507
  setup and finishing, 509
  single casting technique for, 505
  spruing and investing, 504, 518

**T**

T clasp, 141-142, 276-277
Tacky liquid, 234, 242, 247, 249
Talc
  powdered, 119
  in shellac record bases, 96, 97
Tangs, 148
Teaching aids, three-dimensional, 634-658
Telescope crown, 550-553
Template
  mounting, 357
  path, functionally generated, setting artificial teeth to, 354-362
Temporary base, 72
Thermoplastic resin record base, vacuum-adapted, 113-119
Thermoset vinyl custom impression tray, 68-71
Three-dimensional teaching aids, 634-658

Three-prong pliers, 588, 591, 593
Thumb release groove (TRG), 491
Thumb release projection (TRP), 492
Ticonium, 214, 256, 428
Tilting of cast, 160-169
Tinfoil, 101, 106, 125, 126, 127
Ti-Seal, 234, 242
Ti-Wire, 269, 438
Tooth
  additions to, 445-446
  anterior
    arrangement of, 344-345
    replacement of, 152-155
  artificial; see Denture teeth
  chipping or breaking, during removal of record base, 91
  denture; see Denture teeth
  fractured and missing, repair of, 444-445
  porcelain, processed to denture base for posterior tooth replacement, 156
  posterior
    arrangement of, 346-352
    in functionally generated path template, 354-362
    replacement of, 155-158
  replacement, for removable partial denture, 483-485
  resin, processed to denture base for posterior tooth replacement, 156
  selection and arrangement of, 339-362
  tube; see Tube teeth
Tooth undercuts, 166
Torit model 21-A, 269, 284, 285
Torit soldering unit, 428, 429
Transfer splint for tube teeth, 239
Transpalatal appliance, 615, 617-618
Tray, impression; see Impression tray
Trial base, 72
Tripoding, preserving tilt through, 168-169
Tripoli, 397
TRP; see Thumb release projection
Try-in strut, 492
Tube teeth, 239
  for anterior tooth replacement, 152, 153
  for posterior tooth replacement, 157, 239
  transfer splint for, 239
Two-stage pour, beading corrected cast impression with wax and, 42-49

**U**

U clasp, 144, 145
Undercut, 166-168, 200
Undercut gauges, 159, 176
Unilateral distal extension removable partial denture, 131

**V**

Vacuum pump, 640
Vacuum-adapted impression tray, 71
Vacuum-adapted thermoplastic resin record base, 113-119
Vac-U-Vestor/Power Mixer, 12
Vel Mix, 32, 356
Veneer
  labial, 491
  labiogingival tissue acrylic, 491, 509-512
Vent holes, 110
Vinyl Opaquer Pink No. 3527-13, 510
Visual aid, three-dimensional, 634
Vitallium, 214, 496, 505
Vulcanite bur, 407, 410

## W

W-arch appliance, 622-623
Water-cooled impression tray for reversible hydrocolloid impressions, 59
Wax(ing), 253
   beading and boxing corrected cast impression with, 36-41
   beading corrected cast impression with two-stage pour and, 42-49
   beading grip, 36-41
   blockout, formula for, 194
   boxing, 355, 356, 638, 642
   boxing grip, 39
   for construction of silicone molds, 635
   definition of, 228
   elimination of, 372-374
Wax(ing)—cont'd
   framework, 230
      of S/L partial denture, 503
   mandibular casting, 249-253, 254
   maxillary cast, 233-249, 253, 254, 264
   plaster/pumice mix and, boxing corrected cast impression with, 30-35
   for refractory cast, 225-227
   relief, 199, 200
   and spruing, 228-266
Wax-confined dough method of autopolymerizing resin record bases, 91-96
Wax index, lip-support, 491
Wax occlusion rim, 124-128
Wax out, 181
Wax record base, 119-123
Wax-up, framework, 472

Wilhold glues, 636
Wills surveyor, 158
Wire
   for clasps, 268, 269
   orthodontic; *see* Orthodontic wire
   platinum-gold-palladium, for clasp, 268
   reinforcement, 106, 110, 121
Wire cutter with vinyl inserts, 268, 269
Wire-bending pliers, 268-269
Wrought wire alloy, 433-434
Wrought wire clasp, 143-144, 267-292

## Z

Zigzag bend of orthodontic wire, 593
Zinc oxide–eugenol impression paste, record bases stabilized with, 100-106